Diagnostic Procedures
for Bacterial, Mycotic
and Parasitic Infections

DIAGNOSTIC

PROCEDURES *for:*

American Public Health Association
1015 Fifteenth Street NW
Washington, DC 20005

BACTERIAL, MYCOTIC
and
PARASITIC INFECTIONS

Sixth Edition

Albert Balows
William J. Hausler, Jr.
Editors

Interdisciplinary Books & Periodicals
For the Professional & the Layman

Sixth Edition

Copyright © 1981

AMERICAN PUBLIC HEALTH ASSOCIATION, Inc.
1015 15th Street NW
Washington, DC 20005
William H. McBeath, MD, MPH, Executive Director

10M6/81
Library of Congress Catalog Number: 81-68096
International Standard Book Number: 0-87553-086-9

Printed and bound in the United States of America
Typography: Byrd Press, Richmond, VA
Set in: *Times Roman, Helvetica*
Text and Binding: R.R. Donnelley & Sons Company, Crawfordsville, IN

Cover Design: Donya Melanson Assoc., Boston MA

The Editors wish to dedicate
this edition to those who showed
forebearance and patience as we
struggled with this editorial task:
Ann and Mary, our wives, and all of
the authors.

TABLE OF CONTENTS

xiv

CONTRIBUTORS

Donald G. Ahearn, PhD *(51)*
School of Arts and Sciences
33 Gilmer Street
Georgia State University
Atlanta, GA 30312

Libero Ajello, PhD *(53)*
Mycology Division
Centers for Disease Control
Atlanta, GA 30333

William L. Albritton, MD,
　PhD *(31)*
Infectious Diseases
Health Sciences Centre
700 William Avenue
Winnipeg, Manitoba R3E 0Z3
Canada

Stephen D. Allen, MD *(14)*
Department of Clinical Pathology
Indiana University Medical Center
Indianapolis, IN 46202

Carolyn N. Baker *(44)*
Clinical Bacteriology Branch
Bacteriology Division
Centers for Disease Control
Atlanta, GA 30333

Albert Balows, PhD *(29)*
Bacteriology Division
Centers for Disease Control
Atlanta, GA 30333

Allan M. Barnes, PhD *(43)*
Vector-Borne Disease Division
Centers for Disease Control
Atlanta, GA 30333

Marilyn S. Bartlett, MS *(57, 60, 61)*
Clinical Pathology (Allied Health)
Mycology/Parasitology Laboratory
Indiana University School of Medi-
　cine
Indianapolis, IN 46202

James W. Bass *(17)*
Department of Pediatrics
Uniformed Services University of
　the Health Sciences
Bethesda, MD 20014

Joseph H. Blount *(39)*
Venereal Disease Control Division
Centers for Disease Control
Atlanta, GA 30333

Victor D. Bokkenheuser, MD *(20)*
Department of Microbiology
St. Luke's Hospital Center
Amsterdam Avenue at 114th St.
New York, NY 10025

J. Roger Broderson, DVM *(10)*
Scientific Services Division
Centers for Disease Control
Atlanta, GA 30333

George F. Brooks, MD *(24)*
Departments of Laboratory
  Medicine and Medicine
University of California,
  San Francisco
San Francisco, CA 94143

Stuart T. Brown, MD *(39)*
Venereal Disease Control Division
Centers for Disease Control
Atlanta, GA 30333

George H. Brownell, PhD *(23)*
Department of Cell and Molecular
  Biology
Medical College of Georgia
Augusta, GA 30907

G. R. Carter, DVM, DVSc *(34)*
Department of Microbiology and
  Public Health
Michigan State University
East Lansing, MI 48824

Wallace A. Clyde, Jr., MD *(32)*
Infectious Disease Division
Department of Medicine
University of North Carolina
Chapel Hill, NC 27514

Mitchell L. Cohen, MD *(25)*
Enteric Diseases Branch
Bacterial Diseases Division
Centers for Disease Control
Atlanta, GA 30333

Richard H. Conklin, MD *(26)*
University of Texas Medical School
Texas Medical Center
6400 W. Cullen Street
Houston, TX 77025

Jon Counts, MPH, DrPH *(1)*
Arizona Department of Health
Phoenix, AZ 85007

Wallis E. DeWitt *(31)*
Bacterial Immunology Branch
Bacteriology Division
Centers for Disease Control
Atlanta, GA 30333

Robert B. Dienst, PhD *(23)*
Medical College of Georgia
Augusta, GA 30907

Judith K. Domer *(50)*
Department of Microbiology
Tulane University Medical Center
New Orleans, LA 70112

V. R. Dowell, Jr., PhD *(14)*
Enterobacteriology Branch
Bacteriology Division
Centers for Disease Control
Atlanta, GA 30333

Grace Mary Ederer, MS *(46)*
Department of Laboratory Medicine
  and Pathology
University of Minnesota
Minneapolis, MN 55455

Earl A. Edwards, MS *(45)*
Biological Science Division
Naval Health Research Center
Department of the Navy
San Diego, CA 92152

Herman C. Ellinghausen, Jr., PhD
  (30)
Leptospirosis Research
National Animal Disease Center
USDA/ARS
PO Box 70
Ames, IA 50010

John J. Farmer, III, PhD *(25)*
Enterobacteriology Branch
Bacteriology Division
Centers for Disease Control
Atlanta, GA 30333

Martin S. Favero, PhD *(8)*
Phoenix Laboratories Division
Centers for Disease Control
4402 North Seventh Street
Phoenix, AZ 85014

John C. Feeley, PhD *(31)*
Bacterial Immunology Branch
Bacteriology Division
Centers for Disease Control
Atlanta, GA 30333

*Oscar Felsenfeld, MD, MSc   *(18)*
Tulane University
Delta Regional Primate Research
  Center
Covington, LA 70433

John E. Forney, PhD *(3)*
Laboratory Training and Consulta-
  tion Division
Centers for Disease Control
Atlanta, GA 30333

Lorraine Friedman, PhD *(50)*
Department of Microbiology
Tulane University Medical Center
New Orleans, LA 70112

Peter C. Fuchs, MD *(35)*
Department of Pathology
St. Vincent Hospital and Medical
  Center
9205 Southwest Barnes Road
Portland, OR 97225

Mary Ann Gerenscser, PhD *(12)*
Department of Microbiology
West Virginia University Medical
  Center
Morgantown, WV 26505

Robert C. Good, PhD *(40)*
Mycobacteriology Branch
Bacteriology Division
Centers for Disease Control
Atlanta, GA 30333

(* died January 2, 1978)

Norman L. Goodman, PhD *(56)*
Departments of Pathology and Com-
  munity Medicine
University of Kentucky
Lexington, KY 40536

Morris A. Gordon, MD *(54)*
Division of Laboratories
New York State Department of
  Health
New Scotland Avenue
Albany, NY 12201

J. R. Greenwood, PhD, MPH
  (27, 28)
Department of Bacteriology
University of California
Los Angeles, CA 90024

Dieter H. M. Gröschel, MD *(33)*
Microbiology Laboratory
Department of Pathology
Box 168
University of Virginia Medical Cen-
  ter
Charlottesville, VA 22908

Sydney Harvey, PhD *(28)*
US Food and Drug Administration
1521 W. Pico Blvd.
Los Angeles, CA 90015

W. J. Hausler, Jr., PhD
University Hygienic Laboratory
University of Iowa
Iowa City, IA 52242

C. M. Helms, MD *(29)*
Department of Internal Medicine
College of Medicine
University of Iowa
Iowa City, IA 52242

George J. Hermann, DrPH *(22)*
1827 Mason Mill Road
Decatur, GA 30033

Richard L. Hilderbrand, PhD *(45)*
Head, Biochemistry Branch
Biological Science Division
Naval Health Research Center
Department of the Navy
San Diego, CA 92152

Henry D. Isenberg, PhD *(11)*
Long Island Jewish-Hillside
    Medical Center
270-05 76th Avenue
New Hyde Park, NY 11040

W. Johnson, PhD *(29)*
Department of Microbiology
College of Medicine
University of Iowa
Iowa City, IA 52242

James O. Kilburn, PhD *(40)*
Mycobacteriology Branch
Bacteriology Division
Centers for Disease Control
Atlanta, GA 30333

Lawrence J. Kunz, PhD *(38)*
Bacteriology Laboratory
Massachusetts General Hospital
Boston, MA 02114

Herbert L. Lawton, MS *(1)*
Laboratory Management and Con-
    sultation Activity
Centers for Disease Control
Atlanta, GA 30333

Calvin C. Linnemann, Jr., MD
    (17)
Division of Infectious Diseases
231 Bethesda Avenue
Department of Medicine
Cincinnati, OH 45208

Maryls E. Lund *(46)*
3M Center
Minnesota Mining and
    Manufacturing Co.
Hudson Road
St. Paul, MN 55101

Donald C. Mackel, MS, MPH *(9)*
Bacterial Diseases Division
Centers for Disease Control
Atlanta, GA 30333

Sarabelle Madoff *(21)*
Departments of Medicine and
    Bacteriology
The Massachusetts General
    Hospital
Boston, MA 02114

George F. Mallison, MPH *(9)*
Bacterial Diseases Division
Centers for Disease Control
Atlanta, GA 30333

William J. Martone, MD *(36)*
Bacterial Zoonoses Branch
Bacterial Diseases Division
Centers for Disease Control
Atlanta, GA 30333

Michael McGinnis, PhD *(52)*
Department of Hospital Laboratories
North Carolina Memorial Hospital
University of North Carolina
Chapel Hill, NC 27514

K. J. McMahon, PhD *(19)*
Department of Bacteriology
North Dakota State University
Fargo, ND 58102

Dorothy Mae Melvin, PhD *(57, 58)*
Parasitology Training Branch
Laboratory Training and
    Consultation Division
Centers for Disease Control
Atlanta, GA 30333

Robert C. Moellering, Jr., MD *(38)*
Harvard Medical School
Infectious Disease Unit
Department of Medicine
Massachusetts General Hospital
Boston, MA 02114

C. Dwayne Morse, DrPH (5)
Director, Division of Medical Laboratories
Minnesota Department of Health
717 Delaware Street, SE
Minneapolis, MN 55440

Arvind A. Padhye, PhD (55)
Mycology Division
Centers for Disease Control
Atlanta, GA 30333

Barbara G. Painter, PhD (2)
Long Island Jewish-Hillside
  Medical Center
New Hyde Park, NY 11040

Dan F. Palmer, DrPH (6)
Laboratory Training and Consultation Division
Centers for Disease Control
Atlanta, GA 30333

Charlotte M. Patton, MS (36)
Bacterial Zoonoses Branch
Bacterial Diseases Division
Centers for Disease Control
Atlanta, GA 30333

Peter L. Perine, MD (39)
Venereal Disease Control Division
Centers for Disease Control
Atlanta, GA 30333

M. J. Pickett, PhD (28)
Department of Microbiology
Life Sciences 5304
University of California
Los Angeles, CA 90024

Jack D. Poland, MD, PhD (43)
Vector-Borne Disease Division
Centers for Disease Control
Atlanta, GA 30333

Benjamin L. Portnoy, MD (33)
Infectious Disease Consultant
University of Texas Health Science
  Center at Houston Medical
  School
Diagnostic Clinic of Houston
Houston, TX 77030

Harry D. Pratt, PhD (61)
Vector-Borne Disease Control
  Training Service
Training Branch
Centers for Disease Control
Atlanta, GA 30333

Katherine Price, PhD (27)
Department of Microbiology
Cedars-Sinai Medical Center
Los Angeles, CA 90048

Thomas J. Quan, PhD, MPH (43)
Plague Branch
Vector-Borne Disease Division
Centers for Disease Control
Atlanta, GA 30333

Kenneth D. Quist, DVM, MPH (10)
Scientific Services Division
Centers for Disease Control
Atlanta, GA 30333

Horace B. Rees, Jr., PhD (15)
US Army Proving Grounds
Dugway, UT 84022

Edward D. Renner, PhD (19, 29)
Microbiology
Veterans Administration Center
Fargo, ND 58102

John Richardson, DVM, MPH (3, 4)
Office of Biosafety
Centers for Disease Control
Atlanta, GA 30333

Glenn D. Roberts, PhD (49, 53)
Mayo Clinic
220 First Street, SW
Rochester, MN 55901

Stanley A. Rosenthal, PhD (48)
Department of Dermatology
New York University Medical Center
New York, NY 10016

Michael W. Rytel, MD (45)
Section of Infectious Disease
The Medical College of Wisconsin
Milwaukee, WI 53226

Ira S. Salkin, PhD (47)
Division of Laboratories
New York State Department of
 Health
Albany, NY 12201

Ronald L. Schlitzer, PhD (51)
Department of Biology
University Plaza
Georgia State University
Atlanta, GA 30303

Vella Silcox, MS (40)
Mycobacteriology Branch
Bacteriology Division
Centers for Disease Control
Atlanta, GA 30333

Maragarita Silva-Hunter, PhD
 (48)
Columbia-Presbyterian Medical
 Center
622 West 168th Street
New York, NY 10032

Peter Skaliy, PhD (8)
Epidemiologic Investigations
Laboratory Branch
Bacterial Diseases Division
Centers for Disease Control
Atlanta, GA 30333

Bradford P. Smith
Scientific Services Division
Centers for Disease Control
Atlanta, GA 30333

Harry L. Smith, Jr., PhD (42)
Department of Microbiology
Jefferson Medical College of
 Thomas Jefferson University
1020 Locust Street
Philadelphia, PA 19107

J. Kelly Smith, MD (11)
Chief, Department of Medicine
VA Medical Center
Mountain Home, TN 37684

James W. Smith, PhD (24, 57, 58, 59,
 60, 61)
Department of Clinical Pathology
N-440
University Hospital
Indianapolis, IN 46202

Louis D. S. Smith, PhD (13)
3605 Burrchvale Road
Wenatchee, WA 98801

Merlin A. Smith, MS (15)
Environmental Microbiology
Bureau of Laboratories
Utah State Division of Health
44 Medical Drive
Salt Lake City, UT 84113

Peter Byrd Smith, PhD (37)
Clinical Bacteriology Branch
Bacteriology Division
Centers for Disease Control
Atlanta, GA 30333

Frances O. Sottnek (22)
Clinical Bacteriology Branch
Bacteriology Division
Centers for Disease Control
Atlanta, GA 30333

Scott Stewart *(41)*
Rockey Mountain Laboratory
NIAID
Hamilton, MT 59840

Catherine Sulzer, PhD *(30)*
Bacteriology Division
Bureau of Laboratories
Centers for Disease Control
Atlanta, GA 30333

Vera L. Sutter, PhD *(20)*
Research Service, Wadsworth
VA Hospital Center
Los Angeles, CA 90073

William Terranova, MD *(25)*
Enteric Diseases Branch
Bacterial Diseases Division
Centers for Disease Control
Atlanta, GA 30333

Alejandro B. Thiermann, DVM
(30)
USDA Science and Education
Administration
Agricultural Research, North
Central Region
National Animal Disease Center
PO Box 70
Ames, IA 50010

Clyde Thornsberry, PhD *(44)*
Clinical Bacteriology Branch
Bacteriology Division
Centers for Disease Control
Atlanta, GA 30333

Alexander von Graevenitz, MD *(27)*
Department of Medical Microbiology
University of Zurich
CH 8028 Zurich Switzerland

Alwilda L. Wallace *(39)*
Laboratory Training and Consulta-
tion Division
Centers for Disease Control
Atlanta, GA 30333

Kenneth W. Walls, PhD *(57, 60)*
Parasitic Serology Branch
Parasitology Division
Centers for Disease Control
Atlanta, GA 30333

David Weinman, MD *(16)*
Department of International Health
University of California, San
Francisco
San Francisco, CA 94143

Irene Weitzman, PhD *(48)*
Chief of Mycology
Department of Health, City of New
York
Bureau of Laboratories
New York, NY 10016

Joy G. Wells *(25)*
Enteric Disease Laboratory Section
Bacterial Diseases Division
Centers for Disease Control
Atlanta, GA 30333

C. Michael West, MD *(25)*
Hospital Infections Branch
Bacterial Diseases Division
Centers for Disease Control
Atlanta, GA 30333

Geraldine L. Wiggins, MS *(22, 31)*
7145 Cannongat
Dallas, TX 75248

PREFACE TO SIXTH EDITION

The Sixth Edition of *Diagnostic Procedures for Bacterial, Mycotic, and Parasitic Infections* has experienced a protracted and difficult gestation. As a matter of fact, the difficulties have been of such magnitude that there is real concern for the development of subsequent editions. These concerns and difficulties pierce the heart of multiple-author multiple-discipline professional association or organization publications.

In 1975 the Committee on Laboratory Standards and Practices of the American Public Health Association decided that a sixth edition of this manual was essential as a result of the continued refinement and improvement of laboratory techniques for the detection of infectious agents. Co-editors were appointed, an editorial board was approved, and individuals considered outstanding in their field agreed to prepare manuscripts. The goal was to publish the sixth edition in early 1978. It is indeed unfortunate that this goal was not achieved, and actual publication was delayed for 3 years.

These management and organizational difficulties should not in any way detract from the excellence and timeliness of this sixth edition. As in past editions, the manual is organized according to diseases rather than by etiologic agent. In addition to an expanded presentation on quality assurance practices in microbiology, the user will find new chapters on nosocomial and opportunistic infections, legionellosis, campylobacteriosis, and eikenellosis, as well as a discussion of the less common bacterial infections.

This is a working manual for the clinical and public health laboratory as well as a useful textbook for those wishing to expand their understanding of the infectious disease–laboratory interface. When using this manual as a companion to the fifth edition of *Diagnostic Procedures for Viral, Rickettsial and Chlamydial Infections,* the professional will discover almost complete laboratory backup to those diseases presented in the APHA publication *Control of Communicable Diseases in Man.*

The enormous amount of closely coordinated work does permit one to question whether new editions should be considered. Advances in laboratory technology and diagnosis are proceeding at such a rapid pace that it becomes virtually impossible to complete a multi-disciplinary work such as this sixth edition in a timely fashion.

During the latter part of November 1977, Dr. Oscar Felsenfeld submitted his typescript of the chapter on borreliosis to the editors. This manuscript, which was characteristic of Dr. Felsenfeld's work, was excellent and we were delighted that it was submitted on schedule and in good shape. On 2 January 1978 Dr. Felsenfeld suffered a fatal heart attack. As far as we know, this chapter was the last scientific paper he wrote, and it is a fitting tribute to an individual who will be remembered as a scholar, a scientist, and a gentle man.

The editors also wish to acknowledge and express their thanks to all the other authors who, in spite of many adverse situations, continued to doggedly update their manuscripts to meet newly planned publication dates. Their rewards are very minimal but our thanks to them are considerable. There are many others who have agonized through the generation of this edition, but we particularly wish to thank our secretaries, Mrs. Marion Jernigan and Ms. Irene Keating. We also acknowledge the contributions of Mr. Allen J. Seeber, Director of Publications for APHA.

Albert Balows
W. J. Hausler, Jr.

Part One

CHAPTER 1

LABORATORY ADMINISTRATION

Jon M. Counts and Herbert L. Lawton

General Administration in the Laboratory

Introduction

Clinical or public health laboratory management requires the same attention and expertise that traditionally have been expended on the scientific function of the laboratory operation. Therefore, with increasing demands for controlling health costs on the one hand and increasing numbers of sophisticated examinations performed in the laboratory, use of expensive automated equipment, and higher paid personnel on the other, it is essential that laboratory directors develop their administrative capabilities to control effectively the professional and financial management of their laboratory facilities. This section is primarily concerned with managing the public health laboratory.

Management of Laboratory Services

The most pressing problem facing administrators of public health and clinical laboratories is their relative inability to plan their growth and development effectively. Individual laboratory directors, public health commissioners, and state legislators responsible for state health laboratory services must be urged to work together to develop management systems that will assist them in providing the leadership needed to direct such a health program.

For several years, management by objectives (MBO) has been used as a systematic approach to management in the health care industry just as in business and industry. Such a program is an arrangement of interacting factors coordinated to accomplish desired objectives. Among these factors are input (objectives), process (management), output (results), and control (achievements) (1).

With MBO, objectives (or goals) established provide an organizational structure, and a process is followed for achieving results consistent with these goals. It is a system of managing managers and professionals. The set of objectives for each manager or professional individual is consistent with the overall goals of the organization. Each person's performance is evaluated on the basis of attaining the previously agreed-upon goals, i.e., on the basis of results.

3

The MBO process requires that the organization establish a hierarchy of objectives from the top of the institution to the bottom. The objectives at each job level are derived from and complement those established for the previous level. The process of establishing a hierarchy of objectives in the public health laboratory starts with the health department administration. The health department administrator enters into the process of strategic planning to determine the major long-range objectives of the department and the policies that will govern the acquisition, use, and disposition of the resources necessary to achieve the desired public health goals. Strategic planning is always the responsibility of top management.

Once the department's strategic planning has been completed and the long range plans have been defined, the latter must be communicated so that the laboratory director can develop goals consistent with those of the department's administration. Individual department managers must now be able to define the key result areas for their jobs. These areas are the discrete parts of their jobs (expressed in terms of output or result) which justify the existence of the jobs. Key result areas of a laboratory manager's job, include, e.g., the organization of the laboratory, scheduling of personnel and work flow, productivity, and quality and cost control.

The following criteria can be used in determining the importance of a health problem and in establishing priorities for laboratory services.

Magnitude. How wide an effect on people's health does this problem have? Is it of such scope that it affects many people and many communities? If it were solved, what would be the magnitude of the resulting benefits? Would many people or communities benefit or only a few?

Seriousness. Is this problem life threatening in its immediate proportions? Does it create, in turn, other serious or pressing problems?

Urgency. How urgently is the solution to this problem needed? Must a deadline be met? Would the solution to this problem require the prior solution to one or more other problems?

Economic cost. Does this problem cause significant expenditures of public and/or private funds?

Social cost. Does this problem cause significant human deprivation, disability, restricted activity, lost work and school days, loss of income, and reduction of human dignity or quality of life?

Practicality. How practical is it to think that this problem can be solved to any extent? Are there known means of intervention which can be used to solve it? Has anyone else had any success in solving it?

Efficiency. Will work toward solving this problem be more cost effective than if it were applied to another problem? Does this problem lend itself to a solution which requires less investment than others, yet promises at least as great a return in benefits?

Feasibility. Is this a problem which can be solved with presently available resources? When viewed against existing resources (men, facilities, and dollars) and competencies available, is it realistic to attempt to solve this problem?

Preparation for something bigger. Will work toward solving this problem set the stage for solving other problems which derive from it? Will work on this problem establish a foundation for something even bigger or more important?

Coordination potential. Will undertaking the solution of this problem assist in coordinating other programs and activities? Will there be a synergistic effect so that the solution of this problem, coupled with those of others, will have a total effect greater than that of the sum of individual solutions?

Political acceptability. Is work on this problem politically acceptable? Do key officials and decision makers oppose or support work on this problem? Will work on this problem tend to alienate decision makers to the detriment of other future activities? Is it legal to solve this problem?

Good will. Will attempts to solve this problem generate a degree of good will or improved public relations? Do both in-house and public sentiment strongly favor solving this problem?

Composition of Laboratory Services

Many public health laboratories have stopped providing routine laboratory services and are devoting more of their limited resources to epidemiologic and special field studies and to expanding current programs to assure the quality of the tests performed by the private clinical and environmental laboratory sector. Many routine bacteriologic and serologic services now provided by state and local public health laboratories could be discontinued and the funds currently allocated for them could be more appropriately used in other ways. If, in fact, intrastate and interstate laboratory improvement programs (proficiency testing, laboratory licensure, laboratory training activities) are effective, private sector laboratories should be capable of doing routine testing formerly provided in public health facilities.

Many laboratories are also considering providing certain services on a regional basis, e.g., proficiency testing programs and screening the newborn for metabolic disorders. It has been suggested that pooling efforts in other specialty areas might be worthwhile, e.g., such as the diagnosis of rabies and arbovirus infections; highly specialized aspects of bacteria, fungus, and parasite identification; and mycobacterial diagnosis and sensitivity testing (21). A movement in this direction would also reduce the present dependence on the Center for Disease Control for those tests which are required too infrequently to justify having individual state laboratories provide them.

Organization of Public Health Laboratories

Recently Schmidt and Madoff distributed a questionnaire to the directors of the 54 state and territorial public health laboratories asking each one to place his organization into one of the four categories based on functional criteria: central laboratory, single; central laboratory, multiple; university-based laboratory; and the regional laboratory system (31). All but two of the states and territories reported having a central laboratory organization of some sort. A few indicated that they had consolidated their disease control and laboratory services into one functional unit to facilitate coordinating these activities.

Obviously a decentralized public health laboratory has many disadvantages (18), a major one of which is duplication of resources. For example, a communicable or venereal disease control program might operate its own small laboratory or support a network of laboratories in addition to and beyond the control of the primary state laboratory. Such duplication is all too common in the areas of water and air environmental control. For example, the national concern for ecology and protection of the environment has stimulated the development of new or enlarged state environmental protection agencies. In many cases, availability of Federal funding provides a further impetus for states to form such agencies. These agencies in turn have developed laboratory services involving the chemical and microbiological testing of water and air samples, and only occasionally was any agreement made to transfer funds to the traditional public health laboratory for continuing and/or improving these functions. This practice obviously results in fragmented public health laboratory functions. Similar examples can be found in the areas of food and drugs, agriculture, pesticides, highway safety, forensic medicine, occupational health, and preventive medicine screening laboratory services—particularly those provided for crippled children and maternal and child health programs.

In one state, scientific laboratories are operated by at least 14 separate state agencies. The resulting overlap in coordinating activities at the state level often results in inefficiency. Another problem is the difficulty of finding competent laboratory directors and technical staff, many of whom perform nearly identical functions. However, it is only fair to point out that some laboratory directors believe that the advantages of close laboratory contact with other decentralized health department activities far outweigh these disadvantages (31).

Although the centralized state laboratory system—the most common system reported in use—ameliorates these problems, others become prevalent. One major problem is that specimens submitted to a central laboratory must be transported some distance from the site of collection, a situation which affects the quality of the specimen and can delay the production and reporting of results. Various mechanisms for reporting results have evolved, including computerization with 24-hour, on-line feedback mechanisms, messenger services, and telephone calls. This entire area needs to be evaluated further, and the alternative specimen delivery systems similar to those adopted by some major commercial laboratory services should be investigated (31).

Cost Accounting

Introduction

Clinical and public health laboratories (excluding laboratories in physicians' offices) perform approximately 4.5 billion tests annually, at an estimated cost of 13.5 billion dollars, and employ approximately 246,235 technical and nontechnical personnel (2, 24, 28, 29). One group of these laboratories includes the state and territorial public health laboratories (central and branch laboratories), which are represented in the Association of State and Territorial Public Health Laboratory Directors (ASTPHLD). They handle approximately 28,000,000 specimens per year, employ approximately 6,200 persons, and spend more than 98,000,000 dollars annually.

With demands for laboratory services constantly increasing, laboratory directors see a need for more effective management to help them to adequately measure their workload, properly assign costs per work unit, relate effectiveness and effort in the various sections of their laboratories, and accumulate meaningful data to support their efforts to their administrative superiors, their own staff, and their consumers.

One tool which has existed for many years and which can be very helpful to a laboratory director is cost accounting. This portion of the chapter concerns the ways in which the concepts of cost accounting can be applied to internal laboratory transactions.

The cost accounting system we describe is one which has been implemented in 28 state and local public health laboratories in an effort to help the laboratory directors estimate the cost to consumers of specific services provided in their own laboratories. The system also provides cost information for managerial analysis and control, planning future activities, and preparing capital budgets.

Much of the material in this section is also covered in three articles by Duncan (9–11). Additional references are included under General References for those who care to read further on the subject.

Building the Cost Accounting System

The cost accounting system described here operates as follows:

1. The costs (expenses) are identified as closely as possible with the laboratory's technical, administrative, and support sections ("cost centers") in which they are incurred.

2. Those costs which cannot be identified with any particular section are allocated over all sections on a fair-share basis.

3. The cost of operating the sections which provide internal support (such as administrative) are reapportioned to those sections which perform tests and other services on the basis of the percentage of support that they receive. By the end of this step, the total cost for each test- or service-producing section will have been identified.

4. The workload is identified in terms of weighted workload values.

5. The total cost of each laboratory section is allocated over all the tests it did on the basis of weighted workload values it produced.

First, cost centers must be identified. A cost center is a definable activity that produces a product or provides a service and in doing so incurs such costs as salaries, utilities, and postage. (For example, in a public health laboratory, the microbiology cost center is a definable cost center that provides a service or produces a product.) A laboratory support cost center provides such services as maintenance, janitorial work, animal care, media preparation, and glassware processing. Such a cost center provides a service to other cost centers in the laboratory but not to any centers outside the laboratory.

Revenue and nonrevenue producing cost centers

The two categories or types of cost centers are 1) revenue centers and 2) nonrevenue centers. Revenue centers are those that provide services (or products) to users outside the organization and from which revenue can be generated from charges made. For example, a laboratory's microbiology cost center is a revenue center even if there is no direct fee for testing a specimen.

Nonrevenue centers are those activities which support other activities within the organization but which do not directly generate revenue (e.g., laboratory support cost center).

Several criteria should be considered in determining how many cost centers are appropriate. One is that at least one product or service is being provided by the activity designated as a cost center. Another is that services or products that are similar or related in some way should be grouped together and provided by persons in an identifiable organizational unit. Still another is that costs should be identifiable with a reasonable effort. For example, a laboratory's organization chart may show an activity or function entitled "special bacteriology." However, the diagnostic tests in that area may be performed rarely or by different individuals each time so that even the salary costs are difficult to identify. In that case, the special bacteriology subarea is not an appropriate cost center but can be considered part of the microbiology area cost center. A final criterion is that of planning and controlling activities and costs. That is, a cost center should have a continuing program of providing services or products, with a person responsible and accountable for the activity.

Accumulation

After cost centers are designated, their costs can be recorded (accumulated). A major portion of the accumulated costs is labor (salaries). Other costs include those for supplies, travel, and equipment.

Rather than allocating the entire purchase price of an expensive piece of equipment to a cost center for the purchase year (thus raising abnormally the cost of any test done during that year), the item should be depreciated over several years. Depreciation is the decline in value of a real asset over time. Of several methods used for calculating depreciation, the most simple is probably the straight-line method.

The straight-line method assumes that an asset declines at a constant (or linear) rate so that its value is reduced by the same amount each year of its expected life until some predetermined salvage value is reached. Beyond the expected life period, no depreciation expense is charged.

The equation for determining the annual straight-line depreciation is:

$$\text{Annual Depreciation} = \frac{\text{Initial Cost} - \text{Salvage Value}}{\text{Expected Life}}.$$

A document published by the Internal Revenue Service (33) encourages using this method of depreciation. The publication proposes that all equipment for a given type of "industry" be placed in a single class. An American Hospital Association publication (15) contains listings showing that laboratory equipment has an average expected life of 10 years.

The depreciation expense method allows one to use one life expectancy table for all equipment costs instead of having to keep the many files that would be necessary for actual costs and a depreciation life for each piece of equipment.

Allocation

Expenses which cannot be readily assigned to a cost center must be allocated to all cost centers on a fair-share, causal basis. As many costs as possible should, of course, be identified and accumulated by cost center.

In order to allocate a cost, some related fair-share basis must be determined. For example, utility costs could be allocated on the basis of the percentage of floor area located in each cost center. That is, there would seem to exist some causal relationship between the amount of floor space and the utility costs for that space. Thus, if the administrative office has 50% of the floor area, 50% of the utility costs would be allocated to the administrative office. The portions of supplies expenses and of mailing expenses which cannot be identified and accumulated by cost center could be allocated on the basis of the percentage of tests done. If no causal, fair-share basis can be found, the cost can be allocated equally to all cost centers.

Multiple allocation bases could be used for some of the expense categories. For example, $x\%$ of an expense could be allocated to the *nonrevenue* centers based upon estimates, and $(100 - x)\%$ of the expense could be allocated to the *revenue* centers based upon the proportion of tests performed in those cost centers.

The most important aspect of using estimation and judgment as bases for allocation is that valid estimates are based upon evidence and not opinion. The person or persons most knowledgeable about the expense items should determine the allocations. Until all monies can be directly accumulated, a sampling of the actual spending by each cost center is a good basis for making a valid judgment. The sampling should encompass seasonal spending differences and expenses for special or short-term projects. For example, August may be an atypical month in terms of supply purchases if the laboratory does screening for school children. Periodically, the allocation percentages and other allocation bases should be reviewed and revised if necessary.

Reapportionment

When all costs have been accumulated by and allocated to cost centers, the costs previously identified with the nonrevenue centers should be reallocated by accumulation and allocation to the appropriate revenue centers. Thus, the total cost (direct and support) of each revenue center is derived.

The director's office is a nonrevenue cost center, and there may be several others. First, the costs of the director's office must be fairly reapportioned to all of the other cost centers (revenue and nonrevenue). The proportion absorbed by each cost center could be based on the relative amount of service it receives from the director's office. The personnel base of a center represents a service received from the director's office which could serve as the basis for reapportioning the latter's costs.

This reapportionment process continues until all nonrevenue-producing center costs are assigned in some fair-share method to the revenue-producing cost centers.

Cost per Weighted Workload Value Unit

When the cost reapportionment process is completed, the total cost of each revenue center is identified. This cost is allocated to individual procedures performed in that revenue center on an equitable basis. Weighted workload values (WWV) are suggested as such a suitable basis (22). In many laboratories, workload is determined by volume of test results reported; however, published WWV are identified by *procedure* rather than by *reported test results*. Therefore, the procedures used to determine each reported test result must be identified so that all test result reports are assigned a proper workload value. Then the number of WWV produced in each revenue-producing cost center can be calculated.

Determined WWV per reported test result must be revised only as procedures are added or modified. The WWV for a test can be counted as test results are counted, and a total WWV count for each revenue-producing cost center can be identified.

One element of the WWV is the normal batch size, i.e., the number of specimens usually processed concurrently. This batch size must be reviewed at least annually.

The final step of determining the cost of any test has two parts. First, the cost/WWV unit for each revenue center must be determined by dividing the total cost of the revenue center by the WWV produced in a specified amount of time. For example, if the environmental cost center's total cost was $50,000 and that unit produced 35,000 WWV, then the cost per WWV would be:

$$\frac{\$50,000}{35,000 \text{ WWV}} = \$1.43/\text{WWV}$$

To estimate the cost of any test done in that cost center, the cost/WWV is multiplied by the WWV assigned to the test. For example, if basic alkalinity tests are done in the environmental cost center, the cost of one basic alkalinity test (on one specimen) is the cost of producing one WWV in the environmental cost center ($1.43) times the WWV of one basic alkalinity test (0.3), or $0.43 per test result.

Once the cost/WWV is known for each cost center, the cost to perform each test can be estimated. One year's expenditure figures and WWV workload data will produce that year's cost-per-test. Laboratory management may prefer to use the projected budget and a forecasted workload to estimate cost per test for the next year. Cost accounting should be updated at least twice a year: first, to project costs for the upcoming year in order to set prices; second, when the year is over to compare the two sets of figures and determine whether forecasting techniques need to be improved.

Analysis and Use of the Data

Cost data

Several useful analyses can be made from workload and cost data. First, they can be used to estimate the cost of a new test. After the test's WWV has been determined from established procedures, that value is multiplied by the cost/WWV for the cost center in which the test will be done.

The data can also be used in evaluating the relative cost-effectiveness of the revenue centers. Ideally, all cost centers should have about the same cost/WWV, although management cannot control all differences. However, if a cost center has a cost/WWV highly discrepant from the average, further study is indicated.

Intralaboratory comparison of cost/WWV among cost centers is useful. Interlaboratory comparisons are less useful because of environmental differences and differences in pay scales beyond the control of management.

Each cost center should monitor its own cost/WWV over time. A gradual rise each year can be at least partially attributed to inflation and normal business costs, but any excessive rise should be studied.

Productivity data

The total WWV produced in a laboratory divided by total available man hours equals the average laboratory productivity indicator (PI). Comparable PIs can be calculated for individual cost centers.

$$\text{Average Laboratory Productivity Indicator} = \frac{\text{WWV produced in the laboratory}}{\text{Available man hours in the laboratory}}$$

and

$$\text{Productivity Indicator for a Diagnostic Section} = \frac{\text{WWV produced in a particular section}}{\text{Available man hours in a particular section}}$$

Laboratory management could use these productivity figures to detect over- and under-producing sections by comparing those for different laboratory sections, for one cost center over time, and for a section as compared to the overall average for the laboratory. The PI can also reflect over- or under-staffing. For example, the possibility of over-staffing should be considered if the data show a high cost/WWV coupled with a low productivity. Other applications for the PI are explained in the literature listed in the General References.

Cost/WWV and PI data combined should enable the director and his staff to study the two most important resources of an efficient laboratory—money and personnel.

Summary

The cost accounting system which has been described is aimed primarily at identifying costs for specific laboratory functional areas and administrative-support areas, and using these costs and WWV for estimating costs per test and productivity.

The system described proves most useful if cost accounting data are used to project future workload and expenses (e.g., for the next year). Forecasts are also useful in preparing budgets. Quarterly cost accounting on actual expense and workload data can provide short-term information for management. For example, it would be useful to see if actual costs at the end of the first quarter approximate the forecasted costs. If not, the reason for the discrepancy should be determined.

Expense and workload data should come from the same time period. Workload data should be summarized monthly or quarterly and cumulated for the fiscal-year or calendar-year report.

Record Keeping and Reporting

Introduction

Record keeping and reporting have been problems for organizations including laboratories for many years. Requests for information from many sources have exposed weaknesses, particularly in manually kept record keeping and reporting systems. For example, when thousands of items are filed manually in ascending numerical order, it is very difficult to extract items by any other numerical order.

In most laboratories, record keeping and reporting center around financial data (e.g., salaries, supplies, and other fiscal accounting data) and workload data (e.g., numbers of specimens submitted, results of testing, and productivity calculations).

Forms for Data Collection and Reporting

Information on the slip submitted with a specimen supplies the basic data in a laboratory. Each time a piece of paper is handled, the risk of error increases. This problem can be partially solved by color coding all forms and mailing labels by function. Color-coded mailing labels (by function) allow incoming specimens to be routed to the appropriate processing area unopened and obviate the need for a central receiving area. As mailing containers are opened in appropriate laboratory sections, the specimen, the colored form, and the colored mailing label can be visually checked to see whether a specimen intended for one laboratory section was inadvertently misrouted because it was mailed in the wrong container or mailed with the wrong form.

If a central receiving location is used, all specimens can be sorted, opened (except for highly toxic materials or temperature-dependent materials), and delivered to the appropriate specialty laboratories.

Form design is important. The sequence in which the data appear must be planned so that eye and hand movement are natural. For example, the person filling in the form should not have to put one piece of information on the left, the next on the right, then on the top, then on the bottom. Information added in the laboratory should also be sequenced for convenience. Also, adequate space should be provided for any written information required.

Instructions must be carefully worded so that they are clear and elicit the desired information. To this end, forms should always be field tested before they are used. What is clear to the designer may not be clear to the user.

Because the law states that a person's or organization's privacy should not be violated, data of a private nature should not be requested.

All composition must be clear. Characters (numbers, letters, or special printing) that might be confused should not be used. Any constant data or information should be preprinted on all forms.

Printing on both sides of a form would lower supply costs. For example, on the front of a form might be a listing of the abbreviations of reasons why a specimen might be unsatisfactory for testing. There would be a space or box by each abbreviation for the laboratorian to make any check needed. On the back of the form the reasons for a specimen's being unsatisfactory for testing would be written out completely. This information on the back of the form would explain the abbreviations on the front of the form. Code legends on the front would refer the user to the back of the form for more complete definitions of what constitutes an unsatisfactory specimen. For further emphasis, code legends could be set in bold type, surrounded by heavy lines around the printing, or could have shading to highlight the area.

Another way to lower the cost of forms is to print them in-house. If the forms are processed manually, deviations in spacing the data by the customer and the laboratorian should cause little if any trouble. However, if forms are read by data processing equipment, it may be wiser to have them printed by a company with experience in preparing data processing forms. Data processing equipment is designed to tolerate very little deviation in spacing or placement of data. Even forms that are otherwise well designed are useless if they are not printed with lines and spaces precisely located for machine use.

If preprinted forms must be purchased, the cost may be reduced to some extent if stock forms rather than custom-designed ones can be used.

Some question might be raised as to whether so much time, effort, and cost should be spent on forms design. It has been estimated that a clerical cost of $20 is associated with every dollar of forms cost (25). Thus, if forms can be designed so that clerical handling is minimized, a laboratory is saving at the ratio of 20 to 1.

The method described below for effective and efficient study of forms for maximum utilization was developed by Carl E. Stewart, Jr., Laboratory Management Consultation Office, Center for Disease Control. First, the desired size of each form and worksheet to be used or sent from the laboratory must be determined. If the types of work sheets differ in size, the complete cycle of use, reporting, retention, and retrieval was not carefully planned. Among other things, some forms may have been designed without regard to data available on other forms. Some people advocate that all forms in a laboratory be of the same size, which may not be workable or desirable, but as few different sizes as possible should be used. The size of a form should be decided in part by allowing adequate margins so that forms can be mounted on clipboards or in ring binders without risking obscuring any of the data. Also there is the fact that the equipment used to print the forms needs spaces on the head and sides of the form in order to grip the form. These exact measurements can be supplied by your printer.

Filing and mailing are also considerations in determining form size. Ideally, a form should not have to be folded before it is filed (including being mailed). If folding is necessary, the form should be folded once at most before it is filed. If numerous forms must be folded before they are mailed or filed, a mechanical folding machine might be practical. Fold marks should be printed on the form.

The function of a working paper is important. That is, is it a submission form, a report-to-the-client form, an internal work sheet, or some other type? Hopefully, the submission form is also used as the report form. If not, further study may reveal unnecessary typing of extra forms or poorly designed forms.

Next, the type of form should be considered, i.e., is carbon paper used for copies, is it no-carbon-required type, is it a single copy working paper, or is it some other type? Once again uniformity (or standardization) should be considered for ease of handling and simplicity of ordering and stocking.

The number of copies of each form and the manner in which each copy is distributed are key aspects of forms control and usage. Who gets the various copies, where the copies are filled, how the copies are "shuffled" from one office or location to another, and whether the number of copies is correct should be carefully considered.

Examples of things to check are whether a multipart form is still needed with the existing number of copies, whether more copies should be added because extra copies are now being reproduced, and whether the forms can be successfully separated for data capture after the laboratory identification number has been placed on the form and on the specimen. A copy of a form which was at one time needed for some reason may become obsolete. However, if no one questions its presence it will continue to be used.

Using window envelopes for reports mailed back to the submitting agency does away with unnecessary typing of addresses.

What forms must be retained and the length of time a form must be filed should be studied. Usually state law regulates to some degree the keeping of records, and what is to be kept and length of time required may not be clear. These regulations vary from state to state.

Report forms should be carefully monitored to locate any uncalled-for results or handwritten or typed results outside indicated spaces, which could indicate a poorly designed or outdated form. Almost all messages and results from laboratory areas for which forms have been designed can be printed on the form. Thus, the laboratorian simply checks a block next to the result and/or message.

During the process in which the form is stamped into the laboratory, used by the laboratorian, and mailed by the clerical office, any unnecessary handling enlarges the probability of error. All information should be kept on one properly color-coded sheet which is used for receiving and reporting. The laboratorian should record the results; a window envelope should be used for reports; only necessary copies should be kept, and they should be kept only as long as required (which may be for a long period of time).

If forms must be kept longer than 2 years, and if storage space is at a premium, the practicality of microfilm storage should be investigated. The 5 microfilm forms are: spool, cartridge, jacket, fiche, and aperture card. The spool (a roll of microfilm not enclosed in any protective covering) is the least expensive microfilm but may be the most difficult to index. Microfim enclosed in a container, usually plastic, is called a cartridge. The cartridge costs more than the spool, but it offers protection for the microfilm and is perhaps more easily indexed. A jacket is a plastic card which is a holder for flat strips of microfilm. When many micro-images are permanently printed on a plastic sheet, the sheet is called a microfiche. Aperture cards are used for such large presentations as engineering drawings, which are individually microfilmed and placed on one card before they are filed.

Microfilm records obviously save space. Also, with proper equipment and proper indexing techniques data are easily retrieved, and reproduction costs are cheaper than those associated with paper.

Some disadvantages are that special equipment is needed to work with microfilm. Cameras, processors, readers, and printers might be necessary. The cost effectiveness of a microfilm vs. paper system must be evaluated on an individual laboratory basis.

Record Keeping

Efficient record keeping involves both filing and easy retrieval of documents and data. A submitting agency often wants information on work done on a specimen months or years past. The laboratory must be able to locate such data. Thus, proper filing is essential. Some laboratories have separate files of positive and negative results in alphabetical order by patient. Some laboratories file positive and negative results together to avoid having to search two files. Other filing methods include, e.g., alphabetical files organized by requesting physician.

Obviously, the most important aspect of a form is the information it contains. A properly designed data-capture system requires properly designed output forms.

One type of output form is the report slip sent back to the submitting agency. The laboratory and the client should agree on what results and messages should be on the report slip. Then, if possible, all reports and messages should be preprinted so that the laboratorian can simply use check marks for the report. For example, a number of reasons why a specimen was unsatisfactory for testing when it arrived at the laboratory might be printed on the form.

In addition to the data the client wants, the laboratory director must keep in mind what reports must be made to administrative superiors. If reports by age, sex, locality, or agency submitting the request are desired, these data must be available on the report form.

If the data needed must be supplied by the submitting agency, appropriate space must be allocated on the submission side of the slip. If data to be reported by the laboratory to administrative superiors must be organized by the submitting agency and if many of the specimens regularly come from a few submitting agencies (clinics, hospitals, or some other agency), this information (type of submitting agency) could be preprinted on forms. Obviously, the proper forms must be sent to the appropriate agencies.

After all data are accounted for, the submission/report slip can be drawn up, field tested, corrected, and printed.

Automated Data Processing (ADP) Vs. Manual

When record keeping is discussed, the question arises as to whether the system should be manual or automated. The uninitiated visualize fewer people, fewer forms, and reduced costs. However, a computer-based system rarely requires fewer personnel (some might be reassigned to other duties), the number of forms might increase, and the cost of the operation would probably be at least as high as for a manual system.

ADP methodology applied to a data handling situation should allow personnel to perform more creative and challenging tasks after they are relieved of routine, tedious, clerical duties. If properly designed, such a system allows data to be easily retrieved for meaningful analysis for scientific and management purposes.

The submitting agency, the laboratory, and the computer must be interfaced in any ADP system. Data interchange among these elements must be easily conducted. Once again, the basic data form used to transmit data from one element to the others would be the specimen submission form. It must be designed so that the submitting agency can enter all necessary data with minimal effort. When possible, preprinted information and spaces to be checked should be used. The laboratory must have spaces to check or record test results and spaces to check messages preprinted on the form. Finally, the form should be designed so that data can be easily entered into the computer.

As with a manual system, an ADP system must be thoroughly studied, and the data must be defined from beginning to end. First, all laboratory reports to the submitting agency must be designed so that data needed to write the reports and to be entered in the computer are readily identified. The portion of the data to be supplied by the submitting agency and that to be supplied by the laboratory must then be determined. The submission slip can then be designed with a side for data from the submitting agency and one for data from the laboratory.

Not only must data to be used for routine reports be considered. Research studies and known special reports must be considered in terms of data that must be collected.

Personnel Management

Introduction

No company, business, or enterprise exists apart from people. Empty buildings and unused equipment never produce products, make profits, or cure the ill. Discussion of company aims and laboratory policy always must be couched in terms of people. No company earns a profit or assumes a position of leadership in its field independent of the manner in which its employees function. No laboratory serves the health needs of its clientele without productive laboratory personnel.

People in an organization can be success or failure oriented. Guidance, or lack of it, comes from that cadre of an organization called management. This chapter segment contains a brief discussion of some aspects of management as it relates to personnel—the most important aspect of any corporate body.

No claim of originality is made for this material, which is in essence a synthesis of what several members of the Laboratory Management Consultation Office (LMCO), Center for Disease Control, have researched, written about, lectured on, shared orally with me, or of material which has appeared in the literature.

Additional references are included at the end of this section for those interested in further reading.

Organization

Laboratory management must expend much thought and planning before a person is hired and placed in a position. Of major consideration must be the organization into which the person will be brought; there must be a qualified person for every place and a meaningful place for every person.

From a personnel viewpoint, the organizational chart or organizational layout is most important. For the employer's needs, it must include showing where personnel needs exist and helping to identify the type of background prospective employees should have. It shows the prospective employee where he will be located organizationally, where he fits into the laboratory's span of authority, and the pattern of supervisory responsibility.

An organizational layout which might be found in a laboratory is shown in Figure 1.1

Among other things, structured organizational charts such as that outlined in Figure 1.1 aid in identifying areas of responsibility and authority, improving communication channels, clarifying reporting relationships, improving managerial appraisal and training, and eliminating overlaps and conflicts. Unfortunately, a structured organizational chart shows only formal relationships. However, a laboratory manager should be aware that both formal and informal organizational structures probably exist in the laboratory, with the former following established lines of authority and responsibility and the latter following social lines. In order to optimize resources, a laboratory manager must try to make both structures compatible or accommodating, within reason.

Recruitment and Orientation

Despite all efforts by management and labor, problems do arise between employees and employers. The best time to try to avert these problems is during recruitment, placement, and orientation.

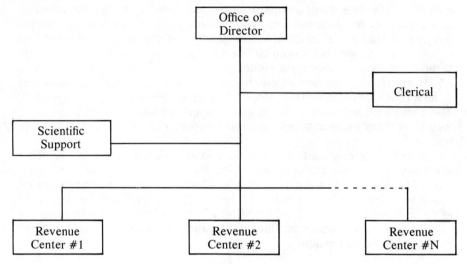

Figure 1.1 Organizational layout.

Unsuccessful recruitment and orientation programs can be extremely costly to an organization. Hiring an inappropriate person is a cost in terms of productivity and/or morale. Dollar costs are also associated with the failure of recruiting and training effort and the necessity to repeat the selection process. Finally, there is loss or cost to a laboratory if an excellent candidate is overlooked and not hired. Work relations will be much smoother if these preplacement criteria are met than if an employee was hired who should not have been or one was inappropriately placed.

Recruitment

Typically, successful recruitment is carried out as follows: planning, preparing to fill the position, screening, and hiring.

Because manpower requirements in an organization change over time, accurate planning should be an ongoing process. Unexpected job openings which occur for various reasons can lead to hasty, costly recruitment.

When a vacancy does occur or a new position is created, job descriptions or classifications, analysis of data on tasks to be performed, and salient personnel specifications must be carefully examined. Current information about the work environment should be used to define further the personnel specifications.

The actual employment process should proceed as follows: first, does any current employee qualify for the position? If so, external recruiting is an unjustified expense. On the other hand, if outside applicants must be located, such sources as schools, professional organizations, professional journals, and general advertisements should be investigated. Third, the qualifications of all the candidates should be evaluated on the basis of information on application blanks, academic and health records, telephone interviews, personal references, test results if applicable, and a personal employment interview. When this process is completed, final selection can be made on the basis of all the available information. If the candidate accepts the offer, efforts should be made to assist in his transition and possible relocation. If the candidate refuses the offer, an attempt should be made to find out why and to reassess the recruitment procedures.

The personal interview of potential employees is a very important part of the recruiting process. Hawk said that the interview is the oldest and most widely used method to appraise job qualifications (19).

From the viewpoint of a supervisor, the purposes of such an interview are to appraise qualifications, form opinions on compatibility, inform applicants of job requirements, indicate supervisor's expectations, and gain information on applicant's goals.

The applicants view the interview quite differently; they wish to learn of job requirements, to form opinions of the supervisor and other employees, to learn about policies and the supervisor's expectations, to appraise the working conditions, and to appraise opportunities for advancement.

Proper preparation and actual practice in effective interview techniques are exceptionally important. The US Civil Service Commission (34) published the following statement on interview preparation:

> The seeming simplicity of the interview has been one of the greatest obstacles to progress in this selection area. So many people interview, so little study is demanded of them, and so little checking of results is made, that many assume that no study and practice are needed. It is a sign of maturity to recognize the employment interview as one of the most complex of all assignments and accordingly, on the one hand, to have humility in reaching conclusions and, on the other, to acknowledge that *thorough preparation* is essential.

Preparation by a supervisor for an employment interview should include: reviewing job requirements and special desirable characteristics, reviewing information on the applicant, noting key points to make and items to be clarified, and preparing a proper physical and psychological interview setting.

Preparation by an applicant for an employment interview might include reading and inquiring about the area of employment, reviewing personal goals, and preparing a list of questions to be asked.

If the interview is to be effective, both interviewer and prospective employee must be unaffected and honest and be able to establish effective communication.

Orientation

The employer should be vitally concerned with the new employee's progress, particularly in his early months, and should insure that a proper orientation program is inaugurated. This program can be relatively simple if the employee was already in the organization but must be more complex if he was not. The new employee may have developed enthusiasm for his new job as a result of the manner in which he was recruited; if so, an orientation procedure is much easier to design and implement.

The supervisor should personally oversee the structured orientation process and ask other employees to assist in it. Orientation must be thorough and continuous because it should constitute the beginning of on-the-job training and career development.

The new employee will obtain some information and form some opinions which cannot be anticipated and may not be accurate. Some new employees become productive and well-adjusted members of the organization without much outside attention, but this progression cannot be relied on. Orientation in its general sense involves defining a desired direction. It should be a carefully structured program and should include instruction on the job to be performed, facilities, company policies, organizational structure, safety regulations and procedures, and personnel benefits and services.

Properly managed recruitment and orientation are essential to screening out potential problems.

Classification and Pay

Job classification and salary scale are areas of personnel management which involve studying and factually describing positions and, according to predetermined standards, assigning a proper level in the work and pay structures.

A competent manager will see to it that there is a meaningful and properly classified position for every employee and a qualified employee in every properly classified position. As stated previously, this process involves a great deal of effort.

Despite the best efforts of management, however, employees may sometimes be inappropriately placed. This error may occur in the context of an employee who is overqualified for a position and is unhappy because of the lack of challenge and opportunity for suitable professional advancement. Conversely, an employee placed in a position in which the demands are beyond his capabilities is likely to become quickly discouraged. Also, inappropriate placement can involve the type of position rather than necessary level of ability, e.g., an employee who likes to work with people and instead is placed in a research position and must work alone most of the time. Finally, management must be ever aware of the necessity to avoid any appearance of making placement decisions on the basis of any factor which could be construed as discriminating against race, sex, color, age, creed, religions, or national origin.

Classification and pay can be effectively used by management to avert employee dissatisfaction, union grievances, and general unrest in the work environment. Ideally, the manager weighs all relevant factors and makes decisions which stimulate a productive work environment in which appropriate persons occupy appropriate jobs.

Productivity

High production, high quality work results, low operating costs, and fair charges for services are all proper and meaningful goals for the laboratory. If they are achieved, both laboratory personnel and consumers benefit.

Productivity levels are dependent upon the proper stimulus applied at the proper time. Elwell attempted to determine whether there was a correlation between workload fluctuation and the productivity of workers (13). One of his study environments had a steady workload with little monthly fluctuation, whereas the second had a varying workload. He found a lower productivity level associated with a steady workload, possibly because the workers had developed a steady and slower work pace. Conversely, apparently a varying workload did not lead to slower work habits being formed. On the basis of his findings, Elwell suggested allowing employees time away from the bench during work lulls to pursue other interests such as continuing education.

In another publication, Elwell examined the problem of leadership and group performance in the laboratory (14). This study centered on leadership situations in which a group either worked on structured tasks (diagnostic testing) or on unstructured tasks (research). Findings showed that a well-liked laboratory supervisor in charge of a group performing structured tasks should be directive, goal oriented, and concerned with efficiency. However, a well-liked laboratory supervisor in charge of a group performing unstructured tasks should be human-relations oriented and should practice participative management.

An unpopular supervisor of a group performing structured tasks should concentrate on displaying an interest in the welfare of group members. An unpopular supervisor in charge of a group performing unstructured tasks should emphasize the task or tasks at hand.

Each health-related laboratory employs valuable and scarce input resources such as personnel, money, equipment, and time to derive meaningful and desirable output data. The common problem is a need for a management tool that would help measure productivity in terms of how effectively and efficiently the input resources were used to produce the output data. There could be up to five areas of concern in a health-related laboratory: administration, biologics production, research, diagnostic services, and laboratory improvement. In the particular case of state public health laboratories a review of consolidated annual reports indicates that approximately 80%-90% of a laboratory's resources are used in the diagnostic services area (7).

The usual custom of reporting laboratory diagnostic workload in terms of numbers of tests performed in a specified period does not provide an accurate measurement of laboratory activity. Such a reporting scheme could be misunderstood by comptrollers and other budgeting personnel not keenly aware of laboratory procedures. A method has been developed which can be used to measure productivity quantitatively (6). This subject is discussed in the Cost Accounting section. However, it should be mentioned here that the number and type of personnel needed to perform examinations could be calculated using weighted workload values (23).

Motivation

As Duncan and Lawton noted, the subject of motivation is of utmost importance because a well-qualified employee who is properly motivated is of inestimable value (8). Since management oversees labor in the production process, it must be aware of the importance of motivation in affecting output.

Webster's New World Dictionary defines motive as "some inner drive, impulse, intention, etc., that causes a person to do something or act in a certain way." Federal and state governments sometimes motivate health-oriented groups to police themselves by threatening them with regulatory laws. According to Myers, there are two types of job-related incentives: motivators and dissatisfiers (27).

> Motivators are those factors about a job that allow an employee to have his needs and aspirations responded to and fulfilled, such as professional training and career development. Dissatisfiers are mostly those factors which are peripheral to the job: work rules, lighting, coffee breaks, fringe benefits, etc. Dissatisfiers are among the inducements applicants look for in today's technologist job market, but motivators are the major considerations and major elements which hold an employee.

In some cases, when employers and employees seem at odds with each other, the employee has misunderstood the expectations of the supervisor, and the manager has misunderstood what the worker expects from the job. For example, an employer might feel that the prime motivator for an employee is money. Ford (16) makes the following observation:

> Once a person has enough income to satisfy adequately one's physiological and security needs, nonmonetary incentives often meet more effectively the needs at higher levels of satisfaction. Money can buy an employee's presence, but not his enthusiasm.

Faulty communication or lack of communication may lead to these misconceptions about sources of motivation and may therefore lead to motivational problems.

Morley and Silver found that the project manager like the film director must depend on four sources of motivation: A sense of professionalism, the basic need to exercise competence, the need for approval and appreciation, and long-term career self-interest (26).

Gelfand states (17):

> The motivation of an employee at any level is strongly related to the supervisory style of his first line supervisor. But this precept is true for all levels of management, and hence it reaches to the top man in an organization. Thus, sound motivation patterns and practices must begin at the top of an organization.

Sometimes a person does not perform satisfactorily because of not understanding the job function or objectives. Communication is a two-way street. Information must be conveyed, but it also must be received. Ideally, in a third step the conveyer and receiver confirm that the information was accurately transferred. The latter is not always feasible, but the person who gives instructions should always try to do so clearly, concisely, and completely. Many times people do not wish to admit that they do not understand, and other times they are not aware of it.

Another problem could arise when output is lagging, but the turnover rate is slow and the manager may believe that his people are happy and contented in their jobs. Thus, he may attribute the low productivity to other factors. The workers actually may be unhappy for several reasons. Sometimes turnover is the not the best sign of job problems, as stated by Ford: "Employees on the job can be unhappy and it will show up in restricted productivity, excessive absenteeism, grievances, and so on" (16).

Some managers do not delegate authority when assigning work. Their employees are given tasks with little or no authority to carry them out—a situation designed to produce frustration. Such a situation could arise, e.g., between a pathologist and a technologist or between a physician and a nurse.

Situations also exist in which a manager does not solicit input from employees. A smart manager is one who acknowledges his fallibility; his employees are certainly aware of it. One who does not ask for and listen to input from employees runs the risk of having the errors he makes gleefully spotted by the employees who might have been able to help to avoid them.

The manager sometimes must deal with the problem of an employee who loses confidence in himself and is unable to produce adequately. Such a situation may result from inordinate use of alcohol, drugs, or emotional disturbance. Granted, laboratory directors should not be expected to be practicing psychologists or psychiatrists, but knowing when to seek professional aid for an employee is very important.

If the lack of confidence on an employee's part is job related, the manager should play a more active role trying to find the source of and alleviate the problem. Such situations as changes in organization or procedures, computer utilization or automated procedures, or a feeling of being eclipsed by younger employees all may contribute to such depression. After the manager has assessed the situation, if he finds no tangible, correctible problem, he should try to arouse the employee's self-involvement, show confidence in the employee and give credit where due and when possible. If on the other hand a situation arises in which the employee believes that his performance is acceptable and the manager does not, it is the manager's responsibility to explain and reemphasize what the employee is expected to accomplish in a given time frame.

It is important to remember that achievement and recognition are both very important to workers and that to a great degree they measure their achievement in terms of the recognition they receive.

Occasionally, a worker promoted to a supervisory position has motivational problems. A supervisor usually is chosen because of professional competence within an academic discipline. Sometimes a good scientist makes a poor supervisor. Too many administrators are still mainly work specialists at heart. Occasionally, for example, a laboratorian feels that it is downgrading to be a manager and wishes to "get back to the bench." Such people do not feel that management is challenging or important (27). By the same token a manager who has little scientific knowledge may sometimes fail to understand problems in a practical laboratory context.

As one author has said, when managers lack the knowledge or skill required to perform the work, they need to know how to share their traditional authority with those who know what has to be done and to motivate them to get results. When managers lack the charisma needed to generate the cooperation of their staffs, they must be able to share their traditional authority with the informal leaders of the group and motivate them to get results.

The point is that in the laboratory there are two basic advancement routes—one technical and the other managerial—and a successful facility must have both types of personnel. In considering the routes, one should be aware of the fact that managers can usually progress to higher levels in an organization than can technologists.

Sometimes a novice manager confuses theory and fact. Often he expects the impossible from his employees and does not understand why they fall short of his goals. A successful manager takes an existing situation and improves it as much as possible.

Experts in the field of motivation have noted some general comments that professional people have been heard to make concerning supervisors such as: "I'm never told what I'm expected to produce or how I'm expected to perform." "I'm not given enough responsibility." "My boss never clarifies his instructions or ideas. I'm always confused." "I don't have the leeway to do my job. I feel too constrained." "I need purpose and direction. Just doing 1,000 specimens a day is no motivation for me." "My boss shows favoritism." "This outfit is interested in you only if you produce, not as an individual. They tell us almost nothing about what's going on." And as Vogel states (35): "If employers recognized worth, unions might not be needed."

Numerous benefits can accompany improved motivation. Among them are increased output and efficiency, lower attrition among personnel, and less waste of time and material. All of the above should lower operating costs.

Several years ago Myers at Texas Instruments conducted a motivational study with startling results (27). Subsequently, organizations looked more closely at the dissatisfiers mentioned earlier. In essence, the study findings showed that people want to work and do not necessarily need to be prodded; they want responsibility on the job; they desire to see the big picture. Motivation seems to stem from the very challenge of the job. Workers want a sense of achievement. Of course, achievement means different things to different people. Part of management's job is to determine the factors involved in allowing each employee to succeed psychologically on the job.

Ford says: "The last third of the 20th century will see greater shortages of competent employees than ever before in our country's history. Being a successful manager is of the utmost importance" (16). Motivation is an indispensable tool for the manager as he utilizes his most valuable resource—people.

Performance Evaluation

An employer must give performance feedback to all employees, including defining the areas in which they exceed expectations and those in which improvement can be made and is expected. In terms of exceeding or failing expectations, there must be a method for comparison and for discussing the comparison—e.g., the employee's performance evaluation procedure.

One authority on personnel management describes evaluating employees as: "The act of estimating the relative worth of employees in order to determine the rewards, privileges, or advantages that should be given or withheld from each" (12). Cavenaugh, Jones, and Brownfield describe performance evaluation as a process by which the supervisor and the employee jointly work toward higher levels of employee achievement (5).

To appraise is inevitable and is a fundamental experience in organizational life. Modern appraisal programs attempt to minimize any bias or inconsistency, establish a format for the review of job performance, and develop a basic method of follow-up to this assessment.

Properly conducted formal performance evaluation programs are expected to help accomplish the following objectives: maintaining acceptable job behavior or improving unacceptable performance, developing improved supervisory relationships, enhancing employee development through evaluation of training opportunities, altering the work environment or redefining a job description to increase responsibility, and determining personnel actions such as transfers, promotions, and dismissals.

Brownfield and Jones categorize the above objectives under Administrative and Self-Improvement, although these categories are not original with them (4). Under Administrative, some possible purposes of performance appraisal programs are: basis for reward, basis for personnel actions, means to help management optimize training and developmental expenditures, basis for certain personnel research, opportunity for stimulation of raters (usually supervisors) to observe and interrelate more constructively, and means to control employee behavior to the extent that organizational objectives are more likely to be realized. Under Self-Improvement, some possible purposes of performance appraisal programs are: opportunity for increased communication and improved supervisor-subordinate relationship, opportunity for job analysis, opportunity for reinforcement of appreciation and identification within the larger organizational unit, opportunity for increased employee understanding and appreciation of organizational mission and activities, and opportunity to effect changes leading to increased job satisfaction.

Appraisal procedures should make an employee aware of personal good points or shortcomings. The rater should have observed performance frequently and discussed it with the employee as often as necessary. Under no circumstances should the outcome of a scheduled, formal performance evaluation come as a total surprise to the employee, especially if it is negative.

Methods introduced over the years for recording and evaluating job behavior have produced a variety of formats. Some examples follow. The ranking method identifies employees in descending order of performance. The rating scale method identifies all employees on some type of scale, perhaps ranging from poor to excellent. The profit performance method is an appraisal of employees by amounts of monetary profit realized in their organizational segment. The objective analyses method appraises employees by degree to which personal and/or organizational goals have been reached.

The job-behavior check list method involves completing a check list for each employee that defines a job in terms of behavior necessary for successful performance. The forced-choice method identifies the most accurate description of each employee from two or more equally desirable phrases. The modified rating-scale method identifies individual employee behavior on scales that have placed proficiency into dimensions of priority.

The person who applies any of these methods should be the one who is most familiar with pertinent job-related behavior—generally the employee's immediate supervisor. However, having the employee and the supervisor work in combination as raters is gaining in popularity. This approach should improve communication in performance appraisal sessions.

In terms of objective, measurable, and achievable work standards, formal judgments, appraisal interviews, and follow-up activities constitute the principal steps in the evaluation process (4). Raters are encouraged to identify factors outside the employee's control which may have affected performance and to avoid the tendency to rate too high (overvalue).

Some suggestions for raters or interviews include: review job specifications and performance standards of employee prior to the appraisal interview; arrange for a suitable environment for the appraisal interview; listen carefully; never discuss another employee; discuss both good and bad points.

If the worker's productivity is indeed down, the supervisor and the employee should agree on courses of action and establish long- and short-term goals which harmonize with organizational objectives. Proposed dates of accomplishment for each goal should be agreed on, and results of these should be followed up. Follow-up activities are important because they provide feedback on progress toward agreed-upon changes, reinforce personal interest, and establish the entire appraisal process as a meaningful instrument. Follow-up may consist of such activities as additional interviews or special visits to the worksite to clarify work assignments.

Personnel Problems

Many define the function of management as planning, organizing, directing, and controlling. Handling personnel problems is part of the controlling function. As stated earlier, the ideal method of handling personnel problems is to prevent them. Since this ideal cannot always be achieved, we offer the following lists of typical personnel problems which Brownfield and Jones classified according to the basic source of dissatisfaction (3).

Personnel problems arising primarily from employee dissatisfaction include: training provided, general working conditions (e.g., heating and lighting), opportunities for advancement, failure to be selected for promotion, and work environment in general.

Personnel problems primarily resulting in employer dissatisfaction include: low productivity, careless work, and being a source of spreading dissatisfaction.

One possible symptom of employee dissatisfaction is a high attrition rate. This aspect of personnel problems is covered by Stewart (32), who lists some of the attendant costs as:

1. Costs incurred in hiring and training each new employee:
   a. Personnel department costs,
   b. Training costs,
   c. Pay to the new employee over and above actual productivity during learning state,
   d. Breakage and wasted materials during the learning period,
   e. Possible costs in accidents while the new employee is being trained.
2. Costs of overtime work which may be required by regular employees to maintain work output until the new employee can be trained to do his share.
3. Loss of production in the interval between the time the former employee is separated and the new employee is fully trained:
   a. Maximum loss until replacement arrives,
   b. Loss in group efficiency during readjustment by group to new employee.
4. Expense from laboratory equipment not being fully utilized during the training period.

Ford states: "A high employee turnover rate is bad enough. However, the turnover rate of employees on the job less than one year is another matter. These employees are just too expensive for any organization" (16).

All managers should have a basic understanding of the categories of problem employees and methods of coping with them (3). The manager should also know where to turn for assistance in dealing with problems. The director of a public health or other laboratory in a Government agency can normally turn to the personnel office for assistance, whereas a hospital laboratory director can expect help from the administrative office.

To be as effective as possible in resolving personnel problems, the supervisor must be informed of currently applicable policies, rules and regulations, precedents established in dealing with similar situations, and of the facts of the problem in question.

Summary

A manager is responsible for working with and through others. Supervisory responsibility is represented in the functions of planning, organizing, directing, and controlling. This brief discussion of personnel management has touched lightly on the manager's role as seen in organization, recruitment and orientation, classification and pay, productivity, motivation, performance evaluation, and handling personnel problems.

References

1. AMOS RE: Should your lab manage by objectives. Medical Laboratory, November:40–43, 1976
2. BROWNFIELD RL and IVES ER: Creating a data base for the laboratory universe. Lab Manage 14:22–26, 1976
3. BROWNFIELD RL and JONES WR: Handling Personnel Problems, Training Material, Laboratory Management Consultation Office, Center for Disease Control, Atlanta, Georgia 30333

4. BROWNFIELD RL and JONES WR: Performance Evaluation Programs, Training Material, Laboratory Management Consultation Office, Center for Disease Control, Atlanta, Georgia 30333
5. CAVENAUGH EL, JONES WR, and BROWNFIELD RL: A supervisor's guide to performance evaluation, Lab Anim 5:26 ff, 1976
6. CENTER FOR DISEASE CONTROL: Diagnostic Workload Measurement: A Relative Value Structure for Public Health Laboratories. Laboratory Management Consultation Office, Center for Disease Control, Atlanta, Georgia 30333, 1973
7. CENTER FOR DISEASE CONTROL: Consolidated Annual Report on State and Territorial Public Health Laboratories. Fiscal Years 1974-1976. Center for Disease Control, Atlanta, Georgia 30333
8. DUNCAN CR and LAWTON HL: Motivation for results. Cadence 4:9-14, 1973
9. DUNCAN CR: Cost accounting for the laboratory. Cadence Sept/Oct: 27-35, 1974
10. DUNCAN CR: Application of cost finding methods to the laboratory. Cadence Jan/Feb: 24-31, 1975
11. DUNCAN CR: Cost accounting in the laboratory—a management tool. South Carolina Bureau of Laboratories Newsletter 9:3, 1977
12. Effective Communication on the Job. American Management Association, Inc, New York, 1973
13. ELWELL GR: Employee productivity: Why do laboratories differ? Lab Manage 13:24-30, 1975
14. ELWELL GR: Leadership and group performance in the laboratory. Lab Med 7:41-42, 1976
15. Estimated Useful Lives of Depreciable Hospital Assets. American Hospital Association, Chicago, Ill
16. FORD RH: Motivation Through the Work Itself. American Management Association, Inc, New York, 1969
17. GELFAND LI: Communicate through your supervisors. Harv Bus Rev 48:101-104, 1970
18. HANLON JJ: Principles of Public Health Administration. 5th edition. The C. V. Mosby Co., St. Louis, 1969, pp 572-573
19. HAWK RH: The Recruitment Function. American Management Association, Inc, New York, 1967
20. JACOBSEN WR: The Diagnostic Marketplace. Medical Marketing and Media, February 1973, pp 1-8
21. KATZ SH, DIAMOND B, PRIER JE, LUKASZCZYK TA, and KEGERRIS JB: Regionalization of laboratory services. Health Lab Sci 10:287-293, 1973
22. LAWTON HL: Diagnostic workload measurement: a relative value structure for public health laboratories. Public Health Lab 31:117-120, 1973
23. LAWTON HL and BROWNFIELD RL: The number of personnel needed to perform examinations. Health Lab Sci 13:118-120, 1976
24. LAWTON HL, DUGAN JB, and ROSSING PH: The national clinical and public health laboratory survey 1977. Am J Med Tech 43:885-895, 1977
25. MARIEN R: Marien on Forms Control, Prentice-Hall, Inc., Englewood Cliffs, N.J., 1962, p 71
26. MORLEY E and SILVER A: A film director's approach to managing creativity. Harv Bus Rev 55:59-70, 1977
27. MYERS MS: Who are your motivated workers? Harv Bus Rev 42:73-88, 1964
28. National Survey of Hospital Clinical Laboratories. Lab Manage 14:18-39, 1976
29. National Survey of Non-Hospital Clinical Laboratories. Lab Manage 14:17-36, 1976
30. ROBINSON D: Cost and Effectiveness of a Program to Prevent Rheumatic Fever. HSMHA Health Rep 86:385-389, 1971
31. SCHMIDT RM and MADOFF MA: The state and territorial public health laboratory: program activities, organization and prospects for the future. Am J Public Health 67:433-438, 1977
32. STEWART CE: Personnel, Training Material, Laboratory Management Consultation Office, Center for Disease Control, Atlanta, Georgia 30333, Chap 3
33. Tax Information on Depreciation. Publ No. 534, Internal Revenue Service, US Department of the Treasury, 1974
34. US CIVIL SERVICE COMMISSION: Employment Interviewing. Personnel Methods, Series No. 5, US Civil Service Commission, Washington, DC, 1956, p 1

35. VOGEL A: Your clerical workers are ripe for unionism. Harv Bus Rev 49:48–54, 1971

General References

AMER DS: Productivity, Personnel, and Problems of Hospital Clinical Laboratories. Bureau of Business and Economic Research, Public Service Grant R01PM00001, Northeastern University, Boston, Mass, 1969

BASSETT GA: Practical Interviewing. American Management Association, Inc, New York, 1965

BATTEN JD: Beyond Management by Objectives. American Management Association, New York, 1966

BENNINGTON JL, WESTLAKE GE, and LOUVAN GE: Financial Management of the Clinical Laboratory. University Park Press, Baltimore, Md, 1974

BLOOM GF: Productivity: weak link in our economy. Harv Bus Rev 49:4 ff, 1971

BONIN P and LAWTON HL: Seattle-King County revisited. Health Lab Sci 13:271–274, 1976

BONIN P, TRONCA EL, and LAWTON HL: A relative value structure for the Seattle-King County public health laboratory. Health Lab Sci 9:112–117, 1972

BOWMAN GW: What helps or harms promotability? Harv Bus Rev 42:6–26, 1964

BROWNFIELD RL and JONES WR: Recruitment and Orientation, Training Material, Laboratory Management Consultation Office, Center for Disease Control, Atlanta, Georgia 30333

BURCH EE: Productivity: its meaning and measurement. Atlanta Economic Review, May-June, 1974

Business Forms. North American Publishing Co., Philadelphia, 1973

Committee on Laboratory Management and Planning: Laboratory Workload Recording Method, 4th edition. College of American Pathologists, Skokie, Ill, 1977

Committee on Unit Values. Canadian Association of Pathologists, Ottawa Civic Hospital, Ottawa, Ontario, Canada: Reevaluation of the Dominion Bureau of Statistics Unit for Clinical Laboratory Procedures, A Report on Canadian Public Health Grant Number 605-7-363, 1968

CONNELLY T: Recruiting: what tactics really work? Medical Lab, United Business Publications, Inc, 1971

Coordinator of Special Studies in Hospital Management, Chicago Hospital Council: A Work Measurement Study of Procedures in Hospital Clinical Laboratories. Chicago Hospital Council, Chicago, Ill, 1965

DALE E: Organization. American Management Association, New York, 1967

DRUCKER PF: The Practice of Management. Harper and Row, New York, 1964

DUNNETTE MD: Personnel Selection and Placement. Wadsworth Publishing, Belmont, Calif, 1966

ELWELL GR and LAWTON HL: A relative value structure helps laboratory management fight the numbers racket. Health Lab Sci 10:203–208, 1973

ELWELL GR, LAWTON HL, and DUNCAN CR: An analysis of cost studies performed in public health laboratories. Health Lab Sci 14:140–144, 1977

FIEDLER FE and CHEMERS MM: Leadership and Effective Management. Scott, Foresman and Co, Glenview, Ill, 1974

FITZGERALD TH: Why motivation theory doesn't work. Harv Bus Rev 49:37–44, 1971

Forms Design and Control. Association for Systems Management, Cleveland, 1970

FRIEDMAN EM: Fringe benefits in the laboratory. Medical Laboratory Observer, May-June, Medical Economics, Inc, Oradell, NJ, 1971

GELLERMAN SW: Management by Motivation. American Management Association, 1971

GILMORE FF: Formulating strategy in smaller companies. Harv Bus Rev 49:71–81, 1971

GRIFFIN DF and GREEBAN GB: The M.T. as supervisor: are you really ready to step into management? Medical Lab, July, 1971

HAINLINE A: The time-skill-frequency (TSF) unit for reporting laboratory workload. Clin Chem 8:665–672, 1962

HARGROVE WR: Better direction to continuing education. Cadence, March-April, 1971

HERZBERG F, MAUSNER B, and SNYDERMAN B: The Motivation to Work, 2nd edition, The World Publishing Co, Cleveland, Ohio, 1966

HICKS HA: Philosophy of laboratory control. Health Lab Sci. 10:268–270, 1973

HORTON FW: Reference Guide to Advanced Management Methods. American Management Association, Inc, New York, 1972

HUTCHINSON JG: Organizations: Theory and Classical Concepts. Holt, Rinehart, and Winston, New York, 1967

Interagency Committee on Laboratory Medicine: A Clinical Laboratory Workload Reporting System. VA Monograph 10-3. Veterans Administration, Washington, DC, 1967

JUCIUS MJ: Personnel Management, 6th edition. RD Irwin, Inc, Homewood, Ill, 1967

KAISER B: Forms Design and Control. American Management Association, New York, 1968

KELLOGG MS: What to do About Performance Appraisal. American Management Association, Inc, New York, 1965

KRUER C: Workload Measurement, A Relative Value Structure. Master of Science Thesis, School of Allied Health Sciences, Georgia State Univ, 1975

LAWTON HL: Development of a relative value structure. Public Health Lab 33:116-122, 1975

LEE JA: Behavioral theory vs. reality. Harv Bus Rev 49:20-ff, 1971

LEVINSON H: Business is Person to Person. Forbes, 1967

LIVINGSTON JS: Myth of the well-educated manager. Harv Bus Rev 49:79-89, 1971

LYNTON RP and PAREEK U: Training for Development. The Dorsey Press, Homewood, Ill, 1967

MARCH, JG: Handbook of Organizations. Rand McNally and Co, Chicago, Ill, 1965

MARTIN BG: The intangible fringes. Medical Laboratory Observer, May-June, Medical Economics, Inc, Oradell, NJ, 1971

MOCKLER RJ: Situational theory of management. Harv Bus Rev 49:146-154, 1971

MOORE RF: AMA Management Handbook. American Management Association, Inc, New York, 1970

MYERS MS: Conditions for manager motivation. Harv Bus Rev 44:58-71, 1966

MYERS MS: Overcoming union opposition to job enrichment. Harv Bus Rev 49:37-49, 1971

Records Management Handbook Forms Design. General Services Administration, National Archives and Records Service, Washington, DC, 1960

ROBINSON RQ and CAVENAUGH EL: Public health laboratories and the future. Health Lab Sci 12:301-304, 1975

ROCHE WJ and MACKINNON NL: Motivating people with meaningful work. Harv Bus Rev 48:97-110, 1970

SIROTA D and GREENWOOD JM: Understand your overseas work force. Harv Bus Rev 49:53-60, 1971

SKINNER W: The anachronistic factory. Harv Bus Rev 49:61-70, 1971

VARDAMAN B: Forms for Better Communication. Effective Communications Series, Van Nostrand Reinhold Co, New York, 1971

WERTLAKE PT: How much employee work time is really available? Lab Manage 12:24, 1974

CHAPTER 2

QUALITY ASSURANCE IN CLINICAL MICROBIOLOGY
Barbara G. Painter

Introduction

Quality assurance can be broadly defined as the adherence to well-prescribed procedures designed to assure the laboratorian that the quality of the work is accurate, reproducible, and reliable. Good quality control practices insure meaningful results which can benefit the patient, the physician, and laboratory personnel. Federal (Clinical Laboratories Improvement Act, 1967) and, in many instances, state and city regulatory agencies have instituted protocols which the clinical microbiology laboratory must follow in order to meet licensing requirements and/or third party payment. Aside from the requirements by law, an ongoing quality control program in the laboratory is necessary from the viewpoint of good practice. Without controls, there is no way to determine whether a test, procedure, or personnel are performing properly and whether the end result is accurate. Any scientific endeavor has always included controls within the experimental design; the clinical microbiology laboratory should not be an exception.

Medical costs continue to rise, making necessary a reduction in personnel and operating costs in many, if not most, hospitals. Concurrently, the need for adequate quality control has not diminished, but rather has escalated. This increased demand for quality assurance in the laboratory obviously requires more technologists' time and increased laboratory expense; thus, an objective of the clinical microbiology laboratory should be to institute simple, inexpensive, but effective methods to maintain an acceptable program of quality control.

General Considerations

A prerequisite requirement for quality control in the laboratory is the degree of qualification and expertise exhibited by the laboratory staff. The construction of a comprehensive program is of minimal value if the bench technologist, media technician, or laboratory aide is not adequately trained and instructed in proper laboratory methodology.

The laboratory should have a procedure manual which is reviewed at appropriate intervals and updated by the supervisor or laboratory director. New personnel should be required to read the manual in order to orient

31

themselves to the established protocol within the laboratory. This practice serves to standardize techniques from individual to individual, thus enabling the supervisor to pinpoint sources of error or breaks in technique. Technical personnel should be encouraged to participate in continuing education programs, and in-house continuing education should be conducted by a microbiologist or other qualified persons on a regular basis. Journals, textbooks, and other references should be available in the laboratory.

Encouraging the technical staff to participate in the quality control program enhances its effectiveness. Thus, problems will be more readily reported to the supervisor, who should take prompt corrective measures. Although each individual contributes to the program in a general way, one person should be responsible for monitoring media, reagents, and equipment. This position can be assumed on a rotation basis, depending upon the individual laboratory structure. The quality control technologist should report to the supervisor or laboratory director.

Accurate records should be maintained in the appropriate quality control log books. These logs should be dated and initialled when the data are entered. The information recorded in the log book should be sufficient to determine the quality of the item being monitored.

Proficiency Testing

Several agencies provide external proficiency testing programs. These include the College of American Pathologists, the American Society of Clinical Pathologists, the Center for Disease Control, and various city and state health departments. Although external proficiency programs may be required for laboratory licensing, the results of this type of testing aid in determining the quality of laboratory performance. Deficiencies in media, reagents, equipment, and personnel can be detected, and appropriate corrective measures can be taken. Specimens from such external sources should be processed in the same manner as patient specimens, but they will probably receive special attention unless introduced into the laboratory as routine cultures. Proficiency cultures often contain organisms infrequently isolated in the laboratory, thereby providing an excellent educational tool. Plate rounds conducted on unusual organisms and discussion of the laboratory results are not only educational but stimulate interest among the staff members.

Internal proficiency testing should be conducted on a weekly basis, because it will most often reflect unbiased overall quality of laboratory performance. These cultures may be submitted as "patient" specimens. In small laboratories with few staff members, the laboratory director may be responsible for issuing internal specimens.

External and internal proficiency testing should not be misconstrued as an exercise in "what's wrong," but rather as a means to educate, learn, and determine "what's right."

Preventive Maintenance

The care and service of equipment in the laboratory must be performed at two levels: (a) The laboratory director or supervisor should assume the responsibility for establishing a maintenance schedule for each piece of equipment. After preparation of this schedule, the facility's maintenance or plant engineering department should be notified when service is required. Occasionally, external service contracts will be needed. Schematic diagrams and the operating manual for all equipment should be accessible to both the maintenance department and to laboratory personnel. (b) Equipment should be cared for and maintained on a daily basis by laboratory personnel. Monitoring equipment at prescribed intervals facilitates the detection of malfunction.

Each morning, the temperatures of refrigerators, freezers, incubators, heating blocks, and water baths should be recorded. Automatic temperature and humidity recording devices for incubators and refrigerators are desirable as is an alarm to alert personnel to malfunction.

Biological safety cabinets should be checked for adequate air flow and for the effectiveness of the ultraviolet light. The ultraviolet lighting fixture should be cleaned with ethyl alcohol weekly and its output monitored at least every 3 months.

Autoclaves should be equipped with automatic temperature recorders. The charts provide a permanent record of the duration and the temperature of each cycle. These charts, along with those from other equipment, should be maintained for 2 years (3). At least once a week, a spore preparation which can be obtained from commercial sources should be included with an autoclave run to monitor the autoclave's effectiveness. This does not preclude careful inspection of the chart after each autoclave cycle.

Anaerobic jars can be monitored by including a "stool pigeon" such as *Clostridium novyi* each time a jar is closed. Fresh catalyst should be used each day.

CO_2 incubators and candle jars can be monitored by including a CO_2-dependent *Neisseria gonorrhoeae* each day. The CO_2 level in the incubator should be checked to assure an adequate supply for the night.

A maintenance log for each piece of equipment can be filed or attached directly to the equipment. Space should be provided for the date, type of service, actual measurement (temperature), comments, and the initials of the person performing the check. Bartlett (1) and Ellis (3) provide detailed maintenance schedules for most laboratory equipment.

Media

Culture media which are prepared in-house should be purchased in dehydrated form from a reliable commercial company, which generally assures consistent performance of the medium from batch to batch, and reduces the amount of quality control procedures—i.e., the testing of raw materials. The bottles of media should be dated upon receipt and again when opened. After they are opened, media bottles should be stored tightly closed to prevent any deterioration. Although a dehydrated medium may be of high quality, it must be carefully prepared if a high-quality finished product is to be obtained. The media technician not only should be well trained in the basic skills required for successful media production, but should understand the necessity for strict adherence to the manufacturer's instructions.

The quality of the final product depends on the following procedures: (a) accurate weighing of dry materials, (b) accurate measurement of water, (c) use of deionized water of good microbiological quality, (d) use of clean glassware, (e) obtaining a homogeneous mixture before dispensing, (f) proper pH of the medium, (g) correct sterilization at prescribed temperature and pressure, (h) careful measurement of additives, and (i) avoidance of prolonged heating before dispensing (5). An automatic volume-controlled dispensing device insures a constant volume and greater reproducibility from plate to plate and reduces costs from those associated with pouring plates manually.

The quality control technologist should select a representative sample from each batch of media to check for sterility by overnight incubation at 35 C. Blood agar should be incubated at room temperature for an additional 24 hr. At least 5% of the tubes or plates should be checked if fewer than 100 are prepared in a batch; for larger volumes, 10–20 tubes or plates may be selected (2). To prevent dehydration, all media excluding thio and thiol should be stored at 4–8 C, the caps on tubed media should be tightly closed (after cooling), and plated media should be stored in plastic bags if they are to be kept for a long period of time. Each batch should be labelled with the date of preparation and description.

After the media are prepared, the quality control technologist is responsible for insuring that that batch functions properly. Samples of the media are inoculated with stock organisms of known physiological and biochemical properties. Test organisms should be selected which will demonstrate the selectivity, inhibitory effects, colonial morphology, growth characteristics, or biochemical reactions for which the medium is intended. Usually, more than one test organism is needed to monitor each medium effectively. Plated media should be inoculated lightly to insure that relatively low numbers of organisms will be isolated. Tubed media should be inoculated according to laboratory procedure. Table 2.1 contains a representative list of commonly used media with their control organisms and expected reactions. When it is not possible to monitor a medium prior to use, additional media from the same batch should be tested concomitantly with the appropriate control organisms.

The results obtained from monitoring the media should be entered in a media quality control log book by the quality control technologist. These data should include the date of preparation, media description, source, lot (control) number, quantity, sterility results, test organism results, the initials of the quality control technologist, and the dates they were tested. If a batch of medium is rejected, this fact should be noted in the log book. The deficient medium must be discarded and the source of error determined.

TABLE 2.1   CONTROLS FOR PLATED MEDIA

MEDIUM	CONTROL ORGANISMS	EXPECTED RESULTS
Blood agar	*Streptococcus pyogenes*	β-Hemolysis
	Streptococcus pneumoniae	α-Hemolysis
Bismuth sulfite	*Escherichia coli*	Inhibited or pale green
	Salmonella typhimurium	Black colonies, metallic sheen
Chocolate agar	*Haemophilus influenzae*	Good growth
	Neisseria gonorrhoeae	Good growth
Corn meal	*Candida albicans*	Growth
Eosin methylene blue	*Escherichia coli*	Lactose positive
	Shigella flexneri	Colorless colonies
	Enterococcus	Inhibition
Hektoen enteric	*Escherichia coli*	Orange colonies
	Salmonella typhimurium	Green colonies, black centers
	Shigella flexneri	Green colonies
MacConkey	*Escherichia coli*	Lactose positive
	Shigella flexneri	Colorless colonies
	Enterococcus	No growth
Modified Thayer-Martin	*Neisseria gonorrhoeae*	Good growth
	Candida sp.	No growth
	Proteus mirabilis	Inhibition of swarming
	Staphylococcus epidermidis	No growth
Mycosel	*Candida albicans*	Growth
	Escherichia coli	No growth
	Aspergillus sp.	No growth
Phenylethyl alcohol	*Streptococcus pyogenes*	Growth
	Proteus mirabilis	Inhibited growth
Sabouraud	*Candida albicans*	Growth
	Escherichia coli	Inhibited growth
Salmonella-Shigella	*Escherichia coli*	Inhibited or no growth
	Salmonella typhimurium	Clear colonies
Selective enterococcus agar	Enterococcus	Colonies with black zone
	Streptococcus mitis	No growth
Staphylococcus 110	*Staphylococcus aureus*	Growth, typical colonies
	Escherichia coli	No growth
XLD	*Escherichia coli*	Yellow or inhibited
	Salmonella typhimurium	Pink-red with black centers
	Shigella flexneri	Pink colonies

Reagents

All chemicals should be dated when received and stored in a cool area. After the containers are opened, the caps must be reclosed tightly. Infrequently used chemicals should be ordered in small quantities to reduce deterioration before use. Reagents should be prepared carefully and stored in opaque bottles at room temperature unless otherwise indicated. The date of preparation and the initials of the person who prepared the reagent should be included on the label. Pre-prepared reagents and those made in-house should be tested with positive and negative control organisms before use (Table 2.2). If a stain or other reagent is used infrequently, a positive and negative control should be run in parallel with the test.

For reagents which require reconstitution such as antisera and coagulase plasma, the manufacturer's instructions must be followed. Reagents should be discarded after the expiration date. The results of the reagent control monitoring should be entered in an appropriate log book with the date, source, and lot numbers of the ingredients and with the initials of the quality control technologist.

Antibiotics

The antibiotic disks used in antibiotic susceptibility testing should be stored with a desiccant at or below −14 C. If minimal storage space is available, the penicillins and cephalosporins should be frozen and the other disks can be maintained at 4–8 C. Each time antibiotic susceptibility testing is performed in the clinical laboratory, control organisms of known susceptibility should be evaluated concurrently. The recommended organisms are *Staphylococcus aureus* (ATCC 25923) for the gram-positive spectrum and *E.*

TABLE 2.2   CONTROL ORGANISMS FOR BIOCHEMICAL MEDIA AND TESTS

MEDIUM	CONTROL ORGANISMS	EXPECTED RESULTS*
Acetate	*Escherichia coli*	Growth, blue
	Shigella flexneri	No growth
Arginine dihydrolase	*Enterobacter cloacae*	Positive
	Proteus mirabilis	Negative
Casein	*Streptomyces paraguayensis*	Hydrolysis
	Nocardia asteroides	No hydrolysis
Cetrimide	*Pseudomonas aeruginosa*	Growth
	Escherichia coli	No growth
Christensen's urea	*Escherichia coli*	No change
	Proteus mirabilis	Pink
Citrate, Simmon's	*Klebsiella pneumoniae*	Growth, blue
	Escherichia coli	No growth
CTA		
Glucose	*Neisseria gonorrhoeae*	Acid
	Branhamella catarrhalis	No change
Maltose	*Neisseria meningitidis*	Acid
	Neisseria gonorrhoeae	No change
Sucrose	*Escherichia coli*	Acid
	Neisseria gonorrhoeae	No change
Cytochrome oxidase	*Pseudomonas aeruginosa*	Positive
	Escherichia coli	Negative
Decarboxylase		
Lysine	*Salmonella typhimurium*	Positive
	Proteus mirabilis	Negative

TABLE 2.2 CONTROL ORGANISMS FOR BIOCHEMICAL MEDIA AND TESTS *(Continued)*

MEDIUM	CONTROL ORGANISMS	EXPECTED RESULTS*
Ornithine	*Salmonella typhimurium*	Positive
	Klebsiella pneumoniae	Negative
Control	*Escherichia coli*	Yellow
	Pseudomonas aeruginosa	No change
DNA (methyl green)	*Serratia marcescens*	Growth with clear zone
	Enterobacter cloacae	No zone
Differential disks		
Bacitracin	*Streptococcus pyogenes*	Zone of inhibition around disk
	Streptococcus mitis	No zone formed
Optochin	*Streptococcus pneumoniae*	16-mm zone of inhibition
	Streptococcus mitis	No zone formed
X & V factors	*Haemophilus influenzae*	Growth between disks
Hippurate	*Streptococcus* Gp. B	Positive
	Streptococcus pyogenes	Negative
Indole	*Escherichia coli*	Positive
	Enterobacter cloacae	Negative
10% Lactose	*Acinetobacter* (var. *anitratus*)	Positive
	Acinetobacter lwoffi	Negative
Malonate	*Klebsiella pneumoniae*	Positive
	Escherichia coli	Negative
Methyl red	*Escherichia coli*	Positive
	Enterobacter cloacae	Negative
Motility	*Escherichia coli*	Positive
	Klebsiella pneumoniae	Negative
Mucate	*Escherichia coli*	Positive
	Shigella flexneri	Negative
Nitrate	*Escherichia coli*	Positive
	Acinetobacter (var. *lwoffi*)	Negative
ONPG	*Escherichia coli*	Positive
	Salmonella typhimurium	Negative
Phenylalanine	*Proteus mirabilis*	Positive
deaminase	*Escherichia coli*	Negative
Pigment media	*Pseudomonas aeruginosa*	Positive
(Pyo, Fluo)	*Escherichia coli*	Negative
OF glucose	*Pseudomonas aeruginosa*	Acid
	Acinetobacter (var. *lwoffi*)	No change
Starch	*Pseudomonas stutzeri*	Hydrolysis
	Pseudomonas aeruginosa	No hydrolysis
Triple sugar iron	*Escherichia coli*	A/AG
	Salmonella typhimurium	K/AG, H_2S
	Pseudomonas aeruginosa	K/NC
Tyrosine	*Streptomyces paraguayensis*	Positive
	Nocardia asteroides	Negative
Voges Proskauer	*Enterobacter cloacae*	Positive
	Escherichia coli	Negative
Xanthine	*Streptomyces paraguayensis*	Positive
	Nocardia asteroides	Negative

*Abbreviations: A/AG, acid/acid and gas; K/AG, H_2S, alkaline/acid gas, hydrogen sulfide; K/NC, alkaline/no change.

coli (ATCC 25922) for the gram-negative battery. Carbenicillin, tobramycin, and gentamicin can be monitored with *Pseudomonas aeruginosa* (ATCC 27853). Zone sizes obtained with the control organisms should be measured and compared to those in the acceptable ranges for the antibiotics (2). If results are not within the prescribed range, the test must be repeated and possible errors in procedure, faulty media, or deficient disks checked for. The results of the control testing should be entered into a log book along with the date and initials of the technologist reading the test.

Antibiotic powders should be stored with a desiccant in the refrigerator. An organism of known susceptibility should be included as a control for each tube dilution test.

Stock Cultures

Media and reagents are quality controlled by testing with organisms of known physiological and morphological characteristics. These stock cultures can be maintained for prolonged periods if frozen below −40 C or if lyophilized. A more convenient method for maintaining stock cultures, particularly for daily use, is inoculating a suitable medium which will preserve the stability and viability of these organisms. Cystine Trypticase agar (CTA), cooked meat medium, or Trypticase soy agar (TSA) can be lightly inoculated and incubated at 35 C until light growth is obtained. Most of these cultures can be stored at room temperature. Fastidious organisms such as *Haemophilus influenzae, Neisseria gonorrhoeae,* and *N. meningitidis* should be maintained on chocolate agar slants. Blood agar slants or plates are recommended for streptococci. Russell describes detailed procedures for maintaining stock cultures (4).

Stock organisms can be obtained from the American Type Culture Collection (ATCC), through a proficiency testing program, or from clinical isolates which have been confirmed by a reference laboratory. Commercial sources such as Difco (Bactrol) and Hyland offer lyophilized quality control stock cultures. Selecting organisms with a variety of biochemical characteristics will reduce the amount of time, labor, and cost involved in maintaining stock cultures.

Summary

An effective quality control program in the clinical microbiology laboratory includes the following basic considerations.

(1) The bench technologists and ancillary personnel should be thoroughly trained and instructed in their duties. Continuing education should be encouraged for all personnel.

(2) All laboratory personnel should participate in external and internal proficiency testing programs. Plate rounds should be conducted for infrequently encountered organisms.

(3) A printed protocol containing all procedures used in the labora-

tory should be accessible to and followed by all personnel.

(4) Quality control log books should be as simple as possible but should contain enough information to allow sources of error to be determined.

(5) Schedules and protocols for each phase of quality control monitoring should be devised and followed carefully. Any problems should be reported to the supervisor or laboratory director.

(6) Procedures should be reviewed periodically by the supervisor or laboratory director and updated when necessary.

(7) As needed, the laboratory should enlist the services of a reference laboratory (e.g., a city, county, or state department of health).

References

1. BARTLETT RC: Functional quality control. *In* Quality Control in Microbiology. Prier JE, Bartola J, and Friedman J (eds.). Univ Park Press, Baltimore, Md, 1975, pp 145-184
2. BLAZEVIC DJ, HALL CT, and WILSON ME: Practical quality control procedures for the clinical microbiology laboratory. *In* Cumitech 3, Balows A (ed.). American Society for Microbiology, Washington, DC, 1976
3. ELLIS RJ: Manual of Quality Control Procedures for Microbiological Laboratories. Center for Disease Control, Public Health Service, US Dept HEW, Atlanta, Ga, 1976
4. RUSSELL RL: Quality control in the microbiology laboratory. *In* Manual of Clinical Microbiology, 2nd edition, Lennette EH, Spaulding EH, and Truant JP (eds.). American Society for Microbiology, Washington, DC, 1974, pp 862-870
5. VERA HD: Quality control in diagnostic microbiology. Health Lab Sci 8:176-189, 1971

CHAPTER 3

LABORATORY SAFETY

John E. Forney and John H. Richardson

Introduction

Hazards exist in the laboratory because of the nature of the equipment, facilities, and materials used in the work area. A safety program in the laboratory encompasses provisions for protection from physical, biological, chemical, and radiological hazards. Physical hazards include mechanical or electrical difficulties; noise, heat, fire, and nonionizing radiation (e.g., ultraviolet light). Chemical and biological hazards exist because of inherent properties such as flammability or toxicity of chemicals and infectivity of biological materials. Radiological hazards are created by the ionizing properties of radioactive materials. By their behavior, workers in the laboratory can introduce additional hazards which can be overcome only by proper attitudes and work habits. Safety in the laboratory can be defined as "a judgment of the acceptability of risks, and risk, in turn, is a measure of the probability and severity of harm to human health. A thing (or act) is safe if its attendant risks are judged to be acceptable" (6).

Administrative Aspects

Laboratory workers are usually well aware of most of the hazards in their work environment and make an effort to minimize them. However, in recent years several Government agencies and professional organizations have set safety standards for laboratories, and many laboratories are subject to inspection by one or several groups.

Government Agencies
Occupational Safety and Health Act of 1970 (OSHA)

The intent of OSHA (9, 14) is to provide every worker in the United States with a safe and healthy work place. Federal, state, county, and municipally operated laboratories are exempt from the provisions of OSHA; however, by administrative directive, Federal laboratories are required to meet the standards established by this act. In states that have not accepted primary enforcement responsibility for OSHA, the state, county, and municipal laboratories are exempt from the provisions of OSHA; however, states that have accepted primary enforcement responsibility must include in their plans a provision for all intrastate Government laboratories to meet the standards of OSHA. One other type of laboratory that is not required to meet the standards of OSHA is a business (laboratory) which is operated solely by the family, i.e., it has no salaried employees. Under the act, the employer is responsible for providing a safe working place and the necessary safety equipment for employees' use. Accident reports and accident records must be maintained, and serious accidents must be reported to OSHA authorities. The employee is responsible for following safe procedures and using the safety equipment prescribed by the employer. The employee is also required to report accidents and unsafe conditions. If working conditions are unsafe, the employee has the right to report such conditions to OSHA authorities, who then are obligated to inspect the premises. If an employer fails to correct hazardous conditions and provide a safe working place, penalties may be assessed by OSHA against the employer. Standards established under OSHA are general in nature; that is, they do not cover in a specific manner the hazards unique to laboratories, such as biological and chemical hazards. Thus, the employer must use his own judgment in determining what constitutes a safe working environment.

Medicare

The Health Insurance for the Aged Program (Medicare) (11) provides that laboratories which are reimbursed for services provided under the program must meet certain standards of operation. Included in these standards are references to safety—particularly in relation to fire, infectious hazards, and hazards from flammable and toxic chemicals. The standards are stated in very general terms and leave the interpretation largely to the Medicare surveyor who visits the laboratory to determine eligibility for reimbursement.

Professional Organizations

Joint Commission on Accreditation of Hospitals (JCAH)

General standards which have been published for the reduction of hazards in a hospital are equally applicable to the hospital laboratory (2). These standards deal principally with preventing fire and evacuating the building in the event of fire; handling toxic and flammable chemicals, including compressed gases; and handling and disposing of infectious materials. Like Medicare standards, the laboratory standards are usually rather general (except, e.g., for those such as the restriction that not more than 10 gallons of flammable solvents may be stored in a laboratory unless they are kept in a flammable storage cabinet).

College of American Pathologists (CAP)

The College of American Pathologists conducts a program of accreditation for medical laboratories (5). As a part of the requirements for accreditation, the safety aspects of the laboratory are reviewed and inspected. The survey manual used by the inspectors contains a checklist of numerous points which are to be investigated. These points are divided into the common subdivisions of the laboratory and are more specific than those of any of the other programs.

American Industrial Hygiene Association (AIHA)

The American Industrial Hygiene Association inspects and accredits laboratories that are performing principally chemical analyses on substances from the environment. These analyses necessitate the handling of volatile and toxic chemicals, so the checklist for the inspectors contains numerous references to these problems (1). The standards of the AIHA are expressed in general terms, but they do cover most of the possible hazards, including employee behavior.

Organization and Responsibilities

Management

Management as represented by the laboratory owner/director is responsible for the following items: a) Establishing a safety policy and assuring that all employees are aware of the prescribed procedures; b) providing a safe working environment; c) assessing the progress of the safety program, including an evaluation of the safety manual and other published information; d) reviewing accident reports: and e) reviewing the safety officer's reports. Funds for administering the safety program must be provided by management.

Safety officer

One individual should be designated as safety officer (or safety supervisor or safety manager). In a small laboratory, this may be an additional duty assigned to one person or, in a large laboratory, it may be a full-time job for one or several individuals. The safety officer should be most knowledgeable about laboratory hazards and ways of alleviating these hazards. This individual should also be aware of the types of safety equipment that are available and should be generally well-informed about safety matters. This person should serve as technical advisor to management and to other employees in the laboratory, and should work with laboratory personnel in developing and incorporating safety procedures into the laboratory procedures. The safety officer should conduct inspections of the laboratory on a regularly scheduled basis. Ideally, such inspections should be made at least every 3 months and certainly not any less often than once a year. These should be formal inspections for which a checklist is used, and every part of every laboratory should be inspected—every cabinet, cupboard, storeroom, drawer, etc. Inspections are best done in the company of a responsible supervisor of the area being inspected so that many deficiencies can be immediately corrected. The safety officer should maintain all records related to safety, for example, records of inspections and accident reports. This person may also serve as the secretary to the safety committee.

Safety committee

The safety committee should have 5 to 10 members who are chosen to represent the various work levels or sections within the laboratory. The term of service should be specified, usually 2 or 3 years, and no member should serve more than 2 consecutive terms. Membership on the safety committee should be rotated so that there are always some experienced members as new members are appointed. The committee is advisory in nature, and matters should be brought to the committee for discussion by the laboratory representatives. Recommendations should be forwarded to management for implementation. Meetings should be held every 1 to 3 months, and an agenda should be prepared before the meeting. Minutes of the meeting should be kept, preferably by the safety officer.

Supervisor

Supervisors are key persons in the safety program just as they are in the overall operation of the laboratory. They should be responsible for most of the training of new employees in the area of safety. This fits in with the overall responsibility for training new employees in the procedures to be followed in the laboratory. Supervisors should maintain continual surveillance of the laboratory's daily operation. They should become accustomed to checking the laboratory when they first come on duty, and during the day when any violations are observed, they should take steps immediately to correct them. They should constantly seek ways to identify and reduce hazards. They are responsible for collecting reports of accidents from the employees and submitting these to management, usually through the safety officer.

Employees

All employees are responsible for following the specified safety procedures, using safety equipment, and reporting any accidents. Employees also should be constantly aware of hazards in the environment; they should report these to a supervisor and make suggestions for reduction or removal.

Safety Manual

A safety manual should be prepared which incorporates the policies and procedures to be followed in the laboratory. Much of the material which should be incorporated in the safety manual is included in this chapter. The following points are examples of what should be covered in the safety manual:

1.0 Policy
2.0 Responsibility and Authority
    2.1 Safety officer
        2.1.1 Duties
    2.2 Safety committee
        2.2.1 Make-up

2.2.2 Term of service
2.2.3 Duties
    2.2.31 Determine and evaluate laboratory hazards
    2.2.32 Review acci-

Physical Hazards

Many physical laboratory hazards are not unique to a laboratory situation. These will not be discussed in great detail since they are subject to common-sense solutions.

Mechanical

Mechanical hazards include obstructed aisles and corridors, unsafe chairs and stools which may tip over, heavy objects placed on overhead shelves, and hazards related to broken glassware. Probably the biggest single hazard in a hospital or public health laboratory is accidental skin puncture by a hypodermic needle. Prevention of such accidents requires constant training and such reminders to personnel, for example, as using needles only for parenteral injection—not as a substitute for pipettes. Needles should be discarded into containers which the point cannot penetrate, autoclaved, and then discarded with solid waste material. Blunted needles or cannulas should be used when possible.

Heat

Laboratory workers frequently are burned by hot equipment such as autoclaves, ovens, and flasks used for melting agar. Such burns can be prevented by providing protective gloves and hot pads and insisting that personnel use them. Instructions should be posted for proper operation of equipment, including safety procedures.

Light

Light rays do not normally present any hazard in the laboratory, either from the standpoint of too high or too low intensity. Light intensity at the bench should be 80 foot-candles. Ultraviolet (UV) light, however, does constitute a hazard, and personnel should be properly protected from any UV light source. Such sources include the illuminating lights for fluorescent microscopy and in spectrophotometers. Unshielded UV radiation may cause skin burns and, more importantly, may damage the eyes, which are very susceptible to radiation at this wavelength.

Noise

Noise levels in laboratories do not constitute an undue hazard. The noise level and pitch of centrifuges, shaking machines, and exhaust fans may be irritating, but are not high enough to constitute a physical hazard to the ears; however, noise can be very distracting and can be the indirect cause of accidents in the laboratory. Noise levels should therefore be kept below the level which is distracting or irritating to personnel. Personal protection plugs or muffs should be provided for short-term exposure and sound absorption devices, etc., for long-term noise problems, particularly when the noise levels are above 90 decibels (the maximum time-weighted average).

Fire

A bad fire in a laboratory is probably the most disastrous event that can occur. A fire not only endangers personnel and causes the direct destruction of property but also frequently results in extensive smoke and water damage. A fire will require a long period of shutdown to repair the damage, and cleaning undamaged glassware and equipment presents a tremendous task. All of these things, in addition to the destruction of irreplaceable records, suggest that all possible means should be taken to prevent fires in the laboratories. Education of personnel in the prevention and control of fire should be a continuous and ongoing program. Personnel should be familiar with the location of fire alarms and fire extinguishers. Every person in the laboratory should be trained in the use of fire extinguishers and should actually discharge one to put out a fire. Fire evacuation routes and procedures should be posted in each laboratory. Fire drills should be scheduled and occasionally held unannounced.

Electrical

Enough electrical outlets should be available in the laboratory so that it is not necessary to use multiple hookups or power cords longer than 6 feet. Grounding circuits should be verified, and all equipment such as motors and heaters which are not double insulated should be provided with a grounding wire. All new equipment should be checked by an electrician for shock hazard before it is installed in the laboratory. Any old equipment which gives any shock to laboratory workers should be unplugged from the power source, checked, and repaired by an electrician. All laboratory personnel should know the location of electrical control panels, and circuits should be clearly marked so that in the event of an electrical accident the circuit can be disconnected promptly.

Chemical Hazards

Chemical hazards in the laboratory are of 3 general types: (a) chemicals which are flammable or combustible, (b) chemicals which produce acute effects on a worker such as severe burns of the skin or lethal effects or severe internal damage after inhalation, ingestion or absorption, and (c) chemicals which will produce damaging effects after long-term, chronic, low-level exposure. These effects also occur after inhalation or skin contamination.

The definitions of "flammable" and "combustible" are stated in National Fire Codes (8). A basic principle to follow in the laboratory is to keep the quantity of flammable chemicals at the lowest possible volume consistent with efficient laboratory operation. OSHA, JCAH, and CAP prescribe maximum quantities of flammable substances allowed in the laboratory outside of a flammable storage cabinet. It is acceptable to use a flammable storage cabinet in the laboratory to store excess stocks of chemicals up to 60 gallons. However, this should not be construed to mean that a flammable storage cabinet should routinely be used for storage of such large volumes of reserve stocks. All reserve stocks of flammable chemicals should be stored in a flammable storage room constructed to meet the specifications of the National Fire Codes (8). The purpose of a flammable storage cabinet as defined in the National Fire Codes (8) is to keep the temperature of its contents below 325 F for 10 min if a fire should occur in the laboratory. If the wall of the cabinet is penetrated with vent holes, the principle for which the flammable storage cabinet is designed is negated. If the cabinet is installed with a mechanical ventilator, intake air should be supplied from outside the laboratory.

Careful attention should be given to the storage of all chemicals. Certain chemicals are considered incompatible because of the possible violent reaction resulting from their being spilled or otherwise accidentally mixed. Chemicals such as perchloric acid, nitric acid, and ethers should be stored in separate areas to prevent the creation of explosive or highly flammable mixtures. Opened cans of ether should be stored on an open shelf or in base cabinets—never in a refrigerator—and should be discarded after 30 days. Chemicals which can produce severe burns include strong inorganic acids and alkalis and some organic compounds such as phenol.

Strong acids and alkalis should be transported from storeroom to laboratory or from one laboratory to another only in a container which shields the bottles from breaking and is large enough to contain the contents of the bottles if they do break. Large containers of such chemicals (5 pounds or greater) should be stored in the laboratory only in base cabinets. They should never be stored on shelves above eye level or permitted to sit on the floor in open areas. Strong chemicals should be poured or buretted over a plastic tray which will contain any spilled material. Materials should be available in the laboratory to neutralize and absorb any chemicals which may be spilled. Appropriate spill clean-up kits should be readily available.

Chemicals which may cause injury to personnel after prolonged exposure include substances such as heavy metals (e.g., lead and mercury) and organic solvents (e.g., carbon tetrachloride, chloroform, xylene, toluene, and organic phosphates). The maximal permissible levels of exposure have been established for many chemicals (13). Environment must be monitored to assure that exposure of personnel does not exceed the maximal permissible levels. Some individuals may be hypersensitive to chemicals and may not be able to tolerate even the generally accepted levels of exposure. Therefore, the guiding principle should be that if a worker is experiencing adverse effects, the level of a chemical in the environment should be reduced. Records should be kept on the exposure of individuals to any toxic chemical and, when indicated, records should also be kept on the concentration of chemical present in the work environment.

Disposal of chemicals

This has become a serious problem as more and more chemicals are used in the laboratory and the standards of the Environmental Protection Agency become more stringent. Strong acids and alkalis in the quantities usually used in a clinical laboratory can be neutralized, and innocuous wastes can be dumped into the sewer system. Small quantities of miscible organics such as alcohol can also be discharged into the sewer system. Nonmiscible organic solvents such as xylene and toluene should not be discarded except in extremely small quantities (no more than a few milliliters). These chemicals must be collected in safety containers and disposed of either in an approved incinerator or in sealed drums which are turned over to a commercial waste disposal company. Mercury and mercury compounds must not be discarded into the sewer system. Substitutes for mercury-containing solutions such as the Schaudinn's fixative should be sought.

Azides contained in some preservatives should not be discarded into metallic drain lines (copper, lead, zinc) because highly explosive metallic azides are formed. Perchloric acid deposits on metal fume hood exhaust ducts are extremely unstable. Hoods used for exhausting perchloric acid must be constructed with special washdown equipment.

Chemical fume hoods

Chemical fume hoods should be provided in any laboratory which handles toxic or flammable chemicals. These should have a face velocity of at least 100 linear feet per minute with the sash in a position that will still permit work in the hood. They should be designed to run continuously as an integral part of the building air exhaust system and should be ducted to the roof of the building by the most direct route. Manifold ducting can be used, but only if the exhaust fan is capable of handling the amount of air required in such a system. These hoods must be monitored with an anemometer to assure that air velocity is being maintained and should have a warning system which will sound if the airflow is reduced or turned off.

Carcinogens

A list of 14 chemicals considered to be carcinogens in man has been published by OSHA (14). Special precautions must be used in handling, storing, and disposing of any chemicals on this list. In addition, there are several hundred potentially carcinogenic compounds which should be handled with care and discretion (13).

Compressed gases

Compressed gases which are distributed in cylinders are hazardous not only because of their inherent flammability or toxicity but also because of the mechanical hazard of the container. They should be stored away from the laboratory in a relatively cool area and be secured in place at all times with the safety cover for the valve also in place. They should be moved from the storage areas to the laboratory only on a suitable wheeled cart. The cylinder should be tightly secured during use in the laboratory and, when empty, should be returned to storage and again tightly secured.

Biological Hazards

Biological agents in the laboratory have been classified according to their hazard level (4). This classification can be used as a guide in planning the level of containment to be set up and followed in the laboratory. Containment is based upon a combination of good microbiological technique and proper construction of spaces, air control, and the use of biological safety cabinets. Control of the air, however, does not replace the necessity for careful handling of biological agents to prevent laboratory infections. Sulkin and Pike (12) and Pike (10) reported the results of almost 50 years of experience with laboratory-associated infections. Routine laboratory procedures such as streaking a plate, transferring liquid cultures, centrifuging, and pipetting may result in the dissemination of organisms into the environment. Unlike the effects of mechanical and chemical accidents which can be observed immediately, an infection resulting from an accident with a biological agent may not develop for several days or several weeks. Therefore, it is extremely difficult to associate infections with laboratory accidents as reported by Pike (10). Because in almost 80% of the cases no direct association could be made, it is assumed that a large number of laboratory-associated infections result from inhaling contaminated particles in the air. Therefore, it is essential that the air in the laboratory be properly controlled. The air-handling system serving the laboratory should be constructed so that the air passes through the laboratory only one time and then is discharged to the outside. This is contrary to the general practice, particularly in office buildings and hospitals, where approximately 80% of the air is recirculated through the facility. Thus, any spill of infectious materials or a chemical with a strong odor can very quickly contaminate other areas of the facility. The airflow can be locally controlled to protect the laboratory worker with various classes of biological safety cabinets (BSC).

Class I negative pressure biological safety cabinets (BSC)

These are open-faced cabinets in which the air is drawn through the opening at 75 linear feet per minute, passes over the work, and is exhausted through the top of the cabinet which contains high-efficiency particulate (HEPA) filters. These filters are designed to entrap 99.9% of particles as large as 0.3 μm in diameter. In most models the air also passes through a plenum containing high intensity UV lights designed to inactivate any organisms which might escape through the HEPA filters. Maintenance of BSC's is discussed in the *Biological Safety Cabinet* (3).

Class II vertical laminar flow biological safety cabinets

Vertical laminar flow cabinets combine some of the advantages of the Class I BSC and the horizontal laminar flow cabinet, which serves as a clean bench. This type of cabinet exhausts only approximately 20% of the air from the cabinet as opposed to the 100% exhausted from the previously described cabinet. The circulated air passes downward over the work and exhausts through slotted grills in the bottom of the cabinet work area to provide a unidirectional flow of high-quality air over the work area. To make up for the air which is discharged from the cabinet, air flows in through the front of the cabinet (which is open to provide access to the work area) at approximately 100 linear feet per minute and provides an air barrier or screen to reduce the possibility of contaminated material passing out into the room and thus exposing the worker. Both types of cabinets must be monitored frequently for proper airflow, frequently cleaned and wiped down with a disinfecting solution, and filters must be replaced when the airflow is reduced below a minimal safe operating velocity. It is imperative that the vertical laminar flow cabinet be checked periodically (approximately every 6 months) to assure that there are no leaks in it or in the filters. The time interval may be extended when the cabinet is used only infrequently. The life of the filters can be extended if the cabinet is turned on only when it is actually used. Leaving the cabinet on all the time only hastens the plugging of the filters to the point where the cabinet needs to be shut down, have its filters replaced, and again be certified as safe to operate. For further information on these operating practices, refer to the National Cancer Institute film "Use of the Laminar Flow Biological Safety Cabinet" (7).

Other types of cabinets provide a higher level of containment, unlikely to be required in a diagnostic laboratory. The Type III BSC is a closed system used only for handling the most hazardous biologic agents.

Inevitably, accidents occur and sometimes cultures are spilled in the laboratory. Almost every time, an aerosol will be created which may infect an exposed individual. If a laboratory has a one-pass air system, the recommended procedure is to leave the room for at least an hour so that the flow of the air can purge the room of any aerosols created when the culture is dropped. When there has been ample time for purging the atmosphere, the area can be cleaned. The person performing this task should assess the hazard level of the organism and, when appropriate, don protective clothing such as a surgical gown, gloves, mask, cap, and booties to cover the shoes. Contaminated areas should be covered with an absorbent material such as paper towels and then flooded with a disinfectant known to be active against the organisms which were probably present in the spilled material. After the disinfectant has had time to inactivate the organisms, the solid material can be cleaned up and placed in a bag or discard pan for autoclaving. The liquid materials should be sponged up with towels, which are also placed in a container for autoclaving.

Contaminated materials from the microbiology laboratory should be discarded in a container with a solid bottom (e.g., a pan or bucket) into which a small amount of disinfectant solution has been placed. Wire baskets and racks should not be used for discarding material because too frequently tubes are upset and spill material which the wire basket or rack will not contain. The building and room number of the laboratory should be indicated on a tag, and a strip of autoclaving tape should be placed on each discard container. Habitually placing contaminated materials in a particular place does not provide an adequate level of safety. Specially-designed plastic bags may also be used for discarding contaminated materials, particularly if they are to be incinerated. All contaminated materials that are not incinerated should be autoclaved long enough to sterilize all the contents of the discard containers completely. Autoclaves should be monitored monthly with a biological indicator such as *Bacillus stearothermophilus*.

Microbiology laboratory workers may be provided additional protection by immunization. However, there are only a limited number of diseases for which immunization procedures are available. These include anthrax, botulism, cholera, diphtheria, Eastern equine encephalitis, measles, plague, poliomyelitis, Q fever, rabies, Rocky Mountain spotted fever, rubella, smallpox, tularemia, typhoid, typhus, Venezuelan equine encephalitis, and yellow fever.

Skin testing may be advisable, particularly for individuals who will be working in an area exposed to mycobacteria. If an individual has had negative tuberculin test results, conversion to positive is a significant indication of infection. Such persons should have chest X rays and other appropriate diagnostic procedures and medical evaluation. Finally, it is advisable to obtain preexposure baseline sera from individuals working in microbiology laboratories, so that if they should later develop an illness that may be laboratory-associated, sera are available to be compared with that obtained during the acute phase of illness.

Radiologic Hazards

Proper monitoring, handling, decontamination, and disposal of radioactive materials in the laboratory are specified and controlled by the U.S. Nuclear Regulatory Commission (NRC). Everyone should read and understand the following parts of the NRC regulations (Title 10 of the Code of Federal Regulations) before working with radioactive materials:

Part 19—Notices, Instructions and Reports to Workers; Inspections

Part 20—Standards for Protection Against Radiation

Part 30—Rules of General Applicability to Licensing of Byproduct Material

Part 33— Specific Licenses of Broad Scope for Byproduct Material

In some states (so-called "agreement states") state health departments have enacted comprehensive radiation control regulations. In these instances the state regulations will apply, and site inspections and enforcement of the regulations will be conducted by state personnel.

Anyone handling radioactive materials in the laboratory should understand the principles of radioactivity and thus the hazard posed by exposure to various levels of radioactivity. On the basis of this knowledge the procedures for protection can then be developed; that is, it can be determined whether time and distance are sufficient to protect the exposed individual or whether appropriate shielding such as lead must be provided for protection. Proper monitoring of personnel and the environment are essential in a laboratory where radioactive materials are handled. Instruments for monitoring the laboratory environment must be available and must be used frequently (generally weekly). Procedures for cleaning up spilled radioactive materials must be developed which are consistent with the nature of the material spilled and the intensity of the radiation, and all laboratory personnel should be familiar with them. Appropriate decontamination procedures must also be available. Disposal of radioactive material is also regulated by the Nuclear Regulatory Commission or the "agreement state." Commercial services, licensed to handle such waste materials, are generally available and should be investigated.

Accidents

Provision must be made for emergency care of injured personnel. Depending upon the training and skills of laboratory personnel, the first aid equipment which should be available in the laboratory may range from supplies for treating minor burns to equipment to arrest hemorrhage or to treat a person in shock. If the laboratory is affiliated with and located in a hospital, emergency care can best be provided by the hospital. However, an independent laboratory or a laboratory not affiliated with a hospital should make arrangements with an emergency room to handle any severe medical or otherwise traumatic emergencies.

A policy regarding the reporting and recording of accidents should be established. All accidents should be reported to the supervisor. Minor cuts, burns, and abrasions should be recorded at the discretion of the supervisor. In a microbiology laboratory even a very insignificant cut or abrasion may cause infection. Any accident resulting in lost time or requiring medical attention should be reported to management and an appropriate record maintained, possibly by the safety officer.

Any accident resulting in time loss, injury, or illness, or resulting in extensive property damage should be investigated. Such an investigation should be made by the safety officer and the supervisor involved. In severe cases, a third person should be included on the investigation board. An attempt should be made to determine what caused the accident, including all contributory factors. A report should be reviewed by the safety committee and by management. Any changes which would prevent the recurrence of a similar accident should be carefully considered and acted upon by management.

Personnel Control

Dress and uniforms

All personnel performing laboratory work and supportive services should wear protective garments over street clothes or uniforms. Before leaving the laboratory to go to administrative or patient care areas, cafeteria, snack bar, or before leaving the building, workers should remove these protective garments.

Smoking

Specific areas in which smoking is allowed should be designated in the laboratory. These areas should not include any laboratory that is handling potentially infectious materials or patient specimens or one where flammable, combustible, or toxic chemicals are being used.

Eating, drinking, and storing food

The restrictions that apply to smoking also apply to eating, drinking, and storing food in the laboratory area.

Pipetting

A mechanical device should be used for pipetting all clinical or infectious materials or toxic chemicals. Hazardous materials should never be pipetted by mouth.

Cosmetics

Cosmetics should not be applied in any part of the laboratory in which hazardous materials are handled.

Contact lenses

When either chemical or infectious material is splattered into the eye of an individual wearing contact lenses, the material tends to be drawn under the lens because of capillary action and is held there in close contact with the cornea. As a result the irritation may be very intense so that it becomes difficult to remove the contact lens. Individuals wearing contact lenses should be warned of this additional hazard and should wear goggles or face shields when handling caustic or infectious materials.

Hand washing

To prevent the ingestion of infectious materials, workers should wash their hands frequently and should always wash them just before leaving the laboratory.

Restricted areas

Traffic through the laboratory should be kept to a minimum. Some parts of the laboratory where particularly hazardous materials are handled should only be entered by personnel actually performing the work. The entire laboratory should be off limits to all but individuals with operational or support duties within the laboratory. Signs should be posted identifying the degree of restriction and the type of hazard area—chemical, biological, or radiological. Warning signs of uniform color and design available from scientific supply houses should be used to indicate both temporarily and permanently restricted areas.

References

1. AMERICAN INDUSTRIAL HYGIENE ASSOCIATION. Site visit questionnaire,
2. BOARD OF COMMISSIONERS OF JOINT COMMISSION ON ACCREDITATION OF HOSPITALS. Functional Safety and Sanitation. Chicago, Ill, December 1975
3. CENTER FOR DISEASE CONTROL. Biological Safety Cabinet. Atlanta, Ga, 1976
4. CENTER FOR DISEASE CONTROL. Classification of Etiologic Agents on the Basis of Hazard. Atlanta, Ga, 1974
5. COLLEGE OF AMERICAN PATHOLOGISTS COMMISSION ON INSPECTION AND ACCREDITATION. Inspection Checklist. CAP, Chicago, Ill. 1976
6. LOWRANCE WW: Of acceptable risk. *In* Science and the Determination of Safety. William Kaufmann, Inc., Los Altos, California, 1976
7. NATIONAL CANCER INSTITUTE. Effective Use of the Laminar Flow Biological Safety Cabinet. Bethesda, Md, undated
8. NATIONAL FIRE PROTECTION ASSOCIATION. Flammable and Combustible Liquid Codes. NFPA No. 30. Boston, 1976
9. OCCUPATIONAL SAFETY AND HEALTH ACT OF 1970. Public Law 91-596. 91st Congress
10. PIKE RM: Laboratory-associated infections: Summary and analysis of 3921 cases. Health Lab Sci 13: 105–114, 1975
11. SOCIAL SECURITY ADMINISTRATION, U.S. DEPARTMENT OF HEALTH, EDUCATION AND WELFARE. Federal Health Insurance for the Aged. Regulations: Conditions for Coverage of Services of Independent Laboratories (20 CFR 405), 1974

12. SULKIN SE and RM PIKE: Survey of laboratory-acquired infections. Am J Public Health 41:769–781, 1951
13. U.S. DEPARTMENT OF HEALTH, EDUCATION AND WELFARE, CENTER FOR DISEASE CONTROL, NATIONAL INSTITUTE FOR OCCUPATIONAL SAFETY AND HEALTH. Registry of Toxic Effects of Chemical Substances. Cincinnati, Ohio, 1977
14. U.S. DEPARTMENT OF LABOR, OCCUPATIONAL SAFETY AND HEALTH ADMINISTRATION, GENERAL INDUSTRY SAFETY AND HEALTH STANDARDS. OSHA 2206 (29 CFR 1910). U.S. Government Printing Office, Washington, DC (Revised January 10, 1976)

General References

Guide for Safety in the Chemical Laboratory. Manufacturing Chemists Association. Van Nostrand Reinhold Co, New York, 1972
Henry RJ, Olitsky I, Lee D, Walter B, and Beattie J: Safety in the Clinical Laboratory. Bio-Science Enterprises, Van Nuys, Calif., 1976
Peterson D: Techniques of Safety Management. McGraw-Hill, Inc., New York, NY, 1971
Safety Guide for Health Care Institutions. A joint publication of the American Hospital Association and the National Safety Council, Chicago, Ill, 1972
Steere NV: Handbook of Laboratory Safety. The Chemical Rubber Co, Cleveland, Ohio, 1971

CHAPTER 4

TRANSPORTATION OF CLINICAL SPECIMENS AND ETIOLOGIC AGENTS

John H. Richardson

Regulations

Clinical specimens and etiologic agents must be transported in the process of obtaining diagnostic services, confirmatory testing, exchange of research materials, proficiency testing, and other activities which are in the national and individual health interests. Inherent in the shipment of these materials is the potential for damage or leakage in transit, resulting in contamination or exposure of personnel and materials. Commonsense packaging procedures which provide containment of infectious materials that may leak or be damaged in shipment also provide the best assurance that transported specimens arrive at their destination in a satisfactory and usable condition. Records maintained at the Office of Biosafety, Center for Disease Control, indicate that although transportation personnel have occasionally been exposed to damaged or leaking shipments of etiologic agents, there is no recorded or anecdotal evidence that they have been infected as a result of such exposures.

Three Federal agencies [Public Health Service (PHS), Department of Transportation, United States Postal Service] and at least one transportation organization (Air Transport Association) have direct input in regulating or specifying conditions under which etiologic agents, diagnostic specimens, and biological products are shipped.

The PHS has been involved in establishing requirements for shipping infectious materials for almost two decades. In 1959, the Interstate Quarantine Regulations administered by the Food and Drug Administration (FDA) were amended to provide for containment packaging and other shipping requirements for etiologic agents. The regulation (42 CFR, Section 72.25) specified 32 etiologic agents for which the following requirements were applicable: that airtight and watertight primary and secondary specimen containers be used; that a maximum volume of 500 ml be allowed in each primary container and an aggregate volume of 1 gallon in a single shipping container; that shipments have "appropriate labeling"; and that the Surgeon General be notified in the event of damage or leakage of specimens in transit. These 32 agents are anthrax, botulism, brucellosis, cholera, Colorado tick fever, Coxsackie viruses, diphtheria, encephalitis (arthropod-borne), glanders, leptospirosis, lymphocytic choriomeningitis, melioidosis, meningococcal meningitis, paratyphoid fever, plague, poliomyelitis, Q fever, rabies, relapsing fever, rickettsial pox, Rift Valley fever, Rocky Mountain spotted fever, schistosomiasis, scrub typhus, smallpox, tetanus, tuberculosis, tularemia, typhoid fever, typhus fever, and yellow fever.

In 1971, the FDA's authority for regulating the interstate shipment of etiologic agents was delegated to the Center for Disease Control, and the regulation was amended, effective July 31, 1972, to incorporate packaging, labeling, volume limitations, and shipping procedures for etiologic agents, diagnostic specimens, and biological products; to expand the list of etiologic agents for which these requirements are applicable; to establish additional procedures for reporting damage or leakage of etiologic agents in transit; and to require notification of receipt of certain etiologic agents. This regulation was subsequently amended in July 1980 expanding the list of etiologic agents and increasing the maximum allowable volume of etiologic agent in a single primary container from 500 ml. to 1,000 ml.

The Department of Transportation (DOT) concurrently developed companion regulations (49 CFR, Section 173.386-7) governing all modes of shipment of etiologic agents, diagnostic specimens, and biological products— i.e., air carriers, motor carriers, rail carriers, and water carriers. The DOT regulations differ from those of the PHS in two principal areas:

1) Section 173.387 specifies environmental conditions, test conditions (water spray, free drop, and penetration), and testing procedures applicable to packages containing etiologic agents; and
2) the authority of the DOT expands the application of their regulations to include the transport of etiologic agents by carriers licensed in interstate commerce regardless of whether material is shipped intrastate or interstate.

The U.S. Postal Service also has requirements applicable to mailing "diseased tissues, blood, serum, and cultures of pathogenic microorganisms." These requirements, compiled in the *Postal Service Manual,* available from Superintendent of Documents, Government Printing Office, Washington, DC, are in general compatible to those of the PHS and the DOT.

The Air Transport Association (ATA), an organization of domestic airline carrriers, publishes and periodically revises Restricted Articles Tariff 6-D (Airline Tariff Publishing Co, Dulles International Airport, PO Box 17415, Washington, DC 20041) which further specifies conditions for air shipping etiologic agents, diagnostic specimens, and biological products. Petitions for revisions in Tariff 6-D are submitted to the Civil Aeronautics Board for consideration and approval. The ATA tariff incorporates the pertinent requirements of the PHS and DOT regulations. It also requires documentation (shippers' certificates) to further identify air-shipped etiologic agents and allows volumes of etiologic agents of <50 ml to be transported on passenger-carrying aircraft. Volumes of >50 ml are relegated to cargo-only aircraft.

Packaging Requirements

Diagnostic specimens and biological products are subject to the minimum packaging requirements described in Section 72.2 of the PHS Interstate Quarantine Regulation (Appendix A) and must "withstand leakage of contents, shocks, pressure changes, and other conditions incident to ordinary handling in transportation." Because of the wide spectrum of materials included in the definition of "diagnostic specimen," a precise description of the variety of packagings that may be needed is impractical. However, the sender is responsible for assuring that packaging will withstand the rigors of "ordinary handling in transit." One packaging system that has proven satisfactory for shipping diagnostic specimens involves commercially available molded polystyrene containers which are taped or enclosed in a cardboard sleeve or container for shipment. These molded containers are available in various sizes and shapes for single or multiple specimens. Several other packaging systems are equally effective for shipping diagnostic specimens. Some are described in *Collection, Handling, and Shipment of Microbiological Specimens,* DHEW Publication No. (CDC) 76-8263 and *Reference Diagnostic Services,* DHEW, PHS, CDC, May 1977, available from the Bureau of Laboratories, Center for Disease Control, Atlanta, Georgia 30333. Organizations such as the National Committee for Clinical Laboratory Standards are also developing standards which include shipping procedures for diagnostic specimens and other clinical materials.

Diagnostic specimens and biological products are not subject to volume limitations of the primary specimen containers or to limitations of the aggregate volume of single shipping containers regardless of the mode of shipment. Special markings and hazard warning labels are not required. Do not place ETIOLOGIC AGENT/BIOMEDICAL MATERIALS on shipment of diagnostic specimens or biological products.

If dry ice is used as a refrigerant for air shipments, the applicable labeling requirements of the ATA Restricted Articles Tariff 6-D apply. Shippers should contact commercial air carriers for current requirements.

Etiologic Agents

Materials known or presumed to contain an agent or its toxin which causes, or may cause, human disease are subject to additional packaging and shipping requirements. Section 72.3 of the Interstate Quarantine Regulations (Appendix A) lists those etiologic agents for which the requirements are applicable and describes packaging, labeling, and shipping requirements.

Packaging requirements for etiologic agents are described in Section 72.3(a)–(d) of the Interstate Quarantine Regulations based on the volume of material in the primary container (i.e., volumes of < 50 ml and volumes of at least 50 ml).

For volumes of etiologic agents of < 50 ml, the commercially available two-part shipping containers illustrated in Figure 4.1 are satisfactory.

Cultures or suspensions of etiologic agents should be placed in a securely closed watertight primary container such as a sealed plastic or glass ampoule; taped, gasketed, screw-capped vial; wheaton bottle; etc. Screw caps should be secured and taped to prevent loosening during shipment. Petri dishes should never be used for transporting cultures.

The space between the *primary* and *secondary* containers should contain enough nonparticulate material to absorb the entire contents of the

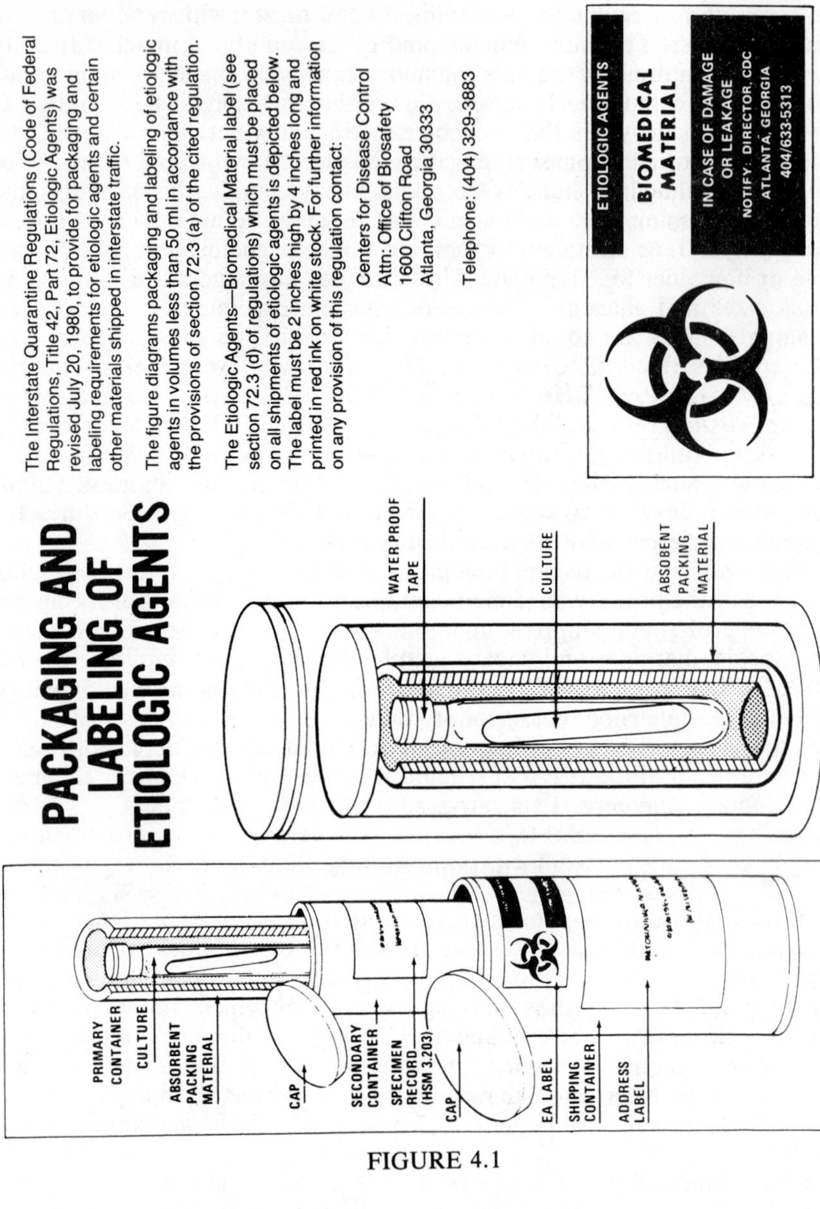
PACKAGING AND LABELING OF ETIOLOGIC AGENTS
The Interstate Quarantine Regulations (Code of Federal Regulations, Title 42, Part 72, Etiologic Agents) was revised July 20, 1980, to provide for packaging and labeling requirements for etiologic agents and certain other materials shipped in interstate traffic.
The figure diagrams packaging and labeling of etiologic agents in volumes less than 50 ml in accordance with the provisions of section 72.3 (a) of the cited regulation.
The Etiologic Agents—Biomedical Material label (see section 72.3 (d) of regulations) which must be placed on all shipments of etiologic agents is depicted below. The label must be 2 inches high by 4 inches long and printed in red ink on white stock. For further information on any provision of this regulation contact:
Centers for Disease Control
Attn: Office of Biosafety
1600 Clifton Road
Atlanta, Georgia 30333
Telephone: (404) 329-3883
ETIOLOGIC AGENTS
BIOMEDICAL MATERIAL
IN CASE OF DAMAGE OR LEAKAGE
NOTIFY: DIRECTOR, CDC
ATLANTA, GEORGIA
404/633-5313
WATER PROOF TAPE
CULTURE
ABSOBENT PACKING MATERIAL
CROSS SECTION OF PROPER PACKING
PRIMARY CONTAINER
CULTURE
ABSORBENT PACKING MATERIAL
CAP
SECONDARY CONTAINER
SPECIMEN RECORD (HSM 3.203)
CAP
EA LABEL
SHIPPING CONTAINER
ADDRESS LABEL

FIGURE 4.1

primary container in the event of breakage or leakage. The screw cap of the *secondary container* should be tightly secured and can be also taped to prevent loosening in transit. Patient and laboratory data forms should be placed between the *secondary container* and the *outer shipping container*—never between the *primary* and *secondary containers*! A label indicating the name and address of the sending and receiving laboratory should be affixed securely to the *outer shipping container*. The ETIOLOGIC AGENT/ BIOMEDICAL MATERIALS label described in Section 72.3(d) must also be affixed to all shipments of etiologic agents. The label must be of the size and color specified in the regulation. Small specimens shipped by airmail or first-class mail are acceptable to the post office and are handled with other letter mail. Specimens sent first-class airmail should also have affixed the NOTICE TO CARRIER label described and illustrated in Appendix B. This label is applicable only to domestic shipments of etiologic agents of < 50 ml which meet all other regulatory requirements and is used instead of the SHIPPERS' CERTIFICATE (Fig. 4.2) specified in the ATA Restricted Articles Tariff 6-D. Specimens so packaged and labeled meet all applicable Federal regulations and carrier tariffs for shipment by all modes including transport on passenger-carrying aircraft.

For shipment of etiologic agents of at least 50 ml, the requirements for the *primary container*, absorbent material, and *secondary container* are the same as for those of smaller volumes. In addition, shock-absorbent material must be placed between the *secondary container* and the *outer shipping container*. Individual *primary containers* shall not exceed 1,000 ml in volume, and the aggregate volume of all *primary containers* in a single *outer shipping container* shall not exceed 4,000 ml.

Shipments of etiologic agents exceeding 50 ml in one or more *primary containers* are relegated to cargo-only aircraft in accordance with the ATA Restricted Article Tariff 6-D. In addition to the ETIOLOGIC AGENT label previously described, such containers to be air shipped must also have two copies of the completed and signed SHIPPERS' CERTIFICATE (Fig. 4.2), as specified in Tariff 6-D, affixed to or accompanying the shipment. If dry ice is used as a refrigerant in shipments of etiologic agents, appropriate markings and labels should be used in accordance with carrier requirements.

The previously cited *Collection, Handling, and Shipment of Micro-biological Specimens and Reference Diagnostic Services* provides descriptions of specimen selection, packaging, and shipment, record keeping and reporting, and other valuable procedures involved in handling clinical laboratory materials.

SHIPPER'S CERTIFICATION FOR RESTRICTED ARTICLES
(excluding radioactive materials)
Two completed and signed copies of this certification shall be handed to the carrier. (Use block letters.)

WARNING: Failure to comply in all respects with the applicable regulations of the Department of Transportation, 49-CFR, CAB 82 and, for international shipments, the IATA Restricted Articles Regulations may be a breach of the applicable law, subject to legal penalties. This certification shall in no circumstance be signed by an IATA Cargo Agent or a consolidator for international shipments.

This shipment is within the limitations prescribed for: *(mark one)*

☐ passenger aircraft   ☐ cargo-only aircraft

Number of Packages	Article Number (int'l only) See Section IV IATA RAR)	Proper Shipping Name of Articles as shown in Title 49 CFR, CAB 82 Tariff 6-D and (for int'l shipments) the IATA Restricted Articles Regulations. Specify each article separately. Technical name must follow in parenthesis, the proper shipping name for N.O.S. items.	Class	IATA Packing Note No. Applied (int'l only)	Net Quantity per Package	Flash Point (Closed cup) For Flammable Liquids
						°C	°F

Special Handling Information:

I hereby certify that the contents of this consignment are fully and accurately described above by Proper Shipping Name and are classified, packed, marked, labelled and in proper condition for carriage by air according to applicable national governmental regulations, and for International Shipments the current IATA Restricted Articles Regulations.

Name and full address of Shipper	Name and title of person signing Certification

Date	Signature of the Shipper (see WARNING above)

Air Waybill No.*	Airport of Departure*	Airport of Destination*

*This box is iptional for completion by issuing carrier.

Figure 4.2

Appendix A

DEPARTMENT OF HEALTH, EDUCATION, AND WELFARE
PUBLIC HEALTH SERVICE
CENTERS FOR DISEASE CONTROL
ATLANTA, GEORGIA 30333
Telephone: (404) 329-3883 (Commercial)
236-3883 (FTS)

42 CFR Part 72—Interstate Shipment of Etiologic Agents[1]

Sec.
72.1 Definitions.
72.2 Transportation of diagnostic specimens, biological products, and other materials; minimum packaging requirements.
72.3 Transportation of materials containing certain etiologic agents; minimum packaging requirements.
72.4 Notice of delivery; failure to receive.
72.5 Requirements; variations.
      Authority: Sec. 215, 58 Stat. 690, as amended, 42 U.S.C. 216; sec. 361, 58 Stat. 703, (42 U.S.C. 264)

§72.1 Definitions.
As used in this part:
"Biological product" means a biological product prepared and manufactured in accordance with the provisions of 9 CFR Parts 102-104 and 21 CFR Parts 312 and 600-680 and which, in accordance with such provisions, may be shipped in interstate traffic.
"Diagnostic specimen" means any human or animal material including, but not limited to, excreta, secreta, blood and its components, tissue, and tissue fluids being shipped for purposes of diagnosis.
"Etiologic agent" means a viable microorganism or its toxin which causes, or may cause, human disease.
"Interstate traffic" means the movement of any conveyance or the transportation of persons or property, including any portion of such movement or transportation which is entirely within a State or possession, (a) from a point of origin in any State or possession to a point of destination in any other State or possession, or (b) between a point of origin and a point of destination in the same State or possession but through any other State, possession, or contiguous foreign country.

§72.2 Transportation of diagnostic specimens, biological products, and other materials; minimum packaging requirements.
No person may knowingly transport or cause to be transported in interstate traffic, directly or indirectly, any material including, but not limited to, diagnostic specimens and biological products which

[1]The requirements of this part are in addition to and not in lieu of any other packaging or other requirements for the transportation of etiologic agents in interstate traffic prescribed by the Department of Transportation and other agencies of the Federal Government.

such person reasonably believes may contain an etiologic agent unless such material is packaged to withstand leakage of contents, shocks, pressure changes, and other conditions incident to ordinary handling in transportation.

§72.3 Transportation of materials containing certain etiologic agents; minimum packaging requirements.
Notwithstanding the provisions of §72.2, no person may knowingly transport or cause to be transported in interstate traffic, directly or indirectly, any material (other than biological products) known to contain, or reasonably believed by such person to contain, one or more of the following etiologic agents unless such material is packaged, labeled, and shipped in accordance with the requirements specified in paragraphs (a)-(f) of this section:

BACTERIAL AGENTS

Acinetobacter calcoaceticus.
Actinobacillus—all species.
Actinomycetaceae—all members.
Aeromonas hydrophila.
Arachnia propionica.
Arizona hinshawii—all serotypes.
Bacillus anthracis.
Bacteroides spp.
Bartonella—all species.
Bordetella—all species.
Borrelia recurrentis, B. vincenti.
Brucella—all species.
Campylobacter (Vibrio) foetus, C. (Vibrio) jejuni.
Chlamydia psittaci, C. trachomatis.
Clostridium botulinum, Cl. chauvoei, Cl. haemolyticum, Cl. histolyticum, Cl. novyi, Cl. septicum, Cl. tetani.
Corynebacterium diphtheriae, C. equi. C. haemolyticum, C. pseudotuberculosis, C. pyogenes, C. renale.
Edwarsiella tarda.
Erysipelothrix insidiosa.
Escherichia coli, all enteropathogenic serotypes.
Francisella (Pasteurella) Tularensis.
Haemophilus ducreyi, H. influenzae.
Klebsiella—all species and all serotypes.
Legionella—all species and all Legionella-like organisms.
Leptospira interrogans—all serovars.
Listeria—all species.
Mimae polymorpha.

Moraxella—all species.
Mycobacterium—all species.
Mycoplasma—all species.
Neisseria gonorrhoeae, *N. meningitidis*.
Nocardia asteroides.
Pasteurella—all species.
Plesiomonas shigelloides.
Proteus—all species.
Pseudomonas mallei.
Pseudomonas pseudomallei.
Salmonella—all species and all serotypes.
Shigella—all species and all serotypes.
Sphaerophorus necrophorus.
Staphylococcus aureus.
Streptobacillus moniliformis.
Streptococcus pneumoniae.
Streptococcus pyogenes.
Treponema careteum, *T. pallidum*, and *T. pertenue*.
Vibrio cholerae, *V. parahemolyticus*.
Yersinia (Pasteurella) pestis, *Y. enterocolitica*.

FUNGAL AGENTS

Blastomyces dermatitidis.
Coccidioides immitis.
Cryptococcus neoformans.
Histoplasma capsulatum.
Paracoccidioides brasiliensis.

VIRAL AND RICKETTSIAL AGENTS

Adenoviruses—human—all types.
Arboviruses—all types.
Coxiella burnetii.
Coxsackie A and *B viruses*—all types.
Creutzfeldt—Jacob agent.
Ctyomegaloviruses.
Dengue viruses—all types.
Ebola virus.
Echoviruses—all types.
Encephalomyocarditis virus.
Hemorrhagic fever agents including, but not limited to, *Crimean hemorrhagic fever (Congo)*, *Junin*, *Machupo viruses*, and *Korean hemorrhagic fever viruses*.
Hepatitis associated materials (hepatitis A, hepatitis B, hepatitis nonA-nonB).
Herpesvirus—all members.
Infectious bronchitis-like virus.
Influenza viruses—all types.
Kuru agent.
Lassa virus.
Lymphocytic choriomeningitis virus.
Marburg virus.
Measles virus.
Mumps virus.
Parainfluenza viruses—all types.
Polioviruses—all types.
Poxviruses—all members.
Rabies virus—all strains.
Reoviruses—all types.
Respiratory syncytial virus.
Rhinoviruses—all types.
Rickettsia—all species.
Rochalimaea quintana.

Rotaviruses—all types.
Rubella virus.
Simian virus 40.
Tick-borne encephalitis virus complex, including *Russian spring-summer encephalitis*, *Kyasanur forest disease*, *Omsk hemorrhagic fever*, and *Central European encephalitis viruses*.
Vaccinia virus.
Varicella virus.
Variola major and *Variola minor viruses*.
Vesicular stomatis viruses—all types.
White pox viruses.
Yellow fever virus.[2]

(a) *Volume not exceeding 50 ml*. Material shall be placed in a securely closed, watertight container (primary container (test tube, vial, etc.)) which shall be enclosed in a second, durable watertight container (secondary container). Several primary containers may be enclosed in a single secondary container, if the total volume of all the primary containers so enclosed does not exceed 50 ml. The space at the top, bottom, and sides between the primary and secondary containers shall contain sufficient nonparticulate absorbent material (e.g., paper towel) to absorb the entire contents of the primary container(s) in case of breakage or leakage. Each set of primary and secondary containers shall then be enclosed in an outer shipping container constructed of corrugated fiberboard, cardboard, wood, or other material of equivalent strength.

(b) *Volume greater than 50 ml*. Packaging of material in volumes of 50 ml. or more shall comply with requirements specified in paragraph (a) of this section. In addition, a shock absorbent material, in volume at least equal to that of the absorbent material between the primary and secondary containers, shall be placed at the top, bottom, and sides between the secondary container and the outer shipping container. Single primary containers shall not contain more than 1,000 ml of material. However, two or more primary containers whose combined volumes do not exceed 1,000 ml may be placed in a single, secondary container. The maximum amount of etiologic agent which may be enclosed within a single outer shipping container shall not exceed 4,000 ml.

(c) *Dry ice*. If dry ice is used as a refrigerant, it must be placed outside the secondary container(s). If dry ice is used between the secondary container and the outer shipping container, the shock absorbent material shall be placed so that the secondary container does not become loose inside the outer shipping container as the dry ice sublimates.

(d)(1) The outer shipping container of all materials containing etiologic agents transported in interstate traffic must bear a label as illustrated and described on page 65.

---

[2]This list may be revised from time to time by Notice published in the Federal Register to identify additional agents which must be packaged in accordance with the requirements contained in this part.

(2) The color of material on which the label is printed must be white, the symbol red, and the printing in red or white as illustrated.

(3) The label must be a rectangle measuring 51 millimeters (mm) (2 inches) high by 102.5 mm (4 inches) long.

(4) The red symbol measuring 38 mm (1½ inches) in diameter must be centered in a white square measuring 51 mm (2 inches) on each side.

(5) Type size of the letters of label shall be as follows:

ETIOLOGIC AGENTS—10 pt. rev.
BIOMEDICAL MATERIAL—14 pt.
IN CASE OF DAMAGE OR LEAKAGE—10 pt. rev.
NOTIFY DIRECTOR CDC, ATLANTA, GEORGIA —8 pt. rev.
404-633-5313—10 pt. rev.

(e) *Damaged packages.* The carrier shall promptly, upon discovery of evidence of leakage or any other damage to packages bearing an Etiologic Agents/Biomedical Material label, isolate the package and notify the Director, Center for Disease Control, 1600 Clifton Road, NE, Atlanta, GA 30333, by telephone: (404) 633-5313. The carrier shall also notify the sender.

(f) *Registered mail or equivalent system.* Transportation of the following etiologic agents shall be by registered mail or an equivalent system which requires or provides for sending notification of receipt to the sender immediately upon delivery:

Coccidioides immitis.
Ebola virus.
Francisella (Pasteurella) tularensis.
Hemorrhagic fever agents including, but not limited to, Crimean hemorrhagic fever (Congo), Junin, Machupo viruses, and Korean hemorrhagic fever viruses.
Herpesvirus simiae (B virus).
Histoplasma capsulatum.
Lassa virus.
Marburg virus.
Pseudomonas mallei.
Pseudomonas pseudomallei.
Tick-borne encephalitis virus complex including, but not limited to, Russian spring-summer encephalitis, Kyasanur forest disease, Omsk Hemorrhagic fever, and Central European encephalitis viruses, Variola minor, and Variola major.
Variola major, Variola minor, and Whitepox viruses.
Yersinia (Pasteurella) pestis.[3]

§72.4 *Notice of delivery; failure to receive.*

When notice of delivery of materials known to contain or reasonably believed to contain etiologic agents listed in §72.3(f) is not received by the sender within 5 days following anticipated delivery of the package, the sender shall notify the Director, Center for Disease Control, 1600 Clifton Road, NE, Atlanta, GA 30333 (telephone (404) 633-5313).

§72.5 *Requirements; variations.*

The Director, Center for Disease Control, may approve variations from the requirements of this section if, upon review and evaluation, it is found that such variations provide protection at least equivalent to that provided by compliance with the requirements specified in this section and such findings are made a matter of official record.

[FR Doc 80-21757 Filed 7-18-80; 8:45 am]

BILLING CODE 4110-86-M

Effective August 20, 1980

Appendix B

SHIPMENT OF ETIOLOGIC AGENTS

The Air Transport Association's (ATA's) Restricted Articles Tariff 6-D, which specifies transportation requirements for hazardous materials shipped by air, was amended June 25, 1977. One of the provisions of this amended tariff, effective September 1, 1977, is that a large shipper's certificate must be used on domestic as well as international air shipments of etiologic agents and other hazardous materials.

This new requirement has prompted a review of applicable regulations and tariffs for alternatives to the use of this large shipper's certificate on small (less than 50-ml) shipments of etiologic agents sent by mail and airmail. The following statement has been reviewed with the U.S. Department of Transportation, the U.S. Postal Service, and the ATA, and it is consistent with the requirements of each of these agencies. In place of the large certificate, the Center for Disease Control (CDC) will use this statement on all domestic shipments of etiologic agents less than 50 ml in volume. Other shippers should consider using the statement in lieu of the large certificate:

NOTICE TO CARRIER

This package contains LESS THAN 50 ml OF AN **ETIOLOGIC AGENT**, N.O.S., is packaged and labeled in accordance with the U.S. Public Health Service Interstate Quarantine Regulations (42 CFR, Section 72.25 (c) (1) and (4)), and MEETS ALL REQUIREMENTS FOR SHIPMENT BY MAIL AND ON PASSENGER AIRCRAFT.

This shipment is EXEMPTED FROM ATA RESTRICTED ARTICLES TARIFF 6-D (see General Requirements 386 (d) (1)) and from DOT HAZARDOUS MATERIALS REGULATIONS (see 49 CFR, Section 173.386 (d) (3)). SHIPPER'S CERTIFICATES, SHIPPING PAPERS, AND OTHER DOCUMENTATION OR LABELING ARE NOT REQUIRED.

Date _____

Signature of Shipper _____

Address _____

CHAPTER 5

SPECIMEN COLLECTION AND HANDLING

C. Dwayne Morse

Introduction

The first and most important consideration in specimen collection and handling is to obtain material that is appropriately matched to the desired analysis and is properly collected. Although this statement may seem to be overly simplified, unsatisfactory and poorly collected specimens are submitted to laboratories entirely too often. An additional important factor is preserving a properly collected specimen in an appropriate container until it reaches the laboratory. Finally, the specimen should arrive at the laboratory with the patient's name and the date of collection on an appropriate laboratory data sheet and on the specimen container.

Safety must always be considered. All of the people involved in collecting and handling laboratory specimens must be familiar with the attendant risks and take steps to minimize or eliminate them.

A public health laboratory is in the unique position of receiving a large percentage of its specimens by mail or through courier services. For this reason it is imperative that every specimen be carefully collected, be placed in the best container available (usually supplied by the laboratory), or be placed in the best preservative or carrier fluid and transported to the laboratory as quickly and reliably as possible.

Since most public health laboratories are at least partly tax supported, the expeditious use of these tax dollars is important to all of us. Thousands of dollars are spent each year to provide mailing containers for laboratory specimens. In addition, considerable time is spent preparing the containers and the laboratory data sheets and sending these specimen collection kits to those who use them. As costs spiral, efforts to conserve and to use our resources wisely (without compromising patient welfare) are very important. Thus, any questions concerning laboratory analyses, types of specimens, specimen collection and shipment, or interpretation or clarification of the report should be directed to the public health laboratory before the fact. Such inquiries can save time and minimize patient risk and discomfort, especially if the type of specimen for an analysis is in question.

Collection Devices, Preservatives, and Storage

Many types of specimen containers are available. The following are guidelines for specimen collection and handling and are based on the most common methods currently used.

Type of Specimens

Blood

Blood or serum specimens are among the most commonly submitted and the most readily rendered unsatisfactory.

Serology. Syphilis and other microbial serologic tests constitute a large proportion of the analyses in a public health laboratory. A clotted blood specimen is usually preferred, and the vacuum collection tube is a convenient, reliable collection container. If a syringe is used to collect the specimen, the needle should be removed before the blood is carefully expelled from the syringe barrel into a sterile, dry tube, which is then securely stoppered. Expelling the blood through the needle can cause hemolysis and make the specimen unsatisfactory for analysis. Certain analyses require paired specimens from the acute and convalescent phases of illness to document a diagnostic rise in titer. Blood specimens must be protected from extremes of heat and cold during transport. Specimens which must be stored temporarily should be refrigerated at about 4 C.

The hazard of serum-transmitted hepatitis must be taken into account when collecting and handling blood samples. Aseptic technique and prevention of aerosols eliminate much of the hazard. Blood specimens should never be pipetted by mouth.

The fifth edition of *Diagnostic Procedures for Bacterial, Mycotic, and Parasitic Infections* contains additional pertinent information about collecting blood specimens (1).

Culture. Although blood for cultures is not often submitted to public health laboratories, such specimens should be very carefully collected and handled because misleading results can be obtained when contaminants are present. This problem can also occur when any normally sterile body fluid is collected for culture. Surface contaminants can be minimized by thoroughly scrubbing the subject's skin with surgical or other soap and removing the soap residue with a sterile applicator or gauze sponge saturated with 70% ethanol. Then a 1%-2% aqueous iodine solution should be applied with a sterile applicator, allowed to dry on the skin, and the residue removed with one or more 70% ethanol-soaked, sterile applicators.

Blood obtained for culturing suspected anaerobes should *not* be exposed to air in any way. Blood should be sent to the laboratory without delay; in fact, most procedures should be initiated immediately. The time required to mail such specimens to the laboratory may render them unsatisfactory.

Feces

A fresh specimen is by far the most desirable; however, when the specimen must be mailed or shipped to the laboratory, it must be treated with a preservative. Stool specimens suspected of containing pathogens should be handled with normal caution.

Culture. A preservative such as buffered glycerol saline helps to prevent the overgrowth of normal flora (20). Multiple specimens for culture should be collected over a 48- to 72-hr period because organisms may be shed intermittently. As is usual with other specimens for culture, the specimen must be obtained before the patient has antibiotics or chemotherapy. Preserved specimens should be kept at room temperature until they are cultured. Stool specimens the size of a walnut can be placed in a 1-ounce, screw-capped jar and mixed with the preservative. *Salmonella, Shigella,* and enteropathogenic *Escherichia coli* can be isolated readily from such specimens. *Compylobacter spp.* can also be isolated; however, other transport media are usually recommended. Please refer to a discussion in another section.

In isolating *Vibrio cholerae* or *V. parahaemolyticus*, the specimen must not be allowed to dry, because the organisms are sensitive to desiccation. Although culture procedures should begin immediately, in cases of unavoidable delay rectal swabs or stool specimens can be placed in a semisolid transport medium such as that of Cary and Blair (2). Regular enteric transport preservative such as buffered glycerol saline should not be used (7). These organisms are discussed further in other chapters.

Parasite identification. Fecal specimens to be used in identifying parasites should not be obtained by using purgatives or laxatives because these compounds can alter the morphology upon which organism identification depends. The two-vial system of preserving specimens is recommended. In one vial the specimen is placed in 5% formalin, and in the other the specimen is placed in polyvinyl alcohol (PVA) (16). The formalin solution preserves protozoan cysts and helminth eggs, whereas the PVA preserves intestinal protozoan's trophozoites. A small portion of the specimen is placed in each vial, and each preservative and specimen are mixed thoroughly with a clean applicator stick. Used sticks should be discarded in the manner of other contaminated material and should *not* be enclosed in the mailing container with the specimens. Vial lids should be tightened firmly so they are not jarred loose during transit. PVA contains mercuric chloride and should be considered a hazardous waste to be handled and disposed of appropriately.

Stool specimens are not needed in diagnosing pinworms. A simple cellophane tape collection method works well. A 2- to 3-inch strip of clear (frosted tape interferes with the microscopic examination) cellophane tape should be held against the patient's rectum when he awakes in the morning and before he moves. The tape is then fixed, adhesive side down, to a glass microscope slide and sent to the laboratory for microscopic examination. These specimens should be carefully handled because the eggs can become airborne; hand-to-mouth transmission is also a hazard.

Sputum

Mycobacteria. Sputum collected for culturing *M. tuberculosis* or other mycobacterial species should be obtained as the patient awakes and should be placed in sterile, leak-proof containers provided by the laboratory. To minimize contamination, the patient should rinse his mouth thoroughly with water before raising the sputum. Disinfectant mouthwash should not be used.

A technique that has not yet gained widespread use but may be useful is placing the sputum in a mixture of cetylpyridinium chloride (CPC) saline during transport (18). The CPC serves as a decontaminant during shipment so that the specimen can be inoculated onto the appropriate medium after simple centrifugation and without further treatment when it arrives in the laboratory. This method is not suitable for sputum specimens believed to contain fungi, which are sensitive to the CPC (17). Sputum for culturing mycobacteria should be refrigerated if it cannot be transported to the laboratory immediately in order to inhibit the growth of normal flora. Every precaution should be taken to prevent the formation of aerosols from sputum thought to contain *M. tuberculosis*.

Fungi. Sputum to be used in culturing fungi can be collected as above, except for the restriction noted. Specimens obtained for diagnosing histoplasmosis should be taken immediately to the laboratory (within 30 to 60 min) (10). Because *Histoplasma capsulatum* soon dies in sputum, if the specimen cannot be taken to the laboratory immediately, it should be inoculated directly onto appropriate culture medium such as cycloheximide chloramphenicol agar (9) before the tubes are sent to the laboratory for incubation and identification.

Sputum contains many contaminants from the throat and mouth. *Candida* and *Aspergillus* species can grow in sputum if specimens are not transported immediately; therefore, the diagnostic significance of isolating such organisms under the noted conditions is questionable.

At the present time sputum or other respiratory tract fluid specimens (except pleural fluids) are not recommended for isolation of *Legionella pneumophila* (14).

Most of the systemic fungi are not transmitted in sputum because it potentially contains the tissue form (noncommunicable stage) of such organisms as *Histoplasma capsulatum, Blastomyces dermatitidis,* or *Coccidioides immitis*. These fungi are infective in the mold form.

As a precaution, all work with mycobacteria, *Legionella pneumophila*, and most fungi should be carried out in a properly functioning biological safety cabinet.

Throat swabs

The procedures for obtaining specimens and culturing beta-hemolytic streptococci should be among the most straightforward bacteriologic techniques; however, in practice far too many liberties or shortcuts are taken in this procedure.

A specimen should be obtained from the back of the throat near the uvula with a cotton- or synthetic-tipped swab and with an attempt to avoid saliva. The type of swab material used has little effect on the recovery of the organisms (5). The swab should be placed in a foil-lined envelope with a packet of a preservative such as silica gel if the specimen is to be mailed to the laboratory. If the specimen is to be processed within about an hour, the swab can be held in a sterile closed container.

Techniques for collecting and handling specimens for isolating *Corynebacterium diphtheriae* and *Bordetella pertussis* are somewhat specialized and are discussed elsewhere in this volume.

Tissue

Such specimens are among the more unusual submitted to public health laboratories; however, tissue submissions have become increasingly important since the isolation and identification of the etiologic agent for Legionnaires' Disease, *Legionella pneumophila*.

Rabies. The most commonly submitted tissue specimen is the animal head sent for rabies diagnosis. *These specimens must be very carefully collected and shipped*. Almost any warm-blooded wild or domestic animal can be rabid, but animals should not be sacrificed without justification. Readers are referred to *Diagnostic Procedures for Viral and Rickettsial Infections* for a more complete treatment of this subject (13).

Culture. Tissue specimens to be used in culturing bacteria or fungi should generally be placed in sterile containers and be kept from drying. The tissue should be collected and handled carefully to avoid contamination. Tissue for culture must remain unfixed.

Immunofluorescence. For *Legionella pneumophila* direct immunofluorescence tests, tissues can be submitted either fresh or fixed. Neutral formalin is considered the best fixative for this purpose (14).

Food

Public health laboratories are asked to analyze food or food products for microbiological or chemical content or for some type of contamination. Even the most conscientious and capable laboratory can provide good results only if such specimens are properly obtained and handled before they arrive at the laboratory. In many cases, correct documentation and chain-of-events data are particularly important because legal actions are involved. The laboratory should be consulted before such samples are submitted because special preparations must often be made for an analysis and because valuable information on the kinds of samples required, shipping methods, etc., can be obtained. A few special considerations are discussed below.

The person submitting the specimen should try to establish the facts in every potential food poisoning or food contamination case. It is very important that stool specimens be obtained from persons involved in a potential foodborne disease outbreak. Depending on the epidemiologic workup these specimens can be cultured for a variety of enteric pathogens and the culture results can then be correlated with the food culture results. All specimens should be collected and labeled in a manner which avoids any possibility of contaminating the specimen before it reaches the laboratory. Food samples should be refrigerated (or on ice) during transport. This is especially necessary when microbiological contamination is suspected and overgrowth is to be prevented. Each container should contain only one specimen.

For more comprehensive information about food microbiology, see the *Compendium of Methods for Microbiological Examination of Food* (3) and the *F.D.A. Bacteriological Manual for Foods* (8).

Culture submitted for identification

The most important aspect of this procedure is that the organisms be cultivated on a medium that will give the best chance of survival during transport. The nature of this material varies with the organism and is discussed in greater detail in the chapters on specific organisms. If there is any doubt about the type of medium or container, the laboratory should be consulted. Generally, specimens should not be submitted in petri plates—especially if fungi are the suspected organisms. Fungal cultures should be sent on a slant of appropriate medium in a vial that has been cotton stoppered and covered with a screw cap.

Miscellaneous

Gonorrhea

The laboratory diagnosis of gonorrhea is a highly important public health consideration. The Public Health Service makes the following recommendations for the laboratory diagnosis of gonorrhea.

For males with purulent urethral discharge, a Gram-stained smear showing typical gram-negative intracellular diplococci is considered presumptively positive. Specimens for cultures should be analyzed to confirm cure or when the disease is suspected in the absence of symptoms.

Cervical culture is recommended as an aid in diagnosing gonorrhea among females. Anyone involved in collecting specimens for gonorrhea diagnosis should obtain specific instruction on preparing smears (in the case of males), obtaining specimens, and inoculating and handling culturing systems. Such information can be obtained from the local public health laboratory or the local venereal disease control organization and from the chapter on gonorrhea in this volume

Gonorrhea is unlikely to be contracted from specimens or cultures, but normal personal hygiene should be practiced.

Although not recommended, if cultures for gonorrhea diagnosis must be shipped two systems are currently widely used. First is the Transgrow system, in which a highly selective culture medium in a small bottle is used (15). The bottle contains 5%–10% carbon dioxide and must be kept upright during inoculation or the CO_2 will be lost. Many strains of *Neisseria gonorrhoeae* require or are stimulated by the presence of the gas. The cap should be tightened firmly after the specimen is inoculated and should be pre-incubated at 36 C before being shipped to the laboratory (the amount of pre-incubation to be noted on the laboratory data sheet). Several common precautions should be taken. Media should be kept cool and should be discarded if dehydration, cracking, mold or bacterial growth is evident or when the expiration date has passed. If the medium is stored in the refrigerator prior to use, it should be allowed to reach room temperature.

A second possibility that would encompass most of the guidelines mentioned above is the newer JEMBEC system (12), in which a clear rectangular plastic compact containing the modified Thayer-Martin medium is used. The container can be opened to expose the medium for inoculation, a small bicarbonate pellet placed in a special depression in one side of the plate, and the lid closed. The bicarbonate pill generates CO_2 in the presence of the moisture on the surface of the medium. The plate is enclosed in a small ziplock plastic bag to keep the gas from escaping. These units can be mailed to the laboratory. Some laboratories have found that a conventional culture dish provides the same benefits if placed in an airtight plastic bag with the CO_2-generating pellet.

Of several other useful media being used [such as the NYC medium (6)], most are probably not widely used in public health laboratories.

Anaerobes

Anaerobes are very sensitive to air, drying, and overgrowth by other organisms. Specimens such as nasal and throat swabs, feces, voided or catherized urine, and vaginal swabs are prone to contamination with normal flora and thus *should not* be cultured to identify anaerobes. Specimens for culturing suspected anaerobes should be taken carefully from the active site of infection, placed under anaerobic conditions immediately, and transported directly to the laboratory (4). Special collection and transport containers are available which contain oxygen-free carbon dioxide. Because CO_2 is heavier than air, the container should be kept upright and only opened long enough to insert the specimen. Some experienced laboratories do not recommend the use of transport media, saline, or other liquid for transporting or enriching specimens (11). Because of the complexity of anaerobes as a group, further reading of the references and the chapters dealing with specific organisms is recommended.

Botulism

Specimens for diagnosing botulism include serum, gastric contents, feces, and food. Laboratory analyses may include isolating *Clostridium botulinum* and/or testing for botulinum toxin. If clinical symptoms are compatible with the disease, the specimens should be sent for analysis without delay. All food specimens should be placed in separate, sterile, leakproof containers; wrapped with packing material; packed with ice in a second leakproof shipping container; and transported as quickly as possible. The laboratory should be notified well in advance about when and how shipment of the specimens is to take place and the projected arrival time and should be given an identification number for the shipment. All clinical specimens should be collected prior to treatment with botulinal antitoxin. Serum (10 ml) for toxin neutralization studies should be separated from whole blood prior to shipment. Serum, gastric contents, feces, and autopsy specimens should be placed in sterile containers and shipped as described above.

Phage or serotyping

Phage typing of *Staphylococcus, Salmonella,* and other organisms is available from some laboratories for epidemiologic, infection, and treatment control. Pure cultures of coagulase-positive *Staphylococcus aureus* or other organisms to be typed are preferred. The laboratory should confirm that the service is offered before specimens are sent. All clinical information necessary to evaluate the outbreak should be provided. Specimens submitted for serotyping should be handled in the same general manner.

Water analysis

Specimens submitted for water microbiological analysis must meet very specific collection and shipment guidelines. Readers are referred to *Standard Methods for the Examination of Water and Wastewater* for a comprehensive treatment of this subject (19).

References

1. BODILY HL: General administration of the laboratory. *In* Diagnostic Procedures for Bacterial, Mycotic and Parasitic Infections, 5th edition. Bodily HL, Updyke EL, and Mason JO (eds.). American Public Health Association, Inc., New York, 1970, pp 1-28.
2. CARY SG and BLAIR EB: New transport medium for shipment of clinical specimens. I. Fecal specimens. J Bacteriol 88:96-98, 1964
3. Compendium of Methods for Microbiological Examination of Foods. American Public Health Association, Washington, DC, 1976
4. DOWELL VR JR and HAWKINS TM: Laboratory Methods in Anaerobic Bacteriology. D.H.E.W. Publication No. (CDC) 74-8272, Atlanta, Ga, 1974
5. FACKLAM RR: Isolation and Identification of Streptococci. Part I. Collection, transport and determination of hemolysis. U.S.P.H.S. (CDC) Laboratory Manual, Atlanta, Ga, 1977
6. FAUR YC, WEISBURD MH, WILSON ME, and MAY PS: A new medium for the isolation of pathogenic *Neisseria* (NYC Medium). I. Formulation and comparison with standard media. Health Lab Sci 10:44-54, 1973
7. FEELEY JC and BALOWS A: *Vibrio. In* Manual of Clinical Microbiology, 2nd edition. Lennette EH, Spaulding EH, and Truant JP (eds.). American Society for Microbiology, Washington, DC, 1974, pp 238-245
8. FOOD AND DRUG ADMINISTRATION. Bacteriological Analytical Manual for Foods, 4th edition. Association of Official Analytical Chemists, Washington, DC, 1976
9. GEORG LK, AJELLO L, and PAPAGEORGE C: Use of cycloheximide in the selective isolation of fungi pathogenic to man. J Lab Clin Med 44:422-428, 1954
10. HALEY LD and STANDARD PG: Laboratory Methods in Medical Mycology, 3rd edition. U.S.P.H.S. (CDC) Publication, Atlanta, Ga, 1973
11. HOLDEMAN LV and MOORE WEC: Anaerobic Laboratory Manual, 2nd edition. The Virginia Polytechnic Institute and State University Anaerobe Laboratory, Blacksburg, Va, 1972
12. HOLSTON JL JR, HOSTY TS, and MARTIN JE JR: Evaluation of the bag-CO_2 generating tablet method for isolation of *Neisseria gonorrhoeae*. Am J Clin Pathol 62:558-562, 1974
13. JOHNSON HN: Rabiesvirus. *In* Diagnostic Procedures for Viral and Rickettsial Infections, 4th edition. Lennette EH and Schmidt NJ (eds.). American Public Health Association, Inc., New York, 1969, pp 321-353
14. JONES GL and HEBERT GA (eds.): "Legionnaires'": the disease, the bacterium and methodology. U.S.P.H.S. (CDC) Laboratory Manual, Atlanta, Ga, 1979
15. MARTIN JE JR and LESTER A: Transgrow, a medium for transport and growth of *Neisseria gonorrhoeae* and *Neisseria meningitidis*. H.S.M.H.A. Health Reports 86:30-33, 1971
16. MELVIN DM and BROOKE MM: Laboratory Procedures for the Diagnosis of Intestinal Parasites. D.H.E.W. Publication No. (CDC) 76-8282, 1975
17. PHILLIPS BJ and KAPLAN W: Effect of cetylpyridinium chloride on pathogenic fungi and *Nocardia asteroides* in sputum. J Clin Microbiol 3:272-276, 1976
18. SMITHWICK RW, STRATIGO CB, and DAVID HL: Use of cetylpyridinium chloride and sodium chloride for the decontamination of sputum specimens that are transported to the laboratory for the isolation of *Mycobacterium tuberculosis*. J Clin Microbiol 1:411-413, 1975
19. Standard Methods for the Examination of Water and Wastewater, 14th edition. Water Pollution Control Federation Publication, Part 900. American Public Health Association, American Water Works Association, 1976
20. VERA HD and DUMOFF M: Culture media. *In* Manual of Clinical Microbiology, 2nd edition. Lennette EH, Spaulding EH, and Truant JP (eds.). American Society for Microbiology, Washington, DC, 1974, p 896

CHAPTER 6

SEROLOGIC PROCEDURES

Dan F. Palmer

Introduction

The serology of infectious diseases apparently continues its transition away from the early opportunism exemplified in seeking evidence of rickettsial infections with *Proteus* antigens or attempting to detect mycoplasma infections with the streptococcal MG-agglutination test. The emergent philosophy in this immunologic field focuses on *"specificity,"* and many of the nonspecific serologic tests so popular in the past are being replaced with procedures in which antigens developed from the suspected etiologic agents are used.

Further, the recent surge of research activity and concomitant technological advances in all areas of immunology have provided a sophisticated array of methods and equipment which can be used to improve both the *sensitivity* and the specificity of serologic assays.

Besides the foregoing scientific advances, several Governmental licensure regulations imposed on the serologist have led to more stringent quality control measures, which can be classified under "accuracy" and "precision." The development and use of reference or standard serologic reagents and the incorporation of certain "internal" control specimens in routine serologic tests have also provided higher possible levels of accuracy and precision. Thus, all four horsemen of the serologic apocalypse (i.e., nonspecificity, insensitivity, imprecision, and inaccuracy) can be combatted.

A survey of the tests routinely used in serodiagnosing bacterial, mycotic, and parasitic diseases reveals that all of the classical approaches of agglutination, precipitation, lysis (including complement-fixation), and neutralization are represented. Tables 6.1, 6.2, and 6.3 list at least some of the tests evaluated and/or used for serodiagnostic purposes. As in most other areas of serology, the classical methods mentioned have been modified to facilitate demonstrating antigen-antibody reactions. Many of the newer modifications are not listed in the tables because they are still being evaluated or are not yet widely used for routine work. Some of these procedural innovations will be discussed later.

The following discussion is included because the serologist needs to understand the nature of the individual immune reactants and the basic principles upon which the various serologic tests are based in order to implement appropriate corrective measures as needed and in order to be able to inter-

TABLE 6.1—SOME ROUTINE TESTS OR THOSE EVALUATED FOR USE IN THE SERODIAGNOSIS OF BACTERIAL DISEASES

BACTERIAL DISEASES	TESTS									
	AGGLUTINATION	BACTERICIDAL	COMPLEMENT FIXATION	INDIRECT FA	TOXIN NEUTRALIZATION	INDIRECT HEMAGGLUTINATION	METABOLIC INHIBITION	LATEX AGGLUTINATION	COUNTERELECTROPHORESIS	OTHER
Actinomycosis				●						
Bacteroides Infection	●			●						
Pertussis	●									
Brucellosis	●									
Cholera	●	●				●				
Diphtheria					●	●			●	
Tularemia	●									
Fusobacterial Infection	●			●						
Gonorrhea										
Leptospirosis	●		●			●				●
Listeriosis	●									
Melioidosis						●				
Mycobacterial Infection										
Mycoplasma Infection			●	●		●	●			●
Neisseria meningitidis Inf.		●		●		●		●		
Paratyphoid Fever	●									
Plague						●				
Propionibacterium acnes Inf.	●			●						
Streptococcal Infection										●
Shigellosis						●				
Syphilis			●	●		●				
Tetanus					●	●			●	
Typhoid Fever	●									
Yersinia Infection	●									

pret test results correctly. Also discussed are some of the control measures required to insure credible interpretations and some pertinent adjunctive procedures for making routine tests more useful.

Elements of the Serologic Reaction

The serologic reaction involves antigen and antibody and the characteristics of their physical interaction. Because the serology of infectious disease cannot be fully understood without detailed knowledge of these elements, this section contains a discussion of them.

TABLE 6.2—SOME ROUTINE TESTS OR THOSE EVALUATED FOR USE IN THE SERODIAGNOSIS OF MYCOTIC DISEASES

MYCOTIC DISEASES	TESTS							
	AGGLUTINATION	COMPLEMENT FIXATION	INDIRECT FLUORESCENT ANTIBODY	LATEX AGGLUTINATION	PRECIPITIN	IMMUNODIFFUSION	COUNTERELECTROPHORESIS	OTHER
Aspergillosis		•				•		
Blastomycosis		•				•		
Candidiasis	•	•		•		•	•	
Coccidioidomycosis		•		•	•	•		
Cryptococcosis	•	•	•	•				•
Histoplasmosis		•		•		•		
Paracoccidioidomycosis		•			•	•		
Sporotrichosis	•			•				

TABLE 6.3—SOME ROUTINE TESTS OR THOSE EVALUATED FOR USE IN THE SERODIAGNOSIS OF PARASITIC DISEASES

PARASITIC DISEASES	TESTS					
	COMPLEMENT FIXATION	BENTONITE FLOCCULATION	INDIRECT HEMAGGLUTINATION	LATEX AGGLUTINATION	INDIRECT FLUORESCENT ANTIBODY	PRECIPITIN
Amebiasis	•		•	•		
Chagas'	•		•		•	
African Trypanosomiasis						•
Leishmaniasis	•		•			•
Malaria					•	
Pneumocystosis Toxoplasmosis	•		•		•	
Ancylostomiasis						
Ascariasis		•	•			
Filariasis	•	•	•			
Toxocariasis	•	•	•			
Trichinellosis	•	•	•	•	•	•
Clonorchiasis	•		•			
Fascioliasis	•		•			
Paragonimiasis	•					
Schistosomiasis	•		•		•	
Cysticercosis	•		•			
Echinococcosis	•	•	•	•	•	

Serologic Antigens

Antigens with which the serologist works are generally proteins or poly-saccharides, usually greater than 10,000 MW, with surface groupings of amino acids (in the case of proteins) or protruding sugar side chains (in the case of polysaccharides) governing their reaction with antibodies. Certain of these surface groupings, termed *"antigenic determinants,"* are sequential or conformational in form. In protein antigens, a sequential determinant usually consists of five or six amino acids linearly arrayed, and a con-formational determinant is one composed of a few amino acid residues juxta-posed in the steric conformation of the native macromolecule but remote from each other in the unfolded polypeptide chain. Ordinarily, protein anti-gens possess relatively few antigenic determinants (approximately one de-terminant per 5000 MW in globular protein) relative to the number of se-quences of immunologically silent polypeptides on the molecule.

Most of the determinants that elicit humoral antibody responses are conformational, and the serologist is well advised to handle antigens care-fully to prevent denaturation or unfolding of the polypeptide chains. When they do unfold, specificity of the serologic test for antibodies directed against the conformational entity is lowered or lost, and the test becomes invalid.

Globular proteins, in which the conformational determinant is pre-dominant, have relatively few repetitive amino acid sequences, and the de-terminants present on macromolecular globular proteins are apt to represent a variety of antigenic or serologic specificities. Antibodies directed against these proteins are correspondingly heterogeneous.

On the other hand, fibrous proteins, which comprise a minority of the serologic antigens, ordinarily have repetitive amino acid sequences along their polypeptide chains, and antibodies directed against such proteins are often less heterogeneous than those directed against antigenically diverse globular protein macromolecules.

Regardless of the chemical nature of antigens involved, infection or dis-ease caused by bacterial, mycotic, or parasitic agents results in the patient's being exposed to numerous antigenic stimuli, which arise both from multiple antigenic determinants on single antigen molecules and from a number of different antigens originating on the surface of the invading organism, its internal components, and its extracellular products. Thus, antigen hetero-geneity is centrally involved in the dynamics of the humoral response to infectious disease, and virtually all serologic tests can only be interpreted validly if scientists are aware of this fact.

Antibodies

Antiserum developed in response to infectious disease almost always consists of a collection of antibody molecules with heterogeneous specific-ities corresponding to the multiple antigens involved in the disease process. Further, several different classes of immunoglobulins (e.g., IgG, IgM) may be present to confound the total antibody picture. However, their presence may be helpful to the serologist, because multiple antibodies often allow crude serologic antigens to be used that could not otherwise be, and the sequential appearance of different immunoglobulin classes during the disease process sometimes enables the scientist to determine whether the antigenic stimuli occurred just before serologic testing, thus providing a basis for diagnosing acute disease.

Traditionally, serodiagnosis of infectious disease has not always been useful because it has often been retrospective. Usually, meaningful results could only be obtained if two or more serum specimens were taken 10–14 days apart and tested simultaneously for evidence of a rise in antibody titer, thus creating a considerable delay before the clinician could make a diagnosis. This requirement still applies in most cases but is gradually being relaxed in instances in which specific IgM can be demonstrated (indicating an early phase of the disease) or in which transient antibodies to an acute-phase antigen can be detected in a single serum specimen. The success of both approaches has been made more likely by recent technological advances in serology.

Antigen-Antibody Interactions

Obviously, another major concern of the serologist is the *in vitro* antigen-antibody interaction. Some of the puzzling occurrences in serologic tests that ordinarily defy interpretation can be resolved by better understanding of one or two relevant immunochemical concepts.

Antigen-antibody interactions *in vitro* are characterized by two stages: the primary binding and the development of some physical manifestation such as precipitation, agglutination, neutralization, or lysis, which signals the serologist that this binding has occurred.

The binding of antigen and antibody results from forces not unlike those of any two unrelated proteins, except that the reaction is very specific. Coulombic, hydrogen bonding, hydrophobic, and Van der Waals forces all are involved at one time or another in the bonding process.

These bonds act in concert to form reversible attachments of various strengths between the antibody and antigen molecules, and the number and total strength of the bonds between an individual antigen binding site and an antigenic determinant can be described in terms of "*affinity*." That is, an antibody molecule with antigen binding sites that "fit" (allow the formation of multiple bonds that are comparatively strong) well with an antigenic determinant is said to have high affinity for that antigen.

A more useful concept for the serologist, however, is that of "*avidity*." This term describes the attachment of the entire multivalent antibody molecule to the antigen and includes all bonds existing among those antigen binding sites on the antibody molecule that have reacted (a maximum of two with IgG) and the antigenic determinants on the antigen molecule. If only one antigen binding site on the antibody molecule is involved in the reaction, the avidity of the attachment is the same as its affinity, and dissociation of the two reactants proceeds on that basis. If both antigen binding sites of a divalent antibody molecule have reacted with antigenic determinants on an antigen molecule, the avidity characterizing the attachment is of the order of 10,000-fold greater than the affinity existing for one site, making dissociation much less likely.

In routine serodiagnostic tests, there is no control for assessing the avidity of antibodies reacting with the serologic antigen used. However, the serologist should bear in mind that antibody titers of serum specimens usually reflect both the concentration of antibody molecules present and their avidity.

The second stage of the antigen-antibody reaction allows numerous serologic testing methods to be used to determine whether specific antibodies are present in serum. Physicochemical phenomena occurring during this stage are (a) the formation of a precipitate; (b) the agglutination of particulate matter bearing surface antigenic determinants; (c) the neutralization of particular biological, physical, or chemical functions ordinarily associated with certain antigenic entities; or (d) the triggering of the complement cascade, which causes lysis of erythrocytes or death of certain gram-negative bacteria.

Precipitation

Conditions favoring the formation of a precipitate during the second stage of an antigen-antibody reaction can be induced, and the resulting precipitate can be detected visually, nephelometrically, or in unusual circumstances by other means. Such tests are called "precipitin tests" and are best exemplified by procedures to detect the formation of visual precipitates in agar gel when the reactants are forced to diffuse toward one another as advancing concentration gradients and precipitate under optimal or near optimal conditions.

Precipitin tests are used in nearly all areas of serology including bacterial, mycotic, and parasitic serology. They are a very specific tool for the serologist but usually are relatively insensitive because a rather large number of molecular complexes must be formed for the reaction to be detected.

Regardless of which technical approach is used to detect the presence of an antigen-antibody precipitate, the test cannot be fully understood or its results properly interpreted without an awareness of the dynamics of various antigen-to-antibody ratios present. This knowledge can best be obtained by studying the "lattice hypothesis" proposed in 1934 by Marrack and quantitatively described by Heidelberger a few years later. The hypothesis includes critical aspects of antigen-antibody interaction and is applicable to the precipitin test and to many other serologic tests.

The lattice hypothesis accounts for the fact that the composition of immune precipitates and the quantity of precipitate vary according to the relative concentrations of antigen and antibody present in the reaction mixture.

The hypothesis states that if increasing amounts of soluble antigen are mixed with a constant amount of antibody, three zones emerge that relate to the quantity of precipitate formed and to the relative composition of antigen and antibody in the precipitate. The first of these, which contains only a little antigen, is referred to as the "zone of antibody excess" and is characterized by no initial precipitation but by a precipitate containing relatively large amounts of antibody which appears as the amount of antigen increases. The amount of precipitate increases as antigen is added until a maximum amount of precipitate forms because of extensive lattice formation. When a maximal or nearly maximal amount of precipitate forms, the "zone of equivalence" has been reached, and the ratio of antigen to antibody in the precipitate reflects the valence of immunoglobulin and antigen involved. This zone does not contain free antigen or free antibody outside the lattice. The third zone, which forms when the amount of antigen is increased beyond that present in the zone of equivalence, is called the "zone of antigen excess" and has a decreasing amount of precipitate forming as antigen concentration increases. This decrease in precipitation results from the lack of uncombined sites available on antibody molecules to allow cross-linking required for lattice formation. Although all of the antigen and antibody form complexes, much of the latter is in small, still soluble molecular complexes (e.g., divalent IgG forms antigen-antibody-antigen triplets) unavailable for inclusion within the precipitate.

Applying the above theory can often resolve many problems which occur in laboratories where precipitin tests are done. For example, there are instances in which specific, precipitable antigen-antibody systems are present in agar gel diffusion test material but do not produce visible precipitate. This situation often results from the fact that the reaction occurs in the zone of antigen excess where little or no precipitate forms. In other words, the specimen which contains the antigen simply overwhelms the reagent which contains the antibody, and either no precipitate line can be seen in the agar or a barely discernible, "washed-out" area develops. Such a situation can be corrected (i.e., moved into the zone of equivalence) by diluting the antigen-containing specimen or, perhaps better, by increasing the concentration of antibody.

Ordinarily, precipitin test reagents are balanced by the test designer or commercial supplier to insure that precipitate will form with normal concentrations of antigen or antibody. However, if a wide range of antigen concentrations is anticipated in unknown specimens, it may be advisable to use several dilutions of the specimens for the precipitin test in order to avoid problems associated with antigen excess.

As is true for all serologic procedures, the precipitin test has many other variables which must be controlled if optimal (or even credible) results are to be obtained (e.g., optimal ranges of time, temperature, molarity of buffer or electrolyte solutions, pH, ionicity, component volume, and concentration). In rare cases, comparatively wide variation of a particular factor is allowable because it affects the final results only slightly, and the desired degree of precision or accuracy is maintained. In most cases, however, optimal ranges of the variables listed are restricted, and persons who perform serologic tests should carefully follow the recommended procedures to obtain credible results and to provide a standardized approach.

As in all serologic tests, control materials must be included in every run to confirm final results. These control materials must include a well-characterized specimen containing a known concentration of the component under assay (two positive controls are preferred—one relatively strong and the other containing the analyte at a concentration just above the threshold of the test's sensitivity). In nearly all instances, a negative control specimen should also be included to confirm the test's ability to detect a negative specimen. Precipitin tests are generally believed to be quite specific and rarely react positively with negative specimens.

Because precipitin tests are relatively insensitive, a number of technical innovations have been made, particularly in agar gel tests. Sensitivity of precipitin reactions can be increased if more antigen and antibody molecules are encouraged to combine in a common reaction arena (rather than allowing large portions to diffuse away from one another, as occurs in double diffusion tests). Thus techniques such as counterelectrophoresis, which overcomes the tendency of antigens and antibodies to diffuse in all directions in gel by electrically driving them toward one another, and rheophoresis, which controls this tendency hydrodynamically, have been designed. In addition to increasing test sensitivity somewhat, these modifications often reduce the time required to obtain results.

Agglutination

The second stage of an antigen-antibody reaction may consist of the aggregation of particles which have surface antigen or antibody which combines with the other reactant to form agglutinated masses under certain conditions. Tests in which particulate antigen or soluble antigen adsorbed to the surface of particulate matter is used are termed "direct" and "indirect" agglutination tests, respectively. The laws governing this type of serologic reaction are not unlike those governing the precipitin reaction. The major distinction between the agglutination test and the precipitin test is the size of the antigenic material involved in the reaction; it is of soluble dimensions in the precipitin test and particulate in the agglutination test.

The agglutination test has been used widely in bacterial, fungal, and parasitic serodiagnosis (see Tables 6.1, 6.2, and 6.3), principally because of historical precedent and because of the rational appeal of agglutinating suspensions of the intact etiologic agent with antibodies from the patient. The technique is also used in identifying unknown cultures by agglutinating the organisms with antibodies of known specificity. The agglutination test is more sensitive than the precipitin test for several reasons, one of which is that fewer antigen and antibody molecules are required to produce a visible aggregated mass (because of the larger size of the antigen). This obvious advantage of greater visibility after reaction with a given amount of antibody led researchers, in early efforts to achieve higher sensitivity, to adsorb soluble antigen onto so-called "inert" particulate matter, which was then induced to agglutinate by small amounts of specific antibody. When soluble antigen is adsorbed onto particulate material in this way and subsequently used in detecting antibodies in a patient's serum specimen, the procedure is called a "passive" or "indirect" agglutination test, because the particulate material is not involved in the immune reaction but is merely a passive vehicle for the antigen. Materials such as charcoal, carmine, and bentonite have been used as the particulate material onto which antigen has been adsorbed, but the most popular particles currently are red blood cells and latex suspensions.

Much of the theory of lattice formation in soluble antigen-antibody precipitation is applicable to the agglutination reaction as well, but additional very important physicochemical theory applying particularly to agglutination (and, to some extent, to precipitation) must be discussed at this point. With an understanding of the relevant factors favoring and opposing agglutination in the test tube (or on the slide), the serologist can more accurately assign causes to the many problems that may occur in agglutination procedures and can take appropriate corrective action.

Since red blood cells are the particles most frequently used in indirect agglutination tests, they are used here to illustrate the theory involved in agglutination. However, principles involved apply equally to all particles used in direct and indirect agglutination tests.

Agglutination of antigen-coated red blood cells by specific antibodies results from interparticulate linkage among cells caused by the reaction between multivalent antibodies and surface-bound antigen. Just as in the precipitin reaction, a lattice is formed. For linkage to occur, however, the cells must be close enough together for antibody molecules to be able to bridge the gap between cells. The size of the gap separating the cells when they are as close to one another as possible under existing conditions is a result of the sum of the forces of attraction and repulsion present in the *in vitro* system of the test. Several possible states can exist. The gap between cells may be too large under certain circumstances for antibodies to effect a linkage, and agglutination does not occur even though specific antibodies are present. Thus a false-negative result is obtained. The gap may be too large for IgG antibodies (approximately 245 Å long) to effect a linkage but small enough for IgM (approximately 1000 Å long) to do so. In this case, only IgM-class antibodies can produce agglutination, and false-negative results will be obtained. The gap may be small enough for all antibodies to bridge the gap between cells and yield a valid result, but cells may approach one another so closely that they "autoagglutinate," i.e., agglutinate in the absence of specific antibody, so that false-positive results are obtained.

The major factor favoring agglutination in a suspension of cells is lowered free energy levels associated with the surfaces of the cells. The second law of thermodynamics states that a system (such as a suspension of red blood cells) is most stable when its level of free energy is lowest. Since systems tend to seek maximal stability, lowering free energy corresponds to the direction of force. Further, since the free energy associated with cell surfaces is diminished when the cells agglutinate (i.e., when parts of their surfaces juxtapose and the free energy associated with those cell surface areas that are touching each other is removed from the system), the tendency is toward agglutination.

On the other hand, since not all cell suspensions immediately agglutinate, obviously some forces must deter agglutination. These opposing forces arise in response to the existence of electric charges on each of the cells in the suspension. All of the cells suspended in an ordinary buffered saline solution have a net negative charge, primarily as the result of ionization of carboxyl groups in sialic acid residues on their surfaces. Because of a natural electromagnetic law that objects with like charges repel one another, the suspended cells, which all have net negative charges, repel one another.

Fortunately, the amount of opposition to agglutination can be controlled by changing the ionic strength or dielectric constant of the medium in which the cells are suspended, by treating the cells with certain enzymes (or other substances), or by adsorbing certain proteins such as antibodies onto the cells. By adjusting the repelling force relative to the attracting forces, a very sensitive system poised at the threshold of agglutination can be created, and agglutination will occur when small amounts of antibody in a patient's serum specimen are added. The reaction will occur more quickly if the test solution is agitated to increase antigen-antibody contact. Control measures required for the agglutination test should include positive and negative reference specimens and preparations of the particulate antigen suspended in the test diluent alone so that any tendency toward spontaneous agglutination in the absence of antibody can be noted. When no agglutination has occurred in this antigen control preparation, it can often be used further as a reading standard with which to compare weak or questionably positive reactions.

Neutralization

In vivo neutralization tests for antibody assay are not popular in bacterial, fungal, and parasitic serology because they require maintaining living host systems (with all the attendant expenses). Further, neutralization tests are often time-consuming, yield imprecise results, and can sometimes be replaced by other serological methods which yield comparable information more efficiently.

Whereas the neutralization concept is quite valid and often is used to reflect the ability of antibodies to prevent disease (especially in virology), no routine diagnostic neutralization tests are yet available for fungal and parasitic diseases. In bacterial serology, occasional tests for antitoxic antibodies are performed in reference laboratories with the technical experience, special reagents, and facilities they require. For example, antibodies directed against *Vibrio cholerae* heat-labile enterotoxin are assayed by neutralization in the ligated rabbit ileal loop, by certain cell cultures, or by the rabbit skin permeability factor test. Titration of diphtheria antitoxin by the rabbit intracutaneous method or assay of tetanus antitoxin by neutralization in mice is also used rarely, but the results obtained with these assays are of little value in the ordinary clinical setting.

Even though the neutralization test is an *in vivo* procedure subject to a number of biological vagaries, results reflect an antigen-antibody proportionality variation analogous to those observed in the precipitation and agglutination reactions. Thus toxin may be overneutralized, in which case an antitoxic antigen-antibody complex is formed, or underneutralized, in which case a toxic complex is formed, depending on whether the neutralization occurs in the zones of antibody excess or antigen excess.

Lysis

The potentiating effect of complement, endowing certain antibodies with the power to lyse (or kill) cells, has led to the development of a number of useful serodiagnostic tests. Tests for bacteriolytic (or preferably, bactericidal) antibodies have been used since the latter part of the 19th century, but they have been replaced to some degree with less cumbersome, less time-consuming procedures. An important exception is the serum bactericidal test for antibodies to *Neisseria meningitidis*, used in studying patients with recurrent meningitis or suspected immune deficiency disease.

The major serologic utility of the lysis phenomenon, however, is not in the dissolution of bacterial cells but rather in providing a basis for the indicator system in the complement fixation (CF) test. Antibodies directed against red blood cells will lyse the cells (which then release hemoglobin) in the presence of complement but not in its absence. The CF test is further predicated upon the fact that when most antigens react with their corresponding antibodies, complement present in the reaction mixture will be consumed or rendered incapable of potentiating any other reaction. It is therefore possible to arrange a series of steps that include first mixing a patient's serum specimen (perhaps containing antibody) with an antigen of interest (e.g., histoplasmin or leptospiral extract) and a standard amount of complement. If specific antibodies are present in the patient's serum specimen, they react with the antigen and consume all or part of the complement present in the mixture. Subsequently, red blood cells and anti-red blood cell antibodies (hemolysin) are added to the mixture. If no complement is available because it was all consumed in the initial antigen-antibody reaction, the red blood cells are not lysed by their corresponding antibody, and a positive reaction is indicated. If, on the other hand, no specific antibodies are present in the patient's serum specimen to react with the antigen initially, complement remains available for the second reaction between red blood cells and their antibodies, and lysis occurs to indicate a negative reaction.

Obviously, the test components (i.e., complement, hemolysin, red blood cells, and diluent) must be carefully balanced quantitatively to insure valid test results. Complement and hemolysin must be titrated so that they can be added in their proper concentration, the required number of red blood cells must be present, and diluent for the test must be correctly prepared to provide a proper milieu for the reactions. These factors and their complicated interrelationships necessitate a number of controls in the CF test to confirm that all components are reacting properly and to provide a basis for analyzing any problems that might occur. As in all serologic assays, positive and negative reference sera must be included in each run, but serum controls should also be included to reflect any reaction of the patient's (or reference) serum with complement in the absence of antigen ("anticomplementary" activity). These serum controls should contain, then, all elements needed for the test except antigen (volume should be made up with test diluent). Further, the activity of complement in the presence of red blood cells, hemolysin, and antigen (no serum) should be ascertained to detect any anticomplementary activity introduced by the test antigen. Activity of complement in the presence of red blood cells and hemolysin only (no antigen or serum) should be determined to rule out excessive variation in this indicator phase of the test. Finally, a control should be run that contains only red blood cells, hemolysin, and diluent to show any cell lysis in the absence of complement.

Because of its relative sensitivity, the CF test has previously been used extensively in parasitic serology, to some extent in bacterial serology, and is currently a major test method in fungal and viral serology. However, since newer, more sensitive methods with equal or better specificity have been developed, the CF method is less widely used. For example, it was long considered a major and definitive test in syphilis serology, but has now been eliminated from the recommended methods in that field.

Other Serologic Systems

Regardless of the basic second stage physicochemical manifestation involved, the immune reaction can be easier to detect by attaching onto antigen or, more often, onto antibody a marker which can be easily and unmistakably detected. In effect, the passive agglutination method in which antibodies are attached to comparatively large particulate material which can be easily seen when aggregated illustrates the principle. A number of other substances used for the same purpose result in various levels of greater sensitivity. For example, antigens or antibodies can be ''tagged'' (linked) with functionally active proteins such as bacteriophage or enzyme, which can subsequently be detected by introducing into the test a suitable host for the phage or substrate for the enzyme. These two tagging substances can provide a marked amplification of the initial antigen-antibody reaction, because the phage can multiply in its host and the enzyme can repeatedly catalyze a substrate conversion. Consequently, the sensitivity of the immune reaction is considerably increased. Antigen or antibody can be tagged with a radionuclide, which results in a very sensitive immunoassay in which a scintillation counter is used. Another substance used to tag the immune reactants is a chemical with the property of spin resonance. This type of reagent has been used in some drug immunoassays. The tagged reactant is detected with an electron spin resonance spectrometer. Ferritin-tagged antibodies are currently used to locate antigens in ultrastructure studies of tissues by electron microscopy, the ferritin being an electron dense material. Finally, antibodies can be tagged with a fluorescent dye such as fluorescein or rhodamine, and results of immunoassays in which these dye-conjugated antisera are used can be obtained visually by ultraviolet microscopy or objectively by fluorometry.

There is considerable commercial interest in developing kits and ancillary instruments to exploit the greater sensitivity levels achieved by using isotope-, enzyme-, and fluorescein-labeled reactants. Some of these methods, however, involve sophisticated instruments and encumber the serologists with the need to insure adequate maintainence of the instruments and control of attendant variables. Further, when a new labeling material is adopted in the serology laboratory, people must be trained to use it, and quality control procedures must be designed specifically for it.

Adjunctive Methods in Serology

The discovery of class-specific immunoglobulins and subsequent elaboration of their functional distinctions provide the opportunity to derive more serodiagnostic data by analyzing the patient's immune response in such terms. For example, the presence of antibody-specific IgM in a patient's serum specimen generally indicates recent infection, but the presence of antibody-specific IgG alone may reflect involvement with the antigen in the remote past. Further, many studies have shown that under normal conditions, only IgG is transferred during gestation from the mother to the fetus, and the presence of antibody-specific IgM or IgA in serum of a newborn normally reflects actual fetal production of these immunoglobulins in response to antigenic stimuli.

Several methods now exist for separating these macromolecular components of the serum. A very convenient method which ordinarily yields comparatively good separation is ultracentrifugation in a gradient of sucrose or similar substance. With this method, immunoglobulins are separated by centrifugal forces which create terminal velocities that vary according to size, shape, mass, and other criteria. The method results in a band of IgM near the bottom of the tube and a band of IgG near the top of the tube. After it is centrifuged, fractions of the specimen are collected, dialyzed if necessary, and serologically analyzed for the antibody of interest. Some data on the class specificity of antibody activity can also be obtained by selective elimination of the reactivity of one or more classes with 2-mercaptoethanol (2-ME) or a similar reagent. Treating serum with this type of reagent theoretically causes a reduction in titer if IgM is contributing to the antibody content, but has little or no effect when all of the specific antibody activity derives from IgG alone. This method is used extensively in brucella serology, but its application is limited because a fourfold or greater reduction in titer is required for significance (indicating an IgM concentration of at least 75%), and specimens are unlikely to contain such a high ratio of IgM to IgG unless obtained quite soon after the subject was exposed to the organism.

A method currently receiving a great amount of attention is the selective adsorption of IgG from the patient's serum with *Staphylococcus* protein A, thereby distinguishing IgM-positive from IgM-negative specimens by the titer remaining after adsorption. Some strains of *Staphylococcus aureus* (e.g., Cowan, I.) will combine with the Fc portion of the human IgG molecule, and the supposition is that serum specimens with antibody titers which cannot be significantly reduced by treatment with the protein A contain mainly IgM and are indicative of recent or current infection with the organism in question. There is considerable evidence that the protein A also adsorbs some IgM, although apparently less than it does of IgG. Regardless of this shortcoming, it appears that the method will make possible some inferences about the presence or absence of IgM. However a "gray" area of inconclusive results still exists, and more definitive methods are needed when specimens yield data which fall in this area.

General References

Barrett JT: Textbook of immunology. An introduction to immunochemistry and immunobiology, 2nd edition. The C. V. Mosby Co, St. Louis, Mo, 1974

Bellanti JA: Immunology. W. B. Saunders Co, Philadelphia, 1971

Day ED: Advanced immunochemistry. Williams & Wilkins Co, Baltimore, 1972

GORDON BL: Essentials of immunology, 2nd edition. F. A. Davis Co, Philadelphia, 1974
HOBART MJ and McCONNELL I: The immune system. A course on the molecular and cellular basis of immunity. Blackwell Scientific Publications, Oxford, 1976
ROITT IM: Essential immunology. Blackwell Scientific Publications, Oxford, 1971
ROSE NR and FRIEDMAN H (eds.): Manual of clinical immunology. American Society for Microbiology, Washington, DC, 1976
SELA M (ed.): The antigens, Vol. I. Academic Press, New York, 1974
WILSON GS and MILES AA: Principles of bacteriology and immunity, 5th edition. Vol. I. Williams & Wilkins Co, Baltimore, 1964

CHAPTER 7

LABORATORY GLASSWARE AND PLASTIC WARE

Bradford P. Smith

Laboratory Glassware and Plastic Ware Usage

The relatively recent increase in availability and continuing proliferation of acceptable plastic and glass disposable laboratory ware have changed the character of glassware and the stocking and preparation procedures associated with it. Before a rational choice can be made between reusable and disposable products, the following must be considered:

1. As disposable plastic and glass items replace reusable glassware, increasingly larger storage areas are required for stock. Therefore, the frequency with which the supplier can deliver becomes important if additional storage area is not available.
2. Conversely, an increase in the use of disposable items leads to a decrease in the amount of glassware washing necessary. Since most disposable items can be purchased packaged and ready for use, no initial preparation is necessary.
3. Depending on the size and scope of the laboratory operation, disposition of disposables back into the environment can become a significant consideration in terms of volume. All discarded materials must be decontaminated before leaving the laboratory. Laboratory management must know the means by which discards are ultimately disposed of (e.g., sanitary landfill or incineration) and must confirm that they are not jeopardizing anyone who must subsequently handle or come in contact with such discarded materials. Additionally, they must determine that the disposal system complies with all local, state, and Federal regulations relative to environmental protection.
4. Initial purchase and materials processing costs of reusables must be carefully weighed against costs of purchase, delivery, and additional storage of disposable ware in deciding whether to supplant reusable items.

The above points must be contemplated quite apart from the advantages of disposables versus reusables to the laboratorian.

Regardless of the mix of wares a laboratory uses, it will always be necessary to prewash and prepare some items. If this process is to be carried out effectively, efficiently, uniformly, and economically the following must be examined:

1. A versatile machine that can wash most types of laboratory glassware is preferable to manual washing.
2. New glassware should be washed before its first use to remove the manufacturer's oily film deposit. "Hand-wash-only" items should be similarly treated.
3. It is a good practice not to sterilize and prepare for delivery more items than are likely to be used in the next 30 days. If a "clean-ready-for-issue" glassware storeroom is used, it must be as free of dust as possible.
4. It is economical and practical to have lower-paid, central service personnel do as much as possible of the preparation of reusable glassware to a "ready-for-use state" rather than expecting laboratorians to do the task.
5. Detergents cannot be universally recommended because of variations in water contaminants and hardness. Detergent manufacturers' representatives should be consulted in the selection and evaluation process.
6. Acid cleaning of new glassware is not recommended. Further, sonic cleaning can be used to replace acid cleaning for all but the most stubborn soils. For any acid cleaning necessary, it is recommended that a commercially prepared acid solution be purchased rather than having a solution made up in the laboratory because the formulation process can be hazardous to personnel.

Used and/or potentially infectious laboratory ware can generally best be decontaminated by being sterilized in an autoclave. In order to insure that all surfaces of vessels, containers, discard pans, and other materials are sterilized, it is necessary to:

1. Loosen all closures to allow air to escape and steam to enter.
2. Place items such as beakers, graduates, flasks, and tubes on their sides to facilitate the removal of air.
3. Put approximately 1 inch of water or other aqueous solution in each discard pan before autoclaving. This not only drives the air up and out of the pan during the beginning of the autoclave cycle, thus permitting live steam to enter the pan and come into contact with all surfaces of the pan contents, but also provides sufficient moisture during the last stage of the autoclave cycle so that material does not become baked on reusable glassware, making it difficult to remove in the subsequent washing process.

Reusable and disposable items should not be placed in the same pan because they must then be sorted before the disposables can be discarded. Sorting introduces the needless hazard of hand cuts and stabs. Heavy items should not be placed on top of light, fragile items in discard pans. Potentially infectious items should be autoclaved as close to the source of origin as possible and not transported through other areas. All autoclaves used for the decontamination of infectious materials should have satisfactory performance confirmed periodically by some accepted method.

Laboratory Safety

Safety orientation and subsequent periodic review of laboratory employees' knowledge retention are the responsibility of the laboratory supervisor and *cannot be delegated*. The necessity for observing safety precautions and the desire to comply must be instilled in every laboratorian. No job should be considered so important that it cannot be done safely.

In its simplest form, the problem of safety is one of application because the state of the science is sufficiently advanced to have evolved excellent techniques and control equipment. Safety training may be a formal or informal function. In either case, part of the training period must be devoted to acquainting employees with specific job-related safety procedures and emphasizing their personal responsibility in preventing accidents and infections.

It is the moral duty of all laboratorians to be knowledgeable about the materials and equipment used and to take due precautions based on this knowledge to protect nonlaboratory personnel. Laboratorians, collectively, are responsible for the safety of all those who enter their facilities, as well as of all those who come in contact with materials generated by the laboratory. This is a grave responsibility and should be treated as such.

CHAPTER 8

STERILIZATION AND DISINFECTION

Martin S. Favero and Peter Skaliy

Introduction

Because sterilization and disinfection are used daily in modern public health laboratories, personnel in such facilities should be familiar with the procedures involved.

Sterilization is the process of destroying all living forms present in the environment treated. Disinfection, on the other hand, reduces the number of harmful microorganisms and, consequently, the risk of infection but does not guarantee sterility. It is obviously important to distinguish between sterilization and disinfection.

In the public health laboratory this distinction is significant from a practical standpoint. Whether a disinfection procedure results in sterilization depends on a number of factors, each of which influences the rapidity and level of antimicrobial action. Among these factors are the nature and number of contaminating microorganisms (especially the presence of bacterial spores), the type and concentration of the disinfectant, length of exposure, amount of organic material present, the type and condition of the material to be disinfected, and the temperature. For example, although a very strong chemical disinfectant may kill bacterial spores exposed to it long enough, the required time may be significantly greater than that required with saturated steam in an autoclave. Thus for practical reasons, sterilization in the public health laboratory is most often effected with physical agents rather than chemicals, and disinfection is performed with either physical agents or chemicals.

Sterilization Procedures

Sterilization by Heat

Dry heat. Dry heat is used to sterilize articles which are corrosively attacked by steam; glassware such as flasks, bottles, and pipettes packed in sealed cans; and anhydrous, dehydrated, or hydrophobic materials that cannot tolerate moist heat. Common examples of materials that are dry-heat sterilized are instruments with cutting edges, surgical gut, ground-glass surfaces, dry chemicals, grease, oil, and glycerol. The primary limitation of dry heat is the time necessary for sterilization. If higher temperatures are used to shorten the sterilization period, fabrics, rubber goods, plastics, and chemicals can be degraded or destroyed. In a dry-heat sterilizer, the hot air should be mechanically circulated to prevent stratification and to insure uniformity of temperature.

The recommended time-temperature relationships for dry heat listed below refer to actual load temperatures and *not* to chamber temperature. Consequently, a recommendation of 170 C for 1 hr does not allow for the time required for the materials being sterilized to reach that temperature. Variations in the load and equipment necessitate that a temperature-sensing device be placed in the center of the load or in that part of the load that is assumed to be the most difficult for heat to penetrate in order to confirm when the material reaches the sterilization temperature. Once the cycle has been established, thermocouples need not be used daily, but it is recommended that the cycle be checked once every month or two. In addition, commercially available spores (*Bacillus subtilis* var. *niger*) should periodically be placed in the centers of loads or into those areas of the loads considered to be the most difficult for heat to penetrate in order to check the sterilization process.

The following time-temperature ratios are listed as guidelines for dry-heat sterilization in a laboratory. These times represent the length of exposure needed after the recommended temperature is reached.

> 170 C (340 F)........ 1 hr
> 160 C (320 F)........ 2 hr
> 150 C (300 F)........ 2.5 hr
> 140 C (285 F)........ 3 hr

Moist heat. Saturated steam under pressure is most frequently used for sterilization. The procedure is based on direct contact with saturated steam, which is a physical entity with properties that can be measured conveniently. All living microorganisms can be rapidly destroyed by pressurized steam. The time-temperature relationships applicable to this type of sterilization are generally agreed upon.

Steam is a readily available store of latent energy liberated simply by change of state, which carries the advantage of rapid heating. When it comes in contact with cold objects, saturated steam condenses, simultaneously heating the object and wetting it, and thus provides two requisites for the rapid thermal destruction of microorganisms.

If this sterilization method is to be effective, air and moisture present in the sterilization chamber must be removed, preferably automatically. Air can be removed from the sterilization chamber by being displaced downward with steam or suctioned with a high-vacuum pump. The high-vacuum method is much more effective because it removes approximately 98% of the air from the chamber and load before the steam is introduced. Steam penetration after air evacuation is almost instantaneous, and the absence of air during heating eliminates the risk of damage to textiles and rubber by oxidation at high temperatures.

The following time-temperature-pressure relationships are recommended for steam sterilization:

15 min at 121 C, 15 psig
10 min at 126 C, 20 psig
3 min at 134 C, 29.4 psig

These times relate only to the period after the materials reach the designated temperature and moisture levels of saturated steam and do not include penetration or heat-up lag. Steam-sterilizer manufacturers have recently developed automatic sterilizers which incorporate new concepts in process and equipment design. Consequently, the modern-day autoclave has progressed from manually operated units to fully automatic, gravity-displacement and high-vacuum, high-pressure sterilizers with integrated time-temperature controls on steam-jacketed vessels with motorized doors. Tables 8.1, 8.2, and 8.3 illustrate the effects of the type of load on the total length of a steam sterilization cycle. These data are guidelines only; actual sterilization cycles should be determined in each laboratory (e.g., with thermocouples and commercially available indicator spores such as *Bacillus stearothermophilus*).

Sterilization by Filtration

The two basic systems for filtering microorganisms from liquid media are depth filtration and screen or membrane filtration.

Depth filtration. Depth filters can be asbestos pads, porcelain candles, and diatomaceous-earth filters. The surface portion of the filter removes large particles, and the center or matrix portion removes the small particles to a rated degree, although never completely. Several factors determine the ability of a depth filter to perform its prescribed function: particle geometry, pore size, surface characteristics, medium velocity, pressure changes, particle migration, and filter-medium migration. The depth filter has a distinct advantage over others in that it can retain a large volume of particulate matter before becoming plugged. Generally speaking, it is best not to reuse depth filters.

Screen or membrane filtration. Screen filters are classified by pore size, which is usually limited to a minimum pore size of 20 μm. Their usefulness is

TABLE 8.1—STERILIZATION TIMES

STERILIZER TYPE	TEMPURA-TURE (°C)	ARTICLE BEING STERILIZED	STERILIZATION TIME (MINUTES)*			
			PENETRA-TION	HOLDING	SAFETY	TOTAL
Downward displacement	121	Instruments	3	12	0	15
		Gloves	5	12	3	20
		Packs	12	12	6	30
High prevacuum	132	Instruments	1	2	1	4
		Gloves	1	2	1	4
		Packs	1	2	1	4

*Measured from the time the autoclave gauge reaches the temperature selected.

TABLE 8.2—STEAM STERILIZATION OF LIQUIDS—EFFECT OF VOLUME/CONTAINER (ERLENMEYER FLASKS) ON TIME REQUIRED TO REACH 121 C (SINGLE CONTAINER LOAD)

SIZE OF CONTAINER (ML)	VOLUME OF LIQUID/ CONTAINER (ML)	CHAMBER TEMP. AT INITIATION OF CYCLE (° C)	LIQUID TEMP. AT INITIATION OF CYCLE (° C)	TIME NEEDED FOR CHAMBER TO REACH 121 C (MINUTES)	TIME NEEDED FOR CENTER OF LIQUID TO REACH 121 C (MINUTES)	TOTAL TIME OF CYCLE (MINUTES)
50	25	110	25	2	4	14
125	75	110	25	2	5	15
200	150	110	25	3	7	17
500	400	110	25	3	10	20
1000	800	110	25	3	14	24
2000	1500	110	25	6	19	29
3000	2500	110	25	7	25	35
5000	4500	110	25	8	33	43
6000	5500	110	25	8	44	54

limited because particles accumulate rapidly. This type of filter is often used as a clarifier rather than in sterilizing liquids.

Membrane filters have been developed with uniform pore sizes that generally range from as large as 14 μm to as small as 10 nm. These filters can be used to sterilize various aqueous media, including serum, water, culture broth, etc. Membrane filters with a rated pore size of no larger than 0.45 μm and ideally 0.22 μm or less should be used for sterilization. This is especially

TABLE 8.3—STEAM STERILIZATION OF LIQUIDS—EFFECT OF VOLUME/CONTAINER AND NUMBER OF CONTAINERS ON TIME REQUIRED FOR LIQUID TO REACH 121 C

LIQUID PER CONTAINER (LITER)	CONTAINERS PER LOAD (NO.)	CHAMBER TEMP. AT INITIATION OF CYCLE (° C)	LIQUID TEMP. AT INITIATION OF CYCLE (° C)	TIME NEEDED FOR CHAMBER TO REACH 121 C (MINUTES)	TIME NEEDED FOR LIQUID TO REACH 121 C (MINUTES)	TOTAL TIME OF CYCLE (MINUTES)
0.5	30	27	29	10	19	29
1.0	20	27	26	12	34	44
1.5	15	56	26	12	36	46
2.0	10	46	27	13	37	47
2.5	10	66	26	15	40	50
3.0	8	46	26	15	43	53
3.5	6	46	26	12	50	60
4.0	5	43	26	12	52	62
4.5	5	44	26	14	58	68
5.0	5	46	26	15	60	70
5.5	5	42	26	17	60	70
6.0	4	42	26	15	62	72

true with reagents or media prepared with water containing high levels of gram-negative water bacteria. With such materials, most of the microorganisms can be removed, but a small portion of the population can pass through an ordinary 0.45 μm membrane filter. The membrane filter offers the advantage that pores are of uniform size and that the filtration rate is faster than with other types of filtration equipment.

Sterilization by Ionizing Radiation

Although the pharmaceutical industry currently sterilizes various medical equipment such as needles, syringes, disposable rubber gloves, and plastic equipment by ionizing radiation, the technique is not practical in the average public health or clinical laboratory. The cost of a cobalt-60 (gamma source) installation or of an electron accelerator for sterilization is prohibitive for all except large-scale commercial applications.

Chemical Sterilization

If the more reliable physical methods are not available or cannot be used, materials can be sterilized with gaseous and liquid germicides. Chemical sterilization, commonly referred to as "cold sterilization," is used primarily for treating heat-sensitive items. Relatively high concentrations of germicidal solutions and prolonged exposure are necessary to assure that all microorganisms are destroyed—particularly the more resistant bacterial endospores.

Aqueous formaldehyde is used as a chemical sterilizing agent. Usually alcohol is added to the solution to retard polymerization of the formaldehyde. An 8%–70% (formaldehyde-alcohol) solution is satisfactory for sterilizing purposes (18 hr of exposure at 25 C).

Glutaraldehyde solutions are broad-spectrum germicides and are used widely in chemical sterilization. With certain items such as instruments with lenses, glutaraldehyde is preferred to formaldehyde because the former is less corrosive. Although glutaraldehyde solutions are relatively stable at low temperatures (4 C), those being used are effective for only 2–4 weeks when stored at room temperature (20–25 C). Glutaraldehyde sterilization usually consists of exposing cleaned items to a 2% solution for 10 hr at 25 C.

Among several important factors which affect the action of chemical sterilizing agents is whether the concentration of the active materials is adequate to destroy the entire microbial population—especially the more resistant bacterial spores.

The time required for sterilization can vary from seconds to hours. The types of organisms and their physical and chemical states determine the length of time necessary for the germicide to destroy them.

The formaldehyde-alcohol and glutaraldehyde solutions are generally applied at room temperature. Such factors as pH, size of the microbial population, surface activity, and the presence of extraneous matter affect the final results obtained with chemical sterilizing agents. *Since proteinaceous material and grease can interfere with the action of the germicidal solution, items being treated must be scrupulously clean, with minimal soil or bacterial contamination.* With complex pieces, the sterilizing chemical must completely penetrate any interstices or small bores to assure sterilization.

Because increasingly more heat-sensitive materials are being used as components of scientific and medical equipment, gas sterilization has come into frequent use. Currently, the biocidal agent of most gas sterilizers is ethylene oxide. Many items damaged by heat can be sterilized with gaseous ethylene oxide (ETO), which is effective against all types of microorganisms. It has excellent penetrating properties and can be used at moderate temperatures and pressures in the closed chamber which confines it. The optimal relative humidity of the gaseous atmosphere is about 50%, and the temperature should be kept between 40 and 60 C. With nonexplosive mixtures of ETO and CO_2 or freon, concentrations of 450–760 mg ETO/liter are readily attainable. For concentrations of $\geq$1000 mg/liter, ETO without a carrier gas is used. Length of the exposure period depends on the type of load and the contaminating microbial population.

Although formaldehyde gas was once used for sterilization, it is now used primarily for fumigation and decontamination. Formaldehyde vapors can be obtained by heating formaldehyde or flaked paraformaldehyde in a relative humidity of at least 70% and at minimum temperature of 20 C. Generally, this gas kills bacterial cells within a few hours, but it takes longer to destroy bacterial endospores.

Commercially available spores should be placed in the centers of loads or in those areas of the load where the least gas penetration is expected to occur in order to monitor sterilization procedures.

Users of ETO sterilization are cautioned that the chemical is toxic to the skin and when inhaled. The gas is highly penetrating; such materials as rubber and plastic can absorb the chemical while being sterilized. Ample time must be allowed for ETO to dissipate after the sterilization cycle is completed. Some sensitive materials must be stored at room temperature in a well-ventilated area for a week after sterilization before they can be safely used. Several manufacturers now produce aeration cabinets designed to increase the rate at which gas is dissipated from sterilized items.

Such factors as temperature, time, concentration, and relative humidity must be precisely controlled to insure an effective sterilization cycle. Although ETO is effective against all types of organisms, the physical state of the microorganisms is an important determining factor in the sterilization process. Extremely dry organisms, particularly bacterial endospores, are highly refractive to the action of ETO. Even with a preconditioning period of high relative humidity before exposure to the gas, some bacterial endospores may not rehydrate to the level necessary for the ETO to act effectively.

Disinfection Procedures

Disinfection refers to the destruction of disease-producing vegetative microorganisms but not ordinarily to that of bacterial spores. The term is generally used to indicate a reduction in the microbial contamination of a particular environment. Literally, disinfection implies a process for destroying agents of infection or disease. In a broader sense, disinfection includes deleterious action against both noninfectious and infectious microbial flora.

Contamination in the laboratory can be minimized or eliminated by good cleaning procedures. Restricting the presence of microbes on inanimate surfaces or physically removing all or a major portion of the microbial populations from objects is usually not difficult.

As an adjunct to physical cleanliness, chemical agents are also widely used in disinfecting procedures. Since it is often difficult to disinfect large objects or surfaces physically, disinfection is most often carried out with chemical substances which have antimicrobial properties.

Chemical germicidal agents are more effective against vegetative microbial cells than against bacterial and fungal spores, tubercle bacilli, and the more resistant viruses. The ultimate action of chemical agents may be either biocidal (the microorganism is killed) or biostatic (growth and multiplication of the microorganism are inhibited).

Of the many different types of chemical disinfectants, only a representative selection of the most common are briefly discussed here.

Chemical Disinfectants

Inorganic and organic mercurials, which are among the oldest types of disinfectants, are not widely used. At present, they are used primarily as fungicides in industrial preservatives. The mercurials are essentially biostatic rather than biocidal, with their biostatic properties being poor even when they are highly concentrated. The presence of organic matter markedly reduces their effectiveness as disinfectants.

Quarternary ammonium compounds are widely used as germicides and are effective primarily against vegetative cells. They are relatively ineffective against tubercle bacilli and bacterial spores. These compounds are good wetting agents because of their strong surface-tension-reducing properties. Because cationic quaternaries are not compatible with soaps, surfaces and objects they are used to treat should be free of soap films. Organic materials such as serum proteins, cork, and cotton fibers also inactivate the compounds. The quaternaries should be diluted carefully, because substances in certain natural waters may affect their germicidal activity adversely. In addition, gram-negative water bacteria can grow in dilute or aged solutions. Thus, freshly prepared solutions are the most effective.

Halogens, chlorine, iodine, and bromine have been widely used as disinfectants. The chlorine-type germicides (sodium hypochlorite, calcium hypochlorite, dichloro- or trichloro-isocyanuric acid) can be used for various decontamination procedures. The presence of organic material reduces the effectiveness of chlorine disinfectants. They are effective against vegetative cells, the tubercle bacilli, and bacterial spores at high concentrations, i.e., 5000 ppm. Disinfection agents which contain chlorine are generally corrosive to inanimate objects and surfaces and are irritating to live tissues.

Tincture of iodine or aqueous iodine preparations are generally used as antiseptics. Iodophors contain iodine and a solubilizing agent and are applied as general disinfectants. The iodophors are stable, relatively stain and odor free, and have the antimicrobial properties of iodine. They are effective against vegetative cells and tubercle bacilli but not against bacterial spores.

Phenol or carbolic acid is infrequently used as a general disinfectant in laboratories. The compound is effective against vegetative bacterial cells, but it has several drawbacks. It is irritating and destructive to skin and tissues, particularly when used at higher concentrations, and it smells unpleasant. Although rarely used in disinfection procedures, phenol continues to be used as a basic standard in laboratory tests for comparison with other types of phenolic preparations.

Synthetic phenols have replaced the original compound as disinfectants. These compounds are similar to phenol but lack its undesirable characteristics. The phenolic derivatives are effective germicides against vegetative bacerial cells and tubercle bacilli but are not very effective against bacterial spores. The compounds are stable and can be inactiviated by organic matter but not by soap. Many of the synthetic phenols are odorless. Since the formulations are compatible with detergents, the synthetic phenols are widely used for general sanitation purposes as disinfectant-detergents.

Ethyl and isopropyl alcohol are commonly used as antiseptics but are sometimes also used as disinfectants. They act rapidly, have a cleansing action, and evaporate quickly. Since alcohols are volatile, no residue remains on treated surfaces; however, this property necessitates that solutions be frequently checked for loss of activity resulting from evaporation.

The alcohols are biocidal against vegetative bacterial cells and tubercle bacilli. The compounds are not effective against bacterial spores and certain viruses (including the hepatitis B virus) and are inactivated by organic matter. Solutions of 70% concentration are generally used as disinfectants. Both ethyl and isopropyl alcohol readily mix with water. The bactericidal activity of isopropyl is slightly greater than that of ethyl alcohol.

Factors influencing activity of chemical disinfectants

In general, the higher the concentration of a chemical disinfectant, the greater is its germicidal activity. To assure lethal action, the chemical agent must be allowed enough time to be absorbed by and to destroy the microorganism. Elevated temperatures may increase the agent's biocidal activity, although some formulations are not stable at higher temperatures. The presence of organic matter interferes with the action of most chemical disinfectants.

The level of contamination must be physically reduced before a disinfectant is applied. No known disinfectant is completely effective against all types of microorganisms, and obviously some are more effective than others against particular microbes. Usually the effectiveness of a chemical disinfectant is stated in terms of selected test strains of microorganisms against which it is best used.

Selecting a chemical disinfectant

A primary consideration in selecting a suitable chemical disinfectant is its purpose. An ideal disinfectant is that with the following characteristics:

a. It should have a wide range of activity, i.e., it should be effective against viral, fungal, rickettsial, protozoan, and bacterial species.
b. It should be stable. Prolonged storage or exposure to moderate temperatures should not decrease its activity.
c. It should not be adversely affected by salts, organic matter, pH, or the hardness of the water used to dilute it.
d. It should not stain or corrode surfaces and objects.
e. It should not be toxic or irritating to tissues and skin.

Part Two

CHAPTER 9

WASTE DISPOSAL IN MICROBIOLOGY LABORATORIES

Don C. Mackel and George F. Mallison

Introduction

All microbiology laboratory personnel are responsible for knowing and strictly practicing laboratory safety procedures. Adequate handwashing is particularly important. In-service training on laboratory safety and handling and disposing of hazardous laboratory materials should be provided on a continuing basis by laboratory management. Specific written rules and procedures should be provided for disposing of pathologic waste, laboratory animals, and chemical, cultural, and radioactive materials. Procedures for handling waste in clinical and research laboratories must be designed not only to protect workers in the laboratory but others in the same building/area and the community at large.

Solid-waste material generated in laboratories is increasing as more disposable items are used (plastic, metal, glass, paper, etc.). After they are contaminated with pathogens, blood, or body wastes, most of these items should be either sterilized or incinerated before disposal.

Microbiologic Waste

Microbiologic wastes include laboratory material or other substances containing bacteria, viruses, fungi, parasites, or human or animal tissues and secretions.

Culture material. All culture media and materials containing or suspected of containing pathogens must be sterilized before being removed from the work area for disposal. In some instances, incineration of these materials may be preferable; presterilization before incineration is not necessary, but *care must be taken* to prevent spread of contamination during transport to a suitable incinerator on the premises. All materials should be placed in impervious biohazard bags designed for this purpose before transporting to the incinerator. Contaminated reusable pipettes, slides, petri plates, volumetric vessels, etc., used in examining or testing biologic specimens must always be sterilized before they are cleaned and processed. These items should be placed into a leak-proof metal container fitted with a lid. Depending on the size of the container, up to 1000 ml of water should be added to a depth of about 1 cm before items are added for sterilization. The container should then be covered but *not hermetically sealed*. During the sterilizing cycle, the added water evaporates into steam and replaces the air in the container; if water were not added, sterilization might not be achieved.

Contaminated disposable or broken glassware, plastic, paper, and metal can either be placed in metal discard containers or in steam autoclavable plastic bags. At least 75 ml of water should be added. Items must be carefully placed into plastic bags so as not to puncture the plastic. Containers should always be filled in a manner to allow the steam to circulate freely around the materials.

All containers with contaminated wastes should be identified with 'biological hazard' labels. Autoclave-indicator tape should also be placed on the containers so that those that have been sterilized can be readily identified.

Clinical specimens. After being examined, all pathologic specimens, and in some instances highly contaminated food and other environmental material, must be sterilized for safe disposal, as described above. Once sterilized, these materials can be disposed of through the municipal solid-waste disposal system. In some cases, it may be better to incinerate solid material, tissues, and some biologically contaminated liquid wastes; these materials do not need to be sterilized before being incinerated, but they *must* be carefully transported to a suitable incinerator.

Liquid wastes (except radioactive material), including blood, are best disposed of by *carefully* pouring down a sewerage drain. For amounts of ≤.5 ml or when a hazard is involved in opening the container, both the container and its contents should be incinerated. These wastes can also be autoclaved, but urine and feces may cause unpleasant odors in the surrounding area.

Laboratory animals and waste. Dead animals, necropsy material, and bedding wastes should be placed in plastic bags or metal leak-proof containers, which should be properly marked and autoclaved prior to disposal or can be sealed successively into two impervious bags (≥3 mil thickness polyethylene) and carefully transported to a suitable incinerator at the location.

Chemical and Radioactive Wastes

Chemicals. Biologically contaminated chemical wastes that contain liquid nontoxic, noncombustible chemicals can be disposed of in the sewerage drain as described above.

Large quantities of unused or outdated liquid chemicals should not be discarded indiscriminately into the sanitary sewer system. Some commonly used laboratory chemicals are flammable or explosive or may react with other substances or metals in the sink drains (e.g., sodium azide becomes extremely explosive). Usually, nonradioactive, and noncombustible, solid or liquid chemicals are best disposed of in the municipal solid-waste disposal system, but not without the approval of the state health department. It is further suggested that the appropriate office of the State or the U.S. Environmental Protection Agency be consulted before disposing of oncogenic chemicals and substances. *These materials must be handled and disposed of very carefully.* Flammable liquids should be held in suitable containers to be disposed of by the local fire department.

Radioactive materials. Radiologic substances must be segregated and handled in accordance with the regulations of the U.S. Nuclear Regulatory Commission.

Noninfectious, Nonhazardous Wastes

Uninoculated liquid media, hot melted agar, unused tissue culture media, etc., can be discarded directly into the sanitary sewer system mixed with hot water running from the faucet. Such materials should be added slowly to avoid clogging the system.

Sterilization and Inactivation of Infectious Materials

Steam autoclaving. Autoclaving with pressurized steam is the safest and least expensive method of sterilizing most contaminated laboratory waste. As mentioned above, materials should be properly contained, but it is also important that the containers be properly loaded into the autoclave. *Steam sterilizers must not be overloaded.* Whatever the nature of the material being sterilized—whether it be liquid or solid—it must be sterilized in a container to which water has been added.

Most laboratory autoclaves are operated at 121 C. The length of time at that temperature is dictated by the size of the load and, in some cases, the resistance of the microorganisms; usually 30 min to 1 hr of autoclaving is indicated after the chamber temperature reaches 121 C.

Chemical sterilization indicators should be used for all containers in each autoclave load, but it should be remembered that they are only designed to indicate exposure to heat; they do not assure sterility of the materials.

The proper functioning of an autoclave should be confirmed at least once a week with biologic autoclave controls *(Bacillus stearothermophilus).* When new types of laboratory wastes are to be sterilized, biologic control tests should be performed even more frequently until an effective cycle time is established. *B. stearothermophilus* controls are commercially available from a number of companies. Results of biological sterility testing procedures must be monitored continuously by persons trained to interpret them.

Incineration. Burning is an effective means of sterilizing infectious material. In some respects, it can be especially desirable because materials can be reduced to ashes and easily disposed of in relatively little space.

Only approved, properly operated and maintained incinerators should be used. Operators must be adequately trained and properly motivated to assure optimal use of the equipment and complete incineration of the materials. Incinerators are banned in certain areas because of pollution regulations.

Chemical sterilization. Chemical sterilization of laboratory and clinical wastes is not recommended because of the intensive monitoring required. Clinically contaminated, heat-sensitive, reusable equipment can be chemically sterilized if the process is properly monitored. The most frequently used chemicals are gaseous ethylene oxide and glutaraldehyde (1, 5-pentanedialdehyde). *Careful* physical cleaning is necessary to remove gross soil before materials are chemically sterilized.

Disposal to sewer. Liquid or suspended biological laboratory wastes can be discarded into a community sanitary sewer system. Solid, noninfectious material can be wet-ground in waste grinders and discharged into the sewer system. Introducing laboratory wastes into a septic tank system in water may be inadvisable because the critical complex biology of the system might be disrupted.

Sanitary landfills. Only sanitary landfills which are approved for specific wastes should be used. Contaminated microbiology laboratory wastes must be sterilized before they are placed in a landfill. Some sanitary landfill authorities will allow dead animals to be disposed of only in certain areas of the landfill; human tissue should not be disposed of in any landfill. Landfills are likely to be located some distance from the laboratory, which means that the contaminated material must be transported.

Transport of wastes. Contaminated laboratory wastes should only be transported in closed, leak-proof containers or in double, impervious plastic bags. All containers should be labeled and contents listed when infectious material is carried outside the laboratory area to an incinerator; it is obviously desirable for an incinerator to be located near the laboratory. Sterile or other laboratory waste should be contained in leak-proof containers when transported to a landfill or incinerator in order to prevent leakage onto the streets and highways.

General References

AMERICAN STERILIZER CO: Sterilization Aids. American Sterilizer Co., Erie, Pa, 1968

BARTLETT RC, GRÖSCHEL DHM, MACKEL DC, MALLISON GF, and SPAULDING EH: Control of hospital-associated infections. *In* Manual of Clinical Microbiology, 2nd edition. Lennette EH, Spaulding EH, and Truant JP (eds.). American Society for Microbiology, Washington, DC, 1974, pp 841–857

BLOCK SS (ed): Disinfection, Sterilization and Preservation, 2nd edition. Lea and Febiger, Philadelphia, 1977

CENTER FOR DISEASE CONTROL: Disposal of Solid Wastes from Hospitals. National Nosocomial Infection Study Report, 4th Quarter. Center for Disease Control, Atlanta, Ga, 1972, pp 24–25 (Issued April 1974)

CENTER FOR DISEASE CONTROL: Laboratory Safety at the Center for Disease Control, HEW (Revised edition 1974). DHEW Publication No. CDC 76-8818. Atlanta, Ga, 1977

INCINERATOR INSTITUTE OF AMERICA: I.T.A. Incinerator Standards. Incinerator Institute of America, New York, 1975

STEERE NV (ed.): Handbook of Laboratory Safety, 2nd edition. The Chemical Rubber Co., Cleveland, 1971

SYKES G (ed.): Disinfection and Sterilization, 2nd edition. JB Lippincott, Philadelphia, 1965

U.S. DEPT. OF HEALTH, EDUCATION, AND WELFARE: National Institutes of Health Biohazards Safety Guide, HEW, GPO No. 1740-00383. Washington, DC, 1977

WENDHOLZ M (ed.): Merck Index, 9th edition. Merck and Co, Rahway, NJ, 1976

CHAPTER 10

LABORATORY ANIMALS

Kenneth D. Quist and J. Roger Broderson

Introduction

The basic information in this chapter on laboratory animals should help persons who are considering using animals in diagnostic and research tests, and the general reading bibliography should help those in well-established animal facilities to solve specific problems.

Laboratory animals used in diagnostic and research procedures have become one of the most costly items in the research institution's budget. Costs have increased dramatically because of the housing and manpower needed to care for the animals and the cost of raising the animals or purchasing them from breeders who use expensive environmental controls.

The Animal Welfare Act of 1966 (PL-89-544; amended in 1970 by PL-91-579) established certain minimum standards for the care of laboratory animals. These standards were published in the *Federal Register* (Vols. 32 and 36). The basic intent of the law is to help regulate the humane treatment, care, and transportation of dogs, cats, nonhuman primates, guinea pigs, hamsters, rabbits, and other warm-blooded animals. The U.S. Department of Agriculture (USDA) administers the Act. By law, USDA periodically inspects animal facilities. All research facilities must be licensed or registered, and annual reports are required for such specific items as animal purchases and standards of care.

On May 14, 1973, the U.S. Department of Health, Education, and Welfare (DHEW) issued a statement regarding animal care which is applicable to all animal research which the Department supported (National Institutes of Health, Food and Drug Administration, and other Federal agencies).

The following statement is from that issuance (DHEW 73.2):

> It is the policy of the Department of Health, Education, and Welfare that institutions using animals in projects or other activities supported with funds from DHEW grants, awards, or contracts shall assure the DHEW in writing that they will evaluate on a continuing basis their animal facilities in regard to the care, use, and treatment of such animals, consistent with the standards established by "Experimental Animals" (Exhibit X1-43-1) and DHEW publication, "Guide for the Care and Use of Laboratory Animals," Fourth Edition. No DHEW grant or contract involving the use of animals will be awarded to an individual without affiliation with an institution which has accepted responsibility for administration of the funds awarded and has filed an assurance with DHEW.

The DHEW "principles" to be applied by grantee institutions require that the work be done under the immediate supervision of a scientist qualified in the scientific area under study. The housing, care, and feeding of all laboratory animals must be supervised by a properly qualified veterinarian or other scientist competent in such matters.

The Facilities

Standards for the construction and use of housing, service, and surgical facilities should be consistent with the recommendations in DHEW publication No. (NIH) 77-23, *Guide for the Care and Use of Laboratory Animals,* or as otherwise required by the U.S. Department of Agriculture's regulations established under the terms of the Animal Welfare Act.

The animal housing portions of older research buildings were often an "afterthought." Present requirements for housing animals are specific and more standardized; they are very much in keeping with requirements in other laboratory areas. There should be no exceptions to the basic environmental requirements of temperature control, ventilation, lighting, and space. The use of space can vary and so, to some degree, can materials.

The facility design of today is more centralized, in that animal housing is located in one building or on one floor, with the ancillary rooms for food preparation and storage, cage washing, and other special needs adjacent to it. The centralized concept permits space and personnel to be used more efficiently. Areas for surgery, radiography, treatment, and necropsy can be shared. Better environmental controls also enhance disease prevention and safety. These factors most often offset the time-distance relationship the researcher wished to optimize by having his office or laboratory next to the animal rooms.

In planning a facility, traffic and airflow should be considered. Rooms and corridors can be designed so that inlet doors lead from cleaner areas and outlet doors lead to corridors used for waste disposal and cage flow to the washing area. Airflow can be directed in a like fashion to aid in disease control and sanitation.

The standard rack size should somewhat determine the linear dimensions of the room, and the number of racks that can be efficiently placed in the rooms should be a criterion for size. However, excessively large rooms should be avoided, and if larger areas are needed, connecting inside doors between the walls should be considered. Generally, experiments require fewer animals than a room is designed to hold, and space is wasted if only large rooms are available. The use of portable soft-wall, enclosed, filtered rack systems can increase flexibility in space utilization. These units provide essentially separate clean air systems which permit multiple species to be housed and multiple experiments to be conducted in the same room.

The general layout of an animal room should be very simple. Unnecessary cabinets should not be present because sanitation cannot be maintained in rooms filled with excess equipment. Often a sink and wall-attached small table are all the fixtures needed. Moveable cans for transporting animal feed and racks and cages are all that should normally occupy floor space.

The larger the animal facility, the greater the need for ancillary rooms to accommodate special activities. Special laboratories or areas contiguous with the animal housing area are needed for such functions as surgery, intensive care, necropsy, radiography, special food preparation, diagnosis, and treatment of laboratory animals. Rooms are needed for storing racks, cages, bedding supplies, food, and equipment. Space for showers, sinks, lockers, and toilets must also be allocated. A rather large area is required for washing cages, and an area for an incinerator or waste removal system is needed.

Incinerators have been the popular means of waste disposal, but many individuals agree that they are fraught with problems. Upkeep, maintenance, and energy needs increase operation costs. Many incinerators are designed to burn waste which contains up to 50% water, but frequently the waste has a much higher water content. If so, there is the problem of driving off water before the material can be burned, which increases the chance of the incinerator's malfunctioning. We suggest storing and removing waste by the "dumpster" system, burning only the material considered unsafe for this type of disposal.

Standards for Caging

The Animal Welfare Act sets standard space requirements for animals held in cages. These standards are periodically reviewed, and the updated listing should be referred to before cages are purchased. Recent increases in floor space requirements made many cages formerly designed to hold large rabbits obsolete.

The two basic designs in caging available for small laboratory animals are the solid cage or "shoe box" design with an open grid top and the mesh-type open floor system. In the shoe-box type, the animal is placed on contact bedding; in the other type, waste material drops from the cage. There are many modifications of these basic designs. Mesh-type caging provides more ventilation, which is desirable, e.g., for rabbits held at higher ambient temperatures. The shoe-box type aids in isolation or disease containment, especially when used with air-filter covers.

Modern animal cages are usually constructed of plastic or metal. Plastic caging is often used for rats and mice and generally costs less than metal caging. However, the cheaper plastic cages are damaged by autoclaving and are not durable. Some types are very sturdy, but they are much more expensive. Plexiglas is really not a plastic material, but the sealant which binds the mat of glass fibers is an acrylic resin. Plexiglas can be used in caging for larger laboratory animals such as dogs and cats.

Metal cages are available in stainless steel, galvanized steel, and aluminum. Stainless steel is the most expensive. Cages made of the proper grade of stainless steel should be considered a long-term investment; they often last for an investigator's working life. Next to the high cost, the greatest disadvantage of purchasing stainless steel caging is the danger of its becoming obsolete. Caging made of galvanized steel, aluminum, or better plastics usually lasts 5 to 7 years. The choice depends upon the special needs of the research laboratory and the designs offered.

Standards for Care

The success of an efficient laboratory animal program rests on the quality of animal care provided. The American Association for Laboratory Animal Science (AALAS), which consists of a diverse group of persons interested in animal research, has promoted quality animal care. Besides providing scientific information concerning laboratory animals, AALAS emphasizes training and recognition of laboratory animal technicians whose performance is of a high quality.

The well-trained animal technician should be able to perform all of the duties involved in care, restraint, and observation applicable to a useful animal experiment. This technician should be aware of common diseases among laboratory animals, and if he sees signs of them in the animals for which he is responsible, he should call them to the veterinarian's attention. The technician's knowledge should enable him to care for many different animal species. He should be able to perform routine procedures (e.g., venipuncture) and to collect tissues at necropsy.

The mission of every facility in which laboratory animals are used must include the training of animal technicians. Assistance in defining the proper curriculum and teaching aids can be obtained through the executive office of AALAS (2317 W. Jefferson St., Joliet, Illinois 60435).

Selection of Animals

The species of animals to be used for disease diagnosis is usually determined by the knowledge of a predictable host response. Information concerning species responses to various disease agents is extensive. The responses can be modified by many factors including strain, sex, age, and environmental conditions. Special genetic stocks of mice and other species are becoming increasingly important as tools in infectious disease and oncology.

Other criteria used in selecting laboratory animals are their size, ease of handling and caging, and certain anatomical peculiarities (e.g., the large ear veins of New Zealand white rabbits make them ideal subjects for hyperimmunization experiments, which require frequent venipuncture).

The researcher needs to know the probable response of an animal to a specific etiologic agent, and he must also be aware of factors that may cause variations from the usual response, such as latent or clinically inapparent infections. For this reason, well-monitored colonies of pathogen-free animals are useful in disease diagnosis.

Breeding Laboratory Animals

Laboratory animal breeding should be maintained as a separate activity, remote from the research animal facility. The average research institution should purchase laboratory animals rather than breed its own. Cost factors and fluctuating needs for many different species make this more feasible. Commercial sources can periodically supply sufficient numbers of uniform animals better than a smaller, self-maintained colony.

The need for rigid isolation, which precludes shipping, or for certain animals not commercially available, may make it necessary to establish a breeding colony.

Some fundamental guidelines must be followed in developing a breeding facility for small rodents and rabbits:

a. The facility must provide proper environmental controls for the necessary species and must serve as an effective barrier against potential disease vectors, including arthropods and wild rodents.

b. Personnel who maintain the breeding colonies must not have contact with other laboratory animals, that is, at the research facility.

c. The animals obtained to start the colony must be from stock with good breeding performance and no known disease agents.

d. Once the colonies are established, no new animals must be allowed to enter them until their pathogen-free status has been established by rigid testing.

e. Visitors must be allowed to enter the facility only under special circumstances.

f. All persons must change to special clothing before entering the facility.

g. All feed, water, bedding, and caging must be sterilized by autoclaving before being put in the rooms in which pathogen-free mice or rats are bred.

h. The microbiological flora and serologic status of animals in the pathogen-free colony must be monitored with special tests at frequent intervals.

Diseases and Disease Control

Every laboratory animal species has some diseases peculiar to it and others which can be transmitted to other animals. Spontaneous intercurrent disease interferes with diagnosis, and the variables associated with it can lead to erroneous data and conclusions.

Viral agents are frequently found among laboratory animals which do not have symptoms of disease. The agent that causes lymphocytic choriomeningitis (LCM) in mice is a good example. Lymphocytic choriomeningitis is passed vertically from mother to young during pregnancy. Baby mice exposed in this way are immune to the virus, but they become lifelong carriers of the agents. When pathogen-free mice are exposed to these carriers, they may develop the disease and many may die from it.

Mouse hepatitis virus (MHV), a coronavirus, is notorious for causing an inapparent infection. Infant pathogen-free mice are often affected with lethal enteritis, whereas adults have hepatic necrosis or demyelinating lesions, depending on the strain of the virus and level of host susceptibility. Mice with immune defects, such as athymic strains, are especially vulnerable.

In addition to LCM and MHV viruses, at least 13 other murine viruses have been identified. These are: the virus that causes epidemic diarrhea in infant mice, Sendai virus, reovirus 3, pneumonia virus of mice, Kilham rat virus, murine encephalomyelitis virus, polyoma virus, ectromelia virus, adenovirus, K virus, minute virus of mice, lactic dehydrogenase-elevating virus, and rat coronaviruses. Many of these viruses do not produce significant overt disease, but they can interfere with finite virologic studies.

Inapparent virus infections apparently affect mice more than they do rats. A rat coronavirus known as sialodacryadenitis (SDA) virus is an interesting exception. Susceptible rats are affected with submandibular swelling and inflammation of lacrimal glands. A severe secondary keratitis with clinical symptoms often results, but the animals usually recover and become carriers. Pathogen-free rats brought into contact with these carriers will become affected, and the pathogen-free colony may be falsely incriminated. Results of serological tests performed 2–3 weeks after the clinical disease often reveal elevated antibody titers to coronavirus.

Control of murine virus disease depends on establishing or procuring pathogen-free stocks. Quality control procedures, including serologic monitoring, must be stringent to insure pathogen-free status. Filter-topped cages are very useful in preventing cross-infection during short-term holding periods.

Except for LCM and cytomegalovirus diseases, very little is known about viral disease in guinea pigs. Serologic evidence implicates groups of viruses similar to those in mice, but clinical disease and isolations have not been correlated. For that reason, no specific viral antigens are available for testing guinea pig sera. Cytomegalovirus infections have been observed in salivary gland tissues from clinically normal guinea pigs.

Viral diseases of consequence in the rabbit are at present limited to the pox and fibroma groups. Rabbit pox is a very rare disease associated with high mortality; it has been reported with and without cutaneous manifestations. The myxoma and fibroma viruses cause cutaneous and subcutaneous growth—most often among wild rabbits.

A great variety of viral diseases occur in nonhuman primates. Isolations of viral agents from tissue used in cell-culture procedures have accounted for the listing and serologic definition of dozens of cytopathogenic viral agents, but there is little evidence of related disease. Of greatest concern to laboratory personnel are those viruses which produce disease in humans. The most notable examples are hepatitis A, herpesvirus simiae (Herpes B), monkey pox, Yaba and Yaba-like virus, and Marburg disease virus. Some of these viruses cause serious diseases which are associated with significant mortality rates in both man and monkeys. Rubeola (measles) outbreaks are quite common in newly imported groups of rhesus monkeys. High mortality rates have been caused by outbreaks of simian hemorrhagic fever on several occasions. *Herpesvirus saimiri*, commonly found in the squirrel monkey, produces a fatal systemic disease in owl monkeys and marmosets. At the Center for Disease Control (CDC), we had an outbreak of an obscure neurologic disease, caused by SV16, which led to a high mortality rate in a colony of rhesus and African green monkeys.

To help avert disease problems, laboratory animal facility personnel should give special attention to species separation and long-term quarantine. They should wear masks to minimize exposure to aerosols, and they should wear protective clothing including gloves and gowns in primate-holding areas at all times. They should also take special precautions to avoid bites and scratches.

Personnel in research laboratories in which dogs and cats are used should be concerned about common viral agents which produce the most serious diseases in these species—namely, canine distemper and feline panleukopenia. Both of these diseases can be prevented by properly timed vaccination. Other viral diseases found among these animals include canine hepatitis, feline calicivirus disease, feline rhinotracheitis, feline infectious peritonitis, and feline leukemia. The reduction of rabies among dogs in the United States has minimized the danger that laboratory animal technicians will be exposed to this disease. In most laboratories, stray dogs are vaccinated against rabies, even though they may already have been exposed to the disease and may be incubating the virus. Under such conditions, vaccination would of course be ineffective in aborting the disease. If stray dogs are used in the laboratory, we strongly recommend that they be quarantined for several months. Individual caging and careful handling can help to avoid exposure to bites. If these recommendations are followed, little will be gained by immunizing dogs against rabies, because when dogs are caged individually they will not be exposed to rabies virus in the laboratory.

Bacterial diseases among laboratory animals are often occult infections which only become apparent after imposed stress. However, the organisms can often be cultured or their effects detected by histologic examination.

Few diseases have been as troublesome to research projects as respiratory disease caused by *Mycoplasma pulmonis*. The disease, which affects rats and mice, causes characteristic pathologic changes which can aid in its diagnosis. It is more chronic among rats, causing bronchiectasis and consolidation of lung parenchyma; these conditions lead to severe animal losses during long-term experiments. Low levels of environmental ammonia in rat cages encourage the development of the disease. In addition, pneumococci and *Corynebacterium kutscheri* can cause sporadic pneumonic disease.

Rabbits frequently have respiratory disease caused by *Pasturella multocida*. This disease, sometimes called "snuffles," is a major problem when rabbits from different stocks are housed together. Rabbits are often seen with conjunctivitis and/or nasal discharge, sneezing, and wet paws. Occasional deaths are caused by acute pneumonia or inflammation of body systems other than the respiratory system. Although *Bordetella* spp. occasionally cause diseases including pneumonia, they are not normally regarded as among the most offending organisms for most laboratory animal species.

The most serious diseases among guinea pigs are caused by *Streptococcus zooepidemicus*. A wide spectrum of diseases including pneumonia, otitis media, peritonitis, myocarditis, nephritis, and lymphadenitis may be seen. This organism causes abscessation of the cervical lymph nodes, a common disease in guinea pigs. Acute infections with *S. zooepidemicus* frequently lead to a mortality rate of over 50%.

Staphylococcal pyoderma is often seen among rats—especially males. The lesions usually originate from bites and scratches of animals held in crowded cages or from fights among breeding-age males caged together.

Salmonella spp. produce disease in all common laboratory species. Certain strains of mice appear to be particularly susceptible. Animals exposed to stressful conditions may have clinically apparent disease, but organisms can frequently be isolated from apparently healthy animals under normal conditions.

Shigellosis is a common serious disease of captive nonhuman primates. This diarrheal disease often causes high mortality among newly imported monkeys, and sporadic outbreaks continue to occur because many animals become carriers.

Mycobacterial infection, including tuberculosis, is still a serious problem in trapped and imported monkeys, especially during the initial quarantine period. The infection rate among newly imported Asian species routinely averages 1% to 2%. Devastating losses can result if all reactors are not removed immediately. We strongly recommend that new monkeys be quarantined for at least 3 months after their arrival at the laboratory facility and that they not be released from quarantine until results of at least three skin tests, obtained at 2-week intervals, are negative. After the monkeys have been released from quarantine, they and all other nonhuman primates should be skin-tested every 3 months. Animals with positive skin tests should be removed from the colony to prevent the possibility of further spread of infection.

Tyzzer's disease, cause by *Bacillis piliformis*, affects a wide variety of animals including rabbits and rodents. The disease, which was first described for mice, is best diagnosed histologically with special stains because the organism will not grow on artificial media. Focal necrotic lesions involving the liver, intestine, and sometimes the myocardium are characteristic of Tyzzer's disease.

Pseudomonas infections are occasionally observed—especially among such suppressed animals as mice in radiation experiments. Acidifiying the water supply reduces exposure to the organism.

Rabbit syphilis (*Treponema cuniculi*) can be a serious problem in breeding colonies.

Ringworm caused by *Microsporum canis* occurs quite frequently among dogs and cats. Young animals are more likely to develop typical lesions. Fungal infections of the hair and skin are also found among rats, mice, and guinea pigs, but lesions are rarely apparent. The investigator should be aware that animals can transmit ringworm to humans. Antifungal agents are effective, but in most cases they are a less practical means of control than removing infected animals from the colony.

Internal and external parasites are still commonly found among laboratory animals. Animals that have been derived by hysterotomy and maintained in a barrier facility are usually free of parasites. Mites are common ectoparasites of rodents. Pinworms are commonly found among mice, hamsters, and rats. The rodent tapeworm, *Hymenolepis nana*, is of special interest because it too has a direct life cycle and can infect man.

Rabbits can be infected with hepatic or intestinal coccidia. The organisms can produce marked epithelial changes in the intestine and bile ducts. However, if control measures are applied, the organisms can be eradicated from a colony. Rabbits from "good" sources should be free of coccidial infections. Recently, domestic cats have been identified as definitive hosts for *Toxoplasma gondii*, a coccidian organism which causes disease in a wide range of species including man. The oocysts, which are periodically shed in feces, represent a health hazard unless wastes are handled in a sanitary manner.

Diagnosing and controlling parasites should be a major concern in facilities housing dogs, cats, and monkeys. These species can be severely debilitated by helminths of many types. Diagnostic testing and vermifuge treatments must therefore be used routinely to control infections.

Postmortem Examinations

Necropsy procedures vary greatly, depending on the species and the thoroughness with which the disease is to be defined. Such essential information as history of previous disease, clinical signs, and epidemic features—including attack rates, morbidity, and mortality—should be recorded. Terminally ill animals which have been euthanized often provide the most useful information because of the lack of postmortem autolysis. Because small-rodent and rabbit tissues autolyze rapidly, these animals should be refrigerated immediately after they die. Ten percent buffered formalin is the best all-purpose fixative. Often, fixation in cold formalin (in the refrigerator) reduces postmortem changes.

Certain safety procedures should be followed during necropsy to avoid injury or the transmission of disease. The carcass should be moistened with disinfectant solution and placed in a pan or on an absorbent pad (such as a bed pad). In certain situations (e.g., when the animal died of tuberculosis), the dissecting should be done in a biological safety cabinet. The dissector should wear disposable gloves, safety glasses, a mask, and a laboratory coat or surgical gown. Although scalpels are more efficient, if etiologic agents or animals (such as nonhuman primates) which pose high risks are involved, blunt-pointed scissors are safer. After the instruments have been used, they should be immersed and stored in a noncorrosive disinfectant solution. When the necropsy is completed, the carcass should be wrapped up, placed in a closed container such as a plastic bag, and incinerated. All sharp objects such as needles and scalpel blades should be placed in special containers so that personnel who handle the refuse will not be injured.

Sources of Animals

High-quality research animals are becoming more readily available. The most comprehensive list of suppliers appears in the publication *Animals for*

Research (Institute of Laboratory Animal Resources, National Research Council, Washington, DC). It can be obtained from the Printing and Publishing Office, National Academy of Sciences, 2101 Constitution Avenue, Washington, DC 20418.

General References

AMERICAN SOCIETY FOR LABORATORY ANIMAL SCIENCE: Manual for Laboratory Animal Technicians. AALAS Publ 67-3, Joliet, Ill, 1970, p 216

AMERICAN SOCIETY FOR LABORATORY ANIMAL SCIENCE: Syllabus for the Laboratory Animal Technologist. AALAS Publ 72-2, Joliet, Ill, 1972, p 462

BARNES CD and ELTHERINGTON LG: Drug Dosage in Laboratory Animals: A Handbook. Univ of California Press, Berkeley, 1966, p 302

BEALL JR, TORNING FE, and RUNKLE RS: A laminar flow system for animal maintenance. Lab Anim Sci 21:206-212, 1971

BRICK JO, NEWELL RF, and DOHERTY DG: A barrier system for a breeding and experimental rodent colony. Lab Anim Care 19:92-97, 1969

BRODERSON JR, LINDSEY JR, and CRAWFORD JE: The role of environmental ammonia in respiratory mycoplasmosis of rats. Am J Pathol 85:115-130, 1976

BRODERSON JR, MURPHY FA, and HIERHOLZER JC: Lethal enteritis in infant mice caused by mouse hepatitis virus. Lab Anim Sci 26 (No. 5): p 824, 1976

CASS JS (ed.): Laboratory Animals: An Annotated Bibliography of Informational Resources. Hafner Publishing Co., New York, 1971, p 316

CHRISTIE RJ ET AL: Techniques used in the establishment and maintenance of a barrier mouse breeding colony. Lab Anim Care 18:544-549, 1968

COMMITTEE ON LABORATORY ANIMAL DISEASE: A Guide to Infectious Diseases of Mice and Rats. Institute of Lab Animal Resources, NAS-NRC, Washington, DC, 1971, p 41

COOK MJ: The Anatomy of the Laboratory Mouse. Academic Press, New York, 1965, p 143

COTCHIN E and ROE FJC (eds.): Pathology of Laboratory Rats and Mice. FA Davis Co, Philadelphia, 1967, p 848

FIENNES R: Zoonoses of Primates. Weidenfeld & Nicholson, London, 1967, p 190

FLYNN RJ: The diagnosis of Pseudomonas aeruginosa infection in mice. Lab Anim Care 13:126-129, 1963

GREEN EL (ed.): Biology of the Laboratory Mouse, 2nd edition. McGraw-Hill Book Co, New York, 1966, p 706

HOFFMAN RA, ROBINSON PF, and MAGALHAES H (eds.): The Golden Hamster: Its Biology and Use in Medical Research. Iowa State Univ Press, 1968, p 545

HULL TG (ed.): Diseases Transmitted from Animals to Man, 5th edition. Charles C Thomas, Springfield, Ill, 1965, p 967

KAUFMANN AF, GARY GW, BRODERSON JR, PERL DP, QUIST KD, and KISSLING RE: Simian virus 16 associated with an epizootic of obscure neurologic disease. Lab Anim Sci 23:812-818, 1973

KRAFT LM: Observations on the control and natural history of epidemic diarrhea of infant mice (EDIM). Yale J Biol Med 31:121-137, 1958

McDOUGALL PR ET AL: Control of Pseudomonas aeruginosa in an experimental mouse colony. Lab Anim Care 17:204-214, 1967

McPHERSON CW: Reduction of *Pseudomonas aeruginosa* bacteria in mouse drinking water following treatment with hydrochloric acid or chlorine. Lab Anim Care 13:737-744, 1963

MELBY EC and ALTMAN NH: Handbook of Laboratory Animal Science. CRC Press, Cleveland, Ohio, 1976, Vol I, p 451: Vol II, p 523; Vol III, p 943

NAPIER JR and NAPIER PH: A Handbook of Living Primates. Academic Press, New York, 1967, p 456

RUCH TC: Diseases of Laboratory Primates. WB Saunders Co, Philadelphia, 1959, p 600

SIMMONS ML and BRICK JO: The Laboratory Mouse, Selection and Management. Prentice-Hall, Englewood Cliffs, NJ, 1970

WAGNER JE and MANNING PJ (eds.): The Biology of the Guinea Pig. Academic Press Inc, New York, 1976, p 317

WEISHBROTH SH, FLATT RE, and KRAUS AL (eds.): The Biology of the Laboratory Rabbit. Academic Press Inc, New York and London, 1974, p 496

CHAPTER 11

THE EPIDEMIOLOGY AND CONTROL OF NOSOCOMIAL AND OPPORTUNISTIC INFECTIONS

Henry D. Isenberg and J. Kelly Smith

Introduction

The various authoritative texts on epidemiology and the control of infections (2, 3, 4, 7, 26, 48) deemphasize the role played by the microbiology services of health care facilities or Governmental agencies. However, it seeems reasonable that success in defining and controlling all epidemics ultimately depends on laboratory results. The complex interactions of all the contributing factors must be determined by health officials, epidemiologists, statisticians, and administrators. In this chapter, we describe how microbiologists can, should, and do contribute to increasing the efficiency and pertinence of their colleagues' efforts and to placing the contributions and conclusions of the specialists on a sound scientific foundation.

For the purpose of this discussion, certain terms must be defined. *Infection* is the overt clinical manifestation of disease resulting from the invasion or excessive presence of microorganisms in or on a given individual; *colonization* is the concentration of microorganisms in various body sites at levels which do not extend beyond or damage mucocutaneous host barriers. *Virulence* is the unique property of a microbial strain which allows it to produce disease in most normal, nonimmune hosts. *Pathogenicity* describes the capability of an admittedly artificially designated species to be involved in disease production in any host. The *normal host resistance* to infection is the capacity of an individual to protect himself against invasion with specific and nonspecific immunological and cellular factors, physical barriers, and mechanical disposal mechanisms. *Microbial resistance* is the ability of a microorganism to survive host resistance, the host's resident microbiota, and/or the action of pharmacological agents administered to the host. The *compromised host* is one whose resistance has been impaired to an extent that even a so-called "nonvirulent" organism can make him ill. The *host-parasite equilibrium* is a complex balance between host resistance factors and the admittedly ill-defined pathogenic propensities of microorganisms. It must be noted on an empirical basis that alteration of host-resistance factors plays the major role in determining infection. *Nosocomial infection* is any infection acquired during hospitalization, even if symptoms become apparent after the patient is discharged. Since the hospitalized patient's resistance is more profoundly impaired by disease and/or treatment, and he is more likely to be exposed to antibiotic-resistant microorganisms in a hospital than elsewhere, nosocomial infection is often actually opportunistic and frequently caused by newly established microorganisms in the hospital environment. *Control* is not only preventing person-to-person transmission of infection but also minimizing the level of infection acquired by immunosuppressed individuals. Successful infection control requires full recognition of the numerous factors in the host-parasite equation. They must (a) preclude the introduction of new, potentially dangerous organisms into the hospital and the community, (b) preclude the colonization of host surfaces by potential pathogens, (c) minimize selective pressures which enhance the overgrowth and/or the resistance of microorganisms, and (d), most importantly, minimize therapy which compromises host resistance.

In the following sections, we present a review of the general principles of infection control and then discuss situations which encourage nosocomial and opportunistic infections. Finally, we offer suggestions for laboratory-based recognition and control.

Infection Control—General Principles

The importance of infection control in the hospital is illustrated by the increasing emphasis placed on nosocomial infections by, e.g., the Joint Commission on Hospital Accreditation and the Center for Disease Control. A program centers around the infection control committee, which is chaired by an expert on infectious disease or epidemiology and includes representatives from medical, paramedical, laboratory, administrative, and purely maintenance services of the hospitals. This group normally serves as an arm of the medical board of the hospital, which in turn can implement regulations passed by the infection control committee. The infection control committee should write and distribute an infection control manual and should meet monthly to record trends in nosocomial infection and to update the manual's policies. In order to set and effect its policies, the committee should include at least one epidemiologist and should maintain active lines of communication with local, state, and Federal public health officials. The ultimate goal of this coordinated effort is to prevent significant disturbances in the host-parasite equilibrium which may result in nosocomial infections.

The first priority in infection control is preventing the introduction of pathogenic, potentially pathogenic, or highly resistant organisms into the hospital. Traditionally, the concern of hospital and public health officials has centered around highly virulent microorganisms that have been associated with community or hospital epidemics or outbreaks and has led to the general practice of strictly isolating patients with proven or suspected anthrax, diphtheria, plague, rabies, smallpox, etc. Patients infected with organisms which are highly contagious if not highly virulent (e.g., *Salmonella*) should also be isolated. Although this practice is a valuable precaution, personnel involved in infection control must recognize that these traditional organisms no longer comprise the greatest threat to the hospitalized patients, largely because of the very effective community control applied over the last four to five decades. Of equal or greater concern today is the failure to recognize organisms which are frequently involved in opportunistic infection and which at the same time may be highly resistant to antibiotics. These include many members of the family

Enterobacteriaceae, the pseudomonads and related gram-negative rods, and, less commonly, resistant staphylococci, various streptococci, neisseriae, and potentially resistant pneumococci. These organisms are often introduced by patients newly admitted to hospitals or nursing homes. Many of these patients have been treated previously with various drugs including antibiotics and have severe underlying disease. Because of the severity of their illnesses, they are often admitted directly to intensive care units containing comparably ill people who are thus at higher risk of infection.

Nurses and physicians who work in admitting areas must be informed about the types of microorganisms which threaten the hospital population. One source of such information is the Center for Disease Control's *Morbidity and Mortality Weekly Report,* which documents local, state, and nationwide trends of infection. They also need information concerning the prevalence and resistance patterns of nosocomial infections and their causes in other area hospitals and nursing homes from which their patients are admitted. It is advisable that patients transferred from other hospitals or from nursing homes be strictly isolated outside intensive care units until their status is evaluated.

The microbiologist and his or her laboratory personnel must also be fully aware of community, state, and nationwide trends of infection. They should immediately communicate with attending physicians and appropriate infection control committee members when a high-risk organism is isolated from inpatients or newly admitted patients. Resistant *Serratia marcescens, Proteus* spp., pseudomonads, etc., should be reported to the physician immediately. Further, it must be appreciated that, besides patients, personnel, visitors, and inanimate or nonhuman animate objects in the hospital can carry infectious organisms (e.g., flowers can carry water and soil bacteria including pseudomonads and the *Serratia* spp.). Because plumbing and water are always potential means of introducing pseudomonads into the hospital, all water sources (particularly sink drains) should be cultured frequently and disinfected as needed.

Although preventing the introduction of infectious organisms into the hospital is doubtlessly the most effective means of controlling nosocomial infections, the second is clearly preventing patients and personnel from being colonized by potentially pathogenic organisms. A major source of contamination with *Enterobacteriaceae* or pseudomonads is the hand contact between hospital personnel and patients. Hands can infect patients (particularly in intensive care or recovery units) directly or through intermediary vectors such as medications, soaps, inhalation equipment, food, shaving equipment, etc., because secretions, excretions, and blood products often contaminate the environment. Since most of the high-risk organisms spread in this fashion are transient skin microbiota, it is possible to eliminate the threat of spread by practicing appropriate handwashing techniques in clean, well-designed facilities. Hands should be washed before and after each contact with each patient (18).

Air currents can also spread infection in the hospital, e.g., those caused by common airborne molds such as the aspergilli and zygomycetes. These fungi can be highly invasive in compromised patients and account for a significant percentage of the deaths caused by infection in hospitalized, immunosuppressed patients. Reliable studies indicate that the risk of these airborne mold infections can be minimized when filtered, mechanically ventilated, non-recirculating air systems are used and when soil and plants which may carry these molds are not allowed in the environment.

Successful infection control must also prevent overgrowth by antibiotic-resistant microorganisms and the development of resistance by micro-organisms. The excessive or otherwise inappropriate use of antibiotics in the community and in the hospital environment is the major cause of this problem (19). Again, the microbiology laboratory must be responsible for documenting and making known antibiotic resistance patterns of microorganisms in the hospital and community. Yearly or twice-yearly reports should be published and distributed to physicians and local public health officials. Unusual resistance patterns should be immediately reported to hospital, community, state, and Federal public health officials. Resistance patterns in the hospital can be correlated with pharmacy records of the use of individual antibiotics. This information serves not only as a guide to treatment and isolation but provides criteria for the institutional control of antibiotic usage. Such committees must recognize the enormous risk of promoting resistance associated with the physical dissemination of antibiotics into the hospital environment.

Finally, efforts must be made to minimize treatments which impair host resistance. The form of manipulation which accounts for most nosocomial infections today is the use of catheters—particularly urinary catheters. In a recent survey of community hospitals by the Center for Disease Control, Atlanta, Georgia, approximately 40% of all nosocomial infections were urinary tract infections, 80% of which were related to urinary tract manipulation (12). Other catheters which are potential sources of infection include indwelling intravenous catheters and peritoneal catheters. Aerosolized bacteria can bypass normal respiratory defense mechanisms and introduce infection into normal or compromised persons. In this circumstance, the infection is generally caused by a gram-negative organism which can survive in water (particularly pseudomonads). In surgery, the skin is opened, giving microorganisms access to deeper tissues. Various immunosuppressive drugs and treatments clearly affect host immune mechanisms enough to leave patients susceptible to infection. When such treatments as the above are necessary, they must be administered carefully and with the threat of environmental microorganisms minimized by various isolation, handwashing, sterilization, housekeeping, and ventilation procedures or systems rather than relying routinely on antibiotic prophylaxis.

Populations at Risk

Opportunistic infections in hospital patients can be categorized as (a) infection occurring in patients whose immunity is impaired by underlying disease or (b) infection occurring in patients whose defense mechanisms are compromised as a result of treatment. Regardless of the manner in which injury is inflicted to the immune system, several types of immune system reactions may be affected. These are shown in Table 11.1, which involves category (a), but they apply to all subsequent discussions of opportunistic infection regardless of the patient category. Disease or treatment may impair the inflammatory re-

TABLE 11.1—INFECTION IN IMMUNODEFICIENT PATIENTS

IMMUNE DEFECT	LIKELY SITE OF INFECTION	LIKELY PATHOGENS	CLINICAL EXAMPLES
Impaired Antibody	Sinuses, middle ear, lung, skin, urine, blood, CNS	*S. pneumoniae, H. influenzae,* Group A streptococci, *S. aureus. Enterobacteriaceae* and pseudomonads (less likely)	Congenital syndromes (Bruton's and Gitlin's agammaglobulinemia), severe combined immunodeficiency (SCID), common variable hypogammaglobulinemia, malignancies (myeloma, chronic lymphatic leukemia)
	Small bowel	*Giardia lamblia*	
Deficient Cell-Mediated Immunity (T lymphocyte, Macrophage Deficiencies)	Skin, mucous membranes, lung, reticuloendothelial system	Intracellular parasites. Viruses (particularly pox and herpes group), fungi (particularly *Candida*), mycobacteria, salmonellae, brucellae, *Listeria monocytogenes, Pneumocystis carinii*	Congenital syndromes, (DiGeorge Nezeloff, Wiskoff-Aldrich, ataxia telangiectasia), chronic mucocutaneous candidiasis, Hodgkin's disease, sarcoidosis, carcinomatosis, chronic renal insufficiency, immunosuppressive therapy
Defective Neutrophil Function			
Defective Intracellular Killing	Skin, lymph nodes, bone, liver, spleen	Catalase-positive bacteria (particularly *Staphylococcus aureus*), *Candida*	Chronic granulomatous disease of childhood, Job's syndrome
Neutropenia	Blood (50%), lungs (25%), mucous membranes and skin	Bacteria, particularly gram-negative (*Enterobacteriaceae,* pseudomonads, and other gram-negative rods), fungi (particularly *Candida*), *Aspergillus,* zygomycetes	Hematological malignancies, particularly leukemia and lymphoma, aplastic anemia, drug toxicities
Deficient Opsonization and Chemotaxis	Skin and mucous membranes	Variable. Frequently *S. aureus* or streptococci	C_1, C_2, C_5 deficiencies, C_3 hypercatabolism
Physical Injury to Mucocutaneous Barrier	Skin, mucous membranes, blood	Environmental microbiota	Third degree burns, exfoliative dermatitis, Stevens-Johnson syndrome

sponse, antibody production, cell-mediated immunity, phagocytosis, opsonization, and cause injury to physical barriers and to physical disposal mechanisms.

This and subsequent tables and discussions are offered as general guides primarily to hospital laboratory personnel who must consider the sources of their specimens and the underlying disease in order to recognize the significance of an organism isolated from a patient. In turn, an understanding of the nature of the immunological deficits of a patient has great predictive value in determining the nature of likely sites of infection and the most prevalent or commonly involved microorganisms. A brief explanation of each of the major immunological compartments follows (9).

The initial response of a nonimmune normal host to an infecting microorganism is characterized by the activation and mobilization of cellular and soluble mediators of inflammation. In the inflammatory response, stimulated leukocytes secrete vasoactive amines (histamine, serotonin), the slowly reactive substance of anaphylaxis (SRS-A), and lysosomal enzymes (cathepsins E and D, basic proteins 1–4, permeability factor, mastocytolytic factor, and proteases) into the environment. Similarly, platelet aggregation may cause them to secrete vasoactive amines and permeability factors and activate the coagulation cascade. Vasoactive amines, SRS-A, and permeability factors enhance the inflammatory response by causing dilation and altered permeability of capillaries and further transudation or exudation of blood products into the area. The reaction may be further increased by the release of large amounts of vasoactive amines from mast cells ruptured by leukocyte mastocytolytic factor. Secreted leukocyte lysosomal proteases can hydrolyze various substrates including the third (C_3) and fifth (C_5) components of complement and kinin. Enzymatic cleavage of C_3 and C_5 causes the release of C_{3a} and C_{5a}, both of which can cause further histamine release (anaphylatoxins), initiate leukotaxis (C_{3a}, $C_{5,6,7}$), and activate the remaining complement cascade. Bacterial endotoxin may also cause the generation of C_3 and C_5 proteases by activating the properdin system (alternate pathway of complement activation). Other biological activities of activated complement include opsonization (immune adherence, C_{3b}) and cell lysis (C_8, C_9). Activation of kinin by leukocyte kininogenases causes the production of vasoactive and pain-producing peptides and permeability globulins which further enhance the inflammatory response. Additionally, some leukocyte enzymes are leukotactic (cathepsin D). Activated Hageman factor (clotting factor XII) may further contribute to the inflammatory process by activating the clotting cascade (intrinsic pathway), the complement system (plasmin activates C_1), and the kinin system (prokallekrein activation).

The inflammatory response is modulated by cyclic nucleotides, cyclic adenosine monophosphate (cAMP), and cyclic guanosine monophosphate (cGMP). Increases in cellular cAMP inhibit inflammation by causing a reduced secretion of soluble mediators. The reverse is true for cGMP. Agents which increase cAMP include histamine, prostaglandin E_1, and beta-adrenergic agents. Prostaglandin F_{2a} and cholinergic agents enhance inflammation by increasing cGMP (47).

The net result of the inflammatory response is an effective but rather indiscriminate destruction of both host and microbial tissues. The ability of the microorganism to survive this and subsequent onslaughts is related to microbial defenses (impedins) which destroy, neutralize, or physically block these host factors and to the inoculum size and the speed and vigor of the host response. The latter is adversely affected by a variety of anti-inflammatory agents (e.g., glucocorticoids, salicylates, indomethicin) and disease processes (Table 11.1) which diminish the quality or quantity of responses of any one of the aforementioned mediators of inflammation.

Should the host and microorganisms survive the initial inflammatory response, specific, or lymphocyte-mediated, immune processes become effectively mobilized in the normal nonimmune host within a week, generally peaking in efficacy 2 to 4 weeks after antigen exposure occurs. In contrast to the primary inflammatory response, the forces of lymphocyte-mediated inflammation are more forcibly and specifically directed against invading microorganisms and other immunologically recognizable materials. There are two major lymphocyte populations in this system—the B and T lymphocytes (8, 14). B lymphocytes best recognize haptenic portions of antigens and are ultimately responsible for the production of immunoglobulins and antibody. T lymphocytes recognize most effectively the carrier portion of antigens and are responsible for initiating the processes of cell-mediated immunity, for regulating the activities of other B and T lymphocytes, and for serving as a repository of immunological memory (the anamnestic response). In turn, T-lymphocyte function is regulated largely through the immune-response, immune-suppressor, and cell-interaction gene loci on chromosome 6 in man. These immune-regulatory genes are located within the major histocompatibility complex. A more detailed explanation of the development and function of lymphocytes is necessary if disorders of specific immunity are to be understood fully.

Immature B cells develop in the bone marrow and undergo a series of cytodifferentiation steps which enable them to produce antibodies and five classes of immunoglobulins. Maturation into an effective IgG, IgA, IgD, IgM, or IgE antibody-producing plasma cell requires the assistance of T-cell subpopulations (referred to as T-helper lymphocytes) and the presence of recognizable antigen. Without T-cell assistance, IgM antibody production can occur but is relatively feeble. B cells normally comprise 20%–25% of peripheral blood lymphocytes and heavily populate the germinal centers of lymph nodes. They have surface receptors capable of binding C_{3b} and the Fc fragment of IgG. They affect immunity only by their production of antibody. In turn, antibody may neutralize certain toxins and viruses, but it affects most microorganisms primarily through fixation and activation of complement (IgG or IgM by the classic pathway; IgA or IgE by the alternate pathway) or by directly enhancing phagocytosis (opsonization) and by "arming" killer lymphocytes.

B-cell deficiencies account for approximately 60% of primary immune-deficiency states. These are often inherited disorders in which B cells either do not develop from the bone marrow stem cells and are therefore absent in the blood and lymph nodes (e.g., Bruton's or sex-linked agammaglobulinemia) or where B cells exist, but their cytodifferentiation of function is arrested, in many cases by suppressor T-cell populations (common variable hypogammaglobulinemia). Acquired disorders of B-cell function in which antibody production is impaired are not uncommon and include multiple myeloma, Waldenstrom's macroglobulinemia, and chronic lymphatic leukemia. Prolonged treatment with certain immunosuppressive drugs can also impair B-cell function. Whatever the cause, impaired antibody production increases host susceptibility to infection, particularly with encapsulated pyogenic bacteria such as *Streptococcus pneumoniae, Haemophilus influenzae, Streptococcus pyogenes,* and *Staphylococcus aureus,* as well as the protozoon *Giardia lamblia.* However, more and more of these infections are caused by members of the family *Enterobacteriaceae,* pseudomonads, and other gram-negative rods in various B-cell deficiency disorders. The usual sites of bacterial infection are the sinuses, middle ear, mastoids, lungs, and skin, and occasionally the blood, central nervous system, and urinary tract. *Giardia lamblia,* of course, infects the small bowel. Patients with primary B-cell deficiencies are more apt to develop cancers, "autoimmune" diseases, and various forms of enterocolitis (13, 16, 21, 40).

T lymphocytes develop in the bone marrow and migrate to the thymus as a functionally immature but antigenically distinct population of cells called prothymocytes. Cytodifferentiation to thymocytes normally occurs in the thymus by action of thymopoietin. Further differentiation of T lymphocytes, first to antigen-reactive cells and then to T-helper, suppressor, or killer lymphocytes, probably takes place in the blood and pericortical areas of lymph nodes. As mentioned, cytodifferentiation of T-cell subpopulations appears to be regulated by chromosome 6 in man. In mice, T-cell subpopulations can be recognized by the presence of specific cell-wall antigens. Human T cells have receptors for sheep erythrocytes which will form rosettes around T lymphocytes *in vitro.* T cells normally comprise 70%–80% of blood lymphocytes. T-suppressor lymphocytes may suppress both B-cell and T-cell function. In addition, T lymphocytes are responsible for initiating inflammatory mediators involved in cell-mediated immunity. Cell-mediated immunity accounts for a number of well-defined immune reactions including delayed cutaneous hypersensitivity, homograft rejection, and graft vs. host reactions, and is essential for the eradication of intracellular microbial infections. T-killer cells can attack and kill target cells directly. Other T lymphocytes may release soluble mediators referred to as lymphokines, some of which are chemotactic for monocytes and can activate blood monocytes and tissue macrophages to a high level of phagocytic and digestive activity. Monocytes and macrophages are the major effector cells in cell-mediated immunity, comprising up to 80% of the cell population in delayed cutaneous hypersensitivity reactions. Other lymphokines increase capillary permeability, have cytotoxic properties, or are capable of stimulating proliferation of lymphocyte populations. Other cells, including monocytes, may release some of these mediators. It is clear that deficiencies in cell-mediated immunity can occur as a consequence of the absence or malfunctioning of T-cell or monocyte populations (1, 4, 27, 30, 40).

Most protista which invade persons with impaired, cell-mediated immunity are those classically considered to be capable of intracellular persistence. These include a variety of fungi (particularly *Candida* spp.), viruses (particularly the herpes and pox group viruses), mycobacteria, salmonellae, brucellae, neisseriae, *Listeria monocytogenes,* and *Pneumocystis carinii.* Primary deficiencies in T cells are often related to a failure of normal thymic development (DiGeorge's syndrome) or lack of bone marrow stem-cell differentiation (severe combined immunodeficiency). T cells may also be adversely affected by acquired diseases such as sarcoidosis, chronic renal failure, carcinomatosis, some hematological malignancies, and by immunosuppressive treatment. Primary monocyte deficiencies probably exist but are rarely documented. Monocyte function may be impaired in the Wiskoff-Aldrich syndrome and chronic mucocutaneous candidiasis and is clearly abrogated by glucocorticoids (30).

A number of deficiencies may occur in cellular and soluble mediators of inflammation which can adversely affect the primary inflammatory responses and lymphocyte-mediated immunity. Perhaps the most striking is defective polymorphonuclear functioning, which, depending on the precise nature of the defect, may predispose to bacterial and fungal infections involving the blood stream and lung, the reticuloendothelial system, or the mucocutaneous barrier. Primary inherent deficiencies in neutrophil function are rare. The most dramatic of these includes the incapacity of neutrophil populations to kill some or all of the ingested microorganisms. Such defects may result in recalcitrant skin, bone, and reticuloendothelial infections, often with catalase-positive bacteria (particularly *Staphylococcus aureus*) and occasionally with fungi (particularly *Candida*). Clinical examples include chronic granulomatous diseases of childhood and Job's syndrome. Deficient function may result from quantitative deficiencies in neutrophils, particularly when total circulating neutrophil counts drop below 1000 cells per mm^3. In these circumstances, sepsis is apt to occur as a consequence of invasion of mucocutaneous barriers by members of the family *Enterobacteriaceae,* the pseudomonads, and related gram-negative organisms, or (in patients given prolonged broad-spectrum antibiotic therapy) by fungi (particularly *Candida, Aspergillus,* and zygomycetes). Diseases which predispose to significant neutropenia include hematological malignancies, particularly leukemias and lymphomas, and aplastic anemia. Eighty percent of fevers occurring in neutropenic leukemic patients are eventually shown to reflect the presence of infection. Stated differently, hospitalized patients with neutrophil counts of 500 cells/mm^3 can anticipate spending 30% of their time being treated for infection; those with neutrophil counts of 100 cells/mm^3 or less can spend 60% of their hospitalization being treated for infection. In one review (10), 70% of infections occurring in severely neutropenic persons were bacterial (70% of which were caused by gram-negative organisms, particularly pseudomonads); 20% were caused by fungi; 50% involved the blood stream; and 25% the lung. Neutrophil function may also be impaired by the absence of appropriate serum opsonins or defective leukotaxis of neutrophils in an area of active infection. The major serum opsonins include antibodies directed specifically against the invading microorganisms and serum complement. Hence, B-cell deficiencies may cause defective opsonization and impaired neutrophil function. The hydrolysis of C_3 into C_{3b} is the most critical feature in opsonization of microorganisms. Therefore, complement may opsonize organisms whether activated by the classic or alternate pathways. Deficiencies in the complement system caused by excessive consumption of complement or by inherited defects in one or more of the complement components may predispose to recurrent bacterial infection involving, in particular, the mucocutaneous barriers and, to a lesser extent, the reticuloendothelial system. Examples include staphylococcal infection and the occurrence of toxic epidermal necrolysis in C_5 deficiencies and, sometimes, in C_2 deficiency states. Additionally, deficient functioning of the complement system may result in impaired chemotaxis of neutrophils. Clinically apparent deficiencies similar to those described in the neutrophil system may occur in the monocyte and macrophage systems. Monocyte and macrophage deficiencies, in addition to potentially influencing the capacity of B- and T-cell populations to respond to specific antigens, also predispose to the persistence of intracellular microorganisms similar to those listed under infectious complications of persons with defective cell-mediated immunity.

Any extensive injury to the mucocutaneous barrier (the skin and the mucous membranes) predisposes to an invasion with environmental microbiota, particularly gram-positive organisms and representatives of the family *Enterobacteriaceae,* pseudomonads and related organisms, and *Candida, Aspergillus,* and zygomycetes. Clinical examples include third-degree burns and severe dermatoses such as Steven-Johnson syndrome and exfoliative dermatitis. Injuries which provide an appropriate reduction in the redox potential also render persons susceptible to invasion by anaerobic organisms.

It seems redundant to state that patients with the diagnoses discussed above should be protected with a type of reverse isolation which insures the least possible exposure to additional colonization by microorganisms found in hospital environments. However, in many instances these infections involve endogenous organisms, which patients may have acquired or harbored before entering the hospital.

Table 11.2 lists the treatments most often involved in infectious complications in the medical facility. It is intended to be only a guide for the laboratory in determining the most common types of microorganisms likely to be found in specimens from patients who have these treatments. Not all infections accompanying such therapy may be clinically apparent. Obviously, it is both the effect of treatment on the host's defense mechanisms and the care exercised to exclude chance microbiota which determine the likelihood of infection. However, our general lack of knowledge concerning the many aspects of infection does not allow the laboratory scientist and the clinician to predict with certainty which of these patients will develop a significant infection (38). The only means of preventing infection in such individuals remains the very careful observation of all of the rules and regulations governing patient treatment and the recognition that an unknown segment of the patient population being treated precisely in the same manner will still manifest with infectious complications. Table 11.2 lists the various manipulations, procedures, or treatments in broad categories. Thus, foreign bodies include a variety of materials which bridge or traverse the mucocutaneous barriers. Of course, the most important of these is the catheter, regardless of the anatomic site in which it is used. In addition, aerosols and tracheostomies are potentially dangerous for precisely the same reason. Another major category includes implants or prostheses. These materials, which serve in areas usually considered sterile or only temporarily contaminated by passing microbial forms, set up a series of as-yet unexplained reactions. Undoubtedly, the nonbiological composition of prostheses prevents their active participation in a defensive fashion. There is also the suggestion that the physical presence of an anatomic abnormality in the form of an implant may allow microbial particles in the blood stream or tissues to find a favorable site for attachment and proliferation.

It may be stretching the category to include surgical procedures as foreign body manipulations. However, surgery, in addition to physically disrupting the cutaneous barriers, usually is accompanied by the use of suture or staple materials which encourage direct colonization by microbiota or sequester microorganisms from the circulation. The environment created by surgery is an excellent nutrient which encourages proliferation of various protista and may cause clinically apparent illness. In addition, surgical procedures are abetted in their host defense embarrassment by the need to apply anesthesia to most of the patients involved. Anesthesia alone can introduce foreign particles into the respiratory tract or circulation, and it may impair host defenses at a time when a large number of challenges are presented to the individual. This contributory factor of anesthesia must be considered—especially if the surgery is prolonged. Postoperative wound infections are most often caused by contamination during surgery. Epidemiological surveillance of hospital patients indicates that occasionally surgical procedures are complicated with microbiota neither introduced into the site at the time of surgery nor part of the endogenous microbiota. The mechanisms of such transmission are poorly understood. Obviously, improper wound handling and care must be questioned, and the need pointed out by Dineen for meticulous patient care outside as well as within the operating room must be emphasized (11).

The second major category of treatments which may cause nosocomial disease includes various immunosuppressive therapies which affect the cellular and humoral host defenses. Certainly, the glucocorticoids impair the inflammatory response and cellular immunity. Cytotoxic agents and radiation therapy diminish or abolish temporarily antibody synthesis as well as phagocytosis. Another category often ignored is splenectomy, which, although a surgical procedure, leads to diminished serum opsonization and an impairment of antibody response to circulating antigens.

Finally, the widespread use of antimicrobial chemotherapy for patients challenged by various other manipulations has profound effects on the patients and on the entire institutional environment. Antibiotics can disrupt the normal host-parasite relationships and allow minority groups of organisms to proliferate as long as they can tolerate the chemotherapeutic agents used. Such agents lead to the replacement of the host's protista by institutional microbiota, which are frequently multiply antibiotic resistant. (Only the most resistant microorganisms survive in medical facilities.) Since antimicrobial therapy kills many members of the patient's normal flora, hospital-acclimated organisms can colonize easily. The reaction of the host to such foreign organisms involves antibody production and the activation of nonspecific defense mechanisms. Since disease frequently impairs such responses, or concomitant treatment may interfere with a normal response, antibiotic-resistant microorganisms present in hospitals are almost sure to complicate a patient's recovery (17, 19).

Table 11.2 also contains some guides to the likely sites of infection associ-

TABLE 11.2—PATIENTS AT RISK DUE TO TREATMENT

MANIPULATION	DEFECT[1] CAUSED BY TREATMENT	LIKELY SITE OF INFECTION	LIKELY MICROORGANISM(S)
FOREIGN BODIES			
Catheters			
Urine	Physically traverses mucocutaneous barriers	Urinary tract	Representative of *Enterobacteriaceae, Pseudomonas,* and other gram-negative rods,[2] enterococci, yeasts
Intravenous	Physically traverses mucocutaneous barriers	Circulation	*Staphylococcus* spp., *Enterobacteriaceae, Pseudomonas,* and other gram-negative rods, yeasts
Peritoneal	Physically traverses barriers	Peritoneum	*Staphylococcus aureus*
Aerosol	Physically traverses mucocutaneous barriers	Respiratory tract, especially lungs	*Pseudomonas* and other gram-negative rods, *Enterobacteriaceae,* especially *Klebsiella Serratia*
Tracheostomy	Physically traverses mucocutaneous barriers	Trachea and bronchi	*Enterobacteriaceae, Pseudomonas,* and other gram-negative rods, *Candida* spp.
Implants (Prostheses)			
Heart Valves	Unknown	At site of implant	*Staphylococcus* spp., *Corynebacterium* spp., *Propionibacterium* spp., *Candida* spp., *Aspergillus* ssp., zygomycetes
Orthopedic	Unknown	Bone/joint	Bacteria including anaerobes; infection may be mono- or polymicrobic
Vascular Graft	Unknown	Blood vessels	*Staphylococcus* spp., *Enterobacteriaceae, Pseudomonas,* and other gram-negative rods, fungi and mycobacteria[3]
Surgery[4]			
"Clean"	Surgically induced anatomic abnormality	Area of procedure	Predominantly *Staphylococcus aureus,* other cocci, some gram-negative rods
"Contaminated"	Surgically induced anatomic abnormality	Area of procedure	Polymicrobic populations including anaerobes
"Postoperative"	Numerous including surgically induced anatomic abnormality	Area of procedure	Polymicrobic populations including anaerobes
IMMUNOSUPPRESSIVE TREATMENT			
Glucocorticoids	Impaired cellular immunity	Anywhere	"Intracellular microbiota"[5]

TABLE 11.2—Continued

MANIPULATION	DEFECT[1] CAUSED BY TREATMENT	LIKELY SITE OF INFECTION	LIKELY MICROORGANISM(S)
Cytotoxic agents & radiation therapy	Impaired antibody production and phagocytosis	Anywhere	Any of the endogenous and/or exogenous microbiota
Splenectomy	Diminished serum opsonins, impaired primary antibody response to circulating antigens	Intravascular	*Streptococcus pneumoniae, Haemophilus influenzae, Neisseria meningitidis, Staphylococcus aureus*
ANTIMICROBIAL CHEMOTHERAPY	Disruption of normal host/parasite relationships	Anywhere across mucocutaneous barriers	Genetically and plasmid-mediated resistant as well as selected microbiota

[1] Defect in host's defense system.

[2] Other gram-negative rods include aerobic and facultative anaerobic bacteria, some with uncertain generic affiliations, such as the genera *Pseudomonas, Alcaligenes, Aeromonas, Plesiomonas, Chromobacterium, Flavobacterium, Moraxella,* and *Acinetobacter.*

[3] Mycobacteria mentioned here are those species associated with certain implants of biological origin, for example, *Mycobacterium chelonei.*

[4] Surgery includes major and minor procedures involving a deliberate incision through the mucocutaneous barrier for medical reasons.

[5] Only nosocomial representatives; however, endogenous, dormant intracellular protista may manifest overtly as the result of this therapy as well.

ated with the manipulations discussed above. Of course, they may only represent the initial areas of involvement because the infections may spread. Certainly, with a urinary catheter, the initial involvement would be in the genitourinary system. Intravenous and peritoneal catheters also affect the areas of introduction. Aerosols and tracheostomies may seed the respiratory tract, whereas implants and prostheses involve the site of insertion. Similarly, surgery affects the surgical site. The initial nidus may be very small and escape detection, whereas bacteremia and metastatic infections may be quite prominent. It is important to determine which manipulations may have compromised the defense mechanisms of patients.

Table 11.2 lists microorganisms likely to complicate the various manipulations discussed. Many times the organisms are those which are part of the human endogenous microbiota, which complicates the judgments which must be made by the laboratorian and the epidemiologist. For example, both the urinary and intravenous catheters can introduce members of the family *Enterobacteriaceae* and a variety of other gram-negative rods. Urinary catheters can also introduce enterococci and certain yeasts—especially *Candida albicans* and *Torulopsis glabrata.* Intravenous catheters, on the other hand, permit the entry of staphylococci—especially *Staphylococcus epidermidis.* Various yeasts besides *Candida albicans* can enter the circulation in this manner. When a specimen is submitted from a patient with complications from peritoneal catheterization, *Staphylococcus aureus* is by far the most frequently found organism. With indwelling catheters, the chances of fungal superinfection are enhanced considerably by the simultaneous systemic or local application of antimicrobial agents. The major decision-making process by the laboratory is the recognition of disease-related organisms which usually are regarded to be environmental contaminants. The epidemiologic history of the patient must be carefully considered when laboratory findings are evaluated. Frequently, the clinical staff must be consulted in order to reach an intelligent conclusion.

The various instruments which deliver aerosols to the respiratory tract tend to introduce bacteria which prefer a moist environment. As a result, many species of *Pseudomonas, Aeromonas,* and *Flavobacterium* may be the major offenders. They are joined by representatives of *Enterobacteriaceae*—especially the genera *Klebsiella, Enterobacter,* and *Serratia.* It is important to reemphasize that these organisms are likely to be encountered. However, there can be no doubt that practically any microbial form may be introduced in this manner. Similarly, tracheostomy may lead to colonization of the trachea and bronchi by any and all members of the family *Enterobacteriaceae* and by a variety of other obligately and facultatively anaerobic gram-negative rods and the many *Candida* species which now colonize the human environment.

When it comes to the various prostheses introduced, certain groups of microorganisms are found more frequently. Heart valves are the sites for implantation, colonization, and in some cases infection by the various *Staphylococcus, Corynebacterium, Propionibacterium, Candida,* and *Aspergillus* species, as well as zygomycetes. Orthopedic prostheses can be infected with a large variety of bacteria. Many times, such complications involve endogenous anaerobic bacteria. Very frequently, the infection may be polymicrobic and/or display a sequential colonization by different microbial forms in response to changes in the antimicrobial therapy to which the patient is exposed. Vascular grafts are complicated by staphylococci, *Enterobacteriaceae* representatives, the gramnegative rods discussed above, and fungi.

"Clean" surgical sites are infected most frequently by *Staphylococcus aureus.* However, other coccal forms including enterococci, group A streptococci, group B streptococci, and numerous gram-negative rods can cause such complications. In "contaminated" surgical sites, the infections frequently are polymicrobic, and, especially associated with bowel surgery, anaerobes may be among the isolates found. With these infections, the culture must be collected properly and submitted to the laboratory immediately. Slides for staining must be prepared when the specimen is secured. The proper stains allow the microbiologist to assess and report with dispatch the probable classification and distribution of the organisms present. The smear also serves as a control on the culture yield for all of the visualized forms. The "postoperative" complications usually involve polymicrobic populations. Anaerobes are not uncommon among these although the predominating bacteria reported in a number of institutions are *Pseudomonas* spp. and representatives of the family *Enterobacteriaceae.*

We have already discussed the microbiota expected to cause complications following immunosuppressive treatment. The immunological effects of splenectomy may predispose to intravascular infection by *Streptococcus pneumoniae, Haemophilus influenzae, Neisseria meningitidis,* and other organisms—particularly gram-negative bacteria—in descending order of frequency. This is especially true if the spenectomized patient has a chronic hemolytic anemia or treated Hodgkin's disease. Specimens from such individuals must be screened especially for these bacteria. The patient should be protected from contacts which might transmit these organisms.

In summary, sick persons are susceptible to infectious complications following microbial colonization regardless of the nature of their disease (6, 15, 33–35, 37, 42). It is only natural to assume also that the hospital environment contains microbial particles originating from lesions and from the normal microbiota of patients, hospital staff, and visitors, which creates an ecosystem that differs qualitatively and quantitatively from the intimate biosphere of each person and certainly from that of the newly admitted patient (21, 22, 24, 25, 31, 39, 41, 43, 45). The conditions listed in Tables 11.1 and 11.2 also underline the fact that the advances in medical science correct or palliate diseases which would have been fatal a few years ago. These great cures and treatments unfortunately compromise the patient's specific and nonspecific defense system and increase the opportunity for complication by microbial residents of the hospital environment in addition to those of the patient's own microbiota. Thus, because hospitalization itself increases the opportunity for disease-passaged microorganisms to join the environmental microbiota, the institutional environment can be regarded not only as a reservoir but as a dynamic system permitting selective and general multiplication of many microorganisms (19).

Laboratory Approaches to Infection Control

Our limited knowledge of the mechanisms of infection (38) often prevents determining the potential epidemiologic significance of the colonization of compromised patients by certain organisms. We do not know whether they threaten only such patients or their noncompromised contacts and the community at large as well. Table 11.3 is an attempt to depict important representatives of the hospital microbiota in terms of their natural habitats, their sources in hospitals, and the actions of individuals who are most likely to transmit these organisms to susceptible patients. Certainly, *Pseudomonas* and related gram-negative rods are important organisms in the hospital environment, although their habitat continues to be water, soil, and vegetation (and they are introduced into the hospital through water- and plant-associated sources). The most probable vehicle of transmission is hand contact of some sort, although foods, contaminated medications, and equipment may also be involved. Primarily at risk among the hospital populations are neutropenic patients as well as those that have had transplants or undergone surgical manipulation.

Despite its name, the family *Enterobacteriaceae* contains organisms not only from feces but also from soil. As a result, Table 11.3 shows the family divided into two major groups, members of both of which are active in the process of nosocomial infection. These organisms can become resistant to various antimicrobics by transferring multiply resistant plasmids.

Another significant group of organisms commonly mentioned as having

TABLE 11.3—THE INSTITUTION AND PATIENT COLONIZATION[1]

MICROBIOTA[2]	NATURAL HABITAT	MAJOR SOURCES IN HOSPITAL	MAJOR VECTORS OF TRANSMISSION		PATIENTS PRIMARILY AT RISK
			PRIMARY	SECONDARY	
GRAM-NEGATIVE RODS					
Pseudomonas and Related Bacteria	Water, soil, vegetation	Sinks, faucets, aerators, toilets, flowers, vegetables	Hands	Foods, medications, patient equipment	Neutropenic, those with foreign bodies and surgical manipulations
Enterobacteriaceae					
Escherichia-Proteus-Klebsiella	Man	Patients	Hands	Food, medications, patient care equipment	Neutropenic, those with foreign bodies and surgical manipulations
Enterobacter-Serratia	Soil and vegetation	Patients	Hands	Medications, patient care equipment	Neutropenic, those with foreign bodies and surgical manipulations
Micrococci					
Staphylococcus aureus	Man	Patients, personnel, visitors	Fomites, hands		Same as above except aerosol treatment; plus phagocytic defects
S. epidermidis	Man	Man	Hands		Intravenous catheters, implants
Yeasts					
Candida spp.	Man	Man	?		Those receiving antibiotic therapy with/without catheters, glucocorticoids, diabetes, defects in cell-mediated immunity; receiving hyperalimentation

Torulopsis glabrata	Man	Man	?	Catheters, diabetes, immuno-suppressive therapy
Others	Varied	?	?	Catheters, diabetes, immuno-suppressive therapy
Filamentous Fungi				
Zygomycetes	Varied	Air conditioners, ventilation systems	Air	Antibiotic-treated leukopenic patients, protracted acidosis, immunosuppressive therapy
Aspergilli	Varied	Air conditioners, ventilation systems plus building materials	Air	Antibiotic-treated leukopenic patients, protracted acidosis, immunosuppressive therapy
Others	Varied	Air conditioners, ventilation systems plus building materials	Air	Antibiotic-treated leukopenic patients, protracted acidosis, immunosuppressive therapy

[1] Selective pressures, procedures, and the degree of patients' compromise enhance or diminish this role.
[2] Only the most common microbiota listed; environmental microbiota is very dynamic. New significant members can appear at any time.
[3] Earlier explanation pertains.

special nosocomial significance are the micrococci, of which the outstanding example is *Staphylococcus aureus*. This bacterium challenges not only the patients threatened by members of *Enterobacteriaceae* already listed but those who have phagocytic defects as well. *Staphylococcus epidermidis*, a bacterium common on the human skin, is transmitted by hands and is of primary concern in patients with intravenous catheters and cardiac prostheses.

Yeasts are another protistal group which take advantage of the compromised patient. Many *Candida* spp., normally commensals in the human body, can complicate the recovery of patients who are given antimicrobial chemotherapy, those with catheters who are given various therapeutic regimens, and those who have underlying diseases such as diabetes. A special new group of individuals now known to be susceptible to attack by various *Candida* spp. includes those exposed to hyperalimentation. *Torulopsis glabrata* can cause problems for patients with indwelling catheters or diabetes, or those who receive immunosuppressive therapy.

The last group listed in Table 11.3, the filamentous fungi, originated from varied sources in nature and inhabit air-conditioning and ventilation systems of many hospitals. They are transmitted by air, and the zygomycetes in particular will attack patients receiving antibiotic therapy and those with leukopenia or protracted acidosis. Aspergilli found in the hospital come from various sources including plants, air-conditioning systems, and stored building materials.

The information conveyed in Table 11.3 should give an indication of the scope and versatility of these hospital-acclimated organisms. As stated at the beginning of the discussion, the table is presented as a guide and does not purport to be an all-inclusive listing.

Opportunistic and nosocomial infections must be controlled by the laboratory on several levels. At the very foundation of these considerations must be an adequate microbiology service which insists on proper control of specimens from the time of collection until they arrive at the laboratory and has the demonstrated ability to isolate, identify, and report the numerous microorganisms which might be found in specimens of various kinds.

Of course, specimens usually contain several types of organisms. The laboratory scientist must rely on clinical information in order to select those most likely to complicate a particular patient's recovery. The laboratory scientist must therefore know or endeavor to ascertain the history, the working clinical impression, and the circumstances of hospitalization of the patient whose specimen is submitted. The presence of a predominating bacterium and leukocytes may justify further analyzing a specimen which would not normally be checked for the presence of such an organism. Thus, one would expect to find *E. coli* in a stool specimen submitted for the isolation of an agent responsible for diarrhea. The absence of any other bacterium and the finding of numerous pus cells in a smear might lead the laboratory to attempt to establish the presence of enterotoxigenic or invasive representatives of this species. Ordinarily, the presence of such an organism in a fecal specimen would certainly not lead to a complete identification workup.

An accurate separate listing of microbiological isolates is helpful in keeping the laboratory updated on potential epidemiologic problems and control measures. Such lists should identify the patient and state his location, the source of the specimen, etc. The lists can be categorized by the type of organism isolated, the underlying disease process, procedures such as catheterization, or some such combination of factors.

Laboratory reports can be immensely valuable not only for deciding on appropriate therapy for a specific patient but for determining what surveillance activities and protective measures are needed throughout the hospital.

Medical personnel responsible for infection control in the hospital must be able to evaluate, in context, past local experience with a particular microorganism, the available history of and diagnosis for the patient in question, the patient's location in the hospital, and the therapy program to be used. They must also be aware of the organisms most likely to be involved in opportunistic or nosocomial infections in their particular facility (Tables 11.1 and 11.2). Many of the scientific, medical, administrative, and governmental factors associated with this problem were outlined elsewhere (18).

In recent years we have learned that random sampling of the hospital environment provides little useful information for implementing effective infection control practices. The role of the environment should be determined only after a common microbial denominator has been identified. Further, laboratory priorities should be based on sound epidemiologic information, and potential "common sources" should be tested regularly in accord with the priorities. The services of the reference laboratory may be used for such procedures as biotyping, serotyping, bacteriophage typing, etc.

A periodic quality assurance environmental program may provide valuable information and serve as an educational tool for the hospital staff. For example, the "in-use" test of equipment (while it is operated for patient care) advocated by Sanford and colleagues (28, 29, 32, 36) can provide an index of changes in the safety status of equipment and the procedures involved in using it with patients.

Other periodic testing which can provide useful information includes that conducted in operating rooms, nurseries, intensive care units, or other areas in which patients are particularly vulnerable to infection. Equipment and fixtures in such locations can be tested with any of a number of established procedures (23, 44, 46).

In this chapter, no attempt has been made to outline the specific methods used in identifying potentially significant etiologic agents of opportunistic or nosocomial infection. This omission was deliberate. First, such procedures are discussed in detail elsewhere in this volume. More important, however, is the recognition of the fact that the dynamic aspects of opportunistic and nosocomial infection do not allow us to state categorically that certain microorganisms will invariably be involved in hospital-associated infection or that others will never be involved. The variables of host response, composition of the hospital environment at any point in time, and degree of adaptation of a particular microorganism to that environment and/or that host must constantly be reevaluated if hospital-acquired infection is to be prevented.

References

1. BACH FH and VAN ROOD JJ: The major histo-compatibility complex—Genetics and biology. N Engl J Med 295:806–813, 872–878, 927–936, 1976

2. BARTLETT RC: Control of hospital-associated infections. Prog Clin Pathol 4:259–282, 1972
3. BENENSON AS: Control of Communicable Diseases in Man, 12th edition. American Public Health Association, Washington, DC, 1975
4. BOYSE EA and CANTOR H: Surface characteristics of T-lymphocyte subpopulations. Hosp Prac 21:81–88, 1977
5. BRACHMAN PS and EICKHOFF TC: Proceedings of the International Conference on Nosocomial Infections. American Hospital Association, Chicago, 1971
6. CALLIA FM, WOLLINSKY E, MORTIMER EA, ABRAMS JS, and RAMMELCAMP CH: Importance of the carrier state as a source of *Staphylococcus aureus* in wound sepsis. J Hyg 67:49–59, 1969
7. CHRISTIE AB: Infectious Disease: Epidemiology and Clinical Practice. Williams & Wilkins Co, Baltimore, Md, 1969
8. CLINE MJ: The White Cell. Harvard University Press, Cambridge, Mass, 1975
9. DAVIS BD, DULBECCO R, EISEN HN, GINSBERG HS, and WOOD WB: Microbiology, 2nd edition. Harper & Row, New York, 1975
10. DILWORTH JA and MANDELL GL: Infections in patients with cancer. Semin Oncol 2:349–359, 1975
11. DINEEN P: Influence of operating room conduct in wound infections. Surg Clin North Am 59:1283–1287, 1975
12. FULKERSON CC: Urinary tract leads in nosocomial infections. Medical Tribune and Medical News 13:3, 1972
13. GEHAR RS, SCHNEEBERGER E, MERLER E, and ROSEN FS: Heterogeneity of "acquired" or common variable agammaglobulinemia. N Engl J Med 291:1–6, 1974
14. GREAVES MF, OWEN JJT, and RAFF MC: T and B Lymphocytes. American Elsevier Publishing Co Inc, New York, 1974
15. HALDEMAN JC: The effect of the hospital environment on the spread of infection. In National Conference on Institutionally Acquired Infections. PHS Publication 1188. US Government Printing Office, Washington, DC, 1964, pp 4–26
16. HOROWITZ S and HONG R: Selective IgA deficiency—Some perspectives. Birth Defects: Original Article Series 11:129–133, 1975
17. ISENBERG HD: Laboratory diagnosis of nosocomial disease. Infect Dis Rev 3:1–21, 1974
18. ISENBERG HD: Significance of environmental microbiology in nosocomial infection and the care of the hospitalized patient. In Significance of Medical Microbiology in the Care of Patients. Lorian V (ed.). Williams & Wilkins Co, Baltimore, Md, 1977, pp 220–234
19. ISENBERG HD and BERKMAN JI: The role of drug-resistant and drug-selected bacteria in nosocomial disease. Ann NY Acad Sci 182:52–58, 1971
20. KATZ DH: Genetic controls and cellular interactions in antibody formation. Hosp Prac 12:85–99, 1977
21. KNIGHT V: Instruments and infection. Hosp Prac 2:82–95, 1967
22. KOMINOS SD, COPELAND CE, GROSTAK B, and POSTIC B: Introduction of *Pseudomonas aeruginosa* into a hospital via vegetables. Appl Microbiol 24:567–570, 1972
23. LENNETTE EH, SPAULDING EH, and TRUANT JP (eds.). Manual of Clinical Microbiology, 2nd edition. American Society for Microbiology, Washington, DC, 1974
24. LITZKY BY and LITZKY W: Bacterial shedding during bed-stripping of reusable and disposable linen as detected by high volume air samples. Health Lab Sci 8:29–34, 1971
25. MANGI RJ and ANDRIOLE VT: Contaminated stethoscopes: a potential source of nosocomial infections. Yale J Biol Med 45:600–604, 1972
26. National Conference on Institutionally Acquired Infections. PHS Publication 1188. US Government Printing Office, Washington, DC, 1964
27. PARKMAN R, GELFAND EW, ROSEN FS, SANDERSON A, and HIRSCHOM R: Severe combined immunodeficiency and adenosine deaminase deficiency. N Engl J Med 292:714–719, 1975
28. PIERRE AR and SANFORD JP: Bacterial contamination of aerosols. Arch Intern Med 131:156–159, 1973
29. REINARZ JA, PIERCE AK, MAYS BB, and SANFORD JP: The potential role of inhalation therapy equipment in nosocomial pulmonary infection. J Clin Invest 44:831–834, 1965
30. RINEHART JJ, SAGONE AL, BALCERZAK SP, ACKERMAN GA, and LoBUGLIO AF: Effects of corticosteroid therapy on human monocyte function. N Engl J Med 292:236–241, 1975

31. ROBERTS FJ, COCKCROFT WH, JOHNSON HE, and FISHWICK T: The infection hazard of contaminated nebulizers. Can Med Assoc J 108:53–56, 1973

32. ROBERTS RB: The anesthetist: cross infection and sterilization techniques. Anaesth Intensive Care 1:400–406, 1973

33. ROSENDORF LL, DAIKOFF G, and BAER H: Sources of gram negative infection after open heart surgery. J Thorac Cardiovasc Surg 67:195–201, 1974

34. ROUNTREE PM and BEARD MA: Sources of infection in intensive care unit. Med J Aust 1:577–582, 1968

35. SALZMAN TC, CLARK JJ, and KLEMM L: Hand contamination of personnel as a mechanism of cross infection with antibiotic-resistant *Escherichia coli* and *Klebsiella-Aerobacter*. Antimicrob Agents Chemother 1967:97–100, 1968

36. SCHULZE T, EDMONSON EB, PIERCE AK, and SANFORD JP: Studies on a new humidifying device as a potential source of bacterial aerosols. Am Rev Respir Dis 96:517–519, 1967

37. SHAFFER JG: Airborne infections in hospitals. Am J Public Health 54:1674–1682, 1964

38. SMITH H and PEARCE JH: Microbial Pathogenicity in Man and Animals. Cambridge Univ Press, Cambridge, 1972

39. Staphylococcal Infections in Hospitals. Central Health Services Council, HMS Stationery Office, London, 1959

40. STIEHM ER and QUIE PG: Recurrent infections: antibody and cellular aspects, phagocytic and complement factors. Forum on Infection 2, 1975

41. TAPLIN D and MERTZ PM: Flower vases in hospitals as reservoirs of pathogens. Lancet 2:1279–1281, 1973

42. THOBURN R, FEKETY FR, CLUFF LE, and MCWIN VB: Infections acquired by hospitalized patients. Arch Intern Med 121:1–10, 1968

43. THOM BT and WHITE RG: The dispersal of organisms from urines. Septic lesions. J Clin Pathol 15:559–562, 1962

44. VESHEY D: Survey of microbiological techniques for recovery from surfaces. *In* Spacecraft Sterilization Technology. National Aeronautics and Space Administration, Washington, DC, 1966, pp 147–154

45. VIRTANEN S and COSTEN O: Contamination of new hospital premises. Hospital environment and personnel or the source of nosocomial infections. Public Health 86:175–181, 1972

46. WALTER CW: Surfaces, their importance and control. *In* National Conference on Institutionally Acquired Infections. PHS Publication 1188. US Government Printing Office, Washington, DC, 1964, pp 27–34

47. WEISSMANN G: The pharmacological control of immunologically induced inflammation. *In* Infection and Immunology in the Rheumatic Diseases. Dumonde DC (ed.). Blackwell Scientific Publications, London, 1976, pp 503–510

48. WILLIAMS REO and SHOOTER RA: Infections in Hospitals: Epidemiology and Control. FA Davis & Co, Philadelphia, 1963

Part Three

CHAPTER 12

ACTINOMYCOSIS

Mary Ann Gerencser

Introduction

Causative Organisms

Four species of the genus *Actinomyces, A. israelii, A. naeslundii, A. odontolyticus,* and *A. viscosus* as well as *Arachnia (Actinomyces) propionica,* cause clinical actinomycosis in man. Of these *A. israelii* is the most common cause of human infections. *Ar. propionica* is probably the second most common cause of human actinomycosis, but infections with other *Actinomyces* species are being reported more frequently (6, 7, 15, 16).

Several *Actinomyces* species also cause infections in animals. *A. bovis* is the common cause of "lumpy jaw" in cattle and may cause infections in other animals. There are no well-authenticated cases of *A. bovis* in humans, but *A. israelii* is occasionally isolated from bovine infections. *A. viscosus* was first isolated from spontaneous periodontal disease in rodents (13) and has been implicated in canine actinomycosis (8).

The concept that other bacteria always accompany *Actinomyces* sp. in actinomycotic lesions and that their presence is necessary for disease production is not supported by recent reports on human disease (4, 16) or by the production of typical lesions in animals with material from pure cultures of *Actinomyces* spp. (9). On the basis of this evidence, it is reasonable to conclude that the *Actinomyces* and *Arachnia* spp. are the etiologic agents of actinomycosis and that the presence of other organisms is not essential for the production of the disease.

Both the *Actinomyces* and *Arachnia* spp. are classified in the family *Actinomycetaceae* in the 8th edition of *Bergey's Manual* (5). In addition to the species already mentioned, three species of uncertain taxonomic status are ascribed to the genus. One of these, *eriksonii*, which causes human disease, has been reclassified as *Bifidobacterium eriksonii* and will not be discussed here.

The *Actinomyces* spp. are gram-positive, non-acid-fast, nonmotile bacteria which often have pleomorphic morphology. In most cases, both diphtheroidal rods and filaments with or without branching are seen microscopically, but some isolates may be entirely coryneform in morphology (Figs. 12.1, 12.2). The *Actinomyces* spp. grow well on most rich culture media used in the laboratory. Growth is often stimulated by the presence of serum in the medium, and that of some isolates is stimulated by Tween 80. The species vary in oxygen requirements, but they can be considered facultative or aeroduric anaerobes. Except for *A. viscosus,* good anaerobic conditions are required for primary isolation, although many isolates of *A. naeslundii* grow well aerobically in the presence of CO_2 after isolation. Both aerobic and anaerobic growth is stimulated by CO_2. The *Actinomyces* spp. obtain energy by fermenting carbohydrates. The major end products of glucose fermentation are acetic, lactic, formic, and succinic acids.

Ar. propionica is morphologically identical to *A. israelii* and was originally classified as *A. propionicus.* It has been placed in a separate genus because of major differences in metabolism and cell wall composition (17). *Ar. propionica* produces propionic acid as a major end product of glucose fermentation. LL-diaminopimelic acid is the diamino acid in the cell-wall peptidoglycan in this species. In contrast, the *Actinomyces* spp. have lysine or lysine and ornithine in the peptidoglycan.

Clinical Manifestations

Actinomycosis is a chronic granulomatous and suppurative disease. The typical lesions are abscesses or indurated masses with fibrous walls surrounding a soft, central area containing pus. The lesions spread directly to contiguous tissue and eventually develop sinus tracts to the skin which discharge pus. The lesions and the discharges contain the organism. In early or acute stages of actinomycosis, the organisms may be found free in the pus as single filaments or small colonies. With longstanding, chronic infection, the organisms

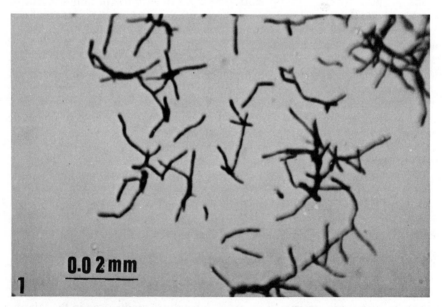

0.02mm

Fig 12.1. *Actinomyces israelii,* Gram stain, 48 hr. Thioglycollate Broth. Filaments with branching.

are usually found in distinct granules ("sulfur" granules). These granules are yellowish and consist of masses of filaments surrounded in some instances by hyaline clubs. *A. naeslundii* is less likely to produce granules than are *A. israelii, A. bovis,* and *Ar. propionica* and is usually found free in the tissues. Less is known about the tendency of *A. viscosus* and *A. odontolyticus* to form granules. *A. viscosus* has produced granules in canine infections (8), and *A. odontolyticus* has been found with and without granules (7).

Draining sinuses and "sulfur" granules are considered characteristic of actinomycosis, but the disease may occur with one or neither of these features (4). It should also be remembered that the presence of granules is not in itself diagnostic of actinomycosis, because several other bacteria can produce similar granules.

Clinically, actinomycosis is usually divided into cervicofacial, thoracic, and abdominal types, of which cervicofacial actinomycosis is the most common. Primary infections can occur in other areas, and secondary spread of the disease can involve almost any tissue or organ. Pelvic actinomycosis associated with the use of intrauterine contraceptive devices is being reported with increasing frequency. A lacrimal canaliculitis with a persistent discharge from the eye and the presence of concretions in the canaliculi is caused by *Actinomyces* and *Arachnia* spp. There is also increasing evidence that the *Actinomyces* spp.—especially *A. naeslundii* and *A. viscosus*—are involved in human periodontal disease (1) and in root surface caries (14).

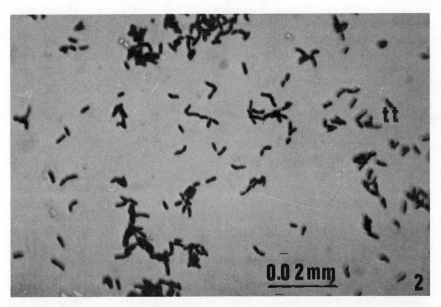

Fig 12.2. *Actinomyces viscosus,* Gram stain, 48 hr. Thioglycollate Broth. Diphtheroidal morphology, short rods.

Epidemiology

Actinomycosis is a disease of endogenous origin. The etiologic agents are normal inhabitants of the mouth of man and animals. They are especially numerous in dental plaque and in gingival crevice debris in man. Gram-positive, facultative and anaerobic bacteria (a large proportion of which are *Actinomyces* spp.) make up 15%–20% of the cultivable bacteria in saliva and on the tongue, 40% of those in plaque, and 35% of those in the gingival crevice (22). *Actinomyces* spp. are also found frequaently in human tonsils (10) when there is no evidence of actinomycosis. The extent to which the *Actinomyces* spp. are present as part of the normal oral flora in animals is not known. *A. bovis* is found in the mouths of cattle (21), and *A. viscosus* has been found in rodents (13).

Actinomycosis results when organisms which normally reside in the oral cavity gain access to the tissue. Cervicofacial infection usually follows tooth extraction or an injury to the mouth or jaw. Pulmonary infection may result from aspirating bits of infectious material from the teeth, saliva, or tonsils into the lungs. Abdominal infections probably result from invasion of the tissue by oral organisms which are swallowed, because the *Actinomyces* spp. have not been found as part of the normal intestinal flora. Abdominal actinomycosis has been associated with abdominal surgery, accidental trauma, or an acute perforative gastrointestinal disease. Cases of actinomycosis which follow human bites support the idea that the normal oral flora causes infections. Secondary lesions may arise in almost any area of the body by direct extension of the primary lesion or less frequently by hematogenous spread. The *Actinomyces* spp. have been found in patients with transient bacteremias following dental manipulations, suggesting that some primary infections may arise from bloodborne bacteria.

There is no evidence of person-to-person (except by bite) or animal-to-person transmission of actinomycosis. The causative organisms are not found on grain, grasses, or elsewhere in nature.

Public Health Significance

Actinomycosis is world-wide in distribution. There is no apparent relationship to race, age, or occupation, but it seems to be more common among males than females. In a recent review, Slack concluded that actinomycosis is neither a rare nor common disease and that the actual incidence of actinomycotic infection may be higher than is generally reported, because actinomycosis is rarely diagnosed clinically unless the physician has a strong basis for suspecting it (4, 19). Because attempts to isolate the *Actinomyces* spp. are frequently unsuccessful, even when actinomycosis is suspected, bacteriologic diagnosis in the absence of clinical suspicion has been uncommon.

Recent evidence associating the *Actinomyces* spp. with human periodontal disease and root surface caries suggests that the public health significance of these bacteria may be greater when they are considered as agents of oral disease rather than as agents of clinical actinomycosis.

Good oral hygiene is probably the most important factor in preventing both clinical actinomycosis and periodontal disease. Oral surgery and other dental manipulations can introduce actinomycetes into the tissue and result in transient bacteremias containing actinomycetes and other oral bacteria.

Collection and Processing of Specimens

The material collected for examination is usually pus but may be pleural fluid or sputum in cases of thoracic infection. Pus should be obtained with a syringe from closed subcutaneous lesions after the skin is carefully cleaned. Pus may be collected from draining sinuses in a sterile tube held at the edge of the lesion. Aspiration with a syringe and an intravenous catheter placed as deeply in the lesion as possible is preferred. If necessary, the walls of the sinus may be washed or curetted. Specimens on swabs should not be used unless absolutely necessary. If a sinus is not draining, pus and granules exuded over an extended period can be trapped in a gauze pad placed over the lesion.

Routine sputum specimens should not be cultured for *Actinomyces*. Expectorated sputum specimens can be used when granules are present or when there is a strong clinical suspicion of actinomycosis. Results of such cultures should be interpreted cautiously, remembering that these organisms are normal inhabitants of the oral cavity.

Diagnostic Procedures

Microscopic Examination

Pus, sputum, or other body fluid is placed in a sterile petri dish and examined for granules. It may help to filter the specimen through a piece of sterile cheesecloth because the granules adhere to the material. Granules are white to yellow, 0.5 to 5.0 mm in diameter, and are usually firm to hard. For examination, the granule should be placed in a drop of water on a slide and pressed out gently under a coverslip. Under lower power and reduced light, the granule has an irregular edge and a definite ray appearance at the periphery. Under higher magnification, filaments surrounded by hyaline clubs can be seen.

Granules should be crushed and used for making smears. If granules are not present, smears should be made from well-mixed pus, the centrifuged sediment of body fluids, or sputum. Smears from each specimen are stained with Gram's stain and an acid-fast stain suitable for the *Nocardia* spp. (Directions for the preparation of media, reagents, and stains are presented in Chapter 46.) The smears are examined under oil immersion for gram-positive, non-acid-fast, diphtheroidal rods and filaments with or without branching.

Selection and Inoculation of Primary Culture Media

Inoculum

Granules should be washed in two or three changes of sterile saline, crushed with a glass rod in a small quantity of saline, and used to inoculate media. If granules are not found, well-mixed pus or exudate or the centri-fuged sediment from body fluids can be used. Sputum specimens should have small, firm particles or concretions or purulent flecks selected and washed free of saliva.

Media for primary isolation

The following media should be inoculated with about 0.1 ml of the speci-men: (a) Fluid thioglycollate broth (BBL or Difco) enriched with 0.2% sterile rabbit serum, (b) two brain heart infusion agar (BHIA) plates, (c) two blood agar plates (BHIA and 5% rabbit or other animal blood).

Brain heart infusion agar and blood agar supplemented with hemin and menadione as recommended for other anaerobic bacteria are also excellent media for growing *Actinomyces* spp. (11).

One BHIA plate and one blood agar plate should be aerobically in-cubated with added carbon dioxide (a candle jar is satisfactory). The other pair of plates should be anaerobically incubated with added CO_2. A GasPak jar (BBL) or a Torbal jar can be used. With the Torbal jar, a freshly reacti-vated catalyst and a gas mixture of 80% N_2, 10% H_2, 10% CO_2 should be used. All cultures should be incubated at 37 C for 7 days.

Identification Procedures

Actinomyces and *Arachnia* spp. must be differentiated from morphologi-cally similar bacteria of the genera *Bifidobacterium, Corynebacterium, Eu-bacterium,* and *Propionibacterium.* Many problems in identifying these bacteria can be avoided by remembering that the actinomycetes are more difficult to isolate in pure culture than are most other bacteria. Contaminating bacteria can be carried in actinomycete cultures for long periods and can cause con-fusing biochemical reactions. Biochemical test results also vary with the me-dium and method used. Reactions described in identification tables may not apply to tests done by different methods and in different media. Even with standard procedures, variations among isolates occur. An attempt has been made to indicate the degree of variation which can be expected among the *Ac-tinomyces* spp. in the identification tables (Tables 12.1 and 12.2). These tables include the characteristics of *A. (Actinobacterium) meyeri,* because it can now be recognized as a distinct species (12, 21) and is being found in clinical mate-rials. *Propionibacterium acnes* and *Corynebacterium pyogenes* are also included because they are easily confused with *Actinomyces* spp.

Examination of primary cultures

BHIA plates should be examined after 24–48 hr with the low-power ob-jective (10×) of a microscope. If filamentous microcolonies are seen, the sec-tion of agar containing a well-isolated colony should be cut out (with an in-oculating needle flattened and sharpened on one edge) and placed in a tube of thioglycollate broth with serum. Plates should be reincubated.

After 5 and again at 7 days, both BHIA and blood agar plates should be examined for colonies resembling *Actinomyces* spp. (see following section) with a stereoscopic microscope. A Gram stain of one colony of each type

TABLE 12.1—CHARACTERISTICS OF *ACTINOMYCES*, *ARACHNIA* SPP., AND RELATED BACTERIA

	MICROSCOPIC MORPHOLOGY[a]	COLONY MORPHOLOGY[b] BHIA 24-48 HOURS	COLONY MORPHOLOGY[b] BHIA 7-14 DAYS	GROWTH IN THIOGLYCOLLATE BROTH	OXYGEN REQUIREMENTS	PRODUCTION OF PROPIONIC ACID FROM GLUCOSE	CELL WALL PEPTIDOGLYCAN CONTAINS LL-DAP
Actinomyces israelii	filaments, branching rods	filamentous	molar-tooth	granular clear broth	Fac. prefers An.	–	–
Actinomyces naeslundii	filaments rods	filamentous dense center	smooth	diffuse	Fac. (best aer. + CO_2)	–	–
Actinomyces viscosus	rods	filamentous dense center or smooth	smooth	diffuse	Fac. (grows aero. without CO_2)	–	–
Actinomyces odontolyticus	rods	smooth	smooth	diffuse	Fac.	–	–
Actinomyces meyeri	rods	smooth	smooth	diffuse	An., Fac.	–	–
Actinomyces bovis	rods	smooth	smooth	diffuse	Fac.	–	–
Arachnia propionica	filaments, branching rods	filamentous	molar-tooth or smooth	granular	Fac.	+	+
Corynebacterium pyogenes	rods	smooth	smooth	diffuse	Fac.	–	–
Propionibacterium acnes	rods	smooth	smooth	diffuse	An.	+	+

[a] Filaments, branching—long, branching filaments common; rods—diphtheroidal rods with V,Y,T forms common.
[b] Most common type listed. Rough isolates of *A. bovis* and *A. odontolyticus* occur as do smooth *A. israelii* colonies. See text for colony descriptions.

TABLE 12.2—BIOCHEMICAL REACTIONS OF *ACTINOMYCES, ARACHNIA* SPP., AND RELATED BACTERIA[a, b]

	A. israelii	A. naeslundii	A. viscosus	A. odontolyticus	A. meyeri	A. bovis	Ar. propionica	C. pyogenes	P. acnes
Catalase	– (0)	– (0)	+ (100)	– (0)	– (0)	– (0)	– (0)	– (0)[c]	+⁻
Indole	– (0)	– (0)	– (0)	– (0)	– (0)	– (0)	– (0)	– (0)	+⁻
Nitrate Red	d (54)	+ (92)	d (87)	+ (98)	–	– (6)	+ (100)	– (0)	+⁻
Esculin Hyd.	+ (97)	+ (93)	+ (95)	d (69)	–⁺	+ (93)	– (0)	–	–
Starch Hyd.[d]	N (50)	N (77)	N (86)	– (14)	– (0)	W (100)	N (56)	– (0)	–
Gelatin Hyd.[e]	– (0)	– (0)	– (0)	– (0)	– (0)	– (0)	– (0)	+ (100)	+⁻ slow
Urea Agar	–	+	+	–		–	–	–	–
Adonitol	– (0)	– (0)	– (0)	– (0)	– (0)	–	d (55)	d (17)	–⁺
Arabinose	d (56)[f]	– (2)	– (0)	d (24)	d (60)	– (7)	– (0)	d (37)	–⁺
Dulcitol	–	– (0)	– (0)	– (0)	–	–	– (0)		
Glucose	+ (100)	+ (100)	+ (100)	+ (100)	+ (100)	+ (100)	+ (100)	+ (100)	+ (100)
Glycerol	– (0)	+ (90)	+ (96)	d (36)	–	d (57)	d (29)	d (47)	d
Inositol	d (80)	+ (93)	+ (90)	– (14)	–	+	d (31)	d (21)	–⁺
Lactose	+ (90)	d (80)	d (86)	d (56)	+ (100)	+ (93)	+ (100)	d (79)	–
Maltose	+ (98)	+ (92)	+ (98)	d (78)	+	d (81)	+ (100)	d (61)	–⁺
Mannitol	d (70)	– (0)	– (2)	– (0)	– (0)	– (10)	+ (100)	– (10)	d
Mannose	d (84)	+ (100)	d (89)	– (8)	– (0)	d (53)	+ (100)	d (43)	+⁻
Raffinose	+ (90)	+ (94)	+ (98)	d (17)	–	– (0)	d (81)		–
Rhamnose	– (9)	d (17)	– (3)	d (55)	–	– (0)	– (0)		–
Salicin	+ (96)	d (79)	d (77)	d (49)	–	d (36)	– (14)	–	–
Sorbitol	– (12)	d (23)	– (0)	– (0)	–	–	d (61)	– (6)	–⁺
Starch	d (40)	d (52)	d (64)	+ (93)	+	+ (96)	d (79)	d (83)	–⁺
Sucrose	+ (99)	+ (100)	+ (99)	+ (98)	+	d (81)	+ (100)	d (44)	–⁺
Trehalose	+ (100)	d (85)	d (86)	d (52)	–	–	+ (100)	d (59)	–⁺
Xylose	+ (94)	– (2)	– (0)	d (70)	+	d (51)	– (0)	d (70)	–⁺

[a] Data compiled from references 5, 11, 12, 18, 20, 21.

[b] + = 90% isolates positive; – = 90% isolates negative; d = different types; symbols used as superscripts indicate occasional reactions. When available, the percentage of isolates reacting positively is indicated in parentheses.

[c] Some isolates of *C. pyogenes* may be weakly catalase positive.

[d] Starch hydrolysis: N = narrow zone (less than 10 mm diameter); W = wide zone (greater than 10 mm diameter).

[e] Liquefaction of gelatin medium such as Thiogel (BBL). If more sensitive methods are used to detect gelatin hydrolysis, some isolates of *A. israelii* and *Arachnia propionica* are positive.

[f] Serotype 1 isolates of *A. israelii* usually ferment arabinose; serotype 2 isolates are negative.

should be prepared and observed. Colonies which contain gram-positive rods or filaments should be picked to thioglycollate broth.

After 48 hr and again at 7 days some of the growth should be removed from the primary thioglycollate culture if the plate cultures are negative. Smears and Gram stains should be prepared. If gram-positive diphtheroidal rods or filaments are seen, material should be subcultured to two BHIA and two blood agar plates, incubated, and examined as for primary plates.

Differential morphological characteristics

Each species of *Actinomyces* and *Ar. propionica* has a typical or most common colony type for the microcolony (24–48 hr) and for the mature-colony (7–14 days) stage. These colonies are often referred to as rough or smooth but actually reflect the degree of filamentation of the culture. Colony type is helpful in recognizing actinomycetes on isolation plates and in differentiating species as one of a battery of identification tests. It cannot be used as a sole criterion for either isolation or identification because of variation within a species.

Microcolony types. 18–24 (sometimes 48) hr; BHIA; 100 ×.

Smooth—Finely granular surface with irregular or dentate edges—no projecting filaments. May have an optically dark center (Fig. 12.3).

Rough—Filamentous or "spider" microcolonies—long, branching filaments which appear to arise from a single point or which cross at the center without a definite center mass (Fig. 12.4). A variant of the "spider" colony has a dense center of tangled filaments with medium-to-long projecting filaments at the edge which may branch (Fig. 12.5).

Typically, *A. bovis, A. meyeri,* and *A. odontolyticus* produce smooth microcolonies; *A. israelii* and *Ar. propionica* produce spider colonies; and *A. naeslundii* and *A. viscosus* produce filamentous colonies with dense centers. Rough (i.e., filamentous) isolates of *A. bovis* and *A. odontolyticus* are found occasionally, as are smooth isolates of *A. israelii.* A fresh isolate of *A. viscosus* usually produces a filamentous microcolony with a dense center, but smooth isolates

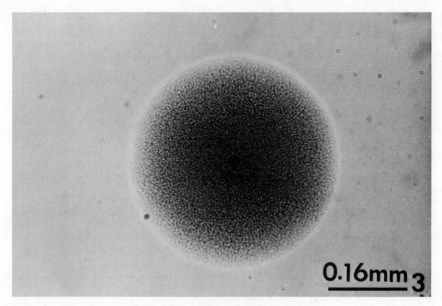

Fig 12.3. *Actinomyces odontolyticus,* Microcolony, 24 hr. BHIA. Granular surface with optically dark center, entire edge.

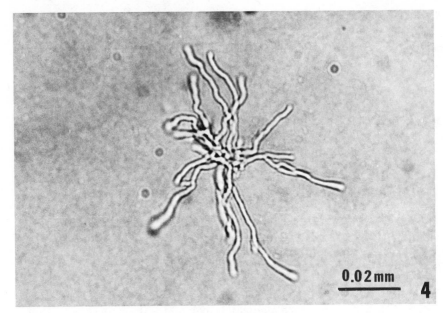

Fig 12.4 *Actinomyces israelii,* Microcolony, 24 hr. BHIA. Filamentous or "spider" colony, little or no center.

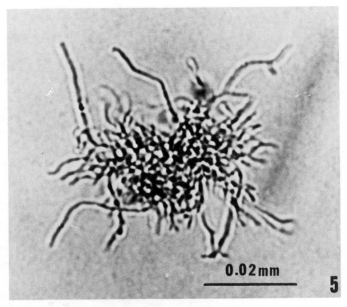

Fig 12.5 *Actinomyces naeslundii,* Microcolony, 24 hr. BHIA. Filamentous colony with dense center of tangled filaments.

of this species are not uncommon. *A. viscosus* isolates frequently begin to produce smooth microcolonies after only a few transfers on artificial media.

Mature colony types. 7–14 days; BHIA or blood agar.

Smooth—Colonies are circular, low convex to umbonate, entire and soft. The surface is smooth but may have a ground-glass appearance (Fig. 12.6).

Rough—Colonies are circular to irregular and have lobate or erose edges. They are umbonate or heaped on the agar and have smooth but convoluted surfaces which have given rise to the descriptive terms "molar-tooth," "bread-crumb," and "raspberry-like." Rough colonies may be hard and may adhere to the medium and be difficult to emulsify (Fig. 12.7).

Species with smooth microcolonies usually have smooth mature colonies. *A. bovis, A. meyeri,* and *A. odontolyticus* produce small (0.5- to 1.0-mm) smooth colonies. Despite their centered filamentous microcolonies, *A. naeslundii* and *A. viscosus* also usually have smooth mature colonies which are somewhat larger than those of *A. bovis. A. israelii* and, to a lesser extent, *Ar. proprionica* produce the rough, molar-tooth colonies often associated with the *Actinomyces* spp.

With one exception, mature colonies on blood agar are identical to those on BHIA. *A. odontolyticus* produces distinctive red colonies on blood agar after 7–14 days. This color may develop during anaerobic incubation or after anaerobically incubated plates are left standing at room temperature in air for

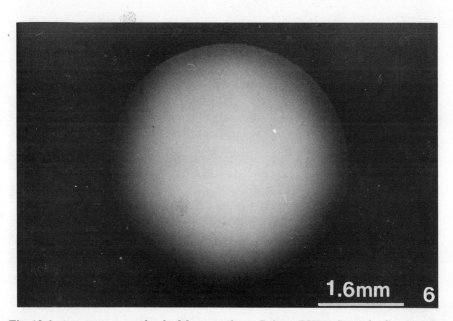

Fig 12.6 *Actinomyces naeslundii,* Mature colony, 7 days, BHIA. Smooth, Convex, entire edge.

several days. *Actinomyces* spp. are not hemolytic except for an occasional isolate of *A. odontolyticus* which may show hemolysis under heavy growth or narrow zones of either alpha or beta hemolysis around individual colonies.

Instructions for biochemical tests

Determination of oxygen requirements. Use a 2- to 3-day-old brain heart infusion broth culture as inoculum. Mix and dilute to barely turbid with sterile broth. Inoculate six BHIA slants in cotton-plugged tubes. Place the tip of a capillary pipette at the bottom of the slant, force out one small drop of inoculum, and draw pipette in a single line from the base to the top of the slant. Incubate slants in duplicate as follows: Aerobically; aerobically with CO_2 (KH_2PO_4-carbonate seal*); anaerobically with CO_2 (pyrogallol-carbonate) seal. After 3 and 7 days at 37 C, record results as 3+ for best growth, 2+ for medium growth in comparison to the best, 1+ for light growth in comparison to the best, and 0 for no growth. In each case, compare the results of growing a single culture under various conditions. Do not compare growth of one strain with that of other strains. If the results of the duplicate tubes do not agree, repeat the test.

Catalase production. This is most useful for separating *Actinomyces* species (except *A. viscosus*) and *Ar. propionica* from morphologically similar bacteria (e.g., *Propionibacterium acnes*) which are catalase positive. Expose anaerobically grown cultures to air for about one-half hour before testing. Test by pouring 3% hydrogen peroxide over growth on a non-blood-containing slant or plate and watching for the presence of a stream of small bubbles. Alterna-

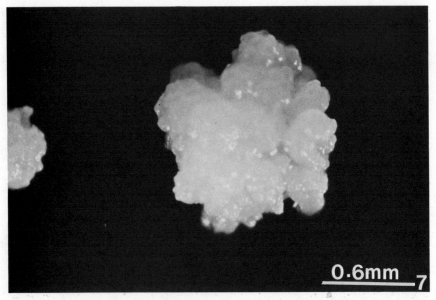

0.6mm

Fig 12.7. *Actinomyces israelii*, Mature colony, 7 days, BHIA. Rough colony, "breadcrumb" type, heaped, knobby surface, lobate edge.

tively, suspend some growth in a drop of hydrogen peroxide on a microscope slide, and add a coverslip. Again, look for the development of a stream of bubbles.

Indole production. Indole-nitrite medium (BBL). Test after 3 and 7 days of incubation by extracting with xylene and adding Erlich's reagent.*

Nitrate reduction. Indole-nitrite medium (BBL). Test after 3 and 7 days with standard nitrate reagents.

Esculin hydrolysis. Incubate esculin broth* for 7 days. Add a few drops of 1.0% FeCl₃ to the top of the tube. Development of a brownish-black color indicates hydrolysis.

Urease. Christensen's urea agar (BBL or Difco). Read after 3 and 7 days.

Starch hydrolysis. Inoculate nutrient starch agar* by placing 1 drop of inoculum on the plate with a capillary pipette and drawing it across the plate. Two isolates can be placed on one plate.

Inoculate duplicate plates and test at 24 hr and 7 days by flooding the plate with 2–4 ml of Gram's iodine. A colorless area around the streak indicates complete hydrolysis of the starch.

Gelatin liquefaction. Thiogel medium (BBL). Inoculate by stabbing medium with a capillary pipette. Incubate test material and an uninoculated tube and observe for liquefaction after 7 and 14 days by placing tubes in the refrigerator until the control tube has hardened.

Carbohydrate fermentation tests. Thioglycollate fermentation base* is suitable for all species of *Actinomyces* and *Arachnia* and does not require an anaerobe jar for incubation. The carbohydrates which are useful in speciating *Actinomyces* are arabinose, glucose, lactose, mannitol, raffinose, salicin, soluble starch, sucrose, trehalose, and xylose.

End products of glucose fermentation. End products of glucose fermentation can be detected in the supernatant of cultures grown in a suitable glucose broth with gas liquid chromatography and the methods described by the Virginia Polytechnic Institute's Anaerobe Laboratory (11). This information can be used to place most isolates in the proper genus on the basis of the test results obtained.

Serologic procedures

Fluorescent antibody techniques have been used extensively in identifying *Actinomyces* and *Arachnia* spp. in clinical materials and in cultures. This technique can be used to differentiate the species of *Actinomyces* and also can be used to identify at least two serovars in each species. Fluorescent antibody (FA) tests can also be used to differentiate between *A. israelii* and *Ar. propionica*. Unfortunately, FA reagents are not yet available for general use.

Miscellaneous procedures

Detection of diaminopimelic acid (DAP). If neither gas liquid chromatographic determination of fermentation end products nor serologic results are available, it may be necessary to use cell-wall DAP to confirm the identity of *Ar. propionica*. This procedure can be easily performed without special apparatus using the whole-cell hydrolysate procedure described by Becker et al. (2).

Grow cells in BHI broth for 5–6 days, centrifuge, wash once with water and once with 95% ethyl alcohol, and air dry. Hydrolyze dried cells (10 mg) in 1.0 ml 6 N HCl for 18 hr at 100 C. Filter the hydrolysate through paper and evaporate until dry on a steam bath. Redissolve in 0.3 ml of water, and dry three times to remove HCl. Take up residue in 0.3 ml of water, and spot 20 μl on Whatman No. 1 filter paper. Chromatograph the sample and appropriate controls with descending chromatography in methanol-water-10 N HCl-pyridine (80:17.5:2.5:10 by volume) overnight. Detect amino acids by dipping in ninhydrin (0.1% in acetone) and then heating at 100 C for 2 min. DAP spots are olive-green fading to yellow. In this procedure, most other amino acids migrate off the paper during the overnight run.

Cell-wall DAP can also be detected with the procedure of Boone and Pine (3).

Antimicrobic Susceptibility and Resistance

Susceptibility testing of *Actinomyces* spp. and *Ar. propionica* can be done with methods recommended for other anaerobic bacteria. *Actinomyces* spp. are susceptible to chloramphenicol, erythromycin, lincomycin, penicillin, and tetracycline (21). Penicillin is usually considered the drug of choice.

References

1. BAKER JJ, CHAN SP, SOCRANSKY SS, APPENHEIM JJ, and MERGENHAGEN SE: Importance of *Actinomyces* and certain gram-negative anaerobic organisms in the transformation of lymphocytes from patients with periodontal disease. Infect Immun 13:1363–1368, 1976
2. BECKER B, LECHEVALIER MP, GORDON RE, and LECHEVALIER HA: Rapid differentiation between *Nocardia* and *Streptomyces* by paper chromatography of whole-cell hydrolysates. Appl Microbiol 12:421–423, 1964
3. BOONE CJ and PINE L: Rapid method for characterization of actinomycetes by cell wall composition. Appl Microbiol 16:279–284, 1968
4. BROWN JR: Human actinomycosis. A study of 181 subjects. Human Pathol 4:319–330, 1973
5. BUCHANAN RE and GIBBONS NE (eds.) Bergey's Manual of Determinative Bacteriology, 8th edition. Williams and Wilkins Co, Baltimore, Md, 1974
6. COLEMAN RM, GEORG LK, and ROZZELL AR: *Actinomyces naeslundii* as an agent of human actinomycosis. Appl Microbiol 18:420–426, 1969
7. GEORG LK: The agents of human actinomycosis. *In* Anaerobic Bacteria: Role in Disease. Balows A, DeHaan RH, Dowell VR, and Guze LB (eds.). Charles C Thomas, Springfield, Ill, 1974
8. GEORG LK, BROWN JM, BAKER HJ, and CASSELL GH: *Actinomyces viscosus* as an agent of actinomycosis in the dog. Am J Vet Res 33:1457–1470, 1972
9. GEORG LK and COLEMAN RM: Comparative pathogenicity of various *Actinomyces* species. *In* The *Actinomycetales*, Jena Inter Symp Taxon. Prauser H (ed.). G Fischer, Jena, Germany, 1970
10. HITOCHI M and SCHWARZ J: Characterization of actinomycotic granules by architecture and staining methods. Arch Pathol 93:392–400, 1972
11. HOLDEMAN LV, CATO EP, and MOORE WEC (eds). Anaerobe Laboratory Manual, 4th edition. Southern Printing Co, Blacksburg, Va, 1977
12. HOLMBERG K and NORD CE: Numerical taxonomy and laboratory identification of *Actinomyces* and *Arachnia* and some related bacteria. J Gen Microbiol 91:17–44, 1975
13. HOWELL A JR: A filamentous microorganism isolated from periodontal plaque in hamsters. I. Isolation, morphology, and general cultural characteristics. Sabouraudia 3:81–92, 1963

14. JORDAN HV and HAMMOND BF: Filamentous bacteria isolated from root surface caries. Arch Oral Biol 17:1–12, 1972
15. MITCHELL PD, HINTZ CS, and HASELBY RC: Molar mass due to *Actinomyces odontolyticus*. J Clin Microbiol 5:658–660, 1977
16. MORRIS JF and KILBOURN P: Systemic actinomycosis caused by *Actinomyces odontolyticus*. Ann Intern Med 81:700, 1974
17. PINE L and GEORG LK: Reclassification of *Actinomyces propionicus*. Int Bull Bacteriol Nomencl Taxon 15:143–163, 1969
18. ROBERTS RJ: Biochemical reactions of *Corynebacterium pyogenes*. J Pathol Bacteriol 95:127–130, 1968
19. SLACK JM: Epidemiology of actinomycosis, a bacterial disease. *In* Epidemiology of Human Mycotic Diseases. Charles C Thomas, Springfield, Ill, 1974
20. SLACK JM and GERENCSER MA: Actinomyces, Filamentous Bacteria: Biology and Pathogenicity. Burgess Publishing Co, Minneapolis, Minn, 1975
21. SMITH L DS: The Pathogenic Anaerobic Bacteria, 2nd edition. Charles C Thomas, Springfield, Ill, 1975
22. SOCRANSKY SS and MANGANIELLO SD: The oral microbiota from birth to senility. J Peridontol 42:485–496, 1971

CHAPTER 13

CLOSTRIDIAL ANAEROBIC INFECTIONS

Louis DS. Smith

Introduction

The genus *Clostridium* is composed of sporeforming anaerobic rods. There are other genera of sporeforming anaerobes—the sporeforming coccus *Sporosarcina* and the sporeforming sulfate reducers *Desulfotomaculum*—but only members of *Clostridium* are found in clinical specimens. Although all belong to the same genus, they vary greatly. Some are aerotolerant; others are among the strictest of the anaerobes. Some can grow with ammonia as the nitrogen source and biotin as the only vitamin, whereas others require more than 20 amino acids and vitamins. Psychrophilic species will not grow at temperatures above 30 C, and thermophiles will grow only above 50 C.

The clostridia found in clinical specimens usually have moderate growth requirements. None of those pathogenic for man is really a strict anaerobe, all are mesophilic in their temperature requirements, and none requires for growth anything that is not found in ordinary bacteriological media. Isolating and identifying the clostridia commonly found in clinical specimens is not difficult. True, one may be alarmed that more than 300 species have been described in the genus *Clostridium*—and the alarm is only slightly mitigated by the fact that 60 species are described in the latest edition of *Bergey's Manual*. However, most of the clostridia found in the clinical laboratory fall into about six species, which simplifies the task of the clinical microbiologist in identifying them.

How often they will be found varies directly with the types of specimens submitted to the laboratory. Blood cultures, soft-tissue abscesses, and pulmonary infections seldom yield clostridia. They are much more frequently found in accidental wounds or associated with abdominal sepsis resulting from perforation of the gut. In wounds of warfare, for example, most of which are contaminated with soil, as many as 85% have contained clostridia; in cases of abdominal sepsis, more than 70% have been found to be infected with clostridia (11). In most such cases, the infecting clostridia did not play any important role in pathogenesis. Thus we can conclude that clostridial infections are neither rare nor usually severe.

Isolation

Because the clostridia found in clinical specimens from man are not highly demanding in their requirements for anaerobiosis, roll tubes or anaerobic chambers are not essential for isolating them. Freshly poured blood agar plates, properly prepared and inoculated, can be incubated in anaerobic jars (7).

The first indication of clostridia in a specimen is the appearance of gram-positive rods, with or without spores, in the Gram stain that is made before culture. The specimen should be inoculated onto freshly poured blood agar plates for aerobic and anaerobic culture, to a plate of egg yolk agar, and to a back-up tube of chopped-meat medium. The blood agar should contain 0.05% cysteine and 0.03% dithiothreitol (5), dithioerythritol, or sodium formaldehyde sulfoxylate. Cultures should be incubated for 2 days at 37 C. One day of incubation is not sufficient for primary isolation, except for *C. perfringens*. Plates should not be taken out of the anaerobe jar at 1 day, examined, and replaced, because the further growth of microcolonies of some strains will be inhibited by this exposure to air.

If the preliminary Gram stain shows a variety of organisms, and the clostridia are particularly desired, the nonsporeformers can be eliminated by heating the tube of chopped-meat medium for 10 min at 80 C before incubating and streaking blood and egg-yolk agar after growth is evident. A milder method and one that is suitable even for spores with slight heat resistance is to suspend the material to be cultured in 50% ethyl alcohol for 1 hr at room temperature, centrifuge, and inoculate blood agar, egg-yolk agar, and chopped-meat medium from the sediment. Media should also be inoculated with unheated material when heat or alcohol treatment is used.

Several media selective for the clostridia have been described. For isolating clostridia from food, media containing sulfite and iron (15) are commonly used. Most of the clostridia reduce sulfite to sulfide, which reacts with the iron to form ferrous sulfide and blackens the colonies. Another semi-selective medium is phenethyl alcohol-blood agar (8). Neomycin, 100 µg/ml, is useful but should only be used in parallel with noninhibitory media, because some strains will be inhibited.

After they are incubated, the plates should be carefully examined to confirm that the agar is not covered by a thin film of one of the swarming clostridia. Often this film is barely perceptible even to the experienced eye. Its presence is easily confirmed by streaking a loop across the uninoculated portion of the plate. The edge of a swarming area should not be picked with the hope of getting a pure culture of the swarmer, for swarmers often carry other bacteria along with them. If swarming is present, isolation should be repeated with a shorter incubation time or, better, by increasing the concentration of agar to 4%–6%. If swarming is not present, colonies should be examined with a dissection microscope or a good hand lens to confirm the isolation. They should be picked to tubes of chopped meat-glucose medium, incubated overnight, and used to inoculate the differential media listed in Table 13.1 and the media for determining antibiotic susceptibility.

TABLE 13.1—DIFFERENTIAL MEDIA FOR THE CLOSTRIDIA

MEDIUM	FOR DETERMINING:
Egg-yolk agar	Lecithinase and lipase production
Chopped meat	Digestion; indole formation
Milk	Digestion
Gelatin	Liquefaction
Glucose broth	Fermentation
Maltose broth	Fermentation
Lactose broth	Fermentation
Sucrose broth	Fermentation
Salicin broth	Fermentation
Mannitol broth	Fermentation

Identification

The shape and position of the spores are useful but not always essential characteristics for identification. Special spore stains are not especially helpful; Gram stain is sufficient. However, phase-contrast microscopy is a useful aid, because spores, within or outside the cell, are much more refractile than are the vegetative cells. Although the clostridia are by definition gram-positive, some readily lose the Gram stain and appear as large, gram-negative rods. If adsorbed sera are used, the fluorescent-antibody technique is valuable for rapidly identifying some of the pathogenic species (3) including *Clostridium chauvoei, C. septicum, C. novyi, C. tetani, and C. botulinum* (19).

It is sometimes necessary to differentiate clostridia from some of the facultative *Bacillus* species, especially when examining food. This is particularly the case with *Bacillus cereus,* which grows well under anaerobic conditions and produces lecithinase on egg-yolk agar. However, it and the other bacilli that may be found produce catalase, whereas the clostridia do not. Catalase production is most easily determined by taking a small amount of growth from the egg-yolk plate (not the blood agar plate, for blood contains catalase) and mixing it with a drop of 3% hydrogen peroxide. A few strains of clostridia break down hydrogen peroxide slowly by means of "pseudo-catalase" but do not do so as rapidly and vigorously as do the bacilli (18).

One of the most useful media for examining clostridia is egg-yolk agar. Some clostridia such as *C. perfringens* produce lecithinase (phospholipase C) that causes a white precipitate to form in the agar around the colonies. Other species produce a lipase that breaks down the fat in the medium, freeing the long-chain fatty acids. This reaction is indicated by a "mother-of-pearl" iridescence around and over the colonies. It is usually difficult to see on 2 days of incubation. If there is doubt, the plate should be re-incubated for another day or so. When reactions are weak, lipase production can be demonstrated by putting a drop of water on the growth on the heaviest part of the plate. If the fat has been broken down with the freeing of the long-chain fatty acids, the drop of water will be covered by a thin, gray film.

Gas liquid chromatography (GLC) is often useful and convenient for identifying metabolic products, because it allows a strain to be identified much more quickly. Procedures for carrying out this determination are described in laboratory manuals on anaerobic bacteriology (7, 13, 21). For laboratories not having this equipment, less expensive thin-layer chromatography can be used (16), but it is less convenient than GLC.

Differential characteristics of some clostridia are shown in Table 13.2. Determining whether toxin is produced by the pathogenic species is often useful in evaluating its possible role in a given pathologic situation. The laboratory animal to use and the conditions for demonstrating toxin production, as well as further information on the clostridia, are discussed elsewhere (18, 20, 23).

Pathogenic Species

Clostridium perfringens

C. perfringens is by far the most frequently encountered clostridium. In one study of the anaerobes in clinical specimens (24), 60 strains of clostridia were found among 1392 anaerobic isolates; 55 of the 60 were C. perfringens. This organism grows rapidly and well, is only slightly sensitive to oxygen, retains the Gram stain, is nonmotile, and seldom forms spores on the usual laboratory media. The optimal temperature for growth is high—44 to 46 C—and should be used when C. perfringens is specifically sought in specimens containing mixed flora such as food, soil, or feces. It is sensitive to cold, so storing cultures or specimens in a refrigerator may cause most of the cells to die (18). Optimal hydrogen ion concentration for growth is pH 6.5 to 6.8. The organism is nutritionally demanding, with eight vitamins and 19 amino acids being required in a chemically defined medium (17).

On blood-agar plates, this organism characteristically forms colonies 2 to 5 mm in diameter, surrounded by a small zone of complete hemolysis which is surrounded by a larger zone of incomplete hemolysis. On egg-yolk agar, the medium under and around the colony contains a whitish precipitate resulting from the breakdown of the lecithin in the egg-yolk (the Nagler reaction). Tentative confirmation can be obtained by making a one-streak inoculation (from a colony showing double zones of hemolysis) across an egg-yolk agar plate, one-half of which has been spread with 1 drop of C. perfringens antitoxin (Burroughs Wellcome C. welchii type A antiserum), and incubating overnight. If the organism is C. perfringens, the Nagler reaction will be inhibited on the side of the plate streaked with the antitoxin. C. bifermentans, C. sordellii, and C. paraperfringens also form lecithinase that is inhibited by C. perfringens antitoxin, but to a lesser extent. These organisms can be readily distinguished from C. perfringens with a few tests (Table 13.2).

C. perfringens is divided into five types on the basis of the production of four lethal toxins as shown in Table 13.3. Most strains are type A; they and those of type C are the only ones important in human disease. The alpha toxin, produced by all types, is a phospholipase C, hydrolyzing lecithin either free or when combined with protein (as in cell membranes). The beta toxin is necrotic for the intestinal mucosa and has lethal central nervous system activity. The

TABLE 13.2—DIFFERENTIAL CHARACTERISTICS OF CLOSTRIDIA

SPECIES	SPORES[a]	MILK[b]	EGG-YOLK AGAR LEC.	EGG-YOLK AGAR LIP.	AEROBIC GROWTH	GELATIN	INDOLE	GLUCOSE	MALTOSE	LACTOSE	SUCROSE	SALICIN	MANNITOL	FERMENTATION PRODUCTS[c]
Toxic, pathogenic														
C. botulinum														
Group I	OS	D	+	+	−	+	−	+	+	−	−	V	−	A, P, B, IB, IV
Group II	OS	−	−	+	−	+	−	+	+	−	−	V	−	A, B
Group III	OS	−	−	+	−	+	−	+	+	−	−	−	−	A, P, B
C. chauvoei	OS	−	−	−	−	+	−	+	+	+	−	−	−	A, B
C. difficile	OS	−	−	−	−	V	−	+	−	−	−	V	+	A, F, L, B
C. haemolyticum	OS	−	+	−	−	+	+	+	−	−	−	−	−	A, P, B
C. histolyticum	OS	D	−	−	+	+	−	−	−	−	−	−	−	A
C. novyi A	OS	−	+	+	−	+	−	+	+	−	−	−	−	A, P, B, V
C. novyi B	OS	D	+	+	−	+	−	+	+	−	−	−	−	A, P, B, V
C. perfringens	OS	−	+	−	−	+	−	+	+	+	+	V	−	A, B
C. septicum	OS	−	−	−	−	+	−	+	+	+	−	V	−	A, B
C. sordellii	OS	D	+	−	−	+	V	+	−	−	−	−	−	A, F
C. tetani	RT	−	−	−	−	+	−	−	−	−	−	−	−	A, P, B
Nontoxic, doubtfully pathogenic														
C. bifermentans	OS	D	+	−	−	+	+	+	+	−	−	−	−	A, F
C. butyricum	OS	−	−	−	−	−	−	+	+	+	+	+	V	A, F, B
C. cadaveris	OT	+	−	−	−	+	+	+	−	−	−	−	−	A, B, IV
C. innocuum	OT	+	−	−	−	−	−	+	−	−	V	+	+	A, F, B
C. limosum	OS	+	+	−	−	+	−	+	−	−	−	−	−	A
C. parapefringens	OS	−	−	−	−	−	−	+	+	+	+	V	−	A, B, L
C. paraputrificum	OT	−	−	−	−	−	−	+	+	+	+	+	−	A, B
C. ramosum	R/OT	−	−	−	−	−	−	+	+	+	+	+	V	A, F
C. sphenoides	R/ST	−	−	−	−	−	+	+	−	V	−	V	+	A
C. sporogenes	OS	+	+	+	−	+	−	+	+	−	−	−	−	A, P, B, IB, IV
C. subterminale	OS	+	−	−	−	+	−	−	+	−	−	−	−	A, B, IB, IV
C. tertium	OT	−	−	−	+	−	−	+	+	+	+	+	+	A, B

[a] O, oval; R, spherical; S, subterminal; T, terminal.
[b] D, digestion; +, clot, digestion.
[c] From glucose broth. A, acetic; B, butyric; F, formic; IB, isobutyric; IV, isovaleric; L, lactic; P, propionic; V, valeric.

TABLE 13.3—MAJOR LETHAL TOXINS OF *CLOSTRIDIUM PERFRINGENS*

		TOXIN TYPES		
A	B	C	D	E
Toxins: alpha	alpha	alpha	alpha	alpha
	beta	beta	epsilon	iota
	epsilon			

epsilon toxin is produced as an inactive prototoxin which is converted to the fully active toxin by trypsin in the small intestine. It increases the permeability of the capillaries in certain parts of the brain. Iota toxin is also activable by trypsin and also causes increased capillary permeability. Infections with types B, D, and E are important only in herbivores. (The few human infections caused by type C are discussed under necrotizing jejunitis later in this chapter.)

The clinical laboratory is seldom asked to type strains of *C. perfringens,* for with very few exceptions strains isolated from human infections have been type A. However, a strain can easily be confirmed as type A by inoculating it heavily into a tube of chopped meat-glucose medium, incubating for 4 to 6 hr at 37 C, and centrifuging. Part of the supernatant fluid is mixed with antitoxin (1.2 ml of fluid, 0.3 ml of type A antitoxin) and let stand for 15 min. Then 0.5 ml is inoculated intraperitoneally into each of two mice. Two control mice are inoculated with the same amounts of culture fluid mixed with rabbit serum or control horse serum. If the culture is a toxigenic type A strain, the control mice will die overnight, and the mice given the antitoxin will survive. (NOTE: Isolates of *C. perfringens* frequently are found that produce too little alpha toxin to be lethal for the control mice. Such strains are still considered to be type A.)

C. perfringens is probably responsible for a wider variety of infections than is any other organism. These include wound infections varying from simple contamination to postabortal sepsis and gas gangrene, necrotizing jejunitis, food poisoning, biliary tract infections, and meningitis. For an authoritative study of infections caused by this organism, see reference 23.

Food poisoning caused by *C. perfringens* is common in the United States and elsewhere. It usually has an incubation period of 8 to 12 hr and involves marked nausea, abdominal cramps, and diarrhea. Vomiting and fever are very rare. It is caused by the ingestion of 10^8 or more living cells of *C. perfringens* that sporulate in the intestine, forming enterotoxin at that time (18). The action of this toxin is similar to that of cholera toxin, which causes fluid to pour into the lumen of the intestine. It is really not an infection, because the intestinal mucosa is not invaded.

C. perfringens food poisoning is almost always associated with eating meat or some other dish prepared with meat such as gravy, thick sauce, soup, chile con carne, casseroles, dressing in stuffed fowl, etc., that has been allowed to stand at room temperature for several hours after cooking and before serving. This association between meat dishes and *C. perfringens* food poisoning is related to three factors: such dishes are within a pH range (nearly neutral) in which *C. perfringens* grows rapidly; they supply the amino acids and growth factors that this organism requires; and these dishes are those apt to be held unrefrigerated for several hours between cooking and serving, during which time the bacteria multiply rapidly. Because *C. perfringens* is found almost everywhere, the source of the strain responsible for any outbreak is not usually considered important.

This organism is incriminated as the cause of a particular outbreak by the isolation of strains of the same serological type from the stools of a number of patients and from the suspected food, if any is available. A more rapid and highly specific method is demonstrating enterotoxin in the stools of patients (9). The population levels of *C. perfringens* in food specimens can be readily determined with plate counts if the food has not been refrigerated, using tryptose-sulfite-cycloserine agar medium, or by documenting the presence of alpha toxin in the food (12).

A much more serious and fortunately much more rare disease caused by *C. perfringens* is necrotizing jejunitis (enteritis necroticans, pig-bel). This disease is found most often in the natives of New Guinea, who contract it following feasts of inadequately cooked pork (14) that is heavily contaminated by strains of type C—a type often carried by swine which produces the beta toxin responsible for the necrotizing jejunitis and the 35% to 40% mortality associated with it. This disease in humans seems to be largely restricted to these people both because they are exposed to a heavy inoculum of type C organisms from the contaminated pork and because they have low levels of trypsin in the intestine. These low levels result from a normally low-protein diet which reduces trypsin production; also, their diet is rich in sweet potatoes, which contain heat-stable trypsin inhibitor. This low level of trypsin activity—to which the beta toxin is extremely susceptible—allows the disease to occur.

C. perfringens wound infections range from simple contamination of wound surfaces to highly fatal and rapidly progressing clostridial myonecrosis (gas gangrene) and postabortal infections. *C. perfringens* has been isolated from 20% of simple wounds that healed without clinical evidence of infection other than a thin seropurulent exudate and a slow rate of healing in some cases. *C. perfringens* is also found in wounds that go on to heal normally. Other clostridia such as *C. novyi*, *C. septicum,* or *C. sordellii* may also be responsible for progressive infection. The diagnosis of clostridial myonecrosis is primarily based on clinical findings, and the patient usually requires prompt surgical treatment (23).

Clostridium tetani

Tetanus continues to be a problem in that part of the population not immunized with toxoid, and mortality continues to be appreciable. The organism is isolated from ante- or post-mortem specimens in only about one-third of the cases and cannot usually be isolated if the patient has been treated with broad-spectrum antibiotics. Because tetanus is readily diagnosed clinically, the laboratory is seldom called upon to isolate this organism from clinical specimens. However, isolating and identifying *C. tetani* are relatively easy, for it will grow readily on blood agar in the anaerobe jar, and it can be tentatively identified with fluorescent antiserum (3) or by the fact that it produces indole and cannot ferment glucose. Although *C. tetani* is described as forming spherical spores, those of some strains are oval. The typical "drum-stick" appearance is found only with cultures containing mature spores which are observed in dried preparations; the cells seen in wet mounts are more wedge-shaped.

Cultures on blood agar generally exhibit "swarming" in a fine film over the surface of the agar, a characteristic that is useful in isolating this organism from a mixed culture. Swarming can be inhibited by using 4%–6% agar, by adding 40–60 units of tetanus antitoxin per ml of medium (22), or can be avoided by incubating blood agar plates for only 1 day. The isolation of *C. tetani* from soil is described in reference 4.

Tetanus toxin can be detected even in mixed culture by inoculating 0.1 ml subcutaneously beside the tails of each of two mice. Protected mice, immunized by intraperitoneal inoculation of 1 unit of antitoxin 2 hr or more previously, should also be inoculated. The next day, the tails of the unprotected mice will curve to the inoculated side, and the leg on that side will also be in spasm. If the culture fluid contains a high concentration of toxin, the unprotected mice will be found dead; the protected mice will continue to live and will have no symptoms.

Clostridium botulinum

Seven toxigenic types of *C. botulinum* are recognized on the basis of antigenically distinct protein toxins. Cases of human botulism are caused by types A, B, or E, or much less frequently by F. Types C and D are frequently involved in outbreaks of botulism among domestic mammals or birds. The three types of human botulism are: foodborne botulism, wound botulism, and infant botulism. For further information, see reference 19.

Food-borne botulism caused by home-preserved foods continues to be a problem in the United States. If food-borne botulism is suspected, specimens should include both serum and feces from the patient and all available incriminated food. State public health laboratories should always be informed of any suspected cases of botulism before specimens are submitted. The process of detecting toxin in food, serum, or feces is that described in the CDC laboratory manual (7).

Wound botulism is much rarer than food-borne botulism. However, more cases have been recognized in recent years. Most of the cases reported to date have been caused by type A, but some were caused by type B. Having a clinical basis for suspecting wound botulism is important because the laboratory can be alerted to look for the organism in clinical materials and to test the patient's serum for botulinal toxin. Egg-yolk agar is a very useful medium for isolating *C. botulinum*. Chopped meat-glucose medium is also used. After 2–4 days of incubation on egg-yolk agar, the colonies of *C. botulinum* show a "mother-of-pearl" iridescence caused by lipase the organism produces. Type A strains and proteolytic type B strains are culturally indistinguishable from *C. sporogenes* and can be identified as *C. botulinum* only on the basis of toxin production.

Although infant botulism has been recognized only recently (2), it is clearly the most frequently encountered form of botulism in the United States. Over 30 cases were diagnosed within a year after the cited report was published. This disease results from the production of toxin in the intestine, where *C. botulinum* somehow becomes implanted during the first weeks of life. The first symptom is constipation, followed by an increasing generalized weakness and paralysis 1 day to several weeks later. Sudden respiratory arrest may occur. Support for the clinical diagnosis can be obtained with electromyography; however, the diagnosis can be confirmed only by identifying *C. botulinum* toxin and organisms in feces of patients. When infant botulism is suspected, both serum and fecal samples should be submitted to the state health laboratory. The accompanying constipation requires that fecal samples be obtained by the aid of a swab carefully inserted into the rectum. Fecal samples should not be allowed to dry out but should be kept moist with sterile water, e.g., water for injection. Saline should not be used.

Other Pathogenic Clostridia

Clostridium septicum

This organism sometimes causes rapidly progressive cases of clostridial myonecrosis associated with severe wounds. Other infections are often associated with malignancy, especially leukemia, the source of the organisms being the patient's own intestinal tract (1). Apparently, *C. septicum* occasionally escapes from this site and is carried by the blood stream to other parts of the body. When body defenses are lowered by the changes accompanying leukemia or by the administration of antimetabolites, steroids, or other immunosuppressive drugs, generalized *C. septicum* infection may result.

This organism grows readily on the usual media and can be identified readily with fluorescent microscopy. It is often a nuisance when present in mixed culture, because it may swarm over the surface of the blood-agar isolation plates. Shortening the incubation period or using hard agar may be necessary to obviate such swarming.

Clostridium difficile

C. difficile has long been known as part of the normal microbial flora of the human gut (10). Recently, however, it has been shown to be the major if not the only cause of pseudomembranous colitis that sometimes follows the administration of antimicrobial agents. Because it may be present in the feces of normal subjects, its demonstration is not necessarily indicative of a pathological condition. Only when the other anaerobes in the intestine are killed or their growth is inhibited by certain antimicrobial agents does *C. difficile* grow in sufficient numbers, and produce a sufficiently great amount of toxin, to cause colitis.

Clostridium novyi

This organism is rarely associated with human infections other than clostridial myonecrosis. Two types can be differentiated either culturally or on the basis of toxin production. Type A strains are much more common than type B strains; the former are the only commonly encountered clostridia that produce both lipase and lecithinase on egg-yolk agar plates. Type B strains, almost unknown in human infections, are among the most sensitive of all clostridia to oxygen. They are primarily a pathogen of sheep.

Clostridium sordellii

This organism is occasionally seen in the clinical laboratory, but most strains isolated from human infections are nonvirulent. Most strains of *C. sordellii* are active producers of urease, which distinguishes them from the non-pathogenic *C. bifermentans*.

References

1. ALPERN RJ and DOWELL VR JR: *Clostridium septicum* infections and malignancy. J Am Med Assoc 209:385–388, 1969
2. ARNON SS, MIDURA TF, CLAY SA, WOOD RM, and CHIN J: Infant botulism. Epidemiological, clinical, and laboratory aspects. J Am Med Assoc 237:1946–1951, 1977
3. BATTY I and WALKER PD: Colonial morphology and fluorescent-labelled antibody staining in the identification of species of the genus *Clostridium*. J. Appl Bacteriol 28:112, 1965
4. BELAND S and ROSSIER E: Isolement et identification de *Clostridium tetani* dans le sol des Cantons de l'Est de la province de Quebec. Can J Microbiol 19:1513–1518, 1973
5. COLLEE JG, RUTTER JM, and WATT B: The significantly viable particle: a study of the subculture of an exacting sporing anaerobe. J Med Microbiol 4:271–288, 1971
6. COLLEE JG, WATT B, FOWLER EB, and BROWN R: An evaluation of the Gaspak system in the culture of anaerobic bacteria. J Appl Bacteriol 35:71–82, 1972
7. DOWELL VR JR and HAWKINS TM: Laboratory Methods in Anaerobic Bacteriology. CDC Laboratory Manual. U.S. Dept. Health, Education, and Welfare, Center for Disease Control, Atlanta, Ga, 1974
8. DOWELL VR JR, HILL EO, and ALTEMEIER WA: Use of phenethyl alcohol in media for isolation of anaerobic bacteria. J Bacteriol 88:1811–1813, 1964
9. DOWELL VR JR, TORRES-ANJEL MJ, RIEMANN HP, MERSON M, WHALEY D, and DARLAND G: A new criterion for implicating *Clostridium perfringens* as the cause of food poisoning. Rev Latino-Am Microbiol 17:137–142, 1975
10. GEORGE RH, SYMONDS JM, DIMOCK F, BROWN JD, ARABI Y, SHINAGAWA N, KEIGHLEY MRB, ALEXANDER-WILLIAMS J, and BURDON DW: Identification of *Clostridium difficile* as a cause of pseudomembranous colitis. Br Med J 1:695–697, 1978
11. GORBACH S, THADEPALLI H, and NORSEN J: Anaerobic microorganisms in intraabdominal infections. *In* Anaerobic Bacteria: Role in Disease. Balows A, DeHaan RM, Guze LB, and Dowell VR Jr (eds.). Charles C Thomas, Springfield, Ill, 1974
12. HARMON SM: Collaborative study of an improved method for the enumeration and confirmation of *Clostridium perfringens* in foods. J Assoc Off Anal Chem 59:606–612, 1976
13. HOLDEMAN LV and MOORE WEC: Anaerobe Laboratory Manual. Virginia Polytechnic Institute and State University Anaerobe Laboratory, Blacksburg, Va, 1975
14. LAWRENCE G and WALKER PD: Pathogenesis of enteritis necroticans in Papua New Guinea. Lancet 1 (7961):125–126, 1976
15. MOSSEL DAA: Enumeration of sulfite reducing clostridia occurring in foods. J Sci Food Agr 10:662–669, 1959
16. PALASUNTHERAM C, BRUCKER DB, and TUXFORD AF: Feasibility of thin-layer chromatography as an inexpensive alternative to gas-liquid chromatography for the identification of some anaerobic gram positive nonsporing rods. J Appl Bacteriol 42:451–453, 1977
17. RIHA WE JR and SOLBERG M: Chemically defined medium for the growth of *Clostridium perfringens*. Appl Microbiol 22:738–739, 1971
18. SMITH L DS: The Pathogenic Anaerobic Bacteria. Charles C Thomas, Springfield, Ill, 1975
19. SMITH L DS: Botulism. The Organism, Its Toxins, the Disease. Charles C Thomas, Springfield, Ill, 1977
20. STERNE M and BATTY I: Pathogenic Clostridia. Butterworths, London, 1975
21. SUTTER VL, VARGO VL, and FINEGOLD SM: Wadsworth Anaerobic Microbiology Manual.

Anaerobic Bacteriology Laboratory, Wadsworth Hospital Center, Los Angeles, Cal, 1975

22. WILLIAMS K and WILLIS AT: A method of performing surface viable counts with *Clostridium tetani*. J. Microbiol 4:639–642, 1970

23. WILLIS AT: Clostridia of wound infection. Butterworths, London, 1969

24. WREN MWD, BALDWIN AWF, ELDON CP, and SANDERSON PJ: The anaerobic culture of clinical specimens: a 14-month study. J Med Microbiol 10:49–61, 1977

CHAPTER 14

ANAEROBIC BACTERIAL INFECTIONS

V. R. Dowell, Jr., and Stephen D. Allen

Introduction

Since the fifth edition of this book was published, procedures for isolating and identifying anaerobes have been simplified, and methods for classifying them have been improved. These advances have made it possible to develop practical systems for identifying anaerobic isolates from clinical materials. As a result of these developments, numerous reports have appeared in the medical literature concerning types of diseases that involve anaerobes, and many clinicians are now requesting the routine performance of appropriate anaerobic bacteriology tests in hospital and public health laboratories.

As discussed elsewhere (61, 68, 88), different authors have defined anaerobic bacteria in various ways. For practical purposes, however, obligately anaerobic bacteria are defined here as those that do not multiply on the surface of nutritionally adequate solid media incubated in air or in a CO_2 incubator (5%–10% CO_2). It is also helpful to group bacteria according to their ability to utilize or tolerate oxygen (as shown in Table 14.1) and to subdivide the obligate anaerobes into moderate and strict groups as described by Loesche (61). Most of the obligate anaerobes associated with human diseases are moderate anaerobes (10, 42, 97, 98). Strict obligate anaerobes are rarely found in properly selected and handled clinical specimens even though these bacteria are components of the normal flora. The anaerobes include all morphologic forms of bacteria—both sporeformers and nonsporeformers. Some are gram-negative and some are gram-positive (Fig 14.1). At least 20 different genera of anaerobes are listed in the eighth edition of *Bergey's Manual of Determinative Bacteriology* (13). In addition, a number of changes in the taxonomic nomenclature of various anaerobes reported in the *International Journal of Systematic Bacteriology* have recently been recommended. These changes will be discussed as appropriate later in this chapter.

Anaerobic bacteria are widely distributed in nature. Their habitats include soil, water (fresh and salt), the food we eat, and the skin and mucous membrane surfaces of humans and other animals; they reside in these sites as part of the normal microbiota. In humans, obligate anaerobes are especially prevalent in the oral cavity and large bowel, where they usually outnumber aerobes and facultative anaerobes. They attach themselves to mucosal epithelial surfaces of the human mouth (40) and are known to associate intimately

TABLE 14.1—DEFINITIONS AND EXAMPLES OF VARIOUS GROUPS OF BACTERIA SEPARATED ON THE BASIS OF THEIR RELATIONSHIP TO OXYGEN*

GROUP	WORKING DEFINITION	EXAMPLE
1. Obligate aerobe	Growth optimal on solid media in room air (use O_2 as electron acceptor in metabolism; unable to generate energy by fermentation).	*Pseudomonas aeruginosa*
2. Facultative anaerobe	Growth under either aerobic or anaerobic conditions on solid media.	*Escherichia coli*
3. Microaerophile	Growth optimal in presence of reduced amounts of oxygen (i.e., in candle jar) but minimal in air (i.e., 21% O_2) or in absence of O_2.	*Campylobacter fetus*
4. Aerotolerant anaerobe	Limited growth on surface of solid media in air or in 5–10% CO_2 but good growth under anaerobic conditions.	*Clostridium tertium*
5. Obligate anaerobe	Will not grow on surface of solid medium (i.e., anaerobe blood agar) in CO_2 incubator (5–10% CO_2) or in room air.	
a. Moderate	Capable of growth at O_2 levels as high as 2–8% (avg. 3%).	*Bacteroides fragilis*
b. Strict	No growth above 0.5% O_2.	*Clostridium haemolyticum*

* Adapted with modifications from McBee et al. (68) and Loesche (61).

with epithelial cells in varous regions of the murine gastrointestinal (GI) tract by attachment or layer formation (16, 17, 84). Localization of microbes within the mucin layers and crypts of Lieberkuhn has been observed in surgical specimens of human colon by histologic methods (75). These microbe-epithelial associations play an important role in the health of an individual and can lead to important pathological consequences when the ecosystem is out of balance (83).

With surgery or other trauma or a tumor arising from a mucosal surface, anaerobes of the normal flora can penetrate the mucosal barrier and enter underlying tissues. Many species of anaerobic bacteria which are members of the normal flora have been identified, and many others await characterization (71), but fortunately only a small number of the latter appear to be associated with disease (7, 20, 21, 52). Some of the more common species of anaerobes indigenous to man and their major endogenous habitats are listed in Table 14.2.

If conditions in the tissues are suitable, anaerobes can invade and multiply in essentially any organ or region of the body (95). According to Gorbach (41), anaerobes of the normal flora have been associated with "90% of intra-abdominal abscess, 95% of the appendiceal abscess, 75% of upper-tract female infections, 90% of aspiration pneumonia, 95% of lung abscess, and 85% of

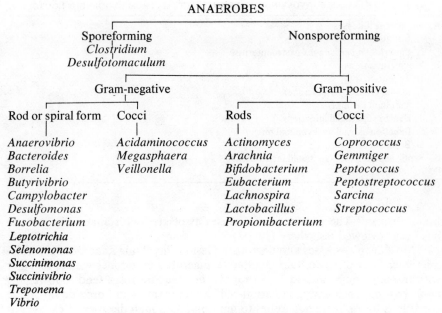

Figure 14.1—Genera of anaerobic bacteria.

TABLE 14.2—MAJOR HABITATS OF ANAEROBES COMMONLY FOUND IN ENDOGENOUS INFECTIONS

SPECIES	ORAL CAVITY	GI TRACT	GU ORIFICES	SKIN
Actinomyces israelii	+			
Arachnia propionica	+			
Bacteroides fragilis group*		+		
Bacteroides melaninogenicus group[†]	+	+	+	
Bifidobacterium eriksonii	+	+	+	
Clostridium perfringens		+		
Clostridium septicum		+		
Eubacterium lentum	+	+		
Fusobacterium nucleatum	+			
Fusobacterium necrophorum	+			
Peptostreptococcus anaerobius	+	+		
Propionibacterium acnes				+

* *Bacteroides fragilis* group includes *B. fragilis*, *B. distasonis*, *B. thetaiotaomicron*, and *B. vulgatus*.

[†] *Bacteroides melaninogenicus* group includes *B. asaccharolyticus* and *B. melaninogenicus* ss *intermedius* (35).

TABLE 14.3—DISEASES INVOLVING ANAEROBIC BACTERIA FROM EXOGENOUS SOURCES

A. Foodborne illnesses
   1. Botulism
   2. *Clostridium perfringens* gastroenteritis
B. Wound infections
   1. Tetanus
   2. Myonecrosis (gas gangrene)
   3. Crepitant cellulitis
   4. Benign superficial infections
   5. Infection caused by an animal bite
   6. Botulism
C. Septic abortion (contaminated instruments)
D. Infant botulism

brain abscess." The incidence of diseases associated with anaerobic bacteria has been reviewed elsewhere (34, 42).

Most deep abscesses and necrotizing lesions involving anaerobes are polymicrobic. They often contain facultative anaerobes or aerobes which, together with trauma, compromised blood supply, or tissue necrosis, tend to lower the tissue oxygen tension and oxidation-reduction potential and provide favorable conditions for obligate anaerobes to multiply. Although diseases of exogenous sources such as botulism and tetanus are certainly significant and are historically well known (Table 14.3), anaerobic infections from endogenous sources (Table 14.4) are far more common.

There are at least two explanations for the rise in the frequency of endogenous anaerobe infections observed in the past decade. Because of improved techniques in anaerobic methodology, many endogenous infections that would have once been misdiagnosed or overlooked are now recognized. Another factor is that more patients are given immunosuppressive drugs and other forms of therapy that compromise host resistance. Infection with anaerobic bacteria commonly occurs in areas where tissue has been damaged, after which bacteremia, tissue invasion with formation of distant tissue abscesses, and an ultimately fatal illness may develop.

In contrast to the time when clostridial infections were in the majority (19), in the 1970's more than 85% of the anaerobes isolated from properly col-

TABLE 14.4—DISEASES INVOLVING ANAEROBIC BACTERIA FROM ENDOGENOUS SOURCES

Abscess of any organ	Myonecrosis (gas gangrene)
Actinomycosis	Necrotizing colitis
Antibiotic-associated colitis	Osteomyelitis
Appendicitis	Otitis media
Cholecystitis	Peritonitis
Crepitant and noncrepitant cellulitis	Thoracic empyema
Dental infections	Septic arthritis
Endocarditis	Sinusitis
Meningitis	Tetanus

TABLE 14.5—DISTRIBUTION OF ANAEROBES ISOLATED FROM HUMAN INFECTIONS AT THE
INDIANA UNIVERSITY MEDICAL CENTER FROM 1972–1978*

GENUS	NUMBER ISOLATED	PERCENTAGE
Bacteroides	3382	39
Fusobacterium	262	3
Peptococcus	1526	18
Peptostreptococcus	443	5
Other cocci	151	2
Gram-positive nonsporeforming bacilli	1944	22
Clostridium	973	11
TOTAL	8681	

* Allen SD, Siders J, and Smith JW, unpublished data.

lected clinical specimens have been nonsporeforming anaerobes. This trend is illustrated in data collected by the Indiana University Medical Center (IUMC) Anaerobe Laboratory (Table 14.5). A number of other clinical laboratories have reported similar results (65, 89, 96).

The most common nonsporeforming gram-negative bacilli associated with human disease include members of the *Bacteroides fragilis* and *B. melaninogenicus* groups and *Fusobacterium nucleatum*. The distribution of species of the *B. fragilis* group isolated from various clinical specimens at IUMC is shown in Table 14.6. These data closely agree with those on *B. fragilis* subspecies referred to the Center for Disease Control (CDC) Anaerobe Section from 1971–1975 (26). The anaerobic bacteria most frequently identified in human clinical materials submitted by laboratories in the United States to the CDC are listed in Table 14.7.

Various other anaerobes are occasionally isolated (23). Some, such as the anaerobic vibrios *Butyrivibrio fibrisolvens, Desulfovibrio desulfuricans,* and *Succinivibrio* spp., have been isolated from specimens from humans only on rare occasions (79, 101), and thus their clinical significance is not known. Detailed information on the clinical significance of anaerobic bacteria has been published elsewhere (34, 42, 88). *B. fragilis* is especially important clinically be-

TABLE 14.6—DISTRIBUTION OF *BACTEROIDES FRAGILIS* SUBSPECIES* ISOLATED FROM CLINICAL
SPECIMENS BY THE INDIANA MEDICAL CENTER ANAEROBE LABORATORY IN 1975

SUBSPECIES	NUMBER	PERCENTAGE
fragilis	203	65
thetaiotaomicron	54	17
vulgatus	16	5
distasonis	14	4
ovatus	1	<1
other (resemble B. fragilis)	25	8
TOTAL	313	

* These former subspecies of B. fragilis now have full species status.

TABLE 14.7—ISOLATES OF ANAEROBIC BACTERIA FROM HUMAN CLINICAL MATERIALS MOST
FREQUENTLY RECEIVED BY THE CDC ANAEROBE SECTION

Clostridium spp.

Clostridium bifermentans	*Clostridium perfringens*
Clostridium butyricum	*Clostridium septicum*
Clostridium cadaveris	*Clostridium sordellii*
Clostridium innocuum	*Clostridium sporogenes*
Clostridium limosum	*Clostridium subterminale*
	Clostridium tertium

Gram-negative bacilli

Bacteroides fragilis	*Bacteroides melaninogenicus* ss *intermedius*
Bacteroides thetaiotaomicron	*Fusobacterium nucleatum*
Bacteroides vulgatus	*Fusobacterium necrophorum*
Bacteroides asaccharolyticus	*Fusobacterium mortiferum*

Gram-positive bacilli

Actinomyces israelii	*Eubacterium alactolyticum*
Actinomyces odontolyticus	*Eubacterium lentum*
Actinomyces naeslundii	*Eubacterium limosum*
Arachnia propionica	*Propionibacterium acnes*
Bifidobacterium eriksonii	*Propionibacterium granulosum*

Gram-positive cocci	Gram-negative cocci
Peptococcus saccharolyticus	*Veillonella parvula*
Peptococcus asaccharolyticus	
Peptococcus prevotii	
Peptrostreptococcus anaerobius	

cause it frequently is isolated from patients with various infections and because it is resistant to various penicillins, tetracyclines, and the aminoglycoside antimicrobics (66, 94). Although *B. fragilis* is the most common species found in clinical specimens, it is the least common member of the *B. fragilis* group found in the feces of North Americans. Holdeman and coworkers (48) found that *B. fragilis* ss *vulgatus (Bacteroides vulgatus,* 14) was the most common (47%) subspecies in the feces of North Americans, followed by intermediate strains (23%), *B. fragilis* ss *thetaiotaomicron (B. thetaiotaomicron)* (17%), *B. fragilis* ss *distasonis (B. distasonis)* (9%), and *B. fragilis* ss *ovatus (B. ovatus)* (3%). The reason for this difference in the frequency of isolation of *B. fragilis* spp. from clinical specimens as compared to fecal samples is not known, but *B. fragilis* may possess virulence factors associated with pathogenicity that the related species (i.e., *B. ovatus)* lack. One group of investigators suggested that the capsule possessed by *B. fragilis* is a unique virulence factor (57, 76) which enables this species to adhere at an infected site (77). On the other hand, Babb and Cummins (6) reported that capsules are not confined to strains of *B. fragilis* and can be detected microscopically by an India ink method in cultures of *B. vulgatus, B. thetaiotaomicron,* and *B. ovatus.*

The steps involved in the laboratory diagnosis of anaerobic bacterial infections include selection, collection, and transport of specimens; gross and direct microscopic examinations; selection of primary isolation media; inoculation of media; use of anaerobic systems; incubation of cultures; inspection and subculture of colonies; presumptive identification and submission of progress reports; antimicrobial susceptibility testing; and definitive identification and submission of the final report (21). The laboratory diagnosis of anaerobic bacterial infections must be properly performed and carefully controlled; otherwise, the laboratory results can mislead the physician and ultimately jeopardize the patient (21). We recommend that laboratories use well-characterized reference cultures of commonly found anaerobes to test the reliability and limitations of their isolation and identification procedures. Once the limitations are known, a system for referring certain anaerobe isolates to a reference laboratory for definitive identification or confirmation should be established. It is unnecessary and unrealistic for all laboratories to attempt to definitively identify all of the anaerobes they isolate. Instead, we recommend that problem cultures be referred to reference laboratories, e.g., the state health department laboratories or the Center for Disease Control, if appropriate, for definitive identification or confirmation. Nonetheless, even smaller hospital laboratories should be capable of isolating anaerobic bacteria in pure culture and presumptively identifying commonly found species. It is essential for hospital laboratory personnel to maintain a close working relationship with the attending physicians and the nursing staff of their institutions. Outlines and information on laboratory services provided by the clinical microbiology laboratory along with detailed instructions on how to properly collect and submit clinical specimens should be made available. It is very important, especially in life-threatening situations, to keep the physician informed throughout the laboratory investigation by telephone calls or by written progress reports; a final report should be submitted when the laboratory tests are completed (21).

Each of the steps in the laboratory diagnosis of anaerobic infections outlined above is discussed in this chapter. Techniques for more detailed characterization of anaerobic isolates along with additional identifying characteristics and tables for identification are available in other publications (23, 49, 95). Procedures for determining the antimicrobial susceptibility of anaerobic bacteria are described in Chapter 44.

Collection of Specimens

The first and probably the most important steps in laboratory diagnosis are collecting and transporting clinical specimens to the laboratory. The samples should be collected from the active site of infection, and precautions must be taken to prevent contamination and aeration of the materials during collection.

Proper Selection of Specimens

With few exceptions, all materials from sites not harboring indigenous microorganisms should be cultured for anaerobic bacteria. Since most anaerobes involved in human infections are normal inhabitants of the oral cavity, gastrointestinal tract, genitourinary orifices, or skin, the following should *not* be routinely cultured anaerobically: (a) throat or nasopharyngeal swabs, (b) sputum or bronchoscopic specimens, (c) feces or rectal swabs, (d) voided or catheterized urine samples, (e) vaginal or cervical swabs (not collected by visualization via a speculum), (f) material from superficial wounds or abscesses not collected properly to exclude surface contaminants, (g) material from abdominal wounds obviously contaminated with feces (e.g., an open intestinal fistula), (h) peritoneal fluid or aspirates taken at the time of emergency or elective abdominal surgery (e.g., repair of knife or gunshot wounds of the abdomen, acute obstruction or infarction of the bowel, etc.) (21).

Skin or mucosal surfaces must be carefully decontaminated if they must be opened to collect samples. Iodine solutions or iodaphores have been suggested as the ideal local antiseptics (18, 39), especially when used in conjunction with alcohol. Many hospitals use tincture of iodine or povidoneiodine (Betadine™) followed by 90% isopropyl alcohol, or vice-versa (8). This technique is also acceptable for preparing phlebotomy sites and other skin surfaces if the iodine is allowed to remain on the skin long enough. Matsen and Ederer (67) recommend at least a 2-min exposure to iodine and alcohol, and Barry (11) recommends a 5-min exposure to iodine for maximum effectiveness.

Suitable Wound and Abscess Specimens

A list of acceptable specimens from various body sites and the methods used for their collection is shown in Table 14.8. The most suitable materials from infected wounds or abscesses are tissue samples and fluid aspirated from the infected area. Swab samples are less satisfactory. Enough material should be collected for microscopic examination, culture studies, and inoculation of animals, if required. In the case of extensive wounds involving large amounts of tissue or multiple lesions, several samples should be taken. If swab samples are obtained, at least two swabs should be used to provide enough material for a complete examination. NEVER ALLOW SWAB SAMPLES TO DRY OUT.

Body Fluids

Body fluids which may yield anaerobes include cerebrospinal fluid, joint fluids, pleural fluid, ascitic fluid, and bile. Aspirated fluid should be placed in a sterile, anaerobic transport tube and centrifuged immediately, and the sediment should be cultured as quickly as possible. It generally is not practical to centrifuge small samples of fluids (i.e., less than 2 ml). Blood samples should be cultured anaerobically as well as aerobically (9, 102). For isolation of anaerobes, 5-10 ml of blood is inoculated into 50-100 ml of liquid media (10% v/v) and the blood cultures are incubated up to 7 days. Several different media which contain 0.025%–0.05% sodium polyanetholsulfonate (SPS) (Liquoid) and an anaerobic or partial CO_2 atmosphere are commercially available. Tryptic (Difco) or Trypticase Soy (BBL) broth, THIOL (Difco), or thioglycollate (BBL) broth and prereduced brain heart infusion broth (Scott) designed for

TABLE 14.8—ACCEPTABLE SPECIMENS FOR ANAEROBIC CULTURE AND METHODS OF
COLLECTION*

SITE	TYPES OF SPECIMENS AND METHODS OF COLLECTION
Central nervous system	Cerebrospinal fluid (especially when turbid); Abscess material; Tissue biopsy.
Dental, ear, nose, throat, and sinuses	Carefully aspirated or biopsied material from oral abscesses after surface decontamination; Needle aspirates and surgical specimens from sinuses in chronic sinusitis.
Pulmonary	Transtracheal aspirate; Percutaneous lung puncture; Thoracotomy specimen; Thoracentesis (pleural fluid).
Abdominal	Paracentesis fluid; Needle and syringe aspiration of deep abscesses; Tissue biopsy; Surgical specimen if not contaminated with intestinal flora; Bile.
Female genital tract	Culdocentesis after decontamination of the vagina; Laparoscopy specimens; Surgical specimens; Endometrial cavity specimen can be obtained with syringe and small plastic catheter after cervical os is decontaminated.
Urinary tract	Suprapubic aspirate of urine.
Bone and joint	Aspirate of joint (in suppurative arthritis); Deep aspirate of drainage material after surgery (e.g., in osteo-myelitis).
Soft tissue	Open wounds—deep aspirate of margin or biopsy of the depths of wound only after careful surface decontamination; Sinus tracts—aspirate by syringe and small plastic catheter after carefully decontaminating skin orifice; Deep abscess, anaerobic cellulitis, infected vascular gangrene, clostridial myonecrosis—needle aspiration after surface de-contamination; Surgical specimens.

*Adapted from Dowell (21), Sutter et al. (95), and Tally et al. (97).

anaerobic blood culture all appear to be equally satisfactory (102, 103). Using
SPS in blood culture media is well-accepted. Although it improves the recovery of certain microorganisms in blood culture (30, 82) an SPS concentration
of 0.025%–0.05% inhibits *Peptostreptococcus anaerobius* (43, 59). However,
SPS inhibition is dependent upon the medium used and can be reversed by the
presence of gelatin (1.2%) (107). Similarly, adding 1.2% gelatin to certain media has been shown to protect *Neisseria meningitidis* from SPS inhibition (31,
80). Although sodium amylosulfate (SAS), another synthetic anticoagulant,
does not inhibit *P. anaerobius* and *N. meningitidis* at a concentration of 0.05%
(59, 80), it is less effective than SPS in neutralizing the bactericidal activity of

human serum (99). Blood cultures should be inspected daily and subcultured to appropriate plating media when there are obvious signs of growth, and blind subcultures should be made after 48 hr and at the end of 5–7 days of incubation (9). In addition to plating on blood agar, it may also be advantageous to subculture to a selective medium which will allow anaerobes in mixed cultures to be detected that might otherwise be overlooked (100).

A bottle of blood culture medium is not a satisfactory transport system for other types of clinical materials. Such an enrichment medium commonly allows fast-growing organisms (e.g., members of the family *Enterobacteriaceae* and *Pseudomonas* spp.) to overgrow anaerobic bacteria and produce misleading results.

Miscellaneous Specimens

Other materials that can be cultured for anaerobes in special situations include vomitus, feces, and foods of various types. In addition, food, serum, and feces specimens may be needed for detecting clostridial toxins. These specimens should always be collected in sterile, covered containers and handled as aseptically as possible to avoid extraneous contamination.

The laboratory diagnosis of foodborne botulism is based on demonstrating botulinal toxin in the serum and the feces of patients as well as in the contaminated food they ingested. This is accomplished by using mice for toxin neutralization tests. It is also useful to culture the feces of patients and food samples for *Clostridium botulinum* (15, 28). Laboratory confirmation of botulism involving an infected wound is made by isolating *C. botulinum* from the wound and by demonstrating botulinal toxin in the patient's serum (15, 23).

The syndrome of infant botulism (5, 72) has usually been confirmed by demonstrating the toxin and/or *C. botulinum* in feces only. So far, of those tested, the serum of only one baby with infant botulism has contained botulinal toxin. Some recent evidence has implicated honey as one possible source of *C. botulinum* for infant botulism (22, 73), but no preformed botulinal toxin has been demonstrated in any food fed to the babies.

When botulism is suspected, serum samples (15–20 ml), stool specimens (50 g), and the suspected food(s) should be collected and sent as soon as possible to a reference laboratory capable of testing for botulism. If infant botulism is suspected, serum (2 ml) and as much passed stool as possible should be collected. At autopsy, samples of serum and intestinal contents (obtained from stomach, small bowel, and colon) should be collected for examination. The Center for Disease Control, Atlanta, Georgia, provides epidemiologic aid and emergency laboratory testing 7 days a week, 24 hr a day (15). To obtain this laboratory service, the attending physician or state epidemiologist must notify CDC in advance so that appropriate action can be taken. During weekdays, the appropriate phone number is (404) 329-3753 (Bureau of Epidemiology), and after 4:30 pm daily and on weekends and holidays, the number is (404) 329-2176.

Methods for Transport of Specimens

Clinical materials to be cultured for anaerobes should be placed in anaerobic transport containers and delivered to the laboratory as soon as possible. Because obligate aerobes and both facultative and obligate anaerobes remain viable under anaerobic conditions, an anaerobic transport container is the only transport system needed when an infection involving obligate anaerobes or obligate anaerobes mixed with aerobes or facultative anaerobes is suspected (36). Satisfactory anaerobe transport containers are widely available from commercial sources, or they can be prepared in the laboratory with a little improvisation. Although in one study (10), a minimal loss of certain anaerobes was shown to occur when relatively large volumes (2 ml or more) of purulent materials were exposed to air for prolonged periods of time (up to 24 hr), viability requirements for other types of specimens may vary. Thus, the maximum time allowable for transporting swabs, surgical specimens, tissue biopsies, and small volumes of fluid samples to the laboratory without loss of viability remains undetermined.

Optimal transport procedures should minimize the following potentially detrimental environmental factors: (a) molecular oxygen, (b) high oxidation-reduction potential (E_h), (c) extremes of pH, (d) lack of moisture, (3) temperature—specimens should be refrigerated if a delay of more than 2 hr is anticipated (70, 95), and (f) overgrowth with aerobes or facultative anaerobes, especially if a significant time elapses before samples are cultured. For the transport of fluid specimens, sterile rubber-stoppered transport vials or tubes containing oxygen-free CO_2 or other oxygen-free gas are commercially available or can be prepared in the laboratory. After any trapped air is carefully expelled into a piece of sterile gauze, specimens aspirated with a needle and syringe can be expelled directly into the transport container. Alternatively, after the air bubbles are removed, the needle can be capped with a butyl rubber stopper, and the syringe itself can be submitted to the laboratory (95). This should be done only if the specimen can be taken to the laboratory immediately and processed without delay. Tissue biopsy specimens should be processed immediately or placed in an anaerobic system for transport to the laboratory. The Anaerobic Culture Set (Marion Scientific Corp, Rockford, IL), which consists of a plastic bag with anaerobic gas generator, catalyst, and indicator, appears quite promising for the transport of tissue specimens. When it is impossible to obtain fluid or tissue, swab samples should be collected and placed in tubes or an anaerobic transport medium such as modified Cary-Blair medium (20, 21, 95, 97) or Port-A-Cul (PAC) medium (BBL, Cockeysville, MD). Helstad and coworkers (46) recently demonstrated excellent recovery of 75 obligate anaerobes from exudates on swabs placed in a modified Cary-Blair medium. The PAC transport tubes and vials were recently evaluated at CDC (70). The number of various obligate anaerobes recovered from simulated swab and fluid specimens was consistently higher from specimens held in the PAC system than from identical specimens exposed to different test conditions. Another type of system recommended by Holdeman and colleagues (49) consists of transport tubes containing oxygen-free CO_2 and a small amount of salts solution with resazurin indicator. Containers of this type (Anaport vials and Anaswab tubes) are commercially available from Scott Laboratories, Fiskville, RI. The laboratory should provide anaerobic transport vials, tubes of transport medium, and instructions for their use to operating rooms, emergency rooms, nursing stations, and other appropriate areas in the hospital. It should also be emphasized that adequate information for identifying specimens and pertinent clinical information must be given on the requisitions accompanying specimens to the laboratory.

Shipment of Specimens for the Detection of Botulinal Toxin and *C. botulinum*

Because botulinal toxins are extremely poisonous, all materials suspected of containing botulinal toxin should be handled *very cautiously*. Only experienced personnel, preferably those immunized with botulinal toxoid, should perform laboratory tests. Food samples in sealed containers should be kept sealed in their original containers, or sterile unbreakable containers should be used. Specimens should be placed in leakproof containers, wrapped with paper or material to cushion them and serve as an absorbent if leaks occur, packed with ice in a second leakproof container, and shipped by the most rapid means available. Serum, gastric contents, feces, and autopsy specimens collected during botulism investigations should be handled in a similar manner. Serum, but not whole blood, is shipped for toxin testing. The receiving laboratory must be notified in advance as to how the specimens are to be shipped, when they should arrive, and of the waybill or shipping number. Additional details related to shipment of a specimen(s) are given in the CDC Laboratory Manual (23). A description of the emergency assistance available as well as information on the epidemiology, diagnosis, and therapy of botulism is provided in the CDC publication *Botulism in the United States, 1899-1977: Handbook for Epidemiologists, Clinicians, and Laboratory Workers, 1979 (15)*.

Bacteriologic Procedures

Microscopic Examination of Clinical Material

The importance of microscopic examination of clinical materials cannot be overemphasized. Direct smears provide information on the cellular characteristics of the specimen and the quantity and morphotypes of microorganisms present. In addition, the direct smear can serve as a quality control measure for the techniques used for isolating and identifying anaerobes. If morphotypes observed in the direct smear were not recovered by culture, isolation procedures may have been defective. A Gram-stained direct smear should be examined from all types of clinical specimens except blood. Phase or bright-field microscopic examination of wet mounts of unstained material is also helpful at times, particularly when "sulfur granules" from patients with actinomycosis are being examined. Acid-fast stains may aid in the presumptive identification of thin branching filaments. *Actinomyces* species are not acid fast with the modified Kinyoun's stain, whereas most strains of *Nocardia asteroides* are (86). Sometimes Giemsa- or Wright-stained smears allow demonstration of bacterial forms that stain poorly with the Gram procedure. Fluorescent antibody (FA) procedures are used routinely by some laboratories for presumptive identification of anaerobes in direct preparations of clinical materials. FA procedures have been used for *C. chauvoei, C. septicum, C. novyi, C. haemolyticum,*

F. necrophorum, A. israelii, A. propionica, and others (26, 86, 88). A polyvalent reagent currently under evaluation at CDC appears promising for direct presumptive identification of *B. fragilis* in clinical specimens.

The information derived from direct microscopic examination must be reported to the attending physician rapidly since it may be 48 hr or longer before anaerobes are detected by culture procedures. The results from microscopic examination of direct smears may be useful in selecting the isolation media to be used (23).

Cultural Procedures

The following procedures are important in the primary isolation of anaerobes: (a) use of nonselective, selective, and enrichment media, (b) use of either fresh media or media that have been reduced under anaerobic conditions, (c) use of a holding jar for uninoculated plates, (d) use of a holding jar immediately after plates are inoculated, (e) incubation in an anaerobic system, and (f) use of a holding jar during inspection and subculture of colonies.

A number of nonselective media for isolating anaerobic bacteria are available. Use of at least the following is recommended for all types of clinical specimens (except blood) regardless of the source: (a) one plate of CDC anaerobe blood agar* incubated anaerobically, (b) one plate of blood agar incubated in a candle extinction jar or a CO_2 incubator, (c) one tube of enriched thioglycollate broth (THIO) incubated anaerobically, and (d) one tube of cooked meat-glucose medium (CMG) incubated anaerobically (20).

Directions for preparing each of these media are given elsewhere (27). CDC anaerobe blood agar contains Trypticase soy agar (BBL) base plus the following: yeast extract, hemin, vitamin K_1, L-cystine, and either sheep or rabbit blood. We have found that this medium supports much better growth of *Fusobacterium necrophorum, Clostridium haemolyticum, Bacteroides melaninogenicus,* certain strains of *Actinomyces israelii,* and *Bacteroides thetaiotaomicron,* and certain thiol-dependent *Streptococcus* species similar to those described by McCarthy and Bottone (69) than does the supplemented rabbit blood Trypticase soy agar (BBL) medium formerly recommended by our laboratory (1, 23). In addition, we have noticed less smooth-to-rough variation of colonies on CDC anaerobe blood agar than that described for colonies on Schaedler blood agar by Starr et al. (93). The plates are wrapped in cellophane bags to retard dehydration and can be stored in a refrigerator (2–4 C) for up to 6 weeks (1, 62). Before they are used, plates are removed from the refrigerator, the agar surface is dried by holding the plates with lids ajar for 5 min at 35 C, and they are held for 4–18 hr in an anaerobic system such as the GasPak (BBL) jar with GasPak generator, an evacuation/replacement jar, or a glove box with an atmosphere of 85% N_2, 5% CO_2, 10% H_2. If the liquid media are not gassed in an anaerobic environment after the autoclaving step as described by Dowell et al. (27), or if they are not prepared by the prereduced, anaerobic-

---

*This medium is prepared as described by Dowell et al. 1977 (27) and is now available commercially (Carr Scarborough Microbiologicals, Inc, Stone Mountain, Ga; Nolan Biologicals, Inc, Tucker, Ga).

ally sterilized (PRAS) technique (49), they should either be held in an anaerobic environment overnight or heated for 10 min in a boiling water bath (to drive off oxygen) and cooled before being inoculated. As currently prepared in our laboratories, the liquid media and some agar media are dispensed in 7-ml quantities into special 15- × 90-mm screwcapped tubes* and autoclaved at 121 C for 15 min. Shelf life is lengthened and the necessity for boiling the medium before use is eliminated by gassing the tubes in an anaerobic glove box after the autoclaving step (27).

The THIO is especially useful for isolating slow-growing, fastidious microorganisms such as *A. israelii*, which may take several days to develop recognizable colonies on solid media. Incubating THIO cultures in an anaerobic system with the caps loosened slightly is recommended to facilitate isolating small numbers of microorganisms which may not grow in the medium if it is incubated in air. If a glove box is used, after the inoculated medium is gassed the caps of the tubes can be tightened, and the tubes placed in a regular incubator. In addition to excluding air, incubation under anaerobic gas (5% CO_2, 10% H_2, 85% N_2) provides sufficient CO_2 to microorganisms which require it.

The CMG medium is an excellent back-up medium and will support the growth of most nonsporeforming anaerobes as well as that of sporeforming anaerobes. It is especially useful for isolating clostridia by a spore-selection procedure [heat or ethanol treatment (60)], for use in identifying clostridial toxins, and as a holding medium for anaerobic cultures. It is also a suitable medium for shipping *Clostridium* cultures to another laboratory if samples are properly packaged in approved mailing containers (23).

Inoculate the primary isolation media as follows:

Fluid specimens—Using a capillary pipette, inoculate the tubes of liquid medium near the bottom with 1 or 2 drops of material. (Capillary pipettes are invaluable for anaerobic culture work). Place 1 drop on each plating medium, and streak with a platinum or stainless steel loop to obtain isolated colonies. Prepare a smear for Gram stain.

Tissue or other solid specimens—Mince with sterile scissors, add sufficient broth such as THIO or buffered gelatin diluent (23) to emulsify the specimen, add sterile sand if necessary, and grind with a sterile mortar and pestle. Treat as described for a liquid specimen above.

Swab samples—Inoculate the liquid media directly with one swab, and use a separate swab to inoculate one-quarter of each plating medium. Streak to obtain isolated colonies as described for liquid specimens. If only one swab is received, prepare a suspension of the material by scrubbing the material from the swab in a small amount of THIO (0.5 ml to 1 ml), and treat as a liquid specimen (23).

In addition to the nonselective media described above, it is advantageous to use selective media for isolating anaerobes when clinical specimens may contain a mixture of microorganisms. The choice of selective media to be used depends on the anatomical source of the specimen and the microscopic appearance of the Gram-stained smear.

Some of the selective media that we have found useful for isolating anaerobes from clinical specimens and the purpose of each are listed in Table 14.9. These include phenethylalcohol blood agar (PEA) (24), kanamycin vancomycin blood agar (KVA) (23, 95), neomycin egg yolk agar (NEYA), and stiff blood agar (Stiff BA) (20, 21). The directions for preparing these media are

---

*Catalog number 949-1040, one-piece white cap, Rochester Scientific Co, Rochester, NY 14624

TABLE 14.9—REPRESENTATIVE SELECTIVE MEDIA FOR ISOLATING ANAEROBIC BACTERIA AND THE PURPOSE OF EACH

MEDIUM	PURPOSE
Phenethylalcohol blood agar	For isolating gram-negative and gram-positive anaerobic bacteria; inhibits facultatively anaerobic gram-negative bacteria such as *Proteus* and other members of the family *Enterobacteriaceae*.
Kanamycin-vancomycin blood agar	For selective isolation of obligately anaerobic gram-negative bacteria (*Bacteroides, Fusobacterium, Veillonella, Acidamincoccus*); essentially all other bacteria found in clinical specimens are inhibited by this medium, including anaerobic gram-positive bacteria.
Neomycin-egg yolk agar	For selective isolation of clostridia and for differentiation of clostridia on the basis of lecithinase or lipase production; inhibits various facultatively anaerobic and obligately anaerobic bacteria.
Stiff blood agar (blood agar prepared with 4%–6% agar instead of the usual 1.5–2.0% agar)	For preventing the swarming of clostridia to allow isolation of clostridia and other microorganisms from mixed cultures.

given in Chapter 46, and each is available commercially (Carr-Scarborough Microbiologicals, Inc, Stone Mountain, Ga; Nolan Biologicals, Inc, Tucker, Ga). Sutter and coworkers described other selective media which are of value in intestinal flora studies (95). Appropriate nonselective media such as anaerobe blood agar should always be used in conjunction with selective media. Examples of the media that are appropriate for clinical specimens from various anatomical sources are given in Table 14.10.

TABLE 14.10—GUIDE FOR SELECTING MEDIA FOR PRIMARY CULTURE OF CLINICAL SPECIMENS FROM VARIOUS ANATOMICAL SOURCES*

SOURCE OF SPECIMEN	AIR	CO_2	ANAEROBIC
Central nervous system	—	BA, CA	BA[†], THIO
Eye, ear, oropharyngeal	MAC	BA, CA, PEA	BA, PEA, THIO
Pulmonary	MAC	BA, CA	BA, PEA, THIO
Intra-abdominal	MAC	BA, PEA, (TM)	BA, PEA, (KV), THIO
Genitourinary	MAC	BA, PEA, TM	BA, PEA, (KV), THIO
Muscle tissue	MAC	BA, PEA	BA, PEA, NEY, CMG
Bone marrow	—	BA, CA	BA, THIO
Miscellaneous body fluids	—	BA, CA	BA, THIO

* Adapted from Dowell (21).
† CDC anaerobe blood agar is recommended for anaerobes.

BA = blood agar.
CA = chocolate agar.
MAC = MacConkey agar.
PEA = phenethylalcohol blood agar.
TM = modified Thayer-Martin medium.

KV = kanamycin-vancomycin blood agar.
NEY = neomycin egg yolk agar.
THIO = enriched thioglycollate medium.
CMG = chopped meat glucose medium.
( ) = optional.

Selective media are also used for enumerating *C. perfringens* in foods and fecal specimens in laboratory investigations of food-poisoning outbreaks (23). Solid plating media used for this purpose include sulfite-polymyxin-sulfadiazine (3), tryptose-sulfite-neomycin (64), Shahidi-Ferguson perfringens (85), tryptose-sulfite-cycloserine agar (TSC) with egg yolk (44), and TSC medium without egg yolk (45). Iron and sulfite ions included in these media permit the detection of sulfite-reducing clostridia which form black colonies, while most other bacteria should either be inhibited or fail to form black colonies. Of the media that have been tested, it appears that TSC agar without egg yolk is best for this purpose (45, 78).

If done properly, treating cultures with heat or alcohol can be useful for isolating sporulating anaerobes for mixed populations. It should be remembered that the spores of various *Clostridium* spp. and strains of the same species vary in their resistance to heat. Not only are the spores of *C. botulinum* type E less heat resistant than those of *C. botulinum* type A, but the spores of the various capsulated types of *C. perfringens* (47) and of other *Clostridium* spp. found in clinical specimens vary considerably in their heat resistance. We recently confirmed that treating specimens with 50% or more ethyl alcohol (23) aids in the selective isolation of sporeforming anaerobes from mixed cultures (60). The alcohol inhibits further growth of vegetative cells but has little effect on the spores. The following procedure, which includes both heat and alcohol treatments, is useful for isolating *Clostridium* spp. from food and feces.

Alcohol treatment

To a 1-ml aliquot of food or fecal suspension in a sterile screwcapped tube, add an equal volume of absolute ethyl alcohol. Incubate the mixture at room temperature for 1 hr with gentle mixing. Remove some of the treated material, and inoculate egg yolk agar and chopped meat-glucose-starch medium (27).

Heat treatment

Heat one tube of reduced (held under anaerobic conditions or heated in a boiling water bath for 10 min) chopped meat-glucose-starch medium in an 80 C water bath for 5 min, and then inoculate it with the sample suspension. Start timing. After 10 min, remove the tube and cool in cold water.

Inoculate an unheated tube of reduced chopped meat-glucose-starch medium and an egg yolk agar plate with untreated sample, and place the egg yolk agar plates under anaerobic conditions as quickly as possible. Also incubate the liquid cultures in an anaerobic system. Incubate plates for at least 2 days and preferably for 3 to 5 days before examining them. Liquid cultures can be examined after 24 hr if growth is evident and can be subcultured at intervals thereafter if necessary.

Anaerobic Systems

Numerous devices have been described for cultivating anaerobic bacteria since the early days of bacteriology (90). The systems most widely used in the United States today are (a) jars (evacuation/replacement and GasPak Jars—BBL), (b) roll-streak tubes with prereduced anaerobically sterilized (PRAS) media, and (c) glove boxes. Killgore et al. (58) and Rosenblatt et al. (81) have shown that jar techniques are comparable to the more sophisticated glove-box and roll-streak tube methods in terms of recovery of anaerobes commonly recovered from properly collected clinical specimens. The choice of which anaerobic systems to use in a clinical microbiology laboratory should be based on the size of the laboratory, availability of laboratory space, specimen workload, cost of the equipment and media, and the technical capabilities of laboratory personnel. Regardless of which system is used, the following are necessary for optimal recovery of anaerobes:

1. proper collection and transport of clinical specimens;
2. processing of specimens with minimal exposure to atmospheric oxygen;
3. use of fresh or properly reduced media;
4. proper use of the anaerobic system with inclusion of an active catalyst to allow effective removal of oxygen.

Anerobic jar techniques

The designs of several different jars (e.g., Brewer, Torbal, and GasPak) are based on the same basic principle to achieve anerobic conditions. Once the jar is sealed, hydrogen is added to the system and in the presence of a catalyst combines with oxygen to form water. The catalyst used with the GasPak system (palladium-coated alumina pellets) is a "cold" catalyst which does not require heating. This is preferable to the palladium catalyst incorporated in the lid of the Brewer jar because the latter requires heating with an electric current to be fully active. "Cold" palladium catalyst is inactivated by hydrogen sulfide and other volatile metabolic products of bacteria. For this reason, we recommend that the catalyst pellets in the lid of the jar be replaced with new or "rejuvenated" pellets each time the jar is used (23). Excessive moisture can reduce the activity of the catalyst. The activity of used catalyst pellets can be restored by heating the pellets in a dry heat oven at 160–170 C for 2 hr. The pellets should be stored at room temperature in a clean, dry container or a desiccator.

Anaerobic conditions can be produced in jar systems with either the evacuation-replacement procedure or with the disposable GasPak hydrogen-carbon dioxide generator (BBL). Both techniques are effective, but the evacuation-replacement procedure is more economical than gas generators, and evacuation of the jar allows anaerobic conditions to be established more rapidly. Any air-tight container (e.g., a GasPak jar with vented lid, a Brewer jar, a Torbal jar, a desiccator, or even a modified pressure cooker) can be used for the evacuation-replacement procedure if a situable gas mixture is used (e.g., 85% N_2, 10% H_2, 5% CO_2) and enough active catalyst pellets are included in the container (23).

An inexpensive device for evacuating and gassing anaerobic systems has recently been described by Whaley and Gorman (104) (Fig 14.2). The device can be used with in-house vacuum and eliminates the need for a vacuum pump during the evacuation-replacement procedure. The procedure is performed as follows:

(a) Remove the used catalyst from the lid of the jar and replace with an equal quantity of new or rejuvenated pellets.

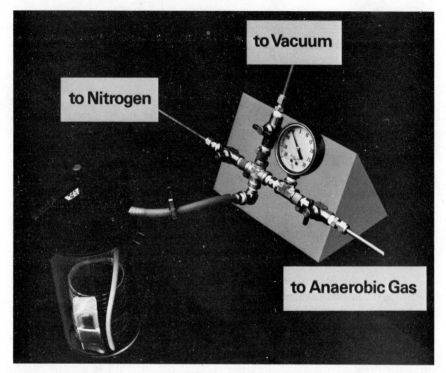

Figure 14.2—Simple set-up for evacuation and replacement procedure in which a
house vacuum is used (104).

(b) Place materials to be incubated inside the jar. Loosen caps of tubes to allow exchange of gasses.

(c) Place in the jar either a methylene blue indicator strip (BBL) or a 15 × 125-mm test
tube containing a few milliliters of methylene blue-NAHCO$_3$-glucose mixture (23).

(d) Fasten a vented lid to the jar with a clamp.

(e) Connect outlet on the jar lid to the evacuation-replacement device as is illustrated
in Figure 14.2.

(f) Evaculate to 20–24 inches (about 50.8 to 60.96 cm) of mercury, and fill the jar with
nitrogen. Repeat this cycle.

(g) Purge the container a third time as before, but this time fill the jar with the gas
mixture (5% CO_2, 10% H_2, 85% N_2).

(h) Clamp the rubber tubing attached to the vent of the jar.

(i) Disconnect the jar from the vacuum gas assembly.

(j) Place jar in the incubator.

The disposable GasPak H_2 and CO_2 generator procedure is done as follows:

(a) Activate the generator envelope by adding 10 ml of water to it. This should result
in the release of H_2 from a tablet containing sodium borohydride and CO_2 from one containing sodium citrate-bicarbonate.

(b) Place the generator in the jar with the inoculated plates and methylene blue indicator.

(c) Seal the lid containing fresh or rejuvenated catalyst. If the lid is not warm within a few minutes, or if condensation does not appear on the inside surface of the jar within 30 min after the generator and jar system have been activated, do not use the jar as set up. Terminate the reaction by opening the jar and discarding the generator. Check the jar and activate another GasPak generator. The three most common causes of GasPak jar failure are failure to include active catalyst, a faulty or defective gas generator, and a poor-sealing gasket which allows escape of gas and influx of ambient air. If the lid and gasket are in good condition, discard the catalyst pellets, and replace with a full bag of new or rejuvenated catalyst (2.5 ± 0.5 g).

An oxidation-reduction potential indicator should always be included in the anaerobic system. One of the simplest and most reliable can be prepared by mixing 400 g of sodium bicarbonate, 100 g of glucose, and a trace of methylene blue chloride (23). Place this mixture to a depth of 0.5 inch in a 15- × 125-mm test tube. Fill the tube to half volume with water, mix by inverting, and place the tube in the jar. The disposable indicator strips (BBL) are also quite satisfactory. The indicator is light blue when oxidized and colorless when reduced. It may take several hours for the indicator to become colorless, but once reduced it should remain colorless as long as the system is anaerobic. It is also wise to check anerobic systems periodically with strict obligate anerobes such as *C. haemolyticum* or *C. novyi* type B. Assure that the medium used for testing the anaerobic system will support the growth of these bacteria. The CDC anerobe blood agar supports good growth of both. The GasPak jar with GasPak generator, when functioning properly, will contain less than 1% oxygen within 30 min after the lid is sealed.

Anerobic glove box

In our experience, the flexible anaerobic glove box developed by Freter and associates at the University of Michigan (4) with certain modifications (23, 56) is a practical, convenient, excellent system for cultivating anaerobic bacteria. This system is now commercially available in various sizes (Coy Manufacturing Co, Ann Arbor, Mich). A number of other companies have recently marketed anerobic glove box systems of various configurations and designs. However, at this writing we are not aware of any published evaluations of any of these new chambers. Detailed instructions for using flexible anaerobic glove boxes are available elsewhere (23, 26).

The roll-streak system

The third major type of anaerobic system was developed by Moore and colleagues at the Anaerobe Laboratory, Virginia Polytechnic Institute and State University (49, 51). This system was modified from the roll-tube technique originally developed by Hungate and associates (53) for culturing anaerobes from ruminants. For the roll-streak system, PRAS media prepared in tubes with butyl rubber stoppers are used. The constituents of these media are combined, boiled to remove dissolved air, and then tubed, autoclaved, and stored in the butyl rubber-stoppered tubes under oxygen-free gas (49). After they are autoclaved, the tubes of PRAS agar media are cooled and allowed to solidify on a rolling machine so that the inner surfaces of the tubes will be coated with the solidified medium. These are the so-called roll-streak tubes. Both the roll-streak agar media and the PRAS liquid media require the addition of a reducing agent (i.e., L-cysteine-hydrochloride) before being sterilize'd. This agent aids in maintaining a low oxidation-reduction potential. Both the liquid and solid PRAS media are inoculated and subcultured in a stream of oxygen-free CO_2 with the aid of a "VPI" inoculating device or a similar apparatus. This device is available commercially (Bellco Glass Corporation, Vineland, NJ). Those interested in further details on the use of the roll-streak system should consult the laboratory manual by Holdeman et al. (49). Both the anaerboic glove box and roll-streak systems have a major advantage over jar techniques; i.e., each of the systems allows inspection and subculture of colonies at any time without exposing the anaerobes to excessive amounts of atmospheric oxygen.

Holding Jar Procedure

After plates of agar media are inoculated, they must not be exposed to ambient air any longer than necessary. If jars are the only anaerobic systems used in the laboratory, we recommend placing the plates in a jar and initiating anaerobic conditions immediately after they are inoculated. However, this is usually not practical in a busy clinical laboratory because specimens for anaerobic culture arrive at various times during the day, and a large number of jars would be required to handle the workload. An alternative approach is to use a holding jar to minimize exposure of inoculated plates to air until there are enough plates to fill a regular jar for anaerobic incubation.

The following modification of the Martin holding jar procedure (65) is an extremely convenient and inexpensive system which allows primary plating, inspection of cultures, and subculture of colonies at the bench with minimal exposure of anaerobic bacteria to oxygen (1). The jars are assembled as illustrated in Figure 14.3. It is convenient to use three holding jars—one to hold reduced uninoculated media, a second for plates containing colonies to be subcultured, and a third for freshly streaked plates of media. The following is a brief description of the modified holding jar procedure:

(a) Use either commercially prepared agar plates or agar media that have been freshly prepared in the laboratory. CDC anaerobe blood agar can be held up to 6 weeks in the refrigerator and gives good quantitative recovery of anaerobes if the plates are packaged in cellophane bags.

(b) Hold the plates to be used during the work day in an anaerobic glove box or an anaerobic jar for 6 to 24 hr before inoculating them.

(c) As needed, place the reduced media in a holding jar, and continuously flush with a gentle stream of nitrogen.

(d) Surface inoculate the plates of reduced media in ambient air. Immediately after they are streaked, place the plates in a second holding jar which is also flushed with nitrogen. Use a third holding jar flushed with nitrogen for any plates containing colonies for subculture which were removed from anaerobic jars after incubation.

(e) As soon as a jar is filled with freshly inoculated plates, seal with a conventional lid (e.g., GasPak), activate the system to produce anaerobic conditions, and incubate at 35 C.

Studies in our laboratory (1) indicate that inexpensive commercial grade nitrogen can be used in the holding jar system. The flow of gas to the holding jars is begun with an initial 20- to 30-sec flush with the regulator on the gas tank set at approximately 4 lb/in^2, followed by a decrease in the flow rate to 1–2 bubbles per second as measured by holding the rubber tubing just under the surface of water in a small beaker. This is equivalent to a flow of 0.25 ft^2/hr or

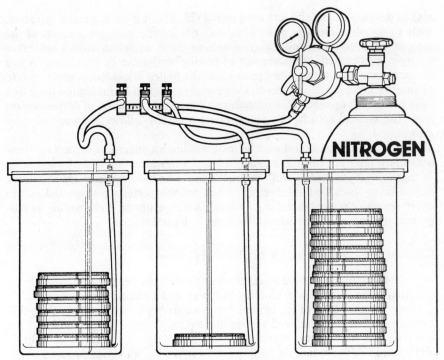

Figure 14.3—Schematic representation of a holding jar system with three jars which are continuously flushed with a gentle stream of nitrogen to minimize exposure of anaerobes to air during and after inspection and subculture of plates.

50–100 cc/min, as measured with a flow meter (Dwyer Co, Michigan City, Ind). It is convenient to regulate the flow of gas to each jar with needle valves of a gang valve with four outlets (commercially available where aquarium supplies are sold). CO_2 passed through a tube of heated copper (Sargeant Furnace) can be used in the holding jars instead of nitrogen (65).

Incubation of Cultures

The most suitable temperature range for cultivating most anaerobic bacteria from clinical specimens is 35–37 C. Enrichment cultures of *C. botulinum* should be incubated at 30 C, particularly if tests for toxin are to be done, since some cultures of *C. botulinum* (e.g., type E strains) may not produce detectable amounts of toxin at higher incubation temperatures (23). *C. perfringens* grows most rapidly at temperatures between 42 and 47 C (64), and incubation of enrichment cultures at a temperature within this range is useful for selective isolation of *C. perfringens* (23). *C. perfringens* grows well in chopped meat glucose medium or thioglycollate broth within 4 to 6 hr when cultures are incubated at 46 C.

Plating media inoculated at the bench and incubated in anaerobic jars should be incubated for at least 48 hr and preferably 72 to 96 hr to allow colonies to develop before the jars are opened (23, 91). If a jar is opened too soon, some of the slow-growing anaerobes may not initiate colonies because of the oxygen exposure. In emergency situations such as when clostridial myonecrosis is suspected, duplicate sets of plating media can be incubated in two different jars. One jar can be opened and the plates inspected as early as 6 to 18 hr after inoculation. However, the second jar should be incubated for 2 to 5 days before it is opened. This procedure allows rapid isolation of *C. perfringens* from the clinical setting of gas gangrene and also allows recovery of slow growers.

Liquid cultures should also be incubated in an anaerobic system to allow maximum recovery of obligate anaerobes. Unless growth is visually apparent in them, THIO or CMG broth cultures should be held a minimum of 1 week before being discarded as negative. When actinomycetes are suspected and in other special circumstances, e.g., when osteomyelitis or endocarditis is suspected, the broth cultures should be held at least 2 weeks.

Colonial Observations and Subculture of Colonies

After incubation under anaerobic conditions, the next step in the primary isolation of anaerobes is examining colonies and isolating pure cultures. If a GasPak or other type of jar is used for incubating plates, the colonies should be examined and subcultured as rapidly as possible after being removed from the jar. This necessitates planning ahead in order to have tubes of reduced THIO and CMG media and plating media available for subcultures when the jars are opened. Only one anaerobic jar should be opened at a time. If available, either an anaerobic glove box or a VPI roll-streak system is ideal for subculture, because both allow inspection and subculture of colonies in the absence of air. If neither is available, a holding jar system as described above can be used.

Examine the plate cultures as follows:

(a) Inspect the colonies with a hand lens and a dissecting microscope by reflected and transmitted light to determine the number of different colony types.

(b) Record the distinctive features of each colony—i.e., the size, shape, elevation, edge, consistency, color, etc.—as described by Dowell and Hawkins (23). Also record hemolysis, fluorescence under ultraviolet light, and reactions on egg yolk-containing media if used.

(c) Using a straight inoculating needle or a sterile Pasteur capillary pipette, transfer each different colony to another anaerobe blood agar plate, and streak to obtain a pure culture. If colonies are well separated on the primary isolation plate, inoculate a tube of enrichment broth such as THIO or CMG to provide a source of inoculum for differential tests and aerotolerance studies to be described below. Chopped meat-glucose is preferred for cultivating clostridia, and the THIO is more suitable for the nonsporulating anaerobes.

(d) If possible, prepare and examine a Gram-stained smear from each colony selected, or examine the morphology of organisms from colonies on the subculture plates. Also examine Gram-stained preparations of the THIO and CMG subcultures.

(e) Incubate the CMG and THIO cultures in an anaerobic jar for 24 to 48 hr. Additional incubation time may be required for some slow-growing, fastidious anaerobes.

(f) If the colonies on the subculture plates are pure as determined with Gram-stained smears and if the THIO or CMG cultures are determined to be pure, use the liquid cultures as a source of inoculum for differential media.

Examine the THIO and CMG enrichment cultures that were inoculated with the original specimen along with the primary isolation plates. If no growth is seen on the primary anaerobic plates or if the colonies isolated fail to account for all the morphologic forms found in the direct Gram-stained smear of the specimen, subculture each broth medium to anaerobe blood agar plates to be incubated anaerobically and to blood agar plates for anaerobic CO_2 incubation. These subculture plates should then be examined as described above.

NOTE: Although the morphology and colony characteristics of some anaerobes are distinctive, some facultative anaerobes often cannot be distinguished from obligate anaerobes without performing aerotolerance tests, even when the CO_2-incubated primary isolation plates show no growth. Therefore a representative of each different colony type must be checked for its relationship to oxygen as described in the next section.

Relationship to Oxygen

The oxygen tolerance of each colony type appearing on anaerobic agar media should be tested by comparing the ability of the microorganisms to multiply on the surface of an agar medium in air, a candle extinction jar or a CO_2 incubator, and an anaerobic system. Aerobic blood agar should be used for air and elevated CO_2 environments and anaerobe blood agar for the anaerobic system. Four to six isolates can be tested on one plate of medium for each atmosphere by streaking only one-fourth or one-sixth of the medium's surface with each. Inoculated plates should be incubated at 35 C for at least 24 hr. The relationship to oxygen can be recorded as obligate anaerobe, aerotolerant anaerobe, microaerophile, or facultative anaerobe as illustrated in Table 14.11. At this point (in a clinical microbiology laboratory), it is worthwhile to send the physician a preliminary culture report describing the microscopic features, Gram reaction, colony characteristics, and relationship to oxygen of the bacteria isolated from the clinical specimen. In some cases, since the microscopic and colony characteristics of certain anaerobes (e.g., *B. fragilis, B. ureolyticus, B. melaninogenicus* group, *F. nucleatum,* and *C. perfringens*) are quite distinctive, it is possible to presumptively identify the organism(s) as well.

Determination of Cultural and Biochemical Characteristics for Identification of Pure Culture Isolates

Characterization

Various characteristics have been used as the basis for the taxonomic classification of anaerobic bacteria. These have included cellular and sub-

TABLE 14.11—GROUPING OF BACTERIA ON THE BASIS OF THEIR RELATIONSHIP TO OXYGEN

	RELATIVE GROWTH* ON BLOOD AGAR IN:		
GROUP	AIR	CO₂ INCUBATOR	ANAEROBIC SYSTEM
Obligate aerobe	4+	2+	± or −
Facultative anaerobe	4+	4+	4+
Microaerophile	± or 1+	4+	± or 1+
Aerotolerant anaerobe	1+	1+	4+
Obligate anaerobe	−	−	4+

* Relative growth usually exhibited by various organisms of each group (4+ = best growth, ± = poor growth, − = no growth).

cellular morphologic features, colony characteristics, relationship to oxygen, various physiological activities, cellular constituents and metabolic products detected by gas liquid chromatography, deoxyribonucleic acid (DNA) guanine + cytosine composition (% G + C) and homology with DNA of other microorganisms, antigenic composition, toxin production, and pathogenicity for laboratory animals (13, 14, 23, 49, 95). Although most of these characteristics and others have been useful in characterization studies, a number of them are impractical for use in identifying clinical isolates.

Identification

The following are characteristics used routinely in the Anaerobe Reference Laboratory at the CDC for definitive identification of anaerobes received from public health laboratories:

Microscopic features—Gram reaction, morphology, cell arrangement, spores, motility, flagella, capsules.

Colony characteristics and hemolysis on blood agar—size, shape, elevation, opacity, margin, consistency, color of colonies, hemolysis of animal erythrocytes (rabbit, sheep, ox, horse).

Oxygen tolerance—ability to multiply on blood agar in air, candle extinction jar, and anaerobic environment.

Growth in enriched thioglycollate broth (THIO)—rapidity of growth, gas production, discoloration, odor, etc.

Fermentation of carbohydrates in CHO carbohydrate media—glucose, mannitol, lactose, sucrose, maltose, salicin, glycerol, xylose, arabinose, rhamnose, trehalose.

Hydrolysis of—casein (milk media), gelatin (Thiogel), esculin (broth and agar), starch (broth and agar).

Production of—indole [indole-nitrite medium and Lombard Dowell (LD) agar], H_2S (H_2S medium and LD esculin agar), catalase (LD esculin agar and LD agar), urease (urea semi-solid medium).

Reactions on egg yolk agar—lecithinase, lipase, proteolysis (modified McClung Toabe and LD egg yolk agar).

Growth on LD bile agar—degree of growth, precipitate in medium.

Acid metabolic products in PYG medium—volatile and nonvolatile acids detected in 48-hr PYG cultures with gas liquid chromatography.

Toxin and toxin neutralization tests—toxins produced in chopped meat glucose (CMG) or chopped meat glucose starch (CMGS) medium as detected in mouse toxin assay and mouse toxin neutralization tests with specific clostridial antitoxins.

Pathogenicity for guinea pigs—pathologic changes resulting from intramuscular inoculation (0.5 ml) of a live CMG culture mixed with sterile 10% calcium chloride (1:1).

Detailed instructions for determining the various differential characteristics used for definitive identification of anaerobes are given by Dowell and Hawkins (23) and by Dowell and Lombard (25). Preparation and storage of the various media required for characterization and identification of anaerobes at CDC are described by Dowell, Lombard, Thompson, and Armfield (27), and the more commonly used media are described elsewhere in this volume. Techniques in which PRAS differential media are used in the characterization and identification of anaerobes are described by Holdeman, Cato, and Moore (49) and Sutter, Vargo, and Finegold (95).

Alternative procedures, including commercially manufactured microsystems (Analytab Products, Inc, Plainview, NY; BBL Microbiology Systems, Cockeysville, Md), which can be used in identifying and biotyping anaerobic bacteria are reviewed by Stargel, Lombard, and Dowell (92) and Dowell et al. (26).

Identification of Anaerobic Bacteria

Sporeforming Bacilli–the Genus *Clostridium*

Practical techniques for isolating and identifying clostridia pathogenic for humans and those commonly found in human clinical materials are described in Chapter 13.

Nonsporeforming Anaerobes

Identification of the nonsporeforming anaerobes is presented in three parts: (a) anaerobic, nonsporeforming gram-negative bacilli, (b) anaerobic, nonsporeforming gram-positive bacilli, and (c) anaerobic cocci.

Anaerobic, nonsporeforming gram-negative bacilli

As shown in Figure 14.1, the rod- and spiral-shaped, gram-negative anaerobes are presently classified in 13 genera (13, 49). Some of the key characteristics for differentiating them are shown in Figure 14.4. It was mentioned previously that only certain members of the genera *Bacteroides* and *Fusobacterium* are commonly isolated from properly collected clinical materials associated with disease in humans. However, we do not intend to imply that members of the other genera cannot be pathogenic for humans under certain circumstances. For example, *Butyrivibrio fibrisolvens,* a normal inhabitant of ruminants, was implicated in an unusual case of endophthalmitis after a farmer's eye was injured by barbed wire (101).

Some key characteristics for identifying the *Bacteroides* and *Fusobacterium* species commonly isolated from human clinical materials are presented in Table 14.12. The selection of these characteristics to aid in identifying the common bacteroides and fusobacteria is based on tests described in the CDC laboratory manual (23) and on new procedures developed during the last few years by Lombard and associates at CDC (25, 27, 92), and by Lombard, Dowell, Thompson, and Armfield (unpublished data). Media required to test an anaerobe isolate for these characteristics include two anaerobe blood agar plates, one Presumpto quadrant plate (LD agar, LD egg yolk agar, LD bile agar, LD esculin agar), one tube of PYG or LD glucose broth, and one tube of urea semisolid medium.

I. Nonmotile or peritrichous flagella if motile:
    A. Butyric acid is a major metabolic product; succinic
        acid is not produced.   *Fusobacterium*
    B. Lactic acid is usually the only major product.   *Leptotrichia*
                                                                        (L. buccalis)
    C. Produces acetic acid and hydrogen sulfide and reduces
        sulfate.   *Desulfomonas*
    D. No butyric acid produced in absence of iso acids; pro-
        duces succinic acid.   *Bacteroides*
II. Polar flagella:
    A. Asaccharolytic.
        1. Produces succinic acid from fumarate.   *Vibrio*
                                                                        (V. succinogenes)
        2. Does not produce succinic acid from fumarate.   *Campylobacter*
    B. Saccharolytic.
        1. Produces butyric acid.   *Butyrivibrio*
        2. Produces succinic acid.
           (a) Spiral-shaped cells.   *Succinivibrio*
           (b) Ovoid cells.   *Succinimonas*
        3. Produces acetic and propionic acids.   *Anaerovibrio*
III. Tufts of flagella on concave side of crescent-shaped cells.   *Selenomonas*
IV. Spiral forms with axial filaments.   *Borrelia* and
                                                                        Treponema

Figure 14.4—Differentiation of anaerobic, nonsporeforming gram-negative bacilli. Adapted with modification from Holdeman, Cato, and Moore (49) and Dowell and Hawkins (23).

    The anaerobe blood agar allows observation of the purity of the isolate, its Gram reaction and morphologic features, colony characteristics, fluorescence with ultraviolet light, pigmentation of colonies, pitting of colonies, reduction of nitrate (disk technique, 106), and growth in the presence of penicillin (2-unit disk), rifampin (15-μg disk), and kanamycin (1-mg disk). Indole, lipase, lecithinase, proteolysis of egg yolk, esculin hydrolysis, catalase, H_2S, growth on bile agar, and formation of a precipitate in bile agar can all be determined with one Presumpto quadrant plate (25). The tube of PYG or LD glucose broth is used in detecting fermentation of glucose (compare the pH of 48-hr culture with that of an uninoculated tube of medium by measuring with a pH meter or a pH indicator such as bromthymol blue solution) and in analyzing for acid metabolic products with gas liquid chromatography (23). The urea medium (27) is used to test for urease production. If urea is hydrolyzed, ammonia is released, the pH of the medium is elevated, and the medium turns bright red (23). The above media are inoculated with a young (18–24 hr preferably) THIO or CMG culture of the isolate as follows:

    1. Place 1 or 2 drops of broth culture on each quadrant of the Presumpto plate and streak about three-fourths of the medium with a capillary pipette.

    2. Place a sterile, blank paper disk, one-fourth inch in diameter, on the LD agar near the outer periphery of the quadrant. This disk is used in the test for indole after the plates are incubated.

3. Evenly inoculate the surface of one anaerobe blood agar plate with a sterile swab which has been dipped in the broth culture.

4. Place the antibiotic disks (penicillin 2 units, rifampin 15 µg, kanamycin 1 mg) on the blood agar with sterile forceps. (Blank disks and the antibiotic disks are available from BBL, Cockeysville, Md.) Evenly space the disks so zones of inhibition will not overlap.

5. Inoculate the second plate of anaerobe blood agar with 1 drop of broth culture, and streak with an inoculating loop to allow development of isolated colonies. Place a nitrate disk (106) on the first quadrant of the plate with sterile forceps.

6. Inoculate the PYG (or LD glucose) and the urea medium each with 1 to 2 drops of the broth culture near the bottom of the medium with a capillary pipette (23). Incubate all of the media, plates, and tubes in an anaerobic system such as an anaerobic glove box or an anaerobic jar (e.g., GasPak jar) at 35 C for 48 hr, or tighten caps of tubes in glove box and remove to regular incubator.

After incubation observe and record results as follows:

Presumpto plate.

(a) *LD agar.* Note and record degree of growth. Test for indole by adding 2 drops of paradimethylaminocinammaldehyde reagent (95) to the blank disk on the LD medium quadrant. Observe for the development of a blue or bluish-green color in the disk within 30 sec, which indicates a positive reaction for indole. Development of another color (pink, red, violet) or no color is negative for indole.

(b) *LD egg yolk agar.* Formation of a zone of insoluble precipitate in the medium around the bacterial growth is a positive reaction for lecithinase production. This zone is best seen with transmitted light. The presence of an iridescent sheen or "pearly layer" on the surface of bacterial growth and the medium immediately surrounding it (best demonstrated with reflected light) is indicative of lipase production. Clearing of the medium in the vicinity of the bacterial growth indicates proteolysis, as exhibited by some proteolytic clostridia.

(c) *LD esculin agar.* A positive result for esculin hydrolysis is indicated by the development of a reddish-brown to dark-brown coloration of the medium surrounding the bacterial growth after exposure of the Presumpto plates to air for at least 5 min. Further evidence for esculin hydrolysis can be obtained by examining the esculin agar quadrant under a Wood's lamp. Esculin agar fluoresces bright blue under the ultraviolet light; this color is not present after the esculin is hydrolyzed. Blackening of the bacterial colonies on esculin agar is indicative of H_2S production. Because the blackening dissipates rapidly after the colonies are exposed to air, the esculin agar quadrant should be observed for blackening of colonies under anaerobic conditions (e.g., in an anaerobic glove box) or immediately after anaerobic jars are opened in air. To test for degradation of hydrogen peroxide as an indication of catalase, the Presumpto plate should be exposed to air for at least 30 min, and the esculin agar quadrant should be flooded with a few drops of fresh, 3% hydrogen peroxide. Sustained bubbling after addition of the H_2O_2 is interpreted as a positive reaction for catalase. In some cases, rapid bubbling may not be evident until 30 sec to 1 min after H_2O_2 is added.

TABLE 14.12—SOME KEY DIFFERENTIAL CHARACTERISTICS OF ANAEROBIC NONSPOREFORMING GRAM-NEGATIVE BACILLI COMMONLY ISOLATED FROM HUMAN CLINICAL MATERIALS

| | COLONIES ON ANAEROBE BLOOD AGAR: | | | GROWTH IN PRESENCE OF: | | | | |
| | FLUO-RESCE RED WITH UV LIGHT* | BROWN TO BLACK[†] | PIT-TED | PENI-CILLIN (2-U DISK) | RIF-AMPIN (15-μG DISK) | KANA-MYCIN (1-MG DISK) | IN-DOLE (LD AGAR) | LI-PASE (LD EYA) |
SPECIES								
Bacteroides distasonis	−	−	−	R	S	R	−	−
Bacteroides fragilis	−	−	−	R	S	R	−	−
Bacteroides thetaiotaomicron	−	−	−	R	S	R	+	−
Bacteroides vulgatus	−	−	−	R	S	R	−	−
Bacteroides asaccharolyticus	+	+	−	S	S	R	+	−
Bacteroides melaninogenicus ss intermedius	+	+	−	S	S	R	+	−[+]
Bacteroides ureolyticus	−	−	+	S	S	S	−	−
Bacteroides CDC F1	−	−	−	S	S	S	−	−
Bacteroides CDC F2	−	−	−	S	S	S	−	−
Fusobacterium mortiferum	−	−	−	R or S	R	S	−	−
Fusobacterium necrophorum	−	−	−	S	S	S	+	+
Fusobacterium nucleatum	−	−	−	S	S	S	+	−
Fusobacterium varium	−	−	−	R or S	R	S	+[−]	−

* Young colonies fluoresce red under long UV light, e.g., Wood's lamp.
[†] Older colonies turn brown to black.
R = growth not inhibited.
S = growth inhibited.
LD = Lombard Dowell.
V = variable reaction.
Superscript = reaction obtained with 11%–25% of strains tested.
+ = positive reaction in 90%–100% of strains tested.
− = negative reaction in 90%–100% of strains tested.
E = growth equal to or greater than growth on LD agar.

TABLE 14.12—Continued

ESCULIN HYDROL. (LD ESCULIN)	CATALASE (LD ESCULIN)	H_2S (LD ESCULIN)	GROWTH ON LD BILE AGAR	PRECIPITATE IN LD BILE AGAR	GLUCOSE FERMENTED	NO_3 REDUCTION	UREASE	GLC ANALYSIS: PYG (48 HR, 35 C)	
								VOLATILE	NONVOLATILE
+	+	−	E	−	+	−	−	A,(P),(IV)	L,S
+	+	−	E	V	+	−	−	A,(P),(IB),(IV)	L,S
+	V	−	E	−	+	−	−	A,(P),(IB),(IV)	L,S
−⁺	−⁺	−	E	−	+	−	−	A,(P),(IB),(IV)	L,S
−	−	−	E or I	−	−	−	−⁺	A,P,IB,B,IV	—
−	−	−	I	−	+	−	−⁺	A,(IB),(IV)	S
−	−	−	I	−	−	+	+	A	S
−	−	−	I	−	−	−	−	A	(S)
−	−	−	I	−	−	+	−	A	(S)
+	−	+	E	−	+	−	−	A,(P),B	—
−	−	+	I	−	+	−	−	A,P,B	—
−	−	−	I	−	+⁻	−	−	A,P,B	—
−	−	+	E	−	+	−	−	A,P,B	—

I = growth inhibited as compared to LD agar.
GLC = gas liquid chromatography.
A = acetic acid.
B = butyric acid.
P = propionic acid.
( )= variable.
IV= isovaleric acid.
L = lactic acid.
S = succinic acid.
IB= isobutyric acid.

TABLE 14.13—ADDITIONAL DIFFERENTIAL CHARACTERISTICS OF *BACTEROIDES* SPP.

Species	Fluoresce Red with UV Light[a]	Brown to Black Colonies[b]	Pitted Colonies[b]	Growth Inhibited by Bile	Catalase LD Esculin Agar	Esculin Hydrol.	Gelatin Hydrol.	Starch Hydrol.	NO₃ Reduction	Indole
B. distasonis	−	−	−	−	+	+	−	V	−	−
B. fragilis	−	−	−	−	+	+	−	V	−	−
B. ovatus	−	−	−	−	+	+	−	V	−	+
B. thetaiota-omicron	−	−	−	−	V	+	−	V	−	+
B. vulgatus	−	−	−	−	−⁺	−⁺	−	V	−	−
B. oralis	−	−	−	+	−	+	−	+	−	−
B. melanino-genicus ss melanino-genicus	+	+⁻	−	+	−	+	+	+	−	−
B. melanino-genicus ss intermedius	+	+	−	+	−	−	+	+⁻	−	+
B. bivius	−	−	−	+	−	−	+	+	−	−
B. disiens	−	−	−	+	−	−	+	+	−	−
B. pneumo-sintes	−	−	−	+	−	−	−	−	−	−
B. asaccha-rolyticus[d]	+	+	−	V	−	−	+	−	−	+
B. ureo-lyticus[e]	−	−	+	+	−	−	−	−	+	−
CDC F-1	−	−	−	+	−	−	−	−	−	−
CDC F-2	−	−	−	+	−	−	−	−	+	−

TABLE 14.13—Continued

GLUCOSE	MANNITOL	LACTOSE	SUCROSE	MALTOSE	SALICIN	XYLOSE	ARABINOSE	TREHALOSE	RHAMNOSE	VOLATILE	NON-VOLATILE	OTHER[c]
+	–	+	+	+	V	+⁻	–⁺	+	V	A,(P),(IV)	L,S	
+	–	+	+	+	–	+	–	–	–	A,(P),(IB),(IV)	L,S	Some isolates produce precipitate in LD bile agar.
+	+	+	+	+	+	+	+	+	+	A,(P),(IV)	L,S	
+	–	+	+	+	V	+	+	V	+	A,(P),(IV)	L,S	Some strains give weak indole reactions.
+	–	+	+	+	–⁺	+	+	–	+	A,(P),(IV)	L,S	
+	–	+·	+	+	–	–	–	–	–	A	L,S	Inhibited by penicillin and rifampin.
+	–	+	+	+	–	–	–	–	–	A,(IB),(IV)	S	Most isolates inhibited by penicillin and rifampin.
+	–	V	V	+⁻	–	–	–	–	–	A,IB,IV	S	Most isolates inhibited by penicillin and rifampin.
+	–	+	–	+	–	–	–	–	–	A,IB,IV	S	Requires hemin for growth.
+	–	–	–	+	–	–	–	–	–	A,IB,IV	S	Requires hemin for growth.
–	–	–	–	–	–	–	–	–	–	A		Very tiny rods, less than 0.3 μm in length.
–	–	–	–	–	–	–	–	–	–	A,P,IV,B,IV		Most isolates inhibited by penicillin and rifampin.
–	–	–	–	–	–	–	–	–	–	A	S	Urease positive, usually inhibited, by penicillin, rifampin and kanamycin.
–	–	–	–	–	–	–	–	–	–	A	(S)	Usually inhibited by penicillin, rifampin and kanamycin.
–	–	–	–	–	–	–	–	–	–	A	(S)	Usually inhibited by penicillin, rifampin and kanamycin.

Column heading groups: FERMENTATION OF: (Glucose, Mannitol, Lactose, Sucrose, Maltose, Salicin, Xylose, Arabinose, Trehalose, Rhamnose); ACID PRODUCTS IN 48-HR PYG CULTURES DETECTED WITH GLC (Volatile, Non-volatile); Other[c]

(Footnotes and key on next page)

(d) *LD bile agar*. The degree of bacterial growth on the LD bile agar should be compared with that on the plain LD agar and recorded as I (growth less than on the LD agar control) or E (growth equal to or greater than on the LD agar control). The presence or absence of an insoluble white precipitate underneath or immediately surrounding the bacterial growth should be determined with transmitted light (if desired, under a stereomicroscope).

Inhibition by antibiotics on anaerobe blood agar. Observe the growth for zones of inhibition around the antibiotic disk and record as follows:

(a) Penicillin, 2-unit disk—record as S (inhibition zone of $\geq$ 12 mm in diameter) or R (inhibition zone of < 12 mm).

(b) Rifampin, 15-μg disk—record as S (inhibition zone of $\geq$15 mm) or R (inhibition zone of < 15 mm).

(c) Kanamycin, 1-mg disk—record as S (inhibition zone of $\geq$12 mm) or R (zone of <12 mm).

---

[a] Young colonies on anaerobe blood agar exhibit a characteristic red fluorescence when viewed with a Wood's lamp.

[b] On blood agar.

[c] Antibiotic susceptibility was tested with the following disk sizes: penicillin, 2 U; rifampin, 15 μg; kanamycin, 1 mg.

[d] Formerly called *B. melaninogenicus* ss *asaccharolyticus;* see Finegold and Barnes (35).

[e] Formerly called *B. corrodens;* see Jackson and Goodman (54).

[f] Hemin is required for succinic acid production by *B. fragilis;* see Macy et al. (63).

Key: + = positive reaction in 90%–100% of strains tested; − = negative reaction in 90%–100% of strains tested; V = variable reaction; superscript = reaction obtained with 11%–25% of strains tested.

GLC (gas liquid chromatography) results: A = acetic acid; B = butyric acid; P = propionic acid; IB = isobutyric acid; IV = isovaleric acid; L = lactic acid; S = succinic acid; ( ) = variable.

TABLE 14.14—ADDITIONAL DIFFERENTIAL CHARACTERISTICS OF *FUSOBACTERIUM* SPP.

SPECIES	GROWTH IN PRESENCE OF: PENICILLIN (2-U DISK)	RIFAMPIN (15-μG DISK)	KANAMYCIN (1-MG DISK)	INHIBITED BY BILE LD BILE AGAR	CATALASE LD ESCULIN AGAR	INDOLE LD AGAR	LIPASE LD EGG YOLK AGAR	ESCULIN HYDROL. LD ESCULIN AGAR
F. gonidiaformans	S	S	S	+	−	+	−	−
F. mortiferum	R or S	R	S	−	−	−	−	+
F. necrophorum	S	S	S	+	−	+	+	−
F. nucleatum	S	S	S	+	−	+	−	−
F. russii	S	S	S	+	−	−	−	−
F. varium	R or S	R	S	−	−	+⁻	−	−

S = sensitive.

R = resistant.

+ = positive reaction with 90%–100% of strains tested.

− = negative reaction with 90%–100% of strains tested.

Superscript = reaction exhibited by 11%–25% of strains.

Purity, microscopic features, Gram reaction, colony characteristics, and nitrate reduction on anaerobe blood agar.

(a) Observe for purity of the culture, colony characteristics, fluorescence under a Wood's lamp, pitting, pigmentation, hemolysis, microscopic features, etc., as described previously (25).

(b) *Nitrate reduction.* Add 1 drop each of sulfanilic acid and 1, 6-Cleve's acid (105), and observe for the development of a pink or red color which indicates a positive reaction for reduction of nitrate to nitrite by the culture. If no color is present after 3 to 5 min, sprinkle a little zinc dust on the disk. The development of a pink to red color after the dust is added is interpreted as a negative reaction, and no color change is presumptive evidence that nitrate has reduced beyond nitrite.

GLC analysis for volatile and nonvolatile acids produced and determination of glucose fermentation in PYG or LD glucose broth culture. This analysis can be made as soon as adequate growth is evident; it usually requires 24 to 48 hr of incubation, but it may take longer with certain slow-growing isolates of *Bacteroides* and *Fusobacterium*. The GLC analysis of volatile and nonvolatile acids is described in detail by Dowell and Hawkins (23), Sutter et al. (95), and Holdeman et al. (49).

Urease production. The technique for detecting urease has been described adequately above. It should be noted that the rate of hydrolysis of urea by cultures can be speeded up by placing a small amount (0.5 ml) of the urea semisolid medium in a sterile test tube, inoculating it heavily from colonies on anaerobe blood agar, and incubating under anaerobic conditions at 35–37 C.

Some additional characteristics of the species listed in Table 14.12 and characteristics of other *Bacteroides* and *Fusobacterium* spp. found less frequently in properly collected clinical materials are shown in Tables 14.13 and

H₂S LD Escu- Lin Agar	FERMENTATION OF:							ACID PRODUCTS DETECTED IN 48-HR PYG CULTURES WITH GLC		OTHER
	GLUCOSE	MANNITOL	LACTOSE	SUCROSE	MALTOSE	SALICIN	MANNOSE	VOLA-TILE	NON-VOLA-TILE	
−	V	−	−	−	−	−	−	A,P,B	None	Highly pleomorphic.
+⁻	+	−	+	+	+	+⁻	+	A,(P),B	None	Highly pleomorphic.
+	+	−	−	−	V	−	−	A,P,B	None	Hemolyzes rabbit but not sheep erythrocytes.
−	V	−	−	−	−	−	−	A,P,B	None	
−	−	−	−	−	−	−	−	A,P,B	None	
+	+	−	−	−	−	−	+	A,P,B	None	

V = variable.   P = propionic acid.
LD = Lombard Dowell.   ( ) = variable.
GLC = gas liquid chromatography.
A = acetic acid.
B = butyric acid.

A. Produces propionic acid.
   1. Catalase usually produced.   *Propionibacterium*
   2. Catalase not produced.   *Arachnia*
B. Propionic acid not produced.
   1. Ratio of lactic acid to acetic acid produced usually greater than 1:1.
      a. Lactic acid usually only major product.   *Lactobacillus*
      b. Succinic acid is a major product.   *Actinomyces*
   2. Ratio of lactic to acetic acid usually less than 1:1.
      a. Produces butyric acid plus other acids or no major acid products.   *Eubacterium* and *Lachnospira**
      b. Butyric acid not produced.   *Bifidobacterium*

* To our knowledge, no isolates of *Lachnospira* from human clinical materials have been reported.

Figure 14.5—Differentiation of anaerobic nonsporeforming gram-positive bacilli. Adapted from Dowell and Hawkins (23).

14.14. For more detailed information on these and numerous other anaerobic, nonsporeforming gram-negative bacilli which have been isolated from various human, animal, and environmental sources, the reader should consult references 12, 13, 23, 49, 50, and 95.

Anaerobic, nonsporeforming gram-positive bacilli

In recent years, numerous changes have been made in the taxonomy of this group and in some of the genus and species names used in the fifth edition of this text (12, 13, 19, 23, 29, 49). The differential characteristics of this group to the genus level are shown in Figure 14.5.

Characteristics we have found to be specially useful in the identification of anaerobic, nonsporeforming gram-positive bacilli include:

1. relationship to oxygen,
2. colony characteristics on anaerobe blood agar,
3. growth in THIO,
4. catalase production,
5. indole production,
6. hydrolysis of esculin,
7. reduction of nitrate,
8. hydrolysis of gelatin,
9. fermentation of certain carbohydrates,
10. acid metabolic products, and
11. reactions with FA reagents.

The characteristics used in identifying the most common non-sporeforming gram-positive bacilli are shown in Table 14.15. Information on various other members of this group that may be found in human, animal, and environmental materials is presented in the manuals by Holdeman, Cato, and Moore (49), Sutter, Vargo, and Finegold (95), and Dowell and Hawkins (23), and in various other publications.

FA procedures have been used successfully for a number of years in reference laboratories at CDC (37) and elsewhere for serotyping and presumptively identifying *Actinomyces, Arachnia, Bifidobacterium,* and *Propionibacterium* spp. (29, 38, 49, 55, 86, 87, 88). However, to our knowledge, none of the FA reagents required for the procedures are available commercially at present.

Whether an isolate of one of the gram-positive, nonsporeforming bacilli is clinically significant can be a perplexing problem. These microorganisms are prevalent in the normal flora of the skin and mucous membranes and tend to associate with other bacteria in polymicrobic infections. Isolates of propionibacteria from blood, cerebrospinal fluid, bone marrow, and joint fluid samples can be especially perplexing. Although *P. acnes,* a normal inhabitant of the skin, is frequently a contaminant of blood, bone marrow, and cerebrospinal fluid cultures, isolating this organism from properly collected specimens can be clinically significant because it has been implicated in endocarditis and other diseases (32, 33, 34). For this reason, it may be worthwhile to biotype multiple isolates of nonsporeforming gram-positive bacilli from such types of clinical materials as described by Dowell et al. (26).

Anaerobic cocci

Anaerobic cocci are commonly found in materials collected from patients for diagnosing various illnesses (34). They can be present in essentially any region or organ of the body. Although there is little doubt that some of the anaerobic cocci isolated from clinical materials are responsible for disease, the pathogenicity of others has not been definitively established. Mixed infections involving anaerobic cocci are common, and it is difficult to ascribe pathogenicity to any one of the microorganisms involved. On the other hand, severe infections involving anaerobic cocci such as crepitant cellulitis and synergistic gas gangrene have been well-documented (2, 34).

The anaerobic cocci are classified in the eighth edition of *Bergey's Manual of Determinative Bacteriology* (13) as follows:
Part 11 Gram-negative anaerobic cocci
  Family I. *Veillonellaceae* Rogosa 1971
    Genus I. *Veillonella* (two species)
    Genus II. *Acidaminococcus* (one species)
    Genus III. *Megasphaera* (one species)

Part 14. Gram-positive cocci
  Family III. *Peptococcaceae* Rogosa 1971
    Genus I. *Peptococcus* (six species)
    Genus II. *Peptostreptococcus* (five species)
    Genus III. *Ruminococcus* (two species)
    Genus IV. *Sarcina* (two species)
More recently, Holdeman and Moore (52) proposed that one new genus *(Coprococcus)* be included in the family *Peptococcaceae,* that two new *Ruminococcus* spp. and a new *Streptococcus* sp. be accepted, and that certain species of *Peptostreptococcus* (as classified in the seventh edition of *Bergey's Manual of Determinative Bacteriology,* 12) be transferred to the genus *Streptococcus.* Since the neotype strain of *Veillonella alcalescens* (ATCC

TABLE 14.15—DIFFERENTIAL CHARACTERISTICS OF ANAEROBIC, NONSPOREFORMING

Species	Relation to Oxygen	Rapidity of Growth	Colonies on Blood Agar Rough	Smooth	Red Colonies on Blood Agar	Growth in Enriched Thioglycollate Broth Appearance	Cell Morphology	Catalase Produced
Actinomyces israelii	M,OA	SLOW	+	(+)	−	DIFF, GRAN	Branching filaments, Diph	−
Actinomyces naeslundii	F	MOD	(+)	+	−	DIFF	Diph, branching	−
Actinomyces odontolyticus	M,OA	MOD	(+)	+	+	DIFF	Diph, branching	−
Actinomyces viscosus	F	RAPID	(+)	+	−	DIFF	Diph, branching	+
Arachnia propionica	M,OA	SLOW	+	(+)	−	GRAN, DIFF	Branching filaments, Diph	−
Bifidobacterium eriksonii	OA	RAPID	−	+	−	DIFF	Thin rods; bifids, bulbous ends	−
Eubacterium alactolyticum	OA	SLOW	−	+	−	DIFF	Thin rods, V-forms, "cross stick" arrangements	−
Eubacterium lentum	OA	MOD	−	+	−	DIFF	Coccoidal rods, Diph	−
Eubacterium limosum	OA	RAPID	−	+	−	DIFF	Plump rods, bulbous and bifid ends	−
Lactobacillus catenaforme	OA	RAPID	−	+	−	DIFF$^{(GRAN)}$	Short rods in chains or singly	−
Propionibacterium acnes	OA^F	MOD	−	+	−	DIFF$^{(GRAN)}$	Diph	+
Propionibacterium avidum	F	RAPID	−	+	−	DIFF	Diph	+
Propionibacterium granulosum	F	RAPID	+	+	−	DIFF	Diph	+

+ = positive reaction for 90%-100% of strains tested.
− = negative reaction for 90%-100% of strains tested.
Superscript indicates reaction given by 11%-25% of strains tested.
V = variable.
( ) = variable.
GLC = gas liquid chromatography.
A = acetic acid.

GRAM-POSITIVE BACILLI COMMONLY ISOLATED FROM HUMAN CLINICAL MATERIALS

| IN-DOLE PRO-DUCED | ESCU-LIN HY-DROL-YSIS | NI-TRATE RE-DUC-TION | H₂S PRO-DUCED | GELA-TIN HY-DROL-YSIS | FERMENTATION OF: | | | | GLC ANALYSIS: ACID PRODUCTS IN PYG CULTURES (48-HR, 35 C) | |
					GLU-COSE	GLYC-EROL	ARAB-INOSE	XY-LOSE	VOLA-TILE	NON-VOLA-TILE
−	+⁻	V	−	−	+	−	+⁻	+⁻	A	L,S
−	+⁻	+⁻	−	−	+	V	−	−	A	L,(S)
−	V	+	−	−	+	V	V	V	A	L,(S)
−	+	+	−	−	+	+⁻	−	−	A	L,S
−	−⁺	+	−	−	+	−⁺	−	−	A,P	L,(S)
−	+	−	−	−	+	−	+	+	A	L
−	−	−	−	−	+	−	−	−	A,B,C	−
−	−	V	V	−	−	−	−	−	A	−
−	V	−	+⁻	−	+	−	−	−	A,B	−
−	+	−	−	−	+	−	−	−	A	L
+⁻	−	+	−	V	+	+	−	−	A,P,(IV)	(L)
−	+	V	−	+	+	+	V	−	A,P	(L)
−	−	−	−	V	+	+⁻	−⁺	−	A,P	(L)

P = propionic acid.
B = butyric acid.
IV = isovaleric acid.
C = caproic acid.
L = lactic acid.
S = succinic acid.
M = microaerophilic.

F = facultative anaerobe.
OA = obligate anaerobe.
MOD = moderate.
DIFF = diffuse.
GRAN = granular.
Diph = diphtheroidal.
PYG = peptone yeast extract-glucose broth.

TABLE 14.16—DIFFERENTIAL CHARACTERISTICS OF ANAEROBIC

	GRAM REAC- TION	CHAINS OF 10 OR MORE CELLS IN THIO	RELA- TION TO OXY- GEN	"CATA- LASE" PRO- DUCED	INDOLE PRO- DUCED	ESCULIN HYDROL- YSIS	NITRATE REDUCED
Peptococcus asaccharolyticus	+	−	OA	−	+	−	−
Peptococcus magnus	+	−	OA	−	−	−	−
Peptococcus prevotii	+	−	OA	−	−	−	−⁺
Peptococcus saccharolyticus	+	−	OA	+	−	−	+
Peptostreptococcus anaerobius	+	+	OA	−	−	−	V
Streptococcus intermedius	+	+	OA,F	−	−	+	−
Veillonella parvula	−	−	OA	V	−	−	+

* Includes *V. alcalescens* and *V. parvula* as classified in the eighth edition of *Bergey's Manual of Determinative Bacteriology* (13).

+ = positive reaction exhibited by 90%–100% of strains tested.

− = negative reaction exhibited by 90%–100% of strains tested.

V = variable.

( ) = variable.

Superscript indicates reaction given by 11%–25% of strains tested.

OA = obligate anaerobe.

F = facultative anaerobe.

"Catalase" = decomposes hydrogen peroxide.

17745) has a high degree of DNA-DNA homology with the neotype strain of *Veillonella parvula,* it is now considered a synonym of *V. parvula* (49).

Only members of the genera *Peptococcus, Peptostreptococcus, Streptococcus,* and *Veillonella* are commonly isolated from properly collected human clinical materials associated with disease. However, most if not all of the others may be found in the normal flora of the oral cavity, gastrointestinal tract,

I. Gram-positive:
   A. Lactic acid sole major acid product. *Streptococcus*
   B. Major acids other than lactic or no major acids produced.
      1. Cells in definite chains (10 or more cells) in liquid medium. *Peptostreptococcus*
      2. Chains not produced in liquid medium. *Peptococcus*

II. Gram-negative: *Veillonella*
 (V. parvula)

Figure 14.6—Differentiation of commonly isolated anaerobic cocci to the genus level.

COCCI COMMONLY ISOLATED FROM HUMAN CLINICAL MATERIALS

| INHIB-ITED BY SPS | FERMENTATION OF: | | | | | GLC ANALYSIS: ACID PRODUCTS IN PYG (48 HR, 35 C) | |
	GLU-COSE	MANNI-TOL	LAC-TOSE	MAL-TOSE	SALI-CIN	VOLATILE	NON-VOLA-TILE
–	–	–	–	–	–	A, B	–
–	–	–	–	–	–	A	
–	–	–	–	–	–	A, (P), B	–
–	+	–	–	–	–	A	–
+	V	–	–	V	–	A, (P), IB, B, IV, IC	–
–	+	–	+	+	+	(A)	L
–	–	–	–	–	–	A, P	–

SPS = sodium polyanethol sulfonate [See Morello and Graves (74) and Wideman et al. (106)].
GLC = gas liquid chromatography.
A = acetic acid.
B = butyric acid.
P = propionic acid.
IB = isobutyric acid.
IC = isocaproic acid.
IV = isovaleric acid.
L = lactic acid.
THIO = enriched thioglycollate broth (27).

genitourinary orifices, or skin. The differential characteristics of the commonly isolated anaerobic cocci to the genus level are shown in Figure 14.6.

Some differential characteristics of seven commonly isolated species of anaerobic cocci are shown in Table 14.16. For more detailed characterization of these species and of various other anaerobic cocci which may or may not be found in human clinical materials, the reader is referred to references 23, 49, 69, 88, and 95.

References

1. ALLEN SD, LOMBARD GL, ARMFIELD AY, THOMPSON FS, and STARGEL MD: Development and evaluation of an improved anaerobic holding jar procedure. Abstr Annu Meet Am Soc Microbiol. Abstract C142, p 59, 1977
2. ALTEMEIER WA and CULBERTSON WR: Acute nonclostridial crepitant cellulitis. Surg Gynecol Obstet 87:206–212, 1948
3. ANGELOTTI R, HALL HE, FOTER MJ, and LEWIS KH: Quantitation of *Clostridium perfringens in foods*. Appl Microbiol 10:193–199, 1962
4. ARANKI AS, SYED A, KENNY EB, and FRETER R: Isolation of anaerobic bacteria from hu-

man gingiva and mouse cecum by means of a simplified glove box procedure. Appl Microbiol 17:568–576, 1969

5. ARNON SS, MIDURA TF, CLAY SA, WOOD RM, and CHIN J: Infant botulism: Epidemiological, clinical, and laboratory aspects. J Am Med Assoc 237:1946–1951, 1977

6. BABB JL and CUMMINS CS: Encapsulation of *Bacteroides* species. Infect Immun 19:1088–1091, 1978

7. BALOWS A: Anaerobic bacteria perspectives. *In* Anaerobic Bacteria: Role in Disease. Balows A, DeHaan RM, Guze LB, and Dowell VR Jr (eds.). Charles C Thomas, Springfield, Ill, 1974, pp 3–6

8. BARTLETT JG, SULLIVAN-SIGLER N, LOUIE TJ, and GORBACH SL: Anaerobes survive in clinical specimens despite delayed processing. J Clin Microbiol 3:133–136, 1976

9. BARTLETT RC: Contemporary blood culture practices. *In* Bacteremia, Laboratory and Clinical Aspects. Sonnenwirth AC (ed.). Charles C Thomas, Springfield, Ill, 1973, pp 15–35

10. BARTLETT RC, ELLNER PD, and WASHINGTON JA: Blood cultures. *In* Cumulative Techniques and Procedures in Clinical Microbiology. Sherris JC (ed.). American Society for Microbiology, Washington, DC, 1974

11. BARRY AL: Clinical specimens for microbiologic examination. *In* Infectious Diseases. Hoeprich PD (ed.). Harper and Row, Hagerstown, Md, 1972, pp 103–117

12. BREED RS, MURRAY EDG, and SMITH NR (eds.): Bergey's Manual of Determinative Bacteriology, 7th edition. Williams and Wilkins Co, Baltimore, Md, 1957

13. BUCHANAN RE and GIBBONS NE (eds.): Bergey's Manual of Determinative Bacteriology, 8th edition. Williams and Wilkins Co, Baltimore, Md, 1974

14. CATO EP and JOHNSON JL: Reinstatement of species rank for *Bacteroides fragilis, B. ovatus, B. distasonis, B. thetaiotaomicron,* and *B. vulgatus: Designation of neotype strains for Bacteroides fragilis* (Veillon and Zuber) Castellani and Chalmers and *Bacteroides thetaiotaomicron* (Distaso) Castellani and Chalmers. Int J Syst Bacteriol 25:230–237, 1976

15. CENTER FOR DISEASE CONTROL: Botulism in the United States, 1899–1977: Handbook for Epidemiologists, Clinicians and Laboratory Workers. U.S. Department of Health, Education and Welfare, Public Health Service, Center for Disease Control, Atlanta, Ga, 1979

16. DAVIS CP, MULCAHY D, TAKEUCHI A, and SAVAGE DC: Location and description of spiral-shaped microorganisms in the normal rat cecum. Infect Immun 6:184–192, 1972

17. DAVIS CP and SAVAGE DC: Habitat, succession, attachment, and morphology of segmented, filamentous microbes indigenous to the murine gastrointestinal tract. Infect Immun 10:948–956, 1974

18. DINEEN P: The choice of a local antiseptic. *In* Drugs of Choice. 1972–1973. Modell W (ed.). C. V. Mosby Co, St. Louis, Mo 1972, p 125.

19. DOWELL VR JR: Anaerobic infections. *In* Diagnostic Procedures for Bacterial, Mycotic and Parasitic Infections, 5th edition. Bodily HL, Updyke EL, and Mason JO (eds.). American Public Health Association, New York, NY, 1970, pp 494–543

20. DOWELL VR JR: Methods for isolation of anaerobes in the clinical laboratory. Am J Med Technol 41:32–40, 1975

21. DOWELL VR JR: Wound and abscess specimens. *In* Clinical Microbiology. How to Start and When to Stop. Balows A (ed.). Charles C Thomas, Springfield, Ill, 1975, pp 70–81

22. DOWELL VR JR: Infant botulism: New guise for an old disease. *In* Hospital Practice, 1978, pp 67–72

23. DOWELL VR JR and HAWKINS TM: Laboratory Methods in Anaerobic Bacteriology. DHEW Publication No. (CDC) 74-8272. Center for Disease Control, Atlanta, Ga, 1974

24. DOWELL VR JR, HILL EO, and ALTEMEIER WA: Use of phenethyl alcohol in media for isolation of anaerobic bacteria. J Bacteriol 88:1811–1813, 1964

25. DOWELL VR JR and LOMBARD GL: Presumptive identification of anaerobic nonsporeforming gram-negative bacilli. Center for Disease Control, Atlanta, Ga, 1977

26. DOWELL VR JR, LOMBARD GL, STARGEL MD, ALLEN SD, THOMPSON FS, and ARMFIELD AY: Biotyping of anaerobic bacteria associated with human disease *In* Biotyping in the Clinical Microbiology Laboratory. Isenberg HD and Balows A (eds.). Charles C Thomas, Springfield, Ill, 1978, pp 47–67

27. DOWELL VR JR, LOMBARD GL, THOMPSON FS, and ARMFIELD AY: Media for Isolation,

Characterization and Identification of Obligately Anaerobic Bacteria. Center for Disease Control, Atlanta, Ga, 1977

28. DOWELL VR JR, MCCROSKEY LM, HATHEWAY CL, LOMBARD GL, HUGHES JM, and MERSON MH: Coproexamination for botulinal toxin and *Clostridium botulinum*. A new procedure for laboratory diagnosis of botulism. J Am Med Assoc 238:1829–1932, 1977

29. DOWELL VR JR and SONNENWIRTH AC: Gram-positive, nonsporeforming anaerobic bacilli. *In* Manual of Clinical Microbiology, 2nd edition. Lennette EH, Spaulding EH, and Truant JP (eds.). American Society for Microbiology. Washington, DC, 1974, pp 396–401

30. ENG J: Effects of sodium polyanethol sulfonate in blood cultures. J Clin Microbiol 1:119–123, 1975

31. ENG J and HOLTEN E: Gelatin neutralizaton of the inhibitory effect of sodium polyanetholsulfonate on *Neisseria meningitidis* in blood culture media. J Clin Microbiol 6:1–3, 1977

32. FELNER JM: Infective endocarditis caused by anaerobic bacteria. *In* Anaerobic Bacteria: Role in Disease. Balows A, DeHaan RM, Dowell VR Jr and Guze LB (eds.). Charles C Thomas, Springfield, Ill, 1974, pp 345–352

33. FELNER JM and DOWELL VR JR: Anaerobic bacterial endocarditis. N Engl J Med 283:1188–1192, 1970

34. FINEGOLD SM: Anaerobic Bacteria in Human Disease. Academic Press, New York, NY, 1977

35. FINEGOLD SM and BARNES EM: Report of the ICSB taxonomic subcommittee on gram-negative anaerobic rods. Proposal that the saccharolytic and asaccharolytic strains at present classified in the species *Bacteroides melaninogenicus* (Oliver and Wherry) be reclassified in two species as *Bacteroides melaninogenicus* and *Bacteroides asaccharolyticus*. Int J Syst Bacteriol 27:388–391, 1977

36. FINEGOLD SM, SUTTER VL, ATTEBERY HR, and ROSENBLATT JE: Isolation of anaerobic bacteria. *In* Manual of Clinical Microbiology, 2nd edition. Lennette EH, Spaulding EH, and Truant JP (eds.). American Society for Microbiology, Washington, DC, 1974

37. GEORG LK: Diagnostic procedures for the isolation and identification of the etiologic agents of actinomycosis. *In* Proceedings of International Symposium on Mycoses, Publication No. 205, Pan American Health Organization, Washington, DC, 1970, pp 71–81

38. GEORG LK: The agents of human actinomycosis. *In* Anaerobic Bacteria: Role in Disease. Balows A, DeHaan RM, Guze LB, and Dowell VR Jr (eds.). Charles C Thomas, Springfield, Ill, 1974, pp 237–256

39. GERSHENFELD L: Iodine. *In* Disinfection, Sterilization and Preservation. Lawrence CA and Block SS (eds.). Lea and Febiger, Philadelphia, Pa, 1968, pp 329–347

40. GIBBONS RJ: Aspects of the pathogenicity and ecology of the indigenous oral flora of man. *In* Anaerobic Bacteria: Role in Disease. Balows A, DeHaan RM, Dowell VR Jr, and Guze LB (eds.). Charles C Thomas, Springfield, Ill 1974, pp 267–286

41. GORBACH SL: Introduction. J Infect Dis 135, Supplement: 52–53, 1977

42. GORBACH SL and BARTLETT JG: Anaerobic infections. N Engl J Med 290:1177–1184, 1237–1245, 1289–1294, 1974

43. GRAVES MH, MORELLO JA, and KOCKA FE: Sodium polyanethol sulfonate sensitivity of anaerobic cocci. Appl Microbiol 27:1131–1133, 1974

44. HARMON SM, KAUTTER DA, and PEELER JT: Improved medium for enumeration of *Clostridium perfringens*. Appl Microbiol 22:688–692, 1971

45. HAUSCHILD AHW and HILSHEINER R: Evaluation and modification of media for enumeration of *Clostridium perfringens*. Appl Microbiol 27:78–82, 1974

46. HELSTAD AG, KIMBALL JL, and MAKI DG: Recovery of anaerobic, facultative, and aerobic bacteria from clinical specimens in three anaerobic transport systems. J Clin Microbiol 5:564–569, 1977

47. HOBBS BC: *Clostridium welchii* as a food-poisoning organism. J Appl Bacteriol 28:74–82, 1965

48. HOLDEMAN LV, CATO EP, and MOORE WEC: Current classification of clinically important anaerobes. *In* Anaerobic Bacteria: Role in Disease. Balows A, DeHaan RM, Guze LB, and Dowell VR Jr (eds.). Charles C Thomas, Springfield, Ill, 1974, pp 67–74

49. HOLDEMAN LV, CATO EP, and MOORE WEC (eds.). Anaerobe Laboratory Manual, 4th edition. Virginia Polytechnic Institute and State University, Blacksburg, Va, 1977

50. HOLDEMAN LV and JOHNSON JL: *Bacteroides disiens* sp. nov. and *Bacteroides bivius* sp. nov. from human clinical infections. Int J Syst Bacteriol 27:337–345, 1977

51. HOLDEMAN LV and MOORE WEC: Roll-tube technique for anaerobic bacteria. Am J Clin Nutr 25:1314–1317, 1972

52. HOLDEMAN LV and MOORE WEC: New genus, *Coprococcus,* twelve new species, and amended descriptions of four previously described species of bacteria from human feces. Int J Syst Bacteriol 24:260–277, 1974

53. HUNGATE RE: The anaerobic cellulolytic bacteria. Bacteriol Rev 14:1–49, 1950

54. JACKSON FL and GOODMAN YE: *Bacteroides ureolyticus,* a new species to accommodate strains previously identified as *Bacteroides corrodens* anaerobic. J Clin Microbiol 28:197–200, 1978

55. JOHNSON JL and CUMMINS CS: Cell wall composition and deoxyribonucleic acid similarities among the anaerobic coryneforms, classical propionibacteria, and strains of *Arachnia propionica.* J Bacteriol 1047–1066, 1972

56. JONES GL, WHALEY DN, and DEVER SM: Use of the Flexible Anaerobic Glove Box. U.S. Department of Health, Education and Welfare, Public Health Service, Center for Disease Control, Bureau of Laboratories, Atlanta, Ga, 1977

57. KASPER DL, HAYES ME, REINAP BG, CRAFT FO, ONDERDONK AB, and POLK BF: Isolation and identification of encapsulated strains of *Bacteroides fragilis.* J Infect Dis 136:75–81, 1977

58. KILLGORE GE, STARR SE, DELBENE VE, WHALEY DN and DOWELL VR JR: Comparison of three anaerobic systems for the isolation of anaerobic bacteria from clinical specimens. Am J Clin Pathol 59:552–559, 1973

59. KOCKA FE, ARTHUR EJ, and SEARCY RL: Comparative effects of two sulfated polyanions used in blood culture on anaerobic cocci. Am J Clin Pathol 61:25–27, 1974

60. KORANSKY JR, ALLEN SD, and DOWELL VR JR: Use of ethanol for selective isolation of sporeforming microorganisms. Appl Environ Microbiol 35:762–765, 1978

61. LOESCHE WJ: Oxygen sensitivity of various anaerobic bacteria. Appl Microbiol 8:723–727, 1969

62. LOMBARD GL, ARMFIELD AY, STARGEL MD, and FOX JB: The effect of storage on blood agar medium on the growth of certain obligate anaerobes. Abstr Annu Meet Am Soc Microbiol. Abstract C95, p 41, 1976

63. MACY J, PROBST I, and GOTTSCHALK G: Evidence for cytochrome involvement in fumarate reduction and adenosine 5-triphosphate synthesis by *Bacteroides fragilis* grown in the presence of hemin. J Bacteriol 123:436–442, 1975

64. MARSHALL RS, STEENBERGEN JF, and MCCLUNG LS: Rapid technique for the enumeration of *Clostridium perfringens.* Appl Microbiol 13:559–563, 1965

65. MARTIN WJ: Practical method for isolation of anaerobic bacteria in the clinical laboratory. Appl Microbiol 22:1168–1171, 1971

66. MARTIN WJ, GARDNER M, and WASHINGTON JA II. *In vitro* antimicrobial susceptibility of anaerobic bacteria isolated from clinical specimens. Antimicrob Agents Chemother 1:148–158, 1972

67. MATSEN JM and EDERER GM: Specimen collection and transport. Human Pathol 7:297–307, 1976

68. MCBEE RH, LAMANNA C, and WEEKS OB: Definitions of bacterial oxygen relationships. Bacteriol Rev 19:45–47, 1955

69. MCCARTHY LR and BOTTONE EJ: Bacteremia and endocarditis caused by satelliting streptococci. Am J Clin Pathol 61:585–591, 1974

70. MENA E, THOMPSON FS, ARMFIELD AY, DOWELL VR JR, and REINHARDT DJ: Evaluation of Port-A-Cul transport system for protection of anaerobic bacteria. J Clin Microbiol 8:28–35, 1978

71. MOORE WEC, CATO EP, and HOLDEMAN LV: Anaerobic bacteria of the gastrointestinal flora and their occurrence in clinical infections. J Infect Dis 119:641–649, 1969

72. Morbidity and Mortality Weekly Report. Follow-up on infant botulism—United States. 27:17–23, 1978

73. Morbidity and Mortality Weekly Report. Honey exposure and infant botulism. 27:249–255, 1978

74. MORELLO JA and GRAVES MH: Clinical anaerobic bacteriology. Lab Manage 15:20–25, 51, 1977
75. NELSON DP and MATA LJ: Bacterial flora associated with the human gastrointestinal mucosa. Gastroenterology 58:56–61, 1970
76. ONDERDONK AB, KASPER DL, CISNEROS RL, and BARTLETT JG: The capsular polysaccharide of *Bacteroides fragilis* as a virulence factor: Comparison of the pathogenic potential of encapsulated and unencapsulated strains. J Infect Dis 136:82–89, 1977
77. ONDERDONK AB, MOON NE, KASPER DL, and BARTLETT JG: Adherence of *Bacteroides fragilis* in vivo. Infect Immun 19:1083–1087, 1978
78. ORTH DS: Comparison of sulfite-polymyxin-sulfadiazine medium and tryptose-sulfite-cycloserine medium without egg yolk for recovering *Clostridium perfringens*. 33:986–988, 1977
79. PORSCHEN RK and CHAN P: Anaerobic vibrio-like organism cultured from blood: *Desulfovibrio desulfuricans* and *Succinivibrio* species. J Clin Microbiol 5:444–447, 1977
80. RINTALA L and POLLOCK HM: Effects of two blood culture anticoagulants on growth of *Neisseria meningitidis*. J Clin Microbiol 7:332–336, 1978
81. ROSENBLATT JE, FALLON AM, and FINEGOLD SM: Comparison of methods for isolation of anaerobic bacteria from clinical specimens. Appl Microbiol 25:77–85, 1973
82. ROSNER R: Effect of various anticoagulants and no anticoagulant on ability to isolate bacteria directly from parallel clinical blood specimens. Am J Clin Pathol 57:220–227, 1968
83. SAVAGE DC: Interactions between the host and its microbes. *In* Microbial Ecology of the Gut. Clarke RTJ and Bauchop T (eds.). Academic Press, New York, NY, 1977, pp 277–310
84. SAVAGE DC, MCALLISTER JS, and DAVIS CP: Anaerobic bacteria on the mucosal epithelium of the murine large bowel. Infect Immun 4:492–502, 1971
85. SHAHIDI SA and FERGUSON AR: New quantitative, qualitative, and confirmatory media for rapid analysis of food for *Clostridium perfringens*. Appl Microbiol 21:500–506, 1971
86. SLACK JM and GERENCSER MA: Actinomyces, Filamentous Bacteria Biology and Pathogenicity. Burgess Publishing Co, Minneapolis, Minn, 1975
87. SLACK JM, LANDFRIED S, and GERENCSER MA: Identification of *Actinomyces* and related bacteria in dental calculus by the fluorescent antibody technique. J Dent Res 50:78–82, 1971
88. SMITH L: The Pathogenic Anaerobic Bacteria, 2nd edition. Charles C Thomas, Springfield, Ill, 1975
89. SOMMERS HM and MATSEN JM: Laboratory Diagnosis of Infectious Disease. Workshop Manual, ASCP-CAP Course No. 704. ASCP Spring Meeting. Miami Beach, Fla, March 1977
90. SONNENWIRTH AC: Evolution of anaerobic methodology. Am J Clin Nutr 25:1295–1298, 1972
91. SPAULDING EH, VARGO V, MICHAELSON TC, KORZENIOWSKI M, AND SWENSON RM: Anaerobic bacteria: Culture and identification. *In* Opportunistic Infections. Prier JE and Friedman H (eds.). University Park Press, Baltimore, Md. 1974, pp 87–104
92. STARGEL MD, LOMBARD GL, and DOWELL VR JR: Alternative procedures for identification of anaerobic bacteria. Am J Med Technol 44:709–722, 1978
93. STARR SE, KILLGORE GE, and DOWELL VR JR: Comparison of Schaedler agar and Trypticase soy-yeast extract agar for the cultivation of anaerobic bacteria. Appl Microbiol 22:655–658, 1971
94. SUTTER VL and FINEGOLD SM: Susceptibility of anaerobic bacteria to 23 antimicrobial agents. Antimicrob Agents Chemother 10:736–752, 1976
95. SUTTER VL, VARGO VL, and FINEGOLD SM: Wadsworth Anaerobic Bacteriology Manual, 2nd edition. Wadsworth Hospital Center, Veterans Administration, Los Angeles, Calif, and the Department of Med UCLA School of Med, Los Angeles, Calif, 1975
96. SWENSON RM, VARGO VL, SPAULDING EH, and MICHAELSON TC: Incidence of anaerobic bacteria in clinical specimens from known or suspected human infections. Abstr Annu Meet Am Soc Microbiol. M67, p 84, 1973
97. TALLY FP, BARTLETT JG, and GORBACH SL: A Practical Approach to Anaerobic Bacteriology in Clinical Laboratories. American Society of Clinical Pathologists Technical Improvement Service. No. 20, 1975

98. TALLY FP, STEWART PR, SUTTER VL, and ROSENBLATT JE: Oxygen tolerance of fresh clinical anaerobic bacteria. J Clin Microbiol 1:161–164, 1975

99. TRAUB WH: Studies on neutralization of human serum bactericidal activity by sodium amylosulfate. J Clin Microbiol 6:128–131, 1977

100. VON GRAVENITZ A and SABELLA W: Unmasking additional bacilli in gram-negative rod bacteremia. J Med (Basel) 2:185–191, 1971

101. WAHL JW: Vibrio endophthalmitis. Arch Ophthalmol 91:423–424, 1974

102. WASHINGTON JA II: Anaerobic blood cultures. *In* Manual of Clinical Microbiology, 2nd edition. Lennette EH, Spaulding EH, and Truant JP (eds.). American Society for Microbiology, Washington, DC, 1974, pp 402–404

103. WASHINGTON JA II and MARTIN WJ: Comparison of three blood culture media for recovery of anaerobic bacteria. Appl Microbiol 25:70–71, 1973

104. WHALEY DN and GORMAN GW: An inexpensive device for evacuating and gassing systems with in-house vacuum. J Clin Microbiol 5:668–669, 1977

105. WIDEMAN PA, CITRONBAUM DM, and SUTTER VL: Simple disk technique for detection of nitrate reduction by anaerobic bacteria. J Clin Microbiol 5:315–319, 1977

106. WIDEMAN PA, VARGO VL, CITRONBAUM D, and FINEGOLD SM: Evaluation of the sodium polyanethol sulfonate disk test for the identification of *Peptostreptococcus anaerobius*. J Clin Microbiol 4:330–333, 1976

107. WILKINS TD and WEST SEH: Medium-dependent inhibition of *Peptostreptococcus anaerobius* by sodium polyanetholsulfonate in blood culture media. J Clin Microbiol 3:393–396, 1976

CHAPTER 15

ANTHRAX

Horace B. Rees, Jr., and Merlin A. Smith

Introduction

Anthrax has been responsible for pandemics of human and animal disease throughout history. It is assumed from Biblical descriptions that anthrax was the Fifth Plague of Egypt that Moses prophesied. In the early Roman Empire, anthrax caused the deaths of half the human and animal populations of Rome. In 1613, approximately 60,000 people in Southern Europe died from this disease—"black bain" (30).

The bacillus of anthrax holds a preemptory position in the sciences of bacteriology and medicine. It was first observed by M. Delafond in 1838, the first bacillus shown to produce a disease by Davaine in 1868, the first pathogen to satisfy Koch's "Postulates" fully in 1877 as Henle had envisioned them earlier, and the first bacterium for which Pasteur produced an effective vaccine in 1881 (30).

Causative Organism

The etiologic agent of anthrax is *Bacillus anthracis*, a large gram-positive, aerobic, nonmotile, sporeforming bacterium. Microscopically it appears usually as a straight, square-ended rod that measures approximately 1.0–1.3 by 3–10 μm. Its oval spores tend to be located centrally to subterminally and produce no detectable swelling of the cell. The microorganism grows well on ordinary laboratory media and produces large, raised, opaque, grayish-white, granular-appearing colonies after incubation at 37 C for 24 hr. Generally, colonies have irregular borders that frequently are described as having "Medusa heads" or "comet tails." On smears prepared from colonies, the rods appear in long chains; however, smears made from animal tissues reveal single cells or short chains. Capsules are demonstrable with specific staining from smears prepared from animal tissues, but not from artificial media unless a special bicarbonate medium is used and the inoculated medium is incubated under increased carbon dioxide tension.

Clinical Manifestations

Anthrax must be diagnosed early from clinical manifestations and history. Frequently, if therapy is to be effective, it must begin without waiting for confirmatory results from the laboratory. Three categories of manifestations are described with the designation pertaining primarily to the route of infection.

The cutaneous or carbuncle form is the most frequently found. Man becomes infected from exposure to infected animals and their by-products. The incubation period ranges from 1 to 12 days, with symptoms usually appearing after 2 to 7 days. The lesion develops as a macular one at first, but becomes papular within a day and is surrounded by a 1- to 2-cm zone of erythema. A large vesicle develops later, and the dark bluish-black fluid discolors the surrounding tissues. After 4 to 6 days, the vesicle ruptures, and a black eschar develops and enlarges before it begins to dry and retract 10 to 14 days later. Lesions that develop in the softer tissues of the face and neck tend to become larger and produce greater toxic sequelae. An important diagnostic feature is the lack of pain associated with the lesion. If pain is present, it is generally caused by pressure from edema or secondary infection.

The localized or cutaneous infection occurs in cattle, swine, horses, dogs, and rabbits. Bacilli concentrate in the cervical lymph nodes and pharyngeal area and produce swelling and hemorrhage with a blood-tinged, gelatinous exudate generally found at the site of the swelling.

Human and animal inhalation, septic, fulminant, or apoplectic anthrax is similar. Sudden onset and rapid fatality characterize this type of infection. Clinically, signs include a mild upper respiratory infection (without a productive cough), fever, headache, nausea, discomfort, and pain in the region around the heart and stomach. After 2 to 4 days the symptoms intensify, with dyspnea, cyanosis, shock, rapid collapse, and death occurring in hours or a few days.

Gastrointestinal anthrax is fulminating in its appearance and may mimic other disorders. It is rapidly fatal. Fever, generalized abdominal pain, and tenderness in the right upper and lower quadrants are present. Lesions and bleeding may occur at the primary site of infection in the upper gastrointestinal tract; vomiting or bloody stools sometimes follow.

Regardless of the portal of entry, the untreated disease appears to follow a similar course after the initial stage. Early in the systemic phase of the disease, the microorganisms are found consistently in the mediastinal lymph nodes. Later, a generalized septicemia and toxemia may develop, and death follows.

The pathophysiology is consistent with the clinical course of the disease. Macrophages transport the microorganism to the mediastinal lymph nodes, where spore germination and multiplication occur. Rapid growth also occurs in the spleen and liver, along with the production of exotoxin—principally in the splenic sinusoids. The potent toxin produces vascular injury. As the concentration of toxin reaches the critical level, injury to the endothelial cells becomes widespread; thrombosis results and is followed with circulatory failure, cyanosis, and death. Walker et al. (59), who studied changes in the blood chemistry of monkeys challenged with anthrax spores, found that most of the pathophysiologic changes occurred late in the course of the disease. Levels of calcium, sodium, and cholinesterase were lowered; levels of potassium, chloride, and phosphate were elevated. Animals were hyperglycemic early in the disease, but became hypoglycemic in the terminal stage.

Epidemiology and Ecology

The frequency and distribution of anthrax in man is determined by his relationship and contact with infected animals or animal products. Persons associated with agriculture—e.g., farmers, butchers, and veterinarians—have the greatest potential for becoming infected. Industrial anthrax is acquired by those working in factories or mills that process wool, mohair, animal hides, or bones infected with anthrax.

It is not surprising that 95%–98% of the human cases of anthrax are cutaneous in origin, because the most frequent type of exposure is direct contact with infected materials. Of the 2400 cases reported from Russia (63) from 1920 to 1959, 94% were cutaneous in origin; 5.2%, intestinal; and 0.7%, respiratory. Brachman (4) reported on 176 cases of human anthrax in the United States from 1955 to 1966 for which the source of infection was known. Cutaneous anthrax was responsible for 168 (95%) of the cases. Respiratory (inhalation) anthrax accounted for 8 (4.5%) of these cases. There were no cases of intestinal anthrax reported in this survey. Of the 168 cases of cutaneous anthrax, 31% of the lesions were found on the head or neck; 54%, on the arms and hands; 0.6%, on the trunk; and 0.5%, on the leg.

The incidence of human anthrax has declined steadily since 1951 (61), when some 60 cases were reported in the United States. Since 1970, however, six or fewer cases have been reported each year (Table 15.1). The reduction in incidence results primarily from improved practices for handling infected materials, better ventilation, and higher standards for cleanliness in the industrial and agricultural sectors.

Industrial cases of cutaneous anthrax arise more frequently in workers handling imported mohair. Of the cases reported in the United States from 1955 to 1969, 33 were associated with wool and 106 with mohair (44). Anthrax

TABLE 15.1—HUMAN MORBIDITY AND MORTALITY FROM ANTHRAX IN THE UNITED STATES,*
1967 TO 1980

YEAR	NO. OF CASES	NO. OF DEATHS
1967	2	0
1968	3	0
1969	4	0
1970	2	0
1971	5	0
1972	2	0
1973	2	0
1974	2	0
1975	2	0
1976	2	1
1977	0	0
1978	6	0
1979	0	0

* Reference 10.

has occurred also in persons whose occupations provide contact with bones or bone meals or the sacks in which these materials are transported (18).

Inhalation anthrax results when anthrax spores in aerosols are deposited in the pharynx and lungs. In 1976, a California weaver who operated a hand loom in his home died from inhalation anthrax. *B. anthracis* spores were isolated from the yarns he used (11, 56). Although inhalation anthrax is rarely seen, its case/fatality ratio is high. Fifteen of the 16 cases of inhalation anthrax reported in the United States from 1900 to 1976 were fatal (34).

Intestinal anthrax occurs even less frequently in the United States than the inhalation variety and is found in persons who consume meats contaminated with the bacillus. Nalin et al. (43) described a case in India in 1975 in which the patient survived an acute intestinal infection.

Livestock losses have ranged from a few animals [e.g., Oklahoma in 1974 (40) or Utah in 1975 (50)] to more extensive mortality [700 head in Louisiana in 1974 (22) or 236 head in Texas during the same year (21)]. In the 8-year period between 1945 and 1953, there were 2785 outbreaks among U.S. livestock herds in which 14,700 head were lost (53).

Anthrax in animals still occurs sporadically in enzootic areas of the United States. The ecologic relationships that perpetuate the disease are not entirely known or understood. The characteristics of the soil in the affected areas seem to be significant. Most of the soils associated with anthrax transmission are derived from or underlain with limestone. They are often found on alluvial plains which are predominantly clay, have a pH of > 6.0, and are poorly drained. Specific climatic conditions also appear to be requisite for the occurrence of anthrax epizootics. The factors apparently needed are cool, moist spring months with above normal precipitation, followed by conditions of drought in the late summer in which temperatures exceed 26 C (50).

Although anthrax spores are known to survive for as long as 60 years in soil held in the laboratory (60), the temperature, pH, and humidity of the soil, as well as the noncompetitiveness of *B. anthracis*, seem to limit its survival in the soil. Davies (15) showed that spore germination occurs optimally in 2 to 3 hr at 39 C. The time required for spores to germinate is increased below 30 C or above 39 C. For endospore formation, relative humidity (RH) is important. At 90%–100% RH, endospores formed within 6 to 12 hr at 37 C. Below 60% RH, spore formation was delayed for 40 to 48 hr. Gonzales y Gonzales (25) found that a pH of 5.1 was lethal for spores after 108 days at any humidity tested.

Spores form more rapidly at temperatures of ≥ 30 C in sanguinous exudates from larger animals and are a source of environmental contamination (57). Spores have been recovered from soils contaminated with sanguinous fluids for 8 months after an animal died from anthrax (28). Within the carcasses of larger animals sporulation occurs more slowly, and the bacillus is overgrown quickly by saprophytes. However, in carcasses of smaller animals such as guinea pigs and rabbits, sporulation occurs more rapidly than in carcasses of sheep and cattle (57). This event may provide a much greater reservoir for contaminating the environment.

It has been suggested that ticks are possible vectors of transmitting anthrax to sheep, cattle, and goats (1, 12, 55). Krinsky (33) suggested that tabanids, house flies, and deer flies transmit anthrax in nature but stated that the extent of the transmission is unknown.

Collection and Processing of Specimens

The persistence of anthrax spores, their ability to propagate naturally in the soil, and the danger of infection heighten the need for extreme care and attention to safety in collecting and processing specimens. More importantly, using good bacteriologic techniques throughout the diagnostic procedures (45) minimizes the possibility of contaminating the specimens with the many saprophytic sporeforming rods that resemble *B. anthracis.*

The order in which specimens are listed below is for both man and animal and can be considered preferential within the guidelines of specimen availability and limitations stated (37). Note that the environmental specimens are discussed separately below.

Clinical Specimens

The protocol for specimen collection must consider whether or not any antibiotic therapy has been given. Penicillin given 6 hr before collection of specimens or broad-spectrum antibiotics given 2 to 5 days earlier eliminate the microorganisms from vesicular fluid of lesions (24). Also, the period in which the bacilli can be found in the blood stream is limited, because they normally appear in the blood only a few hours before death of the victim. In the cases of carcasses, putrification by saprophytic bacteria may eliminate the anthrax bacilli, particularly if atmospheric temperatures are elevated and specimen collection is delayed. In the field, autopsy of animal carcasses should be delayed or eliminated until the examination of microscopic smears rules out the possibility of anthrax. The hazard of infecting veterinary personnel and probable contamination of the environment is reduced if autopsies are done in the field only when absolutely necessary.

Smears for microscopic examination. Several impression slides should be prepared from the clear vesicular fluid of the macular-papular lesions of man or animals and noncoagulating blood from body openings of animal carcasses. Slides should be transported in a plastic petri dish or similar container that can be sealed or taped for airtight closure to minimize environmental contamination while specimens are transported to the laboratory.

Sterile cotton swabs of body fluids. Several swabs should be saturated in the vesicular fluid, blood, etc., and placed in sterile, screw-capped tubes for dispatching to the laboratory. Specimens should be refrigerated in transit unless the volume of fluid collected is small enough to dry on the swab (37).

Blood and tissue. Included in this category are blood taken in the terminal stage of illness and tissues of lymph node or spleen or peritoneal exudate taken by biopsy or at necropsy. Such specimens should be placed in sterile vials or similar containers and frozen or iced for transport to the laboratory. Freezing the specimens is preferred, because it preserves them with a minimal amount of change and affords a greater amount of safety if breakage occurs during handling. (A possible exception for refrigeration rather than freezing specimens exists in one instance, viz., blood collected aseptically in the terminal stage of illness from victims given antibiotic therapy. The plasma fraction should contain demonstrable anthrax toxin, which may be processed for animal inoculation with less difficulty in the absence of lysed erythrocytes.) Repeated freezing and thawing of the specimens should be avoided (37). Large specimens of tissue should be encased in several polyethylene bags and frozen. An excellent alternative suggested by Lincoln el al. (37) is that the specimen be enclosed in a surgical glove which is turned inside out to contain the tissue as the glove is removed. If this method is used, the veterinarian or pathologist should wear two pairs of gloves during the manipulation to avoid contaminating his hands.

For an animal carcass that is not discovered until advanced putrification has occurred, the time-honored custom of removing the ear or other appendage of the animal for possible diagnosis of anthrax by the Ascoli test is discouraged by several authors (10, 37). In addition to the bulkiness of this type of specimen for transport, the possibility of contaminating the environment increases. The extract of these tissues offers little more than confusion to those who must interpret the Ascoli test results [for procedure, see Wright (61)]. A positive precipitin band or ring indicates only that the heat-stable cellular antigens shared by *B. anthracis* and other members of the genus are present. Furthermore, the hyperimmune anthrax serum required for this procedure is not available commercially.

Acute- and convalescent-phase serum samples. Collecting serum specimens in the acute stage of illness and again in convalescence was not recommended in the past, because antibody response to the anthrax bacilli was not specific. To date, publications indicate that the protective antigen of this bacillus is specific and elicits sufficient antibody to be detected by such sensitive serological methods as the diffusion precipitin reaction (48), passive hemagglutination (20), and tests to determine its antigenic combining power (26). These methods, however, are still developmental and are performed only in a few specialized laboratories.

Environmental Specimens

Environmental specimens include all samples collected that do not originate from clinical sources. Hides, hair, bone, fertilizers, soil, water, and samples of airborne particulates from industrial plants are only some of the possibilities. The collection procedures should stress both sterile technique when possible and containment of the samples for transport to the laboratory to avoid infecting handlers and contaminating the environment. Amounts to be collected for each specimen type should approximate 500 g if available (16). Soil samples should be collected to a depth of 15 cm (21). Otherwise, sampling should conform to statistical principles for sample size and randomness as applicable. Large samples, such as hides, hair, or bones, should be placed in double plastic bags, each of which is sealed separately. Smaller samples should be placed in sterile, preferably nonbreakable jars or other containers. Only the liquid samples need refrigeration during transit.

The following procedure has been shown to increase significantly the level of recovery of *B. anthracis* spores from environmental samples of soil when as few as 7 viable spores per 10 g of artificially seeded soil were detected (50). If centrifuge capacity permits, suspensions of about 200 ml should be used as follows.

1. Prepare a 20% suspension of soil or 6% suspension of hide or hair (w/v) in sterile 0.03 mM KH_2PO_4 buffer (pH 7.2) containing 0.25% polyethylene-(20)-sorbitan monooleate ("Tween 80") (3).

2. For preparations that can be homogenized in a mechanical blender, mix the suspension at maximal rpm for 1.5 min *in a bacteriological safety cabinet*. With bone and similar specimens, place the suspension on a mechanical shaker and agitate vigorously for 30 min.

3. Before proceeding, allow the blender or container to stand unopened for 5 min in the safety cabinet to reduce the hazard of infectious aerosol.

4. Transfer the supernatant fluid to an unbreakable centrifuge bottle. If the supernatant fluid contains excessive detritus (the fines of predominantly clayey soils entrap the greatest number of bacterial spores in this operation when compared with those soils composed mainly of humus or sand), centrifuge it at $400 \times g$ for 5 min.

5. Centrifuge the supernatant fluid of the original or clarified suspension at $6000 \times g$ for 30 min.

6. Carefully decant the final supernatant fluid, and discard it into disinfectant [5% hypochlorite or phenol (19)] or to a container that will later be autoclaved.

7. Resuspend the sediment in one-twentieth its original volume or 10 ml of 0.3 mM phosphate buffer without detergent.

8. Mix the suspension thoroughly by hand or mechanically for 2 min, transfer the suspension to a screw-capped tube, secure the cap tightly, and seal the cap to the tube with water-resistant tape.

9. Submerge the entire tube in a 70 C water bath for 10 min, and cool the contents of the tube rapidly. Include a control tube of water with a thermometer or allow sufficient time for the suspension to reach 70 C.

10. Inoculate the suspension to appropriate media and laboratory animals according to the recommendations in a later section.

Water, washings of bone, or hair specimens and samples of air impinged into liquids are more easily concentrated by filtration through sterile, 0.4- to 0.7-μm mean-pore-diameter membrane filters of mixed esters of cellulose or polycarbonate (49). Normally, 100 to 200 ml of water or suspension can be filtered in a reasonable period of time, if the concentration of suspended particles is not too high, or as much as 1 liter of potable water can be filtered. After the filtration procedure, membranes can be placed directly on appropriate media, ground, and processed as above, or subjected to an enrichment procedure before plating to other bacteriologic media as described below.

Devices for sampling the air in factories, processing plants, etc., concentrate airborne particles by impingement either directly on the surface of bacteriological medium [Andersen-type sampler (2)] or into liquid that may be further processed [the large volume slit-type samplers (7, 39)]. An advantage of the Andersen sampler is that it provides information on the range of particle sizes in which the pathogenic spores may occur. Dalldorf et al. (13) showed that particle size of 5 μm or less in diameter is required to infect primates. Disadvantages of this type of sampler are its limited sampling capacity (1 cfm) and the special requirement that a selective or inhibitory medium be used to prevent overgrowth by saprophytes impinged on the surface of the medium (3). In contrast, impingement of airborne particles into liquids by the large volume slit-type sampler offers collection of greater volumes of air (usually at least 1000 liters/min) and affords a variety of procedures for concentrating the trapped spores further; hence, the slit-sampling method is more sensitive for demonstrating anthrax spores.

Diagnostic Procedures

Demonstrating the presence of *B. anthracis* in the laboratory may be very easy or extremely difficult. The portal of entry usually determines the difficulty level. External lesions containing gram-positive, encapsulated rods in the serous fluid provide the information needed for a confirmed diagnosis. Conversely, respiratory or gastrointestinal anthrax mimics various other and more common illnesses and may require considerable testing. The time consumed in performing these procedures is frequently at the expense of the victim, and final diagnosis usually comes after the necropsy. Lack of good bacteriological technique has delayed diagnosis in several instances, because workers considered specimens and cultures "contaminated."

The descriptions and procedures listed below should resolve the diagnostic difficulties, particularly in differentiating between *B. anthracis* and *B. cereus*, a saprophyte distributed abundantly in nature.

Microscopic Examination of Specimens

Smears received or prepared for staining should be fixed in Zenker's fluid for 3 to 5 min or in 10% Formalin for 10 min to inactivate any anthrax spores present. Routine fixation of smears in a flame inactivates few anthrax spores, as Buravtseva demonstrated (8). She found that 20% to 30% of the spores were viable in smears containing 125 million spores/ml even after she had passed the smears through the flame 70 times. Corroboration is presented by Soltys (51), who surmised that a laboratory infection was due to a "heat-fixed" smear of *B. anthracis*.

At least two smears of each specimen should be prepared and inactivated. One should be Gram stained (Giemsa's method or 1% aqueous methylene blue are acceptable substitutes). Feeley and Brachman (19) recommend that the second smear be stained in the fluorescent antibody procedure if possible. Otherwise, smears of tissue, blood, or exudate should be stained with other methods to determine whether cells are encapsulated. Most staining methods for capsules will yield satisfactory results; however, Soltys (52) recommends a modification of Leifson's method. The laboratory that receives only one smear from tissue, exudate, or blood should consider performing a capsule stain. The presence of spores can be demonstrated with any appropriate available method.

B. anthracis is a large, square-ended, gram-positive, sporeforming rod. It measures 1.0 to 1.3 μm by 3 to 10 μm. Spores are oval and located centrally to subterminally and produce no observable swelling of the cell (Figure 15.1). In conjunction with the cellular morphology just described, the presence of encapsulated rods provides sufficient evidence for a tentative diagnosis of anthrax.

Cultural Examination of Specimens

Tissue fragments, blood, sputum, feces, and spinal fluid should be streaked to obtain isolated colonies directly on the surfaces of a routinely used peptone-base agar and 5% blood agar. Blood for the medium must be free of antibiotics, either defibrinated or citrated, and taken from sheep, rabbit, or man (19). Feces and any other specimens likely to contain large numbers of saprophytic microorganisms should also be streaked to selective PLET medium. Incubate plates aerobically at 37 C for 18 hr. All colonies should be examined under good illumination with the light at several different angles to the colonies. A dissecting microscope is helpful. Most colonies of *B. anthracis* are flat, have irregular borders, measure approximately 5 mm in diameter, appear rough in texture, and frequently produce small finger-like outgrowths called commas, comet tails, or "Medusa heads" (Figure 15.2). On blood agar, no hemolysis or very weak hemolysis occurs when colonies are examined after 14 to 18 hr of incubation (32). Noting the hemolytic reaction during the aforementioned time interval is important, because some strains produce questionable hemolysis after longer periods of incubation (35). Colonies with these

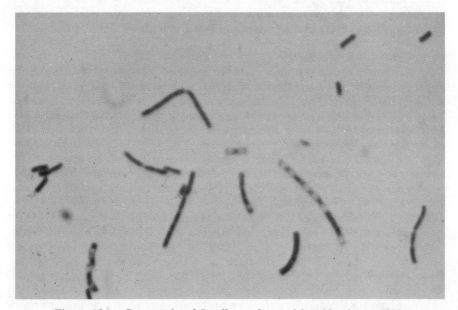

Figure 15.1—Gram stain of *Bacillus anthracis*. Magnification: ×6000.

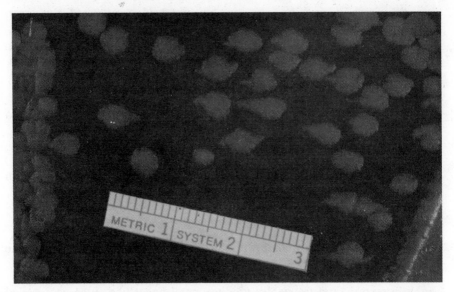

Figure 15.2—Colonies of *B. anthracis* showing comet tail borders of "Medusa heads" on blood agar. Magnification: ×2.

characteristics require further study, and pure cultures inoculated to fresh agar slants should be sent immediately to the state health or veterinary department. The tenacity of cells in the colony should be noted during the step in which colonies are selected for sub-culture. If the edge of a colony is pushed horizontally toward the center of the colony and lifted, colonies of anthrax bacilli may be reshaped and retain the new configuration (Figure 15.3), whereas colonies of *B. cereus* usually will not.

The most decisive and reliable method presently available for differentiating *B. anthracis* from similar but nonpathogenic microorganisms is the gamma phage test. Briefly, the procedure requires the streaking of approximately 0.1 ml of an 18-hr broth culture of the suspected isolate to the dry surface of a peptone-base agar. Similarly, one plate each is streaked with broth cultures of known isolates of *B. anthracis* and *B. cereus* to serve as positive and negative controls, respectively. Two areas on the outside of the dishes should be marked to show one site for deposition of the phage suspension and another for the diluent control. One drop of undilute gamma phage should be placed on the agar in the prescribed area; a drop of sterile broth or saline should be placed in the area marked as the diluent control. Agar surfaces should dry again before the lids of the dishes are secured, and the specimen should be incubated at 37 C. After 18 hr of incubation, the phage sites should be examined for lysis (a zone of little or no bacterial growth) surrounded by luxuriant growth. Lysis, which may be observed as early as 4 hr after incubation begins, for the known *B. anthracis* culture and the unknown isolate, along with absence of lysis for the diluent and *B. cereus* controls, confirms the unknown isolate to be *B. anthracis*. Should a more rapid identification be required, Feeley and Brachman (19) recommend that an extra set of plates as described above be prepared from a suspect colony, but *not* in lieu of testing with an 18-hr broth culture as well. The colony or growth should be emulsified in 1 or 2 ml of broth, diluted with more broth to contain approximately 10^8 cells/ml (equivalent to the No. 1 McFarland nephelometric standard), and streaked as described above.

If gamma phage is not available, other characteristics must be used in identifying *B. anthracis*. One of these traits is lack of motility, although several authors cited by Brown and Cherry (5) report isolating motile strains, and Brown et al. (6) succeeded in inducing motility in 6 of 80 strains with omega phage treatment. A hanging drop of a 12- to 18-hr culture should be used, or motility medium should be inoculated and incubated at 37 C for 4 days.

Another characteristic of *B. anthracis* is its sensitivity to penicillin. This feature permitted developing the "string of pearls" differential test. In this test, a drop of a 12- to 18-hr broth culture is transferred to the surfaces of a nutrient agar containing 0.5 unit of penicillin/ml and to another containing 10 units/ml. After the plates have incubated at 37 C for 3 to 6 hr, a cover slip is placed over the inoculum site on the medium with 0.5 unit of penicillin/ml. Growth under the cover slip is then examined with a microscope under low-power magnification. The presence of large, round cells ("string of pearls") indicates that the culture is *B. anthracis*. Li and Kuo (36) examined 269 strains of *B. anthracis* and found that all the strains produced "a string of pearls," although 4.8% of the strains were judged to be atypical. In contrast, only 8.2% of the 279 nonanthrax strains examined produced atypical forms instead of negative results. After 18 hr of incubation, one should observe little or no growth for *B. anthracis* inoculated to the medium containing 10 units of penicillin/ml.

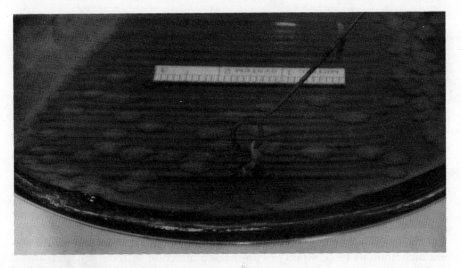

Figure 15.3—Teased colony of *B anthracis* depicting tenacity of cells in colony. Magnification: ×3.

A third method for identifying *B. anthracis* culturally is demonstrating the ability of most virulent strains to encapsulate when cultivated on bicarbonate medium in a candle jar (approximately 2.5% CO_2) at 37 C. A simple medium contains 1 part aqueous, 7% filter-sterilized sodium bicarbonate solution added to 9 parts sterile nutrient agar at 45 C; it is mixed and poured into petri dishes. A more complex medium is described by Meynell and Meynell (41), who developed it when they found that some peptones contain inhibitors that suppress capsule formation. The presence of glucose in the medium also suppresses capsule formation. Their medium buffered the above bicarbonate medium at pH 7.4 for maximal retention of the HCO_3^- and added filter-sterilized bovine serum albumin, fraction V, to a final concentration of 0.7% (w/v). Colonies are examined for a mucoid appearance after incubation at 37 C in a candle jar for 21 to 24 hr. The presence of mucoid colonies is strongly indicative that the isolated unknown is *B. anthracis*. Unfortunately, the absence of mucoid colonies does not exclude *B. anthracis*, because there are nonencapsulating strains of the bacillus.

In the past, differentiating *B. anthracis* from *B. cereus* based on biochemical reactions was stressed; yet the variation in reactions frequently failed to allow an unknown culture to be identified. Testing isolates for biochemical reactions is secondary to determining the susceptibility of the unknown isolate to gamma phage. The principal biochemical reactions for *B. anthracis*, as opposed to *B. cereus*, are: (a) no or very slow reduction in litmus milk within 2 to 3 days or no reduction of methylene blue within 24 hr, (b) no liquefaction of gelatin within 7 days, and (c) no or delayed fermentation of salicin after 24 hr of incubation. Both species usually produce acid but no gas from glucose, maltose, and sucrose; both usually do not produce acid from arabinose, mannitol, and xylose.

Animal Inoculation of Clinical Specimens

Special precautions and strict adherence to safety measures are required when working with animals inoculated with anthrax bacilli. *All operations must be performed in a biological safety cabinet.* Inoculated animals should be housed separately, preferably in safety cabinets as well. All used bedding, cages, syringes, carcasses, etc., must be autoclaved and the disposable items incinerated.

A loopful of an 18- to 24-hr growth from an isolated colony is emulsified with an inoculating loop in a small amount of sterile saline solution. The suspension is diluted with additional saline until no visible turbidity can be detected. Several 18- to 25-g mice are inoculated subcutaneously with 0.2 ml of diluted suspension, or guinea pigs can be inoculated with 0.5 ml of the preparations. Under no circumstances should broth cultures be inoculated, because many *Bacillus* species also produce lethal exotoxins.

Selection of the experimental host should involve considering the apparent dichotomous susceptibility of animals to infection with the microorganism and to resistance to its toxin and vice versa. Lincoln et al. (38) showed evidence to support this hypothesis that animals are resistant to anthrax infection but susceptible to its toxin. Using the terminal number of organisms/ml of blood, amount of toxin in terminal blood, susceptible dose, doubling rate of the organism in the blood, phagocytic inhibition by toxin, etc., these authors rated the susceptibility of the various species. The most susceptible host was the chimpanzee, followed in order by the guinea pig, rabbit, mouse, rhesus monkey, goat, sheep, horse, cow, man, rat, dog, and swine. By reversing the order given, one obtains the sequence for susceptibility to anthrax toxin. Hence, the rat would probably be the most available animal to use in assaying for the presence of toxin in terminal blood.

The dose of *B. anthracis* also influences the time required to produce lethality. Generally, the greater the concentration of the microorganism, the more rapidly clinical signs appear and death occurs. With grossly contaminated specimens, however, deaths of mice and guinea pigs that occur within the first 24 hr after inoculation are frequently caused by microorganisms other than anthrax bacilli. Animals usually die from anthrax 2 to 10 days after being inoculated. For heavily contaminated specimens. Davies and Harvey (16) suggest that suspensions be inoculated into guinea pigs passively immunized with the following antitoxins 24 hr earlier: *Clostridium welchii*, 1000 I.U.; *C. septicum*, 500 I.U.; *C. oedematiens*, 1000 I.U.; and 500 I.U. of tetanus.

Spleens and peritoneal exudates from all necropsied animals should be stained and subcultured to establish the presence of *B. anthracis*.

Environmental Specimens

Two-tenths of a milliliter of the 10-ml suspension processed under "Collection and Processing of Specimens" above is inoculated to each of two plates of 5% blood agar and Knisely's PLET medium. The inoculum is spread over the entire surface of the medium with a sterile rod or loop. The surface is allowed to dry, and specimens are incubated at 37 C. The remaining suspension is halved, and each portion is inoculated subcutaneously into four or five areas on the abdomens of guinea pigs. Animals are checked daily; those which die are necropsied, and the spleens and exudates are processed as described above.

The selective PLET medium aids immeasurably in isolating *B. anthracis* present in specimens contaminated with other sporeforming saprophytes. However, the inhibitors present in this medium reduce significantly the number of spores germinating, as well as the size and roughness of the resulting colonies of anthrax bacilli. A reduction of 28% was noted with a Utah isolate of anthrax when colonies were compared with spores germinating on blood agar (49). Knisely (31) tested 21 strains of *B. anthracis* and found that all of them grow on this medium in 48 hr (20 of 21 grew within 24 hr). Only one of 10 strains of *B. cereus* tested and three of five strains of *B. subtilis* var. *niger* grew on PLET medium. This medium prepared without agar can be used as a selective broth for isolating *B. anthracis* from processed sediments and particles of spores deposited on membrane filters (31).

Suspended particles concentrated on surfaces of membrane filters provide a means for greatly increasing the sensitivity of detecting small numbers of anthrax spores. The thinness of the polycarbonate filter relative to the cellulose variety makes it preferable for use in recognizing colonies of *B. anthracis* (Figure 15.4), although excessive charge of static electricity on the polycarbonate filter makes it more difficult to handle. In addition to placing the membranes directly on the surfaces of blood agar and PLET medium, two other methods involve filters. Mikhailov et al. (42) placed their filters on bicarbonate medium, incubated the medium under increased CO_2 tension for 16 hr at 37 C, and stained the colonies with 1% aqueous safranin solution. Encapsulated colonies of *B. anthracis* were readily identified, because they stained bright yellow. Similarly, Gillissen and Scholz (23) placed membrane filters on the surface of a peptone-based medium containing 100 units of polymyxin B/ml, incubated the plates at 37 C for 24 hr, and transferred the membranes to 5% blood agar for additional incubation before identifying colonies of anthrax based on the hemolytic reaction and colonial morphology.

Serologic Procedures

Staining the smears of blood, tissue impressions, and exudates with fluorescein-labeled antibody rapidly provides presumptive evidence for the presence of *B. anthracis* (19). However, few laboratories possess the specifically labeled antibody or are experienced in using it. The laboratory of the state health department or other governmental reference laboratory can be consulted about examining smears by this staining procedure.

Acute- and convalescent-phase serum samples provide evidence for diag-

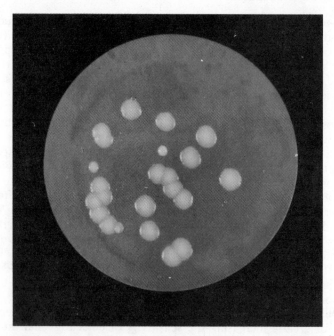

Figure 15.4—Colonies of *B. anthracis* on 47-mm-diameter polycarbonate membrane filter after 24 hr at 37 C on blood agar. Magnification: ×1.5.

nosing anthrax infection when processed with special serological procedures (20, 26, 48) currently being used only in research laboratories. Recently, Kebedjiev and Siromashkova compared the sensitivity of serological tests for detecting the antibody concentrations in the serum of immunized animals and human beings and found that the hemagglutination inhibition technique was considerably more sensitive than the complement fixation procedure (29).

Antimicrobic Susceptibility and Resistance

In its susceptibility to antibiotics and other therapeutics, *B. anthracis* behaves like a typical gram-positive microorganism. Greatest susceptibility is observed *in vivo* when penicillin, streptomycin, or oxytetracycline is administered. Preferred to a lesser degree for effectiveness are chlortetracycline, erythromycin, neomycin, and sulfonamide.

Although reports from several authors (9, 27, 46, 47) state that strains of *B. anthracis* produce penicillinase, there appears to be no evidence that this causes a problem outside the laboratory.

Evaluation of Laboratory Findings

Demonstration of the encapsulated, gram-positive rods in smears of blood and body fluids from persons with clinical signs of anthrax or isolation of gram-positive bacilli that are lysed by gamma phage constitutes the main criterion for diagnosing anthrax. All other observations and tests described are secondary.

Treatment and Prophylaxis

In treating the cutaneous form of anthrax in man, Gold (24) preferred penicillin to the tetracyclines, because of the time required for the microorganisms to disappear from the serous fluid of lesions. He recommended an initial dose of 10,000 to 50,000 units of the crystalline form of penicillin followed by 20,000 to 50,000 units every 3 to 4 hr or 600,000 units of the repository penicillin every 12 to 24 hr. This regimen of therapy was continued until the edema and erythema began to subside, usually in 24 to 48 hr, when the dosage was reduced to 300,000 to 600,000 units daily. Ellingson et al. (17) used total dosages from approximately 1 to 4 million units of penicillin over a 2- to 6-day period in the treatment of 24 cases of cutaneous anthrax in man. The Jarisch-Herxheimer reaction, transient elevation of the patient's temperature within 2 hr after antibiotic therapy begins, should be expected. In untreated, advanced cases, the anthrax toxin must be neutralized if the patient is to survive. Administering hyperimmune antitoxin is the only way to counteract the toxins.

In treatment of laboratory animals infected with *B. anthracis*, Lincoln et al. (37) ranked the preferred treatment for mice given a single injection as follows: penicillin-dihydrostreptomycin combined, followed in order by penicillin alone, dihydrostreptomycin alone, chlortetracycline, and oxytetracycline. Chloramphenicol was only slightly more effective (5% survival) than no treatment for control mice (0% survival) challenged with 100,000 germinated anthrax spores.

Nonviable, protective antigens are available and effective in providing immunization for persons whose occupations may expose them to *B. anthracis* (61). Because these preparations are tolerated well after injection, immunization has been recommended for industrial workers, veterinarians, and scientific personnel who may be exposed to infection. This antigen is available from the Center for Disease Control, Atlanta, Ga, for immunization in the United States. The Ministry of Health in Great Britain provides a similar preparation for distribution throughout the United Kingdom. In Russia, a nonencapsulated spore vaccine which has been administered by the respiratory route as well as the cutaneous one appears to provide significant protection.

Decontamination and Disinfection

The persistence of anthrax spores makes gaseous spaces in laboratories and industry and decontamination of the outside environment particularly difficult. Before beta-propiolactone was shown to be carcinogenic, it was the compound of choice for decontaminating large gaseous enclosures. Presently gaseous formaldehyde applied as sublimated paraformaldehyde or steam or chemically generated solutions of Formalin to sealed buildings at a final concentration of 1.38 to 1.62 mg/liter of air should reduce the viability of anthrax spores tenfold or more (62). If polymerization of the formaldehyde poses a problem in cleaning the rooms after vaporization, 10% methanol should be added to the solution to be aerosolized. For smaller enclosed areas, ethylene oxide is an effective disinfectant. Uchida et al. (58) demonstrated that concentrations of at least 10% ethylene oxide kill anthrax spores in 3 hr. Lesser concentrations, 1.5% at 20 C or 0.5% at 30 C, killed anthrax spores on filter paper and collagen membrane in 72 hr. For clothing, Darlow (14) found that a 4% solution of commercial Formalin that contained 1% cationic or ampholytic detergent killed heavy suspensions of anthrax spores in 4 hr at room temperature.

There has been little success in disinfecting soils contaminated with anthrax spores. Carcasses should be incinerated in situ with fuel oil, discarded lumber, tires, etc., because removing them to distant burning pits substantially increases the probability for contaminating other areas of the pasture, vehicles, and personnel. Chemical disinfection of livestock runs, pastures, and unvegetated soil was attempted by Stellmacher and Zerbe (54), who found that 5.0% aqueous Formalin was effective on sandy soil but ineffective on animal runs of loamy soil or any soil covered with vegetation.

References

1. ANANTHAPADMANABHAN K: An outbreak of anthrax among sheep and goats with particular reference to its possible transmission by ticks. Indian Vet J 39:667–678, 1962. *From* Biol Abstr 43, Entry No. 7126, 1963

2. ANDERSEN AA: New sampler for the collection, sizing, and enumeration of viable airborne particles. J Bacteriol 76:471–484, 1958

3. BIEGELEISEN JZ Jr, CHERRY WB, SKALIY P, and MOODY MC: The demonstration of *Bacillus anthracis* in environmental specimens by conventional and fluorescent antibody techniques. Am J Hyg 75:230–239, 1962

4. BRACHMAN PS: Human anthrax in the United States. Antimicrob Agents Chemother 1965:111–114, 1965

5. BROWN ER and CHERRY WB: Specific identification of *Bacillus anthracis* by means of a variant bacteriophage. J Infect Dis 96:34–39, 1955

6. BROWN ER, CHERRY WB, MOODY MC, and GORDON MA: The induction of motility in *Bacillus anthracis* by means of bacteriophage lysates. J Bacteriol 69:590–602, 1955

7. BUCHANAN LM, DECKER HM, FRISQUE DE, PHILLIPS CR, and DAHLGREN CM: Novel multislit large volume air sampler. Appl Microbiol 16:1110–1123, 1968

8. BURAVTSEVA NP: Effect of fixing smears over a flame on the viability of anthrax spores (Transl. from Russian). In Osobo opasnye infektsii na Kavkaze. Stavropol, 224, 1966. *From* Biol Abstr 49, Entry No. 57451, 1968

9. BURAVTSEVA NP: Role of penicillinase in the mechanism of resistance of Siberian plague to benzylpenicillin (Transl. from Russian). Antibiotiki 16:168–173, 1971. *From* Biol Abstr 54, Entry No. 24335, 1972

10. CENTER FOR DISEASE CONTROL: Annual summary of morbidity and mortality, 1978. Morbid Mortal Weekly Rep 27:54, 1979

11. CENTER FOR DISEASE CONTROL: Epidemiologic notes and reports. Anthrax—California. Morbid Mortal Weekly Rep 25(5):33–34, 1976

12. CHERKASSKII BL and MARCHUK LM: Natural *B. anthracis* infection of mouse-like rodents and ticks in the U.S.S.R. (Transl. from Russian). Zh Mikrobiol Epidemiol Immunobiol 48:45–48, 1971. *From* Biol Abstr 52, Entry No. 139130, 1971

13. DALLDORF FG, KAUFMANN AF, and BRACHMAN PS: Woolsorters' disease: an experimental model. Arch Pathol 92:418–426, 1971

14. DARLOW HM: Decontamination methods for overalls of hide and wool handlers. Proc R Soc Med 63:59–60, 1970

15. DAVIES DG: The influence of temperature and humidity on spore formation and germination in *Bacillus anthracis*. J Hyg 58:177–186, 1960

16. DAVIES DG and HARVEY RWS: The isolation of *Bacillus anthracis* from bones. Lancet 2:86–87, 1955.

17. ELLINGSON HV, KADULL PJ, BOOKWALTER HL, and HOWE C: Cutaneous anthrax. Report of twenty-five cases. J Am Med Assoc 131:1105, 1946

18. ENTICKNAP JB, GALBRAITH NS, TOMLINSON AJH, and ELIAS-JONES TF: Pulmonary anthrax caused by contaminated sacks. Br J Ind Med 25:72–74, 1968

19. FEELEY JC and BRACHMAN PS: *Bacillus anthracis. In* Manual of Clinical Microbiology, 2nd edition. Lennette EH, Spaulding EH, and Truant JP (eds.). American Society for Microbiology, Washington, DC, 1974, pp 143–147

20. FEELEY JC, BUCHANAN TM, HAYES PS, and BRACHMAN PS: Anthrax indirect microhemagglutination test. Bacteriol Proc 126:282–284, 1970

21. FOX MD, BOYCE JM, FEELEY JC, WOOD BT, KAUFMANN AF, and GANGAROSA EJ: Animal anthrax, Falls County, Texas, EPI 75-6-2, 1975

22. FOX MD, KAUFMANN AF, ZENDEL SA, KOLB RC, SONGY CG JR, CANGELOSI DA, and FULLER CE: Anthrax in Louisiana, 1971: epizootiologic study. J Am Vet Assoc 163:446–451, 1973

23. GILLISSEN G and SCHOLZ HG: Die Selektion von Milzbrandbazillen aus Flüssigkeiten mit starker Verunreinigung durch *E. coli.* Zentralbl Bakteriol Parasitenkd Infektionskr Hyg 182:232–237, 1961

24. GOLD H: Treatment of anthrax. Fed Proc 26:1563–1568, 1967

25. GONZALES Y GONZALES G: Viabilidad de los esporos de *B. anthracix* en suelos bajo distintas condiciones. An Edafol Fisiol Veg 9:665–677, 1950

26. GRUBER J and WRIGHT GG: Iodine-131 labeling of purified microbial antigens by microdiffusion. Proc Soc Exp Biol Med 126:282–284, 1967

27. HORODNICEANU T and SASRMAN A: Contribution to the study of bacterial penicillinase. III. Relationships between penicillinase production and susceptibility to penicillin in *Bacillus anthracis* (Transl. from Roumanian). Arch Roum Pathol Exp Microbiol 20:257:262, 1961. *From* Biol Abstr 37, Entry No. 10224, 1962

28. HUGH-JONES ME and HUSSAINI SN: An anthrax outbreak in Berkshire (England). Vet Rec 94:228–232, 1974

29. KEBEDJIEF G and SIROMASHKOVA M: Immunologic study on immunized persons with a past history of anthrax (Transl. from Bulgarian). Probl Zaraznite Parazit Bolesti 3:203–210, 1975. *From* Biol Abstr 66, Entry No. 21634, 1978

30. KLEMM DM and KLEMM WR: A history of anthrax. J Am Vet Assoc 135:458–462, 1959

31. KNISLEY RF: Selective medium for *Bacillus anthracis*. J Bacteriol 92:784–786, 1966

32. KOLYAKOV TE and MELIKHOV AD: The rapid diagnosis of the anthrax bacillus in water (Transl. from Russian). Veterinariya 3:81–84, 1960. *From* Biol Abstr 38, Entry No. 22887, 1962

33. KRINSKY WL: Animal disease agents transmitted by horse flies and deer flies (Dipter; Tabanidae). J Med Entomol 13:225–275, 1976. *From* Biol Abstr 63:Entry No. 59748, 1977

34. LAFORCE FM, BUMFORD FH, FEELEY JC, STOKES SL, and SNOW DB: Epidemiologic study of a fatal case of inhalation anthrax. Arch Environ Health 18:798–805, 1969

35. LEISE JM, CARTER CH, FRIEDLANDER H, and FREED SW: Criteria for the identification of *Bacillus anthracis*. J Bacteriol 77:655–660, 1959

36. LI L and KUO HP: A study of string-of-pearls test of *B. anthracis* (Transl. from Chinese). Acta Microbiol Sinica 11:80–87, 1965. *From* Biol Abstr 49, Entry No. 40917, 1968

37. LINCOLN RE, WALKER JS, KLEIN F, and HAINES BW: Anthrax. Adv Vet Sci 9:3327–368, 1964

38. LINCOLN RE, WALKER JS, KLEIN F, ROSENWALD AJ, and JONES WI JR: Value of field data for extrapolation in anthrax. Fed Proc 26:1558–1562, 1967

39. LITTON SYSTEMS: Model M large-volume air sampler: instruction manual. Report No. 3028. Applied Science Division. Litton Systems, Inc, Minneapolis, Minn, 1966

40. MACVEAN DW and ESPE BH: Occurrence of anthrax in Oklahoma in 1974. Okla Vet 27:18–21, 1975

41. MEYNELL E and MEYNELL GG: The roles of serum and carbon dioxide in capsule formation by *Bacillus anthracis*. J Gen Microbiol 34:153–164, 1964

42. MIKHAILOV B YA, ROZHKOV GI, and TAMARIN AL: A rapid method for the diagnosis and detection of *Bacillus anthracis* (Transl. from Russian). Zh Mikrobiol Epidemiol Immunobiol 31:10–15, 1960

43. NALIN DR, SULTANA B, SAHUNJA R, ISLAM AK, RAHIM MA, ISLAM M, COSTA BS, MAWLA N, and GREENOUGH WB III: Survival of a patient with intestinal anthrax. Am J Med 62:130–132, 1977

44. NATIONAL COMMUNICABLE DISEASE CENTER: Cutaneous anthrax—North Carolina. Morbid Mortal Weekly Rep 18:(56):408, 1969

45. National Institute of Health Safety Guide, 1974. U.S. Dept. of Health, Education and Welfare, Public Health Service. Superintendent of Documents, U.S. Government Printing Office, Washington, DC, 1974

46. PROKUPEK K: The mechanism of arising resistance to penicillin in *Bacillus anthracis* after controlled adaptation (Transl. from Czech). Vet Med (Prague) 13:437–447, 1968. *From* Biol Abstr 50, Entry No. 111242, 1969

47. PROKUPEK K: The penicillinase activity of anthrax and cereus strains (Transl. from Czech). Vet Med (Prague) 13:149–158, 1968. *From* Biol Abstr 50, Entry No. 76564, 1969

48. RAY JG JR and KADULL PJ: Agar-gel precipitin technique in anthrax antibody determinations. Appl Microbiol 12:349–354, 1964

49. REES HB JR and SMITH MA: Enhanced recovery of *Bacillus anthracis* from environmental samples (soils) by membrane filtration of suspensions treated with filter aid. Bacteriol Proc, p. 44, 1977

50. REES HB JR, SMITH MA, SPENDLOVE JC, FRASER RS, FUKUSHIMA T, BARBOUR AG JR, and SCHOENFELD FJ: Epidemiology and laboratory investigations of bovine anthrax in two Utah counties in 1975, Public Health Rep 92:176–186, 1977

51. SOLTYS MA: Anthrax in a laboratory worker, with observations on the possible source of infection. J Pathol Bacteriol 60:253, 1948

52. SOLTYS MA: A new method of demonstrating capsulated *Bacillus anthracis*. J Clin Pathol 13:526–527, 1960

53. STEIN DC: Anthrax in livestock during 1953 and a review of data on incidence from 1945 to 1953. Vet Med 49:277–280, 1954

54. STELLMACHER W and ZERBE J: Disinfection of livestock outdoor runs, pastures and ground (Transl. from German). Source not given, 1971. *From* Biol Abstr 54, Entry No. 53719, 1972

55. STILES GW: Isolation of *Bacillus anthracis* from spinose ear ticks *Ornithodorus megnini.* Am J Vet Res 5:318–319, 1944

56. SUFFIN SC, CARNES WH, and KAUFMAN AF: Inhalation anthrax in a home craftsman. Human Pathol 9(5):594–597, 1978

57. TOSCHKOFF A and VELJANOV D: Sporulation and virulence of *Bacillus anthracis* in opened and unopened animal carcasses (Transl. from Russian). Arch Exp Veterinaermed 24:1153–1160, 1970. *From* Biol Abstr 52, Entry No. 90768, 1971

58. UCHIDA K, TERADA A, TANAKA S, ICHIMAN Y, and NAGANO S: Effect of ethylene oxide sterilization (Transl. from Japanese). Bull Nippon Vet Zootech Coll 21:1–7, 1972. *From* Biol Abstr 56, Entry No. 59913, 1973

59. WALKER JS, LINCOLN RE, and KLEIN F: Pathophysiological and biochemical changes in anthrax. Fed Proc 26:1539–1544, 1967

60. WILSON JB and RUSSELL KE: Isolation of *Bacillus anthracis* from soil stored 60 years. J Bacteriol 87:237–238, 1964

61. WRIGHT GG: Anthrax. *In* Diseases Transmitted from Animals to Man, 6th edition. Hubert WT, McCulloch WF, and Schnurrenberger PR (eds.). Charles C Thomas, Springfield, Ill, 1975, pp 237–250

62. YOUNG LS, FEELEY JC, and BRACHMAN PS: Vaporized formaldehyde treatment of a textile mill contaminated with *Bacillus anthracis.* Arch Environ Health 20:400–403, 1970

63. ZAPOROZHACHENKO AY: Epidemiological and clinical characteristics of anthrax (Transl. from Russian). Zh Mikrobiol Epidemiol Immunobiol 33:111–115, 1962. *From* Defense Documentation Center, Defense Supply Agency, Transl. No. 723, A. D. No. 299067, 1962

CHAPTER 16

BARTONELLOSIS AND ANEMIAS ASSOCIATED WITH *BARTONELLA*-LIKE STRUCTURES

David Weinman

Introduction

Discussed here are three subjects: (1) bartonellosis, a well-defined clinical and microbiological entity caused by *Bartonella bacilliformis*; (2) human anemias wherein the red blood cells are associated with structures resembling *Bartonella*, but in which the erythrocytic structures have not been proved to be microorganisms; and (3) human anemias with unusual erythrocytic bodies which neither resemble *Bartonella* nor have been proved to be microorganisms.

The microorganisms discussed are all prokaryotes. *Bartonella bacilliformis* is a bacterium which infects man, but naturally acquired infection in animals is unknown. The geographical distribution of the organism is extremely restricted. It grows readily on media containing no living cells. *Eperythrozoon* and *Haemobartonella* are mycoplasma-like organisms with no cell walls. Neither occurs in humans despite their very wide host and geographical distribution; neither has been cultivated *in vitro*. Distinguishing features are summarized in Table 16.1.

Bartonellosis

Causative Organism

Bartonella bacilliformis is rod- or ring-shaped and measures about 1–3 by 0.5–0.75 μm. In the blood, the organism is on or within the red cells and also in the plasma. *B. bacilliformis* stains deeply with Romanowsky-type stains (Wright, Giemsa), and its appearance is highly distinctive (Fig 16.1).

B. bacilliformis produces a pathognomonic lesion in the tissues during the anemic phase of Oroya fever. The organism develops massively, often in rounded masses within the cytoplasm of vascular endothelial cells, particularly in the liver, lymph nodes, and spleen. At the peak of this development, the endothelial cells bulge into the lumen of the vessel, where the cells are large enough to be detected at a magnification of 100 to 200 × (Fig 16.2B).

During cutaneous bartonellosis (Verruga peruana), the tissue appears

TABLE 16.1—PROKARYOTES OF POSSIBLE IMPORTANCE IN HUMAN ANEMIAS

	BARTONELLA	*HAEMOBARTONELLA*	*EPERYTHROZOON*
Occurs in man	+	0?	0?
Occurs in other mammals	0?	+	+
Classification	Bacterium	Mycoplasma-like	Mycoplasma-like
Cultivation *in vitro*	+	0	0
Geographical distribution	Very restricted	Widely disseminated	Widely disseminated
Clinical features	1. Anemia 2. Verrucous skin eruption	1. Anemia (frequent) 2. No skin involvement 3. Major control of disease by spleen	1. Anemia (variable) 2. No skin involvement 3. Major control of disease by spleen
Transmission	Phlebotomus	Fleas and lice	Fleas and lice

quite different. *B. bacilliformis* does not develop massively in vascular endothelial cells but is scattered among newly formed cells, where it occurs both intra- and extracellularly (Fig 16.2A). A more detailed description of the pathology of bartonellosis is available elsewhere (28, 29).

In vitro, *B. bacilliformis* can be grown in pure culture by unlimited serial transfers. Tissue cells are not required, but if appropriate cells are present, the microorganism develops both within the cytoplasm and extracellularly. Media containing serum and hemoglobin are used successfully; most widely employed is the semisolid "leptospira medium" of Noguchi et al. (10).

In this medium, growth first appears as a whitish haze about 1 cm below the surface and 1 cm deep. With more growth, spherical colonies 1 to 2 mm in diameter appear. Cultures are frequently incubated at 25 C; at this temperature, 14 to 30 days may pass before growth is evident. At 37 C development is faster, but viability is shortened.

Cultures are also obtained on blood agar slants. The organism does not hemolyze red blood cells *in vitro* nor does it attach to erythrocytes. No distinctive reactions have been obtained with various test compounds added to the medium.

Bartonella has multiple unipolar flagella shown by silver staining or shadowing techniques (16). They have been demonstrated only in culture and never in blood material and are absent from some strains *in vitro*. Although variation in isolates is known, only the species *B. bacilliformis* is recognized.

In electron micrographs, *B. bacilliformis* clearly has a cell wall (16, 20, 27). The organism stains poorly with the customary procedures for bacteria; it does not retain the Gram stain.

Clinical Manifestations

Bartonellosis is a spectacular disease, and its manifestations are unique. There are often two phases to the infection: hematic and cutaneous. These phases never coexist but occur in the sequence stated. First there is Oroya fever, an anemia. Then, in survivors, the anemia improves and bartonellae disappear from the blood, and after an interval, the patient develops a disseminated skin eruption known as Verruga peruana. Bartonellosis is also known as Carrión's disease, after the Peruvian investigator who died of Oroya fever after inoculating himself with verruga and thus greatly strengthened the concept of the unity of the two conditions.

Bartonellosis is a curiosity for the clinician and for the epidemiologist. It is unique not only in the duality of its clinical forms, a duality expressed also in the pathology of each, but it is also distinctive in the interrelation and the opposition between the two forms. These manifestations reflect, in all probability, successive immunological states of the same individual. It is one of the best examples of a geographically restricted bacteriological infection—exclusively tropical and existing only in the mountainous regions of Peru, Colombia, and Ecuador.

Oroya fever is a febrile, hemolytic, macrocytic anemia of rapid evolution, and, if untreated, has a high mortality rate. *Bartonella bacilliformis* is readily visible in stained blood films, increases in numbers with the aggravation of the anemia, and may infect over 90% of the erythrocytes.

The Oroya fever patient is often ill when first seen; if untreated, within a few days it seems amazing that the patient is alive at all. The anemia progresses quickly, and "the erythrocyte count may fall from normal to less than 1,000,000 per ml in 4 or 5 days, more rapidly than in any other condition exclusive of actual hemorrhage" (18).

Pain, fever, and generalized enlargement of the lymph nodes combine with pallor, polypnea, and vertigo to form an entity described in more detail elsewhere (28).

The mortality rate in untreated Oroya fever is about 40% and is substantially reduced by antibiotic therapy. Patients who recover frequently develop the second form of the disease, Verruga peruana.

The verruga eruption may be the initial disease manifestation or follow Oroya fever. Three types of verruga eruption are distinguished: miliary elements, which are small, elevated, and disseminated; nodular elements, which are more deep seated in the skin and fewer in number than the miliary elements; and the mulaire, which are also fewer in number than the miliary elements, deep seated, and grow toward the surface, eventually pushing through the skin.

A florid eruption of miliary verruga is a spectacular sight; the patient appears to be studded with cranberries, the "berries" varying in color from red to purple. Specialists consider it "unique" and "hardly likely to be mistaken for any other disease," whereas the other forms of verruga eruption are less distinctive. The eruptions are not synchronized. All types may occur on the same patient, develop and regress, and persist for many months. Throughout the infection, anemia is never pronounced. *Bartonella* is usually not visible on or in red cells, although it can be cultivated from the blood. The death rate, even when patients are untreated, is probably below 5% in uncomplicated cases.

The pathology of these conditions is described elsewhere (29).

Epidemiology

Bartonellosis is contracted only in northwestern South America, solely in or near the river valleys on the western slopes of the Andes, where the elevation must be less than 9,000 feet but more than 2,500 feet, and, in Peru, usually only at night. This is because the phlebotomus *Lutzomyia verrucarum* which is the Peruvian vector feeds only nocturnally. *L. verrucarum* is restricted to certain zones by its moisture and temperature requirements. Above the upper altitude limits, the night temperatures are too low (50 F or less); below a certain limit, the rainfall is insufficient and conditions too arid (24).

Other factors probably apply, for it is not known why phlebotomi do not transmit bartonellosis along river valleys below the lower altitude limits. In Colombia, the special circumstance of men working in darkened, humid houses is said to permit daylight transmission.

Once introduced to a region, bartonellosis may remain almost indefinitely; in a focus reported in 1630, the infection has persisted for over 300 years (11). Epidemics occur by infection of a previously unexposed and therefore nonimmune population, usually in one of two ways.

A nonimmune population may go into an endemic area; this produces an "internal epidemic" not related to geographical expansion. This apparently occurred in the 1870 Peruvian outbreak, with an estimated 7,000 deaths, when laborers were brought in to build the railway to Oroya (26).

Secondly, there may be actual invasion of new territory, as seems to have been the case in Colombia in 1938, when bartonellosis caused an estimated 4000 deaths (14). As late as 1959, small outbreaks continued to occur, e.g., in 1959 in the Mantaro valley of Peru (5).

Maintenance needs for *Bartonella* appear simple and involve humans and phlebotomi as vertebrate hosts and vectors of the organism. *Bartonella* is transmitted by one or more species of *Lutzomyia* or sandfly indigenous to the endemic area. Known sources of *Bartonella* are limited to man and sandflies almost exclusively, thus the importance of asymptomatic human infections. The 5%–10% of the apparently healthy population in endemic areas which have *Bartonella* circulating in the blood are possible sources of infection for phlebotomi (4, 28). No reservoir other than humans has been found despite prolonged search.

Lutzomyia verrucarum is known to be a vector in Peru; the suspect species in Colombia is *L. colombianus* and in Mantaro (Peru), *L. pescei*. Leishmaniasis, also transmitted by phlebotomus, exists in some parts of the *Bartonella* zone, but the distributions of the two diseases do not coincide.

Public Health Significance

Bartonellosis is primarily a rural disease found in river valleys in the central and western cordilleras of the Andes throughout a zone measuring about 1000 miles from 2 degrees north latitude to 13 degrees south of the equator. The width of the zone in Peru, where the geographical distribution has been most thoroughly investigated, is usually less than 100 miles. Well-entrenched in its homeland, the disease has shown very little tendency to spread (although the outbreak in Colombia may have originated elsewhere).

It is the epidemics which draw attention, and morbidity and death rates cited for interepidemic years are probably incomplete.

Preventive Measures

No effective immunization exists, and prevention centers on limiting the access of sandflies to humans. The houses in the infected valleys are not insectproof, and it would require a considerable expenditure to render them so. However, phlebotomi are susceptible to common insecticides, and DDT has furnished a simple, relatively inexpensive method for community sanitation. The application of residue sprays to the inside of residences and sleeping quarters, to the outside of doors and windows, and to likely breeding spots in the immediate vicinity exerts effective sandfly control (6). Thus far, resistance to DDT by the sandflies has posed no problems. The individual at risk may protect himself by the use of repellents (e.g., dimethyl phthalate), by fine mesh bed nets (25 per square inch), presumably by active antibiotics, and by leaving at night endemic zones where phlebotomi are nocturnal feeders only.

Collection and Processing of Specimens

Oroya fever

Blood is optimally collected before antibiotic therapy and serves for spreads and cultures. The best films are made from fresh drops of blood, not from venous bleedings. Cultures grow more quickly when the erythrocyte infection rate is high but may be positive without visible blood infection. It is advantageous to repeat the cultures for several days.

At autopsy, the spleen, liver, and enlarged lymph nodes (cervical, axillary, mesenteric, etc.) should be taken with aseptic precautions if cultures or inoculations are planned. In any case, multiple impression films should be made and stained with Giemsa or a similar stain and examined for the swollen endothelial cells containing bartonellae. The tissue is advantageously fixed in Regaud's fluid, embedded in paraffin, and stained with Giemsa for tissue sections (Wolbach's modification). Fixation for electron microscopy has been according to standard techniques.

Verruga peruana

Blood cultures are positive during the eruptive phase in the absence of therapy. The verrugas themselves contain bartonellae; however, cultures made from them are frequently contaminated. Verrugas processed in sections can be treated as for Oroya fever tissue.

Inapparent infections

These may occur without history of clinical manifestations, precede or follow Oroya fever or verruga, and are detected by blood culture.

Diagnostic Procedures

As *Bartonella* infections are longlasting, clinical manifestations may occur long after the patient has left western South America. No single item is more

Figure 16.1—*Bartonella bacilliformis* in Oroya fever. From blood films stained with Giemsa after methyl alcohol or May-Grünwald fixation, except as noted. Top row: Human Oroya fever; an intense infection involving erythrocytes and, a most unusual finding, mononuclear leukocytes also. Second row: Human Oroya fever. Left—Reticulocyte and Giemsa stain combined; right—rod and ring forms of *Bartonella*. Third row: Left—Human Oroya fever, Heidenhain's iron hematoxylin stain; right—experimental Oroya fever in a splenectomized *Macaca mulatta*. Fourth row: Human Oroya fever. From left to right, blood films of the same patient taken at intervals during 3 weeks and showing a relapse which coincided with an attack of tertian malaria. Original. Reproduced from *Infectious Blood Diseases of Man and Animals*, Weinman D and Ristic M (eds.). Academic Press, New York, 1968.

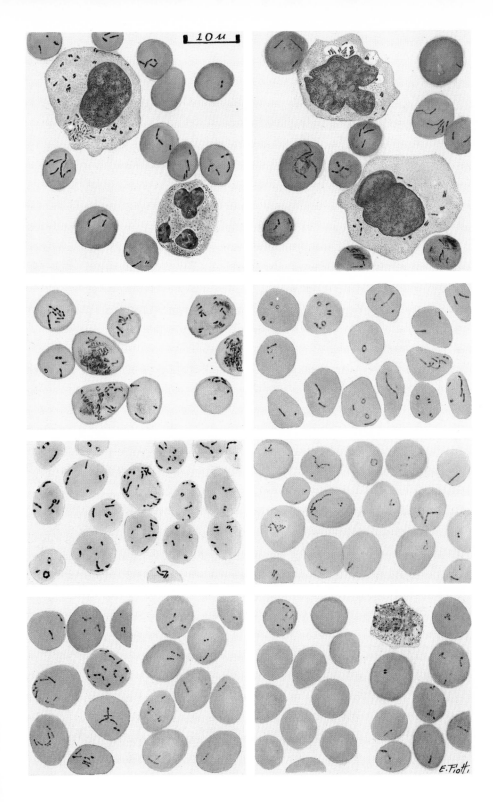

10μ

E.Piotti

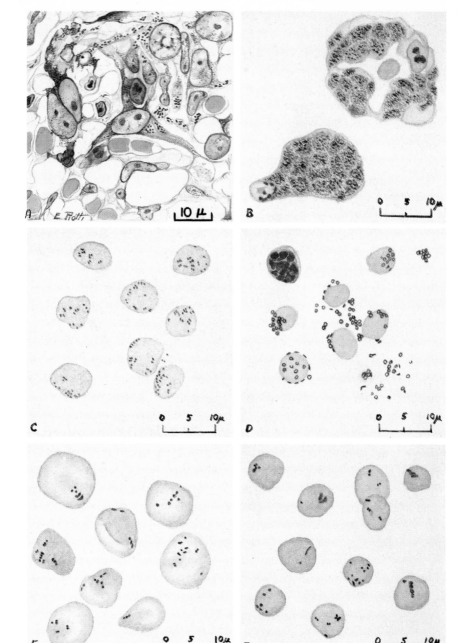

A E. Rott 10 μ

B 0 5 10μ

C 0 5 10μ

D 0 5 10μ

E 0 5 10μ

F RSmith 0 5 10μ

Figure 16.2—(A) Verruga peruana. Section of skin nodule. Regaud fixation. Giemsa stain. *Bartonella* is distinct, bright red, and in some cells clearly intracytoplasmic. Original. Reproduced from *Infectious Blood Diseases of Man and Animals*, Vol. II, Weinman D and Ristic M (eds.). Academic Press, New York, 1968. (B) Oroya fever. Autopsy sections from a patient who died near the peak of the anemia. Regaud fixation. Giemsa stain. Liver (top right). Adrenal (lower left). Bartonellae are within the cytoplasm of vascular endothelial cells. They are red purple, multiple, and frequently cause distention of the endothelial cells which then bulge into the lumen of the vessel. Original. (C) *Haemobartonella muris*. Blood film. Short rods and dotlike forms appear on the erythrocytes and are sometimes free in the plasma. Red purple in color, they may infect the majority of the red cells, which can carry multiple organisms. Original. (D) *Eperythrozoon coccoides*. Blood film. Rounded structures, frequently appearing as rings in blood films. Often multiple on the red cell and free in the plasma. Seen as rods, when on edge, adhering to the periphery of erythrocytes. Original. (E) Erythrocytic structures (case 1989 of Dr. G. Wernsdorfer). Blood film. Red-purple rods and dots, frequently multiple on the erythrocytes. Some are linear in distribution. Resemblance to *Bartonella* or *Haemobartonella* is marked. From a slide furnished by Dr. Wernsdorfer. Original. (F) Structures. Blood film. Multiple red-purple rods on erythrocytes. "Probably related to the *Haemobartonella-Eperythrozoon* group" (Clark). From a slide provided by Dr. Clark. Original.

helpful in diagnosing such an illness than a history of residence in the endemic zone.

Microscopic

The appearance of the blood at the height of infection is illustrated in Figure 16.1. Most red blood cells carry 1 to 6 or more microorganisms. Infections are less severe before and after the anemia peaks and after therapy. If microorganisms are very few, absent, or abnormal in appearance, as occurs at the beginning of recovery, culture results may be necessary before a diagnosis can be made.

Primary culture media

When whole blood is inoculated into leptospira medium and incubated at 25 C, colonies develop usually within 2 to 4 weeks; the time required is roughly proportional to the number of viable organisms inoculated. Red cells can mask the colonies initially; however, these colonies become more evident on subculture. Stained films made at weekly intervals are useful. As stated, isolation can also be made on blood agar and in cultures incubated at 37 C.

Identification procedures

Bartonella typically grows in rounded clumps measuring 25 to 50 μm in diameter. After methyl alcohol fixation and Giemsa staining, these clumps appear dense in the center but show distinct rods measuring 1.3 to 3.0 by 0.75 μm at the periphery. Scattered individual rod and rounded forms are less distinctive.

B. bacilliformis does not retain the Gram stain. Distinctive biochemical reactions have not been described for it, and it is not hemolytic. Grown in appropriate tissue culture, the organism will develop extracellularly and also within the cytoplasm in rounded clumps (19). Tested in rhesus (*M. mulatta*) monkeys by intradermal inoculation in the eyebrow region, many, perhaps most, isolates will produce local verrugas, and blood cultures from these animals will be positive.

Identification depends on isolation of the organism from a patient known to have lived in the endemic areas or from a patient with one of the two forms of the disease. The microorganism thus isolated will develop in leptospira medium, giving the typical appearance described. It grows distinctively in tissue culture medium and is pathogenic for the rhesus monkey, which remains infected for weeks or longer. *B. bacilliformis* is inhibited or killed *in vitro* by a variety of antibiotics (see below).

Serologic procedures and marker systems are not used.

Antimicrobic Susceptibility and Resistance

Many antibiotics provide satisfactory clinical results, whereas arsenicals, effective in the hemobartonelloses, are ineffective in bartonellosis.

Antibiotics control *Bartonella* infection without necessarily eradicating it. A patient treated with antibiotics and recovered from Oroya fever may still have positive blood cultures and develop verrugas. Presumably, the antibiotics restrict the microorganism, a partial immunity develops, and these mechanisms jointly master the disease. Effective antibiotics include penicillin, streptomycin, chloramphenicol, and tetracycline. Antibiotic activity can also be demonstrated *in vitro*.

Choice of antibiotic is regulated by secondary considerations. *Salmonella* infection of Oroya fever patients is not uncommon and the prognosis in such cases is poor. Therapeutic agents which act against both *Salmonella* and *Bartonella* are therefore often preferred. The effective action of chloramphenicol against such combined infections has been reported. It has thus been preferred over other antibiotics, even though *in vitro* activity indicates that it is not the most effective. Resistance of *Bartonella* to antibiotics apparently has not posed any problem.

Evaluation of Laboratory Findings

A blood film showing a majority of red blood cells infected with numerous bartonellae as shown in Figure 16.1 suggests a presumptive diagnosis of Oroya fever. The intracytoplasmic development of *B. bacilliformis* in rounded masses as detected in autopsy or biopsy specimens from Oroya fever cases has not been described in any other disease. Verruga is also distinctive in its histology, and when *B. bacilliformis* is demonstrated within the tissue, it is definitive. In both forms of the disease, blood cultures should be positive; the organisms which grow will have the characteristics described.

Great weight should be attached to the patient's history, the physical findings, and the hematological picture. A characteristic picture in a patient who has passed through or lived in the endemic zone permits a diagnosis of Oroya fever. If the data, historical or laboratory, depart from the "classical" description, the diagnosis may become a research problem, for bartonella-like structures may possibly be involved.

Bartonella-like Structures

Bartonella bacilliformis clearly is an independent living microorganism. But there are structures associated with red blood cells which are not *B. bacilliformis* and which have not been cultivated *in vitro* nor passaged in animals, and for these, the question arises: are they microorganisms or are they produced endogenously?

There are two categories of such structures:

(1) Bodies which resemble *Bartonella* or two similar prokaryotic microorganisms, *Eperythrozoon* and *Haemobartonella*.

(2) Bodies which do not closely resemble known microorganisms, are not constituents of normal blood, and are considered by hematologists to be of endogenous origin and produced under pathological conditions.

Bartonella-like Structures in Man

These usually are reported to resemble *Bartonella, Haemobartonella,* or *Eperythrozoon*.

Haemobartonella occurs in a variety of mammals. Most species are geographically widely distributed and cause anemia. At the peak of the anemia, *Haemobartonella* is in the blood in large numbers, appearing as small rods 1-3 μm by 0.2-0.7 μm. These rods stain purple red with Giemsa. There may be several or many on a single red cell; they are often distributed in a linear arrangement suggesting division. Some of the rods are free in the plasma, and ring and dot forms occur (Fig 16.2C). *Haemobartonella* responds to antibiotics and arsenicals. The method of transmission, when known, involves a blood-sucking arthropod vector.

Eperythrozoon is also widely distributed both as to hosts and geographically. Some species are slightly pathogenic, others markedly so. In blood films, *Eperythrozoon* is round, measures 0.5 to 2.0 μm in diameter, and appears as a biconcave disk shaped like a small erythrocyte. It is found on the red cell surface, in the plasma, or at the red cell margin, where on edge, it appears as a rod or rods which at times encircle part of the red cell. The Giemsa staining is red purple, often with a bluish tinge (Fig 16.2D). Although the disk shape is most commonly observed in films, in phase microscopy *Eperythrozoon* appears as a sphere; presumably, the sphere collapses in blood films which gives the disk appearance. As noted, *in vitro* these microorganisms have not developed, but *E. coccoides* was grown through sixteen serial passages in embryonated chicken eggs (23).

An outstanding immunological feature distinguishes both *Haemobartonella* and *Eperythrozoon*. Animals infected with either do not, in general, show a marked reaction. However, if they are splenectomized, their blood is flooded with large numbers of microorganisms, and at this time maximal pathogenic effects are observed.

Results similar to that of a splenectomy may follow X ray irradiation, inoculation with other microorganisms, or transmissible leukemias, tumor transplants, injection of thorium-x, "chemical splenectomy," etc. If these microorganisms occur in man, they may become evident after splenectomy or under conditions when natural immunity is diminished.

Although neither *Haemobartonella* nor *Eperythrozoon* has been cultivated *in vitro*, they can be passaged in animals.

Suspected human cases are presented in Table 16.2. Four reports of particular interest are summarized.

Wernsdorfer's report (30) is of particular interest. It cites six cases of anemia with red cell bodies seen in 2 months. All of the cases came from the Blue Nile province of the Sudan. One patient was hospitalized, and from this patient tissue sections were obtained.

The patient was a 23-year-old female referred because of fever and an enlarged liver and spleen. Kala-azar was suspected but not confirmed microscopically or by culture, and the patient did not respond to specific therapy. Anemia was marked, and in blood films 80%-90% of the red cells showed dots or rods, often arranged in V or Y shape, or chains of up to four rods.

These bodies are shown in Figure 16.2E from a blood film kindly provided by Dr. Wernsdorfer. The resemblance to microorganisms of the *Bartonella-Haemobartonella* group is apparent.

A microorganism was obtained from blood cultures, but it did not re-

TABLE 16.2*

ERYTHROCYTIC STRUCTURE DESCRIBED AS	SINGLE OR MULTIPLE CASES	WHERE OBSERVED	AUTHOR, DATE, AND REFERENCE	COMMENT
Eperythrozoon(?)	Single	Holland	Schüffner, 1929 (22)	See text
Bartonella sp.	Multiple	Sudan	Wernsdorfer, 1969 (30)	Discussed in text
Haemobartonella-Eperythrozoon	Single	England	Clark, 1975 (3)	See text
Unclassified bacterium	Single	USA	Archer et al., 1979 (1)	See text
Bartonella-like	Multiple	Thailand	Whitaker et al., 1966 (31)	Noncultivable, not infectious for a *M. mulatta*
Bartonella or *Haemobartonella*(?)	Single	USA	Otto and Rezek, 1943 (12)	Rbc structures increased four-fold after splenectomy; noncultivable, did not infect a *M. mulatta*
Haemobartonella-like	Multiple	USA	Kallick et al., 1972 (7)	In systemic lupus erythematosus
Eperythrozoon noguchii	—	—	Lwoff and Vaucel, 1930 (9)	Described from photographs published by Noguchi

* *Haemobartonella* and *Eperythrozoon* have been described from other primates (monkeys); see, for example, Peters et al. (17).

semble *Bartonella bacilliformis* and was reported by the author as "still unidentified." No distended endothelial cells containing masses of *Bartonella* were seen in tissue sections. Wernsdorfer suggests that all six cases from the Blue Nile province were the result of infection with a local *Bartonella*.

In the case described by Clark (3), the red cell structures were said to resemble *Haemobartonella*. The patient had malignant melanoma and, near the end of the illness, fever and pronounced anemia. The erythrocytic bodies occurred in about 13% of the red cells, and upon review similar structures were found in a blood film made seven years earlier. The bodies stained well with Giemsa and "included tiny particles just perceptible by light microscopy, beaded rod-like structures, and coarse clumps of basophilic material."

In Figure 16.2F the bodies are drawn from a slide donated by Dr. Clark.

The structures stained with acridine orange. By electron microscopy, the larger bodies were seen to be clusters or chains of small, rounded or oval organisms approximately 0.2 μm in diameter; a cell wall was not demonstrated. Splenectomized mice were not infected by blood inoculation. Culture attempts were not successful. Transfer of the infection to transfused group O red blood cells did not occur. The anemia was not improved by antibiotics or the arsenical spirotrypan.

A chronic infection lasting at least one year was reported by Archer et al. (1) in a splenectomized adult male. "Small bacterium-like structures were seen on Wright's stain in association with 60 to 80 per cent of the patient's red cells." These bodies were also observed by the writer in a stained blood film kindly furnished by Dr. Archer and were typical of the *Bartonella-Haemobartonella-Eperythrozoon* group in size, distribution on the erythrocyte, and in the red violet color taken after Romanowsky staining. In electron microscopic studies on thawed blood the structures were closely applied to the erythrocytes, but never intracellular; in section the structure was that of a bacterium and different from *Bartonella* (1). The bodies were not grown in culture nor were they transmitted to animals. They stained poorly with Gram's stain "but they appeared to be gram-positive."

The patient, a 49-year-old male, complained of arthralgias, night chills, night sweats, evening temperatures to 39.4 C and purpuric lesions of the feet. He was observed to have generalized lymphadenopathy, purpuric, nodular, tender lesions on both feet, and petechiae on both lower extremities. Hepato- and splenomegaly were not reported. The hemoglobin value was 11.0 g per 100 ml. The relation of this illness to the red cell structures is not known, but successful antibiotic therapy was followed by a coincident clearing of the blood and improvement in symptoms. Chloramphenicol was found particularly effective and cephalexin active.

The splenectomy followed an automobile accident approximately 15 years prior to onset of symptoms. The patient never left the state of Virginia. No co-workers, friends, or family are known to have had a similar disease.

Eperythrozoon possibly caused pseudoleukemic anemia in a child as reported by Schüffner (22). In blood films stained by the Pappenheimer method, red-staining bodies measuring 0.2 to 1.0 μm (often ring-shaped) were seen chiefly in the plasma, sometimes grouped around red cells, but rarely on the erythrocytes. No similar structures occurred in stained experimental precipitates of serum.

Erythrocytic Structures of Presumed Endogenous Origin

Bessis (2) lists eight kinds of inclusions seen in erythrocytes and reticulocytes. Reticulofilamentous substances and siderosomes are not stained by Giemsa. A third kind, the Heinz bodies, is difficult to see with this stain. The remainder are punctate basophilic granules, azurophilic granules (said to result from a pathologic destruction and dispersion of chromatin), Pappenheimer bodies, Cabot rings (possibly from a persistence of spindle fibers), and Howell-Jolly bodies (nuclear remnants). Pappenheimer bodies are described as collections of mitochondria, ribosomes, and degenerate membranes containing iron-bearing particles.

There is also a rare disease, congenital inclusion body anemia. It is characterized by hemolytic anemia, jaundice, pigmenturia, and splenomegaly occurring at birth or in the first years of life. Sheahy (25) summarized the seven cases known at the time and described one patient who was splenectomized.

The inclusion bodies said to occur in 14%–90% of the erythrocytes and to be "large, irregular, usually single bodies measuring 0.5 to 3.0 μm in diameter" stained with Romanowsky-type stains.

Concerning this "endogenous" group, it may be pointed out that, when first described, *Bartonella, Haemobartonella,* and *Eperythrozoon* were considered degenerative structures or artifacts. Successful cultivation and inoculation forced their recognition as microorganisms. Had these procedures failed, they might still be considered of endogenous origin. It is possible then that some of the structures which at present are considered "endogenous" may prove to be independent living organisms, when adequate techniques to demonstrate this are available. Pappenheimer et al. (13) explored this possibility but drew no conclusion.

Particular note should be taken of the Jolly bodies. Certainly they are nuclear remnants in most cases. But they cannot be distinguished from *Anaplasma* with ordinary blood stains. Accordingly, should *Anaplasma* infections, now known only from other animals, also occur in man, and particularly in conjunction with Jolly bodies, they would probably be misdiagnosed. For it would take a high degree of alertness and suspicion and the use of unusual techniques to prove that *Anaplasma* was involved.*

To summarize, throughout the world, patients are seen with unusual structures in the blood, frequently associated with erythrocytes. These bodies cannot be identified with the common red blood cell changes seen in anemia. Their resemblance to known microorganisms is often striking. They occur in sick persons, sometimes in splenectomized ones. The accompanying disease may be causally related to the erythrocytic bodies, the underlying illness may depress immunity so that the supposed microorganisms can infect and/or multiply, or there may be no relationship. In addition to these structures, there are numerous endo-erythrocytic bodies considered to be endogenous and not microbiological in origin.

---

*Concerning this possibility are findings made in cases of systemic lupus erythematosus (8). These observations are primarily immunological whereas cytological evidence is equivocal. Sera used were from *Anaplasma marginale* (*A. m.*) bovines and from systemic lupus erythematosus (SLE) cases. Components, presumably antibodies, from *A. m.* serum fixed on antigen in the basement membrane of the kidney glomeruli of one SLE case. The serum of this person and 21 other lupus cases reacted with *Anaplasma marginale* in an indirect fluorescent antibody test, titers in the SLE cases exceeding those of controls in the range 1 in 40 to 1 in 1,280. *Anaplasma* shares common antigens with *Haemobartonella* and *Eperythrozoon* (8) so that, if microorganisms do cause the reactions described, it is not certain which. It remains to be demonstrated unequivocally that Anaplasmataceae microorganisms are involved and, if so, whether the serological reactions result directly from these infections or are due to antigens shared by SLE patients and the microorganisms.

References

1. ARCHER GL, COLEMAN PH, COLE RM, DUMA RJ, and JOHNSTON CL: Human infection from an unidentified erythrocyte-associated bacterium. N Engl J Med 301:897–900, 1979
2. BESSIS M: Living Blood Cells and Their Ultrastructure. Springer, New York, 1973, 767 pp
3. CLARK KGA: A basophilic microorganism infecting human red cells. Br J Haematol 29:301–304, 1975

4. HERRER A: Carrión's disease; presence of *Bartonella bacilliformis* in peripheral blood of patients with benign form. Am J Trop Med 2:645–649, 1953

5. HERRER A and BLANCAS F: Estudios sobre la enfermedad de Carrión en el valle interandino del Mantaro. I. Observaciones entomológicas. Rev Med Exp 13:27–45, 1959–60 (see Trop Dis Bull 59:28, 1962, abstract)

6. HERTIG M and FISHER RA: Control of sandflies with DDT. US Army Med Dept Bull 88, 97–101, 1945

7. KALLICK CA, LEVIN S, REDDI KT, and LANDAU WL: Systemic lupus erythematosus associated with *Haemobartonella*-like organisms. Nature New Biol 236 (66):145–146, 1972

8. KALLICK CA, THADHANI KC, and RICE TW: Identification of Anaplasmataceae (Haemobartonella) antigen and antibodies in systemic lupus erythematosus. Arthritis Rheum 23:197–205, 1980

9. LWOFF A and VAUCEL M: Les Bartonelloses aigües et les infections mixtes à bartonella et à eperythrozoon. C R Soc Biol 103:973, 1930

10. NOGUCHI H and BATTISTINI T: Etiology of Oroya fever. I. Cultivation of *Bartonella bacilliformis*. J Exp Med 43:851–864, 1926

11. ODRIOZOLA E: La Maladie de Carrión ou la verruga péruvienne. Carré et Naud, Paris, 1898

12. OTTO TO and REZEK P: A new type of *Bartonella* infection in man? J Fla Med Assoc 30:62–66, 1943

13. PAPPENHEIMER AM, THOMPSON DR, and SMITH KE: Anaemia associated with unidentified erythrocytic inclusions, after splenectomy. Q J Med 38, new series 14:75, 1945

14. PATIÑO-CAMARGO L: Bartonellosis en Colombia. Rev Hig (Bogota) 1939 (4):4–37, 1939

15. PETERS D and WIGAND R: Neue Untersuchungen über *Bartonella bacilliformis*; Morphologie der Kulturform. Z Tropenmed Parasitol 3:313–326, 1952

16. PETERS D and WIGAND R: Bartonellaceae. Bacteriol Rev 19:150, 1955

17. PETERS W, MOLYNEUX DH, and HOWELLS RE: Eperythrozoon and Haemobartonella in monkeys. Ann Trop Med Parasitol 68, 47–50, 1974

18. PINKERTON H: *In* Textbook of Medicine, 11th edition. Beeson PB and McDermott W (eds.). Saunders, Philadelphia, 1963, pp 327-329

19. PINKERTON H and WEINMAN D: Carrion's disease. I. Behavior of the etiological agent within cells growing or surviving *in vitro*. Proc Soc Exp Biol Med 37:587–590, 1937

20. RECAVARREN S and LUMBRERAS H: Pathogenesis of the verruga of Carrion's disease: ultrastructural studies. Am J Pathol 66:461–470, 1972

21. RISTIC M and KREIER JP: Hemotropic bacteria (Editorial). N Engl J Med 301:937–939, 1979

22. SCHUFFNER WAP: Eigenaardige vondst in het bloed bij een patientje met anaemia pseudoleucaemia infantum (type van Jaksch-Hayem). Ned Tijdschr Geneeskd 73:3778, 1929

23. SEAMER J: The propagation and preservation of *Eperythrozoon coccoides*. J Gen Microbiol 21:344–351, 1959

24. SHANNON RC: Entomological investigations in connection with Carrion's disease. Am J Hyg 10:78–111, 1929

25. SHEAHY TW: Inclusion body anemia with pigmenturia. Arch Intern Med 114:83–88, 1964

26. STRONG RP, TYZZER EE, SELLARDS AW, BRUES CT, and GASTIABURÚ JC: Report of First Expedition to South America, 1913. Harvard Univ Press, Cambridge, Mass, 1915

27. TAKANO MORON J: Enfermedad de Carrión (Bartonellosis humana). Estudio morfológico de la fase hemática y del periódo eruptivo con el microscopio electrónico. An Programa Acad Med, Univ Nac Mayor San Marcos, Lima 53:44–86, 1970

28. WEINMAN D: Infectious anemias due to Bartonella and related red cell parasites. Trans Am Phil Soc (New Series) 33:243–349, 1944

29. WEINMAN D: Bartonellosis. *In* Infectious Blood Diseases of Man and Animals, Vol II. Weinman D and Ristic M (eds.). Academic Press, New York, 1968, Chap 15

30. WERNSDORFER G: Possible human bartonellosis in the Sudan. Clinical and microbiological observations. Acta Trop 26(3):216–234, 1969

31. WHITAKER JA, FORT E, WEINMAN D, TAMASATIT P, and PANAS-AMPOL K: Acute febrile anemia associated with Bartonella-like erythrocytic structures. Nature 212:855–856, 1966

This report was funded in part by USPHS grant AI 14711.

CHAPTER 17

BORDETELLA INFECTIONS

Calvin C. Linnemann, Jr., and James W. Bass

Introduction

Causative Organisms

In 1900, Bordet and Gengou examined sputum collected at the onset of the first characteristic coughing fit of a 5-month-old child with whooping cough (4). Under the microscope, they observed "an enormous quantity of small ovoid-shaped bacteria, sometimes slightly elongated, sometimes shorter to the point of resembling a micrococcus, but having in general a rather uniform appearance...the vast majority of the microbes were isolated, some were placed by two's end to end. The *Gram* was negative." This was the first clear description of *B. pertussis*, the organism which is the primary cause of whooping cough. The genus *Bordetella*, to which *B. pertussis* belongs, includes two other species, *B. parapertussis* and *B. bronchiseptica*, both of which have been reported to cause disease in humans (6, 10, 14). As originally described, these are small, aerobic, gram-negative coccobacillary organisms, 0.2–0.3 μm by 0.5–1.0 μm. Pleomorphism develops in older cultures, and the organisms undergo phase variations which may be analogous to smooth to rough changes. Capsules have been demonstrated as well as pili-like filamentous appendages.

Initially, Bordet and Gengou were unable to isolate the organism in a gelatin medium with blood which was suitable for the growth of *Haemophilus influenzae*. They also failed to grow the organism on a potato-glycerol medium with blood, later known as Bordet-Gengou (BG) medium, until they examined one of their culture plates with a microscope at the end of several days. Only then were they able to detect the slow-growing colonies of *B. pertussis*. After 2–4 days, *B. pertussis* produces small, smooth-edged, elevated colonies, which are gray, but in reflected light appear silver and have been described as droplets of mercury or bisected pearls. Depending on the blood used in the medium, hemolysis may or may not be present. The growth requirements are limited, but the organism is sensitive to various inhibitors in the media such as unsaturated fatty acids and sulfides (29, 32). Therefore, blood or other absorbents are required to remove these inhibitors. *B. parapertussis* was first distinguished from *B. pertussis* because it grew faster and produced a wider zone of hemolysis (6, 14). *B. bronchiseptica* also grows more rapidly than *B. pertussis* and produces larger colonies. In contrast to *B. pertussis*, the latter two species will grow on a variety of media.

The *Bordetella* share a common heat-stable O antigen and an antigenic heat-labile toxin. Each species has a species-specific, heat-labile agglutinogen. *B. parapertussis* and *B. bronchiseptica* may share common agglutinogens. Other important cellular components which have been identified in *B. pertussis* include protective antigen, lymphocytosis-promoting factor, and histamine-sensitizing factor (28, 30). It has not been determined if these are distinct components. Adjuvant factor(s) in addition to the endotoxin and a hemagglutinin is also present.

Clinical Manifestations

Whooping cough is the classical presentation of *B. pertussis* infection (16, 22, 34). After a 7- to 10-day incubation period, the typical illness begins with nonspecific respiratory symptoms, malaise, anorexia, and sometimes a low grade fever. This prodromal period is traditionally called the *catarrhal stage* and lasts for 1 to 2 weeks. Coughing appears toward the end of this period and becomes progressively worse until the patient is having frequent episodes of paroxysmal coughing. The hallmark of pertussis, the whoop, appears during the *paroxysmal stage*. This occurs at the end of a series of coughs and results from a forced inspiration over a partially closed glottis. Paroxysms of coughing are often followed by vomiting and may be associated with conjunctival hemorrhages, epistaxis, or periorbital edema. The most important laboratory findings are marked leukocytosis and lymphocytosis which appear late in the catarrhal stage and continue in the paroxysmal stage. The appearance of fever or an excessive leukemoid reaction (> 50,000/mm^3) may indicate secondary bacterial infection—including otitis media or pneumonia. After 2–4 weeks, the paroxysms of coughing and vomiting decrease, and the patient enters a *convalescent stage*. Coughing may continue for weeks to months, and exacerbations with whooping may occur with viral infections.

When the typical illness occurs, the clinical diagnosis of pertussis is easy. Approximately 75% of susceptible children who become infected will develop recognizable disease. In infants, both the whoop and the lymphocytosis may be absent, and paroxysms may be followed by a period of cyanosis. In most older children and adults, including those who have been vaccinated or had pertussis in the past, the illness may be atypical. Respiratory symptoms occur with a cough which may or may not be paroxysmal and the whoop is seldom present. Lymphocytosis is usually not found. The only clinical indication that the patient may have a *B. pertussis* infection is the occurrence of typical disease in contacts or in the community.

B. parapertussis may produce typical whooping cough, indistinguishable from that caused by *B. pertussis*, but this occurs in less than 20% of infected children (33). Most patients have a mild cough which lasts less than 3 weeks, and their illnesses are probably diagnosed in most cases as viral infections with bronchitis. Approximately 40% of infected children are asymptomatic. Fatal pneumonias with *B. parapertussis* have been reported, but at least one of these may have been associated with a simultaneous infection with *B. pertussis* (26).

In the few reported cases of *B. bronchiseptica* infection in humans, disease is usually confined to the respiratory tract as with other *Bordetella* organisms (15). Upper respiratory tract disease has been reported in animal handlers, and tracheobronchitis or pneumonia in two patients without animal contact. Whooping cough has been reported in only four patients. It has been suggested that *B. bronchiseptica* may cause endocarditis in humans, but this has not been well documented.

Epidemiology (16)

Man is the only known reservoir of *B. pertussis*, and the organism is transmitted by droplets from an infected individual (16). The high secondary attack rates in susceptible children, ranging from 25%–50% in schools and 70%–100% in households, probably reflect the prolonged and intense exposure to the organism rather than high infectivity of *B. pertussis*. Carriers do not play a significant role in the transmission of the disease (25). Patients with typical or atypical disease can transmit infection. Those who develop typical disease are most dangerous when they are in the catarrhal stage, because they continue to move freely in uninfected populations. Once the whoop develops, the patient is usually isolated and treated with antibiotics. Patients with atypical disease may continue to infect others throughout their illness.

Prior to vaccines, epidemics spread through school populations and were introduced back into the home, so most children were infected at an early age. Because infection produces long-lasting immunity, typical disease was rare in older age groups. Reinfections did occur, but not typical disease. In urban areas, epidemics recurred in 2- to 4-year cycles. In rural areas, epidemics occurred at irregular intervals, depending on reintroduction of infection, and pertussis disappeared among isolated island populations. The seasonal variation seen with many infections is not pronounced in pertussis, although there has been slight predominance in the late summer and early fall in the United States in recent years. In contrast to most infectious diseases, pertussis is reported more commonly in females than males.

Since the introduction of effective pertussis vaccine in the United States in the 1940s, the epidemiology of pertussis has changed (8). The mortality rate was decreasing before vaccine was developed and has continued to decrease since vaccine and antibiotics have been available. A significant decrease in the case rate was not apparent until after introduction of the vaccine. With the subsequent decrease in reported cases, there has been a relative shift in the age of attack, with a higher percentage of reported cases occurring in older children and adults, including those who were previously immunized. One study demonstrated that vaccine is no longer protective 12 years after immunization (21).

In recent years, several studies have suggested that whooping cough is also caused by viruses, particularly adenoviruses. Most of these studies either did not demonstrate the ability to recover *B. pertussis* or did not include appropriate control groups (12). Subsequent studies by investigators experienced with the laboratory diagnosis of *Bordetella* infections have shown that adenoviruses may frequently be recovered from patients with *B. pertussis* infections (20). This suggests that pertussis may increase the excretion of adenoviruses, but not that viruses cause whooping cough. It has not been shown that viruses potentiate the severity of *B. pertussis* infections.

The epidemiology of *B. parapertussis* is probably similar to *B. pertussis*. In

Denmark, Lautrop has shown that epidemics occur every 4 years and alternate with *B. pertussis* epidemics (24). Parapertussis has been reported infrequently in the United States, although one study has reported a significant number of cases occurring at the same time pertussis was occurring (26). Serologic studies have indicated that parapertussis is widespread. The relative mildness of clinical illness probably accounts for the failure to recognize epidemics of *B. parapertussis* in this country.

B. bronchiseptica is frequently found in the respiratory tract of many animals, including rabbits, dogs, cats, and guinea pigs. It has been assumed that only animal-to-man transmission was occurring. One family epidemic has been reported, but since all family members were exposed to animals, man-to-man transmission could not be proven. Recent reports have described infection and disease in situations where animal contact did not occur (15). In the past, *B. bronchiseptica* infections unrelated to animal contacts may not have been identified accurately and were attributed to other gram-negative bacteria.

Public Health Significance

The current public health significance of *Bordetella* infections is difficult to assess with existing data. Before pertussis vaccine was introduced, the significance of *B. pertussis* infections was clearly demonstrated by the morbidity and mortality rates of the disease. Pertussis caused more deaths among children than any other infectious disease except tuberculosis (16). The frequency of reported cases was exceeded only by measles, chicken pox, mumps, and scarlet fever. As discussed above, the number of reported cases has decreased dramatically since the introduction of vaccine, but epidemics continue to occur. The actual morbidity may be markedly underestimated because of the failure to diagnose atypical disease in immunized populations. One specific situation which has been appreciated more in recent years is the transmission of infection among hospital personnel and to patients (27).

Vaccine has been shown to be effective in preventing disease. Because of reactions to the vaccine, questions have been raised as to the need for continuing routine immunization programs, but the persistence of pertussis justifies the continued use of the vaccine. Hopefully, the increasing understanding of *B. pertussis* will provide a basis for an improved vaccine with fewer side effects. Vaccine is not effective if given after exposure to a patient with pertussis, but the susceptible individual may be protected by chemoprophylaxis with erythromycin (3).

B. parapertussis has been reported to be a public health problem in European countries, but data are not available to define the problem in the United States (33). Although parapertussis rarely causes fatal disease, it may be a significant cause of prolonged bronchitis in all age groups. Like parapertussis, the frequency of clinical infection with *B. bronchiseptica* is unknown. One survey in a general hospital reported that two of 1505 clinical isolates over a 1-month period were *B. bronchiseptica* and they recovered the organism 18 times in a 19-week period (15). Because of the animal reservoirs, this organism should also be considered in respiratory tract infections in animal handlers.

Collection and Processing of Specimens

Kind of specimens

A nasopharyngeal swab should be taken for culture (7). *B. pertussis* and *B. parapertussis* are present throughout the respiratory tract from the nasopharynx to the bronchi. There is no blood-stream invasion, so blood cultures are not useful. Traditionally, "cough plates" were collected, but the nasopharyngeal swab has been shown to be more effective because there is less contamination with other organisms. The tip of the swab should be made of cotton or similar substance which has been proven not to be bacteriostatic. Fatty acids on some cotton swabs will inhibit bacterial growth. The swab itself should be a very flexible wire. Suitable commercial swabs are available (Calgiswab, Wilson Diagnostics). The swab is passed through the nose until it touches the posterior nasopharynx, allowed to remain a few seconds, and removed. Then the swab is streaked directly onto BG media and onto glass slides for fluorescent antibody (FA) staining.

If the swab must be transported to a laboratory before inoculation onto culture plates, it should be kept moist by placing it into 0.2 to 0.5 ml of 1% Casamino acids solution or nutrient broth, but not saline. This should be transported immediately and inoculated. Occasionally, there may be a long delay in transporting the swab or it must be mailed to a laboratory for processing. For FA slides, this is simple. After they are air dried, the slides are heat fixed and shipped in a routine mailing container. For culture specimens, this is more difficult. A charcoal agar slant has been evaluated experimentally and shown to support the growth of *B. pertussis* (18). These slants can be stored for a long period of time, in contrast to BG plates. Another transport and enrichment medium has been described recently, but further evaluation is needed (31). Routine BG plates also have been inoculated and mailed to laboratories experienced in recovering the organism. For epidemiologic studies, freshly prepared BG plates can be taken into the field and inoculated directly. These can be transferred back to the laboratory at room temperature.

If it is impossible to pass a swab through the nares because of obstruction, cultures can be obtained by the cough plate method. The culture plate, containing BG media, is uncovered and held several inches from the patient's mouth during a paroxysm of coughing. The cover is replaced and the plate is transported to the laboratory. Successful cultures have also been obtained by peroral nasal swab or by suction of secretions through a sterile tube from the supralaryngeal area.

In contrast to *B. pertussis* and *B. parapertussis, B. bronchiseptica* has been isolated not only from the respiratory tract, but also from blood and urine (15).

Serology is seldom useful in the diagnosis of infection.

Time of Collection

The earlier in the course of pertussis that specimens are collected, the more likely that a positive culture will be obtained. Most studies indicate that less than 50% of untreated patients will be positive after the third week of illness, and 20% or less after the fifth week (7). Specimens for culture should be collected before antibiotic therapy is initiated because cultures and FA smears may become negative very rapidly (Figure 17.1) (3). *B. parapertussis* follows a similar pattern but cannot be recovered as long as *B. pertussis* (33). Presumably, *B. bronchiseptica* would be recovered best early in the illness, but there are no studies to determine the duration of excretion.

Number of Specimens

There are no systematic studies as to the optimal number of cultures needed for diagnosis. It has been suggested that three negative nasopharyngeal cultures examined in an experienced laboratory should exclude *B. pertussis* (23). The question of experience is the most important part of that conclusion. Studies comparing cough plates and nasopharyngeal swabs have shown a slight increase in the total recovery by two cultures, supporting the idea that multiple cultures may be useful.

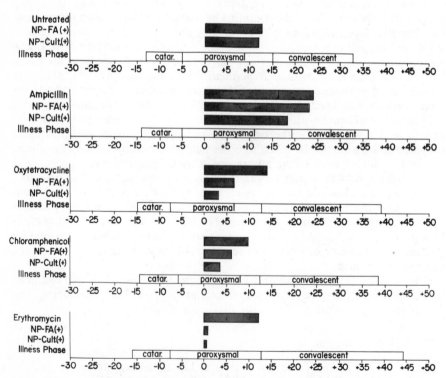

Figure 17.1—Duration of excretion of *B. pertussis* as detected by fluorescent antibody staining and culture and the effect of antimicrobial treatment (from J Pediatr 75:768, 1969).

Diagnostic Procedures

Microscopic Examination

Direct examination of nasopharyngeal secretions by FA staining may provide a presumptive diagnosis (17, 19). A Gram stain is not useful. As described above, the swab can be streaked directly onto a clean slide or placed in 1% Casamino acids solution for transportation to the laboratory. If the latter is done, the swab should be placed back in the solution after inoculation of culture plates and rewashed before making slides for FA staining. The slides are air dried and gently heat fixed. Acetone fixation has been used, but this is not necessary.

The slides are stained with specific antiserum conjugated with fluorescein isothiocyanate. Antisera have been prepared in a variety of animals, most often in rabbits and chickens. Rabbit antiserum may contain *B. bronchiseptica* antibody and has been reported to cross-react with some staphylococci (19). Commercially prepared conjugates of chicken antisera to *B. pertussis* and *B. parapertussis* are available (Difco). Conjugated negative antiserum is not commercially available for controls. Positive and negative slides should be stained with the conjugates. A dilution of the conjugated antiserum which has been shown to produce bright fluorescence of the organisms is used. The fixed smear is covered with the conjugate and placed in a moist chamber for 30 min. The slides are washed several times in phosphate buffered saline (pH 7.0–7.6) for 10 min. After the slide is air dried, buffered glycerol is added and a cover slip placed on the slide.

The slides are examined under a fluorescent microscope for fluorescing organisms which have the morphology typical of *Bordetella*. There should be no fluorescence if a negative antiserum is used as a control. Cross-reactions can occur between *B. pertussis* and *B. bronchiseptica*, and between *B. parapertussis* and *B. bronchiseptica*. Cross-reactions are seldom seen between *B. pertussis* and *B. parapertussis* (17). Because of the rarity of *B. bronchiseptica*, these cross-reactions do not appear to be a problem. It has been suggested that fluorescing organisms are difficult to identify from previously immunized patients.

Selection and Inoculation of Primary Culture Media

The medium of choice for primary isolation of *B. pertussis* is a modified BG medium (23). Other media, such as Lacey's medium, have been shown to be effective for primary isolation, but are much more complex to prepare. BG medium is a potato-glycerol agar to which blood is added. Bordet and Gengou used 50% blood, but it should be decreased to 15%–20%. Sheep, rabbit, horse, and human blood have all been used, but sheep or rabbit blood is used most often because clear hemolysis develops around the colonies. Fresh blood is desirable. The most critical factor is that freshly prepared culture plates are used which are a bright cherry red color at the time of inoculation. Commercial BG agar base is available (BBL, Becton, Dickinson & Co.) with or without peptones. Bordet and Gengou originally left out peptones to decrease the growth of contaminants, and some peptones will inhibit growth of *B. pertussis*. The addition of penicillin has been shown to increase the recovery of *B. pertussis* by decreasing the overgrowth of other organisms (5). Half a unit of penicillin G per milliliter is added to the medium when the plates are poured. Since some strains of *B. pertussis* may be inhibited by the penicillin, it has been recommended that two culture plates be inoculated, one with penicillin and one without. If only one plate is used, penicillin should be used. Other antibiotics such as methicillin have been used instead of penicillin (11). In a recent study, methicillin plates were reported to be subjectively easier to read because of better suppression of other bacterial flora (9).

The culture plate is inoculated directly with the swab. The swab may be streaked across the plate with penicillin and the plate incubated. On the plate without penicillin, an initial inoculation should be made with the swab followed by cross streaking with a wire loop. Then the plates are incubated aerobically at 35 to 37 C. To ensure that the plates do not dry out during the long incubation, they should be taped shut or placed in a sealed container such as a candle jar (no candle).

Both *B. parapertussis* and *B. bronchiseptica* will grow on a variety of media. Since parapertussis will be considered in the same clinical situation as pertussis, BG medium should be used for primary isolation. In contrast, *B. bronchiseptica* may be present in clinical situations in which other gram-negative bacilli are recovered. Routine media used for isolation of gram-negative bacilli are sufficient for the primary isolation of *B. bronchiseptica*.

Identification Procedures

Cultures should be examined daily. Initially, the plates are examined for fast growing organisms that might obscure the presence of *B. pertussis* and, if necessary, these should be cut out of the agar. By the second day, the colonies may begin to appear, particularly if the plate is examined with a hand lens. Colonies are usually present by the fourth day, but the plates should be held for 6 days. The colonies of *B. pertussis* are gray-white, almost transparent, and should be examined in reflected light which brings out the glistening silvery quality. They are not more than 1 mm in diameter and are surrounded by a zone of hemolysis if cultured in modified BG medium as described. *B. parapertussis* and *B. bronchiseptica* produce similar colonies but grow faster. Variation is considerable and thus a definite differentiation cannot be made on growth characteristics on BG medium alone.

Microscopic examination of a Gram stain reveals faintly stained coccobacillary organisms with little pleomorphism in primary culture. *B. parapertussis* tends to be more rod-like and slightly larger than the other *Bordetella* species, and sometimes appears in a palisade arrangement.

Serologic tests are the most important method of identification. A slide agglutination test can be done with colonies selected from the primary culture plate. Suspected colonies are emulsified in 0.85% sodium chloride on one end of a slide. If autoagglutination does not occur, antiserum is placed on the other end of the slide and mixed with the culture suspension. This is observed for agglutination and compared with positive and negative controls. Commercial antisera are available for *B. pertussis* and *B. parapertussis* (Difco). Cross-agglutination does occur on occasion. The FA test is also used for identification of isolates. The culture suspension is placed on a slide, air dried, and heat fixed. This is stained as described above. Sometimes, the slide agglutination and FA stains will not agree. Subcultures may be necessary to obtain sufficient growth for the serologic tests.

The three species of *Bordetella* can be distinguished by cultural characteristics and biochemical reactions (Table 17.1). In practice, the important distinction is between *B. pertussis* and *B. parapertussis*. This can be done by subculture on a peptone agar without blood. *B. pertussis* will not grow, but *B. parapertussis* will grow and produce a brown pigment. Biochemical tests are more important in identifying *B. bronchiseptica*, since it must be differentiated from other gram-negative bacilli. *B. bronchiseptica*, in contrast to the other species of *Bordetella*, is a motile organism which reduces nitrates. It is oxidase positive and, in contrast to *Alcaligenes* species, produces urease.

Serology

Antibodies may develop after infection with *Bordetella* organisms, but the response is variable and antibody tests are not routinely used for diagnosis. The demonstration of a fourfold rise in titer does provide a specific diagnosis, and serology is used to evaluate responses to *B. pertussis* vaccine. Commercial antigens are available (Difco) but reproducibility of tests may be difficult. A variety of assays have been used to measure antibody levels, including agglutination, complement fixation, immunodiffusion, immunofluorescence, opsonic reactions, and bactericidal tests (23). Agglutination tests have been used most often, but the immunodiffusion test may be a simpler approach (1).

Marker Systems

A number of heat-labile agglutinogens have been characterized in *Bordetella*. Serotyping by agglutinogens may be useful for distinguishing various strains of *B. pertussis*. All *B. pertussis* contain antigen 1, but strains vary with regard to antigens 2, 3, 4, 5 and 6. Slide or tube agglutination tests can be performed using adsorbed antisera (13). The antisera must be prepared individually, because there is no commercial source. With this technique, epidemio-

TABLE 17.1—DIFFERENTIAL CHARACTERISTICS OF *BORDETELLA*

	B. PERTUSSIS	*B. PARAPERTUSSIS*	*B. BRONCHISEPTICA*
Growth on blood-free peptone agar	−	+	+
Browning of peptone agar	−	+	−
Motility	−	−	+
Urease production	−	+	+
Citrate utilization	−	+	+
Nitrate reduction	−	−	+

logic patterns may be identified over a number of years. Over the past few decades, there has been a shift from 1.2 or 1.2.3 strains to 1.3 strains in England and from 1.2.3 to 1.3 strains in the United States. Because of the predominance of a few strains, serotyping has not been useful in tracing the spread of individual outbreaks.

Antimicrobial Susceptibility and Resistance

The Kirby-Bauer technique has not been applied to these organisms. *B. pertussis* has been tested for antimicrobial susceptibility on either BG or charcoal medium with disk or plate dilution methods. With the plate dilution technique and charcoal agar, *B. pertussis* isolates from around the United States have been shown to have similar susceptibility patterns (Figure 17.2) (2). The method used two-fold dilutions of antibiotics from 50 μg/ml to 0.01 μg/ml, which were incorporated in the charcoal agar. An inoculum of approximately 10^6 organisms in a 0.1 ml volume was spread evenly over the surface of the medium and the plates were sealed with masking tape. The minimal inhibitory concentration was defined as the lowest dilution of an antimicrobial which produced absolute inhibition of visible growth at 3 days. *B. pertussis* was most sensitive to erythromycin, which correlates with the *in vivo* response (Figure 17.1).

Evaluation of Laboratory Findings

FA results can be reported immediately as showing *B. pertussis* or not. Since most laboratories do the FA infrequently, appropriate control antiserum

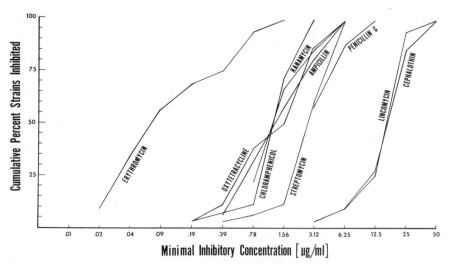

Figure 17.2—Minimal inhibitory concentration of nine antimicrobial agents for *B. pertussis* as determined by a plate dilution technique (from Am J Dis Child 117:276, 1979).

is not easily available, and the specificity of the test is not confirmed by blocking studies, the FA should be reported as a presumptive diagnosis with a note that confirmation by culture is pending. In some patients, a positive FA smear will not be confirmed by culture. This may result from several factors. No viable organisms may be present after transportation of the specimen; the laboratory may lack the expertise to grow and identify the organism; other bacteria may overgrow the plate; the patient may have received antibiotics which inhibit growth but not fluorescence; or there may be fluorescence of non-*Bordetella* organisms. The converse also occurs, in that the FA smear may be negative and the culture positive. Therefore, a negative FA stain does not exclude the diagnosis.

Culture results may be reported by the fourth day as positive for *B. pertussis* or *B. parapertussis,* or negative. Occasionally, a supplemental report will be necessary if the culture becomes positive on the fifth or sixth days. If the culture plate is overgrown with other organisms or if there is scanty growth on the plate, the physician should be informed and repeat cultures obtained. However, he should also be informed that if the patient has been treated with antibiotics appropriate for *B. pertussis,* the cultures may be negative. *B. bronchiseptica* cultures are reported after the appropriate biochemical tests.

References

1. AFTENDELIANS R and CONNOR JD: Immunologic studies of pertussis. J Pediatr 83:206–241, 1973
2. BASS JW, CRAST FW, KOTHEIMER JB, and MITCHELL IA: Susceptibility of *Bordetella pertussis.* Am J Dis Child 117:276–280, 1969
3. BASS JW, KLENK EL, KOTHEIMER JB, LINNEMANN CC, and SMITH MHD: Antimicrobial treatment of pertussis. J Pediatr 75;768–781, 1969
4. BORDET J and GENGOU O: Le microbe de la coqueluche. Ann Inst Pasteur 20:731–741, 1906
5. BRADFORD WL, DAY E, and BERRY GP: Improvement of the nasopharyngeal swab method of diagnosis in pertussis by the use of penicillin. Am J Public Health 36:468–470, 1946
6. BRADFORD WL and SLAVIN B: An organism resembling *Hemophilus pertussis.* Am J Public Health 27:1277–1282, 1937
7. BROOKS AM, BRADFORD WL, and BERRY GP: The method of nasopharyngeal culture in the diagnosis of whooping cough. J Am Med Assoc 120:883–885, 1942
8. BROOKS GF and BUCHANAN TM: Pertussis in the United States. J Infect Dis 122:123–126, 1970
9. BROOME CV, FRASER DW, and ENGLISH JW: Pertussis—diagnostic methods and surveillance. *In* International Symposium on Pertussia. Manclark C and Hill J (eds). U.S. Government Printing Office, Washington, DC, 1979, pp 19–22
10. BROWN JH: *Bacillus bronchisepticus* infection in a child with symptoms of pertussis. Johns Hopkins Med J 38:147–153, 1926
11. CHALVARDJIAN N: The laboratory diagnosis of whooping cough by fluorescent antibody and by culture methods. Can Med Assoc J 95:263–266, 1966
12. CONNOR JD: Evidence for an etiologic role of adenoviral infection in pertussis syndrome. N Engl J Med 283:388–394, 1970
13. ELDERING G, HOLWERDA J, DAVIS A, and BAKER J: *Bordetella pertussis* serotypes in the United States. Appl Microbiol 18:618–621, 1969
14. ELDERING G and KENDRICK P: *Bacillus para-pertussis:* A species resembling both *Bacillus pertussis* and *Bacillus bronchisepticus* but identical with neither. J Bacteriol 35:561–572, 1937
15. GARDNER P, GRIFFIN WB, SWARTZ MN and KUNZ LJ: Nonfermentative gram-negative bacilli of nosocomial interest. Am J Med 48:735–749, 1970

16. GORDON JE, and AYCOCK WL: Whooping cough and its epidemiological anomalies. Am J Med Sci 222:333–361, 1951
17. HOLWERDA J and ELDERING G: Culture and fluorescent-antibody methods in diagnosis of whooping cough. J Bacteriol 85:449–451, 1963
18. JONES GL and KENDRICK PL: Study of a bloodfree medium for transport and growth of Bordetella pertussis. Health Lab Sci 6:40–45, 1969
19. KENDRICK PL, ELDERING G, and EVELAND WC: Fluorescent antibody techniques. Am J Dis Child 101:149–153, 1961
20. KLENK EL, GAULTNEY JV, and BASS JW: Bacteriologically proved pertussis and adenovirus infection. Am J Dis Child 124:203–207, 1972
21. LAMBERT HJ: Epidemiology of a small pertussis outbreak in Kent County, Michigan. Public Health Rep 80:365–369, 1965
22. LAPIN JH: Whooping Cough. Charles C. Thomas, Springfield, Ill and Baltimore, Md, 1943
23. LAUTROP H: Laboratory diagnosis of whooping cough or Bordetella infections. Bull WHO 23:15–35, 1960
24. LAUTROP H: Epidemics of parapertussis. Twenty years' observations in Denmark. Lancet I:1195–1198, 1971
25. LINNEMANN CC Jr, BASS JW, and SMITH MHD: The carrier state in pertussis. Am J Epidemiol 88:422–427, 1969
26. LINNEMANN CC JR and PERRY EB: Bordetella parapertussis. Recent experience and a review of the literature. Am J Dis Child 131:560–563, 1977
27. LINNEMANN CC JR, RAMUNDO N, PERLSTEIN PH, MINTON SD, and ENGLENDER GS: Use of pertussis vaccine in an epidemic involving hospital staff. Lancet II:540–551, 1975
28. MORSE SI: Biologically active components and properties of Bordetella pertussis. Adv Appl Microbiol 20:10–26, 1976
29. PARKER C: Role of the genetics and physiology of Bordetella pertussis in the production of vaccine and the study of host-parasite relationships in pertussis. Adv Appl Microbiol 20:27–42, 1976
30. PITTMAN M: Bordetella pertussis—bacterial and host factors in the pathogenesis and prevention of whooping cough. In Infectious Agents and Host Reactions. Mudd S (ed.). WB Saunders Co, Philadelphia, 1970
31. REGAN J and LOWE F: Enrichment medium for the isolation of Bordetella pertussis. J Clin Microbiol 6:303–309, 1977
32. ROWATT E: The growth of Bordetella pertussis: a review. J Gen Microbiol 17:297–326, 1957
33. VYSOKA B: The epidemiology of pertussis and parapertussis. J Hyg Epidemiol Microbiol Immunol II:196–204, 1958
34 WILKINS J and BASS JW: Pertussis. In Communicable and Infectious Diseases, 8th edition. Top FH Sr and Wehrle PF (eds.). CV Mosby, St. Louis, 1976

CHAPTER 18

BORRELIOSIS

Oscar Felsenfeld

Introduction

Borreliosis is an infection most often carried by arthropods to man and domestic and wild animals, causing principally relapsing fever in man and a febrile disease in some animals. Borreliae have been isolated also from human and animal mucous membranes. The classification of borreliae is not yet fully established. Extensive reviews referring to the diagnosis of human borreliosis are available (2, 4, 6, 7, 8, 10, 11, 12, 14, 17, 19, 22, 23, 24, 25, 26).

Description of Borreliae

The genus *Borrelia* is classified in the family of *Treponemataceae* of the order of Spirochaetales. In older literature and in some publications from other than Anglosaxon countries, the generic designation *Spirocheta (Spirochaeta)* has been frequently used instead of *Borrelia. Borrelia recurrentis* (syn. *obermeyeri)* is carried by the human body and head louse (*Pediculus humanus humanus*). It causes epidemic relapsing fever. Tick-borne relapsing fever is endemic. Primarily tick-borne borreliae, carried by *Ornithodoros* ticks, for instance *B. turicatae* and *B. hermsii*, were sometimes named after the tick that carries them. However, the entire nomenclature of *Borrelia* is arbitrary.

Walters (29) and Felsenfeld (11) believed that *Borrelia* species follow the rules of vector-*Borrelia* species specificity as a rule, but not always. Laboratory experiments must be evaluated carefully because the tick used in transmission studies may already be carrying a strain of *Borrelia*. Burgdorfer (5) showed that borreliae are systemic parasites of argasid ticks and lice.

Ticks conserve and lice propagate borreliae. It is possible that borreliae were originally parasites of small rodents and later were transferred by ticks to man and from man to lice. On the other hand, borreliae may have evolved into different strains with acarinae, with the genetic changes that led to the differentiation of various *Ornithodoros* species. Mammals are only accidental and incidental hosts of borreliae. Davis (8) pointed out that some experimenters injected the borreliae or crushed arthropods into experimental animals, whereas others fed the vectors on infected and on "clean" animals. Different techniques may yield divergent results and conclusions regarding strain-vector specificity.

One may expect that in the future species specificity of borreliae will be questioned. This problem is particularly difficult to resolve because of the antigenic phase variations of the borreliae. Probably under the influence of antibodies, borreliae either develop a new antigenic phase between relapses, or deeper situated antigens emerge and become unmasked. Therefore, borreliae isolated from a later attack do not have the same antigenic structure as do those found in earlier episodes of fever in the same patient. New antibodies also appear in the blood. The antigenic variations of borreliae are cyclical. Some authors have described 20 or more antigenic phases, others only a few (10, 11), according to the particular strain studied. Phase variation is seldom observed in ticks or in Kelly's medium (5). Phase variation may cause false-negative serologic results when sera from late relapses are tested against borreliae isolated from an earlier attack of fever. Conversely, the common antigen may be so readily detectable that cross-reactions become marked. However, the morphology of the borreliae is not influenced by antigenic changes, but borreliae cannot be differentiated on the basis of their morphology.

The dimensions of borreliae are given differently by various authors. The thickness of the microorganisms is determined by the stain used to visualize them. Their length depends on the developmental stage because borreliae that are not separated by full division may appear elongated.

Borreliae are helical microorganisms usually 5 to 25 μm long and 0.2 to 0.5 μm wide, with several coils. The coils are wide and uneven, particularly in smears that have been air dried for a long time. Electron microscopy shows a bundle of about 10 to 20 fibrils coiled around the borreliae between the outer coat and the inner membrane, a cytoplasmic cylinder, and a central axial filament. Fragments of borreliae and very slender forms are often seen in vectors, particularly just after the borreliae have penetrated into the celomic cavity of the arthropod.

Helical rotation, twisting, and corkscrew-like movements are usually seen. The moving borreliae do not show the rigidity of *Treponema*. No "hooks" are observed as in *Leptospira*. No undulating membrane and no flagellum are seen under the optical microscope (Fig 18.1).

Clinical Forms of Borreliosis

Several strains of *Borrelia* cause relapsing fever in man. The incubation time is variable. It seems that 2 to 15 or more days is the usual incubation period; in American relapsing fever it frequently is 5 to 21 days. The first attack begins suddenly with high fever and ends after 3 to 14 days, usually 4 to 7, with lysis. Borreliae circulate in the blood during the first part of the attack and disappear from the peripheral circulation with the beginning of the crisis. Some borreliae survive particularly in lymph nodes, spleen, central nervous system, and heart, and multiply in those organs. There may be only one attack but usually another febrile attack ensues after 3 to 30 days, on the average after 5 to 9 days. In favorable instances these relapses become shorter and milder, and ultimately cease. The number of relapses varies with the epidemic

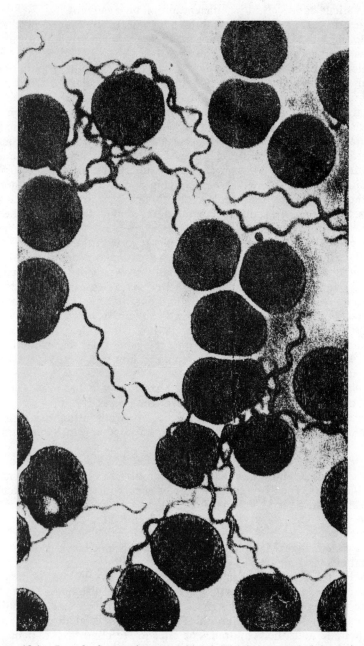

Figure 18.1—*Borrelia hermsii* in mouse blood. Wright—crystal violet stain. ×4,500.

and the geographical location. There are numerous atypical cases, particularly when the patient has received insufficient antibiotic treatment.

Frequently secondary anemia, thrombocytopenia, prolonged prothrombin and clotting times, elevated fibrinogen, often also high serum bilirubin and transaminase values are found.

Atypical clinical forms may be dysentery-like, hepatobiliary, pulmonary, meningeal, and rheumatoid. In many instances, particularly in infections caused by members of the *croidurae* subgroup and by *B. latyschewii*, the disease in man is rather mild and may be misdiagnosed as a "virus infection," or entirely missed. However, complications are not rare. Cardiac and hepatic failure, cerebral edema, shock, and intravascular coagulation are most frequently listed. Antibiotic treatment with one dose of a repository penicillin, and subsequent administration of a tetracycline has reduced the mortality to 0.5% – 5% in treated patients. There is, however, danger of a Jarisch-Herxheimer reaction if the borreliae are destroyed too rapidly and their toxins, together with endogenous pyrogen, are suddenly liberated and deluge the body of the patient.

In animals, borreliosis has been repeatedly reported from rodents. The severity of the disease depends on the age of the particular rodent. Mortality is highest among the young. The disease usually takes a more chronic course than in man, and relapses are uncommon. However, relapses are seen in nonhuman primates. The vector of rodent borreliosis is the *Ornithodoros* tick. Some of the *Ornithodoros* species do not feed on man and therefore they transfer the borreliae only from one rodent to another. Human lice do not feed on other animals as a rule. Therefore epidemic relapsing fever that is carried by human lice does not appear in animals. Monkeys, however, were acceptable to *Pediculus humanus* in laboratory experiments.

B. theileri causes cattle tick fever that resembles piroplasmosis, and also fever with one or two relapses in cattle, sheep, and horses. It has been reported from Africa and Australia. The disease is mild. The transmitting tick is not an *Ornithodoros* but often a *Rhipicephalus*. Perhaps also other arthropods carry *B. theileri*.

B. anserina causes "avian spirochetosis." After 3 to 8 days' incubation the birds become restless and cyanotic, and develop diarrhea, later ataxis and paralysis of the wings. The disease lasts about 2 weeks, with high fever. The mortality rate is high. Several vectors, including *Argas* ticks and *Dermanyssus* mites have been found to carry *B. anserina*. The infection can be transmitted through the feces of sick birds, and by cannibalism. The blood of fowl infected with *B. anserina* is highly infective for other birds but not for man, laboratory rodents, rabbits, and monkeys.

Borreliae from mucous membranes represent a taxonomic problem. *B. vincentii* is believed to be the causative agent of Vincent's angina, with a clinical picture varying from acute gingivitis to peritonsillar abscess and pulmonary lesions, including trench mouth. This fusospirochetal disease is more common in undernourished children. The infection responds well to penicillin, the tetracyclines, and to proper dental and nutritional care. Some authors believe (10, 11, 25) that *Borrelia buccalis* and *Borrelia refringens* from mucous membranes should be classified with other *Treponemataceae* and that the causative agents of diseases ascribed to them are actually *Mycoplasma* and viruses, particularly herpesviruses.

Epidemiology

As already described, the louse-borne *B. recurrentis* causes epidemic relapsing fever, particularly in populations living under hygienic conditions that favor the multiplication of lice. Lice do not tolerate high temperatures. They desert persons with high fever and thrive in heavy clothing worn in the cold.

Masses of people living under bad hygienic conditions are seen during wars, after natural disasters such as earthquakes, in concentration and other prisoner camps, jails, and even in some orphanages. Relapsing fever was rather common in Europe and in the Americas until the end of the 19th century. There were two large outbreaks during and after World Wars I and II. Both of them originated in Northeast Africa. It was believed that louse-borne relapsing fever is endemic among desert tribes in that area but Bryceson et al. (4) showed that the real African focus of borreliosis is Ethiopia, particularly the hilly part. The Central and South American foci, particularly in the high mountains, have been inactive recently. There is no information available about the old foci in China but louse-borne relapsing fever occurred in Northern Vietnam in recent years. No nation is without lice; therefore the danger of louse-borne relapsing fever is a constant menace.

Tick-borne human relapsing fever is limited to areas where the respective *Ornithodoros* ticks live. The range of these ticks is rather small, often only about 20 to 25 meters. They may be carried by rodents into buildings, caves, and burrows, and in the fur of domestic or wild animals from one locality to another. Migrant African laborers often carry *O. moubata* as a good-luck charm. This species of ticks spread to South Africa when carried by such migrants. Because a person has to invade the habitat of ticks to become bitten by them, the infection remains endemic and restricted to visitors of tick-infested areas. Workers, builders, soldiers, hunters, and vacationers are the most frequent invaders of *Ornithodoros*-infested areas and consequently the most frequent victims of tick-borne relapsing fever. Tick-borne relapsing fever has been reported from the Western part of the Americas, in the dry regions of the Mediterranian area, in East, South, and West Africa, and in Asia east to Central Asia. Ticks require a relatively dry and cool climate which they can find in many regions in animal burrows, caves, crevices, and floors of huts. They will not survive in the jungle. *O. erraticus erraticus* followed the route of the Moslem conquest and is found around the Mediterranean. *O. hermsi* prefers higher altitudes. *O. parkeri* is practically restricted to California. *O. turicata* appears to be spreading eastward from the Pacific Coast. *O. moubata* in Africa and *O. turicata* in some parts of Mexico have become domesticated. *O. hermsi* and *O. tholozani* are frequently found in old buildings and huts. Not all strains of *O. talaje* bite man. Most feed only on rodents, transmitting the borreliae from one animal to another. There are also other limitations to the transmission of tick-borne borreliae. The bite of some *Ornithodoros* species is so painful that the victim shakes them off before transmission of borreliae can take place. However, nymphs of *Ornithodoros* and some adults, as for example of the North American species, may have infected salivary glands and transmission of borreliae may take place within a few minutes. Small animals and infants may not be able to rid themselves of a well-attached tick. Hence the infection rate is higher among newborn rodents in burrows inhabitated also by *Ornithodoros*.

B. theileri has been described in Africa and in a few instances in Australia. No proven instances of the disease caused by this organism have been reported from other parts of the world. There is insufficient information concerning its vector. Nevertheless the cattle tick has been found to harbor this *Borrelia*. Man is not susceptible to *B. theileri* infections. Cattle, sheep, goats, and camels may carry *Ornithodoros* ticks in their fur. If such animals are moved from one locality to another, the ticks may become established in a new environment.

B. anserina has been transmitted by several species of ticks and mites, as well as by the feces of infected birds, and by cannibalization of weak and dead fowl. The disease is widespread in the tropics. There are no *B. anserina* infections reported at this time from the United States. Direct transmission of this *Borrelia*, without the mediation of an arthropod vector, has been described in California, India, and Sweden.

Borreliae from mucous membranes are transmitted by direct contact. Airborne infection with oral borreliae and their propagation by soiled linen, food, eating utensils, and other fomites are distinct possibilities. Borreliae living on the mucous membranes of the urogenital tract are usually propagated by sexual intercourse.

The vectors and distribution of commonly encountered *Borrelia* species are summarized in Table 18.1

Public Health Significance

The spread of epidemic relapsing fever in man could be controlled by simple delousing procedures. Unfortunately, lice are becoming increasingly resistant to D.D.T. that has been used, mostly in 5% to 10% powder, to delouse individuals as well as large populations, as in Naples during World War II. Prevention of the spreading of lice by enforcing sanitary measures such as frequent washing of clothing and bathing, as well as the application of dry heat to clothing, is not always practicable. The γ isomer of B.H.C. is widely used for spraying huts and other buildings. Such operations are best carried out at the time when tick larvae hatch, usually in the spring and in the autumn. It is difficult to clean *Ornithodoros* from caves. Visitors, particularly children, frequently come in contact with infected ticks in such caves. Attempts at biological tick control have been carried out but the results are not yet satisfactory for large-scale use.

Relapsing fever in man presents a problem also from the point of view of cost-effectiveness. The disease is not sufficiently frequent in the Americas to stand far enough in the foreground in the medical and laboratory evaluation of patients with "fever of unknown origin." The necessity of maintaining numerous *Borrelia* strains and antisera, as well as the pressure to treat the patient before a blood sample has been collected, coupled with the scarcity of bor-

TABLE 18.1—COMMONLY ENCOUNTERED *BORRELIA* STRAINS AND THEIR VECTORS

STRAIN	VECTOR	GEOGRAPHIC LOCATION OF VECTOR	COMMENTS
Borrelia recurrentis (syn. *Obermeyeri*)	*Pediculus humanus humanus*	World-wide, man only	Epidemic relapsing fever
B. duttonii	*Ornithodoros moubata*	East, West and South Africa Human habitats	African endemic relapsing fever
B. persica	*O. tholozani* (syn. *papillipes*)	Eastern Mediterranean to Central Asia Animal burrows, sometimes buildings	Endemic relapsing fever
B. hispanica	*O. erraticus erraticus*	Mediterranean littoral Usually with animals	Mediterranean relapsing fever
B. latyschewii	*O. tartakowskyi*	Iran to Central Asia Wild rodents	Central Asian relapsing fever
B. caucasica	*O. verrucosus*	USSR to Gulf of Persia Animal burrows, old buildings	Caucasian relapsing fever
B. crocidurae, B. microti, B. merionesi, B. dipodilli	*O erraticus sonrai* and others	North and East Africa, Central Asia With rodents	Cause mild disease in man
B. mazzottii	*O. talaje*	Kansas to Columbia	Not all *O. talaje* bite man
B. turicatae	*O. turicata*	Western part of North America, Canada, Central and South America Sometimes domesticated	American relapsing fever
B. parkerii	*O. parkeri*	Western U.S.	Not very common
B hermsii	*O. hermsi*	Western U.S., Canada highlands. In tree trunks, log cabins	Appears to be spreading
B. venezuelensis (syn. *neotropicalis*)	*O. venezuelensis* (syn. *rudis*)	South America to Texas	South American relapsing fever
B. theileri	*Ripicephalus*	Africa, Australia	Cattle spirochetosis
B. anserina	Numerous, also direct transmission	Old World	Fowl spirochetosis
Borrelia from mucous membranes	No arthropod vector— direct transmission	World-wide	Vincent's angina, ulcers

reliae in the blood of some infected individuals, requiring time-consuming search, makes the establishment of a *Borrelia* section in laboratories a costly and scientifically not always rewarding operation, particularly because the patient is often cured by the blindly administered penicillins and tetracyclines before a diagnosis could be made. It is the Public Health Laboratory system that principally requires fortification to be able to carry out diagnostic procedures in borreliosis. A survey for ticks, particularly for *Ornithodoros* species, and the determination of the proportion of infected ticks is desirable but during this period of disinterest in borreliosis remains a dream of epidemiologists and entomologists alike.

B. theileri infections appear to cause little damage in domestic animals. Dipping cattle to kill their ticks may prove effective. However, "cattle spirochetosis" is most frequent in such parts of Africa in which blood parasites (especially piroplasmata and trypanosomata) as well as bacterial infections are rather common and require more attention.

The United States is fortunate in not having fowl borreliosis at this time. The eradication measures taken in California were strict and effective, even though costly. Extermination of infected flocks, isolation, quarantine, and administration of antibiotics were most helpful in controlling the disease.

Spirochetes of the mucous membranes may present serious problems to the dentist and the laryngologist. It is believed that when proper dental care and adequate nutrition become available to everybody, oropharyngeal spirochetosis will disappear. Urogenital spirochetosis remains restricted to mucous membranes and to ulcers formed as a reaction to other agents. This secondary infection does not represent a problem *per se*, except as a sign of lack of cleanliness and unhygienic habits. Therefore borreliae of the mucous membranes should be appraised from a general rather than from a specific health point of view.

Collection of Specimens

Time of Collection

It is of utmost importance that specimens be collected from infected man and animals before any medication is administered. Thick and thin blood smears, heparinized or citrated blood for animal inoculations and experiments to culture the borreliae, serum for immunological tests, and cerebrospinal fluid (if indicated) should be collected. Borreliae may be sparse in these samples. They often disappear immediately before and during the crisis of the febrile attack. Xenodiagnosis may be performed during the fever period, if this test is feasible for the detection of the respective strain.

If serologic diagnostic studies are contemplated, a second serum specimen should be collected a few weeks (3 to 4) after the first attack. In public health and hospital laboratory practice it is desirable to collect specimens from each attack at least for an attempt to find the borreliae either in smears or in inoculated animals, even if serologic means are not available to differentiate the *Borrelia* species.

Tissue Specimens

Tissue specimens are collected between relapses or postmortem, and searched for borreliae after staining, usually with fluorescent antibody (FA) and a silver impregnation method. In human and animal relapsing fever, the spleen, lymph nodes, less frequently the liver and the central nervous system, are the favorite organs for search for borreliae between attacks and during a postmortem.

Borreliae are very seldom found in the excreta of the patients. However, *B. anserina* is frequently isolated from the feces and the liver of infected birds.

Borreliae from the mucous membranes are collected with a sterile capillary pipette equipped with a rubber bulb. The specimens are used for microscopic and culture examinations, less often for animal inoculations.

Vectors

Vectors are usually studied only in well-equipped specialized laboratories such as the Rocky Mountain Laboratory of the U.S.P.H.S. in Hamilton, Montana. Burghofer (6) recommended that small vectors should be triturated and injected into young mice, the all-around laboratory animal for borreliae. Transmission experiments by feeding suspected vectors on susceptible animals are not always successful and therefore are not recommended for routine use. In lice and larger ticks, amputation of the distal portion of the legs or the separation of an entire extremity from the body will result in an outflow of the hemolymph that can be examined directly. Extirpation of organs for examination for borreliae requires skill. However, several species (e.g., *O. moubata, O. turicata, O. parkeri*) exude coxal fluid after the ventral exoskeleton has been scratched with warmed forceps (6).

Animal Hosts

Animal hosts, particularly wild rodents, are examined for borreliae by studying their blood and, after sacrifice, by direct examination of their organs, as well as by animal inoculation. The handling of wild rodents may be difficult if their blood contains borreliae; the blood that spatters onto the mucosae of the examiner may contain borreliosis. Utmost care must therefore be exercised in dealing with wild (and also laboratory) rodents.

Bacteriological Procedures

Microscopic Examination

For the examination of unstained and stained smears, blood is collected from the fingertip, earlobe, or a vein. Cerebrospinal fluid is handled in the same manner as blood specimens. It is collected usually only in infections with known neurotropic *Borrelia* but the list of such types is yet incomplete. It is recommended therefore that spinal fluid should be examined whenever symptoms of cerebrospinal invasion are present and, as a matter of routine, in patients with high fever of undetermined origin.

Citrated blood specimens (4 ml of blood mixed with 1 ml of 3.8% sterile disodium citrate solution) are used in microscopic tests only for observation of the borreliae with the darkfield microscope, and of the stirring up of groups of red blood cells by motile borreliae. Heparin interferes with azur-eosin stains, causing a diffuse blue coloration, and is therefore avoided in microscopic work even at the lowest (10 IU per ml blood) effective anticoagulant concentration.

Unstained smears

A drop of citrated blood, spinal fluid, or celomic fluid is placed on a scrupulously clean 1 × 3 inch microscope slide and covered with a 20 or 22 mm square coverslip, taking care to prevent the fluid from spreading outside the slide, because of its possible infectiousness. It is not recommended that more than 2 or 3 drops be placed on a single slide. The slides are examined immediately under the dark-field microscope at 400× magnification. The light-field microscope, at the same magnification, will show the movement of the red blood cells that are disturbed in certain areas by the twisting and rotating borreliae. The borreliae themselves are difficult to visualize in unstained preparations except by dark-field and phase microscopy. They remain alive in such preparations usually for 4 to 6 hr, particularly when fingernail polish, paraffin, Carbowax, or some other rapidly solidifying medium has been applied to the edges of the coverslip to prevent evaporation.

Stained smears

Stained smears are permanent records. Since the borreliae may be found with greater ease in thick smears, the preparation of both thick and thin smears is recommended.

Two to three thick smears can be made on each 1 × 3 inch slide. It is customary to follow the same practice as in malaria work and to put one thick and one thin smear from each individual on the same slide. This method requires care in dehemoglobinization of the thick smear and in the fixation of the thin smears. A dividing line may be drawn on the slide between the two smears using a glass-writing pen. This line then serves as a reminder of the need to treat each part of the slide differently.

Thick smears are prepared by collecting a drop of blood on the slide, spreading it out concentrically with a toothpick, wooden applicator, or other instrument, to form a round smear of about 1 to 1.5 cm in diameter, and letting it air dry for about 30 min. Thin smears are prepared by streaking out a small drop of blood using the edge of a coverslip or a slide, as for hematologic examination. The thin smears are also permitted to air dry.

Thick smears can be dehemoglobinized with distilled water. Thick smears that are old or have dried too long require dehemoglobinization with 0.05% acetic acid. Fresh smears may not require treatment at all. They may be stained immediately with a Giemsa-type dye. It is mandatory that the thick preparations be washed immediately after dehemoglobinization using 0.01 M phosphate-buffered saline, pH 6.8, except when immediate staining with Giemsa stain diluted with phosphate-saline follows. The thin smears are fixed with acetone for 1 min or with absolute methanol for 3 min.

Borreliae can be stained with aniline dyes. Azur-eosin dyes are used most frequently, because such preparations also permit a search for other blood parasites that may cause febrile attacks, such as plasmodia, trypanosomata, and others, whereas other human-pathogenic *Treponemataceae* such as *Leptospira* and *Treponema* do not take up azur-eosin dyes.

Stains of the Jenner-Romanowski group are generally used, such as those of Leishman, Giemsa, May-Grünwald, Wright, and others that can be purchased from reliable sources such as Harleco, Gurr, Grübler, and others.

1. In the United States, Wright stain is mostly commonly used, either in prepared solutions or after dissolving the powder according to the manufacturer's directions. The buffer used, 0.01 M phosphate buffer with 0.85% NaCl, pH 6.4 to 6.6, is also available commercially but must be renewed frequently because it is easily contaminated by microorganisms.

The smears are stained with a certain number of drops of Wright stain. After 3 min an equal number of drops of the buffer are added and mixed with the dye by gently blowing on the slide. A metallic scum is formed on the surface. After 1 min the slide is washed with the buffer and dried standing on end.

2. It has been recommended (10) that the slides should be stained after application of the Wright stain using 1% aqueous crystal violet for 10 to 30 sec and then differentiated with distilled water.

3. The fixed slides may be stained with May-Grünwald stain diluted 1:2 with 0.01 M phosphate buffer, pH 6.8, for 6 to 8 min. One ml of stock Giemsa stain (commercial) is diluted with 1 ml absolute methanol and 50 ml of the buffer. The dye solution is put in Coplin jars and the slides immersed for 12 to 18 hr. Differentiation with 0.1% acetic acid may be necessary, followed by thorough rinsing in the buffer.

4. A more rapid staining method is to use Giemsa stain diluted 1:10 with the buffer for 10 min, then washing and, if necessary, differentiating with 0.1% acetic acid.

5. Staining with 1% crystal violet for 10 to 30 sec may also follow the Giemsa stain.

6. Every batch of commercial stains must be tested with "normal" blood smears before being applied to *Borrelia* studies. A satisfactory differentiation of blood platelets and polymorphonuclear leukocytes permits one to expect that borreliae will be seen if present. The additional staining with crystal violet has to be adjusted not only to the batch of stain but also to the personal taste of the examiner.

Personal taste and experience permit also the use of other aniline dyes. Two methods have been found satisfactory (6, 10, 11, 12).

A stain is prepared by mixing 1 volume of saturated solution of methylene blue B in saline with 2 volumes of 10% sodium taurocholate. The stain keeps for about 1 month. The acetone- or methanol-fixed preparation is covered with the stain and a glass or plastic coverslip applied. Examination should be carried out 1 to 2 min after the addition of the stain.

The Ziehl-Neelsen carbolfuchsin stain is applied to the slides for 1 min, followed by washing with distilled water.

Fluorescent antibody method (FA) (1, 6)

For the fluorescent antibody test, blood is collected in citrated saline or isotonic disodium citrate and centrifuged for 5 min at 200 to 300 × *g*. The plasma is separated and 2% formol added to a final concentration of 0.2%. The formolized plasma is then centrifuged for 8 to 10 min at 1000 to 3000 × g. The sediment contains most of the borreliae. Saline with 0.4% formol is used to suspend the sediment. The concentration of the borrelia is adjusted to approximately 50 microorganisms per microscopic field at 400× magnification.

1. Drops of this *Borrelia* suspension are air dried on slides and fixed with acetone for 3 to 5 min.

The serum used in the test is diluted with 4 volumes of phosphate-buffered saline pH 7.2 to 7.3 (PBS, available commercially) and mixed with an equal volume of sonified Reiter's or Nichol's spirochete to absorb the common treponemataceal antibody if present in the serum. The serum-spirochete mixture is kept for 10 min at room temperature. The spirochetes and the antigen-antibody complexes are centrifuged for 30 min at 1000 to 2000 × g. The supernatant may be conjugated with fluorescein isothiocyanate or rhodamine for the direct FA test. It is also possible to conjugate the serum before absorption with the spirochetes.

Known positive and negative control sera also must be used. The titer of a serum of unknown antibody content is routinely checked against that of a homologous rabbit serum of known potency.

2. "Unknown" sera are diluted serially with PBS from 1:5 to 1:400. One drop of each dilution of serum is added to each drop of antigen on a coverslip. After 30 min in the moist chamber at 37 C the slides are washed with PBS. One drop of antihuman rabbit, goat, sheep, donkey, or horse serum labeled with fluorescein isothiocyanate is added to each antigen-antibody mixture. After 10 min the slides are washed again with PBS, mounted in 10% glycerol, and observed under the fluorescent microscope.

This method gives better results than the direct method applying labeled anti-*Borrelia* sera and is more economical because only one serum has to be labeled and not an entire set of specific sera.

3. If the serotype of the *Borrelia* has to be determined, rabbit anti-*Borrelia* sera or globulins are used instead of the "unknown" serum. The procedure is the same as with "unknown" sera. However, the fluorescein-labeled anti-rabbit serum is usually prepared in horses, donkeys, goats, and sheep. Numerous commercial sera are satisfactory. The titers of all sera must be checked periodically.

It is recommended that microscopic observation not be carried out sooner than 10 min after the last washing. If the slide has to be examined later, it must be kept in a refrigerator at 2 to 4 C. It is not recommended to use slides prepared more than 24 hr before examination.

Scrupulous cleanliness of the slides, careful but effective washing with PBS, properly prepared antisera, purchase of commercially prepared sera from a reliable source only, and proper preservation of the sera in small quantities obviating repeated thawing and freezing of the sera are among the prerequisites for successful application of this method.

4. The FA test can also be carried out on tissues. These must be frozen sections. However, formol-fixed tissues from which frozen sections are later made can also be used. The sections are affixed to slides with acetone for 5 min, dried at 37 C, flooded with 1% ammonia water for 3 to 5 min, washed with 3% Tween 80 (polyoxyethylene sorbitan monooleate, Polysorbate 80) in

PBS, blotted dry, treated with rabbit anti-*Borrelia* serum for 30 min at 37 C in a wet chamber, washed with PBS, flooded with fluorescein-labeled anti-rabbit, sheep, goat, horse, or donkey serum for 10 min, washed again with PBS, and mounted in 10% glycerol.

Immunoenzyme test (21)

The indirect method of the immunoenzyme test has been recommended. The antigen is prepared by inoculating mice or rats with borreliae and exsanguinating the animals by cardiac puncture at the peak of the infection. The blood is collected in 10 × volumes of sterile distilled water to destroy red blood cells. The mixture is centrifuged at 200 to 300 × g. The supernatant, containing most of the borreliae, is centrifuged at 3000 to 5000 × g for a few minutes. Drops of approximately 0.01 ml of the sediment containing 50 to 100 borreliae per 400× microscopic field are air dried in marked areas of microscope slides. The slides are fixed with acetone for 5 to 10 min, then stored in a refrigerator.

Anti-human rabbit γ globulin (available commercially) is adjusted to contain 5 mg of protein per ml. The protein content of some commercial γ globulins is marked on the container. If it is not, the protein content is determined by the Lowry, Nessler, Kjeldahl, or other feasible method and the γ globulin solution adjusted with saline to contain 5 mg per ml. Then 12 mg of horseradish peroxidase type VI (Sigma Lab., St. Louis, Mo., or other) are dissolved in each ml of the rabbit globulin solution. Next, 0.05 ml of a freshly prepared aqueous 1% solution of glutaraldehyde is added to each ml under constant stirring. After 2 hr at room temperature, the mixture is dialyzed against PBS in a refrigerator at 2 to 4 C overnight. This conjugate can be kept in a refrigerator until use.

Twofold serial dilutions of the serum to be tested, from 1:2 to 1:64, are prepared using PBS as the diluent. Aliquots of 0.025 ml of these dilutions are added to the smears of borreliae. After 30 min at room temperature, the slides are carefully washed with PBS, and 0.025 ml of the conjugate added. Incubation for 30 min at room temperature follows. Known positive and negative sera and unconjugated rabbit globulin serve as controls.

Staining is carried out with a freshly prepared solution of 5 mg of 3,3'-diaminobenzidine hydrochloride in 10 ml of 0.05 M Tris-HCl buffer, pH 7.6, to which 0.03 ml of 3% hydrogen peroxide has just been added. After 30 min at room temperature the slides are washed with distilled water, dried standing on edge, and examined under the optical microscope at 1000× magnification. Deep brown staining of the borreliae indicates a positive result. Dark scattered granular precipitates may be seen also in negative smears. Yellow coloration of the borreliae is of doubtful significance and should be disregarded in routine laboratory practice.

Silver impregnation (11, 20)

Any silver impregnation method feasible for the demonstration of *Treponema* in tissues can be applied to the studies of borreliae. In this laboratory, the Krajian method modified by Erskine (11) has been used with good results.

Enrichment

Enrichment of the borreliae in blood and other fluids is possible by concentrating them in a microhematocrit tube (16). The tube is filled with citrated or heparinized blood, centrifuged at 100 to 200 × g, then the supernatant removed and placed in another microhematocrit tube. The supernatant is then centrifuged at 1000 × g. The sediment contains the borreliae. When blood that has been laked with distilled water or saponin is used, only one centrifugation at 1000 or more × g is required. The sediment will also contain thrombocytes and fragments of blood cells.

True enrichment is possible only in culture media. Kelly's media are suitable for some borreliae. The medium is inoculated with an equal amount of blood containing 10 to 20 IU of heparin per ml and incubated overnight at 37 C. The supernatant is then centrifuged at 5000 × g. The sediment contains the borreliae.

Culture methods

Noguchi in 1912 was the first to maintain borreliae in a slightly alkaline medium containing ascitic fluid and rabbit kidney, under a liquid paraffin seal. There is considerable controversy concerning the optimal temperature of incubation, but numerous authors agree (6, 19) that 32 to 35 C is favorable for most strains.

The presently recommended media of Wolman and Wolman (31) for *B. recurrentis* and those of Kelly (18, 19, 28) are feasible to maintain certain *Borrelia* strains but are not yet ready for routine diagnostic use. Borreliae are difficult to culture. Their nutritional requirements are little known. Kelly's media are based on recent studies of the nutritional requirements of borreliae. Since it may be expected that these investigations will continue, one of these media that is feasible for the propagation of *B. hermsii* is described elsewhere. Borreliae maintained in liquid cultures may not undergo phase variation. Although morphologic changes as well as loss of virulence may occur, it is believed that this medium should be included in this chapter because it permits maintenance of several *Borrelia* strains without animal inoculation.

Each tube of Kelly's medium is inoculated with 0.05 ml of blood, then incubated for 6 to 7 days at 35 C.

Inoculation of developing chick embryos has served for propagation of borreliae in the past. The most successful method consists of inoculation with blood, spinal fluid, or other liquid containing borreliae of the yolk sac of 9- to 10-day-old chick embryos. The eggs are kept in an egg incubator for 3 to 5 days. Borreliae are collected from the chorioallantoic vessels (10, 11).

Preservation of Live Borreliae

Preservation of live borreliae is desirable not only in diagnostic laboratories but also for shipment of infected materials to a center that is equipped for the diagnosis and classification of these microorganisms.

Culture methods are uncertain. *B. recurrentis* usually remains alive in the medium of Wolman and Wolman (23) at 3 to 5 C for several months. Kelly's medium is feasible for the maintenance of *B. hermsii* and related borreliae if weekly transfers are made (18, 19).

In experimental animals, borreliae survive in mice for only a short time but longer in rats. The brains of guinea pigs inoculated with *B. persica* will remain infective for several months. *B. hispanica* behaves similarly. Infected animals may be difficult to ship, so that other methods have been sought to preserve and to ship borreliae.

Infected ticks carry borreliae during their entire lifespan. No pathology has yet been described in infected *Ornithodoros* ticks, and no phase variation has been observed. The proportion of infected ticks varies with each locality and species. Approximatley 95% of *O. turicata* but only about 0.5% of *O. hermsi* harbor borreliae. It is possible to feed vectors on a patient. The borreliae may be taken up by the *Ornithodoros* but this is not a hard and fast rule.

Ticks are kept in "tickoria," singly, or in small groups in test tubes into which a strip of moist filter paper has been inserted, reaching from the bottom of the tube to below the cotton plug. The cotton plug should be loose but not loose enough to permit escape of the ticks. The tubes are kept in a desiccator the bottom of which is covered with saturated ammonium chloride solution. The ticks are fed at various intervals, preferably on newborn mice. If a "tickorium" is used, a recently killed newborn mouse is dropped into it. If transmission of the borreliae into animals is required, the ticks are fed on the shaved skin of newborn mice or of mice that are just a few days old. The borreliae can be transferred from the blood of the infected mouse into other animals. Not every feeding will be a "take." Frequently ticks refuse to feed because they have recently had a blood meal.

The most convenient method is freezing *Borrelia*-containing blood with or without a final concentration of 5%–10% glycerol in ampules immersed in liquid N_2. The ampules are sealed and kept in the liquid N_2 (3).

Another method is to lyophilize the borreliae in vacuum at −70 to −72 C with 2% lactose in skim milk. The ampules are kept in the deep freeze at −70 C (30).

Repeated freezing and thawing of the ampules containing borreliae is not recommended. Shipment in liquid N_2 is convenient.

The importation and exportation of ticks and *Borrelia* strains are regulated by the U.S. Department of Agriculture and by the U.S. Public Health Service.

Isolation by Animal Inoculation

Mice constitute the all-around laboratory animals for the study of relapsing fever borreliae. Newborn to 2-week-old mice in groups of 5 or 6 animals are usually inoculated intraperitoneally. Blood is diluted with an equal volume of isotonic sodium citrate solution or with one-fourth volume of 2% sodium citrate if the inoculation can be carried out within a short time after the blood was collected. Ten IU of heparin per ml of blood are also useful. The amount injected into the peritoneal cavity of each mouse is most frequently 0.2 ml. The injections can also be given subcutaneously, but larger amounts, 0.4 to 0.5

ml, should be used in these instances. Cerebrospinal fluid received in the laboratory for animal inoculations is usually sparse. It is injected undiluted into the peritoneal cavity.

Beginning on the third day after infection, blood is collected from the tail vein of the infected mice. The preferred method is to snip the end of the tail and collect enough blood for a smear, and to examine the smear after staining. The infection becomes apparent usually in 6 to 7 days, otherwise the mice should be checked for 14 days. If borreliae are found in the blood, it is recommended that the mouse be exsanguinated by cardiac puncture and the blood transferred to a second group of mice and to enrichment media. Several additional smears may be prepared. Frozen blood should be shipped in liquid N_2 to a *Borrelia* laboratory, together with the blood of the patient, or at least with serum collected during and after the attack, as well as available blood smears.

Rats are frequently inoculated to accumulate larger quantities of blood. Guinea pigs, particularly adults, are refractory to *B. duttonii*, most often also to *B. recurrentis*, and to the American borreliae. Other laboratory animals are not recommended for diagnostic tests in relapsing fever (6).

B. anserina cannot be transmitted to rodents. Inoculation of young chicks is recommended. *B. vincentii* is not feasible for testing in animals.

Xenodiagnosis

Xenodiagnosis is most useful in areas where only one *Borrelia* type prevails, for instance in Africa south from the Sahara. A clean (*Borrelia*-free) tick colony is a prerequisite. Five to 10 ticks are fed on the patient during a relapse. After their meal is completed, the ticks fall off the individual and are put into tubes or a "tickorium." Three to 4 weeks later the hemolymph is collected with a capillary tube and examined under the microscope or injected into the peritoneal cavity of mice (6, 31).

Skin Tests

Skin tests have been proposed but they gave disappointing results (6, 11).

Serologic Procedures

Procedures that employ FA and immunoenzyme tests have been discussed. It should be re-emphasized that borreliae are easily transmitted to man not only by their vectors but also with the blood of infected persons and animals; therefore utmost care must be exerted to avoid contamination of laboratory personnel. Borreliae penetrate through wounds, abrasions, and even through intact mucosae. It has been claimed (11) that because of their corkscrew-like motion borreliae may penetrate also intact skin; therefore serum, a potential carrier of borreliae, must also be treated with proper precautions.

Preparation of antisera

Diagnostic antisera are usually prepared in rabbits. It is recommended that a sample of the blood of the rabbit be tested for borreliolysins before the first injection of the antigen. The borreliae to be injected are collected from the blood of mice or rats. This blood is prepared by centrifuging infected citrated blood at 100 to 200 × g, then centrifuging the supernatant at 1000 to 2000 × g to collect the borreliae with the second sediment. The sediment is diluted with 10 volumes of sterile PBS and sonified, then is injected into the ear vein of a rabbit in ascending doses from 0.1 to 1.0 ml. The injections may be given twice a week. The recommended amounts are 0.1, 0.1, 0.25, 0.25, 0.5, 0.5, and 1.0 ml. Then the immobilizine and borreliolytic titers of the serum are determined. Should they be below 1:400, further injections are indicated.

1. When the titer of the serum is satisfactory, the rabbit is exsanguinated under anesthesia, by cardiac puncture. The serum is separated from the coagulated blood and absorbed. It is recommended that the first absorption be with 1/10 volume of sonified blood of the animal whose blood served as a vehicle of the borreliae. Citrated uninfected mouse or rat blood is centrifuged at 200 × g and the supernatant separated by centrifuging at 5000 × g. The sediment is sonified and used to absorb the anti-*Borrelia* rabbit serum for 30 min at room temperature, then centrifuged at 5000 × g. The supernatant is the absorbed serum. Then a second absorption with Reiter's or Nichol's spirochete is carried out. Ten volumes of serum are added to each volume of sonified spirochetes and after 30 min at room temperature again centrifuged. The supernatant is a specific serum that should be kept in ampules at −20 C. Repeated freezing and thawing of the serum is not recommended.

2. It is possible to absorb high titered sera (1:2000 or more) with borreliae belonging to different serotypes and in various phases to obtain highly specific sera. These are useful, however, only in research.

3. Borreliae that multiply in Kelly's medium can be centrifuged off at 2000 or more × g. Rabbit inoculation is carried out as with blood, except that Kelly's medium serves as a diluent. The absorption of the rabbit serum is done first with bovine albumin fraction V, then with Reiter's or Nichol's spirochete. The albumin fraction may be dissolved in the serum. Then it is recommended that the globulin fraction of the serum be separated by precipitation with 50% saturated ammonium sulfate.

The identification of the borreliae

This procedure is carried out with specific sera in the FA and enzyme-labeled staining tests in determinations of immobilizine and lysin titers, and in inoculations of various animals and culture media.

Detection of antibodies

Antibodies can be detected in several procedures. Cross-reactions between borreliae and other *Treponemataceae*, as well as with OX type protei, often occur. Rickettsiae may also show cross-reactions that may be difficult to interpret when louse-borne borreliosis and louse-borne typhus coexist.

The detection of antibodies against borreliae is not a simple task because of the phase variation of these microorganisms with every febrile attack as well as the described cross-reaction with other *Treponemataceae*, protei, and sometimes also *Rickettsia*. Moreover, pure borrelial antigens are difficult to prepare and the antisera are not always specific.

Taxonomic difficulties reflect themselves also in the serology of borreliae. For instance, Dodge (9) found in the same hospital population 2 strains of *B. recurrentis* that reacted differently with the sera of the patients. It appears that the lack of antigen-antibody reaction in these cases was due to greater differences among the strains than to mere phase variation. Therefore, "false"-negatives may also be expected.

The neutralization test is seldom carried out. It is usually performed in mice. Borreliae are separated from blood or a culture medium, then are counted in a chamber and a suspension is made in sterile PBS to contain 50 to 100 borreliae per ml. An equal volume of serum is diluted with sterile PBS 1:5, 1:50, and 1:100, then added to a series of tubes containing 0.3 ml of *Borrelia* suspension each. One-tenth ml of each dilution is injected intraperitoneally into each of 5 mice. *Borrelia* suspensions in PBS instead of a serum dilution, known positive and negative sera, and the tested serum alone are used as controls.

The blood from the tail vein of the mice is examined for borreliae from the third to the 14th day. The sera of infected persons should protect the animals against infection.

The test requires the use of large numbers of mice and should be carried out with several *Borrelia* strains. It may not be specific.

Resistance to superinfection used to be a favorite test for the classification of borreliae during the first half of this century. Young mice and young guinea pigs are used. Guinea pigs are not feasible for tests with *B. recurrentis,* most American borreliae, and the *B. crocidurae* subgroup. The mice are inoculated with 2 or 3 minimal infective doses (MID) of known borreliae. Blood from the tail vein is examined from the third to the 14th day. If negative by that time, the mice are inoculated with 2 to 3 MID of the examined *Borrelia.* If the *Borrelia* used to prime the mice is identical to the tested *Borrelia* strain, no borrelemia develops after the injection of the second *Borrelia.* However, cross-protection may occur and phase variation may permit reinfection with the same *Borrelia* type. Moreover, the one-sided or asymmetric immunity of borreliae described by Geigy and Burgdorfer (15) may lead to false results.

Agglutination-precipitation tests were introduced by Novy and Knapp in 1906. The simple agglutination test may be carried out on a slide on which one drop of a *Borrelia* suspension usually treated with 1% saponin is mixed with a drop of the antiserum. After 10 to 30 min in the wet chamber the agglutination is "read" in the darkfield. The agglutination test may be carried out also in tubes. After mixing 0.25 ml of a saponized or untreated *Borrelia* suspension and 0.25 ml of the serum diluted 1:20 to 1:2560 with PBS in agglutination tubes, the tubes are incubated for 2 hr at 27 C, then overnight at 2 to 4 C. Controls containing only *Borrelia* suspensions and with known positive and negative sera should be included. A slowly forming fluffy sediment is considered the sign of a positive reaction. However, borreliae often display autoagglutination and adherence. The test must therefore be evaluated carefully (6, 10, 21).

Agar gel diffusion by the Ouchterlony method using liver and *B. anserina* renders good results in avian spirochetosis. Strains that cause relapsing fever in man often cross-react with other *Treponemataceae* in this test. Absorbed sera and sonified borreliae give better results by immunoelectrophoresis. This method requires that further purified antigens become available (6, 12).

The adhesion phenomenon is observed during the entire course of the disease. Borreliae cling to red blood cells, to the nuclei of white blood cells, to bacteria, and to glass (10, 21). This phenomenon is complement-dependent. Therefore either fresh serum is used, or the serum is inactivated at 56 C for 30 min, and guinea pig complement is added. The simplest procedure is to prepare a suspension of *Escherichia coli,* approximately 10^4 microorganisms per ml. Equal amounts of this suspension, a suspension containing 80 to 100 borreliae per ml, and fresh serum to be tested are mixed. If the serum has been inactivated, 1:100 diluted guinea pig complement is also added. The mixture is incubated for 20 to 30 min at 30 C. The results are observed in the dark field. This test gives variable results even in the same patient.

Complement fixation tests have also been tried. That of Wolstenhome and Gear (32) used an antigen prepared by injecting 0.4 ml of heart blood of infected mice *(B. duttonii)* into 7-day-old chick embryos. After 1 week at 37 C, the chorioallantoic vessels were opened and permitted to bleed into the allantoic fluid. One-tenth of a ml was used for further egg inoculations. After 10 weekly passages, phenol-saline was added and the antigen used in 1:25 to 1:100 dilutions. Stein (27) prepared the antigen by mixing 1 volume of 2% sodium citrate in saline, 4 volumes of infected rat blood, and 1.3 volumes of 10% saponin. The mixture was centrifuged repeatedly to separate the borreliae. The test proper was usually carried out by mixing 0.1 ml of a *Borrelia* suspension containing approximately 80 borreliae per oil immersion field, 0.1 ml of serum to be tested diluted 1:10 with PBS, 2 units of guinea pig complement in 0.1 ml, and incubation for 30 min at 37 C. Then 0.2 ml of a 5% suspension of sensitized sheep red blood cells with 2 U of antisheep hemolysin were added, reincubated, and read after 10 min. This test is not considered feasible because not all *Borrelia* strains can be adapted satisfactorily to rats or to developing chick embryos. Furthermore, the antigen is frequently anticomplementary.

Immobilizine and borreliolysin tests are the most widely used tests. The immunoglobulin predominantly participating in these reactions is 19S IgM. Perhaps immobilizines and borreliolysins are related and their activities interwoven. Lysins are complement dependent; immobilizines are not. The techniques described here are those of Schuhardt (23) and Felsenfeld (12).

PBS is feasible for both tests. It is recommended that 5 mM calcium chloride be added to the commercial PBS.

In the immobilizine test, serum inactivated for 30 min at 56 C is mixed with an equal volume of a suspension of borreliae in buffer containing 20 to 30 borreliae per 400 × microscopic field. After 10 to 30 min at 37 C in the moist chamber, slides are prepared and a coverslip applied. A *Borrelia* suspension without serum admixture serves as a control. The proportion of immobilized and not immobilized borreliae is obtained by counting at least 20 microscopic fields. The percent of immobilized borreliae is calculated. The control (without antiserum) should not contain more than 20% immobilized borreliae.

Another method consists of using serum diluted serially 1:50 to 1:1600. The highest dilution that immobilizes 50% of the borreliae is considered the end point.

The borreliolysin (lysin) test is performed by mixing an equal volume of inactivated serum with a suspension of borreliae in the buffer. The *Borrelia* suspension should contain 20 to 30 borreliae per 400 × microscopic field. The mixing is usually done in a capillary, using a rubber bulb. The capillary is sealed with clay or wax and kept for 1½ hr at 32 to 33 C. Then one-half volume of guinea pig complement diluted 1:100 in the buffer is added and further incubation for 30 min follows. The contents of the capillary are discharged on a slide, covered with a 20 to 22 mm square coverslip, and the results observed in the dark field. The results are expressed in percent of the borreliae lysed.

The number of borreliae in a preparation containing buffer instead of the serum serves as control. Not more than 20% to 25% of them should be lysed in the absence of antiserum.

It is possible to carry out the entire test on a microscope slide, in which case it is recommended that all ingredients be mixed before the incubation, and the coverslip secured with nail polish, paraffin, or other rapidly solidifying agent to prevent evaporation.

Serum dilutions increasing from 1:50 to 1:1600 may be used on separate slides. The dilution that causes lysis of 50% of the borreliae is considered the titer of the serum.

Evaluating and Reporting Results

Microscopic Examination

When borreliae are not found in at least 60 microscopic fields of a thin smear and in 20 fields of a thick smear, the report of "Borreliae not found in thick and thin smears" should be made. Objects resembling borreliae at 400 × magnification should be verified under oil immersion. Particularly fibrin fibers and the contours of red blood cells in hemolyzed preparations may be mistaken for fragments of borreliae. Broken-up borreliae in the blood are very rare. They may occur only during or shortly before the crisis. Leptospiras and treponemas in the blood do not stain with aniline dyes, so that dark field findings, if not entirely clear, should be confirmed by examination of stained blood smears. If microorganisms with numerous coils (more even in unfixed smears) are seen, the report should be "Microorganisms morphologically resembling borreliae were seen."

Animal Inoculation

The results of animal inoculation are more reliable than are those of the direct examination of smears. It is feasible to include in the report how much blood or spinal fluid was injected into how many animals. Examples: "Five mice were inoculated intraperitoneally with 0.2 ml of citrated blood each. No borreliae were observed in the blood collected from the tail veins for 14 days." "Six young mice were inoculated intraperitoneally with 0.2 ml of heparinized blood each. Microorganisms morphologically resembling borreliae were seen in the blood from the tailveins beginning on the 5th day. These microorganisms are being further studied." Further characterization of the *Borrelia*-like microbes by additional animal inoculations (particularly guinea pigs), use of Kelly's medium, and serologic tests are reported after the respective examinations are finished and evaluated. It is not always recommended to try to report the type of *Borrelia* merely on the basis of mouse and guinea pig inoculation, and attempted growth in Kelly's medium. It is desirable to isolate the *Borrelia* also from the vector with which the patient came in contact, and sometimes from wild rodents handled by the person who became ill with relapsing fever. There is usually little doubt about the type of *Borrelia* isolated from an epidemic in persons covered with lice, but tick-borne types may be difficult to distinguish where several *Ornithodoros* species are infected, as in the western United States and in the Middle East. Xenodiagnosis may not permit pinpointing the vector because several *Ornithodoros* species may be infected in the laboratory with the same type of *Borrelia*.

Serologic Examination

The results of the examination of a single specimen may not give satisfactory information. The collection of paired sera is recommended. The most valuable results are derived from FA, immunoenzyme, immobilizine, and borreliolysin examinations. These are particularly helpful when the titer has increased between the two collections of the blood specimens. However, serological response and serotype etiology are not always related. For instance, cross reactions between American borreliae, and between *B. duttonii* and *B. hispanica* may be confusing.

It is recommended that the physician on the case or the public health official be informed about the titer of the serum giving a positive reaction, or in the case of immobilizines and lysins the percentage of the afflicted borreliae. A fourfold rise in the titer or a 20% increase in the percent of borreliae immobilized or lysed is considered significant in most of the reviewed literature (12). FA tests with 1:1 diluted sera, enzyme-linked tests with 1:8 titers, immobilizine and lysin titers with 1:100 diluted sera or 50% of undiluted sera may be considered "borderline" reactions not necessarily indicative of the *Borrelia* species causing the disease. The immobilizine titer is usually about double that of the lysin titer as determined by using increasing serum dilutions. A specific diagnosis of the *Borrelia* type is not always made easily from the examination of the serum of the infected patient. Many difficulties can be avoided by not attempting to diagnose the *Borrelia* type from the tests carried out with the patient's blood and to report only the titers as well as an explanation: "The tests are negative—doubtful—in the range of significance of a *Borrelia* infection provided that the patient does not have a related treponemataceal or a *Proteus* infection." Recently we have found "positive" *Borrelia* tests in some patients with infectious mononucleosis. Thus general reporting must be carefully done and the numerous difficulties caused by taxonomic, antigenic, and antibody factors must be kept in mind.

References

1. ALLINE M and MARX R: Le diagnostic des borrelioses par immunofluorescence. Ann Inst Pasteur 111 (Suppl. 3):28–35, 1966
2. BOHLS SW and IRONS JV: Laboratory diagnosis of relapsing fever. *In* Symposium on Relaps-

ing Fevers in the Americas. Am Assoc Adv Sci Monogr 18. Am Assoc Adv Sci, Washington, DC, 1942, pp 42–48

3. BOURGAIN H: Contribution à l'étude de la vitalité des spirochètes récurrents. Ann Inst Pasteur (Paris) 73:84–86, 1974

4. BRYCESON ADM, PARRY EHD, PERINE PL, WARRELL DA, VUKOTICH D, and LEITHEAD CS: Louse-borne relapsing fever. Q J Med 39:120–170, 1970

5. BURGDORFER W: Analyse des Infektionsverlaufes bei O. moubata (Murray) der natürlichen Übertragung von Sp. duttoni. Acta Trop 8:193–262, 1951

6. BURGDORFER W: The diagnosis of relapsing fevers. In The Biology of Parasitic Spirochetes. Johnson RA (ed). Academic Press, New York, 1976, pp 225–234.

7. BURGDORFER W: The epidemiology of the relapsing fevers. In The Biology of Parasitic Spirochetes. Johnson RA (ed). Academic Press, New York, 1976, pp. 191–200.

8. DAVIS GE: The spirochetes. Am Rev Microbiol 2:305–334, 1948

9. DODGE RW: Culture of Ethiopian strains of B. recurrentis. Appl Microbiol 25:935–939, 1973

10. FELSENFELD O: Borreliae, human relapsing fever, and parasite-vector-host relationships. Bacteriol Rev 29:46–74, 1965

11. FELSENFELD O: Borrelia. Warren H. Green, St. Louis, Mo, 1971

12. FELSENFELD O: Borreliae. In Methods in Microbiology. Ribbons DW and Norris JR (eds). Academic Press, New York, 8:75–94, 1973

13. FELSENFELD O and WOLF RH: The indirect immunoenzyme test for the detection of antibodies against North American borreliae. Am J Clin Pathol 61:838–848, 1974

14. GEIGY R: Relapsing fevers. In Infectious Blood Diseases of Man and Animals. Weinman D and Ristic M (eds). Academic Press, New York, 2:175–316, 1968

15. GEIGY R and BURGDORFER W: Unterschiedliches Verhalten verschiedener Stämme von Sp.duttoni in der weissen Maus. Acta Trop 8:151–154, 1951

16. GOLDSMITH JM and MAHOUMED M: The use of the microhematocrit technic for the recovery of B.duttonii from blood. Am J Clin Pathol 58:165–169, 1972

17. HINDLE E: Blood spirochaetes. In A System of Bacteriology in Relation to Medicine. British Med Res Council (eds). HM Stat Office, London, 1931, pp 147–184

18. KELLY RT: Cultivation of Borrelia hermsi. Science 173:443–444, 1971

19. KELLY RT: Cultivation and biology of relapsing fever borreliae. In The Biology of Parasitic Spirochetes. Johnson RA (ed). Academic Press, New York, 1976, pp 87–94

20. KRAJIAN AA: Clinical application of the 20-minute staining method of S.pallida in tissue sections. Am J Syph 23:617–620, 1939

21. MOOSER H: Erythrozyten-Adhäsion und Hämagglomeration durch Rückfallfieber-Spirocheten. Zeitschr Tropenmed Parasitol 9:93–111, 1958

22. MOOSER H: Die Rückfallfieber. Ergeb Microbiol Immunitätsforsch Exp 31:184–228, 1958

23. SCHUHARDT VT: Serology of the relapse phenomenon. In Symposium on Relapsing Fevers in the Americas. Am Assoc Adv Sci Monogr 18. Am Assoc Adv Sci, Washington, DC, 1942, pp 58–66

24. SMIBERT RM: Spirochaetales. A review. Crit Rev Microbiol. CRC Press. 2:491–544, 1973

25. SMIBERT RM: Classification of non-pathogenic treponemes. In The Biology of Parasitic Spirochetes. Johnson RA (ed). Academic Press, New York, 1976, pp 121–311

26. SOUTHERN PM and SANFORD JP: Relapsing fever. Medicine 48:129–149, 1969

27. STEIN GJ: The serological diagnosis of relapsing fever. J Exp Med 79:115–178, 1944

28. STOENNER HG: Biology of B.hermsii in Kelly medium. Appl Microbiol 28:540–543, 1974

29. WALTERS JH: Relapsing fever. In Recent Advances in Tropical Medicine, 3rd edition. Woodruff AW and Walters JH (eds). J.H.H. Churchill Ltd, London, 1961

30. WEYER F and MOOSER H: Beobachtungen an Stämmen von Borrelien im Laboratorium. Z Tropenmed Parasitol 8:294–303, 1957

31. WOLMAN B and WOLMAN M: Studies on the biological properties of Sp. recurrentis in the Ethiopian high plateau. Ann Trop Med Parasitol 39:82–93, 1945

32. WOLSTENHOME B and GEAR JHS: A complement-fixation test for the diagnosis of relapsing fever. Trans R Soc Trop Med Hyg 41:513–517, 1948

CHAPTER 19

BRUCELLOSIS

E. D. Renner and K. J. McMahon

Introduction

Brucellosis is an infectious disease of animals which can be transmitted to man. The species infective for humans are *Brucella suis*, the predominant species infecting swine; *B. abortus*, which usually infects cattle; *B. melitensis*, found in goats and sheep; and *B. canis*, a recently recognized pathogen of dogs. *B. neotomae*, isolated from the desert wood rat, and *B. ovis*, the etiologic agent of ram epididymitis, are not known to cause disease in humans.

Brucella is a gram-negative coccobacillus or short rod arranged singly or rarely in a short chain. It is nonmotile, does not form endospores, and does not have capsules. Thiamin, niacin, and biotin are required for growth. It is catalase positive and oxidase positive, but *B. neotomae*, *B. ovis*, and 20% of *B. canis* isolates are oxidase negative. Urea is hydrolyzed to a variable extent. It is aerobic, and growth is often improved by carbon dioxide (5). *B. ovis* and *B. canis* occur normally in the rough form, whereas the other four species have only been found in the smooth form; however, dissociation readily occurs in the laboratory. Colonies appear after 2 days of incubation, reaching 2–3 mm after 4 days. The organism is nonhemolytic, nonpigmented, and has a smooth glistening surface.

The clinical manifestations of human brucellosis are variable. The incubation period can vary from 7 days to 7 months, and the onset can be insidious or abrupt. Brucellosis in man has neither pathognomonic symptoms nor signs. In acute and subacute brucellosis, the predominant symptoms are pyrexia, profuse sweats, chills, weakness, malaise, body ache, joint pains, weight loss, and anorexia (6, 63, 65). Chronic brucellosis (a proven state of infection which has lasted more than 1 year) is usually nonbacteremic and may persist for a number of years. Patients with such illness commonly have a long history of bouts of fever, malaise, headaches, sweating, recurrent depression, inertia, vague pains, sexual impotence, and insomnia. The symptoms are believed related to the hypersensitivity of the patient (43), although this complex disease is not clearly understood.

Subclinical or latent infection is found among apparently healthy individuals whose occupations require frequent contact with animals. Repeated exposure to the infectious agent raises the level of the serum antibodies to what appears to be a diagnostic titer (32).

In 10% to 15% of patients with brucellosis, various complications can occur. The complications can be articular, osseous, visceral, and neurological, with osteomyelitis the most frequent complication in man (25).

The mortality rate in brucellosis is low. Brucellosis was considered a contributing cause of death in 4 of 2356 (0.17%) patients with brucellosis in the United States during 1965–1975 (11). Infective endocarditis is the most frequent cause of death (58).

The severity and duration of brucellosis depend to some extent on the *Brucella* species involved. *B. melitensis* usually results in the most serious and debilitating infection. *B. suis* is highly invasive and tends to localize, causing suppuration and necrosis. *B. abortus* is less invasive, and in general the disease and tissue damage are less severe. Disease caused by *B. canis* in man is mild, and localization with complications is rare (54).

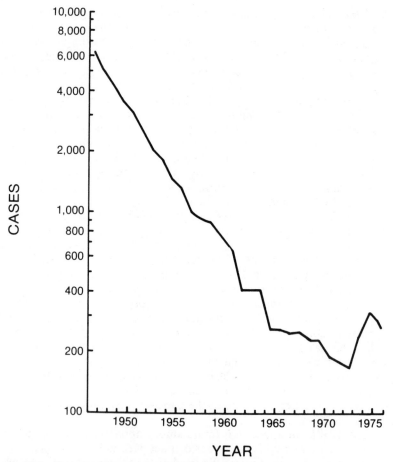

Figure 19.1—Reported cases of human brucellosis in the United States, 1947–1976 (Center for Disease Control, Brucellosis Surveillance).

In the United States there were 6000 reported cases of brucellosis in 1947, a rate which continued to decrease to a low of 175 in 1973. This decrease was a result of compulsory pasteurization of milk and slaughter of infected cattle. However, the incidence increased in 1974–1976 with 246, 328, and 282 cases of human brucellosis reported to the Center for Disease Control (CDC) during those years, respectively (Fig. 19.1) (11, 12). This was followed by a decrease to 241 cases reported in 1977 and 172 reported in 1978.

Most brucellosis in man is the result of direct contact with sick animals. The animals commonly known to serve as sources of human infection are goats, sheep, cattle, water buffalo, and swine. B. canis is transmitted from dogs to man. Human-to-human transmission of the disease is not a problem.

In the United States the disease is largely occupational, affecting those in close contact with cattle or swine (7). In the period 1965–1975, there were 2630 cases of brucellosis reported to the CDC. There were case surveillance reports for 2356 of the cases, including 2188 newly acquired cases and 168 recrudescent infections. Persons working in the meat processing industry (abattoir employees, rendering plant employees, meat inspectors) accounted for 1258 (53%) of these cases, whereas 408 (17%) workers in the livestock industry were counted among those infected (11). The ingestion of unpasteurized dairy products resulted in 215 cases (9%), with 143 attributed to the consumption of dairy products produced outside the United States. Laboratory accidents accounted for 68 cases (3%) either by injection of vaccine (33 cases) or a laboratory-acquired infection (35 cases). Since B. canis was isolated and identified as an etiological agent of contagious abortion in dogs (10), 16 human cases have been reported. Six of these resulted from laboratory infection, six from contact with infected dogs, and four from undetermined sources.

The ratio of males to females in the United States with brucellosis is 6:1, and in 90% of the cases the age is between 20 and 60. This age category reflects the population at greatest risk in the meat packing and livestock industries. This disease is rare in children (1.3% of the cases) but may result from the ingestion of unpasteurized dairy products.

In 1965–1975, brucellae were cultured from clinical specimens from 505 patients. B. suis comprised 52% of the isolates, followed by B. abortus (23%), B. melitensis (11%), and B. canis (2%). The number of cattle-associated brucellosis cases in man increased sharply after reaching a low of 16 in 1971. In 1975 contact with infected cattle resulted in 104 human cases (34%), and contact with domestic swine accounted for 94 cases (30%) (11). This trend continued in 1976 and correlated with an increasing brucellosis reactor rate in market cattle (69).

In addition to the animal hosts mentioned, other animal populations are known to be infected which can transmit the disease to man. In Alaska 12 cases have been associated with the butchering and ingestion of raw meat and bone marrow from caribou and moose. Infected reindeer (with B. suis type 4) are also a menace to the Eskimos because they customarily eat raw liver and bone marrow. Eleven cases of brucellosis have occurred in hunters who killed and butchered feral swine. Two cases have been attributed to the butchering of wild deer, and B. abortus has been isolated from elk, moose, and bison in the United States (51).

Brucellosis in humans can be prevented by eliminating the disease in animal reservoirs. Vaccination of cattle, slaughter of animals with the disease, and pasteurization of milk have decreased significantly the incidence of human brucellosis in the United States. However, the increase in the number of cases in 1974–1976 is evidence that eradicating a disease as well-entrenched as brucellosis is extremely difficult.

Brucellosis infection rates can be reduced in high-risk occupational groups by establishing certain preventive measures and informing people of the modes of transmission of the *Brucella* organisms. For abattoir workers, contact with potentially contaminated animal tissues either by skin cuts or abrasions or conjunctival contact can be prevented by wearing protective gloves, goggles, and masks.

Continued compulsory pasteurization of milk and milk products is necessary to prevent the disease's being transmitted by this route; however, most cases attributed to ingesting unpasteurized dairy products during 1965–1976 in the United States were associated with foreign dairy products.

Water and vegetables contaminated with urine and feces from infected animals are possible sources of infection, but water has not been documented to carry viable *Brucella* organisms. Brucellosis of wild-animal origin is almost always transmitted to man indirectly through domesticated animals.

Vaccinating cattle with attenuated *B. abortus* strain 19 has been effective in controlling bovine brucellosis (46); however, there are no effective vaccines for the prevention of brucellosis in swine or humans.

Collection and Processing of Specimens

Since isolating *Brucella* spp. in cultures is the only way to confirm a diagnosis of brucellosis, multiple blood cultures should be obtained before antimicrobial therapy is begun. Although *B. abortus* can be grown from more than 50% of cases in the acute stage (57), the bacteriological confirmation of brucellosis by positive blood cultures occurs in no more than 20% of the reported cases.

Infected tissues and abscesses should be cultured, as should bone marrow and liver biopsies if available. Rarely cerebrospinal fluid, pleural fluid, peritoneal fluid, urine, and other specimens are submitted to the laboratory for culture. These specimens can be processed with routine procedures, except that a selective medium should be used (next section) if the specimen is highly contaminated, and infected materials should be handled in an approved safety cabinet.

Isolating *Brucella* by inoculating guinea pigs is sometimes helpful in situations in which a few *Brucella* organisms are suspected to be present (milk, cheese). Two or more animals should be inoculated per specimen. The guinea pigs are bled before being inoculated to determine their titers to *Brucella*. The animals can be inoculated intraperitoneally if the material to be inoculated is not contaminated; otherwise, the material should be inoculated intramuscularly or subcutaneously. One of the inoculated guinea pigs should be necropsied 3 weeks and the other 6 weeks after inoculation. Titers of sera obtained during necropsies should be measured. A measurable titer provides presumptive evidence that the organisms were present in the inoculated material, and every attempt should be made to isolate the organism from the animal's tissue.

Serum for serological tests should be obtained when brucellosis is suspected. In patients with acute brucellosis, titers are highest 3 weeks after the onset of symptoms, with seroconversion occurring 1 week after onset of illness (8). Because of the insidious onset of some cases and the difficulty of diagnosing on the basis of clinical symptoms alone, a seroconversion is often difficult to demonstrate. If known causes of cross-reactivity are eliminated (*Francisella tularensis,* cholera vaccination, *Yersinia enterocolitica*), a single high titer against a *Brucella* organism is indicative of a recent *Brucella* infection. The titer will decline in most cases (with and without treatment), and a decrease can be demonstrated during the first 3 months (8). Low-level titers may persist for years. In some cases in which the onset is insidious, antibodies develop slowly. If no other definite diagnosis has been reached, antibody titers should be measured monthly for 5 months.

There have been reports that some positive cultures had no measurable titer (43); however, serological findings can be affected by various unknown factors. Follow-up specimens should be tested in each case, and if serological tests are still negative 5 months after the onset of symptoms, the patient probably did not have brucellosis.

Diagnostic Procedures

Microscopic Examination

Demonstrating *Brucella* organisms in direct stains of tissue specimens with the modified Köster and/or Ziehl-Neelsen methods is not specific or sensitive enough for routine use in diagnosing brucellosis (37). If direct staining of tissues for the organisms is desired, the method of choice is the direct fluorescent antibody technique (2). However, cultures should be prepared in every case, and regardless of the results of the fluorescent antibody test, a positive culture is the only laboratory result for the definitive diagnosis of brucellosis.

Selection and Inoculation of Culture Media

The following media are recommended for primary isolation: a) blood agar (5% sheep blood), b) serum-dextrose agar, c) serum-Trypticase soy or tryptose agar, and d) *Brucella* agar containing 5% serum. The choice of the basal medium depends upon availability and cost. Since most laboratories have easy access to blood agar plates, they are most often used.

The Castañeda technique involves a biphasic (solid and liquid) medium in the same bottle. The Trypticase soy, tryptose, or *Brucella* agar can be used with the solid prepared by adding agar to a final concentration of 2.5%. The Castañeda bottle also should have a final concentration of 5%–10% carbon dioxide added to the air in contact with the medium. The procedure for culturing organisms using the Castañeda bottle is described by Alton et al. (2).

Tissues should be homogenized, and the direct inoculation of the specimen onto appropriate solid media is the preferred method for isolating *Brucella* organisms. When blood and other body fluids are cultured, the Castañeda technique is recommended.

When significant contamination is likely, a selective medium should be inoculated in addition to the basal medium. Adding bacitracin, polymyxin B, and cycloheximide allows *Brucella* to grow but suppresses many other bacterial species. The medium described by Kuzdas and Morse (42) includes circulin in addition to the above antibiotics, and Farrell (23) developed a selective medium that also contains vancomycin, nalidixic acid, and nystatin. The addition of ethyl violet inhibits the growth of dye-sensitive biotypes but has been reported to aid in suppressing contaminants (60). The medium of Kuzdas and Morse has been proven effective in clinical studies (70).

The choice of the basal and selective media is largely a matter of preference, economics, and convenience. However, it is imperative that each laboratory, as part of its quality control program, determine the ability of the culture media to support the growth of *Brucella* organisms. This is best done by inoculating plates with approximately 100 cells of the serum-requiring *B. abortus* biotype 2.

The inoculated plates should be incubated at 35–37 C in an atmosphere of 5%–10% carbon dioxide. Castañeda bottles should also be incubated at this temperature. *Brucella* colonies are generally visible after 3 days of incubation on plated media, but cultures should be held for 10 days. Colonies of *Brucella* can be delayed if selective media are used. Castañeda bottles should be examined twice a week, and if no colonies are apparent on the agar surface the bottle should be tilted so that the broth flows onto the agar slant. The bottle should then be reincubated in the upright position. If colonies are not apparent after 3 weeks of incubation, the bottle can be discarded. If colonies are apparent, they should be subcultured and Gram stained.

Identification Procedures

The six species of *Brucella* and the three biotypes of *B. melitensis,* nine biotypes of *B. abortus,* and four biotypes of *B. suis* are differentiated by susceptibility tests using aniline dyes, and results of biochemical, metabolic, serologic, and bacteriophage tests (Tables 19.1 and 19.2).

Brucella organisms can be tentatively identified by determining the ability of the bacteria to ferment lactose and glucose, by agglutination in *Brucella* antiserum, and by a semiquantitative urease test. Colonies that appear on the initial culture medium should be Gram stained and transferred to a blood agar plate and also used to inoculate glucose and lactose fermentation media. Colonies that are gram-negative coccobacilli, nonhemolytic, do not ferment lactose or glucose, and are oxidase positive (except for *B. ovis, B. neotomae,* and strains of *B. canis*) are tested for urease and agglutination in specific antisera. A semiquantitative urease test is performed by preparing a dense suspension of the organism and placing a loopful of the suspension on the urea agar slant. *B. suis* and *B. canis* will turn the indicator in less than 1 min, whereas *B. abortus* usually takes 5–10 min.

The suspected *Brucella* colonies are emulsified in each of 2 drops of saline on a slide. A drop of anti-*Brucella* serum is added to the first drop and normal serum to the second. The suspensions are mixed and examined for agglutination. The agglutination should be rapid and complete. Dissociated colonies and *B. canis* and *B. ovis* will show a variable degree of agglutination with the anti-smooth *Brucella* serum.

Results described above are sufficient criteria to establish a preliminary identification. *Brucella* organisms should be further differentiated and typed in laboratories that have experience in these identification procedures.

The common criteria for definitive identification of species and biotypes of the genus *Brucella* are: a) requirement for increased carbon dioxide for growth, b) the production of H_2S, c) agglutination in monospecific sera, d) urease production, and 3) growth in the presence of basic fuchsin and thionin in solid media.

Results from these tests can be used in identifying most of the *Brucella* strains as to biotype. However, occasional stains must be tested further to determine biotype. These additional examinations include phage typing and the oxidative metabolic tests (52).

The phage-susceptibility test can be easily adapted to routine use and fits in with conventional typing procedures (63). The metabolic tests, however, are time-consuming and require specialized equipment not readily available in a public health laboratory.

TABLE 19.1—DIFFERENTIAL CHARACTERISTICS OF THE SPECIES AND BIOTYPES IN THE GENUS *BRUCELLA*

Species	Bio-type	Lysis by phage Tb		CO_2 re-quired	H_2S pro-duced	Urease activity	Growth on dyes [a]					Agglutination in sera [b]			Most common host reservoir
		RTD	10^4 × RTD				Basic fuchsin		Thionin						
							II	III	I	II	III	A	M	R	
B. melitensis	1	−	−	−	−	variable	+	+	−	+	+	−	+	−	Sheep, goats
	2	−	−	−	−	variable	+	+	−	+	+	+	−	−	Sheep, goats
	3	−	−	−	−	variable	+	+	−	+	+	+	+	−	Sheep, goats
B. abortus	1	+	+	±	+	1-2 hrs	+	+	−	−	−	+	−	−	Cattle
	2	+	+	+	+	1-2 hrs	−	−	−	−	−	+	−	−	Cattle
	3	+	+	±	+	1-2 hrs	+	+	+	+	+	+	−	−	Cattle
	4	+	+	±	+	1-2 hrs	+	−	−	−	−	−	+	−	Cattle
	5	+	+	−	−	1-2 hrs	+	+	−	+	+	−	+	−	Cattle
	6	+	+	−	±	1-2 hrs	+	+	−	+	+	+	−	−	Cattle
	7	+	+	−	±	1-2 hrs	+	+	−	+	+	+	+	−	Cattle
	8	+	+	+	−	1-2 hrs	+	+	−	+	+	−	+	−	Cattle
	9	+	+	±	+	1-2 hrs	+	+	−	+	+	−	·	−	Cattle
B. suis	1	−	+	−	+	0-30 min	−	−	+	+	+	+	−	−	Pigs
	2	−	+	−	−	0-30 min	−	−	+	+	+	+	−	−	Pigs, hares
	3	−	+	−	−	0-30 min	+	+	+	+	+	+	−	−	Pigs
	4	−	+	−	−	0-30 min	+	+	+	+	+	+	+	−	Reindeer
B.neotomae		−	+	−	+	0-30 min	−	−	−	−	−	+	−	−	Wood rat
B. ovis		−	−	+	−	negative	+	+	+	+	+	−	−	+	Sheep (rams)
B. canis		−	−	−	−	0-30 min	−	−	+	+	+	−	−	+	Dogs

[a] Species differentiation is obtained on trypticase soy or tryptose agar with the following graded concentrations of dyes: 1: 25,000 (I). 1: 50,000 (II). 1: 100,000 (III). Other concentrations may be preferable with other growth media interpretation of results should be controlled with the reference strains of each species. Tests should be conducted in CO_2 for those strains requiring CO_2.

[b] A = monospecific abortus; M = monospecific melitensis; R = anti-rough serum.

Requirement for added carbon dioxide

The strain being examined is inoculated on duplicate tryptose agar slants, and one slant is incubated in air while the other is incubated in 5%–10% carbon dioxide. Tubes should be examined daily for growth. At least a few colonies should grow in air, and growth should be good in carbon dioxide if the latter incubation atmosphere is to be considered adequate.

H₂S production

H_2S production is detected by suspending a lead acetate strip directly over but not touching the inoculated surface of a tryptose agar slant. The strip is examined daily for 4 days, and the strip is replaced with a fresh one each day. Hydrogen sulfide production blackens the strip.

Agglutination in monospecific serum

B. abortus and *B. melitensis* antisera (Difco Laboratories, Detroit, Mich.) are used to examine cultures in their smooth form for the predominant agglutinogen (A or M). A dense suspension of the organism is heated to 65 C for 1 hr in a water bath. A drop each of monospecific *B. abortus* and *B. melitensis*

TABLE 19.2—SUBSTRATE UTILIZATION PATTERN OF THE SPECIES AND BIOTYPES IN THE GENUS *BRUCELLA*

Species and Biotype	D-alanine	L-alanine	L-asparagine	L-glutamate	DL-ornithine	DL-citrulline	L-arginine	L-lysine	L-arabinose	D-galactose	D-ribose	D-xylose
B. abortus types 1-9	+	+	+	+	—	—	—	—	+	+	+	±
B. melitensis types 1-3	+	+	+	+	—	—	—	—	—	—	—	—
B. suis type 1	±	±	—	—	+	+	+	+	+	+	+	+
B. suis type 2	—	—	±	+	+	+	+	—	+	±	+	+
B. suis type 3	+	±	—	±	+	+	+	+	—	—	+	±
B. suis type 4	+	—	—	±	+	+	+	+	—	—	+	—
B. neotomae	+	±	+	+	—	—	—	+	+	+	±	±
B. ovis	+	±	+	+	—	—	—	—	—	—	—	—
B. canis	+	±	—	+	+	+	+	+	±	±	+	—

+ = Oxidized (QO_2 N value greater than 50) by all strains
— = Not oxidized by any strain
± = Oxidized by some strains

antisera are placed on a slide, and a drop of the suspension is added to each and mixed. Agglutination should occur within 1 min with one of the sera. Control cultures of *B. abortus* biotype 1, *B. melitensis* biotype 1, and *B. ovis* or *B. canis* should be used as control cultures for this test. These control cultures should agglutinate in their homologous serum within 1 min without agglutinating in the other sera.

Growth in the presence of thionin and basic fuchsin

The actual concentration of basic fuchsin and thionin (Allied Chemical and Dye Co., New York, NY) to use in these tests must be determined for each lot of dye in combination with the basal medium. The concentration of dyes that differentiates between the control cultures of *B. melitensis, B. abortus,* and *B. suis* biotypes 1 should be used. This concentration is between 10 and 40 μg of dye per ml of medium (1:25,000 and 1:100,000). The actual concentration of dye will depend on the basal medium used and the purity of the dye.

The medium is prepared by heating a 0.1% dye solution in a boiling water bath for 20 min, and then adding the required amount to the melted agar base (tryptose agar, Trypticase soy agar). The agar is mixed and poured into petri dishes. Plate surfaces should be dry before inoculation.

From each pure culture and control strain to be tested, a suspension is made by suspending a loopful of the organism in 1.0 ml of sterile saline. The suspensions should be of equal density.

A sterile cotton swab can be used to inoculate the medium. Six cultures can be tested on each plate including the reference strains. The plates can be incubated under 10% carbon dioxide at 37 C for 3–4 days and examined for growth.

The phage test is particularly useful in distinguishing *B. abortus* biotypes 3–9 from *B. melitensis*. The routine test dilution (RTD) of phage Tbilisi (Tb) will completely lyse smooth cultures of *B. abortus,* but *B. suis* and *B. melitensis* cultures are not affected by this phage dilution (37). *B. suis* is partially lysed by a dilution of 10,000 × RTD, whereas most strains of *B. melitensis* are not lysed by this dilution.

The oxidative metabolic pattern on selected amino acids and carbohydrates is characteristic for each *Brucella* species (Table 19.2) (47, 52). If conventional tests and phage typing do not permit a culture to be typed satisfactorily, it is recommended that the culture be sent to one of the following laboratories for examination:

U.S. Department of Agriculture
Veterinary Services Laboratories
P.O. Box 70
Ames, Iowa 50010

Center for Disease Control
Attn: Data and Specimen Handling
  Activity
Bureau of Laboratories
Atlanta, Georgia 30333

Serologic Procedures on Sera

Isolation and identification of the organism provide definite evidence of *Brucella* infection, but because it is often difficult to achieve these goals, serologic tests are relied upon for routine diagnosis of brucellosis.

The feasibility of using the agglutination test for detecting antibodies to *Brucella* has been studied repeatedly since it was suggested by Wright and Smith in 1897 (72), and it remains the only test in wide use clinically in the United States for detecting *Brucella* antibodies (48). However, it has a number of limitations. Low titers are frequently measured in infected animals and also in animals from which no organisms can be isolated (3). *Brucella* can be agglutinated by nonspecific antibodies in serum (34), and incomplete antibodies are a problem in diagnosing human brucellosis—especially chronic infection (53). Sera from some individuals with brucellosis will not agglutinate *Brucella* but will block the agglutination by other immune sera. This may result in negative tests, prozones of inhibition, and fluctuating titers (27). The presence of a prozone in which agglutination is inhibited in tubes containing the highest concentrations of serum makes interpreting agglutination test results difficult (71). High agglutination titers are often measured for patients with acute brucellosis, but titers may drop or even disappear in people with longstanding or subclinical cases (71). The agglutination test may sometimes fail to detect the presence of 7S antibodies (41)—the type correlated with confirmed cases of acute and chronic brucellosis (59).

Brucella cross-agglutinates with several other microorganisms. Marked cross-agglutination occurs with *Yersinia enterocolitica* type 9 (1). This is regarded as being an important complicating factor in serologic diagnosis and may lead to confusion (36). *Brucella* agglutinins which persist for about 2 years (68) can be produced in high titers in individuals who receive cholera vaccination (21, 22). In early studies on tularemia and brucellosis, researchers found that patients with these two diseases can produce cross-reacting agglutinins (23). However, more recent reports indicate that this cross-reaction is not as important in serologic diagnosis as previously believed (8, 68).

A brucellergen skin test, positive or negative, may cause antibody production in a small percentage of people, but antibodies usually occur in low titer and disappear in a few months (48).

Several serologic tests have been developed and evaluated for use in diagnosing brucellosis. Hall and Manion (28) used 100 human sera in evaluating the tube dilution, rapid macroscopic slide (Huddleson), rapid slide (Castañeda), indirect Coombs antiglobulin, "blocking," centrifugation, and paper chromatographic methods. They found the tube-dilution method to be the most useful, practical procedure for demonstrating *Brucella* agglutinins. Russell et al. (62) concluded that the value of the card test in the presumptive diagnosis of human brucellosis was low and the tube agglutination test was still the method of choice for serologic diagnosis of acute brucellosis. Buchanan et al. (8) suggested that tests other than the standard tube-agglutination test were perhaps best reserved for special studies. In 1956, Spink (65) considered the tube-agglutination test to be the most dependable diagnostic procedure for brucellosis. Edwards et al. (20) compared the indirect fluorescent-antibody test with agglutination, complement fixation, and Coombs test for *Brucella* antibody and concluded that the fluorescent-antibody test appeared to have no particular advantage over others except speed of performance.

The complement-fixation test has been used to a limited extent in the past, but it should be re-evaluated as a diagnostic aid in doubtful cases. Reddin et al. (59) found that the IgG-type immunoglobulin was the distinguishing feature of acute and chronic forms of human infection, and similar results were reported for acute cases by MacDonald and Elmslie (44). Heremans et al. (33) found that these 7S antibodies could be detected by complement fixation. The value of complement fixation lies in its ability to detect antibodies present in cases of chronic brucellosis (38). However, Buchanan et al. (8) found the 2-mercaptoethanol assay to be less complex and more easily standardized than the complement-fixation test as an indicator of disease in patients with chronic symptoms and a positive standard tube-agglutination test.

Glenchur et al. (26) concluded from experimental and clinical data that serum precipitins for *Brucella* indicated active or recent, severe infection and might be a better indication of active infection than serum agglutinins. McMahon et al. (49) used a standardized antigen in an agar-gel immunodiffusion test and reported 97% agreement with the standard tube-agglutination test when the titer was 1:160 or higher. Díaz and Dorronsoro (17) used the immunodiffusion test to detect precipitins to the protein antigen of *Brucella* in human sera, and Díaz et al. (19) used the technique of counterimmunoelectrophoresis in testing sera from persons with clinical brucellosis. An alternate test with antigen other than *Brucella* lipopolysaccharide might be useful in both human and veterinary medicine because of the problem of cross-reaction (19). The lipopolysaccharide antigen is common to *Brucella* and *Yersinia* (35) and plays the most important role in the agglutination, Coombs and Rose Bengal tests for brucellosis (18). Protein antigens from *Brucella* and *Y. enterocolitica* serotype 9 do not crossreact (16, 17, 35).

In 1976 a radioimmunoassay test was suggested for use in diagnosing bovine brucellosis, but its usefulness in routine diagnosis has not yet been determined (14). In 1977, Parrott et al. (56) measured serum antibody against *B. abortus* in the immunoglobulin classes IgM, IgG, and IgA with a radioimmunoassay. They concluded that the technique provided a highly sensitive primary-type assay and had many advantages in attempts to diagnose acute and chronic stages of human brucellosis.

Carlsson et al. (9) used an enzyme-linked immunosorbent assay for detection of *Brucella* antibodies in rabbit sera and found it was from 10- to 100-fold more sensitive than the tube agglutination test.

There is no designated standard serologic test for human brucellosis caused by *B. canis,* but the agglutination test antigen used for detecting antibodies in dogs has been used similarly with human serum (48). Alton et al. (2) indicated that the gel diffusion method described by Myers and Siniuk (55) for detecting antibodies to *B. ovis* could be adapted for diagnosing *B. canis* infection. McCullough (48) suggested that the laboratory which receives only an occasional request should send the specimen to its state laboratory.

Because the agglutination test is still the most commonly used serologic test for detecting *Brucella* antibodies, it will be described.

Standard tube-agglutination test

Antigen. Tube antigen prepared from *B. abortus* strain 1119-3 should be used (67).

Technique of the test (67). Separate serum from the clot and use without inactivation. Place 0.9 ml of saline (containing 0.5% phenol) in the first of a series of 10 tubes (13 × 100 mm) and 0.5 ml of phenolized saline in each of the remaining 9 tubes. Add 0.1 ml of serum to tube 1 with a 1.0-ml serological pipette calibrated to 0.1 ml. Draw up and expel the mixture from the pipette seven or eight times, and transfer 0.5 ml to the next tube. Repeat the process through the tenth tube, discarding the last 0.5 ml. To each tube, add 0.5 ml of standard antigen and mix by shaking. Tube 1 now represents a 1:20 dilution of serum, and the dilution doubles in each succeeding tube; it is 1:10,240 in the tenth tube. Along with test sera, include known positive and negative control sera and an antigen control containing 0.5 ml of saline and 0.5 ml of diluted antigen.

Incubation. Mix by shaking tubes and incubate in a water bath at 37 C for 48 hr.

Reading results. Observe tubes against a dark background with light behind the tubes. In a positive reaction, there is complete clumping of the organisms; the fluid is clear, and gentle shaking does not disrupt the flocculi. In an incomplete reaction, the fluid is partially clear, and gentle shaking does not disrupt the flocculi. In a negative reaction, the fluid is turbid, and no flocculi are evident. Occasionally, partial or no agglutination occurs in the lower serum dilutions. If this prozone makes evaluation of the test difficult, if possible, perform some other kind of test as a confirmatory test. However, this zoning rarely extends beyond a dilution of 1:160 or 1:320 (66). Hall and Manion (28) have reported that the prozone obscured results of tube-agglutination tests in only one of several thousand sera examined in their laboratory.

Interpreting results. The degree of agglutination defined as the endpoint reading varies among laboratories. The exact technique for reporting should be decided and adhered to in the laboratory, and trace reactions should not be taken as an end-point reading (39). It is recommended that the titer be recorded as the reciprocal of the highest serum dilution that shows 50% agglutination of the antigen (8, 30). Patients with acute brucellosis may develop little or no titer during the first 10 days of illness (30), so acute- and convalescent-phase serum specimens, taken 3 to 4 weeks apart, should be tested. A rising titer in the course of illness is significant. It has not been possible for workers to determine the specific titer on a single serum specimen that is diagnostic for *Brucella* infection. Assuming that the possibilities of cross-reactions have been considered, a titer of 160 or higher is indicative of *Brucella* infection but not necessarily of recent infection (30). A titer of less than 160 does not exclude the possibility of *Brucella* infection on the basis of an agglutination test alone. Most patients with proven cases of acute brucellosis have antibody titers of at least 320 or higher (48, 65, 66). However, in groups repeatedly exposed to *Brucella* such as farmers, meat packing plant employees, and veterinarians, high titers lose diagnostic significance, because so many of these persons have titers of 320 or higher without being ill (66).

Rapid slide and plate agglutination tests

According to the National Research Council, Committee on Public Health Aspects of Brucellosis (67), none of the rapid slide and plate agglutination tests have the precision necessary to be recognized as a standard test. The Committee recommended that such tests be carried out only as rapid screening tests and that the reportable titer of all sera should be determined by using the tube agglutination test.

Antigen. Antigens are available commercially for the rapid slide test. If one of these antigens is used, follow the directions supplied with the product. A preferred antigen is *B. abortus* strain 1119-3 plate antigen available from the USDA, National Veterinary Service Laboratories, Ames, Iowa. This antigen is used in the test described.

Technique of test. The test is performed by mixing serum and antigen at room temperature in ruled 1.25-in. (3-cm) squares on a plate that fits into a testing box approximately 17 in. (43 cm) long, 13 in. (33 cm) wide, and 4.75 in. (12 cm) high. Testing boxes are equipped with a light source and a hinged glass cover to prevent rapid evaporation of test materials. Several commercial test boxes are available.

Using a 0.2 ml serological or "Bang's disease" pipette, deliver from left to right 0.08, 0.04, 0.02, 0.01, and 0.005 ml of test serum to the squares of a row on the plate. Mix the contents of the antigen vial by shaking. Using an antigen dropper that delivers 0.03 ml of antigen per drop, place 1 drop of antigen on each quantity of serum. The serum-antigen ratios are considered to yield results approximating those obtained with the tube method at dilutions of 1:20, 1:40, 1:80, 1:160, and 1:320. Mix the serum-antigen mixture in each square with a wooden applicator or toothpick. Mix from right to left to reduce the effect of carryover by the applicator. Lift the plate from the box and rotate to ensure mixing. Replace the plate, and allow it to stand with light off and lid closed for 8 min before reading. However, after approximately 4 min, gently rotate the plate, and replace it in the box. Turn on the light and carefully tilt the box from side to side while reading results. Include known positive and negative control sera and an antigen control along with test sera.

Reading results. Read results macroscopically. Clumps of agglutinated antigen separated by clear liquid represent complete agglutination. Agglutination without complete clearing of the fluid is incomplete, and no evidence of agglutination is a negative reaction.

Interpretation of results. The test is for screening only, and all positive results at any dilution are to be retested by the standard tube-agglutination technique.

Additional serologic techniques

Techniques such as complement fixation, tube mercaptoethanol, and Coombs (antiglobulin) have been described by Alton et al. (2). Blocking antibodies usually do not confuse interpretation of the agglutination test on sera from patients with acute cases (65). Hall and Manion (28) found that only one of more than 200 patients with brucellosis had enough blocking antibody to obscure the results of the tube agglutination test. However, Spink (65) reported that a significant titer of blocking antibodies may be present in sera from patients who have had active disease for a number of years. If a high titer of blocking antibody is present, it may be detected with the Coombs technique or a more simple direct blocking test described by McCullough (48). It has also been suggested that titers of blocking antibodies might be unmasked by heating sera at 56 C for 15 or 30 min (64, 65) or by centrifuging tubes incubated in the regular agglutination test at 2500–4000 rpm for 15 min and then observing for agglutination (28, 65).

Antimicrobic Susceptibility and Resistance

A combination of one of the tetracyclines and streptomycin is currently still regarded as the best treatment for this disease. These drugs are usually administered for 3 weeks. The tetracyclines alone are effective, but the combined therapy is recommended for severe or prolonged cases. Buchanan et al. (6), in analyzing 160 cases of brucellosis, found that the relapse rate for patients receiving antibiotic combinations (tetracycline, sulfonamides) that included streptomycin was significantly lower than for those receiving tetracycline alone or a combination of drugs not including streptomycin.

Most strains of *Brucella* are highly resistant to the penicillins and cephalosporins (29, 61).

Trimethoprim-sulfamethoxazole has given encouraging results in the treatment of brucellosis. Daikos et al. (15) treated 86 patients with brucellosis using this drug for periods ranging from 2 weeks to 4 months. Clinical response was satisfactory in 78 patients.

In vitro studies (61) suggest that kanamycin or gentamicin combined with tetracycline may be more effective than the classical tetracycline/streptomycin regimen.

Routine sensitivity testing of *Brucella* isolates is not necessary. Relapses associated with brucellosis and the progression of some acute cases to chronic brucellosis have not been caused by the emergence of resistant organisms. If resistance to tetracycline or streptomycin is suspected, a standard tube dilution method may be used to determine the susceptibility of the organism (29).

Determining the appropriate antimicrobial therapy for patients with chronic brucellosis is difficult. The patient's symptoms are seldom alleviated by antibiotics; however, trimethoprim-sulfamethoxazole has given encouraging results in the treatment of chronic brucellosis (40).

Evaluation of Laboratory Findings

The isolation of the organism from a clinical specimen is the only irrefutable evidence of a *Brucella* infection. However, since less than 20% of the patients with symptoms of brucellosis have their infections bacteriologically confirmed, the diagnosis must be based on the serologic results.

The initial immunoglobulin response to a *Brucella* infection in man is composed primarily of both IgM and IgG. The IgM usually falls to undetectable levels in 2 to 3 months (47). The IgG often persists for months or years, especially in patients with chronic brucellosis. In longstanding brucellosis, the IgG may assume a nonagglutinating form, and IgA may appear. In acute exacerbations there is a sharp rise in both IgG and IgM. This characteristic temporal evolution of the immune response involving IgM to IgG and IgA forms of antibody has been used with varying success to differentiate acute, subacute, and chronic stages of brucellosis.

The 2-mercaptoethanol test has been used to demonstrate indirectly agglutination by IgM, because this chemical breaks the disulphide bonds of the IgM pentamer while not affecting IgG. However, Díaz et al. (19) found that both IgM and IgG are involved in the agglutination in mercaptoethanol-resistant sera. Several workers (4, 8, 59) have found that antibodies to *Brucella* organisms, as measured in the 2-mercaptoethanol test, could prove useful as an indicator of disease activity in patients with chronic symptoms and positive tube agglutination test results.

The Coombs test measures nonagglutinating IgG and IgA, and titers of >80 are associated with longstanding or chronic brucellosis. A titer of 16 measured with the complement-fixation test is suggestive of active disease.

Attempts are being made to develop refined serological methods, but except for a radioimmunoassay method (56) which appears to be particularly promising in determining stages of brucellosis, most provide little information that is more relevant than that obtained with the standard tube agglutination test.

A standard tube agglutination is sufficient to allow the physician to diagnose acute brucellosis with some confidence in a patient with fever, sweats, fatigue, joint and limb pains, and a history of animal contact. The difficulty arises when chronic brucellosis is considered for a patient who has continued exposure to *Brucella* organisms, e.g., a veterinarian or abattoir worker (31). Such a patient, because of the occupational factor, will frequently have a high titer without acute illness (30, 45), and positive serological results must be carefully and critically assessed in combination with the clinical and epidemiologic findings before reaching a diagnosis.

References

1. AHOVNEN P, JANSSON E, and AHO K: Marked cross-agglutination between brucellae and a subtype of *Yersinia enterocolitica*. Acta Pathol Microbiol Scand 75:291–295, 1969
2. ALTON GG, JONES LM, and PIETZ DE: Laboratory techniques in brucellosis. World Health Organization Monogr Ser No. 55, 1975
3. ALTON GG, MAW J, ROGERSON BA, and MCPHERSON GG: The serological diagnosis of bovine brucellosis: an evaluation of the complement-fixation, serum agglutination and Rose Bengal tests. Aust Vet J 51:57–63, 1975
4. ANDERSON NK, JENNESS R, BRUMFIELD HP, and GOUGH P: *Brucella* agglutinating antibodies. Relation of mercaptoethanol stability to complement-fixation. Sci 143:1334–1335, 1964
5. BUCHANAN RE and GIBBONS NE (eds.): Bergey's Manual of Determinative Bacteriology, 8th edition. Williams & Wilkin Co, Baltimore, Md, 1974
6. BUCHANAN TM, FARBER LC, and FELDMAN RA: Brucellosis in the United States, 1960–1972. Part I. Clinical features and therapy. Medicine 53:403–413, 1974
7. BUCHANAN TM, HENDRICKS SL, PATTON CM, and FELDMAN RA: Brucellosis in the United States 1960–1972. Part III. Epidemiology and evidence for acquired immunity. Medicine 53:427–439, 1974
8. BUCHANAN TM, SULZER CR, FRIX MK, and FELDMAN RA: Brucellosis in the United States, 1960–1972. Part II. Diagnostic aspects. Medicine 53:415–426, 1974

9. CARLSSON HE, HURVELL B, and LINDBERG AA: Enzyme-linked immunosorbent assay (ELISA) for titration of antibodies against *Brucella abortus* and *Yersinia enterocolitica*. Acta Pathol Microbiol Scand Sect C 84:168–176, 1976

10. CARMICHAEL LE and BRUNER DW: Characteristics of a newly recognized species of brucella responsible for infectious canine abortions. Cornell Vet 58:579–583, 1968

11. CENTER FOR DISEASE CONTROL: Brucellosis Surveillance. Annual Summary 1975. U.S. Dept Health, Education, and Welfare, Atlanta, Ga, 1976

12. CENTER FOR DISEASE CONTROL: Brucellosis Surveillance. Annual Summary 1976. U.S. Dept Health, Education, and Welfare, Atlanta Ga, 1977

13. CENTER FOR DISEASE CONTROL: Brucellosis Surveillance. Annual Summary 1978. U.S. Dept Health, Education and Welfare, Atlanta, Ga, 1979

14. CHAPPEL RJ, WILLIAMSON P, MCNAUGHT DJ, DALLING MJ, and ALLAN GS: Radioimmunoassay for antibodies against *Brucella abortus:* a new serological test for bovine brucellosis. J Hyg 77:369–376, 1976

15. DAIKOS GK, PAPAPOLYZOS N, MARKETAS N, MOCHLAS S, KASTONAKIS S, and POPASTERIODIS E: Trimethoprim-sulphamethoxazole in brucellosis. J Infect Dis 128:731–734, 1973

16. DÍAZ R: Valor de la preuba de Rose de Bengala y la demonstracion de anticuerpos antiproteina de *Brucella* en el diagnostico serologico de brucelosis y yersiniosis. Med Clin 63:463–466, 1974

17. DÍAZ R and DORRONSORO I: Contribucion al diagnostico serologico de brucelosis y yersiniosis. I. Utilidad de la reaccion de precipitation en gel. Rev Clin Esp 121:367–372, 1971

18. DÍAZ R and LEVIEUX D: Rôle respectif en sérologie de la brucellose bovine des antigèns et des immunoglobulins G_1 et G_2 dans les tests d'agglutination, de Coombs, et au Rose Bengale ainsi que dans le phénomène de zone. CR Acad Sci Ser D 274:1593–1596, 1972

19. DÍAZ R, MARANI-POMA E, and RIVERO A: Comparison of counterimmunoelectroporesis [sic] with other serological tests in the diagnosis of human brucellosis. Bull WHO 53:417–424, 1976

20. EDWARDS JMB, TANNAHILL AJ, and BRADSTREET CMP: Comparison of the indirect fluorescent antibody test with agglutination, complement-fixation and Coombs test for *Brucella* antibody. J Clin Pathol 23:161–165, 1970

21. EISELE CW, MCCULLOUGH NB, and BEAL GA: *Brucella* antibodies following cholera vaccination. Ann Intern Med 28:833–837, 1948

22. EISELE CW, MCCULLOUGH NB, BEAL GA, and ROTTSCHAEFER W: *Brucella* agglutination tests and vaccination against cholera. J Am Med Assoc 135:983–984, 1947

23. FARRELL ID: The development of a new selective medium for the isolation of *Brucella abortus* from contaminated sources. Res Vet Sci 16:280–286, 1974

24. FRANCIS E and EVANS AC: Agglutination, cross-agglutination and agglutinin absorption in tularemia. Public Health Rep 41:1273–1295, 1926

25. GLASGOW MMS: Brucellosis of the spine. Br J Surg 63:283–288, 1976

26. GLENCHUR H, SEAL US, ZINNEMAN HH, and HALL WH: Serum precipitins in human and experimental brucellosis. J Lab Clin Med 59:220–230, 1962

27. GLENCHUR H, ZINNEMAN HH, and HALL WH: Significance of the blocking antibody in experimental brucellosis. J Immunol 86:421–426, 1961

28. HALL WH and MANION RE: Comparison of the Coombs test with other methods for *Brucella* agglutinins in human serum. J Clin Invest 32:96–106, 1953

29. HALL WH and MANION RE: *In vitro* susceptibility of *Brucella* to various antibiotics. Appl Microbiol 20:600–604, 1970

30. HAUSLER WJ JR and KOONTZ FP: Brucellosis. *In* Diagnostic Procedures for Bacterial, Mycotic and Parasitic Infections, 5th edition. Bodily HL, Updyke EL, and Mason JO (eds.). American Public Health Association, New York, 1970, pp 364–378

31. HENDERSON RJ, HILL DM, VICKERS AA, EDWARDS JM, and TILLETT H: Correlation between serological and immunofluorescence results in the investigation of brucellosis in veterinary surgeons. J Clin Pathol 29:35–38, 1976

32. HENDRICKS SL, BORIS IH, HEEREN RH, HAUSLER WJ JR, and HELD JR: Brucellosis outbreak in an Iowa packing house. Am J Public Health 52:1166–1178, 1962

33. HEREMANS JF, VAERMAN JP, and VAERMAN C: Studies of the immune globulins of human sera. II. A study of the distribution of anti-*Brucella* and anti-diphtheria antibody activities among γss-, γ1M⁻ and γ1A⁻ globulin fractions. J Immunol 9:11–17, 1963

34. HESS WR: Studies on a nonspecific *Brucella* agglutinating substance in bovine serum. 1. The differentiation of the specific and nonspecific agglutinins by heat treatment. Am J Vet Res 14:192–194, 1953

35. HURVELL B: Serological cross-reactions between different *Brucella* species and *Yersinia enterocolitica*. Acta Vet Scand 13:472–483, 1972

36. HURVELL B, AHVONEN P, and THAL E: Serological cross-reactions between different *Brucella* species and *Yersinia enterocolitica*. Agglutination and complement-fixation. Acta Vet Scand 12:86–94, 1971

37. JOINT FAO-WHO EXPERT COMMITTEE ON BRUCELLOSIS: Fifth Report. WHO Tech Rep Ser No. 464, 1971

38. KERR WR, COGHLAN JD, PAYNE DJH, and ROBERTSON L: The laboratory diagnosis of chronic brucellosis. Lancet 2:1181–1183, 1966

39. KERR WR, MCCAUGHEY WJ, COGHLAN JD, PAYNE DJH, QUAIFE RA, ROBERTSON L, and FARRELL ID: Techniques and interpretations in the serological diagnosis of brucellosis in man. J Med Microbiol 1:181–193, 1968

40. KONTOYANNIS PA, PAPAPOULOUS SE, and MORTOGLOUR AA: Co-trimoxazole in chronic brucellosis. A two-year follow-up study. Br Med J 2:480–481, 1975

41. KULSHRESHTHA RC, ATAL PR, and WAKI PN: A study on serological tests for the diagnosis of human and bovine brucellosis. Indian J Med Res 61:1471–1477, 1973

42. KUZDAS CD and MORSE EV: A selective medium for the isolation of brucellae from contaminated materials. J Bacteriol 66:502–503, 1953

43. LAWSON JH: Clinical aspects of brucellosis. Scott Med J 21:128, 1976

44. MACDONALD A and ELMSLIE WH: Serological investigations in suspected brucellosis. Lancet 1:380–382, 1967

45. MANN PG and RICHENS ER: Aspects of human brucellosis. Postgrad Med J 49:523–525, 1973

46. MANTHEI CA, MINGLE CK, and CARTER RW: Duration of immunity to brucellosis induced in cattle with strain 19 vaccine. Proc Am Vet Med Assoc 88:128–134, 1951

47. MCALLISTER TA: Laboratory diagnosis of human brucellosis. Scott Med J 21:129–131, 1976

48. MCCULLOUGH ND: Immune response to *Brucella*. *In* Manual of Clinical Immunology. Rose NR and Friedman H (eds.). American Society for Microbiology, Washington DC, 1976, pp 304–311

49. MCMAHON KJ, RENNER ED, ALLMARAS GW, and ANDERSON DK: An agar-gel immunodiffusion test for detection of *Brucella* antibodies in human serum. Can J Microbiol 25:850–854, 1979

50. MEYER ME: Metabolic characterization of the genus *Brucella*. IV. Correlation of oxidative metabolic patterns and susceptibility to *Brucella* bacteriophage, type abortus, strain 3. J Bacteriol 82:950–953, 1961

51. MEYER ME: Advances in research on brucellosis, 1957–1972. Adv Vet Sci Comp Med 18:231–246, 1974

52. MEYER ME and CAMERON HS: Species metabolic patterns within the genus *Brucella*. Am J Vet Res 19:754–758, 1958

53. MORGAN WJB: The serological diagnosis of bovine brucellosis. Vet Rec 80:612–620, 1967

54. MUMFORD RS, WEAVER RE, PATTON C, FELLY JC, and FELDMAN RA: Human disease caused by *Brucella canis*. J Am Med Assoc 231:1267–1268, 1975

55. MYERS DM and SINIUK AS: Preliminary report of the development of a diffusion in gel method for diagnosis of ram epididymitis. Appl Microbiol 19:335–337, 1970

56. PARROTT D, NIELSON KH, WHITE RG, and PAYNE DJH: Radioimmunoassay of IgM, IgG and IgA *Brucella* antibodies, Lancet 1:1075–1078, 1977

57. PAYNE DJH: Brucellosis. Medicine 36:123–138, 1975

58. PERRY TM and BELTER LF: Brucellosis and heart disease. II. Fatal brucellosis: a review of the literature and report of new cases. Am J Pathol 36:673–678, 1960

59. REDDIN JL, ANDERSON RK, JENNESS R, and SPINK WW: Significance of 7S macroglobulin *Brucella* agglutinins in human brucellosis. N Engl J Med 272:1263–1268, 1965

60. RENOUX G: Sur un milieu selectif pour o'isolement de *Brucella melitensis*. Ann Inst Pasteur 87:325–333, 1954

61. ROBERTSON L, FARRELL TD, and HINCHLIFFE PM: The sensitivity of *Brucella abortus* to chemotherapeutic agents. J Med Microbiol 6:549–557, 1973

62. RUSSELL AO, PATTON CM, and KAUFMANN AK: Evaluation of the card test for diagnosis of human brucellosis. J Clin Microbiol 7:454–458, 1978

63. SCHIRGER A, NICHOLS DR, MARTIN WJ, WELLMAN WE, and WEED LA: Brucellosis: experiences with 224 patients. Ann Intern Med 52:827–837, 1960

64. SCHUHARDT VT, WODDFIN HW, and KNOLLE KC: A heat-labile *Brucella*-agglutinin-blocking factor in human sera. J Bacteriol 61:299–303, 1951

65. SPINK WW: The Nature of Brucellosis. Univ of Minn Press, Minneapolis, Minn, 1956

66. SPINK WW, MCCULLOUGH ND, HUTCHINGS LM, and MINGLE CK: Diagnostic criteria for human brucellosis. Report No. 2 of the National Research Council, Committee on Public Health Aspects of Brucellosis. J Am Med Assoc 149:805–808, 1952

67. SPINK WW, MCCULLOUGH ND, HUTCHINGS LM, and MINGLE CK: A standardized antigen for agglutination technic for human brucellosis. Report No. 3 of the National Research Council, Committee on Public Health Aspects of Brucellosis. Am J Clin Pathol 24:496–498, 1954

68. STANFIELD CA, TAYLOR PW, and MORGAN HR: Some important antigenic relationships in the serologic diagnosis of brucellosis. Am J Clin Pathol 72:211–215, 1952

69. U.S. DEPARTMENT OF AGRICULTURE. Cooperative State-Federal Brucellosis Eradication Program Statistical Tables, FY 1965–1974

70. WEED LA: Use of a selective medium for isolation of *Brucella* from contaminated surgical specimens. Am J Clin Pathol 27:482–485, 1957

71. WILKINSON PC: Immunoglobulin patterns of antibodies against *Brucella* in man and animals. J Immunol 96:457–463, 1966

72. WRIGHT AE and SMITH F: On the application of the serum test to the differential diagnosis of typhoid and Malta fever. Lancet 1:656–661, 1897

CHAPTER 20

CAMPYLOBACTER INFECTIONS

Victor D. Bokkenheuser and Vera L. Sutter

Introduction

Causative Organisms

For many years, the bacteria to be discussed here were assigned to the genus *Vibrio*. Because of numerous phenotypic and genetic differences between *V. fetus* and *V. cholerae*, a new genus, *Campylobacter*, was proposed with *C. fetus* as the type species (38). Bacteria in this genus are gram-negative, slender, curved organisms that move in a characteristic darting fashion propelled by a single, polar flagellum. They grow well in liquid or on solid enriched media incubated in a microaerophilic environment of 5%–7% O_2, 10%–12% CO_2, and the balance N_2. An anaerobic atmosphere is tolerated, but the organisms fail to grow on the surface of media exposed to air. Strains of *C. fetus* are characterized by their biochemical reactions, tolerance to certain inhibitors, including temperature, and their antigenic structure. Of the proposed classifications (Table 20.1), *Bergey's* (13) seems to be the most acceptable. Of the recognized subspecies three are of clinical interest.

1. *C. fetus* subsp. *fetus* causes a venereal disease in cattle often resulting in infertility and occasionally in abortion. It is not pathogenic for humans.

2. *C. fetus* subsp. *intestinalis* is a common inhabitant of the gut of sheep and cattle, frequently causing abortion in sheep and occasionally in cattle. It is pathogenic for humans.

3. *C. fetus* subsp. *jejuni*, also referred to as "related campylobacters," "related vibrios," *C. coli*, and *C. jejuni* (21), is usually found as unobtrusive members of the intestinal flora of many lower animals and birds. *C. jejuni* is pathogenic for both humans and animals.

Clinical Manifestations

Two clinical forms of the disease may be discerned, i.e., a disseminated and a localized (enteric) infection.

Disseminated campylobacteriosis

At least 134 cases have been reported in the literature (7).* They can be divided into the following three categories.

*The list of references 1970–1979 is available from Dr. V. Bokkenheuser.

TABLE 20.1—CLASSIFICATION OF *CAMPYLOBACTER FETUS*

BERGEY'S MANUAL (13)	VERON & CHATELAIN (48)	KING (30)
C. fetus subsp. *fetus*	*C. fetus venerealis*	
C. fetus subsp. *intestinalis*	*C. fetus fetus*	*Vibrio fetus*
C. fetus subsp. *jejuni*	*C. coli & C. jejuni*	Related *Vibrio*

Meningitis and meningoencephalitis. Almost all patients in this group are infants, either born prematurely or with congenital defects of the central nervous system. The syndrome may develop on the day of birth. Onset is usually insidious with a low grade fever, poor appetite, loss of weight, cough, watery diarrhea and then, after 2 to 7 days, signs of meningeal involvement. Cerebrospinal fluid and, occasionally, blood yield growth of *C. fetus*, most often subsp. *intestinalis*. Despite intensive treatment, mortality is about 50%.

Bacteremia in children. Few cases have been reported in this group. Malnutrition is a predisposing factor (37). However, apparently healthy children may also be infected. Onset is usually gradual with frequent loose or liquid, sometimes watery, stools often streaked with blood and mucus. Vomiting, anorexia, and fever are common; in severe cases weight loss and dehydration occur. The symptoms may regress spontaneously, only to reappear a few days later. Blood cultures collected in the symptomatic phases yield growth of *Campylobacter*. Both subspecies pathogenic to humans have been observed. Specific humoral antibodies are present. Complete recovery is either spontaneous or follows antibiotic treatment.

Disseminated infection in adults. More than 80% of disseminated campylobacteriosis occurs in adults, most of whom are debilitated (7). Predisposing disorders are: cardiovascular diseases, hepatorenal and endocrinological disorders, chronic alcoholism, and malignancies (7, 24). In addition, immunosuppressive therapy, and perhaps age (mean for females, 54 years; for males, 52 years; range 21–91 years), likely contribute. Twice as many patients are males as are females

Onset may be gradual or abrupt. In some cases the only sign of infection is a slightly elevated temperature superimposed on an already existing grave disorder. Other patients suffer from brief spells of chills and fever for a day or two accompanied by headache, anorexia, fatigue, and irritability. The disease may also debut with diarrhea (24) or phlebitis of one of the extremities (7). The etiological diagnosis is made by isolating the microorganism. In more than 90% of the cases, *Campylobacter* is recovered from the blood (7); also, it may be isolated from the pericardium, pleura, peritoneum, joints, or placenta. More than 90% of the examined strains are *C. fetus* subsp. *intestinalis*. Specific antibodies are demonstrable in the serum (8).

The infection responds readily to antibiotic treatment which should be continued for 4 weeks to prevent relapse (7).

Enteric infection

Since Dekeyser et al. (19) in 1972 used a filtration technique to demonstrate the presence of *Campylobacter* in the stools of patients with diarrhea, it has become clear that *Campylobacter* enteritis is quite common (14–16). But it was Skirrow's introduction of a selective medium (41) that generated an avalanche of reports on the role of *Campylobacter* in gastroenteritis. Surveys designed to detect both subspecies pathogenic for humans have revealed that *C. fetus* subsp. *intestinalis* is responsible for less than 1% of the cases of *Campylobacter* enteritis (10, 31). The infection has no clear age or sex preference. The incubation period is probably 2–5 days. Some patients become ill with a mild to moderate dysenteric syndrome, with or without fever. The symptoms may linger for weeks. In other cases the clinical syndrome is more severe with vomiting, abdominal cramps, and explosive watery diarrhea with blood and mucus. Polymorphonuclear leukocytes are usually present in the stools (1), indicating that *C. fetus* subsp. *jejuni* is invasive rather than toxigenic. The invasiveness has been confirmed by colonic biopsies of humans but contradicted by findings in experimentally infected dogs (34).

The severity of the infection varies vastly from survey to survey (1, 10, 18, 27). The infection is complicated with bacteremia in less than 1% of the cases (18). The prognosis is generally good. Electrolyte replacement and antibiotic treatment should be instituted on clinical indications (31).

There is considerable uncertainty as to the duration of *C. fetus* subsp. *jejuni* excretion following spontaneous clinical recovery. Karmali and Fleming (27) found that 24 untreated children with acute *C. fetus* subsp. *jejuni* enteritis ceased to excrete the organisms within 4–7 weeks. In another study, Richardson et al. (unpublished observations) showed that of 120 apparently healthy school children examined every 3 months, three excreted *C. fetus* subsp. *jejuni* in their feces for more than a year. The latter observation together with earlier findings (10) indicate that *C. fetus* supsp. *jejuni* occasionally will be isolated from patients in whom it is not the causative agent of diarrhea.

The infection is usually accompanied by a fourfold or greater rise in specific bactericidal antibodies (27). In a few cases, patients believed to have acute *Campylobacter* enteritis do not have changes in antibody levels. The latter patients could be the *Campylobacter* carriers alluded to above.

Epidemiology

Although disseminated campylobacteriosis is observed rarely, cases have been described from most parts of the world (7). Two-thirds of the reported cases are from the United States. Serologic evidence suggests that human infection is relatively common in Southern Africa (9). In 1978 the first cases were reported from that area.

Disseminated campylobacteriosis is almost entirely confined to the very young and the elderly, often with debilitating disorders. It rarely affects persons 2 to 14 years of age, and not a single individual between 15 and 20 has been reported to have the disease.

Campylobacter enteritis has been reported from North America (1, 3, 27, 33, 42, 47), Europe (18, 22, 31, 32, 39), Africa (10, 20), Asia (4), and Australia (44). Most cases seem to occur sporadically. However, small outbreaks have been observed in families and institutions (3, 18, 31); the hitherto largest reported outbreak occurred in Vermont, United States, in the spring of 1978 and involved approximately 2000 cases (47). Reports from Europe suggest that there is an accumulation of cases in the late summer (22, 31).

In developed nations *C. fetus* subsp. *jejuni* is recovered from 4%–7% of patients with diarrhea and from 0%–1% of "normal" individuals. The corresponding figures from underdeveloped areas are 8%–31% and 5%–17%, respectively. This high incidence of *C. fetus* subsp. *jejuni* in asymptomatic individuals makes the interpretation of positive fecal cultures difficult.

Sources of Infection

Disseminated campylobacteriosis is not directly related to animal exposure (7). More likely the infection is secondary to intestinal colonization, whose prevalence and geographical distribution are unknown. Propagation of *Campylobacter* is best considered separately for the two subspecies pathogenic for humans. However, conclusions should be drawn with care, because variations in taxonomy and methods of speciation introduce a measure of uncertainty.

C. fetus subsp. *jejuni* is present in the intestinal tract of most domestic and many wild animals; strangely enough it has not been found in horse and mink (35). It is also present in high numbers in most birds. Allegedly, puppies with diarrhea are a potent source of human infection (2) although there is substantial evidence that the organism is apathogenic for dogs (34). The organism has also been isolated from gallbladders of sheep and cattle slaughtered for commercial purposes (11) and from processed poultry available for human consumption (40, 43). The intestinal contents of more than 80% of broiler chickens sold in a live poultry market in New York City yielded growth of *C. fetus* subsp. *jejuni* with an average of 4.4×10^6 organisms per gram of fecal material (23). At 4 C *C. fetus* subsp. *jejuni* survives in milk, water, and feces for at least 3 weeks (5). Thus, food products contaminated with infected fecal material are potential sources of human infections (1, 2, 36, 46). Contaminated drinking water was implicated as the cause of the Vermont outbreak (18). Whether there is significant transmission to humans from the acutely infected patient or from human carriers is unknown.

The mode of propagation of *C. fetus* subsp. *intestinalis* is less clear. The organism is commonly found in the intestinal flora of cattle and sheep, but it has only been recovered rarely from human feces (16, 31). In view of reports on disseminated *C. fetus* infections following dental extraction and pulmonary *C. fetus* abscess secondary to aspiration, it is conceivable that the organisms also reside in the oral cavity of humans (28, 29, 45). It survives well in artificial mixtures with human fecal flora. It is attractive to speculate that *C. fetus* subsp. *intestinalis* colonizes humans by the same mechanisms as *C. fetus* subsp. *jejuni*, and that the organism is an opportunistic, endogenous invader of the compromised host.

Public Health Significance

It is generally agreed that disseminated campylobacteriosis is grossly underreported (7, 37). With a total of 134 documented cases over a 30-year period, the disease has mustered little public health interest. However, *Campylobacter enteritis* has received much attention since 1973 when Butzler et al.

(14) isolated *C. fetus* subsp. *jejuni* at a higher rate from feces of children with diarrhea than from controls. Since then, *C. fetus* subsp. *jejuni* has been shown to be as common a cause of diarrhea as *Salmonella* and *Shigella* together (1, 33, 42).

Diagnostic Procedures

Transport of Specimens and Cultures

C. fetus subsp. *jejuni* remains viable in stool specimens at 25 C for a few hours, but survives for at least 2 weeks at 4 C in feces, milk, water, and urine (5). Thus, hospital specimens which cannot be processed within a few hours can safely be placed in the refrigerator for a day or two. Swab specimens may be inoculated into Cary-Blair medium which should then be placed at 4 C (50). Pure cultures of *C. fetus* subsp. *jejuni* may be shipped at room temperature in semisolid brucella broth enriched with 10% sheep blood (49).

Selection of Primary Culture Media

Specimens of blood or other normally sterile body fluids should be inoculated into conventional aerobic and anaerobic blood culture media. Fecal specimens can be processed by filtration technique or seeded on selective agar media.

Filtration

This technique has been used by several workers (10, 14, 19). The modification used by Grant et al. (23) is simple and fast. Briefly, 1 g of bulk feces is suspended in 20 ml of saline or brain heart infusion broth. After vigorous agitation, e.g., shaken on a vortex machine for 10–15 sec, the mixture is centrifuged at 650–800 × g for 10 min. Four to five milliliters of the supernatant is aspirated into a syringe and passed through two 25-mm filter chambers. The upper nonsterile chamber is fitted with an 8.0-μm and a 1.2-μm Millipore membrane, while the lower steam sterilized chamber contains a 0.65-μm membrane. Two to four drops of the filtrate are spread onto chocolate agar and incubated. *C. fetus* subsp. *jejuni* colonies grow well and are very characteristic on this medium.

Selective media

These media, now manufactured by at least four commercial companies, consist of blood agar (horse or sheep) supplemented with antibiotics. However, it should be mentioned that media containing cephalothin do not support growth of *C. fetus* subsp. *intestinalis* while many fecal organisms other than *C. fetus* subsp. *jejuni* grow on these plates.

Filtration vs. selective media

The filtration method has several advantages. First, virtually all non-*Campylobacter* organisms are retained by the filters, usually resulting in a plate with either no colonies or a pure culture of *C. fetus* subsp. *jejuni*. Second, *C. fetus* subsp. *jejuni* grows on chocolate agar whether or not it is resistant to the antibiotics in the selective medium. Third, the rapid decay of antibiotics in the medium is not a problem. The drawback of filtration is the preparation of filters; however, it is quite simple and fast, once it has been properly organized.

The obvious advantage of selective media is their easy application to the routine laboratory; the disadvantages are decay of inhibitors and growth of non-*C. fetus* subsp. *jejuni* organisms. Nevertheless, the success of selective media is well documented (31, 39).

Enrichment Media

Enrichment media have been proposed, but their place in the routine diagnosis of *C. fetus* subsp. *jejuni* is far from established. It may be argued that if clinicians reserve treatment for patients with high counts of *C. fetus* subsp. *jejuni*, easily detected by direct plating, then there is little practical use for an enrichment medium.

Incubation

The culture should be incubated in a microaerophilic atmosphere of 5% O_2, 10% CO_2, and 85% N_2. This can be achieved in an anaerobic incubator connected to a vacuum pump and cylinders of CO_2 and N_2. If these are not available, anaerobic jars can be used with commercial gas-generating envelopes designed to create a microaerophilic atmosphere. To increase colony size of *C. fetus* subsp. *jejuni*, the cultures are incubated at 42–43 C. This precludes the isolation of *C. fetus* subsp. *intestinalis*, but they constitute less than 1% of campylobacters recovered from feces (10, 31). If one is confronted with a *C. fetus* subsp. *intestinalis* bacteremia and wishes to look for the organism in the stools, it would be simplest to use filtration techniques.

Although minute colonies often are present on the plates after 24 hr of incubation, most workers prefer an incubation period of 2–3 days.

Identification

For all practical purposes the genus *Campylobacter* is identified by the following criteria: (i) small gram-negative curved rods with occasional "sea gull" forms; (ii) characteristic darting movements under dark-field or phase-contrast microscope; (iii) good growth at 37 C microaerophilically, but not aerobically; (iv) inability to ferment or oxidize glucose; and (v) positive oxidase test. Additional criteria may be found in *Bergey's Manual* (13), but are of little importance to the practicing microbiologist.

The principal tests for subspeciation of strains pathogenic to humans as well as of the nonpathogenic *C. sputorum* subsp. *sputorum* are listed in Table 2. The first six tests are considered adequate by many workers. Temperature tolerance is determined by incubating seeded Muller-Hinton (or similar) agar plates microaerophilically at the appropriate temperature. Hippurate hydrolysis is carried out according to the method described by Harvey (25). The presence or absence of C19-cyclopropane acid in the bacteria is determined by gas-liquid chromatography (6). Until recently, many investigators relied upon

TABLE 20.2—CHARACTERISTICS OF *CAMPYLOBACTER* SPECIES ASSOCIATED WITH HUMANS

CHARACTERISTICS	*C. FETUS INTESTINALIS*	*C. FETUS JEJUNI*	*C. SPUTORUM SPUTORUM*
Catalase	+	+	−
Growth at:			
25 C	+	−	+
37 C	+	+	+
42 C	−	+	−
Nalidixic acid (30-μg disk)	Resistant	Sensitive	
Cephalothin (30-μg disk)	Sensitive	Resistant	
Hippurate hydrolysis	−	+	
C-19 cyclopropane acid	Absent	Present	
Phages I-IV	Sensitive	Resistant	
Phage C	Resistant	Sensitive	

nitrate reduction, growth in 1% glycine and 3.5% sodium chloride, and H₂S production for subspeciation (26).

Phage typing of *Campylobacter* was described by Bryner et al. (12) and appears to be a promising approach (10). Seventy-three percent of strains of recent isolates of *C. fetus* subsp. *jejuni* were lysed by phage C obtained from and propagated in *C. fetus* subsp. *jejuni*. The phage is inactive against *C. fetus* subsp. *fetus* and *C. fetus* subsp. *intestinalis*. Phages I-IV lyse most strains of *C. fetus* subsp. *fetus* and *C. fetus* subsp. *intestinalis* but have no effect on *C. fetus* subsp. *jejuni*. Rare *Campylobacter* strains share antigenic determinants with *C. fetus* subsp. *intestinalis* but are lysed by phage C (10).

The antigenic composition of *Campylobacter* is complex and poorly worked out. The H-antigens are too varied to be of practical importance. The somatic antigens of *C. fetus* subsp. *intestinalis* infecting humans appear to fall in a few main groups (8). Presently at least 15 somatic *C. fetus* subsp. *jejuni* antigens are known, but 75% of the isolates from patients are nonreactive with present antisera (Sabine Lauwers, Belgium, personal communications).

Serology

Of the antigens of *C. fetus* subsp. *intestinalis*, only the determinants of the lipopolysaccharide have the specificity required for a clinically meaningful test (29, 51). In patients with disseminated campylobacteriosis antibodies are demonstrable in a direct agglutination test using heat-killed, washed bacterial suspensions or in the more sensitive indirect bacterial hemagglutination test. Hemagglutination titers of patients range from 400–6400 during the bacteremic phase and decline to 200 or less within 6 months of bacteriologic cure (8).

In sera of patients with *Campylobacter* enteritis, several workers have found rising titers of agglutinins to the homologous strain. With similar patient groups, Karmali and Fleming (27) demonstrated a significant increase in specific bactericidal antibodies, and Blaser et al. (1) corroborated these findings using the indirect fluorescence technique. The tests are not yet suitable for routine investigations due to the lack of standardized antigen suspensions and of reference sera, and the need for autologous isolates.

Antibiotic Susceptibility and Treatment

In vitro antibiotic susceptibility testing results have been reported, and the three subspecies of *C. fetus* generally are susceptible to the aminoglycosides, carbenicillin, chloramphenicol, erythromycin, clindamycin, furazolidone, and tetracycline (10, 15, 17). Many strains are resistant to penicillin and ampicillin. It should be recognized that a standardized method for testing *Campylobacter* does not exist, and therefore the results must be interpreted with caution.

The present tendency is to reserve antibiotic therapy for the disseminated form of the infection and for the severe enteric cases. The drug of choice is erythromycin. Following therapy the organisms disappear from the stools within 48 hr (27). Treatment of disseminated campylobacteriosis should be given for a period of 4 weeks to prevent relapses (7). Similarly, treatment of *Campylobacter* enteritis should be continued for 10 days (15).

Evaluation of Laboratory Findings

Results of laboratory examination of clinical specimens are interpreted as those for enteric fevers: (a) isolation of *C. fetus* subsp. *intestinalis* or subsp. *jejuni* from normally sterile body fluids is significant; (b) isolation of these organisms from stools is consistent with both an acute infection and a carrier state; information on the clinical picture may be helpful; (c) specific antibodies in high titers usually reflect a recent or current infection; rising or falling titers are interpreted conventionally. Hemagglutination titers of less than 80 are of no diagnostic value. Failure to demonstrate antibodies does not entirely exclude a disseminated infection, since a certain variation in determinants is known to exist within the subspecies (8).

References

1. BLASER MJ, BERKOWITZ ID, LaFORCE FM, CRAVENS J, RELLER LB, and WANG WL: *Campylobacter* enteritis: Clinical and epidemiological features. Ann Intern Med 91:179–185, 1979
2. BLASER MJ, CRAVENS J, POWERS BW, and WANG WL: *Campylobacter* enteritis associated with canine infection. Lancet ii:979–981, 1978
3. BLASER MJ, CRAVENS J, RIEPE P, POWERS B, WANG WL, and EDELL TA: *Campylobacter* enteritis. Morbid Mortal Weekly Rep 27:226–227, 1978
4. BLASER MJ, GLASS RI, HUQ IM, STOLL B, KIBRIYA GM, and ALIM ARMA: Isolation of *Campylobacter fetus* ssp. *jejuni* from Bangladeshi children. J Clin Microbiol, 12:744–747, 1980
5. BLASER MJ, HARDESTY HL, POWERS B, and WANG WLL: Survival of *Campylobacter fetus* ss *jejuni* in biological milieus. J Clin Microbiol 11:309–313, 1980
6. BLASER MJ, MOSS CW, and WEAVER RE: Cellular fatty acid composition of *Campylobacter fetus*. J Clin Microbiol 11:448–451, 1980
7. BOKKENHEUSER V: *Vibrio fetus* infection in man. I. Ten new cases and some epidemiological observations. Am J Epidemiol 91:400–409, 1970
8. BOKKENHEUSER V: *Vibrio fetus* infection in man: A serological test. Infect Immun 5:222–226, 1972

9. BOKKENHEUSER V: *Vibrio fetus* infection in man. Occurrence, clinical picture, serology and source of infection. *In* Microorganisms and Infectious Disease. von Graevenitz A and Sall T (eds.). Marcel Dekker, Inc, New York, 1:25–32, 1975

10. BOKKENHEUSER VD, RICHARDSON NJ, BRYNER JH, ROUX DJ, SCHUTTE AB, KOORNHOF HJ, FREIMAN I, and HARTMAN E: Detection of enteric campylobacteriosis in children. J Clin Microbiol 9:227–232, 1979

11. BRYNER JH, O'BERRY PA, ESTES PC, and FOLEY JW: Studies on vibriosis from gallbladders of market sheep and cattle. Am J Vet Res 33:1439–1444, 1972

12. BRYNER JH, RITCHIE AE, BOOTH GD, and FOLEY JW: Lytic activity of *Vibrio* phages on strains of *Vibrio fetus* isolated from man and animals. Appl Microbiol 26:404–409, 1973

13. BUCHANAN RE and GIBBONS NE (eds.): Bergey's Manual of Determinative Bacteriology, 8th edition. Williams and Wilkins, Baltimore, 1974

14. BUTZLER JP, DEKEYSER P, DETRAIN M, and DEHAEN F: Related *Vibrio* in stools. J Pediatr 82:493–495, 1973

15. BUTZLER JP, DEKEYSER P, and LAFONTAINE T: Susceptibility of related vibrios and *Vibrio fetus* to twelve antibiotics. Antimicrob Agents Chemother 5:86–89, 1974

16. BUTZLER JP, DEREUME JP, BARBIER P, SMEKENS L, and DEKEYSER P: L'origine digestive des septicemies a *Campylobacter*. Nouvelle Presse Medicale (Paris) 6:1033–1035, 1977

17. CHOW AW, PATTEN V, and BEDNORZ D: Susceptibility of *Campylobacter fetus* to twenty-two antimicrobial agents. Antimicrob Agents Chemother 13:416–418, 1978

18. COMMUNICABLE DISEASE SURVEILLANCE CENTRE (PUBLIC HEALTH LABORATORY SERVICE) and the COMMUNICABLE DISEASES (SCOTLAND) UNIT: *Campylobacter* infections in Britain 1977. Br Med J 1:1357, 1978

19. DEKEYSER P, GOSSUIN-DETRAIN M, BUTZLER JP, and STERNON J: Acute enteritis due to related *Vibrio*: First positive stool cultures. J Infect Dis 125:390–392, 1972

20. DEMOL P and BOSMANS E: *Campylobacter* enteritis in Central Africa. Lancet 1:604, 1978

21. Editorial: *Campylobacter* enteritis. Lancet 2:135–136, 1978

22. GRAF J, SCHAR G, and HEINZER I: *Campylobacter jejuni* enteritis in Switzerland. Schweiz Med Wochenschr 110(6):590–595, 1980

23. GRANT IH, RICHARDSON NJ, and BOKKENHEUSER VD: Broiler chickens as a potential source of campylobacter infections in humans. J Clin Microbiol 11:508–510, 1980

24. GUERRANT RL, LAHITA RG, WINN WC JR, and ROBERTS RB: Campylobacteriosis in man: pathogenic mechanisms and review of 91 bloodstream infections. Am J Med 65:584–592, 1978

25. HARVEY SM: Hippurate hydrolysis by *Campylobacter fetus*. J Clin Microbiol 11:435–437, 1980

26. HOLDEMAN LV and MOORE WEC (eds.): Anaerobe Laboratory Manual, 3rd edition. Virginia Polytechnic Institute and State University, Anaerobe Laboratory, Blacksburg, 1975

27. KARMALI MA and FLEMING PC: *Campylobacter* enteritis in children. J Pediatr 94:527–533, 1979

28. KILO C, HAGEMAN PO, and MARZI J: Septic arthritis and bacteremia due to *Vibrio fetus*: Report on an unusual case and review of literature. Am J Med 38:962–971, 1965

29. KING EO: Human infections with *Vibrio fetus* and a closely related *Vibrio*. J Infect Dis 101:119–128, 1957

30. KING EO: The laboratory recognition of *Vibrio fetus* and a closely related *Vibrio* from cases of human vibriosis. Ann NY Acad Sci 98:700–711, 1962

31. LAUWERS S, DEBOECK M, and BUTZLER JP: *Campylobacter* enteritis in Brussels. Lancet 1:604–605, 1978

32. LINDQUIST B, KJELLANDER J, and KOSUNEN T: *Campylobacter* enteritis in Sweden. Br Med J 1:303, 1978

33. PAI CH, SORGER S, LACKMAN L, SINAI RE, and MARKS MI: *Campylobacter* gastroenteritis in children. J Pediatr 94:589–591, 1979

34. PRESCOTT JF and BARKER IK: Campylobacter colitis in gnotobiotic dogs. Vet Rec 107:314–315, 1980

35. PRESCOTT JF and BRUIN-MOSCH CW: Carriage of *Campylobacter jejuni* in healthy and diarrheic animals. Am J Vet Res, 42:164–165, 1981

36. ROBINSON DA, EDGAR WJ, GIBSON GL, MATCHETT AA, and ROBERTSON L: *Cam-*

pylobacter enteritis associated with consumption of unpasteurized milk. Br Med J 1:1171–1173, 1979

37. SCHWEITZ I and ROUX E: Campylobacter infections: first reports from Red Cross War Memorial Children's Hospital, Cape Town. S Afr Med J 54:385–388, 1978

38. SEBALD M and VERON M: Teneur en bases de l'ADN et classification des vibrions. Ann Inst Pasteur 105:897–910, 1963

39. SEVERIN WPJ: *Campylobacter* en enteritis. Ned Tijdschr Geneesk 122:499–504, 1978

40. SIMMONS NA and GIBBS FJ: Campylobacter spp. in oven-ready poultry. J Infect 1:159–162, 1979

41. SKIRROW MB: *Campylobacter* enteritis: A "new" disease. Br Med J 2:9–11, 1977

42. SMITH JP, DURFEE K, and MARYMOUNT JH: Incidence of Campylobacter enteritis in the Midwestern United States. Am J Med Technol 46:81–84, 1980

43. SMITH MV II and MULDOON PJ: *Campylobacter fetus* subspecies *jejuni* (*Vibrio fetus*) from commercially processed poultry. Appl Microbiol 27:995–996, 1974

44. STEELE TW and MCDERMOTT S: Campylobacter enteritis in Southern Australia. Med J Aust 2:404–406, 1978

45. TARGAN SR, CHOW AW, and GUZE LB: *Campylobacter fetus* associated with pulmonary abscess and empyema. Chest 71:105–108, 1977

46. TAYLOR PR, WEINSTEIN WM, and BRYNER JH: *Campylobacter fetus* infection in human subjects: Association with raw milk. Am J Med 66:779–782, 1979

47. TIEHAN W and VOGT R: Waterborne *Campylobacter* gastroenteritis. Morbid and Mortal Weekly Rep 27:207, 1978

48. VERON M and CHATELAIN R: Taxonomic study of the genus *Campylobacter* Sebald and Veron and designation of the neotype strain for the type species, *Campylobacter fetus* (Smith and Taylor) Sebald and Veron. Int J Syst Bacteriol 23:122–134, 1973

49. WANG W-LL, LEUCHTEFELD NW, RELLER LB, and BLASER MJ: Enriched brucella medium for storage and transport of *Campylobacter fetus* ss *jejuni*. J Clin Microbiol 12:479–480, 1980

50. WELLS JG, BARRETT TJ, and SOURS HE: A transport media for isolating *Campylobacter fetus* ss *jejuni* from fecal specimens. Annu Meet Am Soc Microbiol, Abstr C175, 1979

51. WHITE FH and WALSH AF: Biochemical and serological relationship of isolants of *Vibrio fetus* from man. J Infect Dis 121:471–474, 1970

CHAPTER 21

CELL WALL DEFECTIVE BACTERIA (L-FORMS)

Sarabelle Madoff

Historical Background

When the first L-form was discovered in 1935, it was thought to be a mycoplasma. Klieneberger isolated tiny colonies resembling the organisms of bovine pleuropneumonia (PPLO) from a culture of *Streptobacillus moniliformis* isolated from a rat (14). These seemed to be growing in symbiosis with the bacillus and were named L₁ (L for Lister Institute). It was not surprising that these colonies were taken for mycoplasma; the colonies were composed of small granular elements embedded in the medium, and a periphery of large bodies surrounded the colonies on the surface. They could not be identified by the usual bacteriological smears, and special methods were devised for staining the colonies in situ. The L-form colonies of all bacterial species are still identified by their characteristic morphologic appearance.

Dienes studied cultures of the *Streptobacillus* and the L₁ and recognized the L₁ as a special growth form of the bacillus occurring spontaneously (4). This concept—the derivation of a mycoplasma-like growth form evolving from a bacterium—was an entirely new one. Twelve years passed before the fact became universally accepted. Proof of the derivation of the L-form came from its reversion and serologic identification with the parent *Streptobacillus* form. Within a few years, L-forms were isolated from several other bacterial species showing spontaneous transformation (8). Bacteria freshly isolated from clinical specimens provided a fruitful source.

An important advance in the study of L-forms was the discovery by Pierce that penicillin induced bacteria to grow as L-forms by interfering with normal synthesis of the cell wall (29). In 1954, Sharp observed that osmotic protection (as provided by increased salt concentration of the medium) is necessary for the development of L-forms from Group A streptococci (34). These fundamental observations led the way to the study of L-forms of a great number of bacterial genera. However, our understanding of the role of the L-forms in the biology of the bacteria is very limited. At the present time, the bacterial L-forms are considered to be products of the laboratory. The concept of an "L-phase of bacteria" has been proposed by many authors, and the terms "L-phase variants" and "L-phase of bacteria" have been used interchangeably with the designation L-forms. However, it is not known whether transformation to the L-form state is a universal property of bacteria, or whether it is confined to individual strains of certain species. It appears to this author that these terms are misleading and the term L-forms should be used exclusively for these microbial forms.

Definition of L-Forms

The L-forms can be defined as the manifestation of the continued growth of a bacterium after alteration or removal of the usual bacterial cell wall. This results in the special growth form of the organisms as small granules and large bodies, in a manner similar to that of the mycoplasma. As a result, bacterial L-colonies can also exhibit the so-called "fried egg appearance." These are the characteristics of the L-forms, and they represent the criteria by which identification is made. When transferred in subculture from agar to agar by the "push-block technique," the growth of the organisms occurs from the small granular elements which develop into large bodies. These also play a role in the reproduction of L-forms (8, 12, 20).

Protoplasts and spheroplasts are not synonymous with L-forms. These are spherical forms produced following partial (spheroplasts) or complete (protoplasts) removal of the bacterial cell walls by enzymatic digestion in a hyperosmolar medium. A major difference from the L-forms is that they are unable to replicate themselves as such, but they may be capable of producing L-forms when transferred to media of the proper osmolarity (10, 13, 15, 16, 38).

Atypical, aberrant, transitional, or variant bacterial forms are bacteria with altered cell wall, usually recovered from clinical specimens. These may grow very slowly at first and have distorted morphology, but they regain the normal growth characteristics after further subculture. They are not to be confused with true L-forms (25, 26, 27).

Induction and Cultivation of L-Forms

In general, the induction of L-forms is accomplished by exposing the bacteria to a penicillin gradient on a suitable agar medium. The physical and chemical properties of the medium are important factors. These include the consistency of the agar gel, the pH of the medium, the presence or absence of animal serum, and the osmolarity. Many gram-negative species can be induced on media containing the normal 0.5% NaCl (6, 8, 9). Most strains of gram-positive and some strains of gram-negative bacteria require increased osmotic protection. Sodium chloride (1–5% w/v) is the usual osmotic stabilizer (21, 28, 34). Other neutral salts are also effective. Sucrose (5–20% w/v) plus Mg^{++} has been used successfully (10, 21). Medium supplemented with PVP (polyvinylpyrrolidine) has also been shown to support the growth of L-forms (17). Often, a slight modification in the concentration of inducing agent or osmotic stabilizer may make a decisive change in the success of the experiment. Anaerobiosis may be necessary for induction; later the cultures can be adapted to aerobic growth. Certain strains of bacteria appear to be impervious to the known methods of induction.

Although the penicillins, with their action on the mucopeptide cross-linkages of bacterial cell wall, are the most effective inducing agents, other antibiotics acting on cell wall (cycloserine, cephalothin, ristocetin, bacitracin, and vancomycin) have been used successfully. High concentrations of a few amino acids (glycine and phenylalanine) have been shown to produce L-forms from some bacterial species. L-forms can be induced by the enzyme lysozyme that digests the murein of the cell wall. The starting material is a suspension of organisms exposed to lysozyme; protoplasts are released which may then produce L-forms when transferred to hyperosmolar media. By similar methods, a phage-associated muralysin has induced L-forms from Group A and other strains of streptococcus (10, 38). In *Salmonella typhi*, exposure of the cultures to antibody and complement resulted in the production of L-form colonies (9). Several publications have reviewed these methods in detail (8, 10, 12, 25, 35, 36).

For the initial induction of L-forms, a rapidly growing bacterial culture is preferred. It is useful to inoculate the culture on a variety of media both with and without osmotic protection. Penicillin is either incorporated into the medium or allowed to diffuse by the gradient technique (25, 32). Transformation of bacteria to L-forms may occur after a variable time of incubation, from several hours to several days. Cultures have to be examined frequently. L-colonies develop in the zone of inhibition, usually at some distance from the penicillin trough (23, 24).

Definitive identification of the L-form colonies is made under oil immersion using the Dienes technique of stained agar preparations (5, 20). This method is indispensable in distinguishing L-forms (as well as mycoplasma) from tiny bacterial colonies and from artifacts. The staining solution is made up by dissolving 2.5 g of methylene blue, 1.25 g of azur II, 10 g of maltose, 0.25 g of Na_2CO_3, and 0.2 g of benzoic acid in 100 ml of distilled water. By means of a cotton applicator, a thin film of Dienes stain is applied to one surface of a coverslip. Many coverslips can be prepared in advance and stored for future use. Suspected L-form colonies are selected by using a hand lens or the low-power objective of a microscope. The area of agar is then cut out, lifted out, and placed face up on a glass slide. The agar block is covered with the Dienes-stained coverslip cut to size with a diamond-point pencil. The preparation is then sealed with melted paraffin, and the preparation is ready for microscopic examination.

L-colonies vary greatly in appearance. They may show a fairly smooth contour, with deeply staining center and a periphery of large bodies, similar to mycoplasma. In general, the fully developed L-colony is larger and contains thicker granules than the mycoplasma colony. Large bodies are a prominent feature of the L-form colonies, and these are found both within and at the periphery of the colonies.

Two types of L-colonies have been described, the A- and B-types (3, 6–8, 25). B-type colonies may grow extremely large (1–5 mm in diameter), and they appear to be composed almost entirely of large bodies. They are known to be highly revertible upon suppression of the inducing agent. By electron microscopy they show the presence of bacterial cell wall which has lost its usual rigidity. Certain bacteria, notably members of the *Enterobacteriaceae,* may produce both A- and B-type L-colonies. Streptococci, staphylococci, and other gram-positive organisms tend to produce A-type colonies almost exclusively. These can occasionally be very small and therefore difficult to distinguish from mycoplasma on a purely morphologic basis. By ultrastructure the A-type colonies show complete absence of cell wall; A-type L-colonies tend to become stabilized very easily and to remain in a non-revertible state.

Significance of the L-Forms in Disease

The role of bacterial L-forms and other cell wall defective organisms in human disease has received attention since the isolation of the Eaton agent on artificial media and its identification as *Mycoplasma pneumoniae* (1, 26, 37). The L-forms resemble mycoplasma in many respects, but there is little information as to their distribution in nature or as to their significance in disease. Their similarity to mycoplasma suggests that a pathogenic role should at least be possible. Important properties such as morphology, mode of replication, nutritional requirements and certain physiological characteristics are similar in the two groups of organisms (3, 6–8). Both are very soft, fragile, and plastic. Mycoplasma and L-forms share a number of other important properties: resistance to penicillin, susceptibility to the broad-spectrum antibiotics, and sensitivity to specific antibody (2, 19, 31). These special properties have created new interest in the role of the L-forms, either as infective agents or as a potential source of recurrent infection. Indeed, they are reported to have been isolated from such diverse conditions as pyelonephritis, endocarditis, and meningeal and gastrointestinal infections. (For a comprehensive review, see Clasener [1]). The growth of atypical bacterial forms from clinical material in hyperosmolar media has been taken as indirect evidence for the involvement of L-forms (27). However, the presence of the "true" L-forms in the disease site has yet to be demonstrated.

Experimental studies in animals have not shown evidence of pathogenicity, except in those instances in which toxins were produced by the L-forms or when reversion to the parent bacterium had occurred (8). It has been shown that L-forms of various strains of streptococci can survive and can produce pathogenic effects in diverse tissue cultures (11, 18, 33). The role of L-forms in disease needs to be elucidated, and the use of new experimental models needs to be investigated. The recent studies by Panos et al. showing enhanced survival of streptococcal L-forms in immunosuppressed mice (30) and my observations on the effect of other bacteria on the growth of *H. influenzae* L-forms (22) represent new avenues of approach and merit further exploration.

Routine attempts to cultivate bacterial L-forms in the clinical laboratory cannot be recommended, as they cannot yet yield the kind of information consistent with the amount of effort involved. Realistically, to undertake L-form cultivation demands the following: (a) careful morphologic studies of the clinical material; (b) proper controls by the use of routine bacteriologic media appropriate for the clinical specimen; (c) special L-form media both without and with a variety of osmotically protective substances; (d) media free of penicillin or other agents acting on bacterial cell wall; (e) aerobic and anaerobic incubation of the cultures; (f) constant awareness of the potential for misinterpretation resulting from the presence of bacteria with defective cell wall showing atypical or aberrant morphology—pleomorphism by itself is not sufficient evidence for the presence of L-forms; and (g) substantial basic knowledge of mycoplasma and L-forms and experience with the techniques of cultivation.

The L-forms of bacteria deserve to be studied for their intrinsic scientific value. The mere fact that a bacterium can, under certain conditions, enter into a wall-less state, that it can survive and reproduce itself in this wall-deficient state, and that it can ultimately revert to its bacterial form—or lose the ability to revert—is in itself a remarkable achievement for a bacterium. This phenomenon cannot be insignificant. The L-forms of bacteria should be studied, therefore, with regard to their fundamental structure, their biochemical function, and their genetic composition. These studies should provide new and exciting information as to the role of the L-forms in the biology of bacteria and as to their potential participation in the infectious disease process.

Acknowledgement

Reproduced by permission of the American Society for Microbiology.

References

1. CLASENER H: Pathogenicity of the L-phase of bacteria. Annu Rev Microbiol 26:55–84, 1972
2. CLYDE WA Jr: Mycoplasma species identification based upon growth inhibition by specific antisera. J Immunol 92:958–965, 1964
3. COLE RM: Some implications of the comparative ultrastructure of bacterial L-forms. In Mycoplasma and the L-forms of Bacteria. S Madoff (ed.). Gordon and Breach Science Publishers, New York, 1971, pp 49–83
4. DIENES L: "L" organism of Klieneberger and Streptobacillus moniliformis. J Infect Dis 65:24–42, 1939
5. DIENES L: Permanent stained agar preparations of mycoplasma and L-forms of bacteria. J Bacteriol 93:689, 1967
6. DIENES L: Morphology and reproductive processes of bacteria with defective cell wall. In Microbial Protoplasts, Spheroplasts and L-forms. Guze LB (ed.). The Williams & Wilkins Co, Baltimore, 1968, pp 74–93
7. DIENES L and BULLIVANT S: Morphology and reproductive processes of the L-forms of bacteria. II. Comparative study of L-forms and mycoplasma with the electron microscope. J Bacteriol 95:672–687, 1968
8. DIENES L and WEINBERGER HJ: The L-forms of bacteria. Bacteriol Rev 15:245–288, 1951
9. DIENES L, WEINBERGER HJ, and MADOFF S: The transformation of typhoid bacilli into L-forms under various conditions. J Bacteriol 59:755–764, 1950
10. GOODER H: Streptococcal protoplasts and L-form growth induced by muralytic enzymes. Microbial Protoplasts, Spheroplasts and L-forms. Guze LB (ed.). Williams & Wilkins Co, Baltimore, 1968, pp 40–51
11. GREEN MT, HEIDGER PM, and DOMINGUE GJ: Demonstration of the pnenomena of microbial persistence and reversion with bacterial L-forms in human embryonic kidney cells. Infect Immun 10:889–914, 1974
12. HIJMANS W, VAN BOVEN CPA, and CLASENER HAL: Fundamental biology of the L-phase of bacteria. In The Mycoplasmatales and the L-phase of Bacteria. Hayflick L (ed.). Appleton-Century-Crofts, New York, 1969, pp 67–143
13. KING JR and GOODER H: Reversion to the streptococcal state of enterococcal protoplasts, spheroplasts and L-forms. J Bacteriol 103:692–696, 1970

14. KLIENEBERGER E: The natural occurrence of pleuropneumonia-like organisms in apparent symbiosis with *Streptobacillus moniliformis* and other bacteria. J Pathol Bacteriol 40:93–105, 1935

15. LANDMAN OE and HALLE S: Enzymatically and physically induced inheritance changes in *Bacillus subtilis*. J Mol Biol 7:721–738, 1963

16. LANDMAN OE, RYTER A, and FREHEL C: Gelatin-induced reversion of protoplasts of *Bacillus subtilis* to the bacillary form: electron microscopic study and physical study. J Bacteriol 96:2154–2170, 1968

17. LAWSON JW and DOUGLAS JT: Induction and reversion of the L-form of Neisseria gonorrhoeae. Can J Microbiol 19:1145–1151, 1974

18. LEON O and PANOS C: The adaptation of an osmotically fragile L-form of *Streptococcus pyogenes* to physiological osmotic conditions and its ability to destroy human heart cells in tissue culture. Infect Immun 13:252–262, 1976

19. LYNN RJ and HALLER GJ: Bacterial L-forms as immunogenic agents. *In* Microbial Protoplasts, Spheroplasts and L-forms. Guze LB (ed.). Williams & Wilkins Co, Baltimore, 1968, pp 270–278

20. MADOFF S: Isolation and identification of PPLO. Ann NY Acad Sci 79:383–392, 1960

21. MADOFF S: L-forms of *Streptococcus* MG: induction and characterization. Ann NY Acad Sci 174:912–921, 1970

22. MADOFF S: The influence of microbial factors on the reversion of L-forms of *Haemophilus influenzae* and streptococci. Abstr Annu Meet Am Soc Microbiol 1974, p 61

23. MADOFF S: Mycoplasma and L-forms: occurrence in bacterial cultures. Health Lab Sci 11:159–166, 1976

24. MADOFF S and DIENES L: L-forms from pneumococci. J Bacteriol 76:245–250, 1958

25. MADOFF S and PACHAS WN: Mycoplasma and the L-forms of bacteria. *In* Rapid Diagnostic Methods in Medical Microbiology. Graber CD (ed.). Williams & Wilkins Co, Baltimore, 1970, pp 195–217

26. MCGEE ZA, ROGUL M, and WITTLER RG: Molecular genetic studies of relationships among mycoplasma, L-forms and bacteria. Ann NY Acad Sci 143:21–30, 1967

27. MCGEE ZA, WHITTLER RG, GOODER H, and CHARACHE P: Wall-defective microbial variants: terminology and experimental design. J Infect Dis 123:433–438, 1971

28. PACHAS WN and CURRID VR: L-form induction, morphology and development in two related strains of *Erysipelothrix rhusiopathiae*. J Bacteriol 119:576–582, 1974

29. PIERCE CH: *Streptobacillus moniliformis*, its associated 1_1 form, and other pleuropneumonia organisms. J Bacteriol 43:780, 1942

30. PRABHAVATHI BF and PANOS C: Persistence, pathogenesis, and morphology of an L-form of *Streptococcus pyogenes* adapted to physiological isotonic conditions when in immunosuppressed mice. Infect Immun 14:1228–1240, 1976

31. PURCELL RH, CHANOCK RM, and TAYLOR-ROBINSON D: Serology of the mycoplasmas of man. *In* Mycoplasmatales and the L-phase of Bacteria. Hayflick L (ed.). Appleton-Century-Crofts, New York, 1969

32. ROBERTS RB and WITTLER RG: The L-form of *Neisseria meningitidis*. J Gen Microbiol 44:139–147, 1966

33. SCHMITT-SLOMSKA J, BOUE A, and CARAVANO R: Induction of L-variants in human diploid cells infected by group A streptococci. Infect Immun 5:389–399, 1972

34. SHARP JT: L-colonies from hemolytic-streptococci: new technique in the study of L-forms of bacteria. Proc Soc Exp Biol Med 87:94–97, 1954

35. SHARP JT (ED.): The Role of Mycoplasmas and L-forms of Bacteria in Disease. Charles C. Thomas, Springfield, Ill, 1970

36. SMITH PF: The Biology of Mycoplasmas. Academic Press, New York, 1971

37. THEODORE TS, TULLY JG, and COLE RM: Polyacrylamide gel identification of bacterial L-forms and Mycoplasma species of human origin. Appl Microbiol 21:272, 1971

38. WYRICK PB and GOODER H: Growth of streptococcal protoplasts and L-colonies on membrane filters. J Bacteriol 646–656, 1971

CHAPTER 22

DIPHTHERIA AND OTHER CORYNEBACTERIAL INFECTIONS

Geraldine L. Wiggins, Frances O. Sottnek, and George J. Hermann

Corynebacterium diphtheriae

Introduction

Causative organism

Corynebacterium diphtheriae, the type species of the genus *Corynebacterium,* is a gram-positive, pleomorphic, nonsporulating, nonmotile, nonacid-fast bacillus. It is facultatively aerobic and grows well on ordinary laboratory media. Optimum temperature range is 34 C to 37 C. Outstanding characteristics include pleomorphic, club-like forms, the "Chinese character" arrangement of cells in smears from growth on Loeffler and Pai media, and the ability to grow on selective media containing potassium tellurite. Lysogenic strains which have prophages with the tox$^+$ gene produce a potent exotoxin. Toxigenic and nontoxigenic strains of *C. diphtheriae* can cause diphtheria.

Clinical manifestations

C. diphtheriae is primarily pathogenic to humans. Symptoms of the infection it causes can consist of local lesions in the nose and throat, and less frequently the infection may be a cutaneous one. Primary infection can also affect such sites as the ear, conjunctiva, umbilicus, and vagina (47). The organism is rarely found in the blood or internal organs. The classic form of disease is characterized by a local pseudomembranous lesion covering the tonsils, pharynx, or larynx, or in the nose. The pseudomembrane can extend into the trachea and completely obstruct the air passages, causing the patient to die of suffocation. Diphtheria toxin produced in the local lesion which is absorbed systemically can damage such distant organs and tissues as the heart, liver, kidney, and nervous system. Such damage, especially to the heart, is often cited as the immediate cause of death from diphtheria.

Epidemiology

The incidence of diphtheria in the United States has declined dramatically to a new low of 65 cases reported in 1979 (12). In comparison, the National Morbidity Reporting System recorded 5048 cases between 1959 and 1970. Additional data, obtained from surveillance forms submitted to the Center for Disease Control (CDC) have been reported for 96% of these cases (11).

The number of cases declined from 671 in 1959 to 145 in 1965 and then steadily increased to 391 in 1970. Most cases were reported in the South (74.4%), with 16.8% in the West and 8.7% in the North. Diphtheria infections were localized in small geographic areas (664 of 3134 counties), with the highest incidence reported among children 1 through 9 years of age. Minority racial groups had attack rates five times as high as that for whites.

From 1971 through October 1, 1977, 1372 cases were reported (12). The number per year ranged from 307 to 128, with attack rates ranging from 0.14 to 0.06 per 100,000. A significant piece of information obtained for this period was that the geographical distribution of cases shifted. The West reported 1104 cases (80.47%), the South reported only 234 cases (17.05%), and the North only 34 cases (2.48%). This shift is accounted for by a decline in the number of cases in the South and outbreaks in Washington State which represented 50% of all the cases reported in the country. The age-group distribution of cases also changed. From 1974 through 1976 most cases per year were reported among the 30–39, 40–49, and 50–59 age groups. This change in pattern is at least partially the result of a persistent epidemic of skin diphtheria reported in a "Skid Row" population in Seattle, Washington (50).

Public health significance

In the United States, diphtheria occurs throughout the year among all age groups. Clinical disease is caused by both toxigenic and nontoxigenic strains (11, 19). Patients with severe diphtheria are almost always infected with toxigenic organisms, whereas patients infected with nontoxigenic strains usually have mild infections. Although nasopharyngeal diphtheria is the form most often seen in this country, cutaneous *C. diphtheriae* infections have been reported in recent epidemics (30, 50).

Morbidity and mortality have declined greatly in the last 50 years, although the fatality rate for nasopharyngeal infections remains approximately 10%. Data obtained on culture-positive, nasopharyngeal diphtheria patients in the United States (1959–1970) suggest that an inadequately immunized population segment and failure to diagnose correctly the cause of illness contribute to the risk of dying (46). At greatest risk were children 0 to 4 years old, persons not immunized with diphtheria toxoid, and patients in small outbreaks. Too often the disease is not recognized until severe illness or death occurs in one or more index cases.

Immunization with diphtheria toxoid does not prevent a person from being a *C. diphtheriae* carrier, and Schick-negative individuals can contract the disease. However, the attack rate and clinical severity are to a large extent a function of the immune status, in that when a fully immunized person has diphtheria, the disease is usually mild and almost never fatal. The most effective control measure still appears to be immunization. It has been suggested that at least 70% of the child population must be immunized to control diphtheria (55). However, Zalma et al. (56) reported that >90% of the overall population might have to be immunized in order to curb clinical diphtheria once an epidemic begins. According to the Immunization Survey in 1976 (48), 49.3% of the children in the United States 0 to 13 years old had four DPT immunizations, 73.1% had three or more, and 3.9% had none. Data on just the lower socioeconomic groups indicate that fewer people in these populations are adequately immunized. Thus, a segment of the total population is still inadequately protected against severe clinical diphtheria and possible death.

Although *C. diphtheriae* is most frequently disseminated by aerosol or direct contact, the organism may be spread on fomites, especially when cutaneous diphtheria is prevalent (4, 30, 50). Once a diagnosis of diphtheria has been confirmed, vigorous epidemiological investigation with laboratory support should be undertaken to identify as many infected individuals as possible. These persons should be treated to eliminate the local focus of infection, and intensive immunization campaigns should be conducted in order to raise the antitoxin level in the community's residents as soon as possible.

Collection and Processing of Specimens

The kind of specimen required

Throat and nasopharyngeal specimens should be taken from patients with symptoms compatible with diphtheria. When a diagnosis has been confirmed, similar specimens should be taken from the patient's contacts. If cutaneous lesions are present, material for cultures can be obtained directly with a dry swab. Swabs are placed onto culture medium as soon as possible after they are collected. When swabs cannot be inoculated directly onto a medium, as in field studies, they can be stored in tubes or packets containing silica gel, a desiccant. Comparative recovery rates for *C. diphtheriae* of 91% (54) and 98% (10) were obtained with direct culture and of 83% (10, 54) from swabs desiccated for 3 to 10 days before they were inoculated onto culture medium.

Reports have been made of isolating *C. diphtheriae* from various environmental sources in homes of infected persons and carriers and in medical facilities where patients are treated (4, 30, 50). Such samples were obtained by moistening the area in question with tap water and swabbing it (30) or by moistening a swab with buffered saline before using it (4). Swabs were immediately placed onto Pai medium. This type of sample may be of value in certain outbreak situations, especially when cutaneous lesions are prevalent.

Time of collection

All specimens should be taken before any antibiotic is administered to the patient.

The number of specimens

Throat and nasopharyngeal specimens should be taken from infected persons and carriers when they are initially evaluated and again after they have therapy. Studies have shown that convalescent patients and carriers may have positive nasopharyngeal cultures and negative throat cultures (34, 51). It has been recommended that infected persons and carriers be isolated until two cultures each from the throat and nose are negative for *C. diphtheriae*. These specimens should be taken ≥24 hr after antibiotic therapy is completed and ≥24 hr apart (5). In one recent study of cultures from treated carriers, 99% were negative 1 and 2 days after therapy; however, 15% of these people had again become carriers when they were retested 2 weeks later. This occurrence led

Miller (42) and Miller et al. (43) to suggest that when the effectiveness of an antibiotic in eradicating the carrier state is evaluated, cultures should be made from material obtained both at the conclusion of therapy and at least 2 weeks later.

Diagnostic Procedures

Microscopic examination

Although at one time examinations of smears made directly from throat or nasopharyngeal swabs were heavily relied upon, the fact that the incidence of diphtheria in the United States has declined greatly means that few bacteriologists have the experience necessary to evaluate such smears.

When *C. diphtheriae* strains are grown on Pai or Loeffler, nutritionally inadequate media, a number of thin spots develop in their walls which result in swelling or bulging (2). The typical morphology of the organism in smears from these media stained with Loeffler's alkaline methylene blue is that of rods of uneven thickness throughout their length. Either end or both ends of the rod may be swollen and appear club-shaped. There may also be swollen areas in the middle of the cell, which usually contain pink to reddish purple granules. Portions of the cell between these granules may absorb the dye poorly, with a resulting beaded or barred appearance. Granules may not be present, and some cells may appear as shorter solid-staining forms. Characteristically V- and L-shaped formations result from the sharp angles at which the cells lie in relation to each other. Groups of V- and L-arrangements produce the "Chinese character" effect often associated with the morphology of *C. diphtheriae* (Fig. 22.1).

Fluorescent antibacterial reagents used in the identification of *C. diph-*

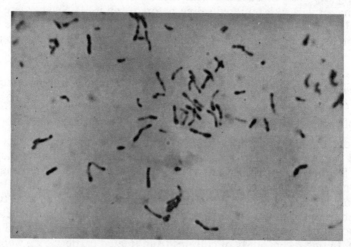

Figure 22.1. Microphotograph of *C. diphtheriae* showing characteristic morphology; stained with Loeffler's methylene blue.

theriae have been described (44). These reagents do not always give satisfactory results on slides made directly from clinical swabs (39) and do not differentiate toxigenic and nontoxigenic strains. Cross-reactions sometimes occur with some strains of diphtheroids and with staphylococci (13).

Selection and inoculation of primary culture media

Loeffler's serum medium was used almost universally for *C. diphtheriae* cultures until Pai (49) described an egg medium which was simple to prepare and gave comparable results. This observation was confirmed by McGuigan and Frobisher (40). Pai medium was later modified by the addition of 8% glycerol (45). Loeffler and Pai media are commercially available. Frobisher (20) reported that it is usually best to inoculate swabs on Loeffler or Pai and incubate overnight before inoculating tellurite medium.

Many media containing tellurite have been developed for the selective isolation of *C. diphtheriae.* Frobisher et al. (21) compared seven plating media and reported that cystine-tellurite-blood agar (CT) and chocolate-blood-tellurite agar gave the best results. Further comparison showed that these two media were similar (22). Colonies of *C. diphtheriae* on CT medium are grayish-black (gunmetal gray). Depending on the biotype, colonies may be small and flat (intermedius) or larger (2 to 3 mm) with raised or convex surfaces (mitis and gravis). When CT medium was compared with a modified Tinsdale medium (MTM) [a tellurite medium upon which *C. diphtheriae* produces hydrogen sulfide, thus creating a distinctive brownish-black zone or halo (tellurium sulphide) under the colony], the two media were equally satisfactory (45). Although other organisms grow on MTM, few others (*C. ulcerans, C. ovis,* and a rare *Staphylococcus* strain) produce halos. Moore and Parsons recommended using MTM because they felt that inexperienced personnel could isolate *C. diphtheriae* more reliably. At the Center for Disease Control (CDC) CT and MTM have been used extensively in isolating *C. diphtheriae* from mixed cultures. When both media were used in carrier surveys, 182 of 185 CT cultures grew *C. diphtheriae,* whereas only 141 of 185 MTM cultures did (10). All 185 strains isolated, however, grew and produced typical halos on MTM when they were subsequently plated from pure culture. We recommend using both media, but if only one tellurite medium can be used we recommend CT.

Identification procedures

Flow charts of steps in isolating and identifying *C. diphtheriae* from suspected diphtheria infections and carrier surveys appear in Figures 22.2 and 22.3. All incubations are at 35 C. Swabs from patients with suspected infections are inoculated onto blood agar and tellurite agar. (If Tinsdale is used, inoculum from the swab should be stabbed into the periphery of the medium during the process of streaking with an inoculating loop.) Finally, the swab is placed onto a Loeffler or Pai slant and allowed to remain during incubation.

Colonies of *C. diphtheriae* are not easily distinguishable from those of other bacteria on blood agar. The blood plate is recommended because occasional strains of *C. diphtheriae* are very sensitive to tellurite and may not grow on the selective medium. The blood plate is also important in detecting the

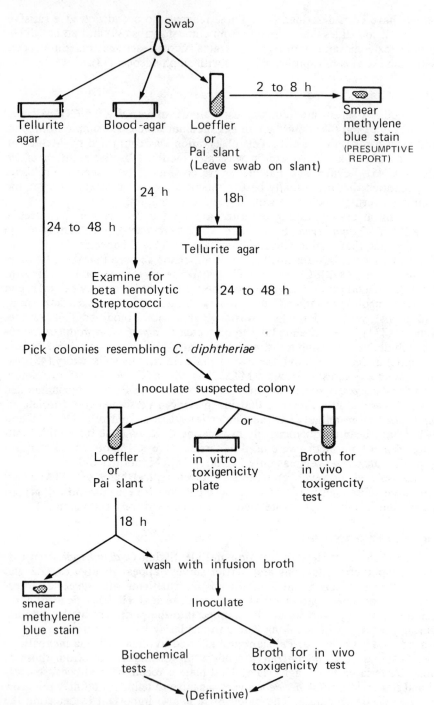

Figure 22.2. Flow chart sequence for isolation and identification of *C. diphtheriae* from suspected cases.

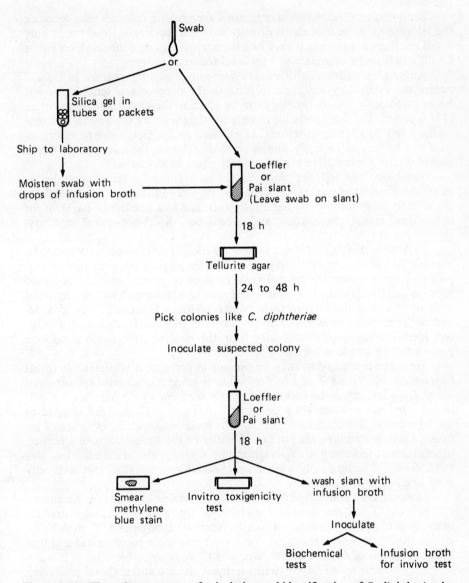

Figure 22.3. Flow chart sequence for isolation and identification of *C. diphtheriae* in carrier surveys.

presence of beta-hemolytic streptococci, which would be missed on the tellurite medium.

If numerous *C. diphtheriae* organisms are present, colonies may grow on the tellurite medium inoculated directly with the specimen. However, if only small numbers are present it may be necessary to incubate the swab on Pai or Loeffler before the organism will grow on tellurite medium.

Although a patient with clinical symptoms of diphtheria must be treated before the laboratory has time to confirm the diagnosis, a tentative report based on microscopic morphology can be given to the physician. Daniel et al. (18) reported that frequently a presumptive diagnosis by smear can be made within 1 to 8 hr after the specimen is incubated on Loeffler. Since other organisms can be morphologically similar to *C. diphtheriae,* the microscopic report provides only presumptive evidence which must be confirmed.

The blood and tellurite plates should be examined after 24 to 48 hr incubation. Suspicious single colonies should be picked to an *in vitro* toxigenicity plate, or to broth for *in vivo* toxigenicity tests, and to a Loeffler or Pai slant for subsequent smear preparation and inoculation for biochemical and toxigenicity tests.

Following this format is not always practical. For example, it may not be possible to fish an isolated colony from the tellurite medium even though suspicious growth is seen in crowded areas or there is typical browning observed in stabs on Tinsdale. In these cases, the area can be swiped and the material used to inoculate the *in vitro* plate (which contains tellurite). If toxin is detected, the presence of either *C. diphtheriae* or *C. ulcerans* is confirmed. Definitive identification must be obtained from the results of biochemical tests on growth from a single colony.

Since fewer organisms may be present in carriers, it is preferable to inoculate the swab on Pai or Loeffler before it is inoculated onto tellurite medium. If swabs cannot be inoculated onto a medium soon after they are collected, they can be stored in a desiccant (silica gel) until they are shipped to the laboratory. Desiccated swabs should be moistened with a few drops of infusion broth before they are put onto Loeffler or Pai slants. Because a portion of organisms, including *C. diphtheriae,* die when swabs are desiccated, this method should be used only when it is not possible to inoculate swabs directly onto Loeffler or Pai.

Nontoxigenic and toxigenic *C. diphtheriae* strains have similar biochemical reactions. These reactions and microscopic appearance, cultural characteristics, and toxigenicity reactions can be used to differentiate *C. diphtheriae* strains from other corynebacteria. Table 22.1 lists some biochemical and toxigenic reactions of *C. ulcerans, C. ovis,* and *C. diphtheriae* biotypes.

All *C. diphtheriae* biotype strains ferment glucose and maltose, producing acid only, and they do not ferment lactose, mannitol, trehalose, and xylose. Sucrose is rarely fermented by strains isolated in the United States. Only the gravis biotype ferments starch and glycogen. Nitrate is reduced by all strains except those referred to here as *C. diphtheriae mitis, belfanti* variety (6, 7). Indole is not formed, urea is not hydrolyzed, and gelatin is not liquefied. In contrast to most corynebacteria commonly found in the nose and throat of man, *C. diphtheriae* strains produce a halo (H_2S) on Tinsdale medium. Strains which produce diphtheria toxin are infected with temperate phage carrying the tox⁺ gene. In the laboratory, nontoxigenic strains of *C. diphtheriae* can be converted to toxigenic strains by lysogenizing them with tox⁺ phage. Barksdale and Arden (3) recently reviewed bacteriophage infection, and Collier (14) reported on the mode of action and structure of diphtheria toxin.

If a strain isolated from a human produces diphtheria toxin, it is either *C. diphtheriae* or *C. ulcerans*. These species can be differentiated biochemically and by intracutaneous tests in animals. Nontoxigenic strains which do not form a halo or ferment glucose, or which hydrolyze urea are not *C. diphtheriae*. Such biochemical and cultural test results should be used to support evidence based on smear examination that the isolate is not *C. diphtheriae*.

Serologic procedures

Serotyping is not routinely used for identifying or confirming *C. diphtheriae*.

TABLE 22.1—SOME BIOCHEMICAL AND TOXIGENIC CHARACTERISTICS OF *C. DIPHTHERIAE* BIOTYPES, *C. ULCERANS*, AND *C. OVIS*

FERMENTATION OF CARBOHYDRATES	*C. DIPHTHERIAE* BIOTYPE				*C. ULCERANS* (36 STRAINS)	*C. OVIS* (PSEUDO-TUBERCULOSIS) (26 STRAINS)
	INTER-MEDIUS	*MITIS*	*MITIS VARIETY BELFANTI*	*GRAVIS*		
Glucose	Aᵃ	A	A	A	A	A
Maltose	A	A	A	A	A	A
Sucrose	−ᵇ	−(A rare)ᶜ	−	−(A rare)	A,Dᵈ or −	− (3A)
Starch	−	−	−	A	A (2−)ᵉ	−
Glycogen	−	−	−	A	A	−
Trehalose	−	−	−	−	D	−
Nitrate	+ᶠ	+	−	+	−	+ (6−)
Urease	−	−	−	−	+	+ (1−)
Catalase	+	+	+	+	+	+
Gelatin	−	−	−	−	−37C +25C	−
Halo on Tinsdale	+	+	+	+	+	+
Natural strains produce diphtheria toxin	+ or −ᵍ	+ or −	+ or −	+ or −	+ or −	−
Lysogenized with tox⁺ phage in the laboratory produce diphtheria toxin	+	+	+	+	+	+

ᵃ Acid produced.
ᵇ Negative results.
ᶜ Only a rare strain isolated in the United States produces acid from sucrose.
ᵈ Acid production is delayed.
ᵉ Number of strains with the reaction in parentheses.
ᶠ Positive results.
ᵍ Some strains positive, some negative.

Several serological tests available for detecting diphtheria antitoxin in serum specimens include a) hemagglutination and b) neutralization procedures in animals, and c) tissue culture (16). Neutralization procedures usually take 2 to 3 days. Even if results could be obtained rapidly with serum from a patient with a suspected infection, interpreting titers is difficult. Ipsen (27) reported that antitoxin levels in diphtheria patients sometimes were ≥0.01 antitoxin units/ml (usually considered to be a protective level) when patients came to be examined. It is not known what antitoxin level in the patient's serum during the acute phase of diphtheria could reliably substitute for antitoxin treatment.

Use of marker systems for epidemiologic investigations

C. diphtheriae can be classified into three broad groups on the basis of colonial morphology and biochemical activity. When originally described (1) the *gravis, mitis,* and *intermedius* types were differentiated by a number of characteristics. However, since that time many strains have been found that do not have all the characteristics of any one type (i.e., they have the colonial morphology of one type and the biochemical reactions of another). At the CDC, *C. diphtheriae* strains that ferment starch and glycogen are categorized as *gravis,* and strains that ferment only glucose and maltose are categorized as *mitis* and *intermedius* on the basis of their colonial morphology. Strains of. *intermedius* produce very small, flat colonies on tellurite media and blood agar. Colonies of this type on modified McLeod's media after 48 hr of growth are usually 0.5 mm in diameter, flat, dry, friable, and have entire or finely crenated edges.

Other marker systems have also been developed for epidemiologic investigation, among them numerous serological typing systems. Two of the most recent articles (25, 33) describe relationships among various systems. Polyacrylamide gel electrophoresis of *C. diphtheriae* has been suggested as a possible epidemiological aid (32). Perhaps the most extensively studied method in use today is the phage typing procedure of Saragea and Maximescu. These workers have used bacteriophage to type strains isolated from many countries (52), including a group of strains isolated from outbreaks in the Southwestern United States (38). Recently, Gibson reported on using diphthericin typing and various other procedures in a numerical analysis of the characteristics of *C. diphtheriae* isolated in Victoria (23).

Toxigenicity tests

Any isolate suspected of being *C. diphtheriae* should be tested for toxigenicity. If toxin is present which is specifically neutralized or precipitated by diphtheria antitoxin, the isolate is confirmed to be either *C. diphtheriae* or *C. ulcerans.* (The latter is seldom found and can be differentiated from *C. diphtheriae* on the basis of its cultural and biochemical characteristics.) Toxigenicity testing (frequently referred to as the virulence test) can be done in several ways, including *in vitro* precipitation, neutralization in tissue culture (31, 53), or *in vivo* procedures. Results can be obtained more rapidly with the *in vitro* test, but it must be carefully controlled because such factors as variability of animal sera, the peptone constituent in the base medium, and purity of the antitoxin can all affect the test results (9). Laboratories which do not frequently analyze *C. diphtheriae* cultures should use an *in vivo* method.

In vivo test

Subcutaneous test. In this procedure, a 48-hr broth culture is prepared by inoculating a pure culture into 10 ml of infusion broth (pH 7.8 to 8.0; contains no dextrose). Two 300- to 400-g guinea pigs and diphtheria antitoxin are also needed.

One guinea pig is injected intraperitoneally with 250 units of diphtheria antitoxin to provide a control. Two hours later both the control and test animals are injected subcutaneously with 4.0 ml of the broth culture. The guinea pig that was injected with only the broth culture is the test animal. If the inoculum contains a toxigenic strain of *C. diphtheriae,* the test animal usually dies within 24 to 96 hr. The control is not affected. If both animals are unaffected, the strain being tested may be a nontoxigenic strain of *C. diphtheriae.* If both animals show ill effects, the organism is not *C. diphtheriae.*

In vitro test

The test is based on a precipitin reaction occurring between diphtheria toxin produced by the test culture and diphtheria antitoxin in the medium. A modification of the Elek method (9) is used at the CDC. Since the *in vitro* test is not recommended for use in laboratories in which *C. diphtheriae* is seldom encountered, this method will not be described in detail here. An *in vitro* plate which has been inoculated with both toxigenic and nontoxigenic strains of *C. diphtheriae* and incubated for 48 hr is shown in Figure 22.4. In reference laboratories, negative *in vitro* results should be confirmed by another method.

Antimicrobic Susceptibility and Resistance

Antibiotics are never given to patients as a substitute for diphtheria antitoxin. Antitoxin is specific therapy for toxin neutralization. Antibiotics are used to eliminate the organism promptly and to treat asymptomatic individuals with positive cultures (carriers). Treatment of carriers reduces their risk of having an active infection and limits the degree to which they spread the organism. Identifying and treating *C. diphtheriae* carriers during outbreaks is thus an important control measure (11, 37, 43). Penicillin and erythromycin are the antibiotics most often recommended.

Antibiotic susceptibility results which involved strains from persons with diphtheria and/or from diphtheria carriers associated with outbreaks in the United States are shown in Table 22.2 (24, 36, 37, 41). These results indicate that *C. diphtheriae* strains are susceptible *in vitro* to various antibiotics, including the two above. These findings are compatible with those of Zamiri and McEntegart (57), who determined the sensitivity to eight antibiotics of 192 strains isolated in Iran and the United Kingdom.

There have been several reports of instances in which *C. diphtheriae* was not completely eradicated in carriers treated with penicillin or erythromycin (37, 43, 56). Although there has been a recent report of two *C. diphtheriae* strains resistant to erythromycin and lincomycin (29), *in vitro* resistance is not

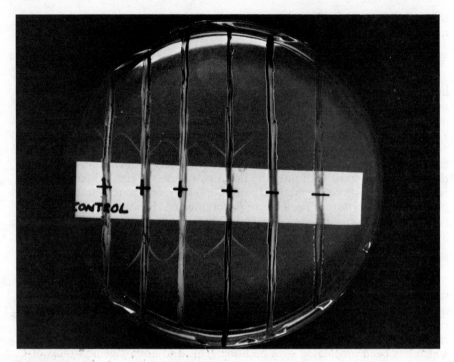

Figure 22.4.   The *in vitro* test for toxigenicity.

a satisfactory explanation for treatment failure in the studies (37, 41) in which *in vitro* susceptibility levels of cultures taken before and after treatment were not markedly different.

Antibiotic susceptibility testing is probably not necessary in cases of isolated infection unless treatment fails to eliminate the organism. Such testing, however, would be prudent before treating a large number of carriers in an outbreak.

Evaluation of Laboratory Findings

Prompt diagnosis of diphtheria in patients with its clinical symptoms is the responsibility of the physician. The bacteriologist should telephone a report to the physician as soon as the presence of *C. diphtheriae* is suspected in specimens submitted to the laboratory. The bacteriologist should emphasize the fact that until toxigenicity tests are completed results are only tentative. Such a report might consist of "Organisms morphologically resembling *C. diphtheriae* seen on smear. Cultural confirmation and toxigenicity tests pending." As soon as a strain is found to produce diphtheria toxin, the report should be confirmed as follows: "Toxigenic *C. diphtheriae* isolated." If the results show that the strain is nontoxigenic, the report can consist of "Nontoxigenic *C. diphtheriae* isolated." When the cultural results are negative the report should be "No *C. diphtheriae* isolated."

Corynebacterium ulcerans

C. ulcerans strains are found in the noses and throats of horses and humans. Human infections usually resemble tonsillitis rather than diphtheria, although some membrane may form in the throat. The disease is usually mild but severity varies (15). Asymptomatic carriers have been reported (35). Strains grow well on tellurite media, with colonies resembling those of C. diphtheriae. Growth on Pai or Loeffler is more luxuriant than that of C. diphtheriae (26). A smear of C. ulcerans from growth on Pai or Loeffler does not resemble C. diphtheriae morphologically. Short rods, coccoid elements, and almost coccal forms with diphtheriae-like rods are sometimes seen in the same microscopic field.

The biochemical reactions of 36 strains tested in the CDC's Special Bacteriology Unit are shown in Table 22.1. The reactions that differ from those of C. diphtheriae strains are: nitrate is not reduced, urea is hydrolyzed, acid is produced from trehalose, and gelatin is liquefied at 25 C. Non-starch-ferment-

TABLE 22.2—ANTIBIOTIC SUSCEPTIBILITY OF STRAINS OF C. DIPHTHERIAE ISOLATED IN THE UNITED STATES

	RANGE OF MINIMAL BACTERICIDAL CONCENTRATION μG/ML (MBC)		RANGE OF MINIMAL INHIBITORY CONCENTRATION μG/ML (MIC)		RANGE OF DIAMETERS OF INHIBITION ZONES AROUND DISKS	
Authors	McCloskey et al. (36)	McCloskey et al. (37)	Gorden et al. (24)	McLaughlin et al. (41)	McLaughlin et al. (41)	
Method	Broth dilution		Agar dilution	Agar dilution	Disk diffusion	
Media	Trypticase soy with fetal		Mueller-Hinton	MH with	MH with	
Number	bovine serum		(MH)	5% blood	5% blood	
of strains	≥84	121	14	136	136	
Antibiotic					Disk	Zone size mm
Penicillin	<0.02–1.0	0.01–1.2	0.05–0.2	0.025–0.5	10-U	24–36
Ampicillin			0.1–0.4			
Oxacillin	1.0–5.0	<0.6–4.8	1.6–3.1			
Methicillin					5-μg	10–25
Erythromycin	<0.5–0.5	0.08–1.2	0.0125–0.05	0.0025–0.01	15-μg	25–40
Tetracycline			0.4–0.8		30-μg	21–36
Lincomycin			0.4–0.8			
Rifampin	<0.01	<0.01	0.0125–0.05	0.001–0.01	30-μg	28–45
Chloramphenicol			0.4–1.6		30-μg	23–43
Cephapirin			0.2–0.4			
Cephalexin	<2–16	1.2–16.0	0.8–1.6			
Kanamycin			0.8–3.1		30-μg	20–38
Gentamicin			0.4–1.6			
Clindamycin	<0.125–1.0	0.08–1.2				
Streptomycin					10-μg	15–28
Cephalothin			0.2–0.4			

ing strains and one which did not hydrolyze urea when first isolated have been reported (28, 35).

Some naturally occurring strains of *C. ulcerans* produce diphtheria toxin in addition to a specific toxic factor. Unlike diphtheria toxin, the latter is not present in sterile filtrates of broth culture. This nonfilterable toxic factor is not neutralized by diphtheria antitoxin. It is present in all strains of *C. ulcerans.*

Lysogenization with diphtheria phage carrying the tox$^+$ gene can cause strains of *C. ulcerans* to produce diphtheria toxin. When this process occurs, the strains maintain their specific morphology and ability to produce urease and continue to produce their own specific toxin (35).

To fully identify *C. ulcerans,* Jebb and Martin (28) recommend both intradermal and subcutaneous tests in guinea pigs. In the intradermal test, a large ulcerating lesion which is not inhibited by the administration of diphtheria antitoxin is produced. In the subcutaneous test, strains of *C. ulcerans* cause a reaction similar to that obtained with strains of *C. diphtheriae.*

Corynebacterium ovis (pseudotuberculosis)

C. ovis strains, which are found in several species of animals including sheep, goats, horses, and cattle, cause ulcerative lymphangitis, abscesses, and purulent infections (17). Of the few human infections reported, most have been animal-associated. Although the pathogenic manifestations of *C. ovis* and *C. diphtheriae* are different, the two species appear to be related (2).

Strains of *C. ovis* grow well on tellurite media. Microscopic morphology of organisms grown on Pai or Loeffler is that of small irregular rods with club forms and metachromatic granules.

The biochemical reactions of 26 strains (including two from humans) tested in the CDC's Special Bacteriology Section are shown in Table 22.1. Unlike *C. diphtheriae,* most *C. ovis* strains hydrolyze urea.

Biberstein et al. (8) reported that two *C. ovis* biotypes exist. Although not absolutely host specific, the biotype that is nitrate negative is usually found in sheep and goats, and that which is nitrate positive usually in cattle and horses. Of the four human infections reported in that study, three isolates were nitrate negative and one was nitrate positive. The strains tested at the CDC which were isolated from humans were nitrate negative.

Most naturally occurring strains of *C. ovis* do not produce diphtheria toxin. However, two strains isolated from Egyptian buffalos and reported to be *C. ovis* based on pathogenicity test results in mice did produce diphtheria toxin (35).

Cell-free filtrates of *C. ovis* strains isolated from natural sources produce a toxin different from diphtheria toxin. However, *C. ovis* strains lysogenized in laboratory experiments with diphtheria phage carrying the tox$^+$ gene can be induced to produce diphtheria toxin (35). Maximescu et al. (35) also reported that 0.1 ml of a 24- to 48-hr broth culture of *C. ovis* kills white mice by any inoculation route, thus distinguishing these strains from those of *C. ulcerans,* which only cause arthritis in white mice. This observation must be confirmed, since Hermann and Parsons (26) reported death in mice within 24 to 48 hr after they were injected with 0.1 ml of a nonfiltered 24-hr broth culture of *C. ulcerans.*

References

1. ANDERSON J, COOPER K, HAPPOLD F, and McLEOD J: Incidence and correlation with clinical severity of *gravis, mitis,* and intermediate types of diphtheria bacillus in series of 500 cases at Leeds. J Pathol Bacteriol 36:169–182, 1933
2. BARKSDALE L: *Corynebacterium diphtheriae* and its relatives. Bacteriol Rev 34:378–422, 1970
3. BARKSDALE L and ARDEN SB: Persisting bacteriophage infections, lysogeny, and phage conversions. Annu Rev Microbiol 28:265–298, 1974
4. BELSEY MA: Isolation of *Corynebacterium diphtheriae* in the environment of skin carriers. Am J Epidemiol 91:294–299, 1970
5. BENESON AS (ed.): Diphtheria. *In* Control of Communicable Diseases in Man, 12th edition. Official Report of the American Public Health Association. 1975, pp 101–105
6. BEZJAK V: Differentiation of *Corynebacterium diphtheriae* of the *mitis* type found in diphtheria and ozaena. I. Biochemical properties. Antonie van Leeuwenhoek J Microbiol Serol 20:269–271, 1954
7. BEZJAK V: Differentiation of *Corynebacterium diphtheriae* of the *mitis* type found in diphtheria and ozaena. II. The rate of rapidity of glucose fermentation by *C. diphtheriae* type *mitis* and *C. belfanti.* Antonie van Leeuwenhoek J Microbiol Serol 21:45–48, 1955
8. BIBERSTEIN EL, KNIGHT HD, and JANG S: Two biotypes of *Corynebacterium pseudotuberculosis.* Vet Record Dec 25, 1971, p 691
9. BICKHAM ST and JONES WL: Problems in the use of the in vitro toxigenicity test for *Corynebacterium diphtheriae.* Am J Clin Pathol 57:244–246, 1972
10. BICKHAM ST, WIGGINS GL, JONES WL, and WEAVER RE: Transport of *C. diphtheriae* specimens on Pai slants and in silica gel packets and subsequent isolation on cystine-telluriteblood and commercial Tinsdale media. (In preparation.)
11. BROOKS GF, BENNETT JV, and FELDMAN RA: Diphtheria in the United States, 1959–1970. J Infect Dis 129:172–178, 1974
12. CENTER FOR DISEASE CONTROL. Morbidity and Mortality Annual Summaries 1959–1978. Morbid Mortal Weekly Rep 26:(40):231, 1976; 28:(51):617, 1980
13. CHERRY WB and MOODY MD: Fluorescent-antibody techniques in diagnostic bacteriology. Bacteriol Rev 29:222, 1965
14. COLLIER RJ: Diphtheria toxin: Mode of action and structure. Bacteriol Rev 39:54–85, 1975
15. COOK GT and JEBB WHH: Starch-fermenting, gelatin-liquefying corynebacteria and their differentiation from *C. diphtheriae* gravis. J Clin Pathol 5:161–164, 1952
16. CRAIG JP: Immune response to *Corynebacterium diphtheriae* and *Clostridium tetani. In* Manual of Clinical Immunology. Rose NR and Friedman H (eds.). American Society for Microbiology, Washington, DC, 1976, pp 324–331
17. CUMMINGS CS: Section 1. Human and Animal Parasites and Pathogens. *In* Bergey's Manual of Determinative Bacteriology, 8th edition. Buchanan RE and Gibbons NE (eds.). The Williams & Wilkins Co, Baltimore, Md, 1974, pp 602–610
18. DANIEL JB, JOHNSON MP, and MACCREADY RA: Laboratory diagnosis of *Corynebacterium diphtheriae:* Early report of positive cultures in 0–8 hours. Can J Public Health 42:185–189, 1951
19. EDWARDS DG and ALLISON VD: Diphtheria in the immunized with observations on a diphtheria-like disease associated with nontoxigenic strains of *Corynebacterium diphtheria.* J Hyg 49:205–219, 1951
20. FROBISHER M: Cystine-tellurite agar for *C. diphtheriae.* J Infect Dis 60:99–105, 1937
21. FROBISHER M, LANKFORD EI, YATES E, and GAY KF: A comparative study of tellurite plating media for *Corynebacterium diphtheriae.* Am J Hyg 48:1–5, 1948
22. FROBISHER M and PARSONS EI: Further studies of tellurite plating media for *Corynebacterium diphtheriae.* Am J Public Health 43:1441–1442, 1953
23. GIBSON LF: Numerical analysis of the characteristics of *Corynebacterium diphtheriae* strains isolated in Victoria from 1962 to 1971. J Hyg 75:413–424, 1975
24. GORDON RC, YOW MD, CLARK DJ, and STEPHENSON WB: In vitro susceptibility of *Corynebacterium diphtheriae* to thirteen antibiotics. Appl Microbiol 21:548–549, 1971

25. GUNDERSEN WB: Investigation on the serological relationships of *Corynebacterium diphtheriae*, type *mitis*, and *Corynebacterium belfanti*. Acta Pathol Microbiol Scand 47:65–74, 1959

26. HERMANN GJ and PARSONS EI: Recognition of *C. diphtheriae*-like corynebacteria (*corynebacterium ulcerans*) in the laboratory. Public Health Lab 15:34–38, 1957

27. IPSEN J: Circulating antitoxin at the onset of diphtheria in 425 patients. J Immunol 54:325–347, 1946

28. JEBB WHH and MARTIN TDM: A non-starch-fermenting variant of *Corynebacterium ulcerans*. J Clin Pathol 18:757–758, 1965

29. JELLARD CH and LIPINSKI AE: *Corynebacterium diphtheriae* resistant to erythromycin and lincomycin. Lancet 1:156, 1973

30. KOOPMAN JS and CAMPBELL J: The role of cutaneous diphtheria infections in a diphtheria epidemic. J Infect Dis 131:239–244, 1975

31. LAIRD W and GROMAN N: Rapid, direct tissue culture test for toxigenicity of *Corynebacterium diphtheriae*. Appl Microbiol 25:709–712, 1973

32. LARSEN SA, BICKHAM ST, BUCHANAN TM, and JONES WL: Polyacrylamide gel electrophoresis of *Corynebacterium diphtheriae*: A possible epidemiological aid. Appl Microbiol 22:885–890, 1971

33. LAUTROP H: Studies on antigenic structure of *Corynebacterium diphtheriae*. Acta Pathol Microbiol Scand 27:443–447, 1950

34. LYMAN E and YOUNGSTROM J: Diphtheria cases and contacts: Is it necessary to take cultures from both nose and throat? Nebr State Med J 41:361–362, 1956

35. MAXIMESCU P, OPRISAN A, POP A, and POTORAC E: Further studies on *Corynebacterium* species capable of producing diphtheria toxin. (*C. diphtheriae, C. ulcerans. C. ovis*). J Gen Microbiol 82:49–56, 1974

36. MCCLOSKEY RV, ELLER JJ, GREEN M, MAUNEY CU, and RICHARDS SEM: The 1970 epidemic of diphtheria in San Antonio. Ann Intern Med 75:495–503, 1971

37. MCCLOSKEY RV, GREEN MJ, ELLER J, and SMILACK J: Treatment of diphtheria carriers: Benzathine penicillin, erythromycin, and clindamycin. Ann Intern Med 81:788–791, 1974

38. MCCLOSKEY RV, SARAGEA A, and MAXIMESCU P: Phage typing in diphtheria outbreaks in the Southwestern United States, 1968–1971. J Infect Dis 126:196–199, 1972

39. MCCRACKEN AW and MAUNEY CU: Identification of *Corynebacterium diphtheriae* by immunofluorescence during a diphtheria epidemic. J Clin Pathol 24:641–644, 1971

40. MCGUIGAN MK and FROBISHER M: Mediums for the study of diphtheria. J Infect Dis 59:22–29, 1936

41. MCLAUGHLIN JV, BICKHAM ST, WIGGINS GL, LARSEN SA, BALOWS A, and JONES WL: Antibiotic susceptibility patterns of recent isolates of *Corynebacterium diphtheriae*. Appl Microbiol 21:844–851, 1971

42. MILLER LW: Diphtheria carriers. Ann Intern Med 82:720, 1975

43. MILLER LW, BICKHAM S, JONES WL, HEATHER CD, and MORRIS RH: Diphtheria carriers and the effect of erythromycin therapy. Antimicrob Agents Chemother 6:166–169, 1974

44. MOODY MD and JONES WL: Identification of *Corynebacterium diphtheriae* with fluorescent antibacterial reagents. J Bacteriol 86:285–293, 1963

45. MOORE MS and PARSONS EI: A study of a modified Tinsdale's medium for the primary isolation of *Corynebacterium diphtheriae*. J Infect Dis 102:88–93, 1958

46. MUNFORD RS, ORY HW, BROOKS GF, and FELDMAN RA: Diphtheria deaths in the United States, 1959–1970. J Am Med Assoc 229:1890–1893, 1974

47. NAIDITCH MJ and BOWER AG: Diphtheria: A study of 1,433 cases observed during a ten-year period at the Los Angeles County Hospital. Am J Med 17:229–245, 1954

48. NATIONAL CENTER FOR DISEASE CONTROL. United States Immunization Survey, 1976

49. PAI S: A simple egg medium for the cultivation of *Bacillus diphtheriae*. Chinese Med J 46:1203–1206, 1932

50. PEDERSEN AHB, SPEARMAN J, TRONCA E, BADER M, and HARNISCH J: Diphtheria on Skid Row, Seattle, Wash, 1972–75. Public Health Rep 92:336–342, 1977

51. RUSSELL WT: The epidemiology of diphtheria during the last forty years. Med Res Counc. Rep No. 247, 1943

52. SARAGEA A and MAXIMESCU P: Phage typing of *Corynebacterium diphtheriae*. Bull WHO 35:681–689, 1966
53. SCHUBERT JH, BICKHAM ST, and WIGGINS GL: Tissue culture method for toxigenicity testing of *Corynebacterium diphtheriae*. Appl Microbiol 16:1748–1752, 1968
54. SINCLAIR MC, BICKHAM S, and SCHUBERT JH: Silica gel as a transport medium for *Corynebacterium diphtheriae*. Southern Med J 65:1383–1384, 1972
55. WORLD HEALTH ORGANIZATION: Diphtheria and Pertussis Vaccination: Part 1, Diphtheria. WHO Tech Rep Series, No. 61, Geneva, 1963, pp 8–21
56. ZALMA VM, OLDER JJ, and BROOKS GF: The Austin, Texas, diphtheria outbreak. J Am Med Assoc 211:2125–2129, 1970
57. ZAMIRI I and MCENTEGART MG: The sensitivity of diphtheria bacilli to eight antibiotics. J Clin Pathol 25:716–717, 1972

CHAPTER 23

DONOVANOSIS

Robert B. Dienst and George H. Brownell

Introduction

The Donovan body, *Calymmatobacterium granulomatis*, is the etiologic agent of donovanosis or granuloma inguinale (1, 2). According to *Bergey's Manual of Determinative Bacteriology* (8th edition), *C. granulomatis* is classified in the family *Brucellaceae*.

Donovanosis is a chronic infection manifested clinically by ulcerating, granulomatous lesions usually located in the inguinal region. The definite venereal origin of donovanosis remains unproved. It is primarily a disease of the skin and corium and occasionally involves the lymphatics. It is a slowly progressive infection and may be adequately controlled by antibiotics (8). The disease is becoming a rarity in locales previously reporting large numbers of cases.

Donovanosis, or granuloma inguinale, is seen throughout the world and is endemic in many areas, including the United States. The infection is encountered chiefly in Negroes and occurs mostly in areas where the climate is warm and humid for several months of the year. The organism is not pathogenic for laboratory animals and has been reportedly isolated from human feces (6). Most researchers support the contention that donovanosis is not a venereal disease but an infection resulting from intimate fecal contamination and poor hygiene (7).

Morphology and Growth

C. granulomatis is a gram-negative, nonmotile, encapsulated coccobacillus often showing bipolar granules following staining with Wright blood stain. The organism does not grow in ordinary culture media, and primary isolation apparently requires a growth factor found in egg yolk (3, 4). Cultivation also requires a reduced oxidation environment for optimal growth at 37 C. Some strains have been adapted to grow on other media (5, 9).

Diagnosis

The most effective means of diagnosing donovanosis is to establish the presence of *C. granulomatis* in lesion exudate. By using a punch forceps or the

335

corner of a glass slide, granulation tissue is removed from the previously cleaned surface of the skin lesion and smeared onto a slide. After air drying, Wright blood stain is applied for 1.5 min, and then the stain is diluted with fresh distilled water (3).

Microscopic examination of the stained smear should reveal typical intracellular Donovan bodies in the cytoplasm of the large mononuclear cells for a positive diagnosis. The intracellular organisms appear as small, straight or dumbbell-curved rods stained dark blue and surrounded by a pinkish capsule. If only extracellular organisms are observed, repeat the smear and stain procedure to confirm the presence of typical intracellular *C. granulomatis.*

References

1. ANDERSON K: The cultivation from granuloma inguinale of a microorganism having the characteristics of the Donovan body in the yolk sac of chick embryo. Science 97:560–561, 1943
2. ANDERSON K, DeMONBREUN WA, and GOODPASTURE EW: An etiologic consideration of *Donovania granulomatis* cultivated from granuloma inguinale in embryonic yolk. J Exp Med 81:25–39, 1945
3. DIENST RB, GREENBLATT RB, and CHEN CH: Laboratory diagnosis of granuloma inguinale and studies on the cultivation of the Donovan body. Am J Syph Gonorrhea Vener Dis 32:301–306, 1948
4. DULANEY AD and PACKER H: Complement fixation studies with pus antigen in granuloma inguinale. Proc Soc Exp Biol Med 65:254–256, 1947
5. DUNHAM W and RAKE G: Cultural and serologic studies on granuloma inguinale. Am J Syph Gonorrhea Vener Dis 32:145–149, 1948
6. GOLDBERG J: Studies on granuloma inguinale. V. Isolation of a bacterium resembling *Donovania granulomatis* from the faeces of a patient with granuloma inguinale. Br J Vener Dis 38:99–102, 1962
7. GOLDBERG J: Studies on granuloma inguinale. VII. Some epidemiologic considerations of the disease. Br J Vener Dis 40:140–145, 1964
8. GREENBLATT RB, BALDWIN KR, and DIENST RB: The minor venereal diseases—their diagnosis and treatment. Clin Obstet Gynecol 2:549–563, 1959
9. RAKE G and OSKAY JJ: Cultural characteristics of *Donovania granulomatis.* J Bacteriol 55:667–675, 1948

CHAPTER 24

EIKENELLA CORRODENS

James W. Smith and George F. Brooks

Pathogenicity

Eikenella corrodens is a small, nonmotile, gram-negative coccobacillus that is facultatively anaerobic or capnophilic and usually produces corroding colonies that penetrate or pit the agar; hence, the species name. Originally, the organism was thought to be a facultative *Bacteroides corrodens* but was subsequently discovered to have biochemical, serologic, and genetic differences. (1, 10, 11, 16). The organisms designated as HB-1 by King and Tatum (12) have been found to be identical to *E. corrodens* (14).

E. corrodens is a member of the flora of the mouth and upper respiratory and gastrointestinal areas. It has been found in 9%–33% of pharyngeal or gingival cultures (1, 13). The organism is isolated from infections, especially abscesses, in tissues adjacent to the above flora-containing areas. *Eikenella* infections are likely to be polymicrobial, especially in combination with various streptococci. Often, abscesses of injection sites of drug abusers, particularly those who inject methylphenidate, contain this organism (1). A variety of other infections due to *E. corrodens* have been described including endocarditis, brain abscess, arthritis, osteomyelitis, meningitis, pneumonitis, and lung abscess (1, 2, 4). Pus from *Eikenella* infections is malodorous, often leading to the clinical impression that the infection is due to anaerobic bacteria and consequently to inappropriate therapy.

Cultural and Biochemical Characteristics

E. corrodens grows well on blood-containing media in air with added carbon dioxide. By incorporation of clindamycin (5 μg/ml final concentration) in Mueller-Hinton agar containing 5% sheep blood (1), a selective medium can be made that will inhibit gram-positive cocci. The medium can be made more selective by adding kanamycin (2.5 μg/ml) in addition to the clindamycin to inhibit the coliforms; however, this slows the growth of *E. corrodens*. If *Eikenella* infection is suspected, a simple approach is to place a clindamycin susceptibility disk on the regular blood or chocolate agar plate to inhibit other organisms in that area of the plate. *E. corrodens* has been shown to grow better on media containing plasma than on media containing serum (11).

E. corrodens colonies typically show pitting or corroding of the agar, although this is actually seen with only about half of the strains (18); the other strains have dome-shaped colonies. A spreading peripheral zone is often present around pitting colonies and may be present around dome-shaped colonies (15). Pitting colonies when young have depressed centers and appear to be penetrating into the agar. Noncorroding dome-shaped colonies may be a pale yellow. In addition to strain variation, pitting is more marked in media with inadequate nutrients and low gel strength (15). Sometimes both domed and corroding colonies are present, and both can be detected on subculture of either type. There is evidence that organisms that form corroding colonies are capable of a type of movement known as "twitching motility" (7, 8, 17). The exact mechanism of this movement is not known, although it is not due to flagella and appears to be related to the presence of polar fimbria (6, 9). Cultures of *Eikenella* have a very distinctive odor of hypochlorite solution. The organisms grow slowly. Pitting strains of *E. corrodens* must be differentiated from the strictly anaerobic *B. corrodens* and from the facultatively anaerobic Tm-1 (5) (Table 24.1) and various *Moraxella* species (9) that also may pit the agar.

E. corrodens is oxidase positive, catalase negative, inactive on carbohydrates, and capable of reducing nitrates to nitrites. It gives positive tests for both lysine decarboxylase and ornithine decarboxylase, and these reactions are quite helpful in differentiating *E. corrodens* from other organisms. Although different serologic groups have been described, typing is not known to be of clinical significance (16).

Antimicrobial Susceptibility

Because the organisms grow slowly, disk antimicrobial susceptibility tests are unsatisfactory, and because the organisms grow very poorly in broth culture, broth dilution tests are also unsatisfactory. The most reliable susceptibility data have been obtained by agar-dilution susceptibility testing (1, 4). A disk test can be used to demonstrate the organism's marked resistance to clindamycin; the organisms will grow up to the clindamycin disk.

TABLE 24.1—CHARACTERISTICS FOR DIFFERENTIATION OF *EIKENELLA CORRODENS*, *BACTEROIDES CORRODENS*, AND TM-1 ORGANISMS

	E. CORRODENS	*B. CORRODENS*	TM-1
Anaerobic growth	+	+	+
Aerobic growth with CO_2	+	−	+
Oxidase	+	+ (weak)	+
Catalase	−	−	−
Acid from glucose	−	−	late
Nitrate	+	+	+ (gas)
Urease	−	+	−
Lysine decarboxylase	+	−	−
Ornithine decarboxylase	+	−	−
Arginine dihydrolase	−	−	−

Eikenella organisms are susceptible to penicillin, cefoxitin, ampicillin, carbenicillin, and tetracycline, and most strains are susceptible to chloramphenicol. They are relatively resistant to aminoglycosides, methicillin, and cephalosporins other than cefoxitin (4); therefore, these drugs should not be used for therapy. They show marked resistance to clindamycin and metronidazole in contrast to *B. corrodens* organisms, which are susceptible to both agents. Penicillin, ampicillin, and cefoxitin are the drugs of choice for therapy. *E. corrodens* abscesses should be drained surgically.

References

1. BROOKS GF, O'DONOGHUE JM, RISSING JP, SOAPES K, and SMITH JW: *Eikenella corrodens,* a recently recognized pathogen: infections in medical-surgical patients and in association with methylphenidate abuse. Medicine 53:325–342, 1974
2. DORFF GJ, JACKSON LJ, and RYTEL MW: Infections with *Eikenella corrodens* a newly recognized human pathogen. Ann Intern Med 80:305–309, 1974
3. GERACI JE, HERMAN PE, and WASHINGTON JA: *Eikenella corrodens* endocarditis: report of cure in two cases. Mayo Clin Proc 49:950–953, 1974
4. GOLDSTEIN EJC, KIRBY BD, and FINEGOLD SM: Isolation of *Eikenella corrodens* from pulmonary infections. Am Rev Resp Dis 119:55–58, 1979
5. HOLLIS DG, WIGGINS GL, and WEAVER RE: An unclassified gram-negative rod isolated from the pharynx on Thayer-Martin medium (selective agar). Appl Microbiol 24:772–777, 1972
6. HENRICKSEN J: Bacterial surface translocation: a survey and a classification. Bacteriol Rev 36:478–503, 1972
7. HENRICKSEN J: The occurence of twitching motility among gram-negative bacteria. Acta Pathol Microbiol Scand Sect B 83:171, 1975
8. HENRICKSEN J: On twitching motility and its mechanism. Acta Pathol Microbiol Scand Sect B 83:187–190, 1975
9. HENRICKSEN J, FROHOLM LO, and BOVRE K: Studies on bacterial surface translocation. 2. Correlation of twitching motility and fimbriation in colony varients of *Moraxella nonliquefaciens, M. bovis* and *M. bengii.* Acta Pathol Microbiol Scand Sect B 30:445–452,1972
10. JACKSON FL, GOODMAN YE, BEL FR, WONG PC, and WHITEHOUSE RLS: Taxonomic status of facultative and strictly anaerobic "corroding bacilli" that have been classified as *Bacteroides corrodens.* J Med Microbiol 4:171–184, 1971
11. JAMES AL and ROBINSON JVA: A comparison of the biochemical activities of *Bacteroides corrodens* and *Eikenella corrodens* with those of certain other gram-negative bacteria. J Med Microbiol 8:59–76, 1975
12. KING EO and TATUM HW: *Actinobacillus actinomycetemcomitans* and *Haemophilus aphrophilus.* J Infect Dis 111:85–94, 1962
13. LABBÉ M, HANSEN W, SCHOUTENS E, and YOURASSOWSKY E: Isolation of *Bacteroides corrodens* and *Eikenella corrodens* from human clinical specimens. Comparative study of incidence and methods of identification. Infection 5(3):159–162, 1977
14. RILEY PS, TATUM HW, and WEAVER RE: Identity of HB-1 of King and *Eikenella corrodens* (Eiken) Jackson and Goodman. Int J Syst Bacteriol 23:75–76, 1973
15. ROBINSON JVA and JAMES AL: Some observations on the colony morphology of "corroding bacilli." J Appl Bacteriol 37:101–104, 1974
16. SCHROTER G: Studies of the antigenic structure of *Eikenella corrodens.* Ann Microbiol (Inst Pasteur) 125B:59–74, 1974
17. SCHROTER G: The demonstration of twitching motility in *Eikenella corrodens.* Med Microbiol Immunol 161:41–46, 1975
18. TATUM HW, EWING WH, and WEAVER RE: Miscellaneous gram-negative bacteria. *In* Manual of Clinical Microbiology, 2nd edition. Lennette EH, Spaulding EH, and Truant JP (eds.). American Society for Microbiology, Washington, DC, 1974, pp 272–274

CHAPTER 25

ENTEROBACTERIACEAE

J. J. Farmer, III, Joy G. Wells, William Terranova, Mitchell L. Cohen, and
C. Michael West

Introduction

It is difficult to treat the *Enterobacteriaceae* as a single group because they have evolved quite differently in their ecology, epidemiology, and pathogenicity (27, 47). Thus, our discussion is divided into five sections. The first section covers the diagnostic procedures used with the *Enterobacteriaceae* as a group. The second deals with the "opportunistic pathogens," the species usually found in soil, water, healthy animals, and humans but which can cause human infections under certain conditions. Sections three through five deal with *Escherichia coli, Shigella,* and *Salmonella-Arizona,* the groups which frequently cause diarrhea in man and animals. A separate chapter covers *Yersinia,* a genus recently added to the family *Enterobacteriaceae,* which differs in many respects and is similar in others.

For a more detailed treatment of *Enterobacteriaceae,* see *Identification of Enterobacteriaceae* by Edwards and Ewing (27) and *Enterobacteriaceae* by Kauffmann (47). For a different approach to a chapter on the *Enterobacteriaceae,* refer to the chapter by Martin and Washington in the *Manual of Clinical Microbiology* (52).

The family *Enterobacteriaceae* is a large group of diverse bacteria with certain common properties. Members are found in almost all environments including soil, water, plants, and the normal flora of most animals. They also cause diseases in plants and animals. Some species occupy a very limited ecologic niche. *Salmonella typhi* is found only in humans and causes typhoid fever. In contrast, strains of *Klebsiella pneumoniae* are widely distributed in the environment and contribute to biochemical and geochemical process. However, *Klebsiella* can also cause human diseases ranging from asymptomatic colonization of the intestinal, urinary, or respiratory tract to fatal septicemia. In this chapter we concentrate on the species which cause human disease, with much of the emphasis on infections in the United States which are often quite

(We submitted this chapter in what we thought was final form in May 1978. That some of the material is not totally up to date is due to many publication delays which were totally beyond our control. The Authors, March 1981)

different from those in other parts of the world, particularly developing nations.

The species which comprise the family *Enterobacteriaceae* have the following properties in common: appear as gram-negative rods; are motile by peritrichous flagella or nonmotile; do not form spores; grow on peptone or meat extract media without additional supplements; grow well on MacConkey agar; grow both aerobically and anaerobically; ferment (rather than oxidize) D-glucose, often with gas production; are catalase positive; are oxidase negative; reduce nitrate to nitrite; and have a 39%–59% range of guanine plus cytosine content of deoxyribonucleic acid (DNA). Although most strains have these properties, occasionally exceptions occur which can be explained by mutation or other genetic mechanisms. The *Enterobacteriaceae* are closely related to other fermentative bacteria in the genera *Aeromonas* and *Vibrio*, but the latter are oxidase positive and have polar rather than peritrichous flagella. From an ecologic, clinical, or public health point of view, *Vibrio* and *Aeromonas* could be included in a discussion of *Enterobacteriaceae* but are treated separately in this volume.

The nomenclature of *Enterobacteriaceae* is always the subject of confusion, controversy, and unfortunately for most of us, of constant change (10, 38). In this chapter we use the nomenclature adopted (10) in the Enteric Section, Centers for Disease Control (CDC), which differs in several important aspects from that previously used. It is beyond the scope of this chapter to repeat the scientific reasons for these changes in nomenclature and classification. The interested reader should consult the CDC publication (10) by Brenner et al. (available without charge; address requests to: Center for Disease Control; ATTN.: Enteric Section, Bldg. 1, Room B-341; 1600 Clifton Road, Atlanta, GA 30333) for a detailed discussion. The most important taxonomic changes are given in Table 25.1. Table 25.2 is given as a "score-card" so that the names used in this chapter can be compared to names used in Ed-

TABLE 25.1—RECOMMENDED CHANGES IN THE NOMENCLATURE AND CLASSIFICATION OF *ENTEROBACTERIACEAE*

OLD DESIGNATION	NEW DESIGNATION
Newly Recognized Species	
Citrobacter freundii, "H_2S^-, indole$^+$ biogroup"	*Citrobacter amalonaticus*
Klebsiella pneumoniae, "indole$^+$ (sometimes gelatin$^+$)"	*Klebsiella oxytoca*
Enterobacter cloacae, "yellow pigmented"	*Enterobacter sakazakii*
Enterobacter aerogenes, "biochemically atypical"	*Enterobacter gergoviae*
Changes in the Classification of Recognized Species	
Enterobacter hafniae	*Hafnia alvei*
Proteus morganii	*Morganella morganii*
Proteus rettgeri, Penner's biogroup 5	*Providencia stuartii*, urea$^+$
Proteus rettgeri, Penner's biogroups 1–4	*Providencia rettgeri*
Providencia stuartii, Ewing's biogroup 4	*Providencia alcalifaciens*

wards and Ewing's *Identification of Enterobacteriaceae* (27), *Bergey's Manual of Determinative Bacteriology* (11), and Cowan and Steel's *Identification of Medical Bacteria* (17).

Since preparation of this chapter was completed, several new species of *Enterobacteriaceae* have been described. *Serratia plymuthica* and *Serratia odorifera* are new species which occasionally occur in clinical specimens (41a).

TABLE 25.2—DIFFERENT NOMENCLATURES USED FOR SPECIES OF *ENTEROBACTERIACEAE*

RECOMMENDATION, THIS CHAPTER	EDWARDS AND EWING (27)	BERGEY'S MANUAL (11)	COWAN AND STEEL (17)
Citrobacter diversus	*Citrobacter diversus*	*Citrobacteri intermedius* biotype b	*Citrobacter koseri*
Citrobacter amalonaticus	*Citrobacter freundii-* Biogroup 2 (H₂S⁻, indole⁺)	*Citrobacter intermedius* biotype a	*Levinea* spp.[a]
Arizona hinshawii	*Arizona hinshawii*	*Salmonella arizonae*	*Salmonella arizonae*
Klebsiella pneumoniae	*Klebsiella pneumoniae*	*Klebsiella pneumoniae*	*Klebsiella pneumoniae*
Klebsiella pneumoniae	*Klebsiella pneumoniae*	*Klebsiella pneumoniae*	*Klebsiella aerogenes*
Klebsiella oxytoca	*Klebsiella pneumoniae-*indole⁺	*Klebsiella pneumoniae*	*Klebsiella oxytoca*
Klebsiella pneumoniae	*Klebsiella pneumoniae*	*Klebsiella pneumoniae*	*Klebsiella atlantae*
Klebsiella pneumoniae	*Klebsiella pneumoniae*	*Klebsiella pneumoniae*	*Klebsiella edwardsii*
Hafnia alvei	*Enterobacter hafniae*	*Hafnia alvei*	*Hafnia alvei*
Enterobacter agglomerans	*Enterobacter agglomerans*	*Erwinia herbicola*	*Erwinia herbicola*
Enterobacter agglomerans	*Enterobacter agglomerans*	*Erwinia stewartii*	*Erwinia herbicola*
Enterobacter agglomerans	*Enterobacter agglomerans*	*Erwinia uredovora*	*Erwinia herbicola*
Serratia liquefaciens	*Serratia liquefaciens*	Not Listed	*Serratia liquefaciens*
Serratia rubidaea	*Serratia rubidaea*	Not Listed	*Serratia rubidaea*
Morganella morganii	*Proteus morganii*	*Proteus morganii*	*Morganella morganii*
Providencia alcalifaciens	*Providencia alcalifaciens*	*Proteus inconstans* Subgroup A	*Proteus inconstans*
Providencia stuartii	*Providencia stuartii*	*Proteus inconstans* Subgroup B	*Proteus stuartii*
Providencia rettgeri	*Proteus rettgeri*	*Proteus rettgeri*	*Proteus rettgeri*

[a] Originally named *Levinea amalonatica*.

Kluyvera (formerly called "Enteric Group 8" by the Enteric Section, CDC) has been redefined as a genus (35a). *Kluyvera* occurs in clinical specimens and appears to colonize the respiratory tract (74a), and can also occur in food and water (49a). *Yersinia intermedia* and *Yersinia frederikensii* were formerly thought to be biogroups of *Y. enterocolitica*, but are distinct species by DNA-DNA hybridization (9a). The two new *Yersinia* species occur in clinical specimens and complicate the identification of true *Y. enterocolitica* strains. *Y. enterocolitica* does not ferment L-rhamnose, raffinose, or melibiose; *Y. frederiksenii* ferments L-rhamnose only, and *Y. intermedia* ferments all three. A fourth *Yersinia* species, which is otherwise very similar to true *Y. entercolitica*, has been named *Y. cristensenii*. Several other new species of *Enterobacteriaceae* have been described—*Enterobacter amnigena, Serratia fonticola, Serratia ficaria, Yersinia ruckerii*, and *Rahnella aquatilis*, and they have occasionally been isolated from clinical specimens.

Enterobacteriaceae—Topics Applicable to the Entire Family

Collection and Processing of Specimens

This subject must be considered in relation to other microorganisms that are likely to be present in specimens. Fortunately, almost all procedures designed for isolating bacterial pathogens are designed to isolate fastidious pathogens (52), insuring that *Enterobacteriaceae* will also be isolated since they survive well and grow on normal plating media. The stool culture is an exception because the procedure is designed primarily to isolate enteric pathogens such as *Salmonella-Arizona, Shigella*, and "pathogenic" *E. coli*. For most specimens, the time of collection and number required are determined by the more fastidious pathogens (52). Thus this discussion is limited to procedures particularly appropriate for *Enterobacteriaceae*.

Enterobacteriaceae can be present in almost any kind of human specimen, including blood, spinal and other body fluids, urine, feces, sputum, and wounds. Because they are also widely distributed in nature, samples from animals, food, water, sewage, soil, and the hospital environment are also likely sources. *Enterobacteriaceae* grow very rapidly which gives them an advantage over slow-growing bacteria in the human or environmental specimen. It cannot be overemphasized that specimens should be returned to the laboratory as soon as possible after collection and plated immediately. If they are not, metabolic or other inhibitory products from *Enterobacteriaceae* are likely to kill more fastidious pathogens. Similarly, fastidious pathogens can be missed on primary plates or in enrichment media because of the sheer number of *Enterobacteriaceae*. In many specimens, *Enterobacteriaceae* are a nuisance because their rapid growth obscures the true etiological agent of disease.

Blood cultures. Blood cultures are usually submitted from patients with a febrile illness of unknown origin, and current blood culture procedures are very efficient in isolating *Enterobacteriaceae* (52). A blood culture positive for *Enterobacteriaceae* is not usually difficult to interpret (as may often be the case with a coagulase-negative *Staphylococcus* or *Corynebacterium*) because they are rarely present on the skin at venipuncture sites. However, it should be remembered that sometimes they colonize the skin and can contaminate a blood culture. An occasional outbreak of "pseudobacteremia" has occurred because of an environmental contaminant introduced into the culturing procedure. *Serratia marcescens* recently caused several outbreaks of pseudobacteremia because it was growing in EDTA tubes used to collect blood (37). The distribution of *Enterobacteriaceae* in a large series (29) of significant bacteremias from England, Ireland, and Wales is shown in Table 25.3. *Escherichia coli* and *Klebsiella pneumoniae* were found in over two-thirds of the positive blood cultures, but many species were rarely or never found. This distribution will no doubt vary by type of institution and geographic location. In this series, *Serratia marcescens* was rarely found, but in the United States it is frequently isolated from blood. These figures should be used only as a rough guide. Because most positive blood cultures contain only one species of *Enterobacteriaceae*, a series of biochemical tests can be inoculated directly from a blood-culture bottle to obtain a preliminary identification. Such an identification would be delayed for 24 hr if a plated subculture were necessary. The results of biochemical tests plus colonial morphology on primary plates should allow a preliminary report 24 hr after the blood-culture bottle becomes turbid.

Spinal fluid. Culture procedures for spinal fluid (CSF) are also efficient in recovering *Enterobacteriaceae* (52). In the newborn, *E. coli* and other *Enterobacteriaceae* are frequent causes of meningitis, but they are not often isolated from meningitis patients in the 2-month to 40-year age group. However, they are found again in the elderly. Table 25.3 shows that *Neisseria meningitis*, *Haemophilus influenzae*, and *Streptococcus pneumoniae* are found much more frequently in CSF than are *Enterobacteriaceae* (29). It also emphasizes that *E. coli* is frequently isolated, in contrast to most other species of *Enterobacteriaceae*. Contamination must be considered if a CSF culture yields one of the *Enterobacteriaceae* rarely associated with meningitis.

Urine. Significant bacteriuria is usually defined as when $> 100,000$ (10^5) organisms per milliliter are present in a (clean void) midstream urine specimen. Since *Enterobacteriaceae* can grow rapidly in urine, specimens should be plated immediately or refrigerated; otherwise initial low-level contamination may give a "false-positive" result because of multiplication. Large numbers of *Enterobacteriaceae* from the feces can contaminate (to yield $> 10^5$ bacteria per ml) a urine specimen unless the perianal area is properly prepared. This is a problem in obtaining specimens from females.

Table 25.3 shows the species and their distribution in a large series (8) isolated from urine. *E. coli, K. pneumoniae,* and *P. mirabilis* most frequently cause urinary tract infections, but other species of *Enterobacteriaceae* can also occur.

Wounds. Material from a previously undrained abscess (if properly collected, transported, and plated) should yield the infecting agent in most instances (52). However, open wounds, ulcers, and sinus tracts can become colonized with endogenous bacteria and also with species found in the environment. Open wounds are frequently colonized with 3–5 species of *Enterobacteriaceae* and with 5–6 other organisms. The microbiologist must decide how many of these different colony types should be isolated and identified. Although techniques are readily available for isolating and identifying all

TABLE 25.3—RELATIVE DISTRIBUTION OF *ENTEROBACTERIACEAE* IN BLOOD, SPINAL FLUID, AND URINE CULTURES[a]

BLOOD		SPINAL FLUID		URINE	
Escherichia coli	1201 (231)[b]	Escherichia coli	64 (21)[b]	Sterile	12,033
Klebsiella pneumoniae	398 (80)	Klebsiella pneumoniae	9 (3)	E. coli	3,268
Salmonella typhi	146	Proteus mirabilis	7 (1)	K. pneumoniae	1,528
Proteus mirabilis	138 (21)	Proteus sp.	5	P. mirabilis	923
Proteus sp.	68 (14)	Enterobacter cloacae	1	Enterobacter sp.	446
Salmonella sp.	54 (15)			Proteus (indole+)	329
Enterobacter cloacae	42 (6)	No Other Enterobacteriaceae Reported		Providencia	95
Salmonella paratyphi A	35				
Salmonella typhimurium	26 (9)	Neisseria meningitidis	571 (45)		
Morganella morganii	25 (4)	Haemophilus influenzae	307 (16)		
Citrobacter freundii	19 (2)	Streptococcus pneumoniae	239 (55)		
Serratia marcescens	15 (1)				
Enterobacter aerogenes	15 (4)				
Salmonella paratyphi B	13				
Enterobacter sp.	12 (2)				
Proteus vulgaris	9 (2)				
Citrobacter diversus	4				
Hafnia alvei	2				

[a] The blood and spinal fluid isolates represent significant bacteremia and meningitis, respectively. The urine isolates were greater than 100,000/ml. Data for bacteremia and meningitis are from reference (29) and include data from England, Wales, and Ireland in 1976. Data for urinary tract infections are adapted from Blazevic, Stemper, and Matsen (8).

[b] The first number gives the number of cases; the number in parentheses gives the number of fatal cases (for blood and spinal fluid only).

of the *Enterobacteriaceae* present, reports of 5–10 different species from a wound are difficult to interpret, leading some to question whether personnel and material are being used wisely (5). Many microbiology laboratories continue to provide this information to physicians.

Respiratory tract. The clinical significance of isolates from most respiratory tract specimens is often unclear (52). *Enterobacteriaceae*, often acquired in the hospital, frequently colonize the nasopharynx and contaminate sputum specimens. Thus they often tend to be more of a diagnostic nuisance than the true agents of pneumonia. Other methods such as transtracheal aspiration, needle biopsy of the lung, needle aspiration of an abscess or empyema cavity, or open lung biopsy are more likely to yield clinically significant results (52). All *Enterobacteriaceae* from these carefully collected specimens should be isolated and identified, but opinion is still divided on how much identification to do on a specimen labeled "sputum" which contains many different species.

Stool culture. Stool cultures are usually submitted with a request to isolate and identify the cause of diarrhea. The groups of *Enterobacteriaceae* usually associated with diarrhea in the United States are *Salmonella-Arizona, Shigella*, and some pathogenic strains of *E. coli*. Table 25.4 lists all the bacteria that have been implicated as causing diarrhea and includes such groups as *Edwardsiella, Citrobacter, Proteus, Klebsiella, Enterobacter, Yersinia*, and *Serratia*. Enterotoxin-producing strains of many of the *Enterobacteriaceae* have now been isolated from people with diarrhea (85), but their etiologic role is not well established. However, it may be necessary to begin issuing reports such as *"Klebsiella pneumoniae* in pure culture (10 of 10 colonies tested)" for stool cultures. Currently, there is no evidence that these newly implicated species are *important* causes of diarrhea in the United States.

TABLE 25.4—*ENTEROBACTERIACEAE* THAT CAN CAUSE DIARRHEA

Inherent Pathogens—Most strains in these groups are *probably* able to cause diarrhea

Salmonella
Arizona
Shigella
Escherichia coli—invasive

Probable Pathogens—These strains have been implicated as the cause of diarrhea throughout the world, but may need "colonization factors" before they can cause diarrhea

Escherichia coli—toxinogenic
Escherichia coli—other pathogenic mechanisms; certain serotypes
Yersinia enterocolitica

Occasional Pathogens—Many or most strains of these groups do not usually cause diarrhea, but occasionally strains have been implicated. Enterotoxins, colonization factors, and perhaps other pathogenic mechanisms are probably involved

Edwardsiella tarda
Proteus, Providencia, Morganella
Klebsiella, Enterobacter, Serratia, Hafnia
Citrobacter

Stool cultures should be plated as soon as possible after they are collected in order to recover fastidious pathogens such as *Shigella*. If rapid processing is not possible, a small portion of the stool (0.2–0.5 g) or a swab coated with feces should be placed in a transport medium until it can be examined in the laboratory. Commonly used transport media include Stuart's, Amies, Cary Blair, and buffered-glycerol saline (32).

There are many different procedures for processing stool specimens (27, 47, 52). Most laboratories are content to isolate *Salmonella* and *Shigella*, but isolation procedures for stools should be designed to include the possible pathogens (see other chapters) listed in Table 25.4. In cases of chronic or severe diarrhea some of the rare pathogens in Table 25.4 should be considered. Table 25.5 lists the pathogens (*Enterobacteriaceae* only) most frequently isolated from feces. Specific points about the isolation and identification of *Salmonella*, *Shigella*, and *E. coli* are considered in subsequent sections.

TABLE 25.5—GROUPS OF *ENTEROBACTERIACEAE* MOST FREQUENTLY REPORTED (13) AS ENTERIC PATHOGENS IN THE UNITED STATES—1977

ORGANISM	NO. OF REPORTED CASES[a]
Shigella sonnei	10,318
Shigella flexneri	3294
Shigella boydii	210
Shigella dysenteriae	126
Salmonella typhi	549
Salmonella typhimurium	9690
Salmonella newport	2187
Salmonella heidelberg	1741
Salmonella enteritidis (1,9,12:g,m:-)	1472
Salmonella infantis	1304
Salmonella agona	1229
Salmonella saintpaul	580
Salmonella montevideo	470
Salmonella oranienburg	440
Other *Salmonella*	7800
Arizona hinshawii	NA[b]
Invasive *Escherichia coli*	NA
Enterotoxinogenic *Escherichia coli*	NA
Other *Enterobacteriaceae*	NA

[a] Includes some extratestinal infections.

[b] NA: not reportable, data not available.

Diagnostic Procedures

Microscopic Examinations

Many specimens are Gram stained and then examined under the microscope. Any gram-negative rod found on microscopic examination can be an *Enterobacteriaceae*, but it can also be any other rod-shaped species that stains gram-negative. However, Table 25.3 indicates that some species are more likely than others to be found in important specimens. For example, a gram-negative rod in a positive blood-culture bottle or spinal-fluid sediment is much more likely to be *E. coli* or *K. pneumoniae* than it is to be *Morganella morganii*. If these data are cautiously interpreted, they can be useful in arriving at a preliminary diagnosis.

Stool specimens should be examined (macroscopically) for the presence of blood and/or mucus. They can also be examined microscopically for leukocytes (64). Small flecks of mucus or stool are mixed with 0.1 ml of Loeffler methylene blue stain on a glass microscope slide. A coverslip is added, and the suspension is examined microscopically for leukocytes. Pickering et al. (64) found leukocytes more frequently in stools which were positive for *Shigella* (24 of 36 or 69% contained leukocytes) than from stools which yielded other pathogens (14%) or no pathogen (17%). None of the stools from four patients with invasive ("*Shigella*-like") *E. coli* had leukocytes. Examination for leukocytes should not be used as a substitute for culturing. The procedure is seldom used in clinical laboratories.

Definitive identification is almost always based on biochemical reactions on pure cultures rather than on microscopic examination. Although identification by fluorescent-antibody staining is theoretically possible for all species, in practice it has been limited to *Salmonella* and to certain serogroups of *E. coli*, and has not been used routinely (52). Serologic cross-reactions with other species of *Enterobacteriaceae* have limited this approach.

Inoculation of primary plates

This topic must be considered from two different points of view. Specimens, except stools, are processed for all pathogens with no particular emphasis on the *Enterobacteriaceae* (52). Culture materials such as urine, sputum, or wound specimens will be plated onto nonselective medium such as blood agar which supports growth of most bacteria and onto a medium such as MacConkey agar [interchangeable throughout this chapter with eosine methylene blue agar (EMB)] which permits growth and some differentiation of *Enterobacteriaceae* and other nonfastidious gram-negative rods. With a few exceptions, *Enterobacteriaceae* will grow on most plating media and form 1- to 3-mm diameter colonies within 18–24 hr.

Identification

There are many different approaches to identifying *Enterobacteriaceae*. In 1968 there was a roundtable—"How Far to Go With the *Enterobacteriaceae*?" (69). Ten years ago the answer was less complicated than today because the basic question was "Which and how many conventional biochemical tests are needed for identification?" Today there are many more methods available (78).

Microbiology laboratories are usually requested to isolate and identify the etiologic agent(s) present in specimens and to determine their susceptibilities to antibiotics. This information would be most useful when the specimen is submitted rather than 2–4 days later. Until a laboratory report is issued, treatment of the patient must be based on clinical and epidemiologic findings. Physicians complain that laboratory results often come too late to benefit the patient. Therefore, preliminary reports (based on limited identification) which occasionally must be modified are more valuable than complete, correct reports which come too late to benefit the patient.

Identification 4–13 hr after the specimen is taken. Until recently the only approaches were to plate the specimen and wait 18–24 hr until bacteria formed visible colonies. It was virtually impossible to obtain identifications before this time. Recently the Auto Microbic System was introduced by Vitek Systems Inc. (595 Anglum Drive, Hazelwood, MO 63042), which partially identifies bacteria in urine without isolating them on plating media. The urine is pipetted into two chambers of a plastic sample holder, diluted, and placed in identification wells. Nine of the wells contain selective media for the five groups of *Enterobacteriaceae* and four other groups most frequently found in urine (*Proteus* spp., *Citrobacter freundii*, *Serratia* spp., *Escherichia coli*, *Klebsiella-Enterobacter*, *Pseudomonas aeruginosa*, yeasts, Group D enterococcus, and *Staphylococcus aureus*). The machine can identify the groups and also give a count of the total number of organisms in the urine. Positive identifications are available within 4–13 hr after inoculation (results for *Enterobacteriaceae* are usually obtained rapidly). Negative results can be reported 13 hr after inoculation. The Auto Microbic System is expensive to purchase and has some advantages and disadvantages. The same technology has been developed for determining antimicrobial susceptibilities, and the system was designed so that it will eventually accommodate other specimens such as sputum, throat swabs, feces, blood, and spinal fluid.

Identification 18–24 hr after specimen is taken. Two different approaches are available. In the first the specimen is plated on different agars and incubated for 18–24 hr until isolated colonies are visible. Two plating media normally used are blood agar and MacConkey agar. Most pathogens grow on the blood agar, but most of the organisms which grow on MacConkey are *Enterobacteriaceae*. *E. coli*, *Klebsiella*, *Enterobacter*, and *P. mirabilis* grown on blood agar, and on MacConkey agar they often have characteristic morphology (Table 25.6) so that a presumptive identification can often be made from their appearance alone.

A report such as "Preliminary Report: *Escherichia coli* present—500,000 organisms/ml" can usually be issued 18–24 hr after the specimen is received. Some laboratories go no further in identifying typical strains of *E. coli*, *K. pneumoniae*, or *P. mirabilis*. Others do various "spot tests" that can be completed the same day to confirm the presumptive identification.

A second identification or partial identification method requiring 18–24 hr is the "specimen culture kit." These commercial products vary in design, but basically incorporate one or more differential media to allow some identification. Most of these kits were designed for urine cultures and give an approximate count of the number of bacteria present and a presumptive identification. The kits probably are most appropriately used in a doctor's office, where otherwise no microbiology would be done.

Identification at 48 hr. This approach seems to be the most popular in hospital laboratories, and also seems the most likely to yield a correct identification; unfortunately, it comes 2 days after the specimen was submitted. A presumptive report based on the organism's appearance on plating media can still be issued at 24 hr and a final identification at 48 hr. One isolated colony of each predominant colony type is picked and used to inoculate a series of biochemical reactions. These reactions can be done with conventional tube tests (27) or with one of the "identification kits" (78) which are commercially available for *Enterobacteriaceae*. The biochemical reactions are incubated for 6–24 hr at 36 C (all reactions given in this chapter are at 36 ± 1 C unless otherwise stated), and the organism is identified on the basis of the reactions. As the number of tests increases, both the likelihood of a correct identification and the cost increase (5).

These examples of methods for identifying organisms illustrate the many different approaches available to the microbiologist. Some are discussed in more detail below.

Conventional biochemical tests in tubes. Until recently this approach was used by almost all clinical and public health microbiology laboratories. Biochemical tests media are prepared, dispensed into glass tubes, and sterilized (27). Although many laboratories prepare their own, most media are also available commercially. Growth from one colony is inoculated into each of the tubes. The tubes are incubated, and the reactions are read at 24 hr (or kept up to 7 days by reference laboratories). An updated chart which contains data for the newly described species can be obtained by writing JJF. Unfortunately, the media and the tests are not well-standardized, and few laboratories use the same tests. Even with so many variables, this approach usually results in correct identification of the more common species of *Enterobacteriaceae*. Figure

TABLE 25.6—APPEARANCE OF THE MOST COMMON *ENTEROBACTERIACEAE* ON BLOOD AGAR AND MACCONKEY AGAR

ORGANISM	MACCONKEY AGAR	BLOOD AGAR
E. coli (Lac$^+$)	Red, usually surrounded with precipitated bile	Smooth 2–3 mm
K. pneumoniae	Pink, mucoid, 3–4 mm	Usually mucoid, 3–4 mm
P. mirabilis } *P. vulgaris* }	Colorless, flat, may swarm slightly	Usually swarms to cover plate
Enterobacter	Pink, not usually as mucoid as *Klebsiella*	Smooth, 3–4 mm
Other *Proteus-Providencia-Morganella*	Colorless, flat, no swarming	Flat, 2–3 mm, no swarming
Salmonella and *Shigella*	Colorless, flat	Smooth 2–3 mm

Figure 25.1. Biochemical reactions of *Enterobacteriaceae* at 48 hr (most occur within 24 hr) in some commonly used.

Organism	1. INDOLE	2. METHYL RED	3. VP	4. CITRATE (SIM.)	5. H₂S-TSI	6. UREA	7. PHENYLALANINE	8. LYSINE	9. ARGININE
PROVIDENCIA ALCALIFACIENS	+	+	−	+	−	−	+	−	−
PROVIDENCIA STUARTII	+	+	−	+	−	⊕	⊕	−	−
PROVIDENCIA RETTGERI	+	⊕	−	+	−	+	+	−	−
MORGANELLA MORGANII	+	+	−	−	−	+	+	−	−
PROTEUS MIRABILIS	−	+	⊕	59	+	⊕	+	−	−
PROTEUS VULGARIS	+	⊕	−	⊕	+	+	+	−	−
SERRATIA RUBIDAEA	−	31	⊕	⊕	−	−	−	61	−
SERRATIA LIQUEFACIENS	−	64	49	⊕	−	−	−	64	−
SERRATIA MARCESCENS	−	⊕	+	+	−	⊕	−	+	−
HAFNIA ALVEI	−	54	65	−	−	−	−	+	⊕
ENTEROBACTER GERGOVIAE	−	36	+	+	−	+	−	64	−
ENTEROBACTER SAKAZAKII	⊕	22	+	+	−	−	50	−	+
ENTEROBACTER AGGLOMERANS	⊕	45	68	67	−	28	28	−	−
ENTEROBACTER AEROGENES	−	−	+	+	−	−	−	+	−
ENTEROBACTER CLOACAE	−	−	+	+	−	65	−	−	+
KLEBSIELLA RHINOSCLEROMATIS	−	+	−	−	−	−	−	−	−
KLEBSIELLA OZAENAE	−	+	−	32	−	⊕	−	48	⊕
KLEBSIELLA OXYTOCA	+	⊕	+	+	−	+	−	+	−
KLEBSIELLA PNEUMONIAE	−	⊕	+	+	−	+	−	+	−
CITROBACTER DIVERSUS	+	+	−	+	−	78	−	−	60
CITROBACTER AMALONATICUS	+	+	−	⊕	−	⊕	−	−	77
CITROBACTER FREUNDII	−	+	−	⊕	⊕	69	−	−	44
ARIZONA HINSHAWII	−	+	−	+	+	−	−	+	⊕
SALMONELLA ENTERITIDIS	−	+	−	⊕	+	−	−	⊕	65
SALMONELLA CHOLERAE-SUIS	−	+	−	−	60	−	−	⊕	−
SALMONELLA TYPHI	−	+	−	+	−	−	−	+	⊕
EDWARDSIELLA TARDA	+	+	−	−	+	−	−	+	−
SHIGELLA SONNEI	−	+	−	−	−	−	−	−	−
SHIGELLA BOYDII	29	+	−	−	−	−	−	−	⊕
SHIGELLA FLEXNERI (SEROTYPE 6)	−	+	−	−	−	−	−	−	−
SHIGELLA FLEXNERI (SEROTYPE 1-5)	62	+	−	−	−	−	−	−	49
SHIGELLA DYSENTERIAE	44	+	−	−	−	−	−	−	−
ESCHERICHIA COLI (INACTIVE)	⊕	+	−	−	−	−	−	⊕	44
ESCHERICHIA COLI (ACTIVE)	+	+	−	−	−	−	−	⊕	⊕

Figure 25.1 continued

BIOCHEMICAL TEST	Escherichia coli (Active)	Escherichia coli (Inactive)	Shigella dysenteriae	Shigella flexneri (Serotype 1-5)	Shigella flexneri (Serotype 6)	Shigella boydii	Shigella sonnei	Edwardsiella tarda	Salmonella typhi	Salmonella choleraE-suis	Salmonella enteritidis	Arizona hinshawii	Citrobacter freundii	Citrobacter amalonaticus	Citrobacter diversus	Klebsiella pneumoniae	Klebsiella oxytoca	Klebsiella ozanae	Klebsiella rhinoscleromatis	Enterobacter cloacae	Enterobacter aerogenes	Enterobacter agglomerans	Enterobacter sakazakii	Enterobacter gergoviae	Hafnia alvei	Serratia marcescens	Serratia liquefaciens	Serratia rubidaea	Proteus vulgaris	Proteus mirabilis	Morganella morganii	Providencia rettgeri	Providencia stuartii	Providencia alcalifaciens
10. ORNITHINE	63	⊖	−	−	−	−	+	+	−	+	+	+	⊖	+	+	−	−	−	−	+	+	−	+	+	+	+	+	−	−	+	+	−	+	−
11. MOTILITY	70	−	−	−	−	−	−	+	+	+	+	+	+	+	⊕	−	−	−	−	+	+	⊕	⊕	+	⊕	+	⊕	⊕	+	+	⊕	+	⊕	+
12. GELATIN-22C	−	−	−	−	−	−	−	−	−	−	−	−	−	−	−	−	+	⊕	−	−	−	34	−	−	−	⊕	+	22	⊕	⊕	−	−	−	−
13. KCN	−	−	−	⊖	−	−	−	−	−	−	−	⊖	⊕	⊕	⊕	+	+	+	+	80	⊕	62	⊕	−	+	⊕	⊕	⊕	+	+	+	+	+	+
14. MALONATE	+	+	−	+	+	−	−	−	−	−	−	+	⊕	+	+	+	+	+	+	+	+	+	+	+	⊕	−	−	+	−	−	+	+	+	+
15. D-GLUCOSE-ACID	+	+	+	+	+	+	+	+	+	+	+	+	+	+	+	+	+	+	+	+	+	+	+	+	+	+	+	+	+	+	+	+	+	+
16. D-GLUCOSE-GAS	⊕	⊕	−	⊕	⊖	+	−	+	−	+	+	⊕	⊕	+	⊕	+	+	+	−	+	⊕	+	+	⊕	+	−	+	+	⊕	⊕	−	⊕	−	⊕
17. LACTOSE	51	⊖	−	−	−	−	−	−	−	−	−	61	39	74	33	+	+	64	−	+	+	41	+	42	−	−	73	+	−	−	−	−	−	−
18. SUCROSE	+	⊖	−	⊖	⊖	−	−	−	−	−	−	⊖	⊕	⊖	+	+	+	24	68	+	+	77	+	+	⊖	+	⊕	+	⊕	⊕	−	⊕	⊕	⊕
19. D-MANNITOL	+	38	+	+	83	+	+	+	+	+	+	+	+	+	+	+	+	+	+	+	+	62	+	+	+	+	+	+	+	−	+	⊕	+	+
20. DULCITOL	37	−	−	−	−	−	−	−	+	+	+	+	60	44	53	+	+	59	+	28	+	64	+	+	−	−	⊕	+	+	−	−	−	−	−
21. SALICIN	−	−	−	−	−	−	−	+	−	−	−	−	−	−	⊖	⊕	+	78	+	21	+	⊕	⊖	+	−	+	⊕	+	+	+	−	+	⊖	⊕
22. ADONITOL	+	⊖	−	−	−	+	−	−	+	−	−	+	−	−	53	+	+	+	+	+	+	⊖	⊕	+	−	+	⊖	+	−	−	−	⊖	⊖	⊖
23. I-INOSITOL	−	−	−	−	−	−	−	−	−	−	38	−	−	−	⊖	⊕	+	+	+	+	+	⊖	+	−	−	+	⊕	⊕	+	−	−	+	+	+
24. D-SORBITOL	⊕	29	−	31	30	42	⊕	−	+	+	+	+	+	+	+	+	+	−	+	+	+	24	72	+	+	56	+	⊕	+	+	−	+	−	−
25. L-ARABINOSE	65	43	−	54	65	54	+	−	+	+	+	+	+	+	+	+	+	+	+	+	+	+	+	−	−	79	64	−	+	−	−	⊕	+	+
26. RAFFINOSE	54	−	−	53	−	−	⊖	−	−	−	⊖	+	⊖	+	−	+	+	60	68	+	+	25	+	+	+	−	⊕	+	−	−	−	⊕	+	−
27. L-RHAMNOSE	62	74	77	−	−	−	−	+	+	+	⊖	⊕	+	+	+	+	+	60	68	⊕	+	⊕	+	+	⊕	−	⊖	+	⊖	−	−	68	−	−

All Results are at 24 or 48 Hours, and are at 36 ± 1 C. (Except Gelatin). Symbols: + = 95% or More of Strains in Taxon are Positive; ⊕ = 80–94.9% Positive; − = 0 to 5% Positive; ⊖ = 5.1 to 20% Positive; Numerals Represent the % Positive. Reactions Positive after 2 Days are not Considered. A more recent chart may be obtained by writing JJF.

25.1 shows the results obtained with the commonly used biochemical tests for some groups of *Enterobacteriaceae*. These data come from the records of the Enteric Section at the Center for Disease Control (CDC) and are based on standard methods described in Chapter 46 of this book. Although other methods may also yield satisfactory results, we caution the reader not to assume that comparable percentages will be obtained with them.

Often we are asked "How many tests are needed to identify *Enterobacteriaceae* correctly?" There is no single answer to this question. Before it can be answered, another question must be asked and answered—"What is the acceptable percentage of incorrect identifications?" Because reference centers must strive for 100% accuracy in identification, 25–50 biochemical tests are done on each culture sent for identification. Other helpful information can be obtained from staining reactions, growth on different media, genus- or species-specific tests, antimicrobial susceptibility patterns, serological typing, and computer analysis. Reference laboratories are not required to obtain results as rapidly as are primary laboratories and can work for 100% accuracy with essentially no time or cost restraints. Obviously a busy hospital microbiology laboratory cannot afford to spend that much time and effort on identification. Most laboratories have developed their own flow charts or abbreviated differentiation charts for identification (5, 69). Since a few species of *Enterobacteriaceae* represent 95%–98% of all those found in clinical specimens, such shortcuts yield acceptable results most of the time. Misidentifications do occur when these schemes are used, because of the biochemical similarity of some species.

"Kits" for identifying Enterobacteriaceae. A "kit" is defined as a series of miniaturized or standardized tests available commercially. A single colony is picked (in some kits additional processing is required) and inoculated into the test system. Samples are incubated, read, and the results are used in making an identification. This approach is similar to the conventional tube method, with the main difference being in the miniaturization, the number of tests available, and the method of analyzing results. Kits have been adopted by over half the U.S. laboratories.

Limited space does not allow discussion of the kits available. However, an excellent review of the kits is available without charge (reference 78; address requests to: Center for Disease Control, Attn: Dr. Peter B. Smith, Bldg. 5, Rm. 210, 1600 Clifton Road, Atlanta, GA 30333). Three basic designs for the kits are:

Design 1—Enterotube and r/b. The Enterotube II (Roche Diagnostic Division, Hoffman-LaRoche, Inc., Nutley, NJ 07110) has 12 compartments in a plastic tube and contains a built-in inoculating needle. An isolated colony is touched with the needle, which is then pulled through the tube to inoculate all the media. The r/b system (Corning Diagnostic, 25 Lumber Road, Roslyn, Long Island, NY 11576) consists of four glass tubes incorporating 14 different biochemical tests. The tubes are inoculated with a straight wire (not furnished) from an isolated colony. Any combination of the tubes could conceivably be used.

Design 2—API and Inolex. In this approach a fixed number of dehydrated substrates which represent some of the more commonly used biochemical tests are used. The API 20E (Analytab Products, Inc., 200 Express Street, Plainview, NY 11803) has 20 plastic cupules which allows 21 or 22 biochemical reactions. The API 10E has 10 cupules in which 11 biochemical tests are done, and the API 50 allows 50 biochemical tests to be done. The Inolex Enteric (Inolex Corporation, 3 Science Road, Glenwood, IL 60425) consists of a plastic card with 20 biochemical tests. A new version called Enteric 20 has 20 tests on one card. With both, a suspension of the culture is inoculated into the cupules with a Pasteur pipette, and the test results are read at the end of the incubation period.

Design 3—Minitec and Pathotec. This approach allows the microbiologist to choose the biochemical tests. Minitec (Bioquest, Cockeysville, MD 21030) consists of a plastic tray and disks impregnated with the biochemical substrates. The user chooses the set of biochemical test disks and inoculates them simultaneously into the plastic tray with a disk-dispenser provided. A colony is suspended in broth and then dispensed into each well of the tray. The Patho-Tec system (General Diagnostic Division, Warner-Lambert Company, Morris Plains, NJ 07950) consists of reagent impregnated paper strips which are placed in small test tubes containing pure cultures of the organism.

Newer "kits" for the identification of *Enterobacteriaceae* include the AIM-4 system (Axford International Inc., P.O. Box 11567, Denver, CO 80211), which is based on conventional media (separated by a plastic divider) in petri dishes. The Micro-ID System (General Diagnostics, Division of Lambert Co., Morris Plains, NJ 07950) provides an identification after 4 hr of incubation in 15 tests (heavy inoculum required). Unlike most systems, it does not require growth of the bacteria in the test compartments. The Micro-Media Quad Enteric Panel (Micro-Media Systems, Inc., San Jose, California) utilizes 20 "standard biochemical" tests in small volumes within a plastic microculture plate, but is otherwise similar to standard biochemical tests previously described (the difference being the miniaturization).

Table 25.7 summarizes some of the characteristics of the kits. Probably the best way to evaluate kits is to use and compare them in the laboratory. The published evaluations are helpful, but personal preferences based on a particular laboratory's needs will probably determine the kit chosen.

Serological Procedures

Isolates. There are two different applications for serological methods on patient isolates. The first is using sera to aid in identification (*Salmonella* and *Shigella* polyvalent sera are examples). Sera can be formulated which agglutinate members of a certain species or serotype but seldom agglutinate other groups of *Enterobacteriaceae*. The second application consists of using antisera to divide a species into serogroups, which can be useful in epidemiologic analysis. These applications are discussed in the appropriate sections.

Serum. The *Enterobacteriaceae* are usually easy to isolate, so this technique is not often used. The one exception is in typhoid fever patients where agglutinating antibodies are often measured. The topic is covered in the *Salmonella-Arizona* section.

TABLE 25.7—CHARACTERISTICS OF SIX BACTERIAL IDENTIFICATION SYSTEMS (78)

| | SYSTEM | | | | | |
PARAMETER	API	ENTERO-TUBE	INOLEX	MINITEK	MICRO ID	R/B
Usual number tests	21	15	20	Variable[a]	15	14[b]
Ease of inoculation;[c] 1 = easiest	2.5	1	3	4	2	1
Manipulation required[c] after incubation; 1 = easiest	3	2	2	3	1	1
Incubation time (hr)	18–24	18–24	18–24	18–24	4	18–24
Versatility;[c] 1 = most	3	4	3	1	2.5	3
Numeric or computer assisted identification available	Yes	Yes	Yes	Yes	Yes	Yes[d]
Conventional media (C) or dried substrate (D)	D	C	D	D	D	C

[a] Any combination of 35 available tests can be used.

[b] Four different tubes are available; 14 tests can be done if all 4 tubes are used.

[c] Based on a subjective scale of 1 to 5.

[d] An electronic device called the "Enteric Analyzer" is also available to assist the identification.

There is another situation in which a patient's serologic response can be useful. Often a clinical specimen yields an isolate of *Enterobacteriaceae* which may or may not be causing infection. If the patient's antibody response is elevated, there is presumptive evidence that the isolate is causing disease. This technique has been used extensively by Neter (60) in his studies on the clinical relevance of *Enterobacteriaceae*. The technique is not used routinely in clinical laboratories but could be used in defining the role of a particular isolate or new species. All serologic results concerning *Enterobacteriaceae* should be interpreted cautiously because it is well-known that antigens are widely shared in the family (27, 47).

Marker systems

Sometimes an organism must be typed to aid in an epidemiologic study. Serotyping is often used because it has several advantages. However, serotyping is not always the method of choice. *Shigella sonnei*, for example, cannot be divided into further serologic types (58). In this and similar instances typing methods, briefly described below, may be used.

1) *Biotyping*. Simple phenotypic properties are determined such as fermentation of D-xylose, production of indole, and growth at 45 C. The procedures can be done in conventional test tubes or with one of the prepackaged kit systems.
2) *Bacteriophage typing*. A standard set of bacteriophages is applied to a series of isolates to determine similarities or differences in their lysis

patterns. Bacteriophage typing of *Enterobacteriaceae* was recently reviewed by Schmidt and Jeffries (74).

3) *Bacteriocin production or bacteriocin sensitivity.* Bacteriocins are inhibitory substances produced by one species which kill or inhibit other strains of the same species. Typing by bacteriocin sensitivity is comparable to bacteriophage typing except that a standard set of bacteriocins is used for typing. When bacteriocin production is used for typing, a strain is grown under such conditions that it produces bacteriocins, which are then tested against a standard set of indicator strains. Bacteriocin typing of several *Enterobacteriaceae* was recently reviewed (36).

Problem strains

Most strains of *Enterobacteriaceae* grow readily on plating media, but there are exceptions. Some strains grow poorly on blood agar but grow much better on chocolate agar incubated in a candle jar. This fact suggests a possible nutritional requirement or a mutation involved with respiration. There are slow-growing strains of *E. coli, K. pneumoniae,* and *Serratia,* but such a metabolic change might occur in any species. Biochemical reactions usually require several days of additional incubation before a typical pattern is obtained and a correct identification possible. A second type of "sluggish" organism is often seen in specimens from patients who have been given antimicrobial agents. Li et al. described such "pleiotropic" mutants in *Serratia marcescens* (53) and *Salmonella.* These strains react atypically in many of the standard biochemical tests and are hard to identify. *Enterobacteriaceae* can lose the ability to transport and catabolize glucose and thus become (by definition) nonfermentative, gram-negative rods. Unfortunately, we do not know how often this change occurs.

Laboratories often isolate strains which grow rapidly but whose biochemical reactions do not fit any of the described species of *Enterobacteriaceae.* At present these cultures can only be reported as "unidentified." In time, the organisms will probably be named as new species which can then be routinely identified (10). By the year 2000, there may be over 200 species of *Enterobacteriaceae,* but most of the newly identified species will rarely be found in clinical specimens. As more data are obtained from taxonomic studies, our identification schemes will have to be modified. An example of this change is the proposal (Table 25.1) to reclassify Penner's Biogroup 5 of *Proteus rettgeri* as *Providencia stuartii* urea$^+$ (38). Although such taxonomic changes are inconvenient, they are indicated for many different reasons (10).

Susceptibility to Antimicrobial Agents

When antibiotics were first introduced, there was only slight resistance among the *Enterobacteriaceae;* however, their resistance has increased. Many strains of *Enterobacteriaceae* isolated from human disease are now antibiotic resistant. There are two different kinds of antibiotic resistance.

Intrinsic resistance. Intrinsic resistance is a genetic property of most strains of a species and evolved long before antibiotic usage by man. Intrinsic resistance can best be shown by studying strains that were isolated and stored in a culture collection before the "antibiotic era." Another way is to study strains from nature that have not been exposed (presumably) to antibiotics. A third way is to collect a large number of strains from a wide variety of sources and study those that have the most sensitive patterns. Table 25.8 illustrates how these approaches have been used to define intrinsic resistance in *Serratia marcescens*. All strains apparently have intrinsic resistance to penicillin G, colistin, and cephalothin. Table 25.9 lists other species of *Enterobacteriaceae* and their resistance patterns.

Nonintrinsic resistance. The middle three isolates shown in Table 25.8 are more antibiotic resistant than those from nature or culture collections. Their additional resistance is probably due to the selective pressure of antibiotic usage in the hospital, a phenomenon which has been well documented in many bacterial species. Many strains of *Enterobacteriaceae* that cause disease have become highly antibiotic resistant through the evolutionary selective pressure of antibiotic usage by man. Genetic studies have shown that much of this antibiotic resistance is plasmid mediated.

The antibiogram as a marker in epidemiologic studies. Antibiotic susceptibility tests are usually done on isolates which are clinically significant, providing an "antibiogram" which can be very useful in comparing isolates in epidemiological studies. When the selective ecologic pressure of antibiotics is changed, the resistance patterns of epidemic (or endemic) strains often change also. These changes have been documented in outbreaks of extended duration (73). Even with these limitations in genetic stability, the antibiogram is one of the most useful laboratory markers in investigating infection problems caused by resistant strains.

TABLE 25.8—ANTIBIOTIC SUSCEPTIBILITIES OF *SERRATIA MARCESCENS*
TAKEN FROM DIFFERENT SOURCES

STRAIN[a]	SOURCE	ZONE SIZE (MM) AGAINST:											
		CL[b]	NA	SD	GM	S	K	TE	C	P	AM	CB	CF
TEV 1	Natural Water, Soil,	7	27	27	23	19	24	17	23	6	15	29	6
TEV 11	Culture Collections	7	26	24	22	19	24	14	26	6	15	26	6
ALE 1		6	25	26	20	18	21	13	25	6	18	24	6
SM 11	Sporadic Cases in	9	6	6	26	12	27	6	19	6	8	23	6
SM 94	Hospitals	6	25	19	23	19	25	6	20	6	6	6	6
SM 41		9	27	19	24	21	27	17	24	6	6	8	6
1680–74	Hospital Outbreaks	6	6	6	23	6	15	6	6	6	6	6	6
5743–72		8	6	6	8	6	6	6	6	6	6	6	6
3377–73		6	29	6	6	6	6	7	6	6	6	6	6

[a] These 9 strains are examples and were chosen from a much larger series (37).

[b] Symbols: CL = colistin, NA = nalidixic acid, SD = sulfadiazine, GM = gentamicin, S = streptomycin, K = kanamycin, TE = tetracycline, C = chloramphenicol, P = penicillin G, Am = ampicillin, CB = carbenicillin, CF = cephalothin

The method used was the standardized (high-potency) single disk method (Kirby-Bauer).

TABLE 25.9—INTRINSIC ANTIMICROBIAL RESISTANCE IN *ENTEROBACTERIACEAE*[a]

SPECIES	MOST STRAINS RESISTANT TO:
Citrobacter freundii	Cepholothin
Citrobacter diversus	Ampicillin, Carbenicillin
Edwardsiella tarda	Colistin
Enterobacter cloacae	Cephalothin
Enterobacter aerogenes	Cephalothin
Hafnia alvei	Cephalothin
Klebsiella pneumoniae	Ampicillin, Carbenicillin
Proteus mirabilis	Polymyxins, Tetracycline, Nitrofurantoin
Proteus vulgaris	Polymyxins, Ampicillin, Cephalothin, Nitrofurantoin
Morganella morganii	Polymyxins, Ampicillin, Cephalothin
Providencia rettgeri	Polymyxins, Cephalothin, Nitrofurantoin, Tetracycline
Other *Providencia*[b]	Polymyxins, Nitrofurantoin
Serratia marcescens[c]	Polymyxins, Cephalothin, Nitrofurantoin

[a] Adapted from von Graevenitz (84).

[b] Most strains of *Providencia stuartii* are also resistant to cephalothin and tetracycline.

[c] *Serratia marcescens* can also have intrinsic resistance to ampicillin, carbenicillin, streptomycin, and tetracycline.

Enterobacteriaceae—The Opportunistic Pathogens

Causative Organisms

At one time or another all of the species of *Enterobacteriaceae* have been incriminated in human disease (27). In the last 30 years our attitude has changed drastically toward "opportunistic" *Enterobacteriaceae*. Members of *Escherichia, Proteus, Providencia, Citrobacter, Klebsiella, Enterobacter, Hafnia,* and *Serratia* are now known to be leading causes of nosocomial infections (infections acquired during hospitalization), and many laboratories now identify all *Enterobacteriaceae* to the species level.

Clinical Manifestations, Epidemiology, and Public Health Importance

Although certain types of infections, such as those of the lower respiratory tract caused by *Klebsiella pneumoniae* have been recognized for many years, the fact that many species of *Enterobacteriaceae* are nosocomial pathogens has been learned only relatively recently. Before antimicrobial therapy was available, most life-threatening infections were acquired outside hospitals. Overshadowed were the proportionately smaller number of patients who acquired nosocomial infections. Most nosocomial infections in the preantibiotic era were caused by *Staphylococcus* or *Streptococcus.*

During the 1950s, both the place in which serious infections were acquired and the types of causative organisms isolated shifted (67). With effective antimicrobial therapy available for many community-acquired infections such as those caused by gram-positive cocci and *Mycobacterium tuberculosis,* relatively fewer patients entered the hospital with a serious infection. In contrast, proportionately more patients developed nosocomial infections, and instead of *Staphylococcus aureus* causing most of these infections, hospitalized patients frequently were infected by *Enterobacteriaceae* and *Pseudomonas aeruginosa*. Some *Enterobacteriaceae,* such a *Serratia marcescens,* which had previously been believed to be benign saphrophytes, were actually causing serious disease.

This shift in the place where serious infections were acquired and in the agents known to cause nosocomial infections was primarily the result of the interplay of advances in medical therapy during the 1950s. Increasing antibiotic usage which led to the development of antibiotic-resistant strains of *Enterobacteriaceae* was probably instrumental in the evolutionary process which continues today. Simultaneous progress in other forms of treatment was also a factor because it gave rise to a population of patients within hospitals who were frequently more susceptible to infection than patients in general had been in the past. Therapy for serious illnesses such as leukemia, diabetes, and pulmonary and renal diseases resulted in a population of patients who were often debilitated by the effects of chronic disorders or treatment for them and were thus susceptible to a superimposed infection. Such medications as corticosteroids, immunosuppressive therapy, and antineoplastic drugs which suppress host defenses were introduced during this period. Treatment with these agents tends to facilitate colonization and subsequent infection, often with gram-negative organisms from the patient's own bacterial flora. Invasive procedures, such as bladder catheterization, assisted ventilation, and intravascular catheterization were also used more often in routine supportive care. These procedures disrupt local epithelial barriers and provide access for invading microorganisms.

Although these changes in medical therapy led to decreased resistance to infection in the patient, the *Enterobacteriaceae* were intrinsically well adapted to become nosocomial pathogens. They are ubiquitous organisms which have numerous potential reservoirs within hospitals. As part of the animate environment (patients and personnel), the *Enterobacteriaceae* normally inhabit the large bowel and less consistently the vagina and pharynx. They are sometimes part of the transient flora of normal skin and can frequently be cultured from the hands of hospital personnel. Another reservoir which is sometimes overlooked in hospital outbreaks is the colonized or infected patient.

In the inanimate environment, the *Enterobacteriaceae* can survive and often multiply in aqueous solutions. They can contaminate (37) intravenous fluids (especially those containing glucose), parenteral medications, irrigating solutions, and even some antiseptics solutions containing hexachlorophene. In fact, gram-negative bacteria can spread so readily in the hospital environment that it may be difficult to determine whether an inanimate reservoir is a primary source of infectious organisms or has become secondarily contaminated, as is often the case with countertops or sink drains in patient-care areas. Routine cultures of the animate or inanimate environment in the absence of a specific patient infection problem are therefore, with few exceptions, unlikely to provide meaningful information and are generally considered to be a waste of infection control resources.

The number of nosocomial infections caused by *Enterobacteriaceae* can only be estimated. Approximately 7% of hospitalized patients develop nosocomial infections, with published rates ranging from 3.5% to 15%. However, no standardized "acceptable" level of nosocomial infections has been set. Nosocomial infection rates vary with the type and size of the hospital; the characteristics of the patient population; the number of acute-care beds; the number and type of surgical procedures performed; the definitions used to distinguish infection from colonization and, particularly, nosocomial from community-acquired infections; the scope and activity of the surveillance program in each institution; and other factors. Through a consistent ongoing program of surveillance each hospital should establish its own baseline nosocomial infection rate.

When a patient develops a nosocomial infection, the potential problem is quite serious. Nosocomial infections are most often acquired by those patients who are least able to tolerate them: the very old, the very young, and the very ill. It has been estimated that each nosocomial infection increases the duration of hospital stay for that patient by an average of 7 days. Besides the increased morbidity and mortality associated with nosocomial infections, the yearly monetary costs associated with them in the United States are in the billions of dollars.

Almost half of all nosocomial infections are caused by *Enterobacteriaceae*. Table 25.10 shows the percentage of nosocomial infections caused by individ-

TABLE 25.10—NOSOCOMIAL INFECTIONS BY SITE OF INFECTION AND PATHOGEN

	SITE OF INFECTION:					
INFECTING ORGANISM	URI-NARY TRACT	POST-OPERATIVE WOUNDS, OTHER CUTANEOUS SITES, AND BURNS	LOWER RESPIRA-TORY TRACT	PRIMARY BACTER-EMIA	ALL OTHER SITES	INFECTIONS CAUSED BY INDIVIDUAL ORGANISMS (%)
Escherichia coli	15.6[b]	4.5	1.1	0.7	0.9	22.8
Klebsiella-Enterobacter-Hafnia	5.7	2.4	2.7	0.7	0.6	12.1
Serratia	1.0	0.4	0.4	0.1	0.2	2.1
Proteus-Providencia-Morganella	4.8	1.9	0.8	0.2	0.4	8.1
Pseudomonas	5.7	2.3	1.7	0.3	0.4	10.4
Staphylococcus aureus	0.5	8.2	2.0	0.6	1.4	12.7
All Other Gram-Positive Cocci	7.0	3.8	1.1	0.9	1.0	13.8
Anaerobes & Fungi	2.8	2.2	0.6	0.7	1.6	7.9
All Other Organisms	2.2	3.0	2.8	0.5	1.6	10.1
Infections at individual sites	45.3	28.5	13.4	4.7	8.1	100

[a] Data are taken from the National Nosocomial Infection Study, Center for Disease Control, 1976.

[b] Each number represents the percent of nosocomial infections by an organism at a given site.

ual pathogens by site of infection. These data were obtained in the National Nosocomial Infection Study (NNIS), an ongoing nationwide surveillance program in U.S. hospitals. The sample consists of 83 hospitals which voluntarily participate and submit monthly information according to a standardized protocol on sites of nosocomial infection, hospital service involved, and organisms isolated.

In 1976 the overall nosocomial infection rate reported by NNIS hospitals was 3.6 infections per 100 patient discharges, which may underestimate the true infection rate by as much as 30%. Gram-negative rods (excluding anaerobes) were associated with 56% of all infections. Of this 56%, 82% (or 45% of all infections) were caused by *Enterobacteriaceae*. The most frequently encountered nosocomial pathogen was *E. coli*, although *Klebsiella* and *Enterobacter* were most often associated with nosocomial infections of the lower respiratory tract.

Both NNIS and other hospitals report that the urinary tract is the most common site of nosocomial infection, accounting for approximately 45% of all such infections (Table 25.10). Most nosocomial urinary tract infections are caused by the *Enterobacteriaceae*, particularly *E. coli*. Of the hospitalized patients who develop a urinary tract infection, approximately 75% have had some type of urologic manipulation. Bladder catheterization is most frequently involved, although other forms of manipulation such as cystoscopy are important as well. An indwelling catheter is more likely to lead to a urinary tract infection than is a single, short-term catheterization. However, the risk of infection with an indwelling catheter can be substantially reduced by maintaining a continuously closed sterile drainage system, rather than having an open system or one which is frequently opened and irrigated (50).

Organisms that cause urinary tract infections in hospitalized patients with catheters enter the bladder in several different ways. If organisms are present in the urethra they can be carried into the bladder on the catheter as it is inserted. Similarly, bacteria which are present in the perianal area probably enter the bladder, through the thin fluid space between the catheter and urethral mucosa. Additionally, if the catheter collecting system is contaminated, bacteria can ascend into the bladder through the catheter (50).

A substantial proportion of community-acquired and nosocomial urinarytract infections caused by *E. coli* are caused by (16) O-antigen groups O4, O6, and O75. Strains of these serogroups colonize the large bowel and often cause infection autogenously, that is, because they are indigenous to the patient's own flora. There is a higher prevalence of these serogroups in stools of hospitalized patients than in stools of individuals in the community. Hospital personnel have a colonization rate similar to that of patients. A similar situation exists with urinary tract infections caused by *Klebsiella pneumoniae*, in which the patient's intestinal tract is an important intermediate reservoir. In this instance, infection is often acquired endogenously; *Klebsiella* which cause urinary tract infection apparently colonize the gastrointestinal tract only after a period of hospitalization. The prevalence of *Klebsiella* colonization in hospital personnel is generally low, and the organism is probably transmitted to patients on the hands of personnel. Antibiotic therapy is a definite factor predisposing to the development of *Klebsiella* intestinal colonization and subsequent urinary tract infection.

In contrast, urinary tract infections with *Serratia* and *Providencia* almost never result from gut infection. In outbreaks caused by these bacteria, the major reservoir is the patients whose urinary tracts are colonized or patients with unrecognized infection. Infection is acquired extrinsically through passive transmission of the organisms from patient to patient on the hands of hospital personnel. Broad-spectrum antimicrobial therapy and catheterization are associated with infection.

Measures for controlling outbreaks of urinary tract infections caused by the *Enterobacteriaceae* are aimed at diminishing or eradicating the reservoir, interrupting the mode of spread, and modifying the factors placing the patients at risk (73). In an epidemic, urine cultures from catheterized patients and limited culturing of solutions and materials which come in contact with genitourinary systems are useful in defining potential animate and inanimate sources. Renewed emphasis on handwashing by personnel and separation of patients with catheters decreases the likelihood of contact transmission. Also, carefully evaluating the need for catheterization and for broad-spectrum antibiotic therapy and emphasizing the principles of good catheter care help reduce the risk of acquiring infection.

After surgical wound and other cutaneous infections, the next most frequent nosocomial infection site is the lower respiratory tract, which accounts for approximately 15% of nosocomial infections in NNIS hospitals (Table 25.10). Almost half of these infections are caused by *Enterobacteriaceae* or *Pseudomonas*. The mortality rate associated with lower respiratory tract infections caused by gram-negative bacteria is high, ranging from 30% to 60%. Most lower respiratory tract infections are probably caused by microorganisms from the pharynx which are spread to the bronchial tree and lungs by inapparent aspiration of oral secretions; however, this has not been demonstrated conclusively (65). Hospitalized patients are more likely than nonhospitalized persons to have pharyngeal colonization with gram-negative bacteria. Chronic or severe illness predisposes to pharyngeal colonization and subsequent lower respiratory tract infection, presumably because of impaired clearance mechanisms in these patients. Antibiotic therapy is also a predisposing factor. Gram-negative microorganisms colonizing the pharynx may come from other patients or from the individual's own gastrointestinal tract.

Although chronic illness coupled with pharyngeal colonization may cause a nosocomial lower respiratory tract infection with gram-negative bacilli, hospitalized patients are frequently exposed to other potential sources of infecting microorganisms. Contaminated respiratory therapy equipment allows potential pathogens to be inhaled directly. Inspired gas mixtures used in respiratory therapy must be saturated with water vapor to keep the respiratory tract mucosa from drying. This saturation can be achieved by either nebulizers or humidifiers. Of the two reservoirs, nebulizers are the more risky because the aerosolized water droplets in which bacteria may be suspended are small enough to be deposited directly in the alveoli. In one hospital, the prevalence of necrotizing pneumonia caused by gram-negative bacteria and seen at autopsy increased 4-fold over a 5-year period after such equipment was introduced and widely used. The rate subsequently returned to baseline levels when a routine program of nebulizer decontamination was instituted. Common-source outbreaks of respiratory tract infection have been caused by contaminated medications and by contaminated water in reservoirs. Multiple-dose vials of medications should not be used and reservoirs should be emptied and refilled every 8–12 hr. Reusable respiratory therapy equipment should be sterilized before it is used, and breathing circuits should be changed every 24 hr. Many strains of *Klebsiella, Enterobacter,* and *Serratia* can multiply in high-quality distilled water, which explains some of the problems with moist environments.

The gram-negative bacteria are also the most common etiologic organisms in nosocomial bacteremias (25). Although bacteremia in hospitalized patients is less common than nosocomial infections at other sites, invasion of the bloodstream by gram-negative organisms carries ominous implications. Associated mortality may approach 90% in certain groups of patients. Outcome is largely dependent on the age of the patient (newborns and the elderly are most likely to have fatal infections) and the severity of the underlying disease. A particularly high mortality rate is associated with septic shock.

Most nosocomial bacteremias are secondary. The organism is transmitted from an identifiable primary infection at another site. The urinary tract is the most common primary site of infection resulting in bacteremia, with less frequent sites being the respiratory tract, gastrointestinal tract, and surgical wounds. With some clinical conditions such as severe burns, secondary bacteremia is almost inevitable. The frequency with which the *Enterobacteriaceae* cause secondary bacteremia reflects their involvement in primary infections at these other sites.

In approximately 20% to 30% of nosocomial bacteremias, there is no readily identifiable focus. These bacteremias are termed primary and have special epidemiologic importance. In some instances, particularly in immunosuppressed or otherwise debilitated patients, organisms enter from an occult portal in the gastrointestinal tract or pharynx. Alternatively, the bloodstream may be seeded during a surgical procedure involving the urinary tract, gastrointestinal tract, or biliary system, or during such procedures as cystoscopy or colonoscopy. Primary bacteremias may also result from contaminated fluids or other materials being introduced into the vascular system. Such was the situation when intravenous fluids contaminated with *Enterobacter agglomerans* and *E. cloacae* caused a large outbreak of bacteremias. Bacteremia associated with intravenous fluid therapy is more likely to result from extrinsic contamination with microorganisms which gain access to the delivery system during the process of preparation and infusion (55). Outbreaks of primary bacteremias have also been caused by parenteral injection of contaminated medications from multiple-dose vials, contamination of infused blood products, particularly platelets, and contamination of intravascular pressure monitoring systems.

Diagnostic Procedures

Most of the diagnostic procedures for the opportunistic *Enterobacteriaceae* were covered in the previous section.

Marker systems

The microbiologist can often provide laboratory data which prove useful during epidemiologic investigations. Important isolates of *Enterobacteriaceae* have usually been identified biochemically and have been tested for anti-microbial susceptibility. Table 25.11 shows how the biochemical profile and antibiograms can be used in epidemiologic analysis. The isolates of *Klebsiella pneumoniae* from patients 1, 2, and 3 are probably the same strain. They all have the same capsule type, unusual biotypes, identical antibiograms, and are highly resistant for this species. Thus several lines of evidence indicate that they are the same strain; however, their API profiles differ because of the Voges-Proskauer test (1 and 2 were positive; 3 was negative). This example shows that slight differences in the biochemical profiles of strains do not necessarily indicate that they are different strains. Many strains of *Enterobacteriaceae* have biochemical reactions which occur after 18–24 hr which explain many of these differences. Similarly, the antibiograms of isolates from the same strain can differ because this marker is influenced by antibiotic usage and other factors. Patients 6 and 7 in Table 25.11 were in the same nursing unit. Their urine isolates have identical biochemical profiles and antibiograms. However, in this instance the laboratory data are not that helpful, because this profile and antibiogram are very common (about 50% of *K. pneumoniae* strains), further emphasizing that although the antibiogram and biochemical profile are very useful markers, data obtained from them must be interpreted cautiously, since serotyping by a reference laboratory showed they were different types.

Marker systems are most useful in differentiating common species, including *E. coli, Proteus mirabilis, Morganella morganii, Providencia rettgeri, Klebsiella, Enterobacter,* and *Serratia.* Marker system are usually not needed for rare species of opportunistic *Enterobacteriaceae,* which include *Edwardsiella tarda, Klebsiella ozaenae, K. rhinoscleromatis, E. agglomerans, Serratia liquefaciens, S. rubidaea, Proteus vulgaris, Hafnia alvei, Providencia,* and *Yersinia.* A cluster of cases caused by one of these rare pathogens is significant and should be investigated.

Specialized or reference methods include serological, bacteriocin, and bacteriophage typing. Although specialized typing methods are very useful in epi-

TABLE 25.11—ANTIBIOGRAMS, BIOCHEMICAL PROFILES, AND CAPSULE TYPES OF 7 ISOLATES OF *KLEBSIELLA PNEUMONIAE* ISOLATED THE SAME WEEK

ISOLATE FROM PATIENT	HOSPITAL LOCATION	SPECI-MEN	SERO-TYPE (CAP-SULE)	API BIO-CHEMICAL PROFILE	RESISTANT TO:
1	Intensive Care	Urine	2	4 214[b] 773	C[a],TE,AM,CB,NA,GM
2	Intensive Care	Urine	2	4 214[b] 773	C,TE,AM,CB,NA,GM
3	Intensive Care	Wound	2	4 215[b] 773	C,TE,AM,CB,NA,GM
4	2 North	Sputum	16	5 214 773	AM,CB
5	3 South	Burn	32	5 205 773	TE,AM,CB
6	7 North	Urine	2	5 215 773	AM,CB
7	7 North	Urine	30	5 215 773	AM,CB

[a] Symbols: C = chloramphenicol, TE = tetracycline, AM = ampicillin, CB = carbenicillin, NA = nalidixic acid, GM = gentamicin.

[b] The fourth digit in the profile is 4 if the Voges-Proskauer Reaction is negative, and 5 if it is positive.

demiological studies, most laboratories should not attempt to do them unless they can allocate the necessary personnel. Setting up typing methods is time-consuming, and the technician must do them often to maintain adequate skill. It is best to refer isolates for typing to a laboratory with the proper expertise and interest.

Serological typing

Many serological schemes have been proposed for typing the *Enterobacteriaceae*. Those used for *Shigella, Salmonella, Arizona,* and *Klebsiella* are standardized by international agreement, but others are poorly standardized. Many of the sera are commercially available. Laboratories should not routinely type the opportunistic *Enterobacteriaceae,* except as part of carefully planned studies or when epidemiologic questions must be answered. When antisera are not available commercially, small laboratories should not attempt to produce them. When sera are available commercially they can be used as the specific circumstances dictate. The monograph of Edwards and Ewing should be consulted for details on serotyping (27).

Sera for typing *Enterobacteriaceae* may eventually become commercially available. Currently it is impractical to use any of them except under very special circumstances. This type of work is best done by specialized laboratories or laboratories with special research interest in serotyping a particular pathogen. The same recommendation holds for bacteriophage and bacteriocin typing.

Escherichia coli

Escherichia coli is a single species, but one which varies considerably in its biochemical reactions, antigens, physiology, ecology, epidemiology, and role in disease (16). It is usually easy to recognize a strain of *E. coli* and identify it correctly, but some strains are closely related to *Shigella* and very difficult to differentiate (some workers would say impossible). As was emphasized previously, *E. coli* is an important opportunistic pathogen, but certain strains may also cause diarrhea.

E. coli as an Enteric Pathogen

Unlike *Shigella, E. coli* is a normal inhabitant of the human gastrointestinal tract and was not recognized as an important intestinal pathogen until the 1940s. At that time, certain strains of *E. coli* were identified as the cause of outbreaks of explosive, severe gastrointestinal illness in infants (27, 48, 63, 71). Over the next 15 years (27), 20–25 strains were shown to cause nursery outbreaks and were termed "enteropathogenic *E. coli*" (EPEC). In recent years, EPEC have seldom been incriminated as important causes of nursery outbreaks of diarrhea in the United States (40), so there is much debate as to whether EPEC are still a significant cause of diarrhea (40, 70). In recent years, however, two mechanisms by which *E. coli* cause diarrhea have been identified: production of enterotoxins and invasion of colonic mucosa (71). However, only a few of the EPEC strains have subsequently been shown to be invasive or toxinogenic (16, 40, 70). It is possible that EPEC were toxinogenic or invasive but have lost these capabilities, or they may have produced disease by a mechanism not yet identified.

Enterotoxinogenic (Tox$^+$) *E. coli* are an important cause of cholera-like diarrhea in adults in India and Bangladesh, of acute diarrhea in children in Brazil, and of travelers' diarrhea in Americans abroad (56, 63, 71). Tox$^+$ *E. coli* have been reported to cause diarrheal outbreaks in the United States, but their role as a cause of endemic diarrhea is not known. Early studies showed that Tox$^+$ strains were important in some geographic areas (41) but not in others (20). In studies on human volunteers, 10^6–10^{10} toxinogenic *E. coli* had to be ingested to cause disease. Perhaps for this reason Tox$^+$ strains seem to play an important role in causing diarrhea only in developing areas of the world where sanitation and potable water systems are poor.

The severe, cholera-like illness seen in adults in Bangladesh and India is characterized by the abrupt onset of watery stools which result in marked dehydration. Stool volume is less than in cholerea, and untreated diarrhea is of shorter duration. Travelers' diarrhea, a syndrome in visitors to developing areas of the world, is characterized by abdominal cramps, anorexia (loss of appetite), malaise, and diarrhea which usually lasts 5–7 days. Vomiting is uncommon and fever is rare. The incubation period is usually 24–48 hr (56, 71).

The worldwide incidence of diarrhea caused by invasive *E. coli* is not known. The organisms have been regularly reported to cause sporadic diarrhea in adults and children in Japan and in children in Brazil (71). In the United States, however, invasive strains have been only rarely associated with sporadic cases, epidemics, or nursery outbreaks of diarrhea. The mechanism and histopathology of disease caused by invasive *E. coli* resemble those of shigellosis (62, 83).

Several recent studies have helped to define the relative frequency of the various infectious agents which cause diarrhea. In most areas of the United States, enterotoxin-producing strains of *Escherichia coli* have been very rare, but in one rural community (White River Apache Indian Reservation) enterotoxinogenic *E. coli* were isolated from 16% of 59 infants with summer diarrhea. The absence of these strains in the United States is in contrast to the situation in a crowded, poorly developed country such as Bangladesh where they were the chief cause (in the summer but not the winter) of diarrhea in the community and an important cause of hospitalization. Data from a 2-year study in Houston, Texas, incriminated a wide variety of organisms from children with diarrhea: *Shigella* (30% of cases), rotavirus (10%), *Giardia lamblia* (7%), *Salmonella* (4%), enterotoxin-producing *E. coli* (4%), invasive *E. coli* (1%). Two surprising organisms were also listed—*Aeromonas* and *Proteus* (strains which produce a positive response in the adrenal cell tissue culture assay, presumably reflecting an enterotoxin or enterotoxin-like activity). In 42% of the diarrheal cases, no infectious agent was identified. Other recent studies have indicated that *Campylobacter* is an important etiologic agent and will comprise a considerable percent of these "diarrheas for which no agent was isolated." Two excellent reviews by Levine and Edelman summarize much of the recent data on diarrhea and its infectious causes (25b, 52a).

E. coli can acquire plasmids which code for two different enterotoxins, called "LT" (the heat-labile toxin) and "ST" (the heat-stable toxin). Strains which produce both ST and LT and strains which produce only ST or only LT have been identified; toxin production in all strains tested has been plasmid mediated (71). K antigens (63) which are necessary for mucosal cell adherence and disease production in animals have not been identified in human enterotoxinogenic strains of *E. coli,* although other similar colonization factors have (30).

Tetracycline lessens the amount of watery diarrhea and shortens its duration, as well as the excretion of toxinogenic *E. coli* in the stools of individuals studied in Bangladesh. This experience suggests that antibiotics should also be effective in treating many cases of travelers' diarrhea. At present, avoiding contaminated food and water is the only proven prophylactic measure against travelers' diarrhea.

Preventing diarrhea caused by *E. coli* with vaccines based on bacterial cellular antigens is considered impractical because of the large number of potentially pathogenic strains. However, evidence indicates that LTs from different strains are immunologically similar and that parenteral immunization protects against intestinal challenge with enterotoxin (71), suggesting that an effective vaccine against disease caused by toxinogenic strains might be developed. Until such a vaccine is available, emphasis must be placed on improving sanitation and potable water systems in developing areas of the world.

Implication of *E. coli* as the Cause of Diarrhea

This topic is the subject of much discussion and controversy today (40, 70, 71). In the past the method most frequently used was to screen for certain O-K serogroups of *E. coli* that had been associated with nursery outbreaks of infant diarrhea (27). Today, strains of *E. coli* can also be tested for 4 virulence mechanisms—production of ST, production of LT, presence of colonization factors, and invasiveness (71). Unfortunately, these four tests are complicated and not readily available for the clinical laboratory.

Two more virulence mechanisms have been postulated for *E. coli.* A cytotoxin, active on the vero tissue culture line, was evaluated by Scotland et al. (74b), who presented evidence that this "pathogenic mechanism" might explain the outbreaks caused by *E. coli* O26:H11. (Strains of O128 were also cytotoxic.) A different mechanism was postulated by Ulshen and Rollo (83a). They described an infant with chronic diarrhea who had overgrowth of *E. coli* in the small intestine which resolved with antibiotic treatment. Small bowel biopsy revealed brush-border damage associated with adherent bacteria, remarkably similar in appearance to *E. coli* O15 infection in the rabbit. There was only rare invasion of the mucosa (as seen with "invasive" *E. coli* strains), and there was no evidence for an enterotoxin. These two reports further indicate that there may be many (a dozen or more?) mechanisms by which *E. coli* can cause diarrhea.

Primary Isolation

Fecal specimens should be plated directly on a nonselective plating medium such as blood agar and on a differential medium of low selectivity such as MacConkey agar. Media of low selectivity which use lactose as the differentiating sugar are best because the proportion of lactose (lac)$^+$ and lac$^-$ colonies can be determined (gram-positive organisms do not form colonies). The disadvantage of the sugar-containing media, however, is that organisms are more likely to be rough (autoagglutinable) in serologic tests if they are grown on a medium which contains sugar. In our own (JGW) laboratory we prefer to use MacConkey agar so that we can select the lac$^+$ and lac$^-$ colonies without additional testing. *E. coli* isolates can be correctly selected with a reasonable degree of accuracy directly from the plating media. Since some *E. coli* strains ferment lactose slowly or are lac$^-$, both lac$^+$ and lac$^-$ colonies should be selected from plating media for additional testing, but most should be lac$^+$. It is generally recommended that 10 colonies be selected, but laboratory resources will dicate how many isolates can be reasonably handled (at least five colonies should be used). For serologic typing, colonies should be transferred to a nonselective medium such as blood agar, blood agar base, or infusion agar. They should not be typed from a sugar-containing media such as triple sugar iron agar (TSI) which can cause the isolate to become rough. Once the *E. coli* colonies have been isolated, there are two basic laboratory approaches to implicate them as the cause of diarrhea: serotyping and assaying for virulence mechanisms.

Screening for Enteropathogenic Strains of *E. coli*

This is the subject of much controversy today, and to understand the problem, it is necessary to understand how certain strains of *E. coli* were incriminated as the cause of diarrhea in infants (27, 48).

Between 1945 and 1950, *E. coli* was implicated as a cause of epidemics of infantile diarrhea, but there was evidence that other microorganisms were also important causes. The classical study which incriminated *E. coli* as an *important* cause of infantile diarrhea was done by Kauffmann and Dupont (48). They showed that *E. coli* strains from outbreaks in several countries belonged to the following O-K-H antigen groups: O55:K59:H2, O55:K59:H6, O55:K59:NM, O111:K58:H2, O111:K58:H12, and O111:K58:NM (NM = nonmotile). These O-K-H combinations had not been observed in the feces of healthy infants or adults. It must be emphasized that they did not say that all *E. coli* strains with O antigen 55 or 111 are enteropathogenic.

In the early 1950s, microbiologists all over the world began to look for the Kauffmann-Dupont strains in epidemics of infantile diarrhea and, often found them. The evidence suggested that these strains were distributed worldwide and were important causes of diarrhea, particularly in nursery outbreaks. Sometimes these specific strains were not found in outbreaks, but other strains of *E. coli* were. Soon it became apparent that other strains of *E. coli* could cause outbreaks of infant diarrhea. It was carefully pointed out that an epidemic was caused by a single strain and that no generalizations could be made until further evidence was available.

After certain strains of *E. coli* were shown to cause diarrhea, commercial companies began to make antisera to screen for the O and K antigens of these strains. Unfortunately, some assumptions were made then which have now come back to haunt us. Although Kauffmann and Dupont carefully showed that the outbreak strains that they studied had characteristic O, H, and K antigens, as well as several biochemical reactions, their definition was ignored. The search began for all *E. coli* strains with O antigens 55 and 111 (and later for other O groups), and the assumption was made that all strains that belonged to these O groups were inherent pathogens. Similarly, as other outbreaks were described, all strains of the same O group were searched for, with the assumption that they would also be inherent pathogens. There is now much evidence that this approach results in many false positives because many strains which have the same O antigen as the epidemic strain are not associated with diarrhea.

We are often asked if we should continue serological screening for the classical EPECs. "Classical EPEC" is defined as a strain of *E. coli* that has one of the O antigens represented in Poly A (O26:K60, O55:K59, O111:K58 and O127:K63) Poly B (O86:K61, O119:K69, O124:K72, O125:K70, O126:K71, O128:K67) or Poly C (O18:K77, O20:K61, O28:K73, O44:K74, O112:K66). (This definition is the one used in most clinical laboratories.) Unfortunately, this question must be answered in each microbiology laboratory on the basis of its own special circumstances and after consultation with local pediatricians, epidemiologists, infectious disease specialists, nursery staff, and other interested parties. The following facts must be considered for the United States:

1. The classical EPECs rarely cause nursery outbreaks today (40).

2. Many of the classical EPECs isolated today have different properties (other H antigens, no K antigens, and different biochemical profiles) from those of the outbreak strains associated with outbreaks in the 1940s and 1950s. Thus there is little evidence that many of these current isolates are inherent pathogens; however some of them probably are.

3. Commercial sera often agglutinate other strains (not implicated as EPEC) of *E. coli* that can result in many false-positive results (27).

4. Many strains of *E. coli* that cause diarrhea are not detected with current serologic screening methods, leading to false-negative results (40).

5. The procedure is costly, and few (if any) clinical laboratories do it correctly.

We think a laboratory is justified in its decision to drop routine screening for the classical EPECs in nonepidemic situations, but we would not argue with a decision to continue serologic screening if it is done correctly and the reports are carefully worded. A laboratory should either do this time-consuming procedure correctly or drop it.

The following discussion is intended for those who have carefully considered the problem and have decided to continue screening for the classical EPECs. All four steps in the procedure must be done to avoid false-positive results (27). Inadequate serotyping can be worse than no serotyping. Some laboratories use only polyvalent sera A and B, but others include polyvalent C. There is no scientific reason to use polyvalent D and E sera produced by one manufacturer (Difco).

Table 25.12 shows the four steps required to determine the O and K antigens of the classical EPEC. If any step is omitted, false positives will result because many *E. coli* strains found in the human gut have antigens that cross-react with the antisera used in the screening procedure. Many strains which are not classical EPEC agglutinate in the polyvalent sera. However, strains which do not agglutinate in the polyvalent sera are probably not classical EPEC (but they can be toxinogenic, invasive, or pathogenic by some other mechanism). If strong agglutination is found with one of the polyvalent sera, the live antigen should then be tested in the individual OK sera that comprise the polyvalent. In step 2 (Table 25.12), the culture agglutinates strongly in the O55:K59 serum. This agglutination could occur because the strain has O antigen 55, K antigen 59, or an O or K antigen which cross-reacts. To avoid false positives, steps 3 and 4 *must* be done. In step 3, both live and heated antigens are tested in O55, and O55:K59. Cultures without K antigens react strongly with both sera whether they are heated or not. However, if the culture has a K antigen, the unheated suspension will not agglutinate in the O serum (Table 25.12). The culture with a K antigen would be reported as "*E. coli* O55:K59" and the other as "*E. coli* O55:K−" ("K−" or "K minus" means that no K antigen was detected). Very few laboratories do step 4 to confirm the O antigen by titrations, but it is *required* to avoid false positives. Some strains of *E. coli* have antigens which cross-react strongly in steps 1–3, and only step 4 will show that they do not belong to the O group of the classical EPECs. In Table 25.12, the *E. coli* O55 strain reacted strongly with dilutions of O55 serum to 1:1280. The strain with the cross-reacting antigen had a titer of only 1:40 and would not be reported as "*E. coli* O55." The classical EPEC strains of *E. coli* were defined on both O and H antigens, so further testing in H antisera (commercial) would further reduce the number of false positive reports. Unfortunately this step is not very practical for the average clinical microbiology laboratory.

There has also been much confusion about the wording of reports for strains which have O antigens of the classical EPEC. Many reports considerably overstate what was actually found by laboratory methods. The following are examples of good and bad reports:

UNACCEPTABLE REPORTS

1. Enteropathogenic *E. coli* isolated
2. Enteropathogenic *E. coli* O111:K58 isolated
3. Enteropathogenic *E. coli*, Poly A, isolated
4. Enteropathogenic *E. coli* identified by fluorescent-antibody techniques

ACCEPTABLE REPORTS

1. *E. coli* O111:K58:H2 isolated
2. *E. coli* O111:K58 isolated
3. *E. coli* O55:K− isolated

A carefully worded report can greatly improve the current state of EPEC screening. One suggested report is:

> This specimen is positive for *E. coli* O111:K58. Certain strains of this O antigen group have caused nursery outbreaks of diarrhea, but other strains with this O group are probably not pathogenic. This particular isolate may or may not be able to cause diarrhea.

At the end of the report, additional comments could also be made to help the physician interpret the report. Contrast these two comments:

> Comment: "This is the first isolate of *E. coli* O111 in the nursery in over 4 months."

or

> Comment: "Five other infants with diarrhea in the nursery are positive for *E. coli* O111, and there have been over 50 cases in the community, mostly in district 3. A reference laboratory has found that the *E. coli* O111 strains from the outbreak cause diarrhea in experimental animals."

We have discussed with many microbiologists the question of whether to continue screening for EPEC. Reactions are mixed. Some are glad to drop the procedure because of the additional work it creates. Others say that pediatricians and physicians believe that it provides useful information and want the procedure continued. Thus there is no answer to the question that can apply uniformly throughout the United States. Each laboratory must evaluate the situation and decide whether to screen for EPEC on this basis (40, 70). Laboratories that continue serologic screening should also include a control group of infants without diarrhea, so that the incidence of EPEC in this group can be compared to the group with diarrhea.

Assays for Pathogenicity

The pathogenicity assays used to implicate *E. coli* as the etiologic agent in diarrhea detect LT, ST, colonization factors, or invasiveness (71). Unfortunately, current methods for detecting enterotoxins are too time-consuming and technically difficult to be used in routine laboratories.

Many assays are available for detecting enterotoxins. Most of those used to detect LT produced by *E. coli* were originally used to detect *Vibrio cholerae* enterotoxin and have been adapted for *E. coli*. Some of the commonly used assays and the enterotoxins which they detect are shown in Table 25.13. The adult rabbit ileal loop, which was the original model used to detect both LT⁺

TABLE 25.12—STEPS IN THE DETERMINATION OF O AND K ANTIGENS IN THE SCREENING PROCEDURE FOR CLASSICAL EPEC

STEP 1—Agglutination of live culture in OK polyvalent sera

Poly A	Poly B	Poly C
++++	–	–

STEP 2—Live culture tested in individual OK sera that comprise the polyvalent serum (Poly A in this case) which strongly agglutinated the culture

O26:K60	O55:K59	O111:K58	O127:K63
–	++++	–	–

STEP 3—Agglutination of live and heated culture in O and OK serum which gave strong agglutination

	Results for Culture with K Antigen			Results for Culture Without K Antigen	
	Serum			Serum	
Antigen	O55:K59	O55	Antigen	O55:K59	O55
Live	4+	–	Live	4+	4+
Heated	4+	4+	Heated	4+	4+

STEP 4—Degree of agglutination of heated antigen with twofold dilutions of O55 serum to confirm O antigen

	DILUTION OF O55 SERUM:						
Antigen	1:40	1:80	1:160	1:320	1:640	1:1280	1:2560
E. coli O55	4+	4+	4+	4+	4+	3+	–
Strain with Cross-reacting Antigen	4+	±	–	–	–	–	–

and ST$^+$ *E. coli,* is still used although not as extensively as it was before some of the newer assays were developed. Maximal fluid accumulation is seen at 6–7 hr for ST and at 18–24 hr for LT. Therefore, injected loops should be observed for both time periods if maximal sensitivity is desired for both LT and ST. A strongly positive loop will have a ratio of volume (in milliliters) to length (in centimeters) of about 2–2.5 depending on the rabbit size. This assay is expensive and time-consuming, and must be carefully controlled because of occasional false positives and false negatives. As a result, most investigators have now turned to less cumbersome assays to detect *E. coli* enterotoxin.

Infant (7–9 days old) rabbits have been used for detecting both LT and ST. The rabbits are challenged by a suspect enterotoxin preparation by inserting it into a plastic tube previously passed into the stomach or by injecting it directly into the small intestine. The animals are killed 6–7 hr later. The entire gastrointestinal tract is removed, and a volume-to-length (of ligated loop) ratio of fluid accumulation is determined (41). Rabbit skin permeability tests can also be used to detect LT$^+$ *E. coli.* Enterotoxin extracts are injected intracutaneously and Evans blue dye is injected intravenously 24 hr later. Areas of induration and blueing are read 1–2 hr later (71). Neither this assay nor the infant rabbit assay is widely used.

The infant mouse assay is usually used to detect ST (20). Mice, 1–4 days old, are inoculated with either culture filtrate or supernatant of *E. coli* cultures to which Evans blue dye has been added. The material is usually injected directly into the stomach, although oral inoculation has also been used. The mice are killed 4 hr after they are inoculated, and fluid accumulation is determined by a ratio of intestine to remaining body weight (56).

Tissue culture assays including the Y-1 mouse adrenal cell assay (22, 71) and the Chinese hamster ovary (CHO) cell (42) have been used extensively in detecting *E. coli* LT, and are the most sensitive. The Y-1 adrenal cells respond to LT by rounding, whereas the CHO cells elongate. Neither cell line responds to ST. The two tissue culture assays have comparable sensitivities.

The Sereny test is used to determine the invasiveness of *E. coli* (64, 75). A 0.05-ml drop of either a suspension or broth culture of an isolate is inoculated into the conjunctival sac of a guinea pig's eye, and the animal is observed for 72 hr for development of keratoconjunctivitis (the eye becomes watery, the eyeball becomes opaque, and the eye begins to swell and often closes completely).

All of these tests must be carefully standardized and controlled. A short review such as this one cannot include extensive details on the subject. The original articles should be consulted, and we strongly recommend that people be trained in a laboratory with expertise in a given method before they use it in their own laboratories.

None of the assays for *E. coli* pathogenicity are suitable for routine use in clinical laboratories. Thus, no practical replacement is available for serotyping, but two approaches look promising. Yolken et al. (89) recently described an enzyme-linked immunosorbent assay (ELISA) for detecting LT$^+$ *E. coli*. If the reagents become readily available, the assay could be used in clini-

TABLE 25.13—ASSAYS FOR ENTEROTOXINS OF *ESCHERICHIA COLI*

ASSAY	HEAT-LABILE ENTEROTOXIN	HEAT-STABLE ENTEROTOXIN
Rabbit ileal loop		
6–7 hr	+[a]	+
18 hr	+	v
Infant mouse (4 hr)	−	+
Infant rabbit	+	+
Rabbit skin	+	−
Y1 mouse adrenal cells	+	−
Chinese hamster ovary cells	+	−
ELISA	+	−

[a] + = positive result in assay, − = negative result. Consult text for exact definition of these terms.

cal laboratories. A second approach, still in the developmental stage, is to test *E. coli* colonies for the presence of colonization factors (30). It may be possible to produce a polyvalent antiserum which will agglutinate strains containing the surface antigens which cause gut colonization. The preliminary evidence indicates that strains must colonize the small intestine to be pathogenic (30).

Biochemical Identification of *E. coli*

This topic is included because many cultures identified as *Shigella* by clinical or even reference laboratories are really *E. coli*. Lactose$^+$, motile, gas producing strains of *E. coli* are easy to identify, but some *E. coli* strains are negative in these tests. The biochemical properties of this group are given in Table 25.14 under "*E. coli* inactive." Many strains which are identified in primary laboratories as *Shigella* are identified by reference laboratories as biochemically inactive strains of *E. coli*. Misidentification often results from the fact that *E. coli* strains cross-react serologically with *Shigella*, and identification is based on agglutination in one of the *Shigella* antisera. A complete set of biochemical reactions would have shown that the organism was *E. coli* rather than *Shigella*. Many of these inactive strains of *E. coli* belong to the *Alkalescens-Dispar* group and were once classified in *Shigella* as *Shigella alkalescens* and *Shigella dispar*. Unlike *Shigella*, these strains are not inherent causes of dysentery in humans; however, they have been implicated in some cases of dysentery. It would be helpful to test such a strain for invasiveness in the Sereny test, which might help resolve its role in the patient's dysentery.

Differentiating *E. coli* from *Shigella*

This process can pose one of the most difficult problems for a laboratory, but fortunately it can be done for most strains. The best approach is to do a *complete* set of biochemical reactions and compare the pattern to that of *E. coli* and to those of all the *Shigella* groups (Table 25.14). The following generalizations are suggested as guidelines:

1. *Shigella* cultures are always nonmotile and lysine negative.

2. With the exception of some *Shigella flexneri* 6, *Shigella* do not produce gas during carbohydrate fermentation (there have been reports of gas production by a few strains of *S. boydii* 13 and 14 and *S. dysenteriae* 3).

3. Cultures which ferment mucate or give an alkaline reaction on acetate or Christensen's citrate are much more likely to be *E. coli* than *Shigella*.

4. *Shigella boydii* and *S. dysenteriae* are very rare in the United States (Table 25.5). Cultures which have been presumptively identified as one of these two species should be carefully checked before any report is made.

It is obvious from this discussion that no definitive rules can be made. Most *Shigella* agglutinate in one of the polyvalent *Shigella* sera and in an individual serum. Although this fact can be very helpful in deciding that a culture is *Shigella*, *E. coli* cultures frequently cross-react in these sera. Because it is very important to differentiate *E. coli* from *Shigella*, complete biochemical and serologic typing should be done in each instance.

TABLE 25.14—BIOCHEMICAL TESTS HELPFUL IN DIFFERENTIATING *ESCHERICHIA COLI* FROM *SHIGELLA*

TEST	E.COLI "NORMAL"	E. COLI INACTIVE	S. DYSEN- TERIAE	S. FLEXNERI GROUPS 1–5	S. FLEXNERI GROUP 6	S. BOYDII	S. SONNEI
Motility	85[a]	0	0	0	0	0	0
Gas from D-Glucose	91	0	0	0	18	0	0
Lactose	90	0	0	0	0	1	2
Indole	99	90	44	62	0	29	0
Mucate	94	25	0	0	0	0	16
Acetate	84	59	0	5	0	0	0
Christensen's (Citrate)	24	NA[b]	0	0	0	0	0
Lysine	88	43	0	0	0	0	0
Arginine	17	2	1.5	0	49	18	1
Ornithine	63	18	0	0	0	3	99
Sucrose	51	11	0	2	0	0	0.1
Salicin	37	3	0	0	0	0	0

[a] Gives the % positive for the test after 48 hr of incubation.
[b] NA = data not available.

Marker Systems

Other techniques besides serotyping have also been used to type *E. coli*. Biotyping can be a useful marker since *E. coli* strains vary in their biochemical reactions (Figure 25.1). One important fact to remember about biotyping is that many of these biochemical reactions occur after 18–24 hr. Otherwise strains will appear to be different biotypes when they are not. Bacteriophage typing and colicin typing can be useful in epidemiologic studies (16), but these techniques are not widely used. They should be reserved for outbreak investigations or for special studies.

Antimicrobic Susceptibility and Resistance

Table 25.9 indicates that, unlike some of the other species of *Enterobacteriaceae*, *E. coli* does not have intrinsic resistance to antimicrobials that are commonly used. Most strains isolated from healthy people (without recent exposure to antibiotics) are multiply sensitive to antibiotics. However, *E. coli* can rapidly become resistant under the selective pressure of antibiotic usage which has been documented when antibiotics have been used prophylactically or to treat infections. Thus, many strains of *E. coli* isolated from domestic animals, hospitalized patients, or patients treated with antibiotics are more resistant to antibiotics than the strains which have not been exposed to antibiotics.

Shigella

Causative Organisms

Organisms of the genus *Shigella* are the most common causes of bacillary dysentery. Before the age of bacteriology, dysentery was regarded as a single, well-defined disease, but between 1875 and 1901 it became apparent that at least two classes of microorganisms were involved: one protozoan, the other bacterial. From 1898 to 1901, Shiga in Japan, Kruse in Germany, and Flexner in the Philippines showed that bacillary dysentery was caused by a bacillus that somewhat resembled the one causing typhoid fever. Since that time, a number of *Shigella* "species" and serologic types which cause dysentery have been described.

Today the four named groups of *Shigella* are *S. dysenteriae* (Group A), *S. flexneri* (Group B), *S. boydii* (Group C), and *S. sonnei* (Group D). There are also strains which are biochemically *Shigella* which cannot be serotyped. The latter groups of *Shigella* are given the status of "Provisional" and each may be added to the *Shigella* schema as a new O group in one of the species. These strains are best called "*Shigella* spp." until they can be further defined. Although the four major groups are given different species names, they are very close genetically and could be considered one species. It should also be remembered that some strains identified as *E. coli* by biochemical tests or serology are more like *Shigella* when pathogenicity is considered (63). Table 25.15 lists the *Shigella* groups isolated in the United States during 1975.

Clinical Manifestations

Shigellosis (14, 86), or "bacillary dysentery" as it is often termed, has an incubation period of 1–7 days. In its most pronounced form, shigellosis begins with fever, cramping, abdominal pain, and diarrhea. The diarrhea initially is often watery, resembling that associated with illness caused by enterotoxin-producing *E. coli* or *Vibrio cholerae*, and may last 1–3 days. This phase may be followed by a second one characterized by frequent, scant stools containing blood, mucus, and pus. Tenesmus (painful, long-continued, and ineffective straining to produce stool) is quite characteristic of the illness at this point. This second phase of shigellosis, most often referred to as "dysentery," may last weeks if untreated. Infection with *S. dysenteriae* serogroup O1 (Shiga's bacillus) often results in the full blown, biphasic syndrome with high morbidity and mortality, especially if untreated or treated inappropriately. The other three *Shigella* species and other serotypes of *S. dysenteriae* cause a wider spectrum of disease including asymptomatic carriage, diarrhea resembling cholera or salmonellosis, and life-threatening dysentery.

Shigellosis is more serious in children than in adults and is often accompanied by high fever and/or convulsions (4). Convulsions can occur in childhood shigellosis regardless of the *Shigella* serotype, the severity of the illness, or the height of fever. Other central nervous system manifestations such as headache, rigidity of the neck, and delirium are often seen (4). Cerebrospinal

TABLE 25.15—SEROTYPES OF *SHIGELLA* ISOLATED IN THE UNITED STATES IN 1976

SEROTYPE		NUMBER[a]	PERCENTAGE[a]	SEROTYPE		NUMBER[a]	PERCENTAGE[a]
S. dysenteriae	1	12	.2	S. flexneri	1a	319	4.0
S. dysenteriae	2	46	.5	S. flexneri	1b	338	4.3
S. dysenteriae	3	21	.3	S. flexneri	2a	771	9.7
S. dysenteriae	4	5	.06	S. flexneri	2b	143	1.8
S. dysenteriae	6	1	.01	S. flexneri	3a	584	7.4
S. dysenteriae	9	1	.01	S. flexneri	3b	98	1.2
S. dysenteriae	10	1	.01	S. flexneri	3c	13	.2
				S. flexneri	4a	195	2.5
S. boydii	1	9	.1	S. flexneri	4b	10	.1
S. boydii	2	62	.8	S. flexneri	5	33	.4
S. boydii	4	8	.1	S. flexneri	6	258	3.3
S. boydii	5	15	.2	S. flexneri			
S. boydii	9	1	.01	Variant X		8	.1
S. boydii	10	24	.3	S. flexneri			
S. boydii	11	1	.01	Variant Y		0	0.0
S. boydii	12	1	.01				
S. boydii	14	4	.05	S. sonnei		4924	62.3
S. boydii	15	1	.01				
				TOTAL		7908	

[a] The values are "adjusted" values obtained by adding the actual number observed to the expected number among the strains that were not actually serotyped.

fluid is usually normal, and the pathogenesis of these neurologic symptoms is not known.

Shigella bacteremia is rare in the immunocompetent host (86); only 101 cases were reported in the world literature before 1964. The one exception now is the strain of *S. dysenteriae* O1 responsible for the Central American epidemic of 1969–72 where about one-third of the cases had bacteremia. Extraintestinal *Shigella* infections are rare in the absence of bacteremia (4), although there is one report of chronic vulvovaginitis caused by *S. flexneri* occurring over a 12-month period in four otherwise well children from an area where *Shigella* is highly endemic (18).

The pathogenesis of shigellosis is not completely understood. In experimentally infected monkeys and human volunteers the mucosal cells in the colon must be invaded before disease occurs (86). The role of enterotoxin has also been shown in the first phase of shigellosis. *S. dysenteriae* O1 produces an enterotoxin which stimulates small bowel secretion of fluid and electrolytes *in vitro,* though not via the adenylate cyclase cyclic AMP system (21). Strains of *S. flexneri* and *S. sonnei* produce an enterotoxin which is antigenically similar to that produced by *S. dysenteriae* 1. Persons infected with *S. flexneri* or *S. sonnei* produce IgM antibodies which neutralize *S. dysenteriae* O1 toxin *in vitro* (49).

Epidemiology

S. sonnei and *S. flexneri* are the most commonly isolated serogroups in the United States (68, Table 25.15). Fortunately, *S. dysenteriae* O1 is rare in this country. It is usually found only among travelers to areas such as the Indian subcontinent, Mexico, and Central America, where it is endemic or occasionally epidemic. Shigellosis is most common in the summer and early autumn months and occurs primarily among children between the ages of 1 and 10. Both sexes are equally affected, except that 20- to 30-year-old women have an incidence twice as high as that found among men of comparable age, probably because of the nursing role women play in caring for ill children.

There are more clinical cases relative to the number of asymptomatic excreters among children than adults (14). In the setting of good personal hygiene, the asymptomatic excreter apparently plays much less of a role in disease than the symptomatic individual (14). Long-term, asymptomatic carriage has been reported, but is very rare. Although immunity is type-specific, evidence obtained in custodial institutions indicates that recent immunity can be overwhelmed by a large inoculum of ingested organisms (68).

Occasionally, shigellosis is widely transmitted in contaminated food or water, but generally illnesses occur sporadically through person-to-person or fomite-to-person transmission. This reflects the fact that if only a few organisms are ingested (on the order of 100 organisms in human volunteer studies) disease results (14, 86).

In the United States, shigellosis not acquired through foreign travel is essentially restricted to populations characterized by poverty, crowded living conditions, inadequate water supplies, poor sanitation, male homosexuality, and/or poor personal hygiene (68). Hence, the areas at greatest risk for *Shigella* epidemics are migrant labor camps, urban ghettos, some American Indian reservations, institutions for the care of the insane and the mentally retarded, and day-care centers. The need for health education and improvement of water supplies and sewage systems in migrant labor camps and Indian reservations will test the imagination and dedication of public health officials in this country. The indiscriminate use of antibiotics in large urban centers and custodial institutions has probably contributed greatly to the increasing antibiotic resistance of *Shigella* (68). Day-care centers have the highest potential for the spread of shigellosis to the general community. Children attending day-care centers are more likely to become ill and more likely to cause secondary spread among their families than children who do not attend day-care centers (68). The importance of concerted hand-washing efforts to prevent and control *Shigella* outbreaks in institutions and day-care centers should be stressed.

Treatment and Prevention

Antibiotics shorten the durations of symptoms and of excretion of *Shigella* in the feces (68), although many strains are now resistant to antibiotics (including ampicillin and tetracycline). The choice of whom to treat and which antibiotic to use have become controversial (87). Generally, the antibiotic susceptibility of the particular strain and severity of the illness are the two major factors affecting this decision. Ampicillin is the antibiotic of choice if the organism is sensitive, but trimethoprim-sulfamethoxazole is effective both *in vitro* and *in vivo,* and resistance to it has not been reported in the United States (68, 87). Antidiarrheal medications such as "Lomotil," which inhibit intestinal motility, are not recommended for shigellosis because they lengthen the durations of diarrhea and carriage (24).

Serotype-specific oral vaccines which looked promising in early European trials proved unsatisfactory in this country because it was necessary to give 4 to 5 doses and frequent boosters (every 4–6 months) and because different serotypes were present in most endemic areas (68). Immunity conferred by the vaccines was easily overwhelmed by large inocula of organisms. Until an effective oral vaccine is produced, insuring safe water supplies and adequate sanitation and stressing good personal hygiene including handwashing will remain the mainstays of shigellosis prevention.

Primary Isolation Procedure

Although the preferred method for maximal recovery of *Shigella* from fecal specimens is direct plating on agar media (57), enrichment of fecal specimens in gram-negative (GN) broth (82) has been reported effective. Selenite broth may also be useful in isolating *S. sonnei.* It is advisable to use plating media of at least two and possibly three levels of selectivity to isolate *Shigella.* Xylose lysine desoxycholate (XLD) agar (intermediate selectivity) is excellent for isolating *Shigella* (57, 81), and should be included. It contains D-xylose as a differentiating agent, and since most *Shigella* do not ferment xylose, they appear as colorless colonies on the plate. However, *Shigella* isolates which ferment xylose rapidly can be missed on this medium. Therefore, additional plating media containing lactose as a differentiating agent should be used in conjunction with XLD agar. A lactose-containing medium of low selectivity such as Tergitol 7, MacConkey, or EMB agar should be included as the second medium used. If laboratory resources permit use of a third plating medium, a more selective agar which contains lactose such as SS, Hektoen enteric (HE), or deoxycholate citrate agar should also be used. Occasional strains of *Shigella* may not grow on some of the more selective media. *S. sonnei* is suppressed more than other species by SS agar (57, 88) and deoxycholate citrate agar (88). *Shigella dysenteriae* O1 is inhibited on SS agar and slightly suppressed by XLD agar, and is best isolated with nonselective media such as Tergitol 7 or MacConkey agar.

Colonies suspected to be *Shigella* should be transferred from the selective agar plates to tubes of nonselective differential agar for preliminary biochemical screening. Two of the media more commonly used for this purpose are TSI and Kligler iron agar (KIA). At least two representatives of each type of suspicious colony should be selected from each plate. Only the center of the colony should be touched, since organisms which are inhibited but do not appear as distinct colonies can still be viable. These contaminants will grow on differential agar stabs and interfere with identification of *Shigella.* Most laboratories in the United States use TSI because it provides information on the ability of the organisms to ferment glucose, lactose, and sucrose, and to produce H_2S and gas. Isolates whose TSI reaction is alkaline/acid, gas⁻ and H_2S^- should be screened serologically with *Shigella* O groups A, B, C, and D antisera and inoculated to a urea-agar slant and motility medium. Urea⁺ or motile cultures can then be discarded. Isolates that are nonmotile, gas⁻, and react serologically may be considered "presumptively positive as *Shigella*." Presumptive positives as well as suspicious cultures which are serologically negative should be tested further biochemically. Biochemically typical *Shigella* isolates (Table 25.14) which agglutinate poorly or not at all should be heated in a water bath at 100 C for 15–30 min. After such treatment, the suspension is cooled and retested for agglutination on a slide.

Marker Systems

The identification to species and O antigen group are the most useful markers for epidemiologic analysis. Unfortunately, many absorbed antisera must be used to differentiate some of the serologic groups such as those in *S. flexneri*. Colicin typing, resistogram (a technique similar to an antibiogram except that antibiotics are replaced with organic or inorganic compounds), antibiogram, and bacteriophage typing have also been used as markers (58, 66). For the rare serotypes these procedures are not necessary, but for the common ones they may add additional information. The results must be carefully interpreted because some of these methods are oversensitive and can give misleading results.

Unlike the other three species, *S. sonnei* cannot be divided into serotypes. Since it is the most common species in most industrialized countries, typing methods can provide useful information in epidemiologic studies. Colicin production is a useful marker in the United States (58), because several colicin types can be identified. Bacteriophage typing has been used for many years to divide strains into many more types (66). However, this technique is more subject to experimental errors and is not as reproducible. The antibiogram can be useful as a marker if differences among strains are interpreted correctly. The resistogram is a new marker that may be more useful than the antibiogram because results are not dependent on the intense selective pressure of antibiotic usage.

Salmonella-Arizona

Causative Organisms

Members of the *Salmonella-Arizona* group are very important in human disease and public health. Because the evolution of the group represents a continuum, it is not surprising that the nomenclature and classification are confusing. We recognize four species, *Salmonella typhi*, *S. cholerae-suis*, *S. enteritidis*, and *Arizona hinshawii*. The pros and cons of this classification are still being debated (33). *S. typhi* and *S. cholerae-suis* do not contain any serotypes, but *S. enteritidis* (the species) contains all of the remaining serotypes of *Salmonella*. According to this nomenclature *Salmonella typhimurium* is a serotype rather than a species and is designated *S. enteritidis* serotype Typhimurium. This nomenclature is more in keeping with modern thoughts about species and the manner in which they are defined. However, to simplify writing the *Salmonella* names, we use the following simplified notation.

1. When "*S.*" precedes *typhi, cholerae-suis,* or *enteritidis,* it means *Salmonella* and is used to describe these as species.

2. When "*S.*" precedes other *Salmonella* serotypes, it means a serotype of *Salmonella enteritidis.* Thus *S. typhimurium* means serotype Typhimurium in the species *S. enteritidis.* This nomenclature saves space and is a compromise between the 2 nomenclatures widely used in the United States. However, one point of possible confusion is that *S. enteritidis* is both a species and a serotype (*Salmonella* strains with the antigenic formula 1,9,12:g,m:−). To avoid confusion we use the following convention:

3. "*S. enteritidis*" (which no antigenic formula following it) refers to the species of *Salmonella* which contains all the serotypes: "*S. enteritidis* (1,9,12:g,m:−)" refers to the individual serotype in this species.

Serotypes of *Salmonella* (formerly called species) are defined on the basis of their antigenic structure and occasionally by an additional biochemical reaction(s). The antigenic formula for *S. typhimurium* is 1,4,5,12:i:1,2. The major antigens are separated by colons, and the components of an antigen are separated by commas. The formula 1,4,5,12:i:1,2 means that serological test results indicate that the strain has O antigen components 1,4,5,12; flagella phase one antigen "i"; and flagella phase two antigen "1,2" (if one of the flagella antigens had been missing it would have been designated by a "−"). Names were given for the *Salmonella* serotypes to avoid having to remember complex antigenic formulas. Thus, if laboratory test results show that a strain has the antigenic formula 1,4,5,12:i:1,2 , *S. typhimurium* is reported. Although over 1800 serotypes of *Salmonella* have been described, most are rarely isolated from human infection.

Clinical Manifestations

Human infections with *Salmonella* can cause various clinical symptoms and involve both intestinal and extraintestinal sites (6, 7, 54, 72). Patients may have intestinal and extraintestinal infections concurrently; however, it is convenient to discuss these separately.

The most common syndrome is that of uncomplicated enterocolitis, in which after an incubation period of 8–48 hr, the typical patient experiences nausea, vomiting, cramps, diarrhea, and fever. Symptoms generally resolve in 2 to 14 days. Severe diarrhea may occur, but death occurs primarily among neonates, the elderly, and patients with underlying diseases. Following recovery, some patients may continue to excrete organisms for weeks or months. Prolonged carriage is more common in infants and in patients treated with antibiotics (1). Carriage for a period of years is uncommon, but is often associated with biliary tract disease when it does occur.

Extraintestinal infections include bacteremia, sepsis, enteric fever, and focal infections. The prognosis for patients with any such extraintestinal infection is related to the site of the infection and to the presence of any underlying disease.

Bloodborne infections may vary in severity and in association with intestinal and extraintestinal syndromes. Bacteremia may occur in patients with enterocolitis without underlying diseases. On the other hand, sepsis with chills and fever, often in the absence of gastrointestinal syndromes, has been reported particularly in adults with underlying disease such as cancer (7). Between 8% and 25% of patients with prolonged bacteremia may develop focal infections (7, 54).

The syndrome of enteric fever includes fever, headache, and prostration which may last days to weeks. The syndrome has been classically associated with *S. typhi* (typhoid fever) and with *S. paratyphi* A, B, or C (paratyphoid fever), but it may be caused by a number of *Salmonella* serotypes. When the causative organism is *Salmonella typhi* the syndrome is more prolonged, has a higher case fatality ratio, and may be complicated by gastrointestinal perforation, bleeding, hemorrhage, or focal infections.

Focal infections may involve almost any site (54), but often occur in certain susceptible individuals. Common associations include meningitis in the neonate, pneumonia and arteritis in the elderly, and osteomyelitis in patients with sickle cell disease (7).

The treatment of salmonellosis depends on the site of the infection and the condition of the patient. Fluid and electrolyte replacement is the treatment of choice in patients with uncomplicated enterocolitis. Antidiarrheal drugs containing components which reduce gut motility may worsen salmonellosis; therefore, these agents should be avoided. Antibiotics are indicated in the treatment of extraintestinal infections but usually not in the treatment of uncomplicated intestinal salmonellosis.

Multiple antibiotic resistance among *Salmonella* is now common and its frequency has increased. Many strains of the more common serotypes isolated in the United States are now antibiotic resistant. The different resistance patterns are often useful for comparing strains in epidemiologic studies.

Chloramphenicol is considered the drug of choice for treating systemic salmonellosis in the absence of sensitivity studies, and until recently chloramphenicol-resistant *Salmonella* isolates were unusual in the United States. However, since 1975 chloramphenicol-resistant *Salmonella* have caused at least five outbreaks. In several of these outbreaks the *Salmonella* were resistant to both chloramphenicol and ampicillin. The increase in antibiotic resistance may result from several factors, including unnecessary treatment of uncomplicated intestinal salmonellosis. Antibiotics in animal feeds may also be a major contributing factor to antibiotic resistance since animals constitute the major reservoir for *Salmonella*.

Epidemiology

Salmonellosis is a primary foodborne disease that is more common in summer and has its highest attack rates among young children. Although it is not possible to explain all of its epidemiologic features, the age-specific incidence may relate to a combination of increased susceptibility and increased exposure among children. Summer temperatures which compound food handling errors and assist the growth of organisms may explain the seasonal incidence.

Transmission of *Salmonella* usually requires a large infectious dose; thus, salmonellosis is primarily a foodborne disease although person-to-person and animal-to-human spread may occur. Poultry and meat products are the most common vehicles of transmission. Eggs, which once were a common source of infection, are now only occasionally associated with outbreaks. Foodborne transmission occurs through either the inadequate preparation of contaminated food or the cross- or re-contamination of adequately cooked foods. Person-to-person spread may occur occasionally in families but has been a serious problem in hospitals and institutions, primarily among neonates and in patients with underlying diseases (2). Direct animal-to-human spread also occurs as in the case of pet turtles.

Over 1800 *Salmonella* serotypes have been reported, but 10 serotypes account for over 70% of those isolates from humans (Table 25.5). Serotypes vary in host specificity, geographic distribution, association with particular vehicle of transmission, infectivity, virulence, and propensity to produce a particular clinical syndrome. Thus, serotyping is a useful marker in epidemiologic studies.

Public Health Significance

Over 20,000 *Salmonella* isolates are reported from humans in the United States each year. Since these isolates are estimated to represent approximately 1% of the people clinically ill with salmonellosis—over 2 million cases of symptomatic salmonellosis may occur annually in the United States (54).

Efforts to prevent human salmonellosis have centered on reducing the contamination of food products, educating consumers to prevent food handling errors, and eliminating sources of high risk (such as banning the interstate shipment of pet turtles). Efforts by industry and government to pasteurize egg products have been associated with a decrease in salmonellosis associated with eggs. On the other hand, outbreaks associated with meat and poultry still occur. The incidence of salmonellosis will only be reduced when the reservoir among food animals is reduced, thus resulting in less overall contamination of food with *Salmonella*.

Primary Isolation

An enrichment broth is recommended for isolating *Salmonella* from fecal specimens even though *Salmonella* colonies are often seen on primary plates of feces from persons who are acutely ill with diarrhea. Enrichment is always indicated to insure the maximal isolation rate. Most enrichment broths for *Salmonella* are highly selective. They allow the growth of *Salmonella* but inhibit growth of other bacteria. The three selective enrichment media most widely used to isolate salmonellae from fecal specimens are tetrathionate broth (59), tetra-thionate broth with brilliant green (46), and selenite F broth (51). Tetrathio-nate brilliant green broth is an excellent medium for recovering most other *Salmonella* (39, 46), but it inhibits *S. typhi*. Many prefer to use either selenite or tetrathionate without the brilliant green dye because neither inhibits *S. typhi*, and both are good for recovering most other *Salmonella* (45, 76). All three selective enrichment broths inhibit certain serotypes of *salmonella*. *Salmonella cholerae-suis* (51, 76, 77), *S. abortusbovis* (76), and *S. paratyphi* A (3) are among the serotypes which have been reported to be inhibited. Strains which are inhibited by the selective enrichment broths are best isolated by di-rect plating or enrichment in a non-selective broth.

Many plating media are used to isolate salmonellae from fecal specimens. These media are differential and vary from slightly selective to highly selec-tive. The media of low selectivity used include MacConkey, EMB, and des-oxycholate agar, but unless a laboratory is screening for one of the more fas-tidious salmonellae, it is generally recommended that the more selective plating media be used. Media of intermediate selectivity such as XLD, des-oxycholate citrate, SS, and HE agar are widely used by laboratories that screen for both *Salmonella* and *Shigella* because they support the growth of both of these groups of organisms. If laboratory resources permit the use of a plating medium for *Salmonella* alone, one of the highly selective media such as brilliant green (BG) or bismuth sulfite agar (BS) is superior to the less selective media (27). Although the media of low and intermediate selectivity suppress growth of some gram-negative bacteria, they are not nearly as selective as BS or BG and allow growth of contaminants which cannot be differentiated from *Salmonella* without further tests. The combination of BG agar and tetrathio-nate brilliant green broth is particularly good for isolating *Salmonella* other than *S. typhi*.

Bismuth sulfite agar is the preferred medium for isolating *S. typhi*, and it is very useful for detecting lactose-fermenting strains of both *Salmonella* and *Arizona*. Bismuth sulfite has been reported to inhibit *Salmonella* serotypes other than *S. typhi* unless is is refrigerated at 4 C for at least 24 hr before use (15, 45). For isolating *S. typhi* however, pour-plates are preferable although streak-plates can be substituted if they are prepared immediately before use. If pour-plates are used, subsurface colonies should be re-streaked (to remove in-hibited bacteria under the colonies) on a nonselective medium such as Mac-Conkey or EMB before biochemical tests are done.

Typical *Salmonella* colonies should be selected from the plating medium and transferred to either TSI or KIA. At least two representatives of each type of suspicious colony should be selected from each plate. Another medium, ly-sine iron agar (LIA) (28), indicates the decarboxylation or deamination of ly-sine and the production of hydrogen sulfide. LIA used in conjunction with TSI agar is particularly helpful in the presumptive identification of *Salmonella*. Both of these media can be inoculated from one colony by first inoculating the TSI in the usual manner and then inoculating the LIA by stabbing the butt of the medium twice and streaking the slant. If results are needed quickly, a trypticase soy tryptose (TST) broth for determining H antigens can also be inoculated from this colony. Otherwise, the TST broth can be inoculated from the TSI culture. If a culture appears contaminated on either the TSI or LIA, it should be replated on nonselective media such as MacConkey or EMB before proceeding. Isolates which react like typical *Salmonella* or *Arizona* on either TSI or LIA (Tables 25.16, 25.17) should be kept for further analysis. If serogrouping is needed they should be examined with the slide test using antisera for the *Salmonella* O group antigens A, B, C_1, C_2, D, E (E_1, E_2, E_3, E_4), and G.

TABLE 25.16—REACTIONS OF *ENTEROBACTERIACEAE* IN TRIPLE SUGAR IRON (TSI) AGAR MEDIUM

TRIPLE SUGAR IRON AGAR[a]				PROBABLE
SLANT	BUTT	GAS	H$_2$S	GENUS AND SPECIES
Acid	Acid	+	−	*Escherichia coli* *Enterobacter* *Klebsiella*
Acid	Acid	−	−	*Salmonella typhi* *Escherichia coli* *Serratia*
Acid	Acid	+	+	*Arizona* *Citrobacter* *Proteus mirabilis* *Proteus vulgaris*
Alkaline	Acid	+	−	*Salmonella* *Citrobacter* *Hafnia alvei* *Escherichia coli* *Morganella morganii* *Providencia*
Alkaline	Acid	−	−	*Salmonella typhi* *Shigella* *Escherichia coli* *Morganella morganii* *Providencia* *Serratia*
Alkaline	Acid	−	+	*Salmonella typhi*
Alkaline	Acid	+	+	*Salmonella* *Arizona* *Citrobacter* *Edwardsiella tarda* *Proteus mirabilis* *Proteus vulgaris*

[a] Alkaline slant indicates lactose and sucrose not fermented. Acid slant indicates lactose or sucrose fermented. Acid butt indicates glucose fermented.

A positive reaction in either the polyvalent H or O group antisera and a typical TSI and LIA reaction indicate a presumptive *Salmonella*. If serotyping information is desired, those cultures positive in the O group antiserum can be screened for H antigens using Spicer-Edwards pooled antisera (26, 79). The Spicer-Edwards pools include seven pools of antisera for determining 17 flagella antigens. Additional absorbed antisera are required for final serotyping. If the serologic screening yields negative reactions, the following tests should be done: urea, indole, lysine decarboxylase, growth in KCN, motility, and fermentation of dulcitol and lactose. Typical *Salmonella* and *Arizona* are urea⁻, indole⁻, lysine⁺, and KCN⁻. Most *Salmonella* ferment dulcitol but not lactose, whereas *Arizona* isolates usually ferment lactose but not dulcitol. If these bio-

TABLE 25.17—REACTIONS OF *ENTEROBACTERIACEAE* IN LYSINE IRON AGAR (LIA) MEDIUM

LYSINE IRON AGAR[a]				PROBABLE
SLANT	BUTT	GAS	H₂S	GENUS AND SPECIES
Alkaline	Alkaline	Variable	+	*Salmonella* *Salmonella typhi*[b] *Arizona* *Edwardsiella tarda*
Alkaline	Alkaline	Variable	−	*Salmonella* *Salmonella typhi* *Arizona* *Hafnia alvei* *Enterobacter aerogenes* *Escherichia coli* *Klebsiella* *Serratia*
Alkaline	Acid	Variable	+	*Salmonella paratyphi* A *Citrobacter* *Morganella morganii*
Alkaline	Acid	Variable	−	*Salmonella paratyphi* A *Shigella* *Citrobacter* *Enterobacter cloacae* *Morganella morganii*
Red	Acid	−	+	*Proteus mirabilis* *Proteus vulgaris*
Red	Acid	−	−	*Proteus mirabilis* *Proteus vulgaris* *Providencia*

[a] Red slant indicates oxidative deamination. Alkaline butt indicates lysine decarboxylation. Acid butt indicates lysine not dexcarboxylated.

[b] A rare culture of *S. typhi* may fail to decarboxylate lysine.

chemical reactions are not characteristic, and *Salmonella* antigens are found, the cultures should be plated on MacConkey agar or EMB to obtain a pure culture, tested biochemically (complete set), or forwarded to a reference laboratory.

Serological Methods for Patient's Serum

A method sometimes used in diagnosing typhoid fever is based on a patient's antibody response to one of the antigens of *S. typhi*, a procedure usually known as the Widal reaction (52). This test measures agglutinating antibodies to O and H antigens of *S. typhi* and is usually used when *S. typhi* can not be isolated. Many consider the antibody titer to H antigen to be of little value because it is much less specific than the O titer, although concurrent rises in H and O titers are supportive. To interpret any febrile agglutination test results, it is necessary to obtain acute-phase and convalescent-phase sera (1 to 2 weeks apart). A $\geq$ 4-fold increase in titer to the O antigen is considered significant by some, but must be interpreted cautiously, since other serologically related (Group D) *Salmonella* could cause the antibody rise. Points to consider in interpreting results of this test are: a) the commercial antigens that are available are poorly standardized; b) patient antibodies to other bacteria with common O and H antigens can cross-react, indicating that a diagnosis of typhoid fever should not be based on this test result alone; c) production of O and H agglutinins may be suppressed by early treatment with chloramphenicol; and d) prior typhoid immunization may be responsible for the patient's antibody titer. An O titer of 1:50 or 1:100 on a single specimen in the first 2 weeks of illness is considered significant by some if the patient has not been vaccinated.

It has also been shown that typhoid carriers may have titers against the Vi antigen; however, the test is difficult to perform, and false-negative as well as false-positive results may be obtained. Both favorable and unfavorable evaluations of this test have been reported.

Marker Systems

Serotyping is the most important marker for *Salmonella* and is very useful in epidemiologic studies. In many countries, including the United States, *Salmonella* isolates are serotyped by regional or national centers. In the U.S. *S. typhimurium* accounts for over 30% of all *Salmonella* infections (Table 25.5); thus additional typing can be helpful in epidemiologic studies (27). The antibiogram can be useful because strains of *S. typhimurium* have many different resistance patterns. A biotyping scheme has been described and used in several countries, but it has not been evaluated in the United States. Bacteriophage typing has provided additional sensitivity for *S. typhimurium* and also for some of the other common serotypes. Unfortunately, bacteriophage typing is a complicated procedure that requires careful standardization, and should be attempted only by a laboratory that can devote considerable time to it. It should only be used in well-defined epidemiologic investigations (a carefully selected control group should be included) where specific questions can be answered with the laboratory data.

References

1. ASERKOFF BA and BENNETT JV: Effect of therapy in acute salmonellosis on Salmonellae in feces. N Engl J Med 281:3–7, 1969
2. BAINE WB, GANGAROSA EJ, BENNETT JV, and BARKER WH: Institutional salmonellosis. J Infect Dis 128:357–360, 1973
3. BANWART GJ and AYRES JC: Effect of various enrichment broths and selective agars upon the growth of several species of *Salmonella*. Appl Microbiol 1:296–301, 1953
4. BARRETT-CONNOR E and CONNOR JD: Extraintestinal manifestations of shigellosis. Am J Gastroenterol 53:234–245, 1970
5. BARTLETT RC: Medical microbiology: How fast to go—how far to go. *In* Significance of Medical Microbiology in the Care of Patients. Lorian V (ed). The Williams & Wilkins Co, Baltimore, 1977, p 15–35
6. BENNETT IL and HOOK EW: Infectious diseases (some aspects of salmonellosis). Annu Rev Med 10:1–20, 1959
7. BLACK PH, KUNZ LJ, and SWARTZ MN: Salmonellosis—A review of some unusual aspects. N Engl J Med 262:813–817, 1960
8. BLAZEVIC DJ, STEMPER JE, and MATSEN JM: Organisms encountered in urine culture over a 10 year period. Appl Microbiol 23:421–422, 1972
9. BLOCK NB and FERGUSON W: An outbreak of Shiga dysentery in Michigan. Am J Public Health 30:43–52, 1940
9a. BRENNER DJ: Speciation in *Yersinia*. Contrib Microbiol Immunol 5:33–43, 1979
10. BRENNER DJ, FARMER JJ III, HICKMAN FW, ASBURY MA, and STEIGERWALT AG: Taxonomic and nomenclatural changes in Enterobacteriaceae. Center for Disease Control, Atlanta, Ga, 1977
11. BUCHANAN RE and GIBBONS NE (eds.): Bergey's Manual of Determinative Bacteriology. 8th edition. The Williams & Wilkins Co, Baltimore, 1974
12. CENTER FOR DISEASE CONTROL: Morbid Mortal Weekly Rep 19:269–270, 1970
13. CENTER FOR DISEASE CONTROL: *Shigella* Surveillance Report No. 39. Annual Summary, 1976, CDC, Atlanta, Ga
14. CHRISTIE AB: Bacillary dysentery. *In* Infectious Diseases: Epidemiology and Clinical Practice, 2nd edition. Churchill Livingstone, London, 1974, pp 122–147
15. COOK CT: Comparison of two modifications of bismuth-sulphite agar for the isolation and growth of *Salmonella typhi* and *Salmonella typhimurium*. J Pathol Bacteriol 64:559–566, 1952
16. COOKE EM: *Escherichia coli* and Man. Churchill Livingstone Co, London, 1973
17. COWAN ST: Cowan and Steel's Manual for the Identification of Medical Bacteria, 2nd edition. Cambridge Univ Press, New York, 1975
18. DAVIS TC: Chronic vulvovaginitis in children due to *Shigella flexneri*. Pediatrics 56:41–44, 1975
19. DE SN, BHATTACHARYA K, and SARKAR JK: A study of the pathogenicity of strain of *Bacterium coli:* from acute and chronic enteritis. J Pathol Bacteriol 71:201–209, 1956
20. DEAN AG, CHING VI-CHUAN, WILLIAMS G, and BARDEN B: Test for *Escherichia coli* enterotoxin using infant mice: application in a study of diarrhea in children in Honolulu, J Infect Dis 125:407–411, 1972
21. DONOWITZ M, NEUSCH GT, and BINDER HT: Effect of *Shigella* enterotoxin on electrolyte transport in rabbit ileum. Gastroenterology 69:1230–1238, 1975
22. DONTA ST and SMITH DM: Stimulation of steriodogenesis in tissue culture by enterotoxigenic *Escherichia coli* and its neutralization by specific antiserum. Infect Immun 9:500–505, 1974
23. DUPONT HL, FORMAL SB, and HORNICK RB: Pathogenesis of *Escherichia coli* diarrhea. N Engl J Med 285:1–9, 1971

24. DuPONT HL and HORNICK RB: Adverse effect of lomotil therapy in shigellosis. J Am Med Assoc 226:1525-1528, 1973

25. DuPONT HL and SPINK WW: Infections due to gram-negative organisms: An analysis of 860 patients with bacteremia at the University of Minnesota Medical Center, 1958-1966. Medicine 48:307-332, 1969

25a. EBRINGER RW, CALDWELL DR, COWLING P, and EBRINGER A: Sequential studies in ankylosing spondylitis: Association of Klebsiella pneumoniae with active disease. Ann Rheum Dis 37:146-151, 1978

25b. EDELMAN R and LEVINE MM: Acute diarrheal infections in infants. II. Bacterial and viral causes. Hosp Pract 15:97-104, 1980

26. EDWARDS PR: Serologic examination of Salmonella cultures for epidemiologic purposes. Center for Disease Control, Atlanta, Ga, 1962

27. EDWARDS PR and EWING WH: Identification of Enterobacteriaceae, 3rd edition, Burgess Publishing Co, Minneapolis, 1972

28. EDWARDS PR and FIFE MA: Lysine-iron agar in the detection of Arizona cultures. Appl Microbiol 9:478-480, 1961

29. EPIDEMIOLOGICAL RESEARCH LABORATORY, CENTRAL PUBLIC HEALTH LABORATORY, COLINDALE: Quarterly Tabulations: Thirteen Weeks 40-52, 1975. Communicable Dis Rpts No. 40-52 (2nd, January 1976). Public Health Laboratory Service, London NW9 5HT, England, 1976

30. EVANS DG, SILVER RP, EVANS DJ JR, CHASE DG, and GORBACH S: Plasmid-controlled colonization factor associated with virulence in Escherichia coli enterotoxigenic for humans. Infect Immun 12:656-667, 1975

31. EWING WH: Isolation and Identification of Escherichia coli Serotypes Associated with Diarrhea Disease. Center for Disease Control, Atlanta, Ga, 1963

32. EWINGWH: Transport methods for Enterobacteriaceae and allied bacteria. Public Health Lab 29:8-23, 1971

33. EWING WH: The nomenclature of Salmonella, its usage, and definition for the three species. Can J Microbiol 18:1629-1637, 1972

34. EWING WH and DAVIS BR: Media and Tests for Differentiation of Enterobacteriaceae. Center for Disease Control, Atlanta, Ga, 1970

35. EWING WH and MARTIN WT: Enterobacteriaceae. In Manual of Clinical Microbiology. Lennette EH, Spalding EH, and Truant JP (eds.). American Society for Microbiology. Washington, DC, 1974, pp 189-221

35a. FANNING R, FARMER JJ III, PARKER JN, HUNTLEY-CARTER GP, and BRENNER DJ: Kluyvera: A new genus in Enterobacteriaceae. Abstr Annu Meet Am Soc Microbiol 1979, Abstr no. I30, p 100

36. FARMER JJ III: Bacteriocin typing of Pseudomonas, Proteus, and Klebsiella-Enterobacter-Serratia. In Opportunistic Pathogens. Prier JE and Friedman H (eds.). University Park Press, Baltimore, 1974, pp 49-63

37. FARMER JJ III, DAVIS BR, HICKMAN FW, PRESLEY DB, BODEY GP, NEGUT M, and BOBO RA: Detection of Serratia outbreaks in hospital. Lancet 2:787-789, 1976

38. FARMER JJ III, HICKMAN FW, BRENNER DJ, SCHREIBER M, and RICKENBACH DG: Unusual Enterobacteriaceae: Proteus rettgeri that change into Providenica stuartii. J Clin Microbiol 6:373-378, 1977

39. GALTON MM, MORRIS GK, and MARTIN WT: Salmonella in Foods and Feeds—Review of Isolation Methods and Recommended Procedures. Center for Disease Control, Atlanta, Ga, 1968

40. GANGAROSA EJ and MERSON MH: Epidemiologic assessment of the relevance of the so-called enteropathogenic serogroups of Escherichia coli in diarrhea. N Engl J Med 296:1210-1213, 1977

41. GORBACH SL and KHURANA CM: Toxigenic Escherichia coli: a cause of infantile diarrhea in Chicago. N Engl J Med 287:791-795, 1972

41a. GRIMONT PAD, GRIMONT F, RICHARD C, DAVIS BR, STEIGERWALT AG, and BRENNER DJ: Deoxyribonucleic acid relatedness between Serratia plymuthica and other Serratia species, with a description of Serratia odorifera sp. nov. (type strain: ICPB 3995). Int J Syst Bacteriol 28:453-463, 1978

42. GUERRANT RL, BRANTON LL, SCHNAITMAN T, REBHUN LI, and GILMAN AG: Cyclic

adenosine monophosphate and alternation of Chinese hamster ovary cell morphology: a rapid, sensitive *in vitro* assay for the enterotoxins of *Vibrio cholerae* and *Escherichia coli.* Infect Immun 10:320–327, 1974

43. HAN T, SOKAL JE, and NETER E: Salmonellosis in disseminated malignant diseases: A seven-year review. N Engl J Med 276:1045–1052, 1967

44. HARRIS JC, DUPONT HL, and HORNICK RB: Fecal leukocytes in diarrheal illness. Ann Intern Med 76:697–703, 1971

45. HOBBS BC and ALLISON VD: Studies on the isolation of *Bact. typhosum* and *Bact. para-typhosum* B. I. Comparison of the selective value of Wilson and Blair (Difco) and desoxycholate citrate agars and four liquid enrichment media including selenite F. Mon Bull Min Health Public Health Lab Serv 4:12–19, 1945

46. KAUFFMANN F: Weitere erfahrungen mit dem kombinierten anreicherungs verfahren fur Salmonellabacillen. J Hyg Infektionskr 117:26–32, 1935

47. KAUFFMANN F: The Bacteriology of Enterobacteriaceae. The Williams & Wilkins Co, Baltimore, 1966

48. KAUFFMANN F and DUPONT A: *Escherichia* strains from infantile gastro-enteritis. Acta Pathol Microbiol Scand 27:552–564, 1950

49. KEUSCH GT and JACEWICZ M: Pathogenesis of *Shigella* diarrhea: VI. Toxin and antitoxin in *Shigella flexneri* and *Shigella sonnei* infections in humans. J Infect Dis 135:552–556, 1977

49a. KLEEBERGER A: Untersuchungen zur taxonomie von Enterobakterien und Pseudomonaden aus hackfleisch. Arch Lebensmittelhyg 30:130–137, 1979

50. KUNIN CM: Detection, prevention and management of urinary tract infections, 2nd edition. Lea and Febiger, Philadelphia, 1974

51. LEIFSON E: New selenite enrichment media for the isolation of typhoid and paratyphoid (*Salmonella*) bacilli. Am J Hyg 24:423–432, 1936

52. LENNETTE EH, BALOWS A, HAUSLER WJ, and TRUANT JP (eds.): Manual of Clinical Microbiology. American Society for Microbiology, Washington, DC, 1980

52a. LEVINE MM and EDELMAN R: Acute diarrheal infections in infants. I. Epidemiology, treatment, and prospects for immunoprophylaxis. Hosp Pract 14:89–100, 1979

53. LI K, FARMER JJ III, and COPPOLA A: A novel type of resistant bacteria induced by gentamicin. Trans NY Acad Sci 36:369–396, 1974

54. LOWENSTEIN MS and GANGAROSA EJ: Nontyphoid salmonellosis. *In* Practice of Medicine, Vol. III, Harper and Row, Hagerstown, Md, 1973, p 4

55. MAKI DG, GOLDMAN DA, and RHAME FS: Infection control in intravenous therapy. Ann Intern Med 79:867–887, 1973

56. MERSON MH, MORRIS GK, and SACK DA: Travelers' diarrhea in Mexico. N Engl J Med 294:1299–1304, 1976

57. MORRIS GK, KOEHLER JA, GANGAROSA EJ, and SHARRAR RG: Comparison of media for direct isolation and transport of shigellae from fecal specimens. Appl Microbiol 19:434–437, 1970

58. MORRIS GK and WELLS JG: Colicin typing of *Shigella sonnei.* Appl Microbiol 27:312–316, 1974

59. MUELLER J: Un nouveau milieu d'enrichissenent pour la recherche du bacille typhique et des paratyphiques. CR Seances Soc Biol 89:434, 1923

60. NETER E: Opportunistic pathogens: Immunological aspects. *In* Opportunistic pathogens. Prier JE and Friedman H (eds.), University Park Press, Baltimore, 1974, pp 37–48

61. NEW HC, CHERUBIN CE, LONGO ED, FLOWTON B, and WINTER J: Antimicrobial resistance and R-factor transfer among isolates of *Salmonella* in the Northeastern United States: A comparison of human and animal isolates. J Infect Dis 132:617–622, 1975

62. OGAWA H, NAHAMURA A, and SAKAZAKI R: Pathogenic properties of enteropathogenic *E. coli* from diarrheal children and adults. Jpn J Med Sci Biol 21:333–349, 1968

63. ORSKOV I, ORSKOV F, JANN B, and JANN K: Serology, chemistry, and genetics of O and K antigens of *Escherichia coli.* Bacteriol Rev 41:667–710, 1977

64. PICKERING LK, DUPONT HL, OLARTE J, CONKLIN R, and ERICSSON C: Fecal leucocytes in enteric infections. Am J Clin Pathol 68:562–565, 1977

65. PIERCE AK and SANFORD JP: Aerobic gram-negative bacillary pneumonias. Am Rev Respir Dis 110:647–658, 1974

66. PRUNEDA RC and FARMER JJ III: Bacteriophage typing of *Shigella sonnei.* J Clin Microbiol 5:66–74, 1977
67. RODGERS DE: The changing patterns of life-threatening microbial disease. N Engl J Med 261:677–683, 1959
68. ROSENBERG ML, WEISSMAN JB, GANGAROSA EJ, RELLER LB, and BEASLEY RP: Shigellosis in the United States: ten-year review of nationwide surveillance, 1964–1973. Am J Epidemiol 104:543–551, 1976
69. ROUNDTABLE: How far to go with *Enterobacteriaceae?* J Infect Dis 119:197–213, 1969
70. ROWE B: *Escherichia coli* in acute diarrhea. *In* Lab Lore (published by Burroughs Wellcome, Research Triangle Park, NC 27709), 7:449–452, 1977
71. SACK RB: Human diarrheal disease caused by enterotoxogenic *Escherichia coli.* Annu Rev Microbiol 29:333–353, 1975
72. SAPHRA I and WINTER JW: Clinical manifestations of salmonellosis in man. N Engl J Med 256:1128–1134, 1957
73. SCHABERG DR, ALFORD RH, ANDERSON R, FARMER JJ III, MELLY MA, and SCHAFFNER W: An outbreak of nosocomial infection due to multiply resistant *Serratia marcescens:* Evidence of interhospital spread. J Infect Dis 134:181–188, 1976
74. SCHMIDT WC and JEFFRIES CD: Bacteriophage typing of gram-negative rod-shaped bacteria. Crit Rev Clin Lab Sci 3:201–246, 1975
74a. SCHWACH T: Case Report. Clin Microbiol Newslett 1(16):4–5, 1979
74b. SCOTLAND SM, DAY NP, WILLIAMS GA, and ROWE B: Cytotoxic enteropathogenic *Escherichia coli.* Lancet 1:90, 1980
75. SERENY B: Experimental *Shigella* keratoconjunctivitis. Acta Microbiol Acad Sci Hung 2:293–296, 1955
76. SMITH HW: The evaluation of culture media for the isolation of salmonellae from faeces. J Hyg 50:21–36, 1952
77. SMITH HW: The isolation of salmonellae from the mesenteric lymph nodes and faeces of pigs, cattle, sheep, dogs and cats, and from other organs of poultry. J Hyg 57:266–273, 1959
78. SMITH PB: Performance of Six Bacterial Identification Systems. Center for Disease Control, Atlanta, Ga, 1975
79. SPICER CC: A quick method for identifying *Salmonella* "H" antigens. J Clin Pathol 9:378–379, 1956
80. STAMM WE: Guidelines for prevention of catheter associated urinary tract infection. Ann Intern Med 82:386–390, 1975
81. TAYLOR WI and HARRIS B: Isolation of shigellae. II. Comparison of plating media and enrichment broths. J Clin Pathol 44:476–479, 1965
82. TAYLOR WI and SCHELHART D: Isolation of shigellae. V. Comparison and enrichment broths with stools. Appl Microbiol 16:1383–1386, 1968
83. TULLOCH EF, RYAN KJ, and FORMAL SB: Invasive enteropathogenic *Escherichia coli* dysentery. Ann Intern Med 79:13–17, 1973
83a. ULSHEN MH and ROLLO JL: Pathogenesis of *Escherichia coli* gastroenteritis in man—another mechanism. N Engl J Med 302:99–101, 1980
84. VON GRAEVENITZ A: Are microbial identification and sensitivity testing necessary for effective chemotherapy? *In* The Clinical Laboratory as an Aid in Chemotherapy of Infectious Disease. Borchi A, Bartola JT, and Prier JE (eds.). University Park Press, Baltimore, 1977, pp 169–179
85. WADSTROM T, AUST-KETTIS A, HABTE D, HOLMGREN J, MEEUWISSE G, MOLLBY R, and SODERLIND O: Enterotoxin-producing bacteria and parasites in stool of Ethopian children with diarrhoeal disease. Arch Dis Child 51:865–870, 1976
86. WEISSMAN JB, GANGAROSA EJ, and BARKER WH: Shigellosis. *In* Tice's Practice of Medicine. Harper and Row Publishers, Inc, Hagerstown, Md, 1974, pp 1–17
87. WEISSMAN JB, GANGAROSA EJ, DUPONT HL, NELSON JD, and HALTALIN KC: Shigellosis: to treat or not to treat. J Am Med Assoc 229:1215–1216, 1974
88. WHEELER KM and MICKLE FL: Antigens of *Shigella sonnei.* J Immunol 51:257–267, 1945
89. YOLKEN RH, GREENBERG HB, MERSON MH, SACK RB, and KAPIKIAN AZ: Enzyme-linked immunosorbent assay for detection of *Escherichia coli* heat-labile enterotoxin. J Clin Microbiol 6:439–444, 1977

CHAPTER 26

ERYSIPELOTHRIX INFECTIONS

Richard H. Conklin

Introduction

Erysipelothrix rhusiopathiae (insidiosa) is the causative organism of erysipeloid, a cutaneous infection of humans, which is probably more common than the literature indicates. The organism was first isolated by Koch in 1880. In 1883, Pasteur and Thuiller isolated the organism and prepared the first live attenuated vaccine. Rosenbach in 1884 named the human infection *erysipeloid* because of its similarity to the cutaneous appearance of streptococcal erysipelas. In 1886, Loeffler presented the first detailed description of the organism (8).

Description

Erysipelothrix is classified in the family *Corynebacteriaceae* with the corynebacteria and *Listeria*. *Erysipelothrix* is a gram-positive rod which is easily decolorized and may appear to be gram-negative. Granules similar to those seen in diphtheroids are often present. It is not acid fast. It is nonmotile, noncapsulated, and nonsporulating.

The cellular morphology of the organism is dependent on the colony type. Initial isolates are usually the smooth colonial form. These are small (0.1–0.5 mm) and may be easily overlooked. They are glistening, clear, circular, convex colonies which become somewhat bluish and opaque with age. On blood agar a small zone of alpha hemolysis is usually seen. The rough colonies are slightly larger (0.5–1 mm), flatter, and more irregular. Intermediate forms may be found. Organisms from smooth colonies appear as slender, short (1–2 μm) rods. They tend to be arranged in short chains and clusters and may look like diphtheroids. The cells from rough colonies are long filaments or in chains. They resemble actinomycetes but do not branch (9). *Erysipelothrix* is a facultative aerobe which grows at a wide range of temperatures (4 to 41 C); 37 C is optimal. The optimum pH for growth is 7.4–7.8. The organism is best grown in 1% glucose broth or *Erysipelothrix* selective broth. Growth in liquid media is enhanced by the addition of serum or Tween 80. The yield of positive cultures is increased when tissue is incubated in glucose broth, tryptose broth, or beef infusion broth at 4 C for 2–5 weeks (6). This is not practical in most clinical situations.

393

One of the most helpful biochemical reactions of *Erysipelothrix* is the acidification of the butt and slant without gas production but with H_2S production in TSI agar. This reaction plus the "test tube brush" appearance in gelatin stabs makes possible the presumptive identification of the organism. Carbohydrate fermentations should be performed using Andrade base with 10% serum (6). *E. rhusiopathiae* is catalase negative and inhibited by potassium tellurite which differentiate it from both *Listeria monocytogenes* and diphtheroids. *Erysipelothrix* is nonmotile, does not have beta hemolysis, does not ferment trehalose or salicin, and is resistant to neomycin. These features help distinguish it from *Listeria monocytogenes*. *Erysipelothrix* also does not hydrolyze esculin or reduce nitrates.

Epidemiology

E. rhusiopathiae has been found as a saprophyte or a pathogen in a wide variety of marine life and in domestic and wild animals (1). Until recently it was thought to persist in contaminated soil for prolonged periods. Wood (8) has found no evidence for this.

Human infection is basically an occupational hazard throughout the world. The population at risk is people handling contaminated animals or products such as meat, fish, shellfish, hides, poultry, or abattoir wastes. The organism is resistant to most food preservation techniques. The risk of infection may be reduced by protection against skin injury, personal hygiene, and treatment of skin breaks. Regular disinfection of instruments and work areas is important in controlling the organism. *E. rhusiopathiae* is readily killed by most common disinfectants (8).

Clinical Disease

Human infection by *Erysipelothrix* causes three distinct clinical entities: 1. erysipeloid, 2. generalized cutaneous infection, and 3. septicemia.

The most common infection caused by *E. rhusiopathiae* is erysipeloid, a localized, cutaneous infection usually on the fingers or hands. It is characterized by a well-demarcated area of violaceous erythema, which spreads peripherally and has central fading. This is associated with local swelling, pruritus, and pain which seems out of proportion to the observed lesion. There is usually no lymphangitis, lymphadenitis, or constitutional symptomatology. The bacteria are introduced through skin wounds or preexisting skin breaks. Erysipeloid appears in 2–7 days after inoculation. The appearance and distribution of the lesions are usually diagnostic for the experienced clinician. The major clinical differential diagnoses are pyogenic infections, dermatitis, and cutaneous anthrax.

In the generalized, cutaneous infection there may be progression from a local lesion or the development of lesions at remote sites. The appearance is similar to the local cutaneous form of infection. Bullae and vesicles may form. Septicemia with or without endocarditis is very rare in nonimmunosuppressed hosts. Endocarditis may occur in patients without preexisting valvular disease. In 40% of the patients cutaneous lesions are also present (2).

Laboratory Diagnosis

In erysipeloid, the appearance of the lesion is often diagnostic; a culture may be unnecessary. If it is necessary to culture cutaneous lesions, the optimal specimen is a full thickness skin biopsy from the advancing border of the lesion (4). Swabs and aspirates are generally less rewarding than a biopsy. When a biopsy is obtained, part of it should be submitted for histopathologic examination with tissue Gram stain. The remainder should be cultured in 1% glucose broth and subcultured on blood agar plates. An alternative or adjunct procedure is mouse inoculation with a suspension of biopsy material (7). For the septicemic form of disease, standard blood culture techniques will yield positive cultures. It is important that *E. rhusiopathiae* is not confused with nonpathogenic diphtheroids or other contaminants.

A fluorescent antibody technique has been reported for the diagnosis of *E. rhusiopathiae*, but it is not available in most clinical laboratories at this time (3).

References

1. CONKLIN RH and STEELE JH: Erysipelothrix Infections. CRC Handbook Series in Zoonoses, Vol. I. Stoenner H and Kaplan W (eds.). CRC Press, Cleveland, 1979, pp 327–337
2. GRIECO MH and SHELDON C: *Erysipelothrix rhusiopathiae*. Ann NY Acad Sci 174:523–532, 1970
3. HEGGERS VP, BUDDINGTON RS, and MCALLISTER HA: *Erysipelothrix* endocarditis diagnosis by fluorescence microscopy. Am J Clin Pathol 62:803–806, 1974
4. HOEPRICH PD: Erysipeloid. *In* Infectious Diseases, 4th edition. Harper and Row, Hagerstown, Md, 1972, pp 753–755
5. REED RW: *Listeria* and *Erysipelothrix*. *In* Bacterial and Mycotic Infections of Man, 4th edition. J.B. Lippincott, Philadelphia, 1965, pp 752–762
6. WHITE TG and SHURMAN RD: Fermentation reactions of *Erysipelothrix rhusiopathiae*. J Bacteriol 82:595–599, 1961
7. WOOD RL: *Erysipelothrix*. *In* Manual of Clinical Microbiology, 1st edition. American Society for Microbiology, Bethesda, Md, 1970, pp 102–105
8. WOOD RL: *Erysipelothrix* Infections. *In* Diseases Transmitted from Animals to Man, 6th edition. Charles C. Thomas, Springfield, Ill, 1975, pp 271–281
9. WOOD RL and SHUMAN RD: Swine erysipelas. *In* Diseases of Swine, 4th edition. Iowa State University Press, Ames, Iowa, 1975, pp 565–620

CHAPTER 27

MISCELLANEOUS GRAM-NEGATIVE RODS

A. von Graevenitz, J. R. Greenwood, and K. Price

Introduction

The bacterial genera and species discussed in this chapter are, according to the 8th edition of Bergey's Manual of Determinative Bacteriology (1), of uncertain affiliation. The new genus *Kingella* is not mentioned in the 8th edition; neither are the bacterial taxa discussed in the Appendix.

The authors have also mentioned G+C (guanine-cytosine) ratios for the various species under discussion. The GC ratio expresses the molar percentage of guanine plus cytosine in the bacterial deoxyribonucleic acid (the percentage of adenine plus thymine making up the rest). Values listed were obtained by thermal denaturation of DNA. The temperature at which 50% of the maximal increase in extinction caused by the DNA is reached—as measured in a spectrophotometer at 260 mμ is called T_m and is related to the G+C ratio by the equation $T_m = 69.3 + 0.41 \cdot GC$.

Chromobacterium

Causative Organism(s)

The genus *Chromobacterium* consists of two species of gram-negative rods with no distinct growth factor requirements: a mesophilic, facultatively anaerobic one (*C. violaceum*) and a psychrophilic, strictly aerobic one (*C. lividum*) (94). The guanine + cytosine (G+C) ratio is 63–72 moles % (T_m). Both species share three unusual features: (a) production of a violet, indole-pyrrole pigment, violacein; (b) motility by one polar flagellum of relatively long wavelength and one to four subpolar or lateral flagella with shorter wavelengths; (c) sensitivity to hydrogen peroxide.

The differential characteristics are listed in Table 27.1. Since only *C. violaceum* has been isolated from human specimens so far, discussion will be limited to this species (G+C ratio 63.4–67.7 moles %) (17).

Clinical Manifestations

C. violaceum is a rare pathogen of animals and humans. Spontaneous disease has been recorded in monkeys, buffaloes, cattle, wild boars, and swine (93). Human infections have been reported from areas with semitropical to

TABLE 27.1—Differential Features of *Chromobacterium* Species [After Sneath (94)]

Test	*C. VIOLACEUM*	*C. LIVIDUM*
Growth at 37 C	+	$-/+^w$
Growth at 4 C	−	+
Acid from trehalose	+	−
Acid from arabinose	−	$+^d$
Esculin hydrolysis	−	+
Casein hydrolysis	+	$-/+^w$

Key: +, positive; −, negative; d, delayed; w, weak.

tropical climates (e.g., Southeast Asia, the Southeastern United States). Characteristic are overwhelming septicemia with pulmonary, liver, and subcutaneous abscesses in previously healthy individuals (14, 61, 106). The case-fatality ratio is high.

Epidemiology

The natural habitats of *C. violaceum* are soil and natural water sources in tropical and nontropical climates. The density is probably low (15). In human infections, the portal of entry is probably a skin lesion, perhaps also the gastrointestinal tract (14, 61, 106). Contact of infected humans with diseased animals has not been reported. No preventive measures have been recommended.

Collection and Processing of Specimens

Specimens include those from the environment (soil, water), human pus, blood, and autopsy tissues. Nothing is known about the effect of transport media, correct collection, and optimal number of specimens.

Diagnostic Procedures (9, 93, 94)

Microscopic examination

Cells of *C. violaceum* are 0.8–1.2 × 2.5–6.0 μm in size and may be pleomorphic in culture. The unique flagellar arrangement is seen best in young cultures on solid media. Lateral flagella are rare in broth cultures.

Primary culture media

C. violaceum grows on ordinary peptone media, blood agar, MacConkey agar, and EMB agar; growth on SS agar is delayed. A special technique for isolation from soil has been described (15). Growth occurs under anaerobic and aerobic conditions between 10 and 40 C; the optimum is between 30 and 35 C.

Identification procedures

Colonies of *C. violaceum* on blood agar are 1–2 mm in diameter after 24 hr of growth at 37 C, round, smooth, low convex, smell of cyanide, and give variable zones of beta hemolysis. Rough colonies may appear after prolonged incubation. Most colonies exhibit the violet pigment, but nonpigmented strains

TABLE 27.2—BIOCHEMICAL REACTIONS OF *CHROMOBACTERIUM VIOLACEUM*

		Acid from:	
Oxidase	+	Adonitol	−
Catalase	+	Arabinose	−
Indole	−	Dulcitol	−
Urease (Christensen)	−/+[d]	Fructose	+
Lysine decarboxylase	−	Galactose	−
Ornithine decarboxylase	−	Glucose	+
Arginine dihydrolase	+	Inositol	−
Phenylalanine deaminase	−	Lactose	−
Gelatinase	+	Maltose	−
Citrate (Simmons)	+/−	Mannitol	−
Triple sugar iron agar	K/A(G) or	Raffinose	−
	A/A(G), H_2S-	Rhamnose	−
Kligler iron agar	K/A(G), H_2S-	Salicin	−
Voges-Proskauer reaction (37 C)	−	Sorbitol	−
Esculin hydrolysis	−	Sucrose	+/−
ONPG	−	Trehalose	+
Nitrate reduction	+	Xylose	−
Gas from glucose	−/(+)		

Key: +, positive; −, negative; d, delayed; ( ), reaction of rare strain; G, gas.

as well as nonpigmented variant colonies are not uncommon. The pigment is not water soluble and thus does not readily diffuse into culture media. Oxygen, and possibly tryptophane, are necessary for its production. Growth at suboptimal temperatures favors its emergence; certain peptones, on the other hand, may be inhibitory. Broth cultures show uniform turbidity and a violet pellicle. Viability of strains on culture media is low.

Biochemical reactions are listed in Table 27.2. Characteristic are positive oxidase and negative indole reactions in a fermentative setting. If pigmentation interferes, the oxidase test may have to be done on anaerobically incubated cultures. Carbohydrate fermentation can be tested in peptone water base media. In the differential diagnosis, rare strains of *Pseudomonas cepacia* forming a violet pigment (96) can be separated by their oxidative metabolism of carbohydrates, whereas other oxidase-positive, nonfastidious fermentative bacilli like *Aeromonas hydrophila*, *Plesiomonas shigelloides*, and *Vibrio* spp. can be separated by tests listed in Table 27.3. Aerogenic strains of *C. violaceum* have only recently been reported (85).

TABLE 27.3—DIFFERENTIAL DIAGNOSIS OF *CHROMOBACTERIUM VIOLACEUM*

TEST	*C. VIOLACEUM*	*AEROMONAS HYDROPHILA*	*PLESIOMONAS SHIGELLOIDES*	*VIBRIO SPP* *
Lysine decarboxylase	−	−/(+)	+	+
Ornithine decarboxylase	−	−	+	+/(−)
Indole	−	+/(−)	+	+
Acid from mannitol	−	+	−	+*
Acid from maltose	−	+	+/(−)	+
Gelatinase	+	+	−	+

Key: +, positive; −, negative; ( ), reaction of rare strain.
* A few strains (halophilic sp.) may be lactose +.

Serologic procedures

C. *violaceum* strains cross-agglutinate extensively (93). No routine serological methods are in use.

Animal pathogenicity

C. *violaceum* strains, regardless of pigmentation, are pathogenic for mice and guinea pigs on intraperitoneal injection (87, 93). The liver is the organ principally affected.

Antimicrobic susceptibility

C. *violaceum* strains tested have been found sensitive in disk tests to tetracycline, chloramphenicol, carbenicillin, nitrofurantoin, and nalidixic acid and resistant to penicillin, cephalothin, ampicillin, and the polymyxins; susceptibility to the aminoglycoside antimicrobials varies (61, 86, 93, 106). It seems necessary to test clinical strains.

Evaluation of laboratory findings

C. *violaceum* is more rarely isolated from human specimens than other soil and water organisms, e.g., *Aeromonas hydrophila* (106). In view of past reports of systemic disease, attention to each strain isolated seems justified.

Flavobacterium

Causative Organisms

The flavobacteria are free-living, saprophytic organisms occurring in soil and water. They are pigmented, nonmotile, gram-negative rods. The majority of flavobacteria isolated from clinical specimens belong in one of these groups: *Flavobacterium meningosepticum*, *F. odoratum* (formerly CDC Group M-4f), *F. breve*, CDC Group IIb, and CDC Group IIf. There are no Linnean binomials for the latter two groups, Complete bacteriological descriptions of these groups are given below.

Clinical Manifestations

Flavobacteria are occasionally found in clinical specimens but seldom have an etiologic role in disease. The important exception to this rule is *Flavobacterium meningosepticum.* This species has caused epidemics of meningitis and septicemia among newborn infants, especially premature infants (8, 47). In the newborn infant, flavobacterial infection presents the typical picture of bacterial septicemia or meningitis of this age group. There is a serious deterioration of the patient's general condition. Symptoms may be loss of appetite, fever, dyspnea, cyanotic spells, bulging fontanels, convulsions, irritability, stiffness of the neck, back or limbs, jaundice, or lethargy. The results in 47 cases of meningitis and/or septicemia were 36 deaths (77%), 7 cases of hydrocephalus (15%), 1 case of retardation (2%), and only 3 recoveries (6%) (21, 54, 77).

Flavobacterium meningosepticum was responsible for an epidemic of postoperative bacteremia in Denmark (62). Eight patients became febrile following major surgery. Blood cultures taken during the febrile episodes grew *F. meningosepticum*. In all cases temperatures returned to normal, and blood cultures became negative in 2 days or less. The patients were treated with penicillin and streptomycin. *F. meningosepticum* is resistant to these drugs *in vitro*, and it is unlikely that they had a significant effect on the outcome of these infections.

F. meningosepticum has also been reported from miscellaneous cases in adults, including meningitis, pneumonia, and endocarditis (47, 99, 108). These patients were suffering from conditions which lowered their resistance to infection.

F. odoratum (M-4f) has been isolated most frequently from urine. Other sources have been wounds, cutaneous ulcers, an amputation stump, gangrenous feet, an ear, sputum, and blood (44, 46, 98). In some of these cases, the organism was judged to be an opportunistic pathogen.

F. breve has been isolated from urine, blood, bronchial secretions, and an eye. It is questionable that any of these isolates were pathogenic (45).

Flavobacteria of CDC Group IIb are encountered in clinical specimens much more frequently than *F. meningosepticum*. They appear to be pathogenic only for a seriously compromised host (4, 70).

Flavobacteria of the CDC Group IIf have been isolated primarily from the genitals and urinary tract. The sources of 86 strains have been reported (63, 65, 98). These include 33 from urine, 43 from male and female genital tracts, two from spinal fluid, two from blood, and one each from an umbilical stump, ear, eye, abdominal cavity, pelvic inflammation, and mastoid process.

Epidemiology

F. meningosepticum has little ability to establish infection in animals and in adult humans, but infection in the newborn is usually fatal. Although cases of meningitis may occur repeatedly in the same nursery, only a small percentage of the nursery population develops serious infection. These victims are the most susceptible infants; about half of them have been premature babies. Simultaneously, the organism can be recovered from the noses and/or throats of healthy babies. This colonization is temporary and may end even without antibiotic therapy (8, 13, 84). The adult nursery personnel do not become colonized. In the cases of postoperative bacteremia mentioned previously, patients recovered quickly although antibiotic treatment did not correspond to the antibiotic sensitivities of the infecting organism (62). From all of these cases a pattern emerges. This pattern of resistance to infection in adults, colonization of some infants, and infection of only a few infants indicates that *F. meningosepticum* is usually removed from the body by the antibacterial defense mechanisms of the normal host.

Possible sources of neonatal infection are: the mother, the nursery personnel, food, and the hospital environment. The epidemic tendency of *F. meningosepticum* meningitis argues against a maternal source of infection. [Olsen and Ravn (63) conclude, "...the female genitals must be considered as possible source of hospital infection with *F. meningosepticum*." We disagree with this opinion because none of their isolates matches King's definition of *F. meningosepticum* (47).] Neither are nursery personnel a likely source since cultural surveys of nursery personnel during epidemics have all been negative (13, 84).

There are no reports in the literature on the isolation of *F. meningosepticum* from food, but isolation of "*Flavobacterium* sp." has been reported many times (12, 56). The environment is a likely source of flavobacteria, including *F. meningosepticum*. Three epidemics have been traced to aqueous reservoirs of the causative organism. In one epidemic the organism was cultured from a sink which had a leaky trap. The epidemic ended when the leaky trap was repaired (13). Plotkin and McKitrick (77) traced two cases to a contaminated saline solution. This solution was used to rinse the eyes of newborn infants following silver nitrate treatment. In the epidemic of postoperative bacteremia (62), the causative organism was isolated from drugs which were administered intravenously during surgery.

Preventive Measures

F. meningosepticum does not pose a threat to normal individuals. It is necessary to protect infants and seriously ill patients from contact with this organism. When a case of neonatal infection by *F. meningosepticum* is suspected or has been confirmed, two steps are recommended: 1) an attempt to identify the reservoir of infection by culture of the environment and of solutions coming in contact with infants; 2) thorough cleaning and disinfection of possibly contaminated delivery room and nursery items, with particular attention to wet areas. Finally, if several cases are related to one institution, cultures of noses and throats of well babies are recommended. Carriers may receive antibiotic therapy. In addition the identification of carriers may help to pinpoint the source of the epidemic.

Collection and Processing of Specimens

Cultures from infants

In meningitis, cerebrospinal fluid (CSF) is the specimen of choice. Culture is positive in almost all cases of flavobacterial meningitis. The bacteria are usually numerous in a Gram-stained smear of the sediment.

Cultures from well babies

Swabs should be made of the nose and throat of each infant. These are streaked onto blood agar plates and incubated for 24 hr. Colonies suspected of being *F. meningosepticum* may be picked directly to media for identification or, if necessary, may be restreaked for isolation in pure culture.

Serum specimens

Serological tests are not usually necessary since cultures are almost always positive. However, in the case of one infant cultures were negative and diagnosis was made serologically (13). Agglutinins have been detected in the sera of convalescent adults (62) seven or more days after the onset of symptoms, but not in the early phase of illness.

Cultures from the environment

Cultures should be taken with particular attention to solutions and wet areas (formula, medications, sinks, faucets, hoses, humidifiers, water baths, refrigerators, etc.).

Diagnostic Procedures

Primary culture media

Media which are routinely used to culture CSF are adequate for *F. meningosepticum*. An atmosphere of elevated carbon dioxide is not required. Blood cultures for *F. meningosepticum* do not require special handling. Swabs from the nose or throat should be streaked onto blood agar plates and incubated for 24–48 hr under routine conditions. MacConkey agar and EMB agar are not recommended. Tatum et al. (98) report that 92% of their strains grow on slants of MacConkey agar, but in our experience very few strains are capable of colony formation on this medium.

Specimens from suspected carriers or from environmental sources should be plated on a selective medium. Selection for *F. meningosepticum* is achieved by the addition of penicillin (50 units per ml) and polymyxin B (400 units per ml) to heart infusion agar (62). Addition of blood is not necessary.

Macroscopic and microscopic morphology

Colonies of *F. meningosepticum* after 24 hr of incubation on blood agar plates are 1.0–1.5 mm. in diameter. They are circular, entire, convex, and smooth. The pigment is of a pale cream color and may not be noticed. In mixed cultures these colonies can be recognized by their unusual appearance under a stereoscopic microscope. "They manifest translucent and opaque streaks, producing a mottled effect..." (47).

After 24 hr colonies of *F. odoratum* range in size from 0.5–4.0 mm in diameter. Larger colonies have raised shiny centers and dull spreading edges; smaller colonies are smooth, shiny, circular, convex, and entire. They produce a bright yellow pigment and a strong fruity odor (44, 46).

Colonies of *F. breve* are 0.25–2.5 mm in diameter after 24 hr, and are circular, entire, smooth, low convex, and pale yellow (45).

Colonies of CDC Group IIb after 24 hr on blood agar plates are 1.0–1.5 mm in diameter. They are circular, entire, convex, and smooth. Their pigmentation is outstanding. It is a dark orange to golden color, but a few strains have only a cream color.

Colonies of CDC Group IIf are very small after 24 hr of incubation. They reach 1.0 mm in diameter by the second day and grow to 7–10 mm after 1 week. They are circular, entire, convex, and mucoid. The pigmentation is pale and cream colored.

Gram stains of these organisms appear very similar. They are gram-negative rods, about 1–3 μm long. The cells have straight axes and parallel sides or may be slightly constricted. Some strains produce short filaments.

Identification procedures

The important features of all three groups of flavobacteria are presented in Table 27.4. They all produce a "nonfermentative" reaction in Kligler iron agar and are easier to identify if they are treated as nonfermentative organisms. The determination of motility in a hanging drop is important. In soft agar media false-positive results may be obtained after 2 or 3 days' incubation. These false positives are probably due to the ability of these organisms to

TABLE 27.4—IMPORTANT FEATURES OF CLINICALLY ISOLATED FLAVOBACTERIA

1. Gram-negative rods
2. "Nonfermentative" in KIA and TSI (i.e., neutral or alkaline butt, no gas, alkaline slant, H_2S-)
3. Nonmotile in hanging drop preparation
4. Pigmented (see text)
5. Positive for: oxidase
        catalase
        gelatinase
6. Negative for: arginine dihydrolase
        lysine decarboxylase
        ornithine decarboxylase
        growth on Simmons' citrate

move on surfaces even though they are nonflagellated. On the other hand, several groups of pigmented nonfermentative bacilli are weakly motile. False-negative results may be obtained if these are tested in soft agar. Correct methodology is important for the indole test also. Only a small amount of indole is produced by flavobacteria. The procedure recommended by King (47) or that of Pickett and Pedersen (76) should be used.

Some, but not all, flavobacteria are saccharolytic. Probably because of their proteolytic activity, acidification of Hugh and Leifson's O/F medium may be delayed as long as 1 to 3 weeks. To obtain final results in the least possible time, we recommend the buffered single substrate method (BBS) (76). Positive results are seen for most strains after 1 or 2 days' incubation, or in rare cases after 5 days' incubation.

F. meningosepticum and CDC Group IIb are similar organisms which differ significantly in their pathogenic potential. Correct identification is obviously important. To distinguish between them, we recommend the use of the four tests shown in Table 27.5. All four tests should be used because of the heterogeneity of CDC Group IIb. We have observed strains of this group which produce cream pigment, or acidify mannitol, or fail to hydrolyze starch (78). Table 27.6 presents the tests which are used for final identification of flavobacteria. *F. breve* is similar to CDC Group IIb, but acidifies fewer carbohydrates, and does not hydrolyze esculin or starch.

The outstanding biochemical characteristics of *F. odoratum* are produc-

TABLE 27.5—TESTS WHICH DIFFERENTIATE *FLAVOBACTERIUM MENINGOSEPTICUM* AND CDC GROUP IIB

TEST	*F. MENINGOSEPTICUM*	IIB
Pigmentation	Cream	Yellow/Orange
Starch hydrolysis	0	96
Lactose acidification	100	0
Mannitol acidification	100	9

Data from reference 68. Numbers show the percent positive.

TABLE 27.6—TESTS FOR IDENTIFICATION OF FLAVOBACTERIA

TEST	F. MENINGO-SEPTICUM	F. BREVE	CDC GROUP IIb	CDC GROUP IIf	F. ODORATUM
Growth at 42 C	−	−	−	+	−
Nitrate reduction	−	−	−(+)	−	−
Nitrite reduction	−	−	−(+)	−	+
ONPG	+	−	+/−	−	−
Indole	+	+	+	+	−
DNase	+	+	+/−	+	+
Urease	−	−	+/−	−	+
Starch hydrolysis	−	−	+	−	−
Esculin hydrolysis	+	−	+	−	−
Phenylalanine deaminase	−	−	+/−	+^{w}	?*
Acid from:					
d-arabinose	+	x	−	−	x
ethanol	+	−	+/−	−	−
glucose	+	+†	+	−	−
lactose	+	−	−	−	−
mannitol	+	−	−(+)	−	−
mannose	+	x	+	−	x
trehalose	+	−	+	−	−
maltose	+	+	+	−	−
xylose	+/−	−	+/−	−	−
G + C (T_m, moles %)	36.1–37.6	31.6–33.1	35.0–38.5	37.0–38.0	31.9–35.1

Key: +, positive; −, negative; x, data not available; +/−, variable; (+) or (−), reaction of rare strains; w, weak. Data from references 12, 22, 44, 45, 46, 64, and 108.

* Conflicting data in the literature (45, 98).

† Some strains produced acid from ammonium salt sugar medium only after incubation at 30 C and not at 37 C (45).

tion of urease, hydrolysis of gelatin, reduction of nitrite but not of nitrate, and lack of saccharolytic activity.

Those organisms which might be confused with *F. odoratum* are *Alcaligenes odorans* and CDC Group IIf. *A. odorans* is also non-saccharolytic, oxidase positive, grows on MacConkey agar, and reduces nitrite but not nitrate. It differs from *F. odoratum* by being motile, nonpigmented, gelatin negative, urease negative, and by growing at 42 C and on Simmons citrate agar. CDC Group IIf differs from *F. odoratum* by its pigmentation, growth at 42 C, production of indole, failure to reduce nitrite, and negative reaction for urease (46).

CDC Group IIf is correctly identified by its lack of saccharolytic activity, growth at 42 C, hydrolysis of gelatin, and production of indole.

Serologic procedures

Six serological groups (A through F) of *F. meningosepticum* have been established, but cross-reactions may occur among them. Some strains of CDC

Group IIb may also cross-react with *F. meningosepticum* antisera (47, 78). Antisera to *F. meningosepticum* (available from Difco Laboratories, Detroit, Mich.) may be used to assist in the screening of unknown cultures. Cultural tests are necessary to confirm the identification of *F. meningosepticum*.

Antimicrobic Susceptibility

Table 27.7 presents antimicrobial sensitivities of the three groups of flavobacteria. The data are all based on the disk diffusion method. The sensitivity pattern of *F. meningosepticum* is unusual for a gram-negative rod. For example, it is resistant to ampicillin, cephalothin, gentamicin, and polymyxin B, but sensitive to erythromycin and vancomycin.

In many cases of neonatal meningitis caused by *F. meningosepticum*, infection has persisted after vigorous antibiotic therapy. Treatment with chloramphenicol, tetracycline, novobiocin, or cephalothin has been unsuccessful. In some cases treatment with erythromycin, vancomycin, or rifampicin has apparently eradicated the infection (27, 35, 51, 77). Three publications (27, 35, 77) recommend the use of vancomycin. Hawley and Gump specifically recommend intravenous vancomycin in a dosage of 40 mg/kg/day (maximum 2 g/day) (35).

The sensitivity patterns of CDC Group IIb, *F. breve*, and *F. odoratum* are similar to that of *F. meningosepticum*. CDC Group IIb is typically heterogeneous, as shown by variable sensitivities to several antimicrobials. Data were not available on the vancomycin sensitivity of *F. breve* or *F. odoratum*. CDC Group IIf is sensitive to many antimicrobials, including penicillin.

TABLE 27.7—ANTIMICROBIAL SENSITIVITIES OF FLAVOBACTERIA

Antimicrobial	*F. MENINGO-SEPTICUM*	GROUP IIb	*F. BREVE*	GROUP IIf	*F. ODORATUM*
Ampicillin	R	R	R	S	R
Cephalothin	R	R	R	S	R
Chloramphenicol	V	V	R	S	R
Colistin	R	R	R	V	R
Erythromycin	S	V	R	S	R
Gentamicin	R	V	R	R	R
Kanamycin	R	R	R	R	R
Nalidixic acid	V	S	MS	S	V
Penicillin G	R	R	X	S	X
Streptomycin	R	V	R	V	R
Sulfonamides	R	V	R	V	V
Tetracycline	V	R	R	S	R
Vancomycin	S	S	X	S	X

R, resistant; MS, moderately sensitive; S, sensitive; V, variable; X, not available. Data from references 2, 12, 28, 44, 45, 46, 47, 64, 76, 84, and 99.

Evaluation of Laboratory Findings

Flavobacteria in patient specimens

The *Flavobacterium* species most frequently occurring in clinical specimens is CDC Group IIb. It should be judged as contributing to a patient's illness only if there is strong supporting evidence such as isolation in pure culture or in large numbers, or in repeated specimens. *F. odoratum*, *F. breve*, and CDC Group IIf also should not be judged significant unless there is supporting evidence. *F. meningosepticum* occurring blood, CSF, sputum or other specimens is significant if its presence is correlated with the patient's disease.

Flavobacteria in the environment

F. meningosepticum, *F. breve*, and CDC Group IIb occur in the environment. *F. meningosepticum* in the hospital environment is a threat to patients. It should not be present in critical sites from which transmission to patients is possible. Isolation of *F. odoratum* or CDC Group IIf from the environment has not been reported.

Gardnerella vaginalis (Haemophilus vaginalis or Corynebacterium vaginale)

Causative Organism

Gardnerella vaginalis is a fastidious, pleomorphic, small gram-negative bacillus. Because of a presumed growth requirement for either X or V factors (hemin or NAD), it was originally placed in the genus *Haemophilus* (26). More recent work has not substantiated these growth requirements, and thus the organism is no longer considered a member of this genus. Other genera including *Corynebacterium* have been proposed for organisms of this description, but they have also been rejected (49). Because the name *H. vaginalis* was not legitimate, it was recently recommended that this organism be transferred to a new genus, *Gardnerella*, which was defined to include catalase- and oxidase-negative, gram-negative to gram-variable bacteria which produce acetic acid as the major end product of fermentation (32). The G+C ratio for the Dukes strain is 41.0–43.0 (T_m) (49).

Clinical Manifestations

The most common clinical manifestation of *G. vaginalis* infection in women is a mild vaginitis with leukorrhea (26). Malodor frequently accompanies the discharge. Bacteremia in newborns and postpartum women has also been reported in the literature (104). Males who harbor *G. vaginalis* are generally asymptomatic, but cases of nongonococcal urethritis and mild prostatitis have been documented (19, 38).

Epidemiology

The epidemiology of *G. vaginalis* infection remains controversial. Because many studies have shown an equal number of symptomatic and asymptomatic culturally positive women, it has been suggested that *G. vaginalis* is part of the normal vaginal flora (24, 52). Others feel that sexual intercourse is the method of transmission. The high recovery rate of *G. vaginalis* from the urethra of consorts of infected women and treatment failures of women whose consorts are not treated simultaneously are given as evidence to support this viewpoint (26).

Public Health Significance

G. vaginalis is considered to be an etiologic agent of what was formerly referred to as "nonspecific" vaginitis. If it is confirmed that this is a sexually transmitted disease, proper public health measures may have to be undertaken.

Collection and Processing of Specimens

Kinds of specimens

Material for vaginal cultures is best obtained with swabs of the posterior fornix of the vagina. Plating media should be inoculated immediately or the swab may be transported to the laboratory in Amies transport medium. A swab in transport medium should be plated within 4–6 hr of collection. Conventional blood culture methods appear satisfactory for initial growth of the organism in cases of suspected *G. vaginalis* bacteremia (104).

Time of collection

There appears to be a specific time for the collection of material for vaginal cultures. However, cultures should not be taken within 24 hr of douching (26). Blood cultures should be taken when the patient is febrile.

Number of specimens

Reculture of women with diagnosed *G. vaginalis* vaginitis is frequently necessary to evaluate the efficacy of antimicrobial treatment.

Diagnostic Procedures

Microscopic examination

G. vaginalis is a pleomorphic, gram-negative rod measuring 0.3–0.5 μm by 1.0–3.0 μm (see Fig 27.1). Occasionally, as with *Neisseria*, some of the cells will stain gram-positive. Direct Gram-stained smears of vaginal material frequently show "clue cells," i.e., epithelial cells covered with numerous small gram-negative rods. Although originally described as diagnostic for *G. vaginalis* infection, the presence of clue cells has recently been shown to lack both sensitivity and specificity for this purpose (1, 92). A diagnosis of *G. vaginalis* infection should not be based on this observation.

Direct fluorescent antibody methods have been described for the identification of *G. vaginalis* in clinical material (81). However, the antisera are not commercially available.

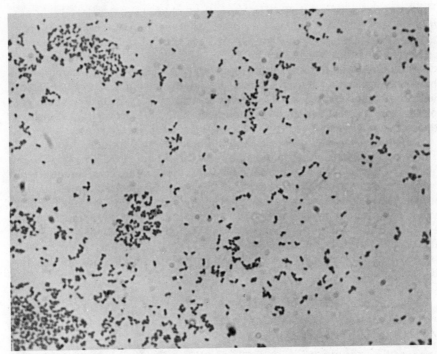

Figure 27.1—*Gardnerella vaginalis* 594. Organisms from a 48–hr culture on vaginalis agar.

Primary culture media

Commercial plates of sheep blood agar, Columbia colistin-nalidixic acid agar (29), or chocolate agar do not provide optimal growth of *G. vaginalis*. After 48 hr of incubation on these media, colonies are generally pinpoint and nondescript. Because of this, it is necessary to plate clinical material on media designed for recognition of *G. vaginalis*. *G. vaginalis* grows aerobically and anaerobically between 28 and 42 C (optimum 35–37 C). All of the plating media listed below should be incubated at 35 C in a humidified CO_2 incubator or candle jar.

Three general types of isolation media for *G. vaginalis* have been described. They are based on:

Recognition of G. vaginalis colonial morphology on peptone-starch dextrose agar (PSD) (18). Forty-eight hour colonies of *G. vaginalis* on PSD agar at 35 C are described as 0.5–2.0 mm in diameter, white, domed, and with a smooth edge. The colonies also are described as having a central "button" at their base. PSD plates are examined with a low-power (40×) dissecting microscope, and colonies fitting this description are subcultured for identification. Although this procedure has been successfully used for many years, recent work has shown that the medium lacks sensitivity and results in frequent subcultures that are not *G. vaginalis* (29, 91).

Fermentation of starch. Two isolation media have been developed that use attack of starch by *G. vaginalis* as a differential feature. Starch agar (91) is a modified PSD medium in which the dextrose is omitted and bromcresol purple is added as an indicator of starch fermentation. Colonies of *G. vaginalis* appear yellow due to starch fermentation. Another starch agar (58) is prepared as an opaque medium with 1 percent corn starch. On this medium, *G. vaginalis* colonies are surrounded by zones of clearing due to hydrolysis of the starch. On both of these media either alpha- or non-hemolytic streptococci may also show attack of the starch.

Unique beta hemolysis. G. vaginalis colonies show a unique, diffuse beta hemolysis on agar containing either human or rabbit blood (see Fig 27.2). Vaginalis agar (34) has been formulated to use this feature to differentiate *G. vaginalis* colonies from other organisms present in vaginal cultures. On this medium, *G. vaginalis* colonies are opaque, domed, entire, and average 0.5 mm in diameter after 48 hr of incubation. This medium facilitates rapid screening of cultures since it is not necessary to examine these plates with a dissecting microscope. Furthermore, diffuse beta hemolysis is an important diagnostic feature which differentiates *G. vaginalis* from vaginal diphtheroids, latobacilli, and streptococci.

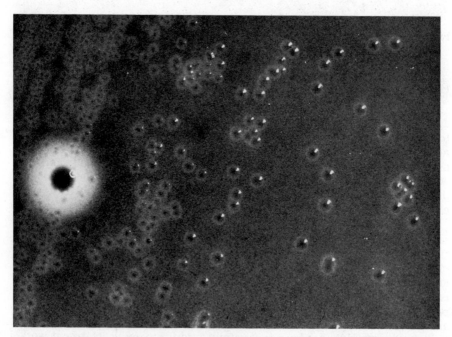

Figure 27.2—Forty-eight-hour colonies of *Gardnerella vaginalis* 594 on vaginalis agar. Large colony on the left is *Streptococcus pyogenes.* Note comparative size and hemolysis.

Identification procedures

Presumptive identification of *G. vaginalis* can be made from vaginalis agar by Gram staining a colony fitting the above description. The combination of a colony with diffuse beta hemolysis, and the Gram stain of a small, pleomorphic, gram-negative rod which fails to show hemolysis on sheep blood agar is presumptive evidence of *G. vaginalis*. If the organism is also oxidase and catalase negative and ferments glucose, maltose, and starch, this confirms the isolate as *G. vaginalis*. The catalase reaction should not be determined from cells that have been grown in the presence of human blood, as false positive reactions have been noted. In liquid thioglycollate media enriched with rabbit serum, puff-ball growth ensues, whereas in heart infusion broth with 1% proteose peptone + 0.5% maltose, full turbidity is seen after 48 hr at 37 C.

Additional biochemical characteristics can be seen in Table 27.8. Fermentation reactions of *G. vaginalis* can be determined in purple broth base (Difco) or heart infusion broth (Difco) supplemented with 5% sterile rabbit serum. It is frequently necessary to incubate these media for at least 48 hr to detect positive fermentation reactions. Cystine trypticase agar (CTA) is not recommended for fermentation studies, as it has recently been shown to lack sensitivity when testing *G. vaginalis* isolates (91).

TABLE 27.8—BIOCHEMICAL REACTIONS OF *GARDNERELLA VAGINALIS*

	SIGN	% +		SIGN	% +
Oxidase	−	0	Acid from:*		
Catalase	−	0	Dextrin	+	100
Indole	−	0	Fructose	+/(−)	81
Urease (Chr.)	−	0	Glucose	+	100
Lysine dec.	−	0	Lactose	−/+	14
Ornithine dec.	−	0	Maltose	+	100
Arginine dih.	−	0	Mannitol	−	0
Gelatinase	−	0	Rhamnose	−	0
Citrate (Si.)	−	0	Salicin	−	0
VPR (35 C)	−	0	Starch	+	100
Esculin hydr.	−	0	Sucrose	−/+	10
ONPG	+/−	53			
NO₃†	−	0			
Egg yolk lipase	−/+	43			
Hippurate hydr.	+/(−)	92			
Hemolysis (beta)					
human blood	+/(−)	96			
sheep blood	−	0			
Growth on 0.01%					
tellurite agar	−	0			

Key: +, positive; −, negative; ( ), reaction of rare strain; VPR, Voges-Proskauer reaction; NO₃, nitrate reduction.

* Carbohydrate fermentations based on reactions with buffered single substrates in 77 strains: other reactions based on 104 strains (31).

† Traditional method.

A rapid buffered single substrate (BSS) method to detect *G. vaginalis* fermentation reactions has also been developed (40). To use this method, a suspected *G. vaginalis* colony is subcultured to a vaginalis agar plate and streaked for maximal growth. Concurrently, a chocolate agar plate is streaked for isolated colonies, and these plates are incubated for 18–24 hr. The hazy growth on the chocolate plate is used as a purity check and for the Gram stain, oxidase, and catalase tests. The vaginalis agar plate is used to inoculate the BSS tests. For the subsequent fermentation tests, 0.1 ml of BSS basal medium is dispensed into four nonsterile 13- × 100-mm tubes. BSS glucose, maltose, and starch are used as substrates. One drop of each substrate is dispensed into three of the tubes; the fourth serves as a substrate-free control. Using a bacteriological loop, inocula are prepared by harvesting the growth on the vaginalis agar plate and transferring this to a fifth tube containing 0.35 ml of basal medium. One drop of this suspension is dispensed with a Pasteur pipette into each of the first four tubes. The inoculated tubes are incubated at 35 C for 3 hr and then scored as positive (yellow) or negative (red). With this method, isolates can be biochemically identified within 72 hr of the initial plating.

Inhibition by H_2O_2 or streptococci (18, 67) is not recommended as a *G. vaginalis* identification method. The tests are non-specific and add little, if any, diagnostic information. There is no growth of *G. vaginalis* on MacConkey agar, SS agar, Thayer-Martin agar, or Rogosa agar (31). Growth on triple sugar iron agar or Kligler iron agar is unreliable.

Serologic procedures

Fluorescent techniques have been described for identification of *G. vaginalis* (16, 81, 105). However, commercial reagents are not presently available. Presently there are no serological tests for serum from patients with *G. vaginalis* infections.

Marker systems

There are no typing systems available for investigations of the epidemiology of *G. vaginalis* infections.

Miscellaneous procedures

Obligately anaerobic strains of *G. vaginalis* have been isolated from vaginal abscesses, Bartholin's cysts, abdominal fluid, and blood (55). Although the prevalence of these strains is unknown, if an anaerobic *G. vaginalis* is suspected (e.g., if no etiologically significant aerobic organism is isolated from such a lesion), proper anaerobic culture techniques should be implemented. The anaerobic strains are reported to have biochemical profiles similar to those of the facultative strains (31, 55).

G. vaginalis is not pathogenic for the usual laboratory animals.

Antimicrobic Susceptibility

G. vaginalis strains are resistant to sulfonamides, colistin, and nalidixic acid (67). Antibiotics to which they are susceptible include chloramphenicol, ampicillin, penicillin, metronidazole, clindamycin, and cephalothin (33, 71).

One of the few antibiotics to show a variable profile is tetracycline, with approximately half of the isolates showing resistance (71). Additionally, erythromycin has recently been shown to be ineffective in treating *G. vaginalis*-associated vaginitis (20).

Evaluation of Laboratory Findings

Reports to the physician should identify the organism and also give an estimate of the number of colonies on the primary plate. This number can be reported in terms of "few," "moderate," or "many" (see also the introductory section for clinical significance).

Actinobacillus

Causative Organisms

The genus *Actinobacillus* consists of facultatively anaerobic, nonmotile, fastidious gram-negative rods with a GC ratio of 38.6–42.6 moles %. The species occurring in human specimens are: *A. lignieresii* (41.8–42.6 moles %), *A. equuli* (very rare; 40.0–41.8 moles %), and *A. actinomycetemcomitans* (39 moles %) (7, 30).

Clinical Manifestations

A. lignieresii causes actinobacillosis in cattle and sheep, manifested by multiple lesions in the subcutis, lymph nodes, the upper gastrointestinal tract ("wooden tongue"), and occasionally in other internal organs. In these lesions, pus and granules are found. A few cases of human actinobacillosis have been reported (meningitis, pneumonia, mesenterial adenitis, conjunctivitis, brain abscess, septicemia) (23, 69). *A equuli* causes suppurative lesions in kidneys and joints of foals and piglets and endocarditis in pigs; a few strains have been isolated from humans (107). Its separate taxonomic status has been questioned, as has the status of the three other species described as animal pathogens: *A. actinoides, A. capsulatus,* and *A. suis* (7, 75). *A. actinomycetemcomitans*, a species *incertae sedis* in the 8th edition of *Bergey's Manual* (75), is a well-described agent of human endocarditis on previously damaged valves (5, 53, 57, 65) and has been found in many cases of actinomycosis—in one series, in 83 of 283 cases together with *Actinomyces israelii*, and in seven cases without it (effect of antibiotics?) (37). Other infections due to *A. actinomycetemcomitans* are rare (10, 48).

Epidemiology

A. lignieresii has been isolated from the oral cavity and rumen of normal cattle and sheep (72, 73). While animal infections seem to be endogenous, transmission from animals accounts for probably all human infections observed (23). *A. equuli* occurs in the oral cavity and in the intestinal tract of normal horses (75). *A. actinomycetemcomitans* is an inhabitant of the normal human oral cavity (37); infections are endogenous. No public health significance has been ascribed to any of these species.

Collection and Processing of Specimens

The majority of specimens from which *Actinobacillus* species are isolated are pus (with or without sulfur granules) and blood, which should be collected and processed in the usual manner. No adverse effects of transport media on actinobacilli are known but the low viability of the organisms outside the body argues for speedy inoculation.

Diagnostic Procedures

Microscopic examination

Actinobacilli are coccobacillary to bacillary gram-negative rods (0.3−0.5 × 0.6−1.4 μm) on solid media containing serum or blood. Coccal elements may be interspersed. Longer bacillary forms may be seen in serum broth and on media containing sugars. There is a tendency towards bipolar staining. Arrangement is single, in pairs, and in chains. In sulfur granules caused by *A. lignieresii*, there is central detritus with a few gram-negative rods, and radially extending gram-negative clubs. In actinomycotic granules, *A. actinomycetemcomitans* is seen in the form of densely packed gram-negative coccobacilli.

Primary culture media

Actinobacilli grow poorly on ordinary peptone media and do not grow on MacConkey or SS agar. Addition of serum or blood in an atmosphere of 5%–10% CO_2 improves growth markedly. Aerobic and anaerobic growth occurs between 20 and 39 C (optimum, 37 C) for *A. lignieresii* and *A. equuli*; for *A. actinomycetemcomitans*, the range is about 30–39 C. *A. lignieresii* has been selected from mixed cultures by addition of antibiotics to primary media: oleandomycin, 29 μg/ml + neomycin, 1.5 μg/ml (100), or oleandomycin, 1 μg/ml + nystatin, 200 μg/ml (73).

Identification procedures

Colonies of *A. lignieresii* and *A. equuli* on blood agar are 0.5−1.5 mm in diameter after 24 hr of growth at 37 C, nonhemolytic, smooth or rough, and sticking to the agar surface. Smooth colonies are dome-shaped and have a bluish hue when viewed by transmitted light. Dwarf and granular colonies may occur also. Colonies of *A. actinomycetemcomitans*, also adherent, show first a central opaque dot which, on further incubation, develops a star-like configuration ("crossed cigars"; 36). In serum broth, actinobacillary growth occurs in granules along the side and the bottom of the tube; sometimes, uniform turbidity prevails. A surface pellicle and a sediment are formed later. Growth in blood culture media is slow (57). Cultures of actinobacilli have a low viability.

Biochemical reactions are listed in Table 27.9. For carbohydrate fermentation tests, 5%–10% serum (or, when a rich peptone is used, 1% yeast extract; 79) should be added to the base, and observation extended up to 10 days (79). Characteristic for *A. lignieresii* and *A. equuli* are positive oxidase and urease reactions in a fermentative setting (which separates them from urease- and oxidase-positive nonfermenters such as *Bordetella bronchiseptica* and *Pseudomonas pickettii*). *A. actinomycetemcomitans* is urease-negative and mostly oxidase-negative. The differential diagnoses of the species are listed in Table 27.10 and Table 27.11. *A. equuli* differs from *A. lignieresii* only in a few charac-

TABLE 27.9—BIOCHEMICAL REACTIONS OF *ACTINOBACILLUS* SPECIES FOUND IN HUMAN SPECIMENS

TEST	A. LIGNIERESII	A. EQUULI	A. ACTINOMYCE-TEMCOMITANS
Oxidase	+	+	$-/(+^w)$
Catalase	+/(−)	+/(−)	+
Indole	−	−	−
Urease (Chr.)	+	+	−
Lysine dec.	−	−	−
Ornithine dec.	−	−	−
Gelatinase	−	$+^d$	−
Citrate (Si.)	−	−	−
TSI	A/A H₂S −	A/A H₂S −	K/A H₂S −
KIA	A/A H₂S −	A/A H₂S −	K/A H₂S −
Esculin hydr.	−	−	−
ONPG	+	+	−
NO₃	+	+	+
Gas from glucose	−	−	−/(+)
Acid from			
Arabinose	+	+/−	−
Dulcitol	−/+	−	−
Fructose	+	+	+
Galactose	+	+	+/−
Glucose	+	+	+
Lactose	+/(−)	+	−
Maltose	+	+	+
Mannitol	+	+/−	+/−
Melibiose	−	+	−
Raffinose	+	+	−
Rhamnose	−	−/+	−
Salicin	−	+/−	−
Sucrose	+	+	−
Trehalose	−	+	−
Xylose	+	+	+/−

Key: +, positive; −, negative; ( ), reaction of rare strain; d, delayed; w, weak; TSI and KIA, triple sugar iron agar and Kligler iron agar; NO₃, reduction of nitrate.

TABLE 27.10—DIFFERENTIAL DIAGNOSIS OF OXIDASE +, UREASE +, FASTIDIOUS FERMENTATIVE GRAM-NEGATIVE RODS

TEST	A. LIGNI-ERESII	A. EQUULI	PASTEU-RELLA UREAE	PASTEU-RELLA PNEUMO-TROPICA	PASTEU-RELLA "GAS" (107)
Indole	−	−	−	+	+
Gelatinase	−	+^{d}	−	−	+/−
Catalase	+/(−)	+/(−)	+^{w}/−	+	+
Acid from:					
Mannitol	+	+/−	+	−	−
Trehalose	−	+	−	+	+
Xylose	+	+	−	+	−

Key: +, positive; −, negative; ( ), reaction of rare strain; d, delayed; w, weak.

teristics; also, sodium hippurate is reported to be hydrolyzed by *A. equuli* but not by *A. lignieresii* (75).

Serologic procedures

Six antigenic types and two subtypes, differing in heat-stable antigens, have been defined in *A. lignieresii* (74). Type 1 occurs in cattle, and types 2, 3, and 4, in sheep. Antisera are not routinely used (or available) for identification. Agglutination tests on patient sera are not useful because of the presence of normal agglutinins (68). *A. equuli* strains are antigenically related to *A. lignieresii* (102). In *A. actinomycetemcomitans*, 24 antigenic patterns have been detected; all strains possess at least one of the antigens (80).

Marker systems

Eight different biotypes of *A. actinomycetemcomitans* have been identified on the basis of galactose, mannitol, and xylose fermentation (79).

Animal pathogenicity

Actinobacilli are not pathogenic for rabbits or guinea pigs by the subcutaneous, intraperitoneal, or intravenous route (69, 75). Pathogenicity of *A. lignieresii* for mice is questionable (59).

Antimicrobial Susceptibility

A. lignieresii and *A. equuli* strains have not been examined systematically for antimicrobial susceptibility. Sensitivity to chloramphenicol and variable susceptibility to tetracycline, streptomycin, and erythromycin, as well as resistance to penicillin have been reported (59, 102), *A. actinomycetemcomitans* strains have been tested more thoroughly (53, 66, 100). They have been reported sensitive to chloramphenicol, tetracycline, kanamycin, streptomycin, gentamicin, and polymyxin B. Susceptibility to ampicillin was variable; penicillin was usually ineffective. Susceptibility testing seems indicated for every clinically significant strain.

TABLE 27.11—DIFFERENTIAL DIAGNOSIS OF OXIDASE − (OR WEAKLY +), UREASE −, FASTIDIOUS FERMENTATIVE GRAM-NEGATIVE RODS

Test	A. ACTINO-MYCETEM-COMITANS	H. APHRO-PHILUS	HB-5	G. VAGI-NALIS	S. MONILI-FORMIS	DF-1
Catalase	+/(−)	−(+^{w})	−	−	−	−
Indole	−	−	+^{w}	−	−	−
NO$_3$	+	+	+	−	−	−/+
Esculin hydrolysis	−	−	−	−	+^{w}	v*
Acid from:						
Lactose	−	+	+	−	−	+
Maltose	+	+	−	+	+	+
Sucrose	−	+	−	−/+	−	+
Pigment	−	−	−	−	−	+†
Gliding	−	−	−	−	−	+‡

Key: +, positive; −, negative; w, weak; ( ), rare strain.
* v, Variable data from different laboratories (60, 109).
† Yellow-orange.
‡ See text.

Evaluation of Laboratory Findings

A. lignieresii and *A. equuli* are probably significant in every case of isolation from human material while *A. actinomycetemcomitans* would be clinically significant (as the sole isolate) only outside the gastrointestinal tract, and would be significant, in addition, if found together with *Actinomyces israelii* for which it provides invasive factors (37).

Cardiobacterium

Causative Organism

The genus *Cardiobacterium* (50) consists of one species, *C. hominis*, a facultatively anaerobic, nonmotile, fastidious gram-negative rod with a G+C ratio of 58.7–60.2 moles %.

Clinical Manifestations

C. hominis is an agent of endocarditis on previously damaged or on previously healthy heart valves (review: 83).

Epidemiology

The natural habitat of *C. hominis* is the upper respiratory tract of man; it has also been isolated from human stools (90). Endocarditis follows entry of the organisms into the bloodstream, e.g., after dental procedures (83). Pre-

TABLE 27.12—BIOCHEMICAL REACTIONS OF *CARDIOBACTERIUM HOMINIS*

Oxidase	$+/+^w$	KIA	K/A or NG	Acid from:	
Catalase	−		H_2S-	Glucose	+
Indole	$+/+^w$	Esculin hydrolysis	−	Inositol	−
Urease (Chr.)	−	ONPG	−	Lactose	−
Lysine dec.	−	NO_3	−	Maltose	$+/(-)$
Orinithine dec.	−	Gas from glucose	−	Mannitol	$+/(-)$
Arginine dih.	−	Acid from:		Raffinose	−
Gelatinase	−	Adonitol	−	Rhamnose	−
Citrate (Si)	−	Arabinose	−	Salicin	−
TSI	A/A or NG	Dulcitol	−	Sorbitol	+
	H_2-	Fructose	+	Sucrose	+
		Galactose	−	Trehalose	−
				Xylose	−

Key: +, Positive; −, negative; w, weak; ( ), rare strain; NG, no growth.

ventive measures would presumably include those taken to prevent endocarditis due to other oral bacteria, e.g., viridans streptococci (penicillin prophylaxis in rheumatic patients).

Collection and Processing of Specimens

This would follow rules applicable to blood culture collection and processing.

Diagnostic Procedures

Microscopic examination

Cells of *C. hominis* are 0.5–0.75 × 1.0–3.0 μm in size, arranged singly, in pairs, short chains, or rosette-like clusters, and may have bulbous ends. In media containing yeast extract, pleomorphism is less marked than in those without yeast extract (83). Crystal violet may be partially retained by *C. hominis* cells.

Primary culture media

Growth on tryptic digest agars with or without blood is usually satisfactory but will be markedly improved by high humidity or an atmosphere of 5%–10% CO_2. The temperature range is 20–41 C. Growth in broth is improved by addition of 5%–10% serum. On these media, aerobic as well as anaerobic growth is observed, but there is no growth on MacConkey agar or on SS agar.

Identification procedures

On blood agar, colonies have a diameter of 0.5 mm after 24 hr of growth at 37 C, and a diameter of 1–2 mm after 48 hr. They are circular, opaque, butyrous, and nonhemolytic.

Biochemical reactions are listed in Table 27.12. The indole reaction may

TABLE 27.13—DIFFERENTIAL DIAGNOSIS OF OXIDASE +, UREASE −, FASTIDIOUS FERMENTATIVE GRAM-NEGATIVE RODS

TEST	C. HOMINIS	KINGELLA KINGAE	K. INDOLOGENES	K. DENITRIFICANS	HB-5	EF-4	DF-O-2	P. MULTOCIDA	P. HAEMOLYTICA	E. CORRODENS
Catalase	−	−	−	−	−	+	+	+	+	−
Growth on MacConkey agar	−	−	−	−	−	+/−	−	−	+/−	−
Indole	+/+^{w}	−	+	−	+^{w}	−	−	+	−	−
NO$_3$	−	−/+^{w}	+	G	+	+/+, G	−	+	+	+
Acid from:										
Glucose	+	+	+	+	+	+	+	+/−	+	−
Mannitol	+/(−)	−	−	−	−	−	−	+	+	−
Sucrose	+	−	+	−	−	−	−	+	+/−	−
Susceptibility to colistin	+	+	+	−	?	+	−	+	+	+

Key: +, positive; −, negative; w, weak; ( ), rare strain; G, gas.

TABLE 27.14—BIOCHEMICAL REACTIONS OF *KINGELLA* SPECIES

TEST	K. KINGAE	K. INDOLOGENES	K. DENITRIFICANS
Oxidase	+	+	+
Catalase	−	−	−/(+)
Indole	−	+	−
Urease (Chr.)	−	−	−
Lysine dec.	−	−	−
Ornithine dec.	−	−	−
Arginine dih.	−	−	−
Gelatinase	−/+	−/+	−
Citrate (Si.)	−	−	−
TSI	NG or N or A or K/N, H_2S-	NG or N or A or K/N, H_2S-	NG or N or A or K/N, H_2S-
KIA	as for TSI	as for TSI	as for TSI
Esculin hydrolysis	−	−	−
ONPG	−	−	−
NO_3	$-/+^w$	−	G
Gas from glucose	−	−	−
Acid* from:			
Fructose	−	+	−
Glucose	+	+	+
Maltose	+	+	−
Sucrose	−	+	−

* Often delayed. No fermentation of other carbohydrates is observed.
Key: +, positive; −, negative; w, weak; G, gas; N, neutral; NG, no growth.

be weak or may be detected only after extraction with xylene or isoamylalcohol. Carbohydrate fermentations, determined in liquid peptone media with 5% serum, are often delayed (107). The differential diagnosis of oxidase +, urease −, fastidious gram-negative fermenters is listed in Table 27.13.

Serologic procedures

Genus specificity has been demonstrated in *C. hominis* by agglutination and fluorescent antibody techniques (89, 90). For the demonstration of *C. hominis* in mixed cultures, the fluorescent antibody technique is superior to nonselective culture (90). Antibodies in individuals known to harbor the organism normally have not been detected (90) but sera of patients with *C. hominis* endocarditis agglutinated the infective strains (101).

Animal pathogenicity

C. hominis is not pathogenic for laboratory animals (101).

Antimicrobic Susceptibility

All strains tested so far have been sensitive to penicillin, ampicillin, carbenicillin, cephalothin, tetracycline, chloramphenicol, streptomycin, kanamycin, gentamicin, erythromycin, and colistin (83). In view of the potential dam-

TABLE 27.15—BIOCHEMICAL REACTIONS OF GROUPS HB-5, EF-4, and DF/O-2

TEST	HB-5	EF-4	DF-2	DF-1
Oxidase	$+^w/-$	$+^w/-$	+	−
Catalase	−	+	+	−
Indole	$+^w$	−	−	−
Urease (Chr.)	−	−	−	−
Lysine dec.	−	−	−	−
Ornithine dec.	−	−	−	−
Arginine dih.	−	+/−	−	ND
Gelatinase	−	$-/+^d$	−	−/+
Citrate (Si.)	−	−	−	ND
TSI	A/A (G)	K/A or K/N	NG or N/N	K or N/N or A
KIA	as for TSI	as for TSI	as for TSI	as for TSI
Esculin hydr.	−	−	+	v
ONPG	−	−	+	ND
NO₃	+	+/+, G*	−	−/+
Gas from glucose	+/−	−	−	−
Acid from:				
Fructose	+	−	−/+	+
Glucose	+	+	+	+
Lactose	−	−	+	+
Maltose	−	−	+	+
Mannitol	−	−	−	v
Sucrose	−	−	−	+

Key: +, positive; −, negative; d, delayed; w, weak; v, variable, depending on laboratory (60, 109); ND, no data available; G, gas; N, neutral; NG, no growth.

* G in heart infusion base only (98).

age *C. hominis* can elicit, testing of individual strains from the blood is recommended.

Evaluation of Laboratory Findings

At present, *C. hominis* is only known as an agent of endocarditis. Isolates from the upper respiratory tract, from stool, or from the genital tract seem insignificant (88, 90).

Kingella

Causative Organisms

The proposed genus *Kingella* (41) includes fastidious, nonmotile, fermentative gram-negative rods with a G+C ratio of 47.3–54.8 moles % (T_m). Three species have been proposed (95): *K. kingae* [formerly classified as *Moraxella kingii* (40) but different from the genus *Moraxella* in failing to exhibit catalase, and in saccharolytic activity], *K. indologenes*, and *K. denitrificans* [formerly called TM-1 (43)].

Clinical Manifestations

Reports of isolation of *Kingella* species are rare. *K. kingae* has been isolated from purulent lesions, from blood, and from the respiratory tract (39, 40), *K. indologenes* from the eye [corneal abscess (97), angular conjunctivitis (103)], and *K. denitrificans* from the normal pharynx (43).

Epidemiology

The natural habitat of *K. kingae* and *K. denitrificans* is probably areas of the upper respiratory tract of man; the habitat of *K. indologenes* is not known. Transmission and importance for public health remain to be determined.

Collection and Processing of Specimens

Nothing specific known at this time.

Diagnostic Procedures

Microscopic examination

K. kingae and *K. denitrificans* are coccoid to medium-sized (0.4 × 1-3 μm), gram-negative rods with square ends, occurring in pairs and short chains. There is some tendency to resist decolorization. *K. indologenes* cells are longer and stain more evenly.

Primary culture media

Growth on ordinary peptone media is scarce. On blood agar, in a humid atmosphere, one colony type of *Kingella* is 0.1-0.5 mm in diameter after 24 hr of growth at 37 C and is translucent and smooth. Another colony type shows pitting of the medium and, later, spreading edges; it is associated with fimbriation, twitching motility, and pellicle formation in broth. Pitting and spreading may get lost; pitting without spreading has also been described (25). A CO_2 atmosphere is not required for growth. The majority of *K. indologenes* and some *K. denitrificans* strains grow at 20 C; only *K. denitrificans* seems to be able to grow up to 42 C. Both aerobic and anaerobic growth are observed, although anaerobic growth may be very scarce. *K. kingae* is markedly beta-hemolytic. *K. indologenes* may produce greening or diffuse lysis, while *K. denitrificans* produces greening or no change on blood agar. None of the species grows on MacConkey agar or on SS agar. Viability on culture media is low. The pitting and spreading characters resemble those of *Eikenella corrodens*.

Identification procedures

Biochemical reactions of *Kingella* species are listed in Table 27.14. There is very scant growth on O/F media; therefore, carbohydrate fermentation (most often weak and delayed) should be tested in supplemented media. Addition of serum, however, may lead to splitting of maltose and, consequently, false-positive reactions for maltose fermentation (42). The differential diagnosis of the species is listed in Table 27.13. As mentioned, "corroding" strains may be initially confused with *Eikenella corrodens* or *Bacteroides corrodens* (if grown anaerobically), but the two latter species are nonsaccharolytic. *K. denitrificans* may be confused with those *Neisseria* species that are able to grow on Thayer-Martin agar: *N. gonorrhoeae, N. meningitidis,* and *N. lactamica.* Microscopic morphology and gas formation from nitrate serve as differential criteria.

Antimicrobic Susceptibility

K. kingae and *K. indologenes* strains are sensitive to penicillin, streptomycin, chloramphenicol, erythromycin, and tetracycline (40, 103). *K. denitrificans* strains have not been systematically examined for susceptibility; they are at least resistant to vancomycin and to colistin (43).

Evaluation of Laboratory Findings

At present, detailed case studies evaluating the pathogenic potential of *Kingella* species are lacking. *K. denitrificans* is one of the few bacteria able to grow on Thayer-Martin agar.

Other Fastidious Fermentative Gram-Negative Rods

The HB-5 Group (98)

Bacteria belonging to this group are nonmotile, coccoid to coccobacillary rods, gram-negative, which probably require capneic conditions for growth. Colonies are 0.5–1.0 mm in size after 24 hr of growth on blood agar at 37 C, smooth, sometimes mottled, and give rise to greening or to no hemolysis at all. There is poor growth on normal peptone media, and no growth on MacConkey agar, SS agar, or in O/F medium. Biochemical reactions are listed in Table 27.15. The oxidase reaction is often weak, and indole has to be extracted. For carbohydrate fermentations, 5% serum has to be added to the basal medium. Differential diagnostic considerations are mentioned in Tables 27.11 and 27.13. HB-5 bacteria have been isolated from the human genital tract and from wounds. Nothing has been published so far about their antimicrobial susceptibility, their pathogenic potential, or their habitat.

The EF-4 Group (82, 98)

Bacteria belonging to this nonmotile group are short, coccoid to bacillary shaped, gram-negative rods. Occasionally, longer rods and chain formation are seen. Colonies are 1–2 mm in diameter after 24 hr of growth at 37 C, circular, entire, opaque, with sometimes a slight yellow to tan pigment and greening around the colonies on blood agar. There is aerobic and anaerobic growth, and some strains will grow on MacConkey agar, albeit late. No growth is seen on SS agar. Biochemical reactions are listed in Table 27.15; differential diagnostic considerations, in Table 27.13. For carbohydrate fermentations, peptone bases suffice, and EF-4 strains grow on O/F media as well. Reactions on TSI are quite variable.

The EF-4 bacteria have been isolated from the oral cavity of normal dogs, and from human wounds due to dog or cat bites (82). Antimicrobials effective against EF-4 bacteria include ampicillin, chloramphenicol, gentamicin, nitrofurantoin, tetracycline, and polymyxin B. Susceptibility to penicillin, cephalothin, and lincomycin is variable (82).

The DF-2 Group (6, 11)

These nonmotile, fastidious gram-negative rods are 1–3 μm long or longer. Serum or blood and 5%–10% CO_2 are probably required for growth. Colonies on blood agar are punctate after 24 hr of growth at 37 C, enlarging to 1–2 mm after 48 hr. There is no growth on MacConkey agar or SS agar, and in many instances none on TSI. For carbohydrate fermentations, beef extract has been used as an additive to a broth base. Acidification occurs slowly. Biochemical data are given in Table 27.15; the differential diagnosis, in Table 27.13.

These organisms have been isolated from 18 patients (6, 11), of whom 7 had cellulitis, 4 had bacteremia without localized signs, 4 had meningitis, and 3 had endocarditis. Fourteen had underlying diseases. In 10, the illness had been preceded by dog bites. Sensitivity was recorded to penicillin, ampicillin, cephalothin, tetracycline, chloramphenicol, erythromycin, clindamycin, carbenicillin, and sulfamethoxazole-trimethoprim; there was resistance to kanamycin, gentamicin, and colistin. The reservoir of the agent is unknown (animals?).

The DF-1 Group (*Capnocytophaga ochracea*) (60, 109)

These fastidious, nonmotile, straight, fusiform gram-negative rods, previously described as *Bacteroides ochraceus* (109), are of various lengths and often show granules. The G+C ratio is 39.6–41.1 moles % (109). Growth on blood agar requires 5%–10% CO_2 and may only become apparent after 2–3 days at 37 C. Colonies are yellow-orange and most often show gliding, macroscopically visible as radial colony extensions, microscopically as continuous movement following the long axis of the cells. This type of surface translocation, however, may not be apparent on all media or even on all blood agar plates. There is no growth on enteric media. For carbohydrate fermentation tests, supplemented media have to be used. Results of biochemical tests are given in Table 27.15; the differential diagnosis is given in Table 27.11. Some reactions have varied from laboratory to laboratory (60). *C. ochracea* strains have been isolated from the oral cavity of healthy individuals; its main reservoir seems to be this biotype. The organism is a potential agent of juvenile periodontitis. Septicemia has been seen in patients with malignancies and/or granulocytopenia associated with oral ulcerations (60). *C. ochracea* is sensitive to penicillin, ampicillin, carbenicillin, clindamycin, erythromycin, tetracycline, and chloramphenicol, but resistant to aminoglycoside antibiotics. Susceptibility to cephalosporins has varied.

References

1. AKERLUND M and MARDH PA: Isolation and identification of *Corynebacterium vaginale (Haemophilus vaginalis)* in women with infections of the lower genital tract. Acta Obstet Gynecol Scand 53:85–90, 1974

2 ALEXANDER AD: *Actinobacillus. In* Manual of Clinical Microbiology, 2nd edition. Lennette EH, Spaulding EH, and Truant JP (eds.), American Society for Microbiology, Washington, DC, 1974, pp 320–322

3 ALTMANN G and BOGOKOVSKY B: *In vitro* sensitivity of *Flavobacterium meningosepticum* to antimicrobial agents. J Med Microbiol 4:296–299, 1971

4. BAGLEY DH, ALEXANDER JC, GILL VJ, DOLIN R, and KETCHAM AS: Late *Flavobacterium* species meningitis after craniofacial exenteration. Arch Intern Med 136:229–231, 1976

5. BLOCK P, YORAN C, FOX AC, and KALTMAN AJ: *Actinobacillus actinomycetemcomitans* endocarditis: report of a case and review of the literature. Am J Med Sci 266:387–392, 1973

6. BOBO RA and NEWTON EJ: A previously undescribed Gram-negative bacillus causing septicemia and meningitis. Am J Clin Pathol 65:564–569, 1976

7. BOHACEK J and MRAZ O: Basengehalt der Desoxyribonukleinsaeure bei den Arten *Pasteurella haemolytica, Actinobacillus lignieresii,* and *Actinobacillus equuli.* Zentralbl Bakteriol Parasitenkd Infektionskr Hyg Abt I Orig 202:468–478, 1967

8. BRODY JA, MOORE H, and KING EO: Meningitis caused by an unclassified Gram-negative bacterium in newborn infants. Am J Dis Child 96:1–5, 1958

9. BUCHANAN RE and GIBBONS NE (eds.): Bergey's Manual of Determinative Bacteriology, 8th edition. Williams & Wilkins Co, Baltimore, 1974

10. BURGHER LW, LOOMIS GW, and WARE F: Systemic infection due to *Actinobacillus actinomycetemcomitans.* Am J Clin Pathol 60:412–415, 1973

11. BUTLER T, WEAVER RE, RAMANI TKV, UYEDA CT, BOBO RA, RYU JS, and KOHLER RB: Unidentified gram-negative rod infection. A new disease of man. Ann Intern Med 86:1–5, 1977

12. BYROM NA: The Adansonian taxonomy of some cannery flavobacteria. J Appl Bacteriol 34:339–346, 1971

13. CABRERA HA and DAVIS GH: Epidemic meningitis of the newborn caused by flavobacteria. I. Epidemiology and bacteriology. Am J Dis Child 101:289–295, 1961

14. CENTER FOR DISEASE CONTROL: Multiple abscesses and death due to *Chromobacterium violaceum.* Morbid Mortal Weekly Rep 23:387, 1974

15. CORPE WA: A study of the widespread distribution of *Chromobacterium* species in soil by a simple technique. J Bacteriol 62:515–517, 1951

16. CRISWELL BS, LADWIG CL, GARDNER HL, and DUKES CD: *Haemophilus vaginalis:* vaginitis by inoculation from culture. Obstet Gynecol 33:195–199, 1969

17. DE LEY J and VAN MUYLEN J: Some applications of deoxyribonucleic acid base composition in bacterial taxonomy. Antonie van Leeuwenhoek J Microbiol Serol 29:344–358, 1963

18. DUNKELBERG WE JR, SKAGGS R, and KELLOGG DS JR: Method for isolation and identification of *Corynebacterium vaginale (Haemophilus vaginalis).* Appl Microbiol 19:47–52, 1970

19. DUNKELBERG WE JR and WOOLVIN SC: *Haemophilus vaginalis* relative to gonorrhea and male urethritis. Mil Med 128:1091–1101, 1963

20. DURFEE MA, FORSYTH PS, HALE JA, and HOLMES KK: Ineffectiveness of erythromycin for treatment of *Haemophilus vaginalis*-associated vaginitis: possible relationship to acidity of vaginal secretions. Antimicrob Agents Chemother 16:635–637, 1979

21. EECKELS R, VANDEPITTE J, and SEYNHAEVE V: Neonatal infections with *Flavobacterium meningosepticum.* Report of two cases and a review. Belg. Tijdschr. Geneesk. 21:244–256, 1965

22. EYKENS A, EGGERMONT E, EECKELS R, VANDEPITTE J, and SPAEPEN J: Neonatal meningitis caused by *Flavobacterium meningosepticum.* Helv Paediatr Acta 28:421–425, 1973

23. FLAMM H and WIEDERMANN G: Infektionen durch den *Actinobacillus lignieresii* beim Menschen. Z Hyg 148:368–374, 1962

24. FRAMPTON J and LEE Y: Is *Haemophilus vaginalis* a pathogen in the female genital tract? J Obstet Gynaecol Br Commonw 71:436–442, 1964

25. FROHOLM LO and BOVRE K: Fimbriation associated with the spreading-corroding colony type in *Moraxella kingii*. Acta Pathol Microbiol Scand B 80:641–648, 1972

26. GARDNER HL and DUKES CD: *Haemophilus vaginalis*. Am J Obstet Gynecol 69:962–976, 1955

27. GEORGE RM, COCHRAN CP, and WHEELER WE: Epidemic meningitis of the newborn caused by flavobacteria. II. Clinical manifestations and treatment. Am J Dis Child 101:296–304, 1961

28. GILARDI GL: Antimicrobial susceptibility as a diagnostic aid in the identification of non-fermenting gram-negative bacteria. Appl Microbiol 22:821–823, 1971

29. GOLBERG RL and WASHINGTON JA II: Comparison of isolation of *Haemophilus vaginalis (Corynebacterium vaginale)* from Peptone-Starch-Dextrose agar and Columbia colistin-nalidixic acid agar. J Clin Microbiol 4:245–247, 1976

30. GOODMAN YE: Bacterial identification: clues from computer and chemistry. Can J Med Technol 34:2–16, 1972

31. GREENWOOD JR and PICKETT MJ: Salient features of *Haemophilus vaginalis*. J Clin Microbiol 9:200–204, 1979

32. GREENWOOD JR and PICKETT MJ: Transfer of *Haemophilus vaginalis* (Gardner and Dukes) to a new genus, *Gardnerella: G. vaginalis* (Gardner and Dukes) comb. nov. Int J Syst Bacteriol 30:170–178, 1980

33. GREENWOOD JR, PICKETT MJ, and MACK EG: *Haemophilus vaginalis* vaginitis: Current methods for diagnosis and treatment. Am J Obstet Gynecol (in press)

34. GREENWOOD JR, PICKETT MJ, MARTIN WJ, and MACK EG: *Haemophilus vaginalis (Corynebacterium vaginale):* Method for isolation and rapid biochemical identification. Health Lab Sci 14:102–106, 1977

35. HAWLEY HB and GUMP DW: Vancomycin therapy of bacterial meningitis. Am J Dis Child 126:261–264, 1973

36. HEINRICH S and PULVERER G: Zur Aetiologie und Mikrobiologie der Aktinomykose. II. Definition und praktische Diagnostik des *Actinobacillus* actinomycetem-comitans. Zentralbl Bakteriol Parasitendk Infektionskr Hyg Abt I Orig 174:123–135, 1959

37. HEINRICH S and PULVERER G: Zur Aetiologie und Mikrobiologie der Aktinomykose. III. Die pathogene Bedeutung des *Actinobacillus actinomycetem-comitans* unter den "Begleitbakterien" des *Actinomyces israelii*. Zentralbl Bakteriol Parasitenkd Infektionskr Hyg Abt I Orig 176:91–101

38. HELTAI A and TALEGHANY P: Nonspecific vaginal infections. A critical evaluation of *Hemophilus vaginalis*. Am J Obstet Gynecol 77:144–148, 1959

39. HENRIKSEN SD: Corroding bacteria from the respiratory tract. I. *Moraxella kingii*. Acta Pathol Microbiol Scand 75:85–90, 1969

40. HENRIKSEN SD and BØVRE K: *Moraxella kingii* sp.nov., a haemolytic, saccharolytic species of the genus Moraxella. J Gen Microbiol 51:377–385, 1968

41. HENRIKSEN SD and BØVRE K: Transfer of *Moraxella kingae* Henriksen and Bøvre to the genus *Kingella* gen.nov. in the family Neisseriaceae. Int J Syst Bacteriol 26:447–450, 1976

42. HOLLIS DG, RILEY PS, and WEAVER RE: Serum supplementation as a cause of false positive maltose reactions: Emended description of *Kingella denitrificans*. Abstr Annu Meet Am Soc Microbiol, 1979, p 317

43. HOLLIS DG, WIGGINS GL, and WEAVER RE: An unclassified gram-negative rod isolated from the pharynx on Thayer-Martin medium (selective agar). Appl Microbiol 24:772–777, 1972

44. HOLMES B, SNELL JJS, and LAPAGE SP: Revised description, from clinical isolates, of *Flavobacterium odoratum* Stutzer and Kwaschnina 1929, and designation of the neotype strain. Int J Syst Bacteriol 27:330–336, 1977

45. HOLMES B, SNELL JJS, and LAPAGE SP: Revised description, from clinical strains, of *Flavobacterium breve* (Lustig) Bergey et al. 1923 and proposal of the neotype strain. Int J Syst Bacteriol 28:201–208, 1978

46. HOLMES B, SNELL JJS, and LAPAGE SP: *Flavobacterium odoratum:* a species resistant to a wide range of antimicrobial agents. J Clin Pathol 32:73–77, 1979

47. KING EO: Studies on a group of previously unclassified bacteria associated with meningitis

in infants. Am J Clin Pathol 31:241–247, 1959

48. KING EO and TATUM HW: *Actinobacillus actinomycetemcomitans* and *Haemophilus aphrophilus.* J Infect Dis 111:85–94, 1962

49. LAPAGE SP: *Haemophilus vaginalis. In* Bergey's Manual of Determinative Bacteriology, 8th edition. Buchanan RE and Gibbons NE (eds.). Williams & Wilkins Co, Baltimore, 1974, pp 368–370

50. LAPAGE SP: Genus *Cardiobacterium* Slotnick and Dougherty 1964. *In* Bergey's Manual of Determinative Bacteriology, 8th edition. Buchanan RE and Gibbons NE (eds.). Williams & Wilkins Co, Baltimore, 1974, p 368

51. LEE EL, ROBINSON MJ, THONG ML, and PUTHUCHEARY SD: Rifamycin in neonatal flavobacteria meningitis. Arch Dis Child 51:209–213, 1976

52. LEOPOLD S: Heretofore undescribed organism isolated from the genitourinary system. US Armed Forces Med J 4:263–266, 1953

53. MACKLON AF, INGHAM HR, SELKON JB, and EVANS JG: Endocarditis due to *Actinobacillus actinomycetemcomitans.* Br Med J 1:609–610, 1975

54. MADRUGA M, ZANON U, PEREIRA GMN and GALVAO AC: Meningitis caused by *Flavobacterium meningosepticum.* The first epidemic outbreak of meningitis in the newborn in South America. J Infect Dis 121:328–330, 1970

55. MALONE BH, SCHREIBER M, SCHNEIDER NJ, and HOLDEMAN LV: Obligately anaerobic strains of *Corynebacterium vaginale (Haemophilus vaginalis).* J Clin Microbiol 2:272–275, 1975

56. MCMEEKIN TA, PATTERSON JT, and MURRAY JG: An initial approach to the taxonomy of some gram-negative, yellow pigmented rods. J Appl Bacteriol 34:699–716, 1971

57. MEYERS BR, BOTTONE E, HIRSHMAN SZ, SCHNEIERSON SS, and GERSHENGORN K: Infection due to *Actinobacillus actinomycetemcomitans.* Am J Clin Pathol 56:204–211, 1971

58. MICKELSON PA, MCCARTHY LR, and MANGUM ME: A new differential medium for the isolation of *Corynebacterium vaginale.* J Clin Microbiol 5:488–489, 1977

59. MRAZ O: Vergleichende Studie der Arten *Actinobacillus lignieresii* und *Pasteurella haemolytica.* I. *Actinobacillus lignieresii* Brumpt, 1910, emed. Zentralbl Bakteriol Parasitenkd Infektionskr Hyg Abt I Orig 209:212–232, 1969

60. NEWMAN MG, SUTTER VL, PICKETT MJ, BLACHMAN U, GREENWOOD JR, GRINENKO V, and CITRON D: Detection, identification, and comparison of *Capnocytophaga, Bacteroides ochraceus,* and DF-1. J Clin Microbiol 10:557–562, 1979

61. OGNIBENE AJ and THOMAS E: Fatal infection due to *Chromobacterium violaceum* in Vietnam. Am J Clin Pathol 54:607–610, 1970

62. OLSEN H, FREDERIKSEN WC, and SIBONI KE: *Flavobacterium meningosepticum* in 8 nonfatal cases of postoperative bacteremia. Lancet 1:1294–1296, 1965

63. OLSEN H and RAVN T: *Flavobacterium meningosepticum* isolated from the genitals. Acta Pathol Microbiol Scand Sect B 79:102–106, 1971

64. OWEN RJ and LAPAGE SP: A comparison of strains of King's group IIb of *Flavobacterium* with *Flavobacterium meningosepticum.* Antonie van Leeuwenhoek J Microbiol Serol 40:255–264, 1974

65. OWEN RJ and SNELL JJS: Comparison of group IIf with *Flavobacterium* and *Moraxella.* Antonie van Leeuwenhoek J Microbiol Serol 39:473–480, 1973

66. PAGE ML and KING EO: Infection due to *Actinobacillus actinomycetemcomitans* and *Haemophilus aphrophilus.* N Engl J Med 275:181–199, 1966

67. PARK L, FAUBER M, and COOK CB: Diagnosis of *Haemophilus vaginalis.* Am J Clin Pathol 51:412–415, 1968

68. PATHAK RC and RISTIC M: Detection of an antibody to *Actinobacillus lignieresii* in infected human beings and the antigenic characterization of isolates of human and bovine origin. Am J Vet Res 23:310–314, 1962

69. PAUČKOVÁ V, LÁSKOVÁ H, and KRAKOVIČ B: *Actinobacillus lignieresii* human infection. Zentralbl Bakteriol Parasitenkd Infektionskr Hyg Abt I Orig A 224:489–491, 1973

70. PEDERSEN MM, MARSO E, and PICKETT MJ: Nonfermentative bacilli associated with man: III. Pathogenicity and antibiotic susceptibility. Am J Clin Pathol 54:178–192, 1970

71. PHEIFER TA, FORSYTH PS, DURFEE MA, POLLOCK HM, and HOLMES KK: Nonspecific vaginitis: role of *Haemophilus vaginalis* and treatment with metronidazole. N Engl J

Med 298:1429–1434, 1978

72. PHILLIPS JE: The commensal role of *Actinobacillus lignieresii*. J Pathol Bacteriol 82:205–208, 1961

73. PHILLIPS JE: Commensal actinobacilli from the bovine tongue. J Pathol Bacteriol 87:442–444, 1964

74. PHILLIPS JE: Antigenic structure and serological typing of *Actinobacillus lignieresii*. J Pathol Bacteriol 93:463–475, 1967

75. PHILLIPS JE: Genus *Actinobacillus* Brumpt 1910, 849. *In* Bergey's Manual of Determinative Bacteriology, 8th edition. Buchanan RE and Gibbons NE (eds.). Williams & Wilkins Co, Baltimore, 1974, pp 373–377

76. PICKETT MJ and PEDERSEN MM: Characterization of saccharolytic nonfermentative bacteria associated with man. Can J Microbiol 16:351–362, 1970

77. PLOTKIN SA and MCKITRICK JC: Nosocomial meningitis of the newborn caused by a flavobacterium. J Am Med Assoc 198:662–664, 1966

78. PRICE K: A study of the taxonomy of flavobacteria isolated in clinical laboratories. Ph.D. Dissertation, University of California, Los Angeles, 1977

79. PULVERER G and KO HL: *Actinobacillus actinomycetem-comitans:* fermentative capabilities of 140 strains. Appl Microbiol 20:693–695, 1970

80. PULVERER G and KO HL: Serological studies on *Actinobacillus actinomycetem-comitans*. Appl Microbiol 23:207–210, 1972

81. REDMOND DL and KOTCHER E: Comparison of cultural immunofluorescent procedures in the identification of *Haemophilus vaginalis*. J Gen Microbiol 33:89–94, 1963

82. SAPHIR DA and CARTER GR: Gingival flora of the dog with special reference to bacteria associated with bites. J Clin Microbiol 3:344–349, 1976

83. SAVAGE DD, KAGANE RL, YOUNG NA, and HORVATH AE: *Cardiobacterium hominis* endocarditis: description of two patients and characterization of the organism. J Clin Microbiol 5:75–80, 1977

84. SELIGMANN R, KOMAROV M, and REITLER R: *Flavobacterium meningosepticum* in Israel. Br Med J 2:1528–1529, 1963

85. SIVENDRA R: Unusual *Chromobacterium violaceum*: aerogenic strains. J Clin Microbiol 3:70–71, 1976

86. SIVENDRA R, LO HS, and LIM KT: Identification of *Chromobacterium violaceum*: pigmented and nonpigmented strains. J Gen Microbiol 90:21–31, 1975

87. SIVENDRA R and TAN SH: Pathogenicity of nonpigmented cultures of *Chromobacterium violaceum*. J Clin Microbiol 5:514–516, 1977

88. SLOTNICK IJ: *Cardiobacterium hominis* in genitourinary specimens. J Bacteriol 95:1175, 1968

89. SLOTNICK IJ and DOUGHERTY M: Further characterization of an unclassified group of bacteria causing endocarditis in man: *Cardiobacterium hominis* gen. et sp.n. Antonie van Leeuwenhoek J Microbiol Serol 30:261–272, 1964

90. SLOTNICK IJ, MERTZ JA, and DOUGHERTY M: Fluorescent antibody detection of human occurrence of an unclassified bacterial group causing endocarditis. J Infect Dis 114:503–505, 1964

91. SMITH RF: New medium for isolation of *Corynebacterium vaginale* from genital specimens. Health Lab Sci 12:219–224, 1975

92. SMITH RF, RODGERS HA, HINES PA, and RAY RM: Comparisons between direct microscopic and cultural methods for recognition of *Corynebacterium vaginale* in women with vaginitis. J Clin Microbiol 5:268–271, 1977

93. SNEATH PHA: A study of the bacterial genus *Chromobacterium*. Iowa State J Sci 34:243–500, 1960

94. SNEATH PHA: Genus *Chromobacterium* Bergonzini 1881,153. Nom. gen. cons. Opin. 16, Jud. Comm., 1958, 152. *In* Bergey's Manual of Determinative Bacteriology, 8th edition. Buchanan RE and Gibbons NE (eds.). Williams & Wilkins Co, Baltimore, 1974, pp. 354–357

95. SNELL JJS and LAPAGE SP: Transfer of some saccharolytic *Moraxella* species to *Kingella* Henriksen and Bøvre 1976, with descriptions of *Kingella indologenes* sp.nov. and *Kingella dentirificans* sp.nov. Int J Syst Bacteriol 26:451–458, 1976

96. STANIER RY, PALLERONI NJ, and DOUDOROFF M: The aerobic pseudomonads: a taxonomic study. J Gen Microbiol 43:159–271, 1966

97. SUTTON RGA, O'KEEFFE MF, BUNDOCK MA, JEBOULT J, and TESTER MP: Isolation of a new *Moraxella* from a corneal abscess. J Med Microbiol 5:148–150, 1972

98. TATUM HW, EWING WH, and WEAVER RE: Miscellaneous gram-negative bacteria. *In* Manual of Clinical Microbiology, 2nd edition. Lennette EH and Spaulding EH (eds.). American Society for Microbiology, Washington, DC, 1974, pp 270–294

99. TERES D: ICU-acquired pneumonia due to *Flavobacterium meningosepticum*. J Am Med Assoc 228:732, 1974

100. TILL DH and PALMER FP: A review of actinobacillosis with a study of the causal organism. Vet Rec 72:527–534, 1960

101. TUCKER DN, SLOTNICK IJ, KING EO, TYNES B, NICHOLSON J, and CREVASSE L: Endocarditis caused by a *Pasteurella*-like organism. N Engl J Med 267:913–916, 1977

102. VALLÉE A, THIBAULT P, and SECOND L: Contribution à l'étude d'*A.lignieresii* et d'*A. equuli*. Ann Inst Pasteur 104:108–114, 1963

103. VAN BIJSTERVELD OP: New *Moraxella* strain isolated from angular conjunctivitis. Appl Microbiol 20:405–408, 1970

104. VENKATARAMANI TK and RATHBUN HK: *Corynebacterium vaginale (Hemophilus vaginalis)* bacteremia: Clinical study of 29 cases. Johns Hopkins Med J 139:93–97, 1976

105. VICE JL and SMARON MF: Indirect fluorescent-antibody method for the identification of *Corynebacterium vaginale*. Appl Microbiol 25:908–916, 1973

106. VICTORICA B, BAER H, and AYOUB EM: Successful treatment of systemic *Chromobacterium violaceum* infection. J Am Med Assoc 230:578–580, 1974

107. WEAVER RE, TATUM HW, and HOLLIS DG: The identification of unusual pathogenic gram-negative bacteria. Center for Disease Control, Public Health Service, Dept of HEW, Atlanta, Ga, 1972

108. WERTHAMER S and WEINER M: Subacute bacterial endocarditis due to *Flavobacterium meningosepticum*. Am J Clin Pathol 57:410–412, 1972

109. WILLIAMS BL, HOLLIS D, and HOLDEMAN LV: Synonymy of strains of Center for Disease Control group DF-1 with species of *Capnocytophaga*. J Clin Microbiol 10:550–556, 1979

CHAPTER 28

HAEMOPHILUS INFECTIONS

J. R. Greenwood, Sydney Harvey, and M. J. Pickett

Introduction

Description of Genus

The genus *Haemophilus* is composed of small nonmotile, gram-negative rods or coccobacilli which may be pleomorphic. They are strict parasites with *in vitro* growth requirements for hemin or other porphyrins (X-factor) and/or NAD (V-factor) or other definable coenzyme-like factors (45). The genus presently encompasses 19 species which meet this definition. Of these 19, seven will be considered here: *Haemophilus influenzae, Haemophilus parainfluenzae, Haemophilus haemolyticus, Haemophilus ducreyi, Haemophilus aphrophilus, Haemophilus paraphrophilus,* and *Haemophilus segnis*. Strains previously designated *Haemophilus aegyptius* are included as a biotype of *Haemophilus influenzae*. *Haemophilus vaginalis (Corynebacterium vaginale)* is not considered a member of the genus (17) and is discussed in another chapter of this volume. All hemophilic bacteria to be treated here, with the exception of *H. segnis,* have been implicated in human disease. Information about other species in the genus may be obtained by consulting *Bergey's Manual of Determinative Bacteriology,* 8th edition, or Kilian's taxonomic study (30).

Clinical Manifestations

H. influenzae, the type species of the genus, requires both X and V factors for growth and occurs in both capsulated and noncapsulated forms. The capsular forms are designated as antigenic types a, b, c, d, e, and f. Although both capsulated and nonencapsulated forms can cause human disease, *H. influenzae* type b is most frequently involved. Severe infection due to *H. influenzae* occurs more commonly in children and infants than in adults. Clinical disease may appear as pharyngitis, sinusitis, epiglottitis, endocarditis, pneumonia, meningitis, otitis media, and conjunctivitis (6, 16, 22, 26, 27, 35, 43). Septic arthritis in infants and children has also been described (21). Epiglottitis, characterized by a cherry red markedly edematous epiglottis, can rapidly cause laryngeal obstruction. This may necessitate prompt tracheotomy to prevent asphyxia. Meningitis is one of the most frequently seen manifestations of *H. influenzae* infection and may be fatal unless promptly diagnosed and treated. In contrast to

431

other forms of *H. influenzae* disease, otitis media and conjunctivitis are predominantly caused by nonencapsulated strains (20). Since it is thought that the pathogenic potential of *H. influenzae* for humans is related to the presence of a capsule, it is difficult to evaluate the primary pathogenesis of these strains. The majority of strains isolated from conjunctivitis are those formerly referred to as *H. aegyptius* (Koch-Weeks bacillus) (30) and many of these can effect *in vitro* hemagglutination of human erythrocytes.

H. parainfluenzae is part of the normal oropharyngeal flora in humans. It requires V factor, is found in both capsulated and nonencapsulated forms, and is only rarely associated with disease. Although isolation of *H. parainfluenzae* is reported from cases of endocarditis, meningitis, puerperal bacteremia, and neonatal sepsis (1, 8, 12, 23, 44, 47), definitive identification is frequently lacking in these case reports.

H. haemolyticus is nonencapsulated, requires X and V factors, and is hemolytic when grown on horse or rabbit blood agar. *H. haemolyticus* is part of the normal flora of the upper respiratory tract of humans (18, 31). Rare cases of subacute bacterial endocarditis have been reported.

H. ducreyi, an X-requiring member of the genus, is the etiological agent of chancroid. The clinical manifestations of this disease include ulcerations ("soft chancre") of the penis, labia majora, and the clitoris. Painful inguinal lymphadenopathy frequently appears several days after onset of the chancre.

H. aprophilus is a member of the normal oral flora and is also found in dental plaques (32). When clinically significant, it is most frequently associated with endocarditis and brain abscesses (3). Cases of sinusitis, cholecystitis, and respiratory tract infections have also been reported (14, 24, 37). *H. aprophilus* was considered by some workers to require X factor for initial growth, but others have disputed these findings (37). Thus, it is not a true *Haemophilus* as the genus is presently defined.

H. paraphrophilus is a V-requiring member of the normal flora of the oral cavity. Infrequently, it may cause brain abscesses, subacute endocarditis, or laryngo-epiglottitis (13, 28). It was originally described as requiring increased CO_2 for growth (46), but not all isolates are this demanding (30).

H. segnis is a recently described, V-requiring member of the normal oral flora. A pathogenic role for this organism has not been demonstrated (30).

Epidemiology

From a clinical and bacteriological viewpoint, *H. influenzae* type b is the most important member of the genus. Since it is found as normal flora in the nasopharynx, diseases caused by this organism have worldwide distribution. Meningitis, the most serious of these infections, has predisposing factors which include low socioeconomic status, middle infancy, and acute upper respiratory tract infections with middle ear involvement. It is estimated that there are 8000 cases of type b meningitis annually, making *H. influenzae* the leading cause of bacterial meningitis (15). Seasonal variation has been noted, with the greatest number of cases usually occurring in the late fall or early winter. *H. influenzae* pneumonia is a frequent sequela to viral influenza and other viral respiratory diseases, with infants and the aged comprising the populations at risk. Bacterial conjunctivitis caused by *H. influenzae* biotype III (*H. aegyptius*) also has a worldwide distribution, although infection in warmer climates is more common. Person-to-person spread and possibly flies have been implicated in transmission.

In comparison to *H. influenzae, H. parainfluenzae, H. paraphrophilus,* and *H. aphrophilus* rarely cause illness. When they do, it has been shown that underlying illness such as leukemia, or surgical or dental manipulations are frequently associated with these *Haemophilus* infections. Chancroid, caused by *Haemophilus ducreyi,* is a sexually transmitted disease. Rarely reported in the United States, it is more commonly found in tropical and subtropical countries.

Public Health Significance

As with any infectious disease, rapid isolation and identification of *H. influenzae* is necessary in cases of meningitis or pneumonia. This is particularly important since increasing numbers of *H. influenzae* have been shown to be ampicillin resistant. In certain high-risk situations, when *H. influenzae* disease occurs in day care centers or in families with children under 6 years old, prophylaxis with antimicrobials may be warranted (40). Because chancroid is a sexually transmitted disease, contacts to these cases should be followed.

Collection and Processing of Specimens

Kinds of Specimens

Throat swabs, sputum, spinal fluid, middle-ear exudates, and blood can all yield *Haemophilus* species. Depending on the clinical entity, one or several of these specimen sources should be considered. In systemic disease, cerebrospinal fluid (CSF) and serum can be collected for detection of capsular antigen (polyribophosphate) with countercurrent immunoelectrophoresis, latex particle agglutination, or enzyme-linked immunosorbent assay (ELISA) (see below).

To obtain specimens for isolation of *H. ducreyi* from genital lesions, first clean the ulcer base with a gauze pad moistened in normal saline. The sample should be taken from the cleaned base with a cotton swab moistened in normal saline. Selective media should be inoculated immediately (19) (see below).

Time of Collection

Material for culture should be taken as soon as an infectious process is suspected.

Number of Specimens

It is frequently necessary to obtain follow-up cultures to properly evaluate antibiotic therapy. This is particularly important in cases of meningitis, bacteremia, and obstructive laryngotracheal infection.

Diagnostic Procedures

Microscopic Examination

Microscopic examination of Gram-stained smears of *Haemophilus* species reveals small (0.3–0.5 μm × 0.5–2.0 μm), pleomorphic, gram-negative bacilli. Threadlike fragments and bipolar staining are also frequently observed. Smears of CSF should be prepared from the sediment of a centrifuged specimen. Generally, 10–15 min at 2500 rpm is sufficient to sediment the bacteria and white blood cells (WBCs). Smears from purulent CSF can be prepared without centrifugation of the specimen. Examination of the Gram-stained CSF should be done with great care. An improperly decolorized stain can cause *Listeria monocytogenes* or *Streptococcus pneumoniae* to resemble *Haemophilus*. Organisms in positive spinal fluids may be typed directly using either direct fluorescent antibody techniques or a capsular swelling (Quellung) reaction (see below).

Swab material of chancroid-like lesions should also be Gram stained and examined for small gram-negative bacilli. The swab should be gently rolled over the slide to preserve the clustered or parallel growth (so-called "school of fish") of *H. ducreyi*. Diagnosis of chancroid, however, should not be made from Gram-stain results. Genital lesions frequently have a mixed microbial flora, and other organisms present, such as *Bacteroides* species, can resemble *H. ducreyi*. Material from the ulcer should also be examined by dark field for possible *Treponema pallidum,* a far more comon cause of genital lesions in the United States.

Bacteriologic Procedures

Culture

All material suspected of containing *Haemophilus* species should be incubated at 35 C in a humidified CO_2 incubator or a candle jar lined with a water-saturated paper towel. These conditions will not only enhance the growth of *H. influenzae* but also allow the growth of the moisture- and CO_2-demanding hemophilic bacteria.

The primary consideration for *Haemophilus* plating media is that they contain adequate levels of X and V factors. These levels can be obtained in a properly prepared chocolate agar medium. On chocolate agar at 24 hr, type-specific *H. influenzae* colonies are 1–2 mm in diameter, smooth, grayish, and mucoid. Capsulated organisms produce more mucoid and larger colonies than the unencapsulated strains. Another medium useful for demonstrating capsulated strains of *H. influenzae* is Fildes enrichment agar. Capsulated strains produce iridescent colonies on this medium after 24 hr of incubation. *H. influenzae* biotype III is generally described as being smaller than the other biotypes of *H. influenzae*. The other species of *Haemophilus* have colonial morphologies similar to that of *H. influenzae*. Thus, most workers would find it difficult to distinguish species by colonial morphology alone. A chocolate plate should be incubated for at least 48 hr before it is discarded as showing no growth.

A sheep blood agar plate should be inoculated concurrently with the chocolate agar. Because hemophilic bacteria grow poorly or not at all on sheep blood agar, growth on chocolate but not sheep blood agar is presumptive evidence that one is dealing with *Haemophilus*. Inclusion of sheep blood agar also has the advantage that hemolysis can be determined on a non-*Haemophilus* isolate (e.g., *Streptococcus* or *Listeria*). A MacConkey plate and/or anaerobic media can be used in addition to the media described if *Enterobacteriaceae* or anaerobes are also suspected.

Because some *Haemophilus* species are important etiologic agents of bacteremia and endocarditis, blood cultures are a frequent necessity. Brain heart infusion blood culture medium (GIBCO) and tryptic soy broth (GIBCO or Difco) have been shown to be superior for this purpose (34).

The isolation of *H. ducreyi* presents special problems. Because of the fastidious nature of this bacterium and the fact that it occurs in mixed flora, even enriched chocolate agar is not a suitable plating medium. Although no single method can be recommended, techniques are available to attempt the isolation of *H. ducreyi*. One method relies on heating a clot of the patient's blood to 56 C for 30 min, cooling, and then inoculating this material as an enrichment medium (4). The clot is incubated at 35 C and then subcultured daily to rabbit blood agar plates prepared especially for *H. ducreyi*. This method is, however, subject to overgrowth by contaminants. A more recent approach that shows some promise is the use of chocolate agar supplemented with 3 μg of vancomycin per ml. These plates are inoculated directly with swabs of clinical material and then streaked for isolation. Plates are incubated at 33 C in a 5%–10% CO_2 water vapor saturated atmosphere. After 48 hr of incubation, the plates are examined for nonmucoid yellow-gray translucent colonies. Plates should be incubated for up to 9 days before being discarded as negative (19).

Identification

Hemophilic bacteria are speciated primarily by their growth factor requirements and their hemolytic properties. Subspecies are determined by biochemical reactions. Table 28.1 lists the differential characteristics of the commonly encountered *Haemophilus* species. The following methods are available to determine these features:

X and V factor growth requirements. Several methods are available to test the X and V requirements of an isolate suspected of being *Haemophilus*. Perhaps the easiest method is to test for satellite growth around commercially prepared disks of X and V factors (Difco or BBL). This test is performed by emulsifying a 24-hr colony in 1 ml of sterile distilled water. A dilute suspension of organisms is used to prevent possible carryover of X factor. A plate of brain heart infusion agar (Difco) is inoculated for confluent growth with a swab saturated in the suspension. X and V disks are placed on the plate approximately 5 mm apart. After 24 hr of incubation the plate is examined for growth around and between the disks. Growth between the disks denotes a requirement for both X and V factors; growth around a disk is indicative of a requirement for that factor only.

Conversion of D aminolevulinic acid (ALA) to porphyrins. This test has been recommended by Kilian as an alternative method of testing for the X re-

TABLE 28.1.—DIFFERENTIAL FEATURES OF *HAEMOPHILUS* SPECIES

	H. influenzae					*H. parainfluenzae*	*H. haemolyticus*	*H. ducreyi*	*H. aphrophilus*	*H. paraphrophilus*	*H. segnis*
	I	II	III	IV	V						
Growth factors required:											
X	+	+	+	+	+	−	+	+	−	−	−
V	+	+	+	+	+	+	+	−	−	+	+
ALA → porphyrin	−	−	−	−	−	+	+	−	+	+	+
Hemolysis	−	−	−	−	−	d	+	+sl	−	−	−
Indole	+	+	−	−	+	−	d	−	−	−	−
Urease	+	+	+	+	−	d	+	−	−	−	−
Ornithine decarboxylase	+	−	−	+	+	d	−	−	−	−	−
Glucose	+	+	+	+	+	+	+	−	+	+	+w
Lactose	−	−	−	−	−	−	−	−	+	+	−
Sucrose	−	−	+	−	+	+	+	−	+	+	+w
Catalase	+	+	+	d	+	d	+	−	−	−	+w
Oxidase	+	+	+	d	+	+	+	−	−	+	−

Symbols: +, 90% (or more) of strains positive; −, 10% (or less) of strains positive; d, different reactions with different strains, 11%–89% positive; +sl, slightly positive; +w, weakly positive. ALA = δ-aminolevulinic acid.

Biotypes I-V of Kilian (30); biotype III = *H. aegyptius*.

quirement of an isolate (29). It avoids the potential difficulties of X factor carryover or low levels of X contamination in a basal medium used in satellite testing. To perform the test, a heavy suspension of a 24-hr plate culture is made in 0.5 ml of the ALA reagent. The tube is incubated for 2 to 4 hr and then examined in a darkened room with a long wave-length fluorescence light (Wood's lamp). The tube will fluoresce red if the test is positive. Organisms that can convert ALA to porphyrins (positive test) do not require X factor for growth.

In the absence of commercially prepared disks, X and V factor requirements can be determined by comparing satellitism around streaks of *Staphylococcus aureus* and *Streptococcus faecalis*. To perform the test, a plate of brain heart infusion agar is inoculated for confluent growth as above. Next, using a relatively large inoculum, streak *S. aureus* across the plate as a cord about 2 cm from the center. Streak *S. faecalis* as a cord 4 cm from and parallel to the first streak. Incubate the plate for 24–48 hr and then examine the area around the streaks for evidence of satellite growth. Both X and V factors diffuse from *S. aureus*, while only V factor is released from *S. faecalis*. Thus, satellite growth around both streaks denotes a V-requiring isolate, while growth only around the *S. aureus* signifies an X and V requirement.

Hemolysis. The hemolysis of an organism may be tested on rabbit blood agar or horse blood agar (supplemented with V factor). Isolated colonies should be observed after 24 and 48 hr of incubation.

Indole production. A 48-hr Levinthal broth culture is tested with Kovacs' reagent. For a more practical test, we have also used spot indole reagent. The test is performed by smearing 24-hr colonies on a piece of filter paper saturated with the spot indole reagent. A positive test is shown by a blue-green color, while negatives show no change or turn the paper yellow.

Decarboxylation of ornithine. A heavy suspension of a 24- to 48-hr plate culture is made in 1 ml of Møller ornithine decarboxylase medium. The results are recorded after 48 hr of incubation.

Production of acid from carbohydrates. Several methods are presently available. Kilian (30) uses a phenol red broth base (Difco) supplemented with hemin and NAD. A more practical approach for smaller laboratories is to heavily inoculate tubes of Cystine Trypticase Agar. A commercial XV disk is then aseptically pushed into the semisolid medium. Tubes are incubated in air at 35 C and examined daily for evidence of acid production. The Minitek System (BBL) has also been used to demonstrate acid production from carbohydrates (2). These last two methods allow smaller laboratories routinely to biotype *H. influenzae* isolates.

Detection of urease activity. Heavily inoculate a tube of urea broth. Incubate at 35 C in air for up to 4 days before discarding as negative. A urease-producing strain turns the broth from yellow to red.

Oxidase. The oxidase reaction of an isolate can be determined by rubbing a loopful of 24-hr cell paste onto a moistened strip of filter paper previously saturated with a solution of 1% tetramethyl-p-phenylenediamine dihydrochloride in 0.2% ascorbic acid. Development of a purple color within 10 sec is scored as positive for cytochrome *c* oxidase.

Serologic Procedures

On the isolate

H. influenzae isolates can be serotyped by six methods, and all of these procedures use antisera that are commercially available (Difco and Hyland).

Slide agglutination. A heavy suspension of a 24-hr chocolate agar culture is prepared in 1 ml of 0.85% NaCl containing 0.5% formaldehyde. A loopful of this suspension is placed on a microscope slide and then mixed with a loopful of *H. influenzae* polyvalent antiserum. The slide is rocked gently for 1 min and observed for agglutination. If agglutination occurs with the polyvalent antiserum, the test should be repeated with type-specific antiserum. It is probably best to use type b first since this is the most common serotype isolated.

Quellung capsular swelling reaction. A suspension of organisms is prepared as above, and the turbidity is then adjusted to a density of approximately 25 to 100 organisms per oil immersion field. A loopful of this suspension is placed on each end of a microscope slide. To one loopful of the suspension add a drop of *H. influenzae* antiserum and a drop of Loeffler methylene blue, mix, and cover with a cover slip. The other end of the slide is treated in the same manner, except that normal serum is substituted for *Haemophilus* antiserum. This end of the slide is used as a control for capsule size. The slide is examined under oil immersion, and an increase in capsular size is recorded as a positive reaction. A slide should be observed for 30 min before it is recorded as negative. If a spinal fluid is observed to have organisms morphologically compatible with *H. influenzae,* a direct Quellung reaction may be performed on the CSF with the same technique outlined above.

Fluorescent antibody techniques. Reagents are available for serotyping *H. influenzae.* These techniques are rapid and efficient when used in laboratories with fluorescent microscopy capabilities. It is best to use the manufacturer's recommended procedures supplied with the fluorescent antisera.

Three other methods for serotyping are countercurrent immunoelectrophoresis, latex agglutination, and antiserum agar. All of these methods give results comparable to those outlined above (25).

In all of these procedures, it is important to remember that *H. influenzae* antisera can cross-react with other bacteria. *Escherichia coli* (some strains), *Staphylococcus aureus, Bacillus subtilis,* and several of the pneumococcus types have been shown to have these cross-reacting antigens (5).

On sera and body fluids from the patient

Countercurrent immunoelectrophoresis and coagglutination with specific antibody-coated staphylococci are two immunological methods available to detect *Haemophilus* antigens in CSF or other body fluids. These methods rely on detection of the soluble polyribophosphate capsular antigen of *H. influenzae* type b and are extremely sensitive and rapid. They have been shown to be useful adjuncts to direct Gram stain and cultural techniques (9, 11, 36, 41).

Marker Systems

Other than the serological typing methods listed above, there are no other marker systems available for epidemiological investigations.

Miscellaneous Procedures

Selective media have been developed for isolation of *Haemophilus* species. Most of these media contain 5 units of bacitracin per ml of basal medium (10, 47), and although they have proven useful in normal flora studies, they are probably of less value in routine clinical use.

It is extremely important that each lot of chocolate agar be tested for quality control with a strain of *H. influenzae.* In this way it will be known if the primary plating medium will support the growth of an organism requiring both X and V factors.

Antimicrobic Susceptibility

Within the last few years, there have been numerous reports of ampicillin-resistant, beta-lactamase-producing isolates of *H. influenzae* (38). Because ampicillin has generally been the drug of choice in treating meningitis, the importance of *in vitro* susceptibility testing of *H. influenzae* has increased markedly. Both broth and agar dilution methods are available for susceptibility testing, and they can be found in Chapter 44 of this book. Additionally, several rapid methods of detecting beta-lactamase-producing strains have also been described (7, 39). At this time, and with few exceptions (33), *H. influenzae* isolates are susceptible to chloramphenicol and the tetracyclines, which can be used as alternative drugs for therapy. Cephalosporins show excellent in vitro activity against *H. influenzae* type b, *H. parainfluenzae,* and *H. aprophilus.* If clinical trials substantiate results, cephalosporins may be used for *Haemophilus* infections such as otitis media in patients who are allergic to ampicillin (42).

H. aprophilus is generally susceptible to aminoglycosides, tetracyclines, and chloramphenicol. Variable susceptibility has been reported with lincomycins and the penicillins (3). Good susceptibility data are not available on *H. paraprophilus* because of this organism's generally poor growth characteristics.

Several antimicrobials have been used to eliminate nasopharyngeal colonization by *H. influenzae.* These have included ampicillin, trimethoprim and sulfamethoxazole, or rifampin. At present, rifampin seems to be most effective (40).

Evaluation of Laboratory Findings

The species, serotype if known, and the clinical source of *Haemophilus* isolates should be reported to the physician. Susceptibility testing should be performed on all isolates from cases of meningitis, otitis media, endocarditis, and epiglottitis.

References

1. BACHMAN DS: *Haemophilus* meningitis: comparison of *H. influenzae* and *H. parainfluenzae.* Pediatrics 55:526–530, 1975
2. BACK AE and OBERHOFER TR: Use of the Minitek System for biotyping *Haemophilus* species. J Clin Microbiol 7:312–313, 1978
3. BIEGER RC, BREWER NS, and WASHINGTON JA II: *Haemophilus aprophilus:* a microbiologic and clinical review and report of 42 cases. Medicine 57:345–355, 1978.

4. BORCHARDT KA and HOKE AW: Simplified laboratory technique for diagnosis of chancroid. Arch Dermatol 102:188–192, 1970
5. BRADSHAW MW, SCHNEERSON R, PARKE JC JR, and ROBBINS JB: Bacterial antigens cross-reactive with the capsular polysaccharide of *Haemophilus influenzae* type b. Lancet 1:1095–1097, 1971
6. BUCK LL and DOUGLAS GW: Meningitis due to *Haemophilus influenzae* type e. J. Clin Microbiol 4:1381, 1976
7. CATLIN BW: Iodometric detection of *Haemophilus influenzae* beta-lactamase: rapid presumptive test for ampicillin resistance. Antimicrob Agents Chemother 7:265–270, 1975
8. CHOW AW, BUSHKELL LL, YOSHIKAWA TT, and GUZE LB: *Haemophilus parainfluenzae* epiglottitis with meningitis and bacteremia in an adult. Am J Med Sci 267:365–368, 1974
9. COLDING H and LOND I: Counterimmunoelectrophoresis in the diagnosis of bacterial meningitis. J Clin Microbiol 5:405–409, 1977
10. CRAWFORD JJ, BARDEN L, and KIRKMAN JB JR: Selective culture medium to survey the incidence of *Haemophilus* species. Appl Microbiol 18:646–649, 1969
11. CROSSON FJ JR, WINKELSTEIN JA, and MOXON ER: Enzyme-linked immunosorbent assay for detection and quantitation of capsular antigen of *Haemophilus influenzae* type b. Infect Immun 22:617–619, 1978
12. DAHLGREN J, TALLY FP, BROTHERS G, and RUSKIN J: *Haemophilus parainfluenzae* endocarditis. Am J Clin Pathol 62:607–611, 1974
13. DESILVA M, RUBIN SJ, LYONS RW, LISS JP, and ROTATORI ES: *Haemophilus paraphrophilus* endocarditis in a prolapsed mitral valve. Am J Clin Pathol 66:922–926, 1976
14. ENCK RE and BENNETT JM: Isolation of *Haemophilus aphrophilus* from an adult with acute leukemia. J Clin Microbiol 4:194–195, 1976
15. FRASER DW, GEIL CC, and FELDMAN RA: Bacterial meningitis in Bernalillo County, New Mexico: a comparison with three other American populations. Am J Epidemiol 100:29–34, 1974
16. GERACI JE, WILKOWSKE CJ, WILSON WR, and WASHINGTON JA II: *Haemophilus* endocarditis—report of 14 patients. Mayo Clin Proc 52:209–215, 1977
17. GREENWOOD JR and PICKETT MJ: Transfer of *Haemophilus vaginalis* (Gardner and Dukes) to a new genus, *Gardnerella: G. vaginalis* (Gardner and Dukes) comb. nov. Int J Syst Bacteriol 30:170–178, 1980
18. HABLE KA, WASHINGTON JA II, and HERRMANN ER: Bacterial and viral throat flora. Comparison of findings in children with acute upper respiratory tract disease and in healthy controls during winter. Clin Pediatr 10:199–203, 1971
19. HAMMOND GW, LIAN CJ, WILT JC, and RONALD AR: Comparison of specimen collection and laboratory techniques for isolation of *Haemophilus ducreyi.* J Clin Microbiol 7:39–43, 1978
20. HARDING AL, ANDERSON P, HOWIE VM, PLOUSSARD JH, and SMITH DH: *Haemophilus influenzae* isolated from children with otitis media. *In Haemophilus influenzae.* Sell SHW and Karzon DT (eds.). Vanderbilt Univ Press. Nashville, Tenn. 1973, pp 21–28
21. HARLOW M, CHUNG SMK, and PLOTKIN SA: *Haemophilus influenzae* septic arthritis in infants and children. Clin Pediatr 14:1146–1150, 1975
22. HODGE JLR and BREMNER DA: *Haemophilus* endocarditis and the isolation of haemophilic bacteria in blood culture. Case report NZ Med J 79:824–825, 1974
23. HOLT RN, TAYLOR CD, SCHNEIDER HJ, and HALLOCK JA: Three cases of *Haemophilus parainfluenzae* meningitis. Clin Pediatr 13:666–668, 1974
24. HUCK W and BRITT MR: *Haemophilus aphrophilus* cholecystitis. Am J Clin Pathol 69:361–363, 1978
25. INGRAM DL, COLLIER AM, PENDERGRASS E, and KING SH: Methods for serotyping nasopharyngeal isolates of *Haemophilus influenzae:* slide agglutination, Quellung reaction, counter-current immunoelectrophoresis, latex agglutination, and antiserum agar. J Clin Microbiol 9:570–574, 1979
26. JOHNSON RH, KENNEDY RP, MARTON KI, and THORNSBERRY C: *Haemophilus* endocarditis: new cases, literature review, and recommendations for management. South Med J 70:1098–1102, 1977
27. JOHNSTONE JM and LAWY HS: Acute epiglottitis in adults due to infection with *Haemophilus influenzae* type b. Lancet 2:134–136, 1967

28. JONES RN, SLEPACK J, and BIGELOW J: Ampicillin-resistant *Haemophilus paraphrophilus* laryngo-epiglottitis. J Clin Microbiol 4:405–407, 1976

29. KILIAN M: A rapid method for the differentiation of *Haemophilus* strains. The porphyrin test. Acta Pathol Microbiol Scand Sect B 82:835–842, 1974

30. KILIAN M: A taxonomic study of the genus *Haemophilus,* with the proposal of a new species. J Gen Microbiol 93:8–62, 1976

31. KILIAN M, HEINE-JENSEN J, and BULOW P: *Haemophilus* in the upper respiratory tract of children. Acta Pathol Microbiol Scand Sect B 80:571–578, 1972

32. KRAUT MS, ATTEBERY HR, FINEGOLD SM, and SUTTER VL: Detection of *Haemophilus aphrophilus* in the human oral flora with a selective medium. J Infect Dis 126:189–192, 1972

33. MANTEN A, VAN KLINGEREN B, and DESSENS-KROON M: Chloramphenicol resistance in *Haemophilus influenzae.* Lancet 1:702, 1976

34. SCHELL RF, LeFROCK JL, BABU JP, and ROBINSON DB: Recovery of *Haemophilus influenzae* from twenty-three blood culture media. J Clin Microbiol 9:84–87, 1979

35. SELL SHW: The clinical importance of *Haemophilus influenzae* infections in children. Pediatr Clin North Am 17:415–426, 1970

36. SUKSANONG M and DAJANI AS: Detection of *Haemophilus influenzae* type b antigens in body fluids, using specific antibody-coated staphylococci. J Clin Microbiol 5:81–85, 1977

37. SUTTER VL and FINEGOLD SM: *Haemophilus aphrophilus* infections: clinical and bacteriologic studies. Ann NY Acad Sci 174:468–487, 1970

38. THORNSBERRY C and KIRVEN LA: Antimicrobial susceptibility of *Haemophilus influenzae.* Antimicrob Agents Chemother 6:620–624, 1974

39. THORNSBERRY C and KIRVEN LA: Ampicillin resistance in *Haemophilus influenzae* as determined by a rapid test for beta-lactamase production. Antimicrob Agents Chemother 6:653–654, 1974

40. WARD JI, FRASER DW, BARAFF LJ, and PLIKAYTIS BD: *Haemophilus influenzae* meningitis. A national study of secondary spread in household contacts. N Engl J Med 301:122–126, 1979

41. WARD JI, SIBER GR, SCHEIFELE DW, and SMITH DH: Rapid diagnosis of *Haemophilus influenzae* type b infections by latex particle agglutination and counterimmunoelectrophoresis. J Pediatr 93:37–42, 1978

42. WATANAKUNAKORN C and GLOTZBECKER C: Comparative susceptibility of *Haemophilus* species to cefaclor, cefamandole, and five other cephalosporins and ampicillin, chloramphenicol, and tetracycline. Antimicrob Agents Chemother 15:836–838, 1979

43. WEINSTEIN L: Type b *Haemophilus influenzae* infections in adults. N Engl J Med 282:221–222, 1970

44. WORT AJ: *Hemophilus parainfluenzae* meningitis. Can Med Assoc J 112:606–607, 1975

45. ZINNEMANN K: Report of the subcommittee on the taxonomy of *Haemophilus.* Int J Syst Bacteriol 17:165–166, 1967

46. ZINNEMANN K, ROGERS KB, FRAZER J, and BOYCE JMH: A new V-dependent *Haemophilus* species preferring increased CO_2 tension for growth and named *Haemophilus paraphrophilus,* nov. sp. J Pathol Bacteriol 96:413–419, 1968

47. ZINNER SH, McCORMACK WM, LEE Y-H, ZUCKERSTATTER MH, and DALY AK: Puerperal bacteremia and neonatal sepsis due to *Haemophilus parainfluenzae:* report of a case with antibody titers. Pediatrics 49:612–614, 1972

CHAPTER 29

LEGIONELLOSIS (LEGIONNAIRES' DISEASE)

A. Balows, E. D. Renner, C. M. Helms, and W. Johnson

Introduction

Causative Organism

Legionellosis was first recognized in association with the epidemic of Legionnaires' disease pneumonia which occurred in Philadelphia, Pennsylvania, in July 1976 (39). Shortly thereafter, the etiologic agent, a previously unrecognized bacterium subsequently named *Legionella pneumophila,* was isolated by McDade et al. (6, 63) from lung tissues of patients who died of Legionnaires' disease. Since then, six serogroups of *L. pneumophila* have been recognized (7, 28, 65, 66). In addition, five other species within the genus *Legionella* have been identified and proposed (Table 29.1): *L. micdadei, L. bozemanii, L. dumoffii, L. gormanii,* and *L. longbeachae* (5, 49, 64, 68). The term "legionellosis" will be used to refer to any infection caused by bacteria of the family *Legionellaceae,* but it should be understood that our current knowledge stems largely from disease caused by *L. pneumophila.*

L. pneumophila is a gram-negative rod approximately 0.5–0.7 μm wide and 2–20 μm or more long. Growth appears in 2 to 5 days on enriched media containing L-cysteine and a supplemental source of ferric iron. Organisms grown on agar media are usually longer than those observed in tissue, and as cultures age, filamentous forms, swollen rods, and bizarre forms are frequently seen. The organism can be demonstrated in lung tissue, respiratory tract secretions, and other clinical specimens by direct immunofluorescence (DFA) with specifically prepared fluorescein isothiocyanate conjugates (15) and nonspecifically with a modification of Dieterle's silver impregnation procedure (13, 89, 91). The organism will stain only rarely with standard tissue Gram stains such as Brown-Brenn, Brown-Hopp, and MacCallum-Goodpasture procedures. Smears from cultures will "Gram stain" lightly unless the contact time of safranin is extended to at least 2 min or carbol-fuchsin is used as the counterstain. Hematoxylin and eosin usually will not stain the organism, and the Gimenez stain is unsatisfactory for most clinical specimens, even though the latter stain is successfully used for infected guinea pig tissues or yolk sac.

L. pneumophila is usually weakly oxidase positive by Kovac's method and strongly catalase positive when 72-hr cultures grown on charcoal-yeast extract (CYE) agar are tested (31). *L. pneumophila* produces a soluble pigment that re-

TABLE 29-1—PROPOSED CLASSIFICATION OF THE FAMILY *LEGIONELLACEAE,* GENUS
LEGIONELLA

PREVIOUS DESIGNATION OR TRIVIAL NAME	PROPOSED NOMENCLATURE	ATCC No.	YEAR FIRST ISOLATED
OLDA, Legionnaires' Disease Bacterium	*L. pneumophila*	33152	1947
TATLOCK, HEBA, PPA[a] (Pittsburgh pneumonia agent)	*L. micdadei*	33218	1943
WIGA, M1-15, GA-PH	*L. bozemanii*	33217	1959
NY-23, TEX-KL, ALLO₄	*L. dumoffii*	33297	1979
LS-13, ALLO₃	*L. gormanii*	33242	1979
Long Beach-4	*L. longbeachae*	33462	1981

[a] *L. pittsburgensis* has been proposed for PPA (75).

sults in brown coloration of the clear Feeley-Gorman (F-G) agar medium (32), liquefies gelatin, and does not appear to ferment carbohydrates, reduce nitrates, or hydrolyze urea (91). The amino acids required for growth have been described (43). The organism grows on suitable laboratory media at a pH of 6.9. Although growth occurs in ambient air, better growth is obtained in a candle jar or in an atmosphere containing 2.5% CO_2. Cultures on CYE agar may be incubated without added CO_2. The bacterium grows slowly at 25 C and rather well at 35–42 C when inoculated on CYE agar. The optimum temperature for growth in the laboratory is 35 C, but organisms have been isolated from water with temperatures ranging from 5.7–63 C (34). It does not grow anaerobically. More than 80% of the fatty acids of the organism are branched-chain acids (69). Flagella have been demonstrated on many strains of *L. pneumophila* with a modified Leifson flagella stain (81).

Species within the genus *Legionella* have similar phenotypic characteristics (Table 29-2). Initial growth on CYE and F-G agar, colony color on CYE agar containing bromocresol purple and bromothymol blue (90), hippurate hydrolysis (47), fluorescence of colonies with ultraviolet light (48), and synthesis of β-lactamase (85) are of particular value in differentiating the *Legionella* species but are insufficient alone.

The cellular fatty acid composition of *Legionella* is unusual for gram-negative bacteria because of the large amount of total branched-chain acids. The major acid in *L. pneumophila* is i-16:0, whereas an i-15:0 is the major acid in the other recognized species except *L. longbeachae,* which apparently shows some variation. *L. micdadei* differs from other *Legionella* in that this species contains small amounts of an a-17:1 acid (49).

The role of cell surface antigens and extracellular toxins in the pathogenesis of legionellosis has not been fully elucidated. A high-molecular-weight cell surface antigen responsible for the serogroup specificity of *L. pneumophila* has been isolated (55, 56). This antigen is the major antigen detected by the indirect fluorescent antibody (IFA) test and has been shown to induce significant levels of protection against infection with *L. pneumophila* in guinea pigs (26, 55). *L. pneumophila* produces proteolytic enzymes (70). An exotoxin caus-

TABLE 29-2—PHENOTYPIC CHARACTERISTICS OF THE *LEGIONELLACEAE*, SIX SPECIES OF THE GENUS *LEGIONELLA*

CHARACTERISTIC	L. PNEUMOPHILA	L. BOZEMANII	L. DUMOFFII	L. MICDADEI	L. GORMANII	L. LONGBEACHAE
Growth on:						
CYE	+	+	+	+	+	+
F-G	+	−[b]	−[b]	−[b]	−	−
Blood agar	−	−	−	−	−	−
Color on dye containing CYE[a]	white-green	green	green	blue-grey	green	ND[c]
Browning on F-G agar[d]	+	+	+	−	no growth	no growth
Fluorescence	dull-yellow	blue-white	blue-white	dull-yellow	blue-white	dull yellow
Gram stain	−	−	−	+	−	−
Acid-fast in tissue	−	−	−	+	−	ND
Flagella	+	+	+	+	+	+
Oxidase	+	−	−	+	−	W[e]
Catalase	+	+	+	+	+	+
Urease	−	−	−	−	−	−
Gelatinase	+	+	+	+	+	+
β-Lactamase	+	+	+	−	+	V[e]
Nitrate reduction	−	−	−	−	−	−
Hippurate hydrolysis	+	−	−	−	−	−
Carbohydrate fermentation	−	−	−	−	−	−[f]
Major fatty acid	i-16:0	a-15:0	a-15:00	a-15:00	a-15:00	ND
Guanine and cytosine content of DNA (%)	38.8 ± 0.9	40.4 ± 0.7	40.4 ± 0.7	44.3 ± 0.7	ND	ND

[a] CYE containing 0.001% bromocresol purple and bromothymol blue (see reference 42).
[b] Adapted growth can be obtained after several transfers on CYE agar.
[c] ND = not determined.
[d] Both L. gormanii and L. longbeachae grow and produce browning on medium containing 1% yeast extract, 0.025 ferric pyrophosphate soluble, 0.04% L-cysteine HCl, 0.04% tyrosine, and 1.7% agar.
[e] W = weakly positive. V = variable with different strains.
[f] Not distinguishable from L. pneumophila.

ing lysis of guinea pig and rabbit red blood cells (2) and a cytotoxin which causes inhibition of growth and the death of Chinese hamster ovary cells (41) have been reported.

Clinical Manifestations

L. pneumophila infection has been recognized in two clinical forms: as an acute pneumonia (39) and as an acute febrile non-pneumonic illness (44). Pneumonia has been the more commonly reported of the two forms.

L. pneumophila pneumonia begins 2 to 10 days after exposure with a brief prodrome of malaise, myalgia, and headache, followed rapidly by prostration, high fever, and rigors. Cough, dyspnea, pleuritic and abdominal pain, vomiting, diarrhea, and unexplained encephalopathy are often seen. On physical examination there are no specific findings. Routine sputum cultures and Gram stains are nondiagnostic. Specific attention should be given to examinations with DFA conjugates, and sputum specimens should be cultured on suitable media and carefully observed. Leukocytosis with a shift to the left of the granulocyte series, an elevated sedimentation rate, proteinuria, hematuria, and abnormal serum enzyme determinations are common. Radiographic progression of pneumonia with consolidation occurs with a substantial proportion of patients. Pulmonary cavitation has been reported in compromised hosts. Renal failure with and without rhabdomyolysis has also been seen. Mortality is significant, with the most common cause of death being respiratory failure or shock or both.

Histopathology in *L. pneumophila* pneumonia occurs primarily in the lungs. An acute fibrinopurulent pneumonia with a dense intra-alveolar infiltrate of neutrophils, macrophages, fibrin, and often erythrocytes is usually seen (13, 92). *L. pneumophila* organisms are found within leukocytes or free within the alveolus. Hematogenous and lymphatic spread of the organism to lymph nodes, spleen, bone marrow, liver, and kidney occur in about 25% of fatal cases (92). Extrathoracic inflammatory lesions have been infrequently described (20).

The non-pneumonic illness (Pontiac fever) begins 24 to 36 hr after exposure. Malaise, myalgia, and headache rapidly progress to prostration—usually within 12 hr of the onset of symptoms. As with the pneumonia, high fever, chest pain, abdominal pain, and gastrointestinal symptoms often are present, although rigors and cough are less prominent. Confusion, bizarre dreams, irritability, and photophobia suggest central nervous system involvement. Pneumonia is not observed, and reports of laboratory determinations have not been specific. The acute illness lasts 2 to 5 days, and no fatalities or serious sequelae have been reported (38, 44).

Legionella species other than *L. pneumophila* have also been associated with human disease. *L. bozemanii, L. micdadei, L. dumoffii,* and *L. longbeachae* have been isolated from human lung tissue in cases of pneumonia (5, 18, 49, 54, 59, 64, 71, 74, 75, 82, 83). *L. micdadei* has also been grown from blood of a patient with Fort Bragg fever (79) and another patient with suspected pityriasis rosea (4). Although *L. gormanii* has not been isolated in human disease, serologic evidence suggests that it may be a human pathogen (68).

Because the full spectrum of illness associated with legionellosis is not known with certainty, it would behoove clinicians and laboratory personnel alike to be alert for other unexplained clinical syndromes which may be associated with *Legionella* infection.

Epidemiology

L. pneumophila infection is neither new nor geographically limited. The earliest known case occurred in 1947 (62), and cases have occurred worldwide. The preponderance of disease, based on an analysis of 1000 sporadic cases, is caused by serogroup 1 (27).

L. pneumophila infection has occurred in large common-source epidemics, in smaller clusters in presumed hyperendemic areas, and sporadically in isolated cases. Cases occur more frequently in males than in females, and there is an increasing incidence with age (27). Cases in children, although reported, are uncommon. Risk factors include immunosuppression, renal failure or transplantation, cancer, smoking, chronic bronchitis, travel to endemic areas, and exposure to construction and excavation sites (27, 80). The disease is seasonal, with most epidemics and sporadic cases occurring in the summer and autumn (12, 27, 38, 39, 52).

L. pneumophila infection is probably transmitted by the airborne route (37). *L. pneumophila* has been isolated from water from air-conditioning cooling towers and evaporative condensers in association with epidemics (9, 10, 11, 16, 19). Drift from contaminated air-conditioning heat-rejection devices has been implicated in airborne dissemination of the organism (19, 60). Contaminated shower heads have been found in the environment of nosocomial cases of *L. pneumophila* infection, suggesting potable water as a source of infection (17, 88).

Organisms antigenically related to *L. pneumophila* have also been observed in soil-dwelling animals (15). *L. pneumophila* has been isolated from creek water, wet sand, mud, and freshwater ponds (9, 35). Growth of *L. pneumophila* is facilitated in the presence of some algal species (87).

On the basis of available data, it is reasonable to conclude that *L. pneumophila* resides in water and possibly in soil, that it contaminates the immediate human environment by waterborne and airborne mechanisms, and that infection in humans may occur by either route or after additional dissemination by environmental control systems. Further confirmatory information regarding transmission and the ecological distribution of *L. pneumophila* and other legionellae is needed.

The epidemiology of infections caused by *Legionella* species other than *L. pneumophila* is not well understood. Available evidence suggests that the organisms reside in water (18). Aerosol nebulizers used in respiratory therapy are a potential focus of nosocomial *L. micdadei* infection (45).

Public Health Significance and Preventive Measures

An estimated 1%–4% of "nonbacterial" pneumonias in the United States are caused by *L. pneumophila* infection (36, 63, 76). The incidence of *L.*

pneumophila pneumonia is estimated at 4 to 28 sporadic cases per 100,000 population per year (36). Case-fatality ratios have ranged from 7 to 19% (12, 27, 39, 52). As with other bacterial pneumonias, case-fatality ratios among elderly individuals, those with underlying medical illness, and among compromised hosts are greater than ratios among young and previously healthy persons. The public health significance of infections caused by *Legionella* species other than *L. pneumophila* is not known as yet.

Measures for the prevention of epidemics and clusters of *L. pneumophila* infection have not been tested. Given the association of contaminated air-conditioning cooling towers and evaporative condensers with dissemination of infection, however, it would be wise to subject all suspect apparatus to decontamination or cleaning procedures. Some guidance on procedures which may be effective in controlling *Legionella* in water is available (77).

Although person-to-person transmission of *Legionella* infection has not been documented, in view of the limited clinical experience, it would be prudent to handle respiratory secretions from suspected cases with caution, especially in the vicinity of compromised patients.

Collection and Processing of Specimens

All specimens suspected of containing *Legionella* should be processed in a biological safety cabinet. Specimen preparations or suspended cultures should be centrifuged in tightly sealed centrifuge cups with an O-ring seal.

Lung tissue obtained at autopsy or by biopsy is optimally selected from areas of dense consolidation or necrosis. A representative portion of the specimen should be placed in 10% neutral formalin for subsequent DFA and histopathological studies. If initial isolation efforts are unsuccessful and further studies are warranted, additional tissue should be cultured directly on bacteriologic media and the remainder stored at −70 C as reference material or for *in vivo* isolation with guinea pigs and embryonated hens' eggs.

Pleural fluid, transtracheal aspirates, and other lower respiratory specimens that are relatively free from oral-pharyngeal flora are satisfactory for DFA studies and culturing. Representative portions of these specimens should be stored at −70 C as reference material.

Isolation of *L. pneumophila* from specimens containing human pharyngeal flora may be difficult since it has been shown that some pharyngeal isolates of *Streptococcus* and *Staphylococcus* may inhibit the growth of *L. pneumophila* (33). Sputum and bronchial washings are satisfactory for DFA studies or guinea pig inoculation. However, a selective medium should be used for direct isolation (22). Successful isolation from pleural fluid, respiratory tract specimens, and blood has been reported (21, 23, 58).

Specimens to be shipped to a reference or central laboratory should be packaged and mailed according to Interstate Quarantine Regulations (42 Code of Federal Regulations, Part 72) for shipping etiologic agents. Unfixed specimens should be packaged with sufficient dry ice to remain frozen during shipment. Tissues submitted for pathological and DFA studies should be fixed in neutral formalin only and should not be refrigerated during transport.

Acute-phase serum should be collected during the first week of illness and convalescent-phase serum 3–5 weeks after onset. Ideally, for interpretative purposes, only paired sera should be examined for antibodies to *Legionella*. If acute-phase serum is not available, a convalescent antibody titer of ≥256 to *L. pneumophila* serogroup 1 is presumptive evidence of an infection at an undetermined time. When titers of ≥256 are obtained on single serum specimens, it may be desirable to determine subsequent titers 3, 6, and 12 months after onset of illness in order to detect a possible decrease in titer. However, the significance of declining titers is not clearly understood.

Samples of water and soil to be tested for *Legionella* should be collected aseptically in sterile containers and refrigerated at 4 C until analyzed.

The recognition of six serogroups of *L. pneumophila* and five additional *Legionella* species and the possible recognition of other groups clearly indicate the need to maintain clinical specimens for future reference if preservation is possible. Isolates should be stored at −70 C and paired sera, at −20 C.

Diagnostic Procedures

A confirmed diagnosis of legionellosis is based on one of the following procedures:

1. Isolation and identification of *Legionella* from clinical specimens either on artificial media or by guinea pig inoculation followed by passage in embryonated hens' eggs.

2. Demonstration of a four-fold or greater rise in antibody titer from acute-phase to convalescent-phase serum by the IFA test. Other serologic tests have been developed (25, 30, 53), but additional information on the sensitivity and specificity of these methods is required before their diagnostic value can be determined.

3. Demonstration of the organism in clinical specimens by DFA when epidemiological, clinical, microbiological, and pathological data are also considered.

Demonstration of *L. pneumophila* antigens or organisms in respiratory tract secretions (86) or urine (3) with an enzyme-linked immunosorbent assay (ELISA) is reported to be useful but requires additional evaluation before acceptance as a diagnostic test. These tests have not been used for detecting antigen from other *Legionella* species.

Microscopic Examination

The histologic pattern of the pulmonary tissue reaction in patients with *L. pneumophila* pneumonia is similar to the pattern associated with lobar pneumonia. Histologically, however, the pathology is best described as that of a bronchopneumonia. Cellular infiltration of the air spaces, primarily by macrophages, and the large amount of intra-alveolar fibrin are distinctive features of this disease (13, 92). In paraffin-embedded tissue sections, bacteria which stain dark brown to black with the modified Dieterle silver impregnation stain, but stain only rarely with standard tissue stains for bacteria or fungi (Brown-

Brenn, Brown-Hopp, and MacCallum-Goodpasture), are presumptively *Legionella*. *Legionella micdadei* will stain acid fast in tissue but does not retain this characteristic when grown on CYE medium (50).

Selection and Inoculation of Primary Culture Media

The artificial medium first used for the isolation of *L. pneumophila* was Mueller-Hinton agar supplemented with 1% hemoglobin and 1% IsoVitaleX (MH-1H) (63). Two media incorporating ferric pyrophosphate (soluble) and L-cysteine instead of hemoglobin and IsoVitaleX have also been described (31, 32). These media, F-G (32) and CYE (31) agars are recommended for primary isolation of *Legionella*. A semiselective medium containing polymyxin B and vancomycin has been described (22) and should be used with the above media if the specimens are heavily contaminated with other flora. With the addition of 0.001% bromocresol purple and 0.001% bromothymol blue to CYE agar, *L. micdadei* can be readily differentiated from the other *Legionella* species and most other clinical isolates (90). If isolation of the organism from blood is attempted, a biphasic CYE medium is recommended (23).

Tissue specimens can either be ground with a mortar and pestle or sliced so that a freshly cut surface of the tissue can be slid over the surface of the media. The latter procedure is preferred for tissue specimens obtained from patients who have received antibiotic therapy. If the former procedure is used, a 10% suspension of ground tissue is prepared by grinding 1.0 g of tissue in 9.0 ml of sterile distilled water with a sterile mortar and pestle using 60 mesh alundum. The supernatant suspension is decanted into two sterile screw-capped tubes. One tube is quick frozen in dry ice and 95% ethanol and stored at −70 C as reference material and, if necessary, for guinea pig inoculation. The supernatant fluid in the other tube is used to inoculate two plates each of F-G and CYE agars. Approximately 0.1 ml of this supernatant fluid is placed directly on duplicate plates of F-G and CYE media. One set of media is spot inoculated, with the inoculum spread over a small area but not streaked. The inoculum on the other set of media is streaked for isolation. An additional 0.1 ml of the supernatant fluid is added to 4.9 ml of sterile distilled water, and this 0.2% suspension is used to streak an additional set of F-G and CYE media for isolation.

Pleural fluid and transtracheal aspirates are inoculated directly onto the media, as described for the 10% tissue suspension.

Routine bacteriological media, including 5% sheep blood and chocolate and MacConkey agars, should also be inoculated with the above specimens. The inoculated media are incubated in candle jars or 2.5% CO_2 at 35 C for 2 weeks and examined daily. CYE agar can be incubated without additional CO_2.

Identification Procedures

On CYE agar growth usually appears in 2–3 days in areas of heavy inoculum and several days later in areas of light inoculum. Isolated colonies may reach a diameter of 3–4 mm and are glistening, convex, and circular, with an entire edge. Colonies of *Legionella* look like ground glass when viewed with oblique light at about a 10° angle. On F-G media, colonies of *L. pneumophila* will darken the agar (1). *L. bozemanii, L. dumoffii,* and *L. micdadei* will only grow on F-G agar after several transfers on CYE agar, and only the first two organisms will produce a browning of the medium. *L. longbeachae* has not been grown on F-G agar. On CYE agar *L. bozemanii, L. dumoffii,* and *L. gormanii* will give a blue-white fluorescence under long-wave (366 nm) ultraviolet light.

Colonies suspected of being *Legionella* are subcultured to tryptic digest of soy, 5% sheep blood, and CYE agars. Test cultures which grow on 5% sheep blood and Trypticase soy agars are probably not *Legionella* species. Isolates that grow on CYE, but fail to grow on commonly used laboratory media, and have characteristic morphology and biochemical properties may be reported as presumed *Legionella.* Presumptive speciation of the isolates can be accomplished by utilizing tests delineating the phenotypic differences listed in Table 29-2. Such isolates can be confirmed by demonstrating serologic reactivity with DFA reagents.

Organisms that have properties similar to those of *Legionella,* but do not react serologically, may represent different species or serogroups and should be sent to a reference laboratory for confirmation. Species described after *L. pneumophila* were determined by differences in antigenic composition, gas-liquid chromatographic fatty acid profiles, and ultimately DNA relatedness determinations.

Most strains of *L. pneumophila* will remain viable for 4 weeks when stored on CYE medium at room temperature; *L. micdadei* and *L. dumoffii* will remain viable for at least 16 weeks under the same conditions. Strains of *L. bozemanii* are variable in their survival at room temperature; some remain viable for 16 weeks whereas others remain viable for only 2 weeks (46).

Serologic Procedures

Direct immunofluorescence microscopy

The DFA test adds a dimension of serologic specificity not present in other stains. Formalin-fixed tissue, fresh or fresh-frozen tissue, pleural fluids, and lower respiratory tract secretions such as sputum, transtracheal aspirates, and bronchial washings are stained for diagnostic DFA tests by the procedure of Cherry et al. (15). The test may also be used to examine culture smears. It appears to be highly specific but should be used in conjunction with culture of the organism whenever possible. Laboratory reports of DFA test results should indicate the species of *Legionella* and serogroup of *L. pneumophila* identified. Reagents for this procedure are not available commercially as yet, but a limited quantity can be obtained from the Centers for Disease Control (CDC) or prepared in the laboratory.

Direct FA procedure (14)

1. *Specimen preparation.* Specimens from the lower respiratory tract are smeared within 1.5-cm-diameter circles on slides designed for fluorescent procedures. Tissue imprints are made from fresh or fresh-frozen tissue by pressing

the cut surface of the tissue against the slide. These specimens are then air-dried, heat-fixed, and fixed in 10% neutral formalin for 10 min. The slides are then briefly rinsed in distilled water. Scrapings from formalin-fixed tissue are placed directly on the slide, air-dried, and gently heat-fixed. Tissue sections can be stained after sections are de-paraffinated.

2. *Staining procedure*

a.   Specimen preparations are covered with 1–2 drops (0.05 ml) of specific conjugate. Negative control conjugates, if available, should be used on duplicate smears. Currently, a polyvalent conjugate for *L. pneumophila* serogroups 1, 2, 3, and 4 and monovalent conjugates for *L. pneumophila* serogroups 1–6, *L. bozemanii*, *L. micdadei*, *L. dumoffii*, *L. gormanii*, and *L. longbeachae* are available from the Centers for Disease Control (CDC).

b.   Slides are incubated in a moist chamber for 20 min.

c.   Excess conjugate is removed by rinsing smears with phosphate-buffered saline (PBS). Slides are then immersed in PBS for 10 min.

d.   Slides are then dipped in distilled water and air-dried.

e.   Buffered glycerol, pH 9.0, is added and a cover slip is placed on the slide.

3. *Reading of slides.*   Slides are screened with the 10× or 40× objective of a fluorescence microscope. Bacteria will be visible as intra- or extracellular short rods. Morphology of the organisms is confirmed by using the 100× oil immersion objective. The number of fluorescing bacteria per smear should be reported along with the specific conjugate used to stain the organism.

Indirect immunofluorescence microscopy

The IFA test is now the most commonly used test for serodiagnosis of *Legionella* infections (62, 94, 97). Experience with the IFA test for *Legionella* infections other than *L. pneumophila* is limited. The recognition of six serogroups of *L. pneumophila* and five additional species of *Legionella* requires that more than one antigen be used for serologic testing. Reagents for the IFA test are not as yet commercially available. They can be prepared in the laboratory or, in limited quantities, may be obtained upon written request to CDC.

IFA procedure (94)

Reagents:

Preparation of antigen.   Cultures of representative strains of each serogroup are inoculated heavily on a CYE agar slant and incubated in a candle jar at 35 C until growth occurs (2–4 days). Two milliliters of sterile distilled water is added to the tube, and the growth is gently scraped off the slant with a Pasteur pipette. The cell suspension is transferred to a screw-capped test tube and placed in a boiling water bath for 15 min. The screw cap is loosened during the boiling process and then tightly sealed. (A CYE and a blood agar plate are streaked to determine the sterility of the samples. The plates are observed for growth for at least 10 days.) The tube is then placed in a centrifuge cup with an O-ring seal cap and centrifuged for 5 min at 1600 × *g*. The supernatant fluid is discarded, and the packed cells are resuspended in 2 ml of sterile distilled water. Working dilutions of the antigen suspension are prepared in

0.5% normal yolk sac suspension so that the suspension will contain approximately 500 cells per field at 315×. Optimal antigen dilutions have ranged from 1:20 to 1:80, with most suspensions optimal at about a 1:50 dilution. For screening purposes, antigen suspensions of *L. pneumophila* serogroups can be combined, and sera with positive titers to this polyvalent antigen should be reexamined using individual antigens.

Antihuman fluorescein-labeled globulin.   The globulin fraction of rabbit or goat anti-human serum is labeled with fluorescein isothiocyanate. This reagent is available from several commercial sources. The conjugate working dilution should be obtained by titering the conjugate against *L. pneumophila*-positive human serum of a known titer obtained by using standard antigen and conjugate (available from CDC upon written request). For adequate sensitivity, the conjugate must detect IgG, IgM, and IgA (93, 95).

Normal hens' egg yolk sac.   Homogenize a suspension of yolk sac in PBS, pH 7.2, to give a 3% suspension (w/v). Add sodium azide to a final concentration of 0.05% and store at 4 C.

Preparation of antigen slides
1. Evenly suspend the antigen by shaking.
2. Apply antigen to wells on multiwell slides (Cel-line Associates, P.O. Box 213, Minotola, NJ 98341).
3. Air-dry slides for 30 min.
4. Fix the slides in acetone for 15 min at room temperature.
5. Air dry.

Control sera.   A positive human serum that gives an IFA titer of at least 1:256 is required. Standardized human control sera can be obtained from the CDC. The negative control can be any human serum that gives less than 1+ fluorescence at a dilution of less than ≤1:128.

Dilution of sera
1. Prepare a 1:16 dilution of the positive and negative controls and patient's paired sera in 3% normal yolk sac.
2. Make additional two-fold dilutions of 1:64 to 1:2048 in PBS, pH 7.6. Dilutions of the negative control to 1:128 are sufficient.
3. Place the 1:64 through 1:2048 dilutions of the positive control sera and the dilutions of the patient's sera in their designated antigen wells.
4. Incubate slides in a moist chamber at 35–37 C for 30 min. Rinse briefly with PBS, and place in PBS for 10 min. Air-dry the slides or very gently blot them dry.
5. Add antihuman conjugate, adjusted to the predetermined dilution, to each well. Incubate at 37 C for 30 min. Rinse briefly with distilled water. Allow slides to air-dry or gently blot them dry.
6. Add glycerol mounting medium to each slide, and use a #1 coverslip to cover the wells. Examine the slides with an appropriately equipped fluorescence microscope.

Reading of slides.   Record brightness of staining at each dilution. The staining intensity recorded is based on the overall appearance of the smear:

4+   Maximum or brilliant yellow-green
3+   Bright yellow-green

2+	Definite but dim yellow-green
1+	Barely visible yellow-green
Negative	Complete absence of specific fluorescence

The serum titration end-point (titer) is the highest dilution given a 1+ fluorescence of at least half the *Legionella* per field. The titer is the end-point dilution factor.

Microagglutination (MA) test (30)

In the MA test, a steam-killed, safranin-stained suspension of *L. pneumophila* is used. Because of the test's relative simplicity, it can be more readily performed in clinical laboratories than the IFA test. However, the MA test is less sensitive than the IFA, and sera pretreated with 2-mercaptoethanol and then tested by MA showed that IgM is primarily responsible for positive MA titers (29).

Preparation of antigen:
1. Grow the *L. pneumophila* on CYE agar plates for 48 hr at 35 C.
2. Harvest growth by flooding each plate with 3–5 ml of PBS, pH 7.2. Remove growth by scraping the surface with a bent rod.
3. Pool the cells from four to five plates, and place in an autoclave for 1 hr at 101 C.
4. Centrifuge the heat-killed cells in a graduated conical centrifuge tube for 30 min at $1600 \times g$. Wash the packed cells twice in sterile PBS, pH 7.2. Use cups with O-ring seal caps for all centrifugation.
5. Prepare the stock antigen suspension by adding 2 ml of sterile PBS, pH 7.2, to each 0.1 ml of packed cells. Store the suspension at 4 C. It can, however, be used immediately after it is prepared.
6. Initially determine the proper dilution of stock antigen for use in the MA test by diluting the antigen to an optical density reading of 0.155 on a Coleman Junior spectrophotometer at 420 nm. Prepare the working suspension of antigen by diluting the stock suspension of antigen with PBS, pH 6.4, containing 0.005% safranin.

The MA test is performed in rigid polystyrene U plates. Using 0.025 ml microdilutors, the sera to be tested are diluted 1:10, and 0.05 ml of each serum is added to the first well in each row. After the sera have been diluted, a 0.025-ml volume of the working suspension of antigen is added to each well. The plates are then placed on a vertical vibrator for 15 sec to mix the reagents. The plates are then sealed and incubated at room temperature for 16–20 hr and then for 2 hr at 4 C. The end point is the highest dilution of serum at which no distinct button forms in the bottom of the well. A positive and negative control serum should be included in all MA tests. The positive control is important, since data on the storage life of the stock antigen suspension are not available. If the titer of the positive control serum drops, a new stock antigen suspension may have to be prepared. Equivocal MA test results or results that are at variance with the clinical findings indicate that the sera should be tested with IFA. Further evaluation of this test is needed to determine the extent to which it can be applied in the serologic diagnosis of legionellosis.

Other serological tests

Hemagglutination (25) and counterimmunoelectrophoresis (53) tests have been described for detecting *L. pneumophila* antibodies. These tests deserve further evaluation.

A slide agglutination test has been shown to be a good alternative method to DFA staining for serogrouping of *L. pneumophila*. The antigen for the slide agglutination test is prepared by suspending growth from a 2-day culture of *L. pneumophila* in 2.5 ml of neutral formalin for 5 min. One drop of antigen suspension is mixed with one drop of serogroup-specific antiserum. This procedure has been shown to correctly identify the serogroups of 38 isolates of *L. pneumophila* (96).

Specific immunohistochemical stains for *L. pneumophila* employing glucose oxidase and immunoperoxidase have been described that appear to be as specific and sensitive as immunofluorescence methods (8, 78).

Miscellaneous Procedures

Guinea pig inoculation (61)

Since guinea pigs are relatively resistant to many bacterial infections, they serve as a "selective medium" for isolating *Legionella* from clinical specimens that may be contaminated with, or may contain, other microbial agents.

A piece of fresh or unpreserved human lung tissue approximately 2 cm square is ground in a sterile tissue homogenizer or with a mortar and pestle. The minced tissue is suspended in enough PBS, pH 7.2, to make a 10% suspension. If guinea pigs are not immediately available, the tissue suspension can be stored at −70 C until it is processed. Four male guinea pigs (600 g each) are inoculated intraperitoneally with 1 ml of the tissue suspension. The guinea pigs are examined daily for signs of illness, and their rectal temperatures are recorded. Any guinea pigs showing evidence of fever (rectal temperature of ≥39 C) are sacrificed 2 days after the onset of fever. Since *Legionella* may be killed or injured by chloroform and ether, the guinea pigs are sacrificed by exposure to CO_2 vapor. Spleens of the infected guinea pigs are aseptically removed and ground in a tissue homogenizer or with a mortar and pestle with sufficient PBS, pH 7.2, to make a 10% suspension. The suspension is plated on CYE and F-G agars for growth of *Legionella* and on blood agar and Trypticase soy agar to check for the presence of organisms other than *Legionella*. Aliquots of the spleen suspensions should be quick frozen and stored at −70 C for other possible tests.

Egg inoculation (61)

The cultivation of *Legionella* from guinea pig spleen may not always be successful, and passage in embryonated eggs may be necessary. Twelve 6- to 7-day-old embryonated hens' eggs from antibiotic-free flocks are used. The eggs are candled and numbered. The guinea pig spleen suspension is diluted 1:10 in PBS, pH 7.2, and 0.5 ml is injected into the yolk sac. The eggs are incubated at 35–37 C in an egg incubator for 10 days. The eggs are candled each day, and any embryos that die within the first 3 days are discarded. Embryos that die between the 4th and 10th days are harvested by aseptically removing the yolk sac membrane. A piece of the membrane is removed and blotted on sterile gauze to remove excess liquid. This piece of membrane is used to make smears on glass slides. The slides are air-dried, heat-fixed, and stained by the Gimenez method. The remainder of the harvested yolk sac is plated on Trypicase soy, blood, and CYE agars. The plates are incubated at 35–37 C and checked for growth daily for 10 days. Any suspected colonies of *Legionella* are screened by DFA examination of smears or slide agglutination and other tests as indicated.

Isolation from environmental samples (67)

At present, water or mud represent the most likely sources for isolation of *Legionella* from the environment. Preliminary screening of both water and mud samples is done by DFA analysis of concentrated water samples and aqueous suspensions of mud. Environmental samples should be screened for all known *Legionella* species. The mud suspension is prepared by adding about 10 g of mud to 90 ml of sterile distilled water containing 0.5% Tween 60. The suspension is vigorously shaken for 30 min, and the aqueous layer is then removed. Each sample is diluted 10^{-1} to 10^{-4}, and 0.1 ml of each dilution is plated in triplicate on CYE agar and incubated at 35 C. After the plates have been incubated for 3 days, the growth on each plate is graded for bacterial growth other than *Legionella* as low ($<10^4$ colony-forming units [CFU]/ml), moderate (10^4 to 10^6 CFU/ml), or high ($>10^6$ CFU/ml). Additionally, the plates are observed for up to 10 days for the appearance of colonies resembling *Legionella*. Most strains show growth within 6 to 8 days. Colonies suspected of being *Legionella* should be confirmed by using tests previously described.

Tests in guinea pigs may aid in selecting *Legionella* from heavily contaminated specimens and may make it easier to isolate the organisms when they are present in samples in low numbers, but not less than about 10^2/ml. If the colony counts of water samples are low, the sample is concentrated by centrifugation at high speed. The supernatant fluid is discarded and the sediment is suspended in 6 ml of sterile distilled water. Each of two guinea pigs is inoculated intraperitoneally with 3 ml of the suspended sediment. If the plate count of the sample is moderate, each guinea pig is inoculated with 3 ml of the untreated sample. If the plate count is high, each guinea pig is inoculated with 3 ml of the high-count sample diluted to yield approximately 10^6 CFU/ml.

Aqueous suspensions of mud samples are initially processed as previously described. The aqueous layer is centrifuged at 400–600 $\times$ g for 5 min to remove large particulate matter. The supernatant fluid is removed and centrifuged at 2900 $\times$ g for 30 min. The supernatant fluid is discarded, and the sediment is resuspended in 10 ml of sterile distilled water. The total CFU/ml is determined on the final suspension, and the preparation is inoculated into each of two guinea pigs. When the CFU/ml is $\leq 10^6$, 3.0 ml is injected. When the CFU/ml is $>10^6$, the preparation is diluted with sterile distilled water to 10^6 CFU/ml, and 3.0 ml is injected. The guinea pigs are observed daily and rectal temperatures are recorded. Guinea pig spleen is processed for culture and egg passage as previously described.

Antimicrobic Susceptibility and Resistance

Given the preliminary nature of our knowledge of the antibiotic suscepti-bility of *L. pneumophila* and the absence of controlled studies on the efficacy of antibiotic therapy for *L. pneumophila* infection, antibiotic susceptibility testing should be performed on each isolate for correlation with the clinical outcome only by microbiologists with experience in testing legionellae for antibiotic susceptibility profiles. Even under this circumstance the test should be inter-preted with reservation as a standardized method is not available. A number of isolates of *L. pneumophila* have been tested for susceptibility to 22 antibiot-ics *in vitro* by agar dilutions (84). All isolates were susceptible to rifampin, ce-foxitin, erythromycin, the aminoglycosides, minocycline, doxycycline, chlor-amphenicol, ampicillin, penicillin G, carbenicillin, colistin, and trimethoprim-sulfamethoxazole on the basis of accepted minimal inhibitory concentration breakpoints. The only antibiotic to which there was clearcut resistance *in vitro* was vancomycin. Rifampin has also been shown to be significantly more effec-tive than erythromycin and tetracycline in plaque reduction tests of *L. pneumophila* in monolayer cultures of primary chick embryo cells (73).

Injections of erythromycin, rifampin, and minocycline, begun after fever appeared, have been shown to protect guinea pigs following lethal intra-peritoneal challenge with virulent *L. pneumophila* (40, 72). Penicillin, chloram-phenicol, tetracycline, and the aminoglycosides have no protective effect in guinea pigs (72). These results parallel the limited clinical information avail-able on antibiotic efficacy (39). *In vitro* tests with legionellae do not correctly predict the choice of drugs for therapy, but accumulated experience indicates that erythromycin, rifampin, and doxycycline may be used empirically.

A β-lactamase produced by *L. pneumophila* has been described (85). The activity is directed primarily against cephalosporins, but some effect on pen-icillins is also seen. The activity of this enzyme may account for the failure of β-lactam antibiotics in the treatment of patients with *L. pneumophila* pneu-monia. *L. bozemanii*, *L. gormanii*, and *L. dumoffii*, but not *L. micdadei*, also produce β-lactamase. All *Legionella* species have thus far been susceptible to erythromycin.

Evaluation of Laboratory Findings

Interpretation of the DFA test and culture results is straightforward. Other bacteria such as staphylococci may fluoresce in the DFA test. One strain of *Pseudomonas fluorescens* and 3 of 53 strains of *Bacteroides fragilis* tested were specifically stained by the diagnostic dilution of the DFA conjugate to *L. pneumophila* serogroup 1 (24). The DFA test should be used in conjunction with histopathological staining and, when possible, culture methods.

Organisms that conform morphologically and biochemically to *Legion-ella*, but do not react serologically with DFA reagents prepared against known species or serogroups of *Legionella*, should be sent to reference laboratories for further study.

A four-fold or greater increase in titer to at least 128 from acute-phase to convalescent-phase sera, as determined by the IFA test, is indicative of a recent infection with *Legionella*. A standing or single titer of ≥256 is presumptive evidence of infection at an undetermined time.

The upper limit of normal microagglutination titers for *L. pneumophila* serogroups 1, 2, 3, and 4 is 1:8 to 1:16. For a single serum sample, a titer of 1:32 is the lowest suggestive of infection, not necessarily of disease (51, 57). The specificity of a single convalescent microagglutination titer of ≥1:32 in the diagnosis of legionellosis is >93% (51).

There is little information available at the present time to allow interpretation of titers obtained by other serologic methods, especially the specificity of the tests in differentiating infections caused by serogroups and species of *Legionella*.

References

1. BAINE WB, RASHEED JK, FEELEY JC, GORMAN GW, and CASIDA LE JR: Effect of supplemental L-tyrosine on pigment production in cultures of Legionnaires' disease bacterium. Curr Microbiol 1:93–94, 1978

2. BAINE WB, RASHEED JK, MACKEL DC, BOOP CA, WELLS JC, and KAUFMAN AF: Exotoxin activity associated with the Legionnaires' disease bacterium. J Clin Microbiol 9:453–456, 1979

3. BERDAL BP, FARSHY CE, and FEELEY JC: Detection of *Legionella pneumophila* antigen in urine by enzyme-linked immunospecific assay. J Clin Microbiol 9:575–578, 1979

4. BOZEMAN FM, HUMPHRIES JW, and CAMPBELL JM: A new group of rickettsia-like agents recovered from guinea pigs. Acta Virol 12:87–93, 1968

5. BRENNER DJ, STEIGERWALT AG, GORMAN GW, WEAVER RE, FEELEY JC, CORDES LG, WILKINSON HW, PATTON C, THOMASON BM, and SASSEVILLE KRL: *Legionella bozemanii* species nova and *Legionella dumoffii* species nova: Characterization of two additional species of *Legionella* associated with human pneumonia. Curr Microbiol 4:111–116, 1980

6. BRENNER DJ, STEIGERWALT AG, and McDADE JE: Classification of the Legionnaires' bacterium: *Legionella pneumophila*, genus novum, species nova, of the family *Legionellaceae*, familia nova. Ann Intern Med 90:656–658, 1979

7. BRENNER DJ, STEIGERWALT AG, WEAVER RE, McDADE JE, FEELEY JC, and MANDEL M: Classification of the Legionnaires' disease bacterium: An interim report. Curr Microbiol 1:71–75, 1979

8. BUSCHBAUM P, CLEARY T, SALDANA M, and CASTRO A: Immunoperoxidase staining for the serotype specific demonstration of *Legionella pneumophila*. N Engl J Med 304:613, 1981

9. CENTERS FOR DISEASE CONTROL: Isolates of organisms resembling Legionnaires' disease bacterium from environmental sources, Bloomington, Indiana. Morbid Mortal Weekly Rep 27:283–285, 1978

10. CENTERS FOR DISEASE CONTROL: Isolates of organisms resembling Legionnaires' disease bacterium—Tennessee. Morbid Mortal Weekly Rep 27:368–369, 1978

11. CENTERS FOR DISEASE CONTROL: Isolates of organisms resembling Legionnaires' disease bacterium—Georgia. Morbid Mortal Weekly Rep 27:415–416, 1978

12. CENTERS FOR DISEASE CONTROL: Legionnaires' disease—United States. Morbid Mortal Weekly Rep 27:439–441, 1978

13. CHANDLER FW, HICKLIN MD, and BLACKMON JA: Demonstration of the agent of Legionnaires' disease in tissue. N Engl J Med 296:1218–1220, 1977

14. CHERRY WB and McKINNEY RM: Detection of Legionnaires' disease bacteria in clinical specimens by direct immunofluorescence. *In* Legionnaires': The Disease, the Bacterium, and Methodology. Jones GL and Hebert GA (eds.). Center for Disease Control, Public Health Service, U.S. Dept. of Health, Education, and Welfare, Atlanta, Ga, 1979, pp 93–103

15. CHERRY WB, PITTMAN B, HARRIS PP, HEBERT GA, THOMASON BM, THACKER BL, and WEAVER RE: Detection of Legionnaires' disease bacteria by direct immunofluorescent staining. J Clin Microbiol 8:329–338, 1978

16. CORDES LG, FRASER DW, SKALIY P, PERLINO CA, ELSEA WR, MALLISON GF, and HAYES PS: Legionnaires' disease outbreak at an Atlanta, Georgia, country club: Evidence for spread from an evaporative condenser. Am J Epidemiol 111:425–431, 1980

17. CORDES LG, WIESENTHAL AM, GORMAN GW, PHAIR JP, SOMMERS HM, BROWN A, YU VL, MAGNUSSEN MH, MEYER RD, WOLF JS, SHANDS KN, and FRASER DW: Isolation of *Legionella pneumophila* from hospital shower heads. Ann Intern Med 94:195–197, 1981

18. CORDES LG, WILKINSON HW, GORMAN GW, FIKES BJ, and FRASER DW: Atypical *Legionella* like organisms: A group of fastidious water-associated bacteria pathogenic for humans. Lancet 2:927–930, 1979

19. DONDERO TJ, RENDTORFF RC, MALLISON GF, WEEKS RM, LEVY JS, WONG EW, and SCHAFFNER W: An outbreak of Legionnaires' disease associated with a contaminated air-conditioning cooling tower. N Engl J Med 302:365–370, 1980

20. DORMAN SA, HARDIN NJ, and WINN WC: Pyelonephritis associated with *Legionella pneumophila,* serogroup 4. Ann Intern Med 93:835–837, 1980

21. DUMOFF M: Direct in vitro isolation of the Legionnaires' disease bacterium in two fatal cases. Cultural and staining characteristics. Ann Intern Med 90:694–696, 1979

22. EDELSTEIN PH and FINEGOLD SM: Use of a semiselective medium to culture *Legionella pneumophila* from contaminated lung specimens. J Clin Microbiol 10:141–146, 1979

23. EDELSTEIN PH, MEYER RD, and FINEGOLD SM: Isolation of *Legionella pneumophila* from blood. Lancet 1:750–751, 1979

24. EDELSTEIN P, MCKINNEY R, MEYER R, EDELSTEIN M, KRAUSE C, and FINEGOLD S: Immunologic diagnosis of Legionnaires' disease: Cross-reactions with anaerobic and microaerophilic organisms and infections caused by them. J Infect Dis 141:652–655, 1980

25. EDSON DC, STIEFEL HE, WENTWORTH BB, and WILSON DL: Prevalence of antibodies to Legionnaires' disease. A seroepidemiologic survey of Michigan residents using the hemagglutination test. Ann Intern Med 90:691–693, 1979

26. ELLIOTT JA, JOHNSON W, and HELMS CM: Ultrastructural localization and protective activity of a high-molecular-weight antigen isolated from *Legionella pneumophila.* Infect Immun 31:822–824, 1981

27. ENGLAND AC, FRASER DW, PLIKAYTIS BD, TSAI TF, STORCH G, and BROOME CV: Sporadic Legionelllosis in the United States: The first thousand cases. Ann Intern Med 94:164–170, 1981

28. ENGLAND AC, III, MCKINNEY RM, SKALIY P, and GORMAN GW: A fifth serogroup of *Legionella pneumophila.* Ann Intern Med 93:58–59, 1980

29. FARSHY CE, CRUCE DD, KLEIN GC, WILKINSON HW, and FEELEY JC: Immunoglobulin specificity of the microagglutination test for Legionnaires' disease bacterium. Ann Intern Med 90:690, 1979

30. FARSHY CE, KLEIN GC, and FEELEY JC: Detection of antibodies to Legionnaires' disease organisms by microagglutination and microenzyme-linked immunosorbent assay tests. J Clin Microbiol 7:327–331, 1978

31. FEELEY JC, GIBSON RJ, GORMAN GW, LANGFORD NC, RASHEED K, MACKEL DC, and BAINE WB: Charcoal-yeast extract agar: Primary isolation medium for *Legionella pneumophila.* J Clin Microbiol 10:437–441, 1979

32. FEELEY JC, GORMAN GW, WEAVER RE, MACKEL DC, and SMITH HS: Primary isolation media for Legionnaires' disease bacterium. J Clin Microbiol 8:320–325, 1978

33. FLESHER AR, KASPER DL, MODERN PA, and MASON EO: *Legionella pneumophila:* Growth inhibition by human pharyngeal flora. J Infect Dis 142:313–317, 1980

34. FLIERMANS CB, CHERRY WB, ORRISON LH, SMITH SJ, TISON DL, and POPE DH: Ecological distribution of *Legionella pneumophila.* Appl Environ Microbiol 41:9–16, 1981

35. FLIERMANS CB, CHERRY WB, ORRISON LH, and THACKER L: Isolation of Legionnaires' disease bacteria from non-epidemic aquatic habitats. Appl Environ Microbiol 37:1239–1242, 1979

36. FOY HM, HAYES PS, COONEY MK, BROOME CV, ALLAN I, and TOBE R: Legionnaires' disease in a prepaid medical-care group in Seattle 1963–75. Lancet 1:767–770, 1979

37. FRASER DW: Legionellosis: Evidence for airborne transmission. Ann NY Acad Sci 353:61–66, 1980

38. FRASER DW, DEUBNER DC, HILL DL,, and GILLIAM DK: Nonpneumonic, short-incubation-period Legionellosis (Pontiac fever) in men who cleaned a steam turbine condenser. Science 205:690–691, 1979

39. FRASER DW, TSAI T, ORENSTEIN W, PARKIN WE, BELCHAM HJ, SHARRAR RG, HARRIS J, MALLISON GF, MARIN SM, MCDADE JE, SHEPARD CC, BRACHMAN PS, and the FIELD INVESTIGATION TEAM: Legionnaires' disease. I. Description of an epidemic of pneumonia. N Engl J Med 297:1189–1197, 1977

40. FRASER DW, WACHSMUTH IK, BOPP C, FEELEY JC, and TSAI T: Antibiotic treatment of guinea pigs infected with agent of Legionnaires' disease. Lancet 1:175–178, 1978

41. FRIEDMAN RL, IGLEWSKI BA, and MILLER RD: Identification of a cytotoxin produced by Legionella pneumophila. Infect Immun 29:271–274, 1980

42. GARRITY GM, BROWN A, and VICKERS RM: Tatlockia and Fluoribacter: Two new genera of organisms resembling Legionella pneumophila. Int J Syst Bacteriol 30:609–614, 1980

43. GEORGE J, PINE L, REEVES M, and HARRELL W: Amino acid requirements of Legionella pneumophila. J Clin Microbiol 11:286–291, 1980

44. GLICK TH, GREGG MB, BERMAN B, MALLISON G, RHODES WW JR., and KASSANOFF I: Pontiac fever. An epidemic of unknown etiology in a health department. I. Clinical and epidemiologic aspects. Am J Epidemiol 107:149–160, 1978

45. GORMAN GW, YU VL, BROWN A, HALL JA, MARTIN WT, BIBBS WF, MORRIS GK, MAGNUSSEN MH, and FRASER DW: Isolation of Pittsburg pneumonia agent from nebulizers used in respiratory therapy. Ann Intern Med 93:572–573, 1980

46. HEBERT GA: Room temperature storage of Legionella cultures. J Clin Microbiol 12:807–809, 1980

47. HEBERT GA: Hippurate hydrolysis by Legionella pneumophila. J Clin Microbiol 13:240–242, 1981

48. HEBERT GA, MOSS CW, MCDOUGAL LK, BOZEMAN FM, MCKINNEY RM, and BRENNER DJ: The rickettsia-like organisms Tatlock (1943) and HEBA (1959): Bacteria phenotypically similar to but genetically distinct from Legionella pneumophila and the WIGA bacterium. Ann Intern Med 92:45–52, 1980

49. HEBERT GA, STEIGERWALT AG, and BRENNER DJ: Legionella micdadei species nova: Classification of a third species of Legionella associated with human pneumonia. Curr Microbiol 3:255–257, 1980

50. HEBERT GA, THOMASON BM, HARRIS PP, HICKLIN MD, and MCKINNEY RM: "Pittsburgh pneumonia agent": A bacterium phenotypically similar to Legionella pneumophila and identical to the Tatlock bacterium. Ann Intern Med 92:53–54, 1980

51. HELMS CM, JOHNSON W, RENNER ED, HIERHOLZER WJ, WINTERMEYER LA, and VINER JP: Background prevalence of microagglutination antibodies to Legionella pneumophila serogroups 1, 2, 3, and 4. Infect Immun 30:612–614, 1980

52. HELMS CM, VINER JP, RENNER ED, CHIU LC, and WEISENBURGER DD: Legionnaires' disease among pneumonias in Iowa (FY 1972–78). II. Epidemiologic and clinical features of 30 sporadic cases of L. pneumophila infection. Am J Med Sci 281:2–13, 1981

53. HOLLIDAY MG: The diagnosis of Legionnaires' disease by counterimmunoelectrophoresis. J Clin Pathol 33:1174–1178, 1980

54. JACKSON EB, CROCKER T, and SMADEL JE: Studies on two rickettsia-like agents probably isolated from guinea pigs. Bacteriol Proc 1952, p 119

55. JOHNSON W, ELLIOTT JA, HELMS CM, and RENNER ED: A high molecular weight antigen in Legionnaires' disease bacterium: Isolation and partial characterization. Ann Intern Med 90:638–641, 1979

56. JOHNSON W, PESANTI E, and ELLIOTT J: Serospecificity and opsonic activity of antisera to Legionella pneumophila. Infect Immun 26:698–704, 1979

57. KLEIN GC, JONES WL, and FEELEY JC: Upper limit of normal titer for detection of antibodies to Legionella pneumophila by the microagglutination test. J Clin Microbiol 10:754–755, 1979

58. LATTIMER GL, MCCRONE C, and GALGON J: Diagnosis of Legionnaires' disease from transtracheal aspirate. N Engl J Med 299:1172–1173, 1978

59. LEWALLEN KR, MCKINNEY RM, BRENNER DJ, MOSS CW, THOMASON BM, and BRIGHT RA: A newly identified bacterium phenotypically resembling, but genetically distinct

from, *Legionella pneumophila:* An isolate in a case of pneumonia. Ann Intern Med 91:831–834, 1979

60. MALLISON GF: Legionellosis: Environmental aspects. Ann NY Acad Sci 353:67–70, 1980
61. MCDADE JE: Primary isolation using guinea pigs and embryonated eggs. *In:* Legionnaires': The Disease, the Bacterium and Methodology. Jones GL and Hebert GA (eds.). Center for Disease Control, Public Health Service, U.S. Dept of Health, Education and Welfare, Atlanta, Ga, 1979, pp. 69–76
62. MCDADE JE, BRENNER DJ, and BOZEMAN FM: Legionnaires' disease bacterium isolated in 1947. Ann Intern Med 90:659–661, 1979
63. MCDADE JE, SHEPARD CC, FRASER DW, TSAI TR, REDUS MA, DOWDLE WR, and the LABORATORY INVESTIGATION TEAM. Legionnaires' disease. Isolation of a bacterium and demonstration of its role in other respiratory disease. N Engl J Med 297:1197–1203, 1977
64. MCKINNEY RM, PORSCHEN RK, EDELSTEIN PH, BISSETT ML, HARRIS PP, BONDELL SP, STEIGERWALT AG, WEAVER RF, FIN ME, LINDQUIST DS, KOPS RS, and BRENNER DJ: *Legionella longbeachae* sp. nov., another agent of human pneumonia. Ann Intern Med 94:734–743, 1981
65. MCKINNEY RM, THACKER L, HARRIS PP, LEWALLEN KR, HEBERT GA, EDELSTEIN PH, and THOMASON BM: Four serogroups of Legionnaires' disease bacteria defined by direct immunofluorescence. Ann Intern Med 90:621–624, 1979
66. MCKINNEY RM, WILKINSON HW, SOMMERS HM, FIKES BJ, SASSEVILLE KR, YUNGBLUTH MM, and WOLF JS: *Legionella pneumophila* serogroup six: Isolation from cases of legionellosis, identification by immunofluorescence staining, and immunological response to infection. J Clin Microbiol 12:395–401, 1980
67. MORRIS GK, PATTON CM, SKALIY P, and FEELEY JC: Method for isolating Legionnaires' disease bacterium from soil and water samples. *In* Legionnaires': The Disease, the Bacterium and Methodology. Jones GL and Hebert GA (eds.). Center for Disease Control, Public Health Service, U.S. Dept of Health, Education, and Welfare, Atlanta, Ga, 1979, pp 85–90
68. MORRIS GK, STEIGERWALT A, FEELEY JC, WONG ES, MARTIN WT, PATTON CM, and BRENNER DJ: *Legionella gormanii* sp. nov. J Clin Microbiol 12:718–721, 1980
69. MOSS CW, WEAVER RE, DEES SB, and WONG WB: Cellular fatty acid composition of isolates from Legionnaires' disease. J Clin Microbiol 6:140–143, 1977
70. MÜELLER HE: Proteolytic action of *Legionella pneumophila* on human serum proteins. Infect Immun 27:51–53, 1980
71. MYEROWITZ RL, PASCULLE AW, DOWLING JN, PAZIN GJ, PUERZER M, YEE RB, RINALDO CR, and HAKALA TR: Opportunistic lung infection due to "Pittsburgh pneumophia agent." N Engl J Med 301:953–958, 1979
72. NASH P, SIDEMAN L, PIDCOE V, and KLEGER B: Minocycline in Legionnaires' disease. Lancet 1:45, 1978
73. ORMSBEE RA, PEACOCK MG, LATTIMER GL, PAGE LA, and FISET P: Legionnaires' disease: Antigenic peculiarities, strain differences and antibiotic sensitivities of the agent. J Infect Dis 138:260–269, 1978
74. PASCULLE AW, MYEROWITZ RL, and RINALDO CR: New bacterial agent of pneumonia isolated from renal-transplant recipients. Lancet 2:58–61, 1979
75. PASCULLE AW, FEELEY JC, GIBSON RJ, CORDES LG, MYEROWITZ RL, PATTON CM, GORMAN GW, CARMACK CL, EZZALL JW, and DOWLING JN: Pittsburgh pneumonia agent: Direct isolation from human lung tissue. J Infect Dis 141:727–732, 1980
76. RENNER ED, HELMS CM, HIERHOLZER WJ JR, HALL N, WONG YW, VINER JP, JOHNSON W, and HAUSLER WJ JR: Legionnaires' disease in pneumonia patients in Iowa. A retrospective seroepidemiologic study, 1972–1977. Ann Intern Med 90:603–606, 1979
77. SKALIY P, THOMPSON TA, GORMAN GW, MORRIS GK, MCEACHERN HV, and MACKEL DC: Laboratory studies of disinfectants against *Legionella pneumophila.* Appl Environ Microbiol 40:697–700, 1980
78. SUFFIN SC, KAUFMANN A, WHITAKER B, MUCK K, PRINCE G, and PORTER D: *Legionella pneumophila:* Identification in tissue sections by a new immunoenzymatic procedure. Arch Pathol Lab Med 104:283–286, 1980
79. TATLOCK H: A rickettsia-like organism recovered from guinea pigs. Proc Soc Exp Biol Med 57:95–99, 1944
80. THACKER SB, BENNETT JV, TASI TF, FRASER DW, MCDADE JE, SHEPARD CC, WILLIAMS

KH JR, STUART WH, DULL HB, and EICKHOFF TC: An outbreak in 1965 of severe respiratory illness caused by the Legionnaires' disease bacterium. J Infect Dis 138:512–519, 1978

81. THOMASON BM, CHANDLER FW, and HOLLIS DG: Flagella on Legionnaires' disease bacteria: An interim report. Ann Intern Med 91:224–226, 1979

82. THOMASON BM, EWING EP, and HICKLIN MD: Tatlock bacterium (Pittsburgh pneumonia agent) presumptively identified in five cases of pneumonia. Ann Intern Med 92:510, 1980

83. THOMASON BM, HARRIS PP, HICKLIN MD, BLACKMON JA, MOSS CW, and MATTHEWS F: A Legionella-like bacterium related to WIGA in a fatal case of pneumonia. Ann Intern Med 91:673–676, 1979

84. THORNSBERRY C, BAKER CN, and KIRVAN LA: In vitro activity of antimicrobial agents on Legionnaires' disease bacterium. Antimicrob Agents Chemother 13:78–80, 1978

85. THORNSBERRY C and KIRVEN LA: β-Lactamase of the Legionnaires' bacterium. Curr Microbiol 1:51–54, 1978

86. TILTON RC: Legionnaires' disease antigen detected by enzyme-linked immunosorbent assay. Ann Intern Med 90:697–698, 1979

87. TISON DL, POPE DH, CHERRY WB, and FLIERMANS CB: Growth of Legionella pneumophila in association with blue-green algae (Cyanobacteria). Appl Environ Microbiol 39:456–459, 1980

88. TOBIN JO'H, DUNNILL MS, FRENCH M, MORRIS PJ, BEARE J, FISHER-HOCK S, MITCHELL RG, and MUERS MF: Legionnaires' disease in a transplant unit: Isolation of the causative agent from shower baths. Lancet 2:118–121, 1980

89. VAN ORDEN AD and GRIER PW: Modification of the Dieterle spirochete strain. J Histotechnol 1:51–53, 1977

90. VICKERS RM, BROWN A, and GARRITY GM: Dye-containing buffered charcoal-yeast extract medium for differentiation of members of the family Legionellaceae. J Clin Microbiol 13:380–382, 1981

91. WEAVER RE and FEELEY JC: Cultural and biochemical characterization of the Legionnaires' disease bacterium. In: Legionnaires': the Disease, the Bacterium and Methodology. Jones GL and Hebert GA (eds.). Center for Disease Control, Public Health Service, U.S. Dept of Health, Education, and Welfare, Atlanta, Ga, 1979, pp 19–25

92. WEISENBURGER DD, HELMS CM, and RENNER ED: Sporadic Legionnaires' disease. A pathologic study of 23 fatal cases. Arch Pathol Lab Med 105:130–137, 1981

93. WILKINSON HW, CRUCE DD, and BROOME CV: Validation of Legionella pneumophila indirect immunofluorescence assay with epidemic sera. J Clin Microbiol 13:139–146, 1981

94. WILKINSON HW, CRUCE DD, FIKES BJ, YEALEY LP, and FARSHY CE: Indirect immunofluorescence test for Legionnaires' disease. In Legionnaires': The Disease, the Bacterium and Methodology, Jones GL and Hebert GA (eds.). Center for Disease Control, Public Health Service, U.S. Dept of Health, Education and Welfare, Atlanta, Ga, 1979, pp 111–116

95. WILKINSON HW, FARSHY CE, FIKES BJ, CRUCE DD, and YEALY LP: Measure of immunoglobulin G-, M-, and A-specific titers against Legionella pneumophila and inhibition of titers against nonspecific, gram-negative bacterial antigens in the indirect immunofluorescence test for legionellosis. J Clin Microbiol 10:685–689, 1979

96. WILKINSON HW and FIKES BJ: Slide agglutination test for serogrouping Legionella pneumophila and atypical Legionella-like organisms. J Clin Microbiol 11:99–109, 1980

97. WILKINSON HW, FIKES BJ, and CRUCE DD: Indirect immunofluorescence test for serodiagnosis of Legionnaires' disease: Evidence for serogroup diversity of Legionnaires' disease bacterial antigens and for multiple specificity of human antibodies. J Clin Microbiol 9:379–383, 1979

Chapter 30

Leptospirosis

Herman C. Ellinghausen, Jr., Alejandro B. Thiermann, and Catherine R. Sulzer

Introduction

Causative Organism

Microscopic morphology

The approximately 160 leptospiral serotypes (serovars), which are subdivided into 21 serogroups, are generally morphologically similar and are best observed by dark-field microscopy at magnifications of 100× to 600×. These spirochetes are slender, averaging 0.05 to 0.1 μm in diameter, as judged by the best available estimates established with specimens treated with the negative staining technique used in electron microscopic studies (77, 78, 79). Leptospires usually vary in length from 6 to 20 μm, which aids in observing their rather distinctive motility, but in some instances are as short as 4 μm or as long as 40 μm. When organisms in a culture or strain are, in general, of comparable length, they are frequently in the log phase of growth. With adverse environmental conditions (e.g., inadequate nutrients, incubation temperatures above 30 C, toxic conditions, presence of antibody), they tend to move languidly and to elongate and synthesize protoplasm without undergoing the process of cell division and forming septa. Leptospires are the most tightly coiled of the *Spirochaetales* and have elongated structures with terminal segments that may curve to resemble the letters C, S, and J. Some cells are hooked at both ends, which makes the terminus appear to have a larger diameter than the rest of the cell; some have one hooked and one relatively straight end; some appear at 100× to 600× to have partially bent, straighter, or pointed ends. However, such morphological observations do not provide a basis for differentiating members of a group. Although other methods such as phase-contrast microscopy are available for observing leptospires, dark-field microscopy is by far the most universally accepted and is essential in such studies as those in which, for example, leptospires are used for diagnostic whole cell antigens in the microscopic agglutination microtitration (live antigen) test. Dry-dark-field and conventional objectives (10×, 25×, 63×) are preferable for general observation, and a long working distance objective, L 10×/0.22 with iris diaphragm, is preferable for viewing the microtitration reaction. Using 10×-high eyepoint periplan eyepieces is helpful to laboratory workers who wear eyeglasses. Beyond a magnification of 630×, there is not usually sufficient light to observe most preparations with conventional equipment.

The motility of leptospires can be observed in body fluids, tissue homogenates, and liquid and semisolid (0.2% agar) cultures. Typically in fluid media they are quite motile, rotating rapidly on a longitudinal axis, and are usually characterized by their spinning, generally hooked ends. There are cultures, however, in which the organisms are very languid, a characteristic which is not necessarily related to viability or degree of infectivity. Such strains as just described are frequently fastidious in their nutritional demands and have long lag periods (1–8 days) before the onset of progressive logarithmic growth (9 to 14 days) (Figs 30.1 and 30.2). In semisolid media, motility diminishes greatly, and movement is of a serpentine, boring action. When observed under a coverslip preparation in which cells are in the more fluid portion of the semisolid medium, there is a wide variation in motility. There is a tendency toward diminished motility in kidney, liver, and brain homogenates, and in urine, which should not be construed as diminished infectivity. Recent studies on the increased translational motion of leptospires in viscous environments (57) suggest that the infectious process is aided by their ability to travel through the viscous fluids, mucosal surfaces, and intracellular spaces of human and animal hosts.

Dark-field examination cannot be relied upon in judging the purity of a leptospiral culture. Contamination may be present because of improperly prepared media. Contaminants may be carried along in culture media, aided in their survival by the lower incubation temperature used for cultivating leptospires. Media should be sterility tested at 25 C, 30 C, and 37 C. Difficulties occur when another organism, such as free-living *Spirochaeta aurantia* is simultaneously present with leptospires. This organism is capable of continuous growth in leptospiral media at a ratio of spirochaeta to leptospiral cells of 2×10^6/ml to 600×10^6/ml. *S. aurantia* can be separated from the leptospire by streaking the culture on Trypticase soy agar. Electron microscopy (79) (Fig 30.3), has shown three major anatomical structures: an outer sheath or envelope, independent axial filaments originating individually from opposite ends of the cell, and a cytoplasmic membrane beneath these filaments. The results of other studies (78) indicate a wide diversity of membrane elaborations, coils derived from the outer membrane and/or slime layer, axial filament and accessory structures, and cell-free coiled structures.

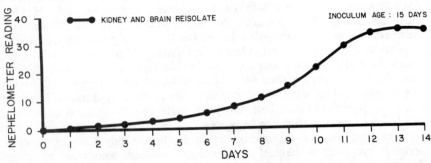

Figure 30.1—Growth of kidney or brain hamster reisolate of a human isolate of *Leptospira hardjo* in bovine albumin polysorbate 80 medium.

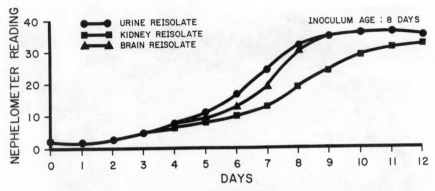

Figure 30.2—Growth of urine, kidney, or brain hamster reisolate of a human isolate of *Leptospira hardjo* in bovine albumin polysorbate 80 medium.

Growth patterns

Liquid, semisolid (0.2% agar), and solid (1.0% agar) plating media can all be used for specific applications for leptospiral cultures. Liquid media are employed for cultivating whole cells to be used as antigens in the microscopic agglutination test, growth inhibition test, pathogenicity studies, production of bacterins and plate antigens, and *in vitro* testing of antibiotics and cell masses for extraction of antigen used in the hemolytic and indirect hemagglutination tests and the complement-fixation test. Semisolid media are most useful in isolation attempts, maintenance of stock cultures, preservation of virulence, and pretests of agar quality. Solid plating media have been used in cloning, attempts to detect colony types, and sometimes in isolation and purification procedures.

Growth patterns in liquid media are important when propagating cells to be used as live antigens in the microscopic agglutination test. Nephelometry is a technique well adapted to measuring the light scattering of leptospires in albumin lipid, synthetic, or in serum-enriched media. In 1967 Roessler (81) developed a reference turbidity standard against which, more recently (31), secondary standards have been calibrated and made available to leptospiral investigators on an international basis. Nephelometric standards provide a reference for adjusting antigens to reproducible density, Petroff-Hauser counting of diluted cells, and in testing whether liquid media can adequately support the growth of diluted cell preparations. Cultures on which cell counts are being done should be initially diluted to give a turbidity value of 25 measured with a standardized nephelometer (31), which correlates with about 200×10^6 cells/ml. With a 1:10 dilution prepared from the adjusted culture, one can count between 80 and 110 cells in the chamber, an ideal number for accuracy and precision. A laboratory can evaluate leptospiral turbidity using data obtained with light-transmission instruments [see Table 30.1 in which standardized nephelometer readings (31) are compared to light transmittance values obtained with other instruments]. Readings were obtained by suspending leptospires in a water-clear diluent which had little light absorbing character-

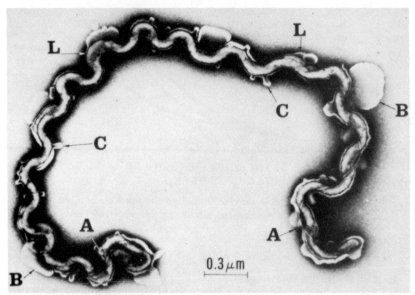

Figure 30.3—A leptospiral cell (strain Canada BW-2) mounted in potassium phospho-
tungstate negative stain. Its independent axial filaments (A) are attached
at the poles and extend backward along the protoplasmic cylinder for a
distance of less than one-third of the cell's length. The outer envelope/
slime layer is marked by large blebs (B) and small projections (C)
formed by their underlying coiled structures. Two large areas of the protoplasmic cylinder contain lamellar bodies (L) that represent internal
membranous organelles. (Courtesy of A. E. Ritchie, National Animal
Disease Center.)

istics and thereby made use of blue wavelengths of light more practical. Minor
color variations or light scattering in liquid media must be taken into account
with either nephelometric or transmittance determinations. When severely hemolyzed serum enrichments are used, a less sensitive and therefore less efficient wavelength such as 500 or 600 nm must be used. There is no absolute
uniform correlation of cell count with nephelometer reading for all strains
(Table 30.2). Generally, at a standard turbidity, the shorter the average cell
length, the higher is the cell count/ml. Once the relationship of cells/ml to turbidity reading is established and the organism is growing well, the count needs
to be redetermined only periodically.

Serologic diagnosis of leptospirosis still predominantly relies on the microscopic agglutination test with live antigens, a procedure which is generally
accepted as the standard reference method for demonstrating leptospiral antibodies (1). Published reports on growth patterns for leptospires in serum media (22, 23) as measured directly by turbidity and more recent reports on leptospires grown in albumin polysorbate 80 media (24, 29, 31) can be used as
guidelines in clinical diagnostic and public health laboratories. Every laboratory which uses the live antigen microscopic agglutination microtitration test

TABLE 30.1—COMPARISON OF TURBIDIMETRIC VALUES OF SUSPENSIONS OF *LEPTOSPIRA POMONA* IN 0.005 M PHOSPHATE BUFFER*

NEPHELOS		PERCENT TRANSMITTANCE		
NEPHELOM-ETER	KLETT-SUMM. NO. 42 FILTER	COLEMAN-6A JR· SPECTROPHO. 420 NM	BAUSCH & LOMB SPECTRONIC-20 400 NM	BECKMAN-DU 400 NM
5	97.0	95.2	97.0	97.9
10	92.0	91.0	89.0	85.8
15	91.3	89.3	85.5	82.5
20	85.9	85.5	82.0	78.6
25	81.5	81.0	75.0	71.8
30	80.0	78.5	71.0	68.0
35	75.0	72.0	66.0	62.8
40	73.3	70.2	64.0	59.0
45	72.1	69.8	61.8	56.5

* Nephelometer; Coleman 7 or 9 adjusted to scale reading of 54 with turbidity standard (Proceedings of the U.S. Animal Health Association, 1976, pp 126-141).

naturally prefers to use its own readily available glassware for culture propagation. Again, leptospires are aerobic and grow well in an environment in which they have free access to air. Aerated cultures can be grown conveniently in 19- × 150-mm steel-capped culture tubes (Figs 30.4 and 30.5) under static or shake culture conditions (180 rpm) or in cotton-stoppered, nephelo-culture flasks (24).

TABLE 30.2—CORRELATION BETWEEN NEPHELOMETER READING, PER CENT TRANSMITTANCE, CELL COUNT, AND BACTERIAL DENSITY OF STANDARDIZED SUSPENSIONS OF VARIOUS LEPTOSPIRES

SEROTYPE		NEPHELOMETER READING	400 NM %T	CELL COUNT × 10⁶/ML	MG/100 ML SUSPENSION	µG /ML
L. icterohaemorrhagiae		31	56	208	7.23	72.3
L. grippotyphosa	I	29	62	169, (U) 76, (H)	6.82	68.2
	II (A)	30	63.2	—	6.84	68.4
	(B)	30	63.1	—	6.66	66.6
L. ballum		30	64	190	6.83	68.3
L. hyos		30	63	144	6.79	67.9
L. pyrogenes		30	61.5	218	6.52	65.2
L. sejroe		30	59	218	6.24	62.4
L. australis		32	60	234	6.05	60.5
L. autumnalis		29	56.5	247	5.85	58.5
L. pomona J		29	66	280	4.71	47.1
L. mini		30	60.5	250	—	—
L. hardjo S-91		31	56	200	—	—
L. bataviae		32	61.5	230	—	—

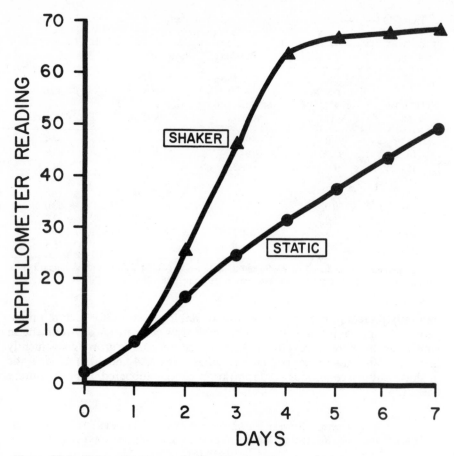

Figure 30.4—Tube culture growth of antigen strain of *L. hardjo* using shaker and
static growth conditions.

The turbidity of leptospires in liquid cultures must be checked at least
macroscopically if the organisms are to be grown effectively. Leptospires in
fluid cultures in the log phase of growth and in pure cultures have a shot-silk,
minutely fine turbidity when viewed in front of a light. Leptospires have a
lesser tendency to settle out of suspension than other bacteria. By checking
cultures frequently, one can: (a) be alert to a marked change in turbidity which
might indicate contamination; (b) detect when the leptospires are granular,
making them less useful as live antigens; and (c) note when turbidity first appears after liquid media are inoculated with various dilutions of cells. The latter can be extremely useful in assessing the relative quality of media if a turbi-
dity-measuring instrument is not available. Frequent subculture every 4 to 6
days in adequate medium provides the greatest assurance of obtaining rapidly
growing, homogeneous cultures of leptospires.

Factors which influence the quality of semisolid cultures (0.2% agar) are the choice of method used to inoculate the surface of the agar, the quality (31) of the agar used, the number of organisms in the inoculum, the nutritional adequacy of the medium, and the degree of nutritional fastidiousness of the strain. The most useful form for isolating organisms, semisolid medium must be checked by inoculating it with cells diluted from 200×10^6 to 20 cells/tube/ 10 ml of semisolid. Although the subsurface growth of leptospires can be observed macroscopically (31), cultures should be examined periodically with a dark-field microscope so that the presence of leptospires can be reported as soon as possible. Zones of subsurface growth in semisolid agar vary widely among serotypes, strains, and isolates. In homogeneously dispersed agar medium intensified areas of growth can be observed if the culture is held in front of a concentrated light source. Some growth zones have sharp, clearly defined lines, others are diffuse and irregular, and others appear as dispersed microcolonies. Laboratory-adapted cultures usually grow at a predictable rate, but clin-

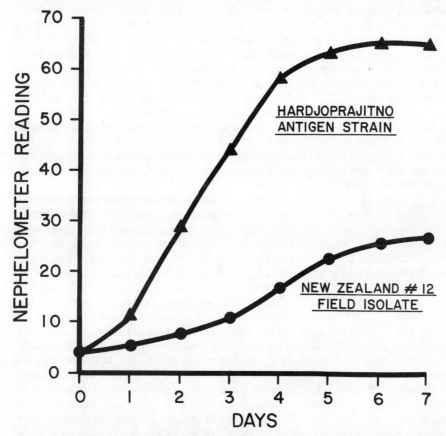

Figure 30.5—Shaker culture flask growth of *L. hardjo* laboratory-adapted antigen strain and nonadapted field isolate.

ical isolates may grow extremely slowly (30 days ± 20). Cultures can be stored for as long as 12 months at 25 C. When transferred from storage there may be an absence of a clearly visible growth zone. At least 2.0 ml of the stored culture should be transferred to a tube (10.0 ml) of semisolid medium (28).

Most clinical diagnostic laboratories and public health laboratories elect not to use solid medium (1% agar) for leptospiral cultures because insufficient data are available on the colony types that can be reliably reproduced in different laboratories. We do not intend to discourage investigators who wish to obtain more suspension-stable antigens by cloning, who wish to differentiate serotypes in an isolation, or who wish to find virulence markers.

Some agreed-upon points concerning using a solid medium are: (a) The inoculum, whether pure culture or specimen, must be diluted (29) to 10^{-10} in order to obtain single colonies (Fig 30.6). (b) Most researchers agree that agar concentration is critical, but insufficient attention has been paid to agar quality (31). (c) Thick plates (30 ml/plate) work best. (d) Evaporation should be prevented in some manner (e.g., taping). (e) Saprophytic, free-living leptospires (biflexa types) can usually be grown much more easily than pathogenic leptospires. (f) Plate surfaces should be dry when diluted inoculum is added. (g) Veils (growth from large number of cells) and individual colonies (from 50 to 5 cells per plate) grow beneath the surface of the agar. (h) Colonies to be picked must be chosen very carefully and must be far enough apart to ensure purity of the culture and absence of subsurface growth. (i) Widely varying generation times of 8 to 40 hr might preclude a colony arising from one cell.

Currently, solid media offer no advantages over conventional semisolid media for primary isolation of pathogenic leptospires from infectious material. In fact, it is very doubtful that an all-purpose, selective, solid plating medium will be developed because leptospires grow so slowly in plates. Although pure culture plates can be prepared, dilution extinction and selective membrane filtration work equally well.

Growth requirements. An understanding of the nutritional requirements of leptospires is important in preparing live diagnostic antigens in quality control of culture media, and in isolation attempts from humans and animals. Growth requirements of leptospires have been defined in investigations in which serum-enriched, albumin-lipid, and synthetic, chemically characterized media were used. Several reseachers (22, 23, 38, 47–49, 55, 62, 83, 102) reported the following: (a) that unextracted rabbit albumin supported growth and that thiamine must be added; (b) that growth response to serum was linear; (c) that the nutrient complex in serum could not be dialyzed, carbohydrate was not used, and protein nitrogen did not disappear; (d) that rabbit serum was a respiratory stimulant; (e) that fatty acid oxidation occurred; (f) that the globulin fraction of serum provided lipid; (g) that serum ultrafiltrate could be replaced with NH_4Cl and thiamine; and (h) that long-chain fatty acids were required.

More definitive growth requirements of leptospires were determined with bovine albumin polysorbate medium (25, 26, 29, 33–35, 54). It was found that: (a) NH_4Cl supplied nitrogen, (b) long-chain fatty acids or surfactant polysorbate supplied carbon, (c) glucose stimulated growth of some strains, (d) only half the thiamine molecule (thiazole fragment) was needed, (e) in some instances growth was continuous when triple deleted media (polysorbate 80, NH_4Cl, and 1-cystine) were used in conjunction with vitamin B_{12} and thi-

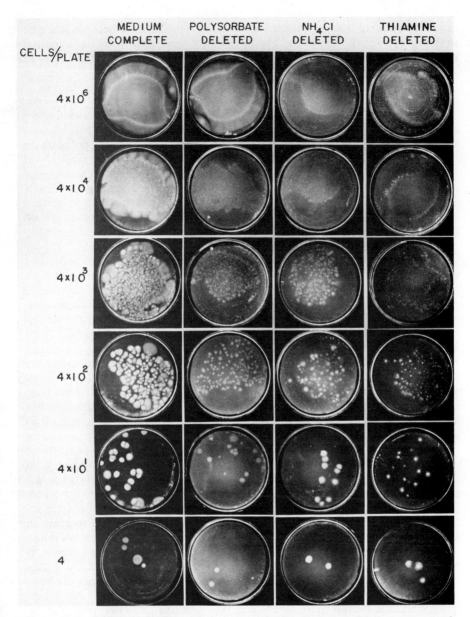

Figure 30.6—Effect of inoculum dilution upon the development of *L. pomona* growth on various media containing 1% agar (Ann. Microbiol. [Inst. Pasteur] 124B:477-493, 1973).

amine, and (f) saprophytic and pathogenic leptospires required different lipids.

Studies with nonprotein, chemically characterized (8, 87, 90, 103) media have been aimed at emphasizing the metabolic potentials of leptospires. It is generally believed that organisms grown in these media have become resistant to the lytic action of fatty acids. The media have been used with only a limited number of leptospiral strains and only rarely outside of the laboratories in which they were developed.

Outstanding characteristics

Leptospires are temperature sensitive *in vitro*, although the exact effect which elevated temperatures have on them is not entirely clear (28). Various effects of temperature on growth in serum-enriched and albumin polysorbate media have been described (23, 25, 28, 50). Leptospires probably multiply in hosts at 37 C or higher. A correlation has not been found between virulence and the ability to initiate or grow continuously at 37 C from an impaired state. Saprophytic leptospires are more capable of growing in lower temperature ranges (15 to 20 C) than pathogens (28, 50). Thus, in initial attempts to isolate leptospires and in further efforts to identify them definitively, it is probably good practice to incubate cultures at 13, 15, 29, and 37 C.

Leptospires are sensitive to the hydrogen ion. In various serum-enriched and albumin-based media they grow best when the pH is 7.0 to 7.4 ± 0.2.

Leptospires are currently treated as two major groups: the pathogenic parasitic leptospires classified under *Leptospira interrogans* (serotypes *icterohaemorrhagiae, canicola, pomona, grippotyphosa, hardjo, szwajizak, autumnalis*, etc.) and the apparently free-living serologically heterologous, "saprophytic" water leptospires called *Leptospira biflexa*. A major difference between organisms in the two groups is that the parasitic pathogens infect the proximal convoluted tubule of the kidney and can cause acute, febrile, systemic disease of man and other mammalian species. Recently *biflexa* has been isolated from cell cultures (98), deionized water used in leptospiral media (9), carrier rats in Israel (88), and horses in Argentina (68). How such organisms are related to the immunological response of man and animals remains to be seen.

Numerous attempts have been made to differentiate the pathogens from the saprophytes on the basis of nutritional requirements (5), bacteriostatic action of divalent copper ions (39), 8-azaguanine (52), aniline dyes (11), temperature tolerances (50), cytopathogenic effects in tissue culture (73), lipolytic activity (40), hemolytic activity (74), oxidase activity (41), ability to grow in CO_2-deficient air (107), lipid content (51), and lytic action of asbestos-filtered medium (27). However, despite all these attempts, the pathogenic leptospires are still classified on the basis of distinct agglutinogenic characteristics. Microscopic-agglutination (85) and agglutination absorption techniques are the serologic methods available for specific identification. The currently used taxonomic scheme is essentially that which Wolff and Broom (106) published in 1954. There are approximately 160 serotypes (serovars) and 21 serogroups, and attempts are being made to subdivide some of the larger serogroups (Hebdomadis). Serotypes are assembled into serogroups based on "major antigenic relationships as disclosed by cross-agglutination tests." In addition to agglutinogens, leptospires contain other antigens which can be extracted chemically and which are more commonly distributed among the diverse leptospiral serotypes (14, 82). Some of the antigens have been used in genus-specific serologic tests (19, 86, 97).

Clinical Manifestations

The fact that leptospirosis can cause death in humans was extensively reviewed by Szyfres (96) in a recent appraisal of the public health problem it presents in Latin America and the Caribbean area. Persistent reports in the literature that this disease is always accompanied by jaundice should be corrected. It is outside the scope of this chapter to deal extensively with the symptoms of leptospirosis; this information can be found elsewhere (4, 20, 36). The numerous names used for years to describe leptospirosis (Weil's disease, 7-day fever, cane-cutter's disease, swineherd's disease, swamp fever, autumnal fever, and others) advanced the assumption that leptospirosis encompassed a group of separate diseases caused by diverse serotypes. This view is no longer held. We now know that with appropriate host exposure and susceptibility, any of the pathogenic leptospires can cause varying degrees of illness. With any febrile illness of unknown origin and particularly if the patient may have been exposed to leptospires, a diagnosis of leptospirosis should be considered and appropriate laboratory procedures performed.

Contrary to common belief, leptospires are easily cultivated. Since the shelf-life (24 months) of media for such purposes has been adequately documented (30, 31), any clinical diagnostic laboratory should have the expertise to analyze specimens from patients with aseptic meningitis-like or nonparalytic poliomyelitis-like leptospirosis infections. A portion of this effort should include attempts to determine the extent and quality of leptospiral antibodies with the most sensitive procedures available.

Leptospirosis can be a mild or severe disease and relapses can occur. Its initial symptoms can be quite nonspecific, appearing abruptly after an incubation period of about 10 days. Shivering or rigor is often the first symptom. The patient may have a temperature of 38.9 to 40.6 C, constantly or at intervals, for 2 to 12 days or more (an average of 6 to 8 days). Early symptoms include headache (severe and persistent), myalgia, malaise, prostration, retro-orbital pain, conjunctival suffusion, muscle tenderness, and lung involvement (46). Blood and cerebrospinal fluid can be culture positive. Detection of agglutinating antibodies sometimes is difficult.

During the early phases the leucocyte count may range from 4,400 to 13,000/μm^3 in nonicteric cases. If the patient becomes jaundiced, the leucocyte count may be as high as 35,000/μm^3. Neutrophilia and proteinuria may be present, and the patient may have otherwise normal renal functions. The patient usually has signs of meningeal involvement which often become pronounced during the second week and which frequently dominate the clinical picture in benign leptospirosis infections. Spinal fluid culture and a determination of increased pressure and lymphocytic pleocytosis should be considered in the first 10 days. One report (46) cited aseptic meningitis, infectious hepatitis, and fever of unknown origin as predominant initial clinical impressions.

Until 1948 nearly all leptospirosis infections reported in the United States were accompanied by jaundice. Heath (46) analyzed clinical data from patients diagnosed as having the disease between 1949 and 1961 and reported that jaundice was associated with 43% of the cases. Although the disease was known and described in the 1920's, the environments and health status of humans and animals have changed greatly. Szyfres (96) relates the severity of the disease as seen in Latin American and the Caribbean area to the nature of developing countries. He notes that half of the population lives in rural areas in close contact with animals and that most labor is done manually, so that the people are in continuous physical contact with an environment contaminated with animal urine. The scarcity of diagnostic laboratories and immunogens and the tropical or subtropical climates all contribute to the fact that leptospirosis infections are usually severe in such countries.

Patients with mild infections usually recover uneventfully, with fever disappearing along with disappearance of leptospires from the blood and other symptomatic improvements occurring as early as the sixth to eighth day of illness. However, some patients have a second bout of fever which is usually accompanied by asymptomatic or clinical meningitis. At this point, patients usually develop agglutinating antibodies, and leptospires can no longer be cultured from blood and cerebrospinal fluid. A fast rising antibody titer and a fever probably associated with some destruction of leptospires produces an allergic type reaction including skin rash, meningitis, and nephritis. Leptospiral meningitis usually appears 12 to 24 hr after the temperature returns to normal the first time and when antibodies can first be detected. Headaches sometimes recur with such intensity that the patients must be treated specifically for them. In this period there is spinal fluid pleocytosis, predominantly neutrophils, little changes in protein level and normal sugar values. Signs of spinal fluid pleocytosis are infrequently observed during the leptospiremic stage. Most of these anicteric meningeal forms are benign, those of late meningitis onset tend to remain symptomatic.

Patients with severe infections may have relapses if antibiotic therapy has not been properly administered. Leptospires may be shed in urine constantly or intermittently during the first weeks after symptoms disappear, with some animals shedding the organisms in urine for the rest of their lives. Because of the manner in which leptospires localize in the kidney and thus are protected from antibody, they can remain indefinitely without being found unless daily urine isolation attempts are made. Severe infections leading to death during the first week of illness are usually associated with vascular collapse, hemorrhage, or myocardial disease. Renal and hepatic failure are major causes of death in later weeks. Kidney involvement ranges from a mild, transient proteinuria, which is commonly associated with benign leptospirosis, to severe nephritis with hematuria, casts, and diminished or no urinary output.

Patients who are jaundiced may also have nephritis. The jaundice usually appears in the middle or latter part of the first week. The liver becomes enlarged and tender. Hemorrhages may occur in skin, mucous membranes, and gastrointestinal tract.

Epidemiology

Laboratory personnel must be conversant with the epidemiology of leptospirosis in order to place test results properly into context for an accurate diagnosis. Humans are infected by leptospires in the environment, frequently through contact with infected animals that are shedding the organism in their urine or whose blood, livers, kidneys, or brains contain the organisms (20, 93).

Animals involved are the Norway rat, regarded as the principal maintenance host, as well as domestic swine, cattle, and dogs. Many animal species are known to be permanent, temporary, or chronic carriers and to remain asymptomatic as they shed leptospires in urine throughout the year (Table 30.3). Man may come in contact with leptospires by partial or total immersion in water of ponds, creeks, rivers and other impoundments contaminated by animals. Leptospires penetrate abraded skin or mucous membranes of the eye, nasopharynx, or oropharynx.

Predicting the persistence and intensity of leptospiruria is difficult and depends to a large extent on the host and the serotype. The Norway rat infected with *icterohaemorrhagiae* may shed profuse numbers of leptospires for the rest of its life (Fig 30.7), although *canicola* apparently persists for shorter periods of time in the kidneys of rats. Leptospiruria is less persistent in dogs, ruminants,

TABLE 30.3—VARIOUS LEPTOSPIRAL SEROTYPES AND HOSTS FROM WHICH THEY HAVE BEEN ISOLATED

SEROGROUP	SEROTYPE	HOSTS
icterohaemorrhagiae	*icterohaemorrhagiae*	Rat, dog, man, cattle, mouse, raccoon, fox, muskrat, skunk, opossum, nutria, marmot.
	copenhageni	Man, cattle, dog, raccoon.
	dakota	River water.
canicola	*canicola*	Dog, man, cattle, pig, skunk, raccoon, armadillo.
ballum	*ballum*	Mouse.
	arborea	Mouse, opossum, rat.
	undetermined	Rat, mouse, shrew, fox, bobcat, skunk, rabbit, snake.
pyrogenes	*zanoni*	Deer.
	myocastoris	Nutria.
autumnalis	*Fort-Bragg*	Man.
	autumnalis	Opossum, raccoon.
	Orleans	Nutria.
	Louisiana	Armadillo.
pomona	*pomona*	Cattle, pig, man, horse, dog, skunk, raccoon, opossum, bobcat, goat, fox, deer, woodchuck, armadillo, mouse.
australis	*australis*	Raccoon, opossum, fox, skunk.
grippotyphosa	*grippotyphosa*	Cattle, raccoon, skunk, fox, mole, opossum, mouse, squirrel, dog.
hebdomadis	*hardjo*	Cattle.
	Georgia	Man, raccoon, opossum, skunk.
	szwajizak	Cattle.
bataviae	*paidjan*	Raccoon, nutria, opossum.
tarassovi	tarassovi	Skunk, opossum.
	bakeri	Skunk, opossum.
	atlantae	Opossum, raccoon, skunk, fox.
	atchafalya	Opossum.

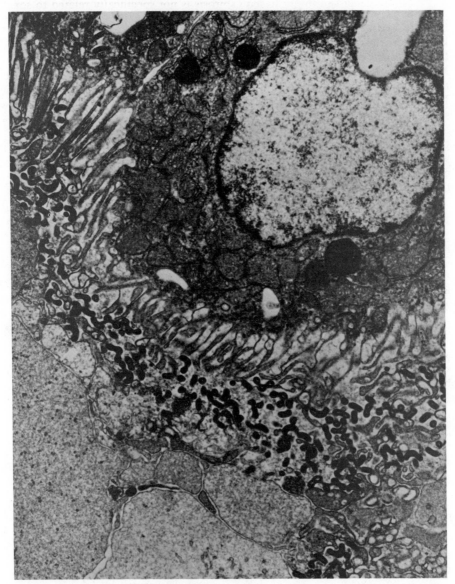

Figure 30.7—Section of proximal kidney tubule from a wild caught *Rattus norvegicus* showing localization of *Leptospira icterrohaemorrhagiae* near the brush border of the tubular epithelium. (Courtesy of C. R. Sterling and A. B. Thiermann, Wayne State University.)

and swine, although there have been reports of asymptomatic dogs shedding leptospires. The fact that a human or animal host is seronegative does not mean it is not shedding leptospires. Seropositive rats may or may not shed the organisms, as may seronegative rats.

Although susceptibility to leptospirosis is not specifically related to sex, more men than women are infected because they have more frequent occupational contacts with contaminated environments. No evidence has been found to indicate a natural resistance to leptospirosis. Although people 20 to 30 years old have the highest reported leptospiral attack rate, recent reports indicate that children frequently have the disease (13).

The interested reader is referred to a report published by the Center for Disease Control on the epidemiologic trends of leptospirosis in the United States from 1965–1974 (13). In it the authors indicate that our knowledge of this disease is still incomplete.

Public Health Significance

Generally leptospirosis is not transmitted from person to person, but leptospirosis contracted during pregnancy can lead to the death of the human fetus, as indicated by reports of spontaneous abortion attributed to *canicola* and *icterohaemorrhagiae* (15). Cited in this report were data which suggested a high rate of abortion and miscarriage associated with leptospiral infections in rice-growing areas of China. People who work in sewers, mines, or other rat-infested premises; personnel in fish processing plants, meat markets, and slaughterhouses; and those involved in agricultural activities related to rice, cane, or flax are all at risk of acquiring leptospirosis. Increased use of recreational water facilities, ponds, streams, and rivers may contribute to the incidence of leptospirosis (20). Jungle streams and swamps are extremely effective sources of infection (6, 60, 63).

We cannot argue that leptospirosis is a major health problem in the United States; however, many cases may not be correctly diagnosed, and a substantial number of those that are diagnosed may not be reported. Also, such factors as the high degree of mechanization in agriculture, increased urbanization, and improved standards of household and community sanitation contribute to the fact that leptospirosis is less prevalent in the United States than in some other parts of the world.

In the continental United States leptospirosis is primarily of concern to veterinarians. This is currently evidenced by widespread use of leptospiral bacterins containing three serotypes (*pomona, grippotyphosa,* and *hardjo*), which are given to cattle, and those composed of *canicola* and *icterohaemorrhagiae*, which are given to dogs. The advisability of using pentavalent bacterins is being considered. In a recent review (45) of leptospirosis in domestic animals, the authors discuss the serotypes that have been isolated: (a) from cattle—*pomona, hardjo, szwajizak, grippotyphosa, canicola,* and *icterohaemorrhagiae;* (b) from swine—*pomona, grippotyphosa, icterohaemorrhagiae* and *canicola*; serologic evidence of exposure to *autumnalis, ballum, and tarrasovi*; (c) from horses—*pomona* and an unexplained serologic reaction to *autumnalis*; (d) from sheep—*pomona*; and (e) from dogs—*canicola, icterohaemorrhagiae, pomona,* and *grippotyphosa*. The disease tends to be enzootic and to occur cyclically. The incidence of clinical infection decreases as the population becomes immune from the naturally occurring disease or the application of vaccines. Thus, leptospirosis is not actually a problem of the individual animal but a problem of a population (see *Proceedings of the U.S. Animal Health Association*).

It has never been the practice to vaccinate humans against leptospirosis in the United States. However, high-risk occupational groups should be informed of the danger of infection and told what preventive measures to practice. Also, the incidence of human infection can be lowered by controlling the disease in animal populations (i.e., domestic animals should be immunized, rat population control should be implemented, and newly acquired animals should be quarantined).

Collection and Processing of Specimens

Kinds of Specimens

Blood, spinal fluid, and urine specimens can be used in tests for leptospirosis, but the timing in obtaining the different types of specimens is critical. Blood is extremely useful because it can be easily obtained aseptically and because it can be used in establishing the presence or absence of leptospiral antibodies. Although relatively few leptospires are usually found in the blood, with careful dark-field examination they can be detected in suspensions containing 20,000 to 2 million cells/ml. However, the blood itself inhibits leptospiral growth, so that samples may contain early antibody at levels which cannot be detected. Blood specimens should be taken during the leptospiremic phase of disease (between the 2nd and 8th days) (95), though isolations have been made as late as the second week of the disease. If few of the organisms are present in a sample, it should be inoculated undiluted into multiple tubes of media (1 drop/10 ml). If the sample was collected too soon for early antibody to be detected, it should be diluted 1:10 through 10^{-5} and 1-ml amounts inoculated drop by drop onto semisolid media. The blood specimens used can be either untreated or mixed with anticoagulants such as heparin or oxalate. If the blood to be analyzed is clotted, the clot can be aseptically broken up and used in leptospiral cultures. If blood must be sent away for analysis, it should be protected from excessive heat or cold from the time it is collected until it is processed.

Although there have been no reports of comparative studies on leptospires with sodium polyanethol sulfonate (Grobax) added to media or blood, the possibility of using this compound should be considered. (Any laboratory which expects to culture leptospires routinely from blood should do comparative quality control studies with normal human blood containing anticoagulants inoculated with diluted suspensions of leptospires.)

At the time cultures are initiated, weanling hamsters should be inoculated intraperitoneally with concentrated blood. Although this procedure probably does not yield results sooner than cultures, if the hamsters die of leptospirosis the strain can be reported as highly pathogenic, and if the hamsters survive, blood serum is available for serologic analysis. The presence of subsurface growth in cultures should be carefully monitored visually, but its absence does not necessarily mean that the culture is negative for leptospirosis.

Though little has been published on using 2-mercaptoethanol (2-me) with serum which has detectable agglutinins in the microscopic agglutination test (32), the possibility should be considered. It may thus be possible to establish the presence of IgM antibody. Human sera apparently must be diluted at least 1:5 before equal volumes of 0.2 M 2-me are added and held for 2 hr before testing with living antigen. The possibility of being able to determine the level and persistence of antibody titers and whether they are resistant to 2-me merits further study.

Cerebrospinal fluid may contain leptospires during the first 2 to 5 days after the patient becomes ill (or into the second week of illness). It can be cultured directly or after it has been centrifuged to concentrate the leptospires.

Urine can also be used to test for leptospirosis. The patient should be alkalinized, and the specimen should be collected as aseptically as possible. The pH of the specimen should be adjusted to neutral or slight alkalinity as needed, and the specimen should be centrifuged to concentrate the leptospires. Cultures can be made in semisolid medium (with or without inhibitors) directly or with the specimen diluted 10^{-4}, or the specimen can be inoculated intraperitoneally into weanling hamsters. Attempts to isolate from urine can be spread over a much longer time period (2–3 months after infection) than can attempts from blood or cerebrospinal fluid. Urine which is not cultured immediately should be diluted and stored at 10 C to prevent other bacterial growth. Because it is difficult to collect urine specimens aseptically, they cannot be in transit to the laboratory as long as blood can.

Postmortem specimens used to check for the presence of leptospires can be obtained from kidney, liver, brain, and blood. Tissues can be examined with fluorescent antibody (FA) techniques and silver stain impregnation methods.

When domestic and small laboratory animals are being examined, two factors must be considered: (a) If the animal died, was it the result of leptospirosis? (b) If the animal survived, was it the result of the fact that it was infected with a strain whose virulence had diminished? When the animal dies, it is wise to demonstrate the presence of the organism in as many body fluids and tissues as possible to obtain an impression of the virulence level of the infecting strain. Kidney tissue can be examined with FA or silver staining techniques (Fig 30.8). When the animal survives, blood should be taken for serologic studies, and urine, kidney, and brain tissue cultures may be informative. In the examination of wild animals, kidney tissue and blood samples should be obtained (from rats, also urine).

Isolation from water presents a problem in specimen preparation. Concentration, filtration, and animal inoculation methods should be adapted to the specific situation.

Persons attempting to isolate leptospires from various tissues and fluids first must be knowledgeable about the organisms' ability to survive. There are reports (65, 101) that leptospires have survived in coagulated or defibrinated uncontaminated blood kept at room temperature (25 C). However, reports of the survival of leptospires (31, 58, 69, 70) in urine indicate that specimens must be properly collected and processed and must be analyzed as soon as possible. Survival time of leptospires in sterile urine is measured in terms of hours, even if the urine is left undiluted.

Protective diluents can be added to homogenized tissue which is to be further diluted and cultured. Bovine serum albumin protects leptospires (28, 31, 84) in diluted urine, dilute suspensions, and when stored at −75 C. Viable cultures have been obtained from diluted blood and kidney suspensions stored 40 to 60 days at 25 C. If 0.005 M phosphate buffer with 1% bovine albumin is used to supplement such preparations, 10 cells/ml of leptospires can be maintained for 7 days (28) at 25 C.

Survival time of leptospires can be gauged to some degree by checking tissues of slaughtered animals; some reported times range from 33 hr at 5 C to 3 to 12 days at 3 to 5 C (43, 65, 104). If unmacerated tissues are stored at −80 C, they can later be thawed, homogenized, and used in leptospiral cultures (although growth is extremely slow). Coghlan et al. (16) reported that they preserved leptospiral suspensions cooled slowly to −79 C and reviewed the findings of seven other studies on leptospiral preservation. Data indicate that if such specimens are frozen rapidly and maintained at −70 C, isolates can survive for as long as 5 years in cultures and in infected blood and tissues. Even more drastic measures (75) such as rapid freezing and storage in liquid nitrogen refrigerators have been used in attempts to preserve some viability and virulence of leptospires for prolonged periods. At a concentration of about 5%, such cryoprotective substances as glycerol and dimethylsulfoxide have been used in attempts to preserve specimens or cultures frozen and stored at dry ice or liquid nitrogen temperatures (59, 75).

Some veterinarians are concerned about whether leptospires can survive in semen. Limited study results (56) have documented that pomona cells have survived at −190 C for 31 days in bovine semen extender on the basis of leptospiremia and serologic response in guinea pigs. Much more work is needed in this area.

The possibility of adding antibiotics to specimens should not be overlooked. Tetracycline, erythromycin, ampicillin, Cleocin, Minocin, Lincocin, and streptomycin are bactericidal. Colimycin, Vibramycin, Doxycillin, Terramycin, Garamycin, Geopen, and Kantrex are quite bacteriostatic. Chloromycetin, Keflex, Furadantin, polymyxin, neomycin, Keflin, Unipen, and Mysteclin F are very weakly bacteriostatic. Albamycin, vancomycin, Furoxone, rifampin, and ethambutol are noninhibitory.

Neomycin, 5-fluorouracil (53), and furazolidone (67) have been added to media in attempts to inhibit contaminating bacteria. Although such efforts are to be encouraged, results obtained when these drugs are present must be carefully evaluated before such procedures are adopted routinely in a diagnostic laboratory. The composition of the medium used in leptospiral cultures could greatly influence the effectiveness of an added inhibitor. Myers (67) found that 5-fluorouracil was effective in Fletcher's semisolid rabbit serum medium. However, Ris (76) believed that 5-fluorouracil was not effective in sheep serum.

Leptospires can be separated from other bacteria by filtration because of their size (80). Although many common bacteria can be filtered from contaminated urine with readily available 0.8-, 0.45-, and 0.2-μm filters, many of the leptospires are also removed. With 0.8-μm filters, at least 10 to 10,000 leptospires/ml are necessary to support leptospiral growth, and at least 10^5 leptospiral cells/ml are necessary to obtain successful cultures from sterile urine processed through 0.45-μm filters (69).

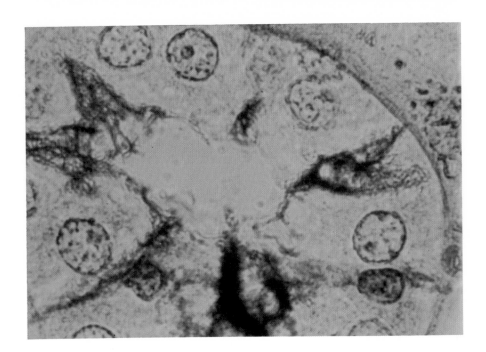

Figure 30.8.—Rat kidney tubule (magnification 1000X); kidney from a chronically infected wild rat; stained according to the Steiner and Steiner silver staining method (J. Lab. Clin. Med. 29:868-871, 1944; note numerous leptospires residing in the tubular lumen. (Courtesy of A. B. Thiermann, Wayne State University.)

Diagnostic Procedures

Direct Microscopic Examination

The morphology of leptospires grown in pure culture was described earlier. Because it is very difficult to find leptospires in blood, urine, and tissue suspensions with a dark-field microscope, this method should not be relied on in attempts to diagnose leptospirosis. Although leptospires may in fact be present in specimens examined, many times they bear little resemblance to those seen in pure culture. Artifacts present in blood can be extremely confusing. Direct examination of tissue suspensions and urine can be used for a presumptive diagnosis on the basis of typical morphology and motility but with extreme caution. Cultural and serologic confirmation are mandatory. With small numbers, detection is not possible and failure to see the organism does not mean it is not present. Cells can be found in kidney suspensions from wildlife, urine from some domestic animals, and tissues and fluids harvested from laboratory-infected animals such as the hamster.

Silver staining (10, 37, 95) and fluorescent staining (61) methods have been extensively used with leptospires, but such results should also be confirmed serologically and culturally. The methods are useful: (a) when leptospirosis has been fatal and the causative organisms can be found in sections of kidney, liver, and brain tissue, and (b) when cultures are not informative (e.g., with aborted bovine fetuses). Serotypes cannot be differentiated with either method.

Use of Culture Media for Isolation

Semisolid medium (0.2% agar) is generally preferred for isolating leptospires. However, personnel in clinical diagnostic laboratories and public health laboratories must remember that: (a) the medium should be pretested (27, 28, 30, 31) to confirm its ability to support the growth of diluted inocula of pathogenic strains (preferably of varying degrees of fastidiousness) of leptospires; (b) the quality of the agar and the enrichment should be confirmed; (c) the practical shelf life of the medium should be known; (d) the medium should be readily available and properly shipped; (e) manufacturer's instructions accompanying the medium on how and when to use it should be carefully followed.

Quality control procedures should be applied consistently in order to avoid reporting false-negative results. In many cases, serologic results may strongly indicate that leptospires are present when they cannot be isolated in cultures. Laboratories should attempt to improve their isolation procedures rather than to blame diagnostic failures on inferior specimens.

Laboratories may use commercial media or prepare their own, but both must be pretested. Media supplemented with bovine albumin and polysorbate (34) and those supplemented with buffered salts enriched generally with rabbit serum (e.g., Fletcher's, Korthof's, or Stuart's) can be used. Modified versions (50) of the basic albumin polysorbate medium (34) are available from various commercial sources. Because no one medium can be used to isolate every serotype found in man and in a wide variety of animal hosts, it is helpful to know which serotypes are most common to the area in which the infection occurred so that appropriate media can be used for cultures.

Four materials (blood, spinal fluid, urine, and tissue) can be used at various times in attempts to isolate leptospires:

Blood

Leptospires can be isolated from blood in the first 2 weeks after infection, preferably before antibiotic treatment has begun. Blood either can be untreated or treated with anticoagulants. The smallest possible amount of inoculum should be added to 10 ml of semisolid medium in order to try to avoid possible growth inhibition of leptospires by the blood and to avoid having so much blood that it masks the development of subsurface growth in the form of a Dinger's zone. To culture a large volume of blood, a greater number of tubes should be inoculated with 1 to 4 drops on the surface of each tube of semisolid medium. For control, pure cultures diluted to 20 cells/ml can be inoculated in 1-ml amounts on the surface of semisolid media; however, even with laboratory-adapted strains macroscopic evidence of growth may not appear until 20 to 30 days of incubation. Growth can be determined before the appearance of growth rings in suspect cultures by examining small volumes (0.05 ml) by dark-field microscopy. In some cultures, leptospiral growth never becomes visible without the aid of dark-field examination. As soon as growth is deemed adequate, the isolate should be transferred from the blood-containing medium to fresh semisolid medium.

If a serum-enriched medium is used, its effective shelf life should be determined. Albumin-based media, if protected from dehydration, can be stored for at least 36 months and still retain their ability to grow leptospires (30, 31).

The above-mentioned procedures should be used in cases in which the laboratory is in close proximity to the patient. If samples must be shipped to the laboratory, medium can be provided to physicians or hospital laboratories on request and inoculated at the patient's bedside, with cultures packaged so that they are protected against extremes in temperature.

Spinal fluid

Such specimens should be obtained in the same time frame as blood and can be analyzed with the same techniques used for the latter, except that spinal fluid specimens can be centrifuged to concentrate the number of leptospires.

Urine

Urine culture specimens should always be diluted (as high as 10^{-6} with 1% BSA diluent) to minimize the likelihood of bacterial contaminants and of urine's toxic effect on leptospires. The pH of the urine should be adjusted to neutral. By subculturing urine to a general purpose peptone medium one can get some idea of the effects of competing bacteria. Urine specimens can be sedimented at $11,000 \times g$ for 60 min and the sediment washed and cultured. Because urine specimens must be diluted, the media used must be of excellent quality if accurate results are to be obtained.

Such compounds as 5-fluorouracil (53), neomycin (67), and furazolidone (67) can be added to the semisolid medium. Urine can also be inoculated intraperitoneally into weanling hamsters and its effects monitored. If the animals die, blood, urine obtained by bladder tap (64, 66), kidney, liver, and brain should be cultured. If the animals survive, urine, kidney, and brain should be cultured and blood taken for serology.

Tissues

Tissue specimens should be taken aseptically, homogenized, and diluted. When tissues from small animals such as hamsters or guinea pigs are used for serologic analysis or direct cultures, the five types of specimens discussed below can be taken whether the animal dies of its infection or is sacrificed. If the animal has not been dead very long, it can be washed off with 70% alcohol. Blood then taken by cardiac puncture should be diluted from 1:10 to 10^{-4} with a 1% solution of bovine albumin solution. These dilutions should be inoculated in 1-ml amounts onto the surface of semisolid medium (10 ml per 20- X 125-mm screw-capped tube). When the postmortem examination is begun, the first organ seen is the liver, which is impressive in its size and position. With sterile forceps and scissors, a piece of tissue is obtained and placed in the barrel of a 3.0-ml disposable syringe, the plunger replaced, and the syringe set aside. The bladder can sometimes be tapped with a 1-ml tuberculin syringe and needle, but if it has collapsed, it should be flushed with 1.0 ml of 1% BSA diluent and the fluid withdrawn into 10 ml of 1% BSA and set aside. The less-accessible kidneys should be cultured next in the manner similar to liver tissue. The animal should then be turned over, the cranial area washed with 70% alcohol, the outer skin removed, the skull opened, and the brain removed and deposited in a disposable syringe. Samples from as many as 25 hamsters can be taken in this manner before cultures in semisolid medium are made from them. From each diluted blood and urine specimen, 1 ml is added to each tube containing 10 ml of semisolid medium for culture. Kidney, liver, and brain tissues are then expressed through the 3-ml syringe into 10 ml of 1% BSA diluent, shaken, and set aside for as little as 30 min or as long as 6 hr. One-ml quantities are inoculated in semisolid media. Viable cultures have been obtained from diluted hamster blood and kidney suspensions even after 40–60 days at room temperature (25 C).

With man and larger animals the size of the organs makes sampling more complicated (although the procedure described above can be used for homogenizing, diluting, and inoculating the surface of semisolid media). To obtain bovine kidney tissue specimens (approximately 0.5 X 0.5 X 2.0 cm) the surface should be disinfected with 70% alcohol, the capsule stripped, and the organ bisected longitudinally with an extremely sharp sterile knife. Sterile forceps and scissors should be used in obtaining multiple samples from cortical, medullary, and cortico-medullary junction areas at 12 locations in the kidney. These tissues are placed in the barrels of 3-ml disposable syringes, the plungers replaced, and the tissues expressed into 1% BSA diluent, shaken, set aside, and subsequently cultured. Because kidneys are more fibrous, pressure must be exerted on the syringe to express tissue through the orifice. Liver and brain tissue can be obtained and processed in the same manner. In culturing 136 kidney samples taken from 10 cows experimentally infected with *L. hardjo* and diluted 1:10, 55 pure cultures, 77 contaminated cultures, and 4 negative cultures were obtained. At 1:100 dilution 115 pure cultures, 17 contaminated cultures, and 4 negative cultures were obtained. Finally, from the 1:1000 dilution, 132 pure cultures and 4 negative cultures were obtained. Obviously some judgement must be used in determining whether a tissue specimen is suitable for culture.

If tissues must be shipped to a laboratory for culturing, they should be frozen without first being homogenized. In the laboratory, frozen samples can be thawed rapidly and then homogenized. At each step of analysis, sterility tests in nonleptospiral media can provide valuable information as to whether the specimen is contaminated with organisms other than leptospires.

If only badly degenerated tissues are submitted for analysis, they can be inoculated into hamsters, since it is almost impossible to find leptospires with the microscope in such material. With all specimens it is good practice to use a combination of serologic techniques, direct observation, cultures, and animal studies in testing for the presence of leptospires.

Animal inoculation

Controversy still prevails on whether the use of small animals leads to a higher recovery rate of leptospires than can be obtained with direct cultures.

Weanling hamsters are most often used in attempts to recover leptospires, partially because they can be infected by numerous serotypes (105). When cultures are repeatedly nonrewarding, some other laboratory animal [such as the gerbil used in isolating *grippotyphosa* (44)] can be used as a source of *in vivo* enrichment. Laboratory animals can serve five functions in attempts to isolate leptospires: (a) organisms inoculated into them are concentrated; (b) inoculated specimens are decontaminated; (c) the animals' reactions provide information on the leptospiral strain's killing capacity; (d) provide serum for serologies; and (e) suggest the status of the agent as pathogenic or saprophytic. Blood, urine, and tissue all can be intraperitoneally inoculated in hamsters in 0.5- to 1.0-ml amounts. The material should be diluted to minimize inhibitory action and at least three hamsters should be inoculated with each dilution.

Not all animals thus inoculated will have "typical" clinical infections. Blood obtained by cardiac puncture early in the first 10 days of infection should be diluted 1:10 and inoculated onto semisolid culture medium. Although some workers attach importance to such things as weight loss and fever, the infecting agent must be isolated before a diagnosis is confirmed. Death of the laboratory animal can be as early as 3 to 5 days and as late as 2 weeks ± 4 days (35). In the report just cited, the authors stated that when they used a highly virulent strain of *canicola* in doses of 20 cells/hamster, 13 out of 20 animals died. The organisms were in such high number that the tissue homogenates yielded growth when diluted as much as 1×10^{-8}. The animals sometimes died soon after inoculation and had no definitive premonitory signs, though many of them bled from the nostrils and the anus. Animals thus infected may have greatly enlarged, blood-engorged kidneys, or the organs may be pale and shrunken depending upon the strain's virulence. They may have petechial hemorrhages in the intestinal tract; livers may be friable; there may be numerous or few hemorrhages in the lungs; the animals may or may not be jaundiced.

If the hamster survives for more than 14 days, it should be sacrificed, blood should be taken for serology, and urine, kidney, and brain specimens should be taken for isolation attempts. Some serotypes apparently can be isolated only from urine and kidney specimens from hamsters. Others such as *hardjo* can be isolated from the brain as often as from the kidney, even when blood cultures are negative.

When a laboratory animal dies within 24 to 48 hr after inoculation, the cause should be questioned (89). If animals do not die until 14 to 21 days after inoculation, a diagnosis of leptospirosis should be confirmed by cultural isolation. Since hamsters can appear active one hour and die the next, they must be closely observed. If animals die during the night, attempts to isolate the causative organism can still be made the next day. To avoid contamination, 1:100 and 1:1000 dilutions should be used. Once isolated, the leptospiral strain can be titrated to determine its minimal lethal or infectious dose in conjunction with nephelometry and Petroff-Hauser counting (35).

Guinea pigs (150 to 200 g) can also be used in the analytical procedures described above. Any laboratory animal selected should be known to be free of infection (e.g., apparently healthy mice frequently harbor leptospires). One- to 2-day-old chicks and the chicken embryo have been used in isolating leptospires.

Maintenance of Cultures

The use of leptospiral cultures as diagnostic antigens requires proper quality control. Such cultures should include those grown in liquid media and those grown and subsequently stored in a semisolid medium (28). The latter is the most widely accepted, proven, useful form in which to preserve both viability and virulence of leptospires (28, 29, 35, 71, 72).

Quality control procedures for liquid media have already been discussed. A liquid medium adequate for microscopic agglutination antigen production is not necessarily satisfactory when converted to a semisolid form. If inocula are used at a concentration of less than 20×10^6 cells/ml, growth will be less rapid and may not occur at all with inferior media. If a particular liquid medium does not produce successful cultures consistently, the cause should be determined. Since liquid antigens are not readily purified, good fundamental transfer techniques must be practiced. Antigens being used regularly should be tested each week for the presence of other bacteria. Standardized inocula (31) and growth curves of antigens establish the frequency with which they should be transferred. The agglutinogenic properties of active, liquid-propagated cultures should be tested against homologous and heterologous antisera and sera of known reactivity. Serologic procedures using live antigens require good precision and careful record keeping of the number of transfers in liquid media to detect any evidence of partial, gradual, or complete loss of antigenicity.

Purification of contaminated cultures has been reviewed by Turner (100), Alexander (3), and Sulzer (95). Laboratory management should continue to emphasize the necessity for continued testing to confirm that liquid antigens are pure. Duplicate liquid cultures can be minimally inoculated and stored in static conditions at 25 C so that growth of the strain can be re-initiated without reverting to stock cultures. The purification of liquid cultures by selective membrane filtration (0.8, 0.45, and 0.22 μm diameter), dilution extinction, plating, and intraperitoneal inoculations of animals require considerable time before purity can be re-established (7, 72).

Serologic Procedures

Several blood samples should be obtained during the period of infection in order to demonstrate seroconversion or a rise in titer. Seropositivity may be detected as early as the end of the first week after infection with the microscopic agglutination test, although measurable titers with the indirect hemagglutination test may be present even sooner in human serum. Agglutinins may persist at various levels for several months and may still be detectable for more than a year after infection (in some cases as long as 10 years: personal communication). There is not currently available a serologic test with which to distinguish between an infectious and an exposure titer against leptospires, and titer levels do not necessarily correlate directly with severity of infection. Serum separated from clots can be filtered through 0.45 μm disposable filters and aseptically stored at -80 C. If preservatives must be added to specimens, 1 part glycerol to 1 part serum or 1 part 1:1000 aqueous Merthiolate solution to 9 parts serum can be used. If possible, lipemic serum should be avoided. Serum samples should be shipped frozen.

Microscopic agglutination test

The live-antigen microscopic agglutination test has been the most widely used procedure for detecting leptospiral antibodies and will probably become more widely used as it is adapted to microtitration methods (17). It is generally accepted as the standard reference test against which all other proposed tests have been evaluated. The test is highly sensitive and specific and can be used for both animal and human sera. It is, however, highly serotype-specific, and to ensure that antibodies produced by different serotypes can be detected, a battery of antigens that encompass most of the known cross-reactions of leptospires must be used. It is not a genus test. The diagnostic or public health laboratory using the procedure should be familiar with the pattern of local isolations and should be informed of surveillance data (12). Up-to-date information on incidence of infection, serotypes which should be used in the agglutination test, epidemiologic features of leptospirosis, geographical distribution, sources of infection, and clinical features can be very useful in laboratory attempts to diagnose leptospirosis.

In the microscopic agglutination test, which is partially serotype specific, agglutinins elicited by leptospires of a particular serotype often agglutinate leptospires of other serotypes in the same serogroup and of related serotypes in other serogroups. The test can be used not only in diagnosing human infections but also in diagnosing infections in domestic animals when epidemiological information indicates that an antibody response was elicited many months previously. In principle, the serotype of an infecting strain can be determined with certainty only by isolation and cross-agglutination absorption studies. However, results of absorption studies on serum from an infected individual can indicate at times the most probable infecting serotype. Those serotypes currently used routinely in the microscopic agglutination test in the leptospiral reference laboratory of the Center for Disease Control are listed in Table 30.4.

The microscopic agglutination test involves: (a) growing the antigen, (b) manipulating the antigen, (c) selecting the number of serotypes to be used, (d) having WHO reference antisera and secondary antisera available, (e) performing the test with the required equipment, (f) interpreting results, and (g) reporting results.

In the following paragraphs, the means of conducting agglutination-microtitration live antigen tests for leptospiral agglutinins are described in detail. Other tests are mentioned later and are discussed in more detail in two other reports (3, 95).

The media used for, growth pattern of, and standardization of cell mass for antigen propagation have been discussed. Table 30.1 shows the correlation between nephelometer reading, percent transmittance, cell count, and bacterial density (dry weight). The optimal antigen density (31) for this test is believed to be that of a cell mass equivalent to a nephelometer reading of 25 ± 5. For all known serotypes, this reading represents a range of 180×10^6 to 300×10^6 cells/ml depending on cell size. The Roessler (81) primary and National Animal Disease Center (NADC), Ames, Iowa (31), secondary turbidity stan-

TABLE 30.4—SEROTYPE ANTIGENS USED IN THE MICROSCOPIC AGGLUTINATION TEST AT THE LEPTOSPIRAL REFERENCE LABORATORY, CENTER FOR DISEASE CONTROL

SEROGROUP	SEROTYPE AND STRAIN
Icterohaemorrhagiae	copenhageni, M20
Icterohaemorrhagiae	mankarso
Canicola	canicola, Hond Utrecht IV
Pomona	pomona, Pomona
Grippotyphosa	grippotyphosa, Andaman
Autumnalis	autumnalis, Akiyama A
Autumnalis	fort bragg, Fort Bragg
Autumnalis	djasiman, Djasiman
Hebdomadis	wolffi, 3705
Hebdomadis	georgia, LT 117
Hebdomadis	borincana, HS 622
Bataviae	bataviae, Van Tienen
Ballum	ballum, S102
Pyrogenes	pyrogenes, Salinem
Australis	australis, Ballico
Tarassovi	tarassovi, Pereplicin
Pyrogenes	alexi, HS 616
Javanica	javanica, Veldrat Bataviae 46
Celledoni	celledoni, Celledoni
Cynopteri	cynopteri, 3522C
Cynopteri	butembo, Butembo
Panama	panama, CZ 214K
Andamana	andamana, CH 11

dards may be used interchangeably. The secondary standards were determined against the Roessler primary standard thus allowing the live antigen used in the test to be readily standardized in any U.S. laboratory. Information on available standards and an anodized cuvette holding dry well can be obtained from the NADC.

The medium currently preferred in the CDC leptospiral reference center is bovine albumin polysorbate 80 as originally described (34) or a commercially available modification (see Chapter 46). In Table 30.5, the standardized nephelometer reading of 25 is related to antigen-diluent ratios for cultures with readings above 25. Microcolonies (breed nests, excessively large aggregations) of leptospires seem to be characteristic for some strains, older cultures, and those not media-adapted. A practical solution is to search out strains which have little tendency to nest or aggregate. Centrifugation at 1500 to 2000 × g for 15 to 30 min may cut down on the number of antigen clumps.

Reference antisera in small amounts can be obtained from CDC, but laboratories should prepare their own primary supplies or obtain them commercially (Difco Laboratories, Detroit, Mich). The latter preparations should be compared with those from CDC because there is no uniform code of standards which is accepted worldwide. Some generally accepted points are: (a) rabbits (8 to 9 pounds) in good health whose sera have been pretested in 1:10 dilutions for the presence of detectable agglutinins are used; (b) four successive injections should be made at 5–7 day intervals in the marginal ear vein; (c) live cultures should be used; (d) an initial test sample can be taken after the third injection; (e) material used for the injections is from the rich growth zones of semisolid young cultures; (f) injection doses should be progressively larger (0.5, 1.0, 2.0, and 4.0 ml); (g) organisms derived from bovine albumin polysorbate 80 media (34) give results similar to those obtained from cultures of rabbit serum in Fletcher's semisolid medium (95).

If the homologous titer is at least 6400, the blood is removed by cardiopuncture. A 0.45 μm filter is used to sterilize 10-ml serum samples. One-milliliter samples are a convenient size to freeze at −20 C and below. Serum can be

TABLE 30.5—DILUENT VOLUMES FOR ADJUSTMENT OF LEPTOSPIRAL ANTIGEN SUSPENSIONS TO A NEPHELOMETER READING (N.R.) OF 25

N.R.	N.R./25	CULTURE VOL (ML) 10 ML/F	DILUENT VOL (ML) 1% BSA
100	4F*	2.5	7.5
90	3.6	2.8	7.2
80	3.2	3.1	6.9
70	2.8	3.6	6.4
60	2.4	4.2	5.8
50	2.0	5.0	5.0
40	1.6	6.2	3.8
30	1.2	8.3	1.7

* F = N.R. of actual culture divided by 25 N.R. (desired suspensions turbidity; Coleman 7 or 9).

freeze-dried or treated with glycerol or Merthiolate. Because live, virulent cultures are always a potential infection hazard, some laboratories use Formalin- or heat-killed cultures (2).

Samples submitted for analysis may or may not be pretested, depending on such factors as facilities available, testing load, mission of laboratory, available staff, and availability of paired sera. If the test is performed at maximum sensitivity, a 1:5 dilution of serum in phosphate buffered saline (95) can be used. When 0.05-ml microdiluters are used, 0.1 ml of the 1:5 serum dilution is placed in the first well of a 96-well microtitration dish. When 0.025-ml microdiluters are used, 0.05 ml is placed in the well. In each of 11 other wells, 0.05 or 0.025 ml of saline diluent is placed (#12 as antigen control). This represents a 1:5120 serum dilution in the 11th well. Adding an equal volume of standardized antigen to each well produces a serum dilution sequence of 1:10 to 1:10240. The antigen-serum dilutions are covered and incubated at 25 C for 2 hr ± 30 min.

The length of incubation should be determined carefully (e.g., some leptospiral strains begin to clump after 2 hr of incubation). The degree of agglutination in each well is read with a dry dark-field microscope equipped with a 10×/0.22-long working distance objective and 10× eyepieces. If laboratory workers wear eyeglasses, periplan eyepieces can be used. Flat-bottomed microtitration dishes are used after their outer edges have been removed with a milling machine or an acrylic sheet cutting tool. Many microtitration dishes are 14 mm high, and after removal of the outer edge are approximately 12.5 mm high thus allowing critical focusing with the long working distance objective. An alternative is to mill out an area on the underneath side of the microscope stage to allow for condenser movement and obviating the need to modify the height of each microtitration dish.

Agglutination patterns vary and must be interpreted by an experienced observer. The textbook picture of an intense black background with masses of leptospires of various sizes where the morphological identity of the leptospiral cell has been obliterated can be easily seen. Antigens must be carefully controlled. Some antigens reacting homologously appear as described above, and others agglutinate in a lacy, less compact pattern. The intensity of blackness of the background, the degree to which cells agglutinate, and the number of freely moving cells are all evaluated. The intensity of this reaction has been read 1+, 2+, 3+, 4+ and the end point reported as the last dilution showing a 2+ 25% to 50% agglutination (2, 3, 17, 95). In an attempt to overcome the subjectivity of the 2+ reaction, other workers (32) modified the reading procedure as follows: reactions are still read as 4+, 3+, 2+, and 1+ as they relate to 100%, 75%, 50%, and 25% agglutination, but the 1+ reaction to a perfect antigen control is designated as the end point. All reactions in the 11-well series are rated 4+, 3+, 2+, or 1+. This procedure requires that the antigens be propagated rapidly, that they be free of clumping, and that they be stable for 2 hr of incubation.

The use of Formalin-fixed antigens has been described (3, 95). The basic steps involve fixation, centrifugation, standardization against antisera, adjustment of proper antigen density, and storage at 5 C. Such an antigen is stable for 1 to 2 weeks.

Macroscopic plate test

The other procedure relying on agglutination is a macroscopic plate test. Two types of commercially available antigens can be used in different procedures. One (42) is a slide screening test for serodiagnosing leptospirosis (designed primarily to be used with human sera) in which standardized concentrations of washed, Formalin-fixed cells are used. Twelve serotypes are pooled in groups of three. Specific instructions for performing the test are provided by the manufacturer. Stability of the antigen, use of control sera, and the fact that the test is less sensitive than the microscopic agglutination test are all factors to be considered. A second system (91) is one in which single antigens are used in the reagent. A laboratory which cannot develop the live antigen system (the microscopic agglutination test) can use the macroscopic plate test but should be aware of its limitations.

Other serologic procedures proposed for detecting leptospiral antibodies include complement-fixation, hemagglutination, and hemolytic tests and fluorescent antibody techniques.

In the complement-fixation test, as in the hemolytic test, a *L. biflexa* antigen is used; the test is genus-specific (92, 99). The leptospires are killed with Merthiolate in saline preserved by 1:1000 sodium azide and stored at 4 C. This test may be useful in detecting current and recent past infections in humans.

The hemolytic test (18) is conducted with an antigen which consists of a 50% ethyl alcohol-insoluble, 95% ethyl alcohol-soluble extract from leptospiral cells (2, 95). *L. biflexa* strains provide antigens which remain active when freeze-dried. The antigen dilution for sensitizing red cells is predetermined with standard antiserum. The antigen-sensitized cells are washed, resuspended at a concentration of 1%, and added with guinea pig complement to serial dilutions of sera. Reaction mixtures are incubated at 37 C for 1 hr. The lysis of the sensitized erythrocytes indicates a positive reaction. Cox et al. (19) reported that titers of sera obtained during the convalescent phase of illness were generally greater than 1000 and ranged as high as 100,000. This test can be used in detecting antibodies in human sera regardless of the infecting serotypes. It has been used very little with animal sera. In a simplified form of the test, sensitized erythrocytes are fixed with glutaraldehyde (7) or pyruvic aldehyde (7, 94). The test has excellent genus specificity and sensitivity for detecting antibodies in early stages of disease. Negative results may be obtained a few weeks after convalescence.

Serologic procedures with isolates

The only leptospiral reference laboratory in the United States is located at the Center for Disease Control (CDC) in Atlanta, Georgia, although any clinical diagnostic or public health laboratory has the facilities to provide partial identification of an isolate. Isolates can be tested against different WHO reference antisera of various serotypes which are available in limited quantities from CDC. When the serogroup to which the isolate belongs has been established, it can be tested further with antisera against serotypes in its serogroup. Reciprocal agglutinin-absorption tests can be used in attempts to identify the isolate definitively. If necessary, 80 ml of the culture and its hyperimmune

TABLE 30.6—COMPARISON OF THE ANTISERA REACTIONS OF 3 LEPTOSPIRAL SEROTYPES AS FIELD ISOLATES SUBSEQUENTLY IDENTIFIED, AND LABORATORY-ADAPTED ANTIGENS*

ANTISERA	HARDJO		SZWAJIZAK		POMONA	
	ISOLATE	ANTIGEN	ISOLATE	ANTIGEN	ISOLATE	ANTIGEN
Copenhageni	10	20	—	—	1280	80
Coxi	10	10	—	—	—	20
Canicola	10	20	20	20	160	40
Pyrogenes	—	—	—	—	10	10
Butembo	10	20	—	—	10	ND
Autumnalis	—	40	—	—	320	320
Pomona	10	40	10	10	10,240	10,240
Grippotyphosa	—	—	—	—	10	10
Szwajizak (CDC)	80	160	10,240	10,240	10	10
Szwajizak (NADC)	640	1280	10,240	10,240	20	20
Hardjo (Prajitno)	5120	10,240	160	40	320	20
Hardjo (Downey)	10,240	10,240	320	320	ND	10
Hardjo (BV$_6$)	1280	1280	320	160	320	10
Hardjo (Wint 5)	2560	5120	80	80	ND	20
Hardjo (KAP 249)	5120	5120	80	40	ND	10
Wolfii (3705)	10,240	5120	80	160	ND	ND
Bataviae	—	—	—	—	10	—
Tarasovi	—	—	—	—	10	—

*Cross agglutination pattern of virulent field isolates and laboratory-adapted antigens (reciprocal titers).
ND = not done.

antiserum can be submitted to the CDC reference typing laboratory. Table 30.6 contains a comparison of data on antisera of three leptospiral isolates and three similar laboratory antigens of known identity. Agglutination patterns obtained with the microtitration test are shown in Figure 30.9. Supplementary information developed by the diagnostic laboratory can frequently speed the work of the CDC reference laboratory.

Antimicrobic Susceptibility and Resistance

Very little information has been published on the antibiotic-resistant patterns of leptospires. The antibiotics which have been used in *in vitro* testing were listed earlier.

Evaluation of Laboratory Findings

Isolation of leptospires from human blood, cerebrospinal fluid, or urine is reliable laboratory confirmation of a clinical diagnosis of current illness.

Leptospires isolated from human urine have usually been obtained from people infected within recent months. We know very little about how long humans continue to shed leptospires in urine. Different animals shed the organ-

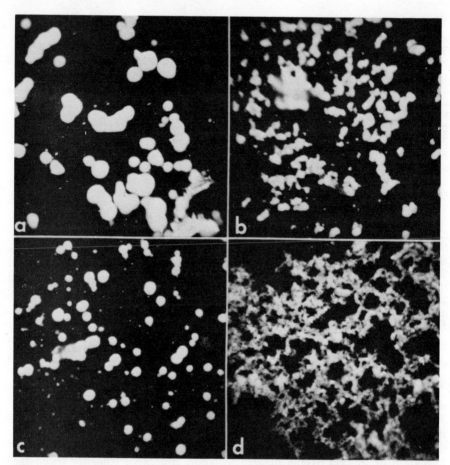

Figure 30.9—Patterns of agglutination in the microscopic agglutination microtiter test:
(a) 4+ clearing, outer periphery smooth, hard ball agglutination in a
1:640 positive reacting serum; (b) 4+ clearing, smaller particles, agglutination in a 1:80 positive reacting serum; (c) 3+ clearing, smaller particles, agglutination in a 1:640 positive reacting serum; (d) 4+, loose, lace-
work agglutination pattern, in a 1:80 positive reacting serum.

ism for various lengths of time, making it difficult to determine when they
were originally infected. Negative culture results indicate that no infection is
present only if tests are performed on multiple specimens which were collected
in the correct manner at the proper times and if the patient continues to be
serologically negative for leptospires.

It is often impossible to determine whether titers against leptospires are
the result of current or past infection. In addition, it is not yet possible to differentiate in animals whether a titer has been induced by vaccination and by
infection. Serological results must be interpreted in accord with available clini-

cal and epidemiologic data. With data obtained from serologic tests it is not always possible to identify the infecting serotype (95) and rarely possible to reach a definitive diagnosis of leptospirosis in the first week of infection (2).

Low and high titers against leptospires indicate only that the animal or person has been exposed to the organism at some time and do not necessarily indicate that active infection occurred. Conversely, the absence of a titer against leptospires does not necessarily indicate that the animal or person has not been infected by them, particularly if specimens are taken during the early stages of infection. Paired sera obtained at the proper times are much more useful than a single serum specimen. When such specimens are analyzed, results usually follow a pattern of: (a) a significant rise in titer between early and later samples (usually at least a fourfold rise obtained with the microscopic agglutination test—a level which exceeds the experimental error with this procedure); (b) positive results but no rise in titer; or (c) negative results from all tests.

If positive serologic results are obtained and there is no accompanying rise in titer, the animal or person may have been exposed to leptospires in the past, the test antigens may not have been the proper serotypes, or a rise in titer did not show up because specimens were collected after the titer reached its peak.

There is no substitute for the isolation and identification of the agent. The identity of a serotype should be reported as confirmed only on the basis of agglutinin-absorption test results. Serologic results are even more difficult to report and explain, and use of terms such as *infected, significant titer,* and *reactor* are discouraged. The test antigens used should be listed in any report.

There is a need for improved laboratory procedures dealing with better sero-diagnosis emphasizing agglutinin-absorption, differentiation of current infection and past exposure, evaluation of IgM and IgG antibodies, and a medium in which leptospires will grow more rapidly (i.e., after 2 to 4 days of incubation).

Safety Precautions for Laboratory Workers

All laboratory workers should be taught how to handle the leptospiral antigens used in the microscopic agglutination test. Although practically all of the antigens used in the microscopic agglutination test have lost their virulence, they should be viewed as pathogens. All specimens submitted for analysis should be treated as if they are potentially infectious. For this reason, no culture should be pipetted by mouth.

Extreme care should be taken when inoculating laboratory animals with materials suspected of containing leptospires. Many infections have occurred as the result of laboratory workers being inoculated with leptospires while replacing needle guards or while inoculating rabbits in the marginal ear vein in the production of hyperimmune sera. Some workers are now using heat-killed antigens (60 C for 15 min) for the production of hyperimmune sera.

When cultures are being examined, some disinfectant should always be available for flushing skin areas exposed to leptospires. Persons who homogenize tissue specimens should wear protective gloves and have their forearms covered. The homogenization should be performed in a biological safety cabinet.

The normal serologic profile of laboratory workers involved with leptospires should be recorded and reference serum from each stored at −80 C. If a worker is accidentally inoculated with or otherwise exposed to infectious material, the area of exposure should be flushed with disinfectant, blood should be taken for serologic analysis (an immediate and a follow-up sample), and antibiotic treatment might be indicated. If the worker develops an infection despite such measures, attempts should be made to isolate the causative organism, the amount of tissue involvement should be evaluated, and the patient should receive supportive therapy.

Although there have been numerous reports that antibiotics do not alter the course of leptospirosis, aggressive treatment should be initiated in an attempt to avoid allowing the cells to be deposited in the kidneys.

Additional safety procedures are outlined in the *Federal Register,* Part II, Recombinant DNA Research, N.I.H., Department of Health, Education, and Welfare, Bethesda, MD 20014 (Page 27913, paragraph 2; *Fed. Register* Vol. 41, #131, July 7, 1976) and in *Classification of Etiologic Agents on the Basis of Hazard,* Center for Disease Control, Atlanta, GA 30333.

Leptospirosis: Media and Reagents

Media for growing leptospires can be prepared from individual ingredients in the laboratory or obtained commercially. In either case quality control practices must be adhered to carefully if attempts to propagate and isolate leptospires are to be successful.

Either albumin polysorbate 80 or serum-enriched media can be used. Both can be prepared as liquids, semisolids, or solids. The albumin-based media differ only in their degree of solidity, with different names used for the various forms: Stuart's for the liquid, Fletcher's for the semisolid (0.2% agar), and Cox's for the solid (1.0% agar). These three media have different formulas. No one medium will suffice for every purpose or grow every leptospiral isolate.

The processes for preparing media are described in Chapter 46.

ACKNOWLEDGEMENTS. The authors wish to acknowledge the assistance of Dr. Barbara Kingscote, Animal Pathology Laboratory, Guelph, Canada, who supplied the strain used in Figure 30.3; Mssrs. Wayne Romp, Tom Glasson, and Gene Hedberg of the NADC photography laboratory; Miss Teri McClannahan of the Bacteriological and Mycological Research Laboratory of NADC; Dr. Charles Sterling, Comparative Medicine, Wayne State University, Detroit, Michigan; and Mr. Tom Kelly, Chief of the Arts and Graphics Section of the Atomic Energy Laboratory.

References

1. ABDUSSALAM M, ALEXANDER AD, BABUDIERI B, BOGEL K, BORG-PETERSON C, FAINE S, KMETY E, LATASTE-DOROLLE C, and TURNER LH: Research needs in leptospirosis. Bull WHO 47–113, 1972
2. ALEXANDER AD: Serological diagnosis of leptospirosis. *In* Manual of Clinical Immunology.

Rose NR and Friedman H (eds.). American Society for Microbiology, Washington DC, 1976

3. ALEXANDER AD, GOCHENOUR WS, REINHARD KR, WARD MK, and YAGER RH: Leptospirosis. *In* Diagnostic Procedures for Bacterial, Mycotic and Parasitic Infections. American Public Health Association, New York, 1970

4. ALSTON JM and BROOM JC: Leptospirosis in Man and Animals. E&S Livingstone, Edinburgh, 1958

5. BABUDIERI B and ZARDI O: Studies on the metabolism of leptospirae. I. Vitamin B_{12} as a growth factor. Z Vitam Horm Fermentforsch 11:299–309, 1960

6. BAKER HJ: Leptospirosis in Malaysia. Mil Med 130:1101–1102, 1965

7. BAKER LA and COX CD: Quantitative assay for genus-specific leptospiral antigens and antibody. Appl Microbiol 25:697–698, 1973

8. BASEMAN JB, HENNEBERRY RC, and COX CD: Isolation and growth of leptospira on artificial media. J Bacteriol 91:1374–1375, 1966

9. BRENDLE JJ and ALEXANDER AD: Contamination of bacteriological media by *Leptospira biflexa.* Appl Microbiol 28:505–506, 1974

10. BRIDGES CH and LUNA L: Kerr's improved Warthin-Starry technic. Study of the possible variations. Lab Invest 6:357–367, 1957

11. CACCHIONE RA, CASCELLI ES, BULGINI MJD, and MARTINEX ES: Colorantes inhibidores en el D'Esarrole de las leptospires su empleo en la diferenciacion de las leptospiras de las biflexas. Rev Invest Agropecu 1:1–9, 1964

12. CENTER FOR DISEASE CONTROL: Leptospirosis Surveillance Report: Annual Summary 1975. U.S. Dept. Health, Education, and Welfare, Atlanta, Ga, 1976

13. CENTER FOR DISEASE CONTROL: Bacterial diseases—epidemiologic trends of leptospirosis. Vet Public Health, 1977

14. CHANG RS and MCCOMB DE: Erythrocyte-sensitizing substance from five strains of leptospirae. Am J Trop Med Hyg 3:481–489, 1954

15. COGHLAN JD and BAIN AD: Leptospirosis in human pregnancy followed by death of the foetus. Br Med J 1:228–230, 1969

16. COGHLAN JD, LUMSDEN WHR, and MCNEILLAGE GJC: Low temperature preservation of leptospira. J Hyg 65:373–379, 1967

17. COLE JR, SULZER OR, and PURSELL AR: Improved microtechnique for the leptospiral microscopic agglutination test. Appl Microbiol 25:976–980, 1973

18. COX CD: Standardization and stabilization of an extract from *Leptospira biflexa* and its use in the hemolytic test for leptospirosis. J Infect Dis 101:203–209, 1957

19. COX CD, ALEXANDER AD, and MURPHY LC: Evaluation of the hemolytic test in the serodiagnosis of human leptospirosis. J Infect Dis 101:210–218, 1957

20. DIESCH SL and ELLINGHAUSEN HC JR: The Leptospirosis. *In* Hull's Diseases Transmitted from Animals to Man, 6th edition. Charles C. Thomas, Springfield, Ill, 1975

21. ELLINGHAUSEN HC JR: Nephelometry and a nephelo-culture flask used in measuring growth of leptospires. Am J Vet Res 20:1072–1076, 1959

22. ELLINGHAUSEN HC JR: Further observations on some cultural characteristics of *Leptospira pomona.* Bacteriol Proc 18:33, 1960

23. ELLINGHAUSEN HC JR: Some observations on cultural and biochemical characteristics of *Leptospira pomona.* J Infect Dis 106:237–244, 1960

24. ELLINGHAUSEN HC JR: The effect of aeration upon the growth of *Leptospira* serotypes. Am J Vet Res 27:975–979, 1966

25. ELLINGHAUSEN HC JR: Cultural and biochemical characteristics of a leptospire from frog kidney. Bull Wildlife Dis Assoc 4:41–50, 1968

26. ELLINGHAUSEN HC JR: Stimulation of leptospiral growth by glucose. Am J Vet Res 29:191–199, 1968

27. ELLINGHAUSEN HC JR: Death and lysis of leptospirae when cultured in asbestos-filtered growth media. Appl Microbiol 26:959–968, 1973

28. ELLINGHAUSEN HC JR: Growth temperatures, virulence, survival, and nutrition of leptospires. J Med Microbiol 6:487–497, 1973

29. ELLINGHAUSEN HC JR: Virulence, nutrition, and antigenicity of *Leptospira interrogans* serotype *pomona* in supplemented and nutrient-deleted bovine albumin medium. Ann Microbiol 124B:477–493, 1973

30. ELLINGHAUSEN HC JR: Nutrition of leptospires in bovine albumin polysorbate medium. Proceedings of the 1st International Symposium on the Biology of the Pathogenic Spirochetes. Academic Press, New York, 1976

31. ELLINGHAUSEN HC JR: Variable factors influencing the isolations of leptospires and testing. Proceedings of the U.S. Animal Health Association, 79th Annual Meeting, Portland, 1976, pp 126–141

32. ELLINGHAUSEN HC JR, DEYOE BL, and NERVIG RM: Leptospirosis in perspective. Proceedings of the U.S. Animal Health Association, 81st Annual Meeting, 1978, pp 161–182

33. ELLINGHAUSEN HC JR and MCCULLOUGH WG: Nutrition of *Leptospira pomona* and growth of 13 other serotypes: a serum-free medium employing oleic albumin complex. Am J Vet Res 26:39–44, 1965

34. ELLINGHAUSEN HC JR and MCCULLOUGH WG: Nutrition of *Leptospira pomona* and growth of 13 other serotypes: fractionation of oleic albumin complex and a medium of bovine albumin and polysorbate 80. Am J Vet Res 26:45–51, 1965

35. ELLINGHAUSEN HC JR and PAINTER GM: Growth, survival, antigenic stability and virulence of *Leptospira interrogans* serotype *canicola*. J Med Microbiol 9:29–37, 1976

36. ELLINGHAUSEN HC JR and TOP FH: Leptospirosis. *In* Communicable and Infectious Diseases, 8th edition. CV Mosby, St. Louis, 1976

37. FENNESTAD KL and BORG-PETERSEN C: Fetal leptospirosis and abortion in cattle. J Infect Dis 102:227–236, 1958

38. FULTON JD and SPOONER DF: The metabolism of *Leptospira icterohaemorrhagiae in vitro*. Exp Parasitol 5:154–177, 1956

39. FUZI M and CZOKA R: Die Differenzierung der Pathogen und saprophytischen Leptospiren mittels eines Kupfer Sulfattestes. Zentralbl Bakteriol Parasitenkd Infektionskr Hyg Abt 1: Orig 179:231–237, 1960

40. FUZI M and CZOKA R: An egg yolk reaction test for the differentiation of leptospirae. J Pathol Bacteriol 82:208–212, 1961

41. FUZI M and CZOKA R: Rapid method for the differentiation of parasitic and saprophytic leptospirae. J Bacteriol 81:1008, 1961

42. GALTON MM, POWERS DK, HALE AD, and CORNELL R: A rapid macroscopic slide screening test for the serodiagnosis of leptospirosis. Am J Vet Res 19:505–512, 1958

43. GSELL OR: Epidemiology of leptospirosis. Walter Reed Army Medical Research Center, Washington, DC, Med Sci Pub No 1:34–55, 1952

44. HANSON LE, ELLINGHAUSEN HC, and MARLOWE R: Isolation of *Leptospira grippotyphosa* from a cow following an abortion. Proc Soc Exp Biol Med 117:495–497, 1964

45. HANSON LE, GLOSSER JW, STOENNER HG, DIESCH SL, SMITH RE, and MORTER RL: Leptospirosis of domestic animals. Superintendent of Documents, U.S. Govt Printing Office, #001-000-0371-1, 1976

46. HEATH CW, ALEXANDER AD, and GALTON MM: Leptospirosis in the United States. N Engl J Med 273:857–864, 915–922, 1965

47. HELPRIN IJ and HIATT CW: The effects of fatty acids on the respiration of *Leptospira icterohaemorrhagiae*. J Infect Dis 100:136–140, 1957

48. JOHNSON RC and GARY ND: Nutrition of *Leptospira pomona*. I. Studies on a chemically defined substitute for the rabbit serum ultrafiltrate. J Bacteriol 83:668–672, 1962

49. JOHNSON RC and GARY ND: Nutrition of *Leptospira pomona*. II. Fatty acid requirements. J Bacteriol 85:976–982, 1963

50. JOHNSON RC and HARRIS VG: Differentiation of pathogenic and saprophytic leptospires. I. Growth at low temperatures. J Bacteriol 94:27–31, 1967

51. JOHNSON RC, LIVERMORE BP, WALBY JK, and JENKIN HM: Lipids of parasitic and saprophytic leptospires. Infect Immun 2:286–291, 1970

52. JOHNSON RC and ROGERS P: Differentiation of pathogenic and saprophytic leptospires with 8-azaguanine. J Bacteriol 88:1618–1623, 1964

53. JOHNSON RC and ROGERS P: 5-Fluorouracil as a selective agent for growth of leptospirae. J Bacteriol 87:422–426, 1964

54. JOHNSON RC and WALBY JK: Cultivation of leptospires: fatty acid requirements. Appl Microbiol 23:1027–1031, 1972

55. JOHNSON RC and WILSON JB: Nutrition of *Leptospira pomona*. J Bacteriol 80:406–411, 1960

56. JONES RK: Study of the viability of *Leptospira pomona* in frozen extended bovine semen. Am J Vet Med 133:216–218, 1958

57. KAISER GE and DOETSCH RN: Enhanced translational motion of *Leptospira* in viscous environments. Nature 255:656, 1975

58. KIRSCHNER L and MAGUIRE T: Survival of leptospira outside their hosts. N Z Med J 6:385–391, 1957

59. LINSCOTT WD and BOAK RA: Protective action of glycerol in the freezing of leptospirae. J Bacteriol 80:573, 1960

60. MACKENZIE RB, REILLY CKG, ALEXANDER AD, BRACKNER EA, DIERCKS FH, and BEYE HK: An outbreak of leptospirosis among U.S. Army troops in the Canal Zone. 1. Clinical and epidemiological observations. Am J Trop Med Hyg 15:57–63, 1966

61. MAESTRONE G: The use of an improved fluorescent antibody procedure in the demonstration of leptospira in animal tissue. Can J Comp Med 27:108–112, 1963

62. MARSHALL PB: Measurement of aerobic respiration in *Leptospira icterohaemorrhagiae*. J Infect Dis 84:150–152, 1949

63. MCCRUMB FR JL, STOCKARD JL, ROBINSON CR, TURNER LH, LEWIS DO, MAISEY CW, KELLEHER MF, GLEISER CA, and SMADEL JE: Leptospirosis in Malaya. 1. Sporadic cases among military and civilian personnel. Am J Trop Med Hyg 6:238–256, 1957

64. MENGES RW, GALTON MM, and HALL DD: Diagnosis of leptospirosis from urine specimens by direct culture following bladder tapping. J Am Vet Med Assoc 132:58–60, 1958

65. MISHRA A: Studies on survival of *Leptospira pomona* in body fluids and tissues outside the animal host. Indian Vet J 41:446–453, 1964

66. MONZON OT, ORY EM, DOBSON HL, CARTER E, and YOW EM: A comparison of bacterial counts of the urine obtained by needle aspiration of the bladder, catheterization and midstream voided methods. N Engl J Med 259:764–767, 1958

67. MYERS DM: Efficacy of combined furazolidine and neomycin in the control of contamination in *Leptospira* cultures. Antimicrob Agents Chemother 7:666–671, 1975

68. MYERS DM: Serological studies and isolations of serotype *hardjo* and *Leptospira biflexa* strains from horses of Argentina. J Clin Microbiol 3:548–555, 1976

69. NERVIG RM and ELLINGHAUSEN HC JR: Recovery of leptospires from filtered swine urine. Annual Proceedings of the American Association of Laboratory Diagnosticians, 19th Annual Meeting, 1976, pp 57–64

70. NERVIG RM and ELLINGHAUSEN HC JR: Viability of *Leptospira interrogans* serotype *grippotyphosa* in swine urine and blood. Cornell Vet 68:70–77, 1978

71. NERVIG RM, ELLINGHAUSEN HC JR, and CARDELLA MA: Growth, virulence, and immunogenicity of *Leptospira interrogans* serotype *szwajizak*. Am J Vet Res 38:1421–1424, 1977

72. PAINTER GM and ELLINGHAUSEN HC JR: Immunizing potency of *Leptospira interrogans* serotype *canicola* after heat inactivation at different temperatures. J Med Microbiol 9:487–492, 1976

73. PARNAS J and PINKIEWICZ H: The influence of leptospirae and their toxins on tissue culture and the possibility of differentiation of serotypes. Zentralbl Veterinaermed 13B:369–376, 1966

74. PENTEK-JUHASZ M: Untersuchungen über die hämolytische Eigenschaft von *Leptospira biflexa*-Stammen. Acta Vet Acad Sci Hung 10:233–237, 1960

75. RESSELER R, VAN RIEL J, and VAN RIEL M: Conservative des leptospires après refroidissement ou lyophilisation. Ann Soc Belge Med Trop 46:213–222, 1966

76. RIS RD: Limitations of the use of 5-fluorouracil as a selective agent for the isolation of leptospirae. Appl Microbiol 27:270–271, 1974

77. RITCHIE AE: A Brief Consideration of Anatomical Features of the Spirochetes as Revealed by Electron Microscopy. Proceedings of the 5th National Congress of the Italian Society of Parasitology. Leonardo Edizioni Scientifiche, Trieste, Italy, 1968

78. RITCHIE AE: Morphology of leptospires. Proceedings of the 1st International Symposium on the Biology of the Pathogenic Spirochetes. Academic Press, New York, 1976

79. RITCHIE AE and ELLINGHAUSEN HC JR: Electron microscopy of leptospires. I. Anatomical features of *Leptospira pomona*. J Bacteriol 89:223–233, 1965

80. RITTENBERG MB, LINSOTT WD, and BALL MG: Simple method for separating leptospirae from contaminating microorganisms. J Bacteriol 76:669, 1958

81. ROESSLER WG and BREWER RR: Permanent turbidity standards. Appl Microbiol 15:1114–1121, 1967

82. ROTHSTEIN N and HIATT CW: Studies on the immuno-chemistry of leptospires. J Immunol 77:257–265, 1956

83. SCHNEIDERMAN AM, GREENE RR, SCHIELER L, MCCLURE LE, and DUNN MS: A chemically defined basal medium containing purified rabbit serum albumin. Proc Soc Exp Biol Med 78:777–780, 1951

84. SCHUBERT JH and SULZER CR: Preservation of *Leptospira* by storage at −75°C versus transferring every three months. Bacteriol Proc 20, 1970

85. SCHUFFNER W and MOCHTAR A: Versuche zur Abteilung von Leptospirenstammen mit einleitenden Bemerkungen über den Verlauf von Agglutination und Lysis. Zentralbl Bakteriol Parasitenkd Infektionskr Hyg Abt 1: Orig 101:405–413, 1927

86. SHARP CF: Laboratory diagnosis of leptospirosis with the sensitized erythrocyte lysis test. J Pathol Bacteriol 76:349–356, 1958

87. SHENBERG E: Growth of pathogenic *Leptospira* in chemically defined media. J Bacteriol 99:1598–1606, 1967

88. SHENBERG E, LINDENBAUM I, DIKKEN H, and TORTEN M: Isolation of a "saprophytic" leptospiral serotype *andamana* from carrier rats in Israel. Trop Geogr Med 27:395–398, 1975

89. STALHEIM OHV and HEDDLESTON KL: Isolation of *Pasteurella multocida* from the urine of steers. Vet Rec 87:135–136, 1970

90. STALHEIM OHV and WILSON JB: Cultivation of leptospirae. I. Nutrition of *Leptospira canicola.* J Bacteriol 88:48–54, 1964

91. STOENNER HG and DAVIES E: Further observations on leptospiral plate antigens. Am J Vet Res 28:259–266, 1967

92. STURDZA N, ELIAN M, and PULPAN G: Diagnosis of human leptospirosis by the complement-fixation test with a single antigen. Arch Roum Pathol Exp Microbiol 19:572–582, 1960

93. SULZER CR: Leptospiral serotype distribution list according to host and geographic area: July 1966 to July 1973. Center for Disease Control, Atlanta, Ga, 1975

94. SULZER CR, GLOSSER JW, ROGERS F, JONES WL, and TRIX M: Evaluation of an indirect hemagglutination test for the diagnosis of human leptospirosis. J Clin Microbiol 2:218–221, 1975

95. SULZER CR and JONES WL: Leptospirosis methods. *In* Laboratory Diagnosis. Center for Disease Control, Atlanta, Ga, 1973

96. SZYFRES B: Leptospirosis as an animal and public health problem in Latin America and the Caribbean area. Bull Pan Am Health Organ 10:110–125, 1976

97. TAN DK: The importance of leptospirosis in Malaya. Med J Malaya 18:164–170, 1964

98. TUMILOWICZ JJ, ALEXANDER AD, and STAFFORD K: On the contamination of cell cultures by *Leptospira biflexa.* In Vitro 10:238–242, 1974

99. TURNER LH: Leptospirosis. II. Serology. Trans R Soc Trop Med Hyg 62:880–889, 1968

100. TURNER LH: Maintenance, isolation, and demonstration of leptospires. Trans R Soc Trop Med Hyg 64:623–646, 1970

101. UHLENHATH P and FROMME P: Zur Aetiologie der sogenannten weilschen Krankheit (Ansteckende gelbuscht). Berl Klin Wochenschr 54:269–273, 1916

102. VAN ESELTINE WP and STAPLES SA: Nutritional requirements of leptospirae. I. Studies on oleic acid as a growth factor for a strain of *Leptospira pomona.* J Infect Dis 108:262–269, 1961

103. VOGEL H and HUTNER SH: Growth of leptospira in defined media. J Gen Microbiol 26:223–230, 1961

104. WESSELINOFF W, DELTSCHEFF C, and BAILOSOFF D: Über die Lebensdauer der Leptospieren in tierschen Geweden. Berl Münch Tierärztl Wochenschr 75:184, 1962

105. WOLFF JW: The Laboratory Diagnosis of Leptospirosis. Charles C. Thomas, Springfield, Ill, 1954

106. WOLFF JW and BROWN JC: The genus *Leptospira noguchi,* 1917. Problems of classification and a suggested system based on antigenic analysis. Doc Med Geogr Trop 6:78–95, 1954

107. YANAGAWA R, HIRAMUNE T, and AKAIKE Y: Growth of saprophytic and pathogenic leptospirae on solid medium in carbon dioxide-free air. J Bacteriol 85:953–954, 1963

General References

ALEXANDER AD: Serological diagnosis of leptospirosis. *In* Manual of Clinical Immunology. American Society for Microbiology, Washington, DC, 1976, pp 352–356

ALSTON JM and BROWN JC: Leptospirosis. *In* Man and Animals. E. and S. Livingstone, Edinburgh, 1958

BERMAN SJ, TSAI CC, HOLMES K, FRESH JW, and WATTEN RH: Sporadic anicteric leptospirosis in South Vietnam. A study of 150 patients. Ann Intern Med 79:167–173, 1973

CENTER FOR DISEASE CONTROL. Bacterial diseases—epidemiologic trends of leptospirosis in the U.S. 1965–1974. Vet Public Health, 1977

CENTER FOR DISEASE CONTROL. Leptospirosis Surveillance Report: Annual Summary 1975. U.S. Dept. Health, Education, and Welfare, Atlanta, Ga, 1976

DIESCH SL and ELLINGHAUSEN HC JR: The leptospiroses. *In* Diseases Transmitted from Animals to Man, 6th edition. Charles C. Thomas, Springfield, Ill, 1975, pp 436–462

EDWARDS GA: Clinical characteristics of leptospirosis. Observations based on a study of twelve sporadic cases. Am J Med 27: 4–17, 1959

ELLINGHAUSEN HC JR and TOP FH: Leptospirosis. *In* Communicable and Infectious Diseases, 8th edition. C. V. Mosby Co, St. Louis, 1976, pp 395–409

FOLIA FACULTATIS MEDICAE, Univ Bratislava, Smolenice, Czechoslovakia. Proceedings of the International Symposium on Leptospirosis, 12:1–300, 1974

HANSON LE, GLOSSER JW, STOENNER HG, DIESCH SL, SMITH RE, and MORTER RL: Leptospirosis of domestic animals. Superintendent of documents, U.S. Govt Printing Office, #001-000-035711-1, 1976

HEATH CW, ALEXANDER AD, and GALTON MM: Leptospirosis in the United States. N Engl J Med 273:857–864, 915–922, 1965

SULZER CR and JONES WL: Leptospirosis—methods in laboratory diagnosis. Center for Disease Control, Atlanta, Ga, 1973

SZYFRES B: Leptospirosis as an animal and public health problem in Latin America and the Caribbean area. Bull Pan Am Health Organ 10:110–125, 1976

TURNER LH: Leptospirosis I. Trans R Soc Trop Med Hyg 61:842–855, 1967

TURNER LH: Leptospirosis II. Serology. Trans R Soc Trop Med Hyg 62:880–899, 1968

TURNER LH: Leptospirosis III. Maintenance, isolation and demonstration of leptospires. Trans R Soc Trop Med Hyg 64:623–646, 1970

VAN THIEL PH: The Leptospiroses. Univ of Lieden, The Netherlands, 1948

WOLFF JW: The Laboratory Diagnosis of Leptospirosis. Charles C. Thomas, Springfield, Ill, 1954

WONG ML, KAPLAN S, DUNKLE LM, STECHENBERG BW, and FEIGIN RA: Leptospirosis: a childhood disease. J Pediatr 90:532–537, 1977

CHAPTER 31

LISTERIOSIS

W. L. Albritton, G. L. Wiggins, W. E. DeWitt, and J. C. Feeley

Introduction

Causative Organism

Listeria monocytogenes, the causative agent of listeriosis, is a short, motile, gram-positive, nonsporeforming rod (Fig 31.1), exhibiting characteristic gram-positive cell wall structure by electron microscopy. The organism is a facultative anaerobe, and can grow over a wide temperature range on ordinary media. Isolates from clinical cases produce a narrow zone of β-hemolysis around or beneath the colonies on blood agar (Fig 31.2). Characteristic tumbling motility in a hanging drop preparation is more pronounced after growth at 20–25 C than at 37 C, and a typical umbrella-type growth is observed in semisolid motility medium (Fig 31.3).

Clinical Manifestations

A wide variety of clinical manifestations have been described with infections caused by *L. monocytogenes* (27.). Most infections reported in the United States (22), however, occur in one of three clinical settings:
Nonspecific "flu-like" illness during pregnancy or puerperal sepsis
Neonatal sepsis (early-onset disease) or meningitis (late-onset disease)
Sepsis or meningitis in immunocompromised hosts
Although other infections are reported less frequently, there appear to be no sufficiently characteristic manifestations to distinguish any infection caused by *L. monocytogenes* from a similar one caused by other organisms. Thus, diagnosis must depend on appropriate bacteriological findings.

Epidemiology

L. monocytogenes is ubiquitous in nature, and strains have been isolated in association with disease in a wide variety of fish, birds, and mammals (11, 33). Asymptomatic carriage in apparently healthy people and animals has been reported with increasing frequency. Ralovich, in summarizing data from several studies and population groups in Hungary, reported the overall rate of fecal carriage as 2.2% (26). Gregorio and Eveland (13) reported a carriage rate of 1.75% in 400 patients hospitalized in Michigan with diagnoses other than listeriosis. Significantly higher carriage rates have been reported in other studies (8, 17). The age distribution of human cases reported in the United States is not uniform, with most cases occurring at the extremes. Neonatal listeriosis constitutes the largest group of identified infections, and among infants appears to share similarities with infections caused by the Group B streptococcus (1, 29). Factors responsible for the increasing incidence with advancing age have been poorly characterized. Between these extremes of age, listeriosis occurs primarily in association with pregnancy or underlying immune deficiency states, particularly lymphoreticular malignancies. There are, however, well documented cases in otherwise healthy individuals (20). Primary cutaneous listeriosis is apparently an occupationally related disease in individuals (e.g., veterinarians) who handle infected animal material (6).

Public Health Significance

The ubiquitous nature of the organism and the sporadic nature of the disease in the United States make it unlikely that most preventive measures will have a significant impact on the reported incidence of listeriosis. Proper handling of potentially infected material from either human or animal sources and prompt treatment of recognized maternal listeriosis are the best potential preventive measures. Infected hospitalized patients should be isolated in an at-

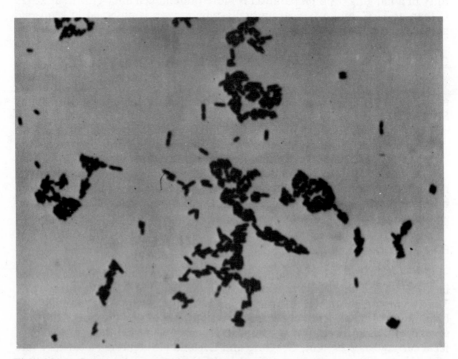

Figure 31.1. Gram-stain morphology of *Listeria monocytogenes.*

tempt to limit nosocomial transmission. Practicing physicians and veterinarians should carefully document and report infections to provide further understanding of the epidemiology of listeriosis.

Collection and Processing of Specimens

Kind of Specimen Required

Appropriate specimens for culture vary with the clinical syndrome, but *L. monocytogenes* is readily isolated from the usual sources such as blood, cerebrospinal fluid, amniotic fluid, and genital tract secretions. In some laboratories, primary isolation from biopsy material and placental or fetal tissue has been successful. Although present serological techniques for the diagnosis of

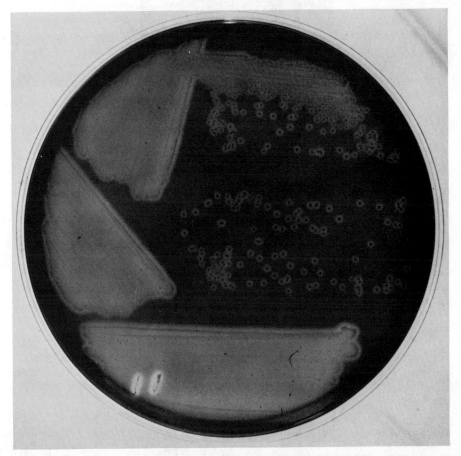

Figure 31.2. *Listeria monocytogenes* colonies on HIA with 5% rabbit blood after 18–24 hr incubation at 35 C.

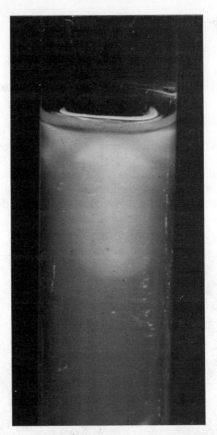

Figure 31.3. Umbrella-type formation of *Listeria monocytogenes* in motility medium.

listeriosis are inadequate, acute and convalescent sera may be of value in selected patients (28) and, when possible, paired sera from bacteriologically confirmed cases should be forwarded to the National *Listeria* Typing Center, Center for Disease Control (CDC), Atlanta, GA 30333, for future epidemiologic
use and test evaluation.

Time of Collection

Appropriate specimens should be obtained whenever clinically indicated,
preferably before any antibiotics have been administered. Serum specimens
should be obtained as early as possible in the illness and at 2–3 week intervals
thereafter.

Number of Specimens

Multiple specimens for culture from a variety of sources will, in general,
improve the rate of positive isolations. Likewise, serial serum specimens at 2-

week intervals for 6–8 weeks may improve serodiagnosis since the optimum interval between specimens has not been established.

Diagnostic Procedures

Microscopic Examination

Direct examination of the Gram-stained sediment of centrifuged cerebrospinal or amniotic fluid is useful in establishing a tentative diagnosis and planning further diagnostic procedures. Examination of hanging-drop preparations of such specimens for the characteristic tumbling motility of *L. monocytogenes* may be helpful. Specific immunochemical staining with fluorescent antibody (FA) may also be helpful in preliminary identification of organisms seen on Gram stain from normally contaminated sources such as stool, the female genital tract, and the respiratory tract (3). Every attempt should be made to confirm FA-positive specimens by cultural procedures.

Selection and Inoculation of Primary Culture Media

Although a number of investigators have recommended a variety of selective media for primary isolation of *L. monocytogenes* (26, 27), most clinical isolations are made on conventional media. Heart infusion agar plates containing 5% sheep or rabbit blood, brain heart infusion broth, and various commercial blood culture media have all been satisfactory. The inoculum should be stabbed into the agar as well as streaked for isolation. The β-hemolysis is usually marked in the stab at 18–24 hr, whereas hemolysis surrounding individual colonies may be weak. Cold enrichment procedures have occasionally improved isolation rates from tissue sources and contaminated specimens (12).

Identification Procedures

L. monocytogenes strains from pathological sources appear as round translucent colonies showing narrow-zone, β-hemolysis (serotype 5 organisms show wide-zone hemolysis) on blood agar plates or appear blue-green on clear agar plates when examined with oblique light (10). Gram stains of colonies from solid media reveal short, gram-positive coccobacilli with occasional short chains and are frequently confused with various streptococci. Gram stains of broth cultures generally reveal longer gram-positive bacilli with the more typical palisade formation characteristic of diphtheroids. Occasionally, uneven staining and excessive decolorization leads to confusion with gram-negative, pleomorphic organisms such as *Haemophilus*. Presumptive biochemical identification of *L. monocytogenes* can be made on the basis of the differentiating characteristics shown in Table 31.1. Some strains such as *L. monocytogenes* serotype 4f, *L. grayi*, and *L. murrayi* are not β-hemolytic. These strains are usually nonpathogenic and are isolated from sources other than blood or cerebrospinal fluid. Separate species designation as *L. bulgarica* has recently been proposed for *L. monocytogenes* serotype 5 strains (15). These strains have been

TABLE 31.1—BIOCHEMICAL CHARACTERISTICS OF STRAINS OF *LISTERIA*

SPECIES	GRAM STAIN	HEMOL-YSIS	UMBRELLA MOTILITY	CATA-LASE	V.P.[a]	NITRATE REDUC-TION	LITMUS MILK	ACID PRODUCTION IN ENTERIC BASE FROM				
								GLU-COSE	MAL-TOSE	RHAM-NOSE	XY-LOSE	MANNI-TOL
L. monocytogenes Usual serotypes from clinical sources	gram-positive coccobacilli (+)	Beta	+	+	+	−	IR[b]	+	+	+	−	−
Serotype 5[c]	+	Wide-zone beta	−/+	+	+	−	IR	+[e]	+[e]	−[e]	+[e]	−[e]
L. grayi[d]	+	Not beta	+	+	+	−	IR	+	+	−	−	+
L. murrayi[d]	+	Not beta	+	+	+	+	IR	+	+	−	−	+

[a] Method of Coblentz.
[b] Indicator reduction.
[c] Recently proposed as a separate species *L. bulgarica* (15).
[d] Taxonomic status for both species and genus not definitely established (30, 35).
[e] Serum must be added to the base to enhance growth.

reported from several countries and are isolated predominantly from veterinary sources. They are distinguished from other strains of *L. monocytogenes* by a wide zone of β-hemolysis and poor growth in unmodified medium (4). Recent taxonomic studies indicate that *L. murrayi* may be a biovar of *L. grayi* (35) and separate genus status has been proposed for these species (30). Definitive serological identification requires serotyping of both somatic (O) and flagellar (H) antigens. Isolates presumptively identified as *L. monocytogenes* should be submitted through the state health department to: National *Listeria* Typing Center, Bacterial Immunology Branch, CDC, Atlanta, GA 30333.

Serologic procedures

(i) Although *L. monocytogenes* somatic (type 1, type 4, and polyvalent) and control antigens and directions for a rapid slide and tube agglutination test are available commercially (Difco), in general, isolates should be submitted to CDC through the state health department for more definitive serotyping.

(ii) Despite extensive attempts to develop serological techniques for diagnosing listeriosis, none has proved satisfactory and few centers attempt serodiagnosis. A standardized agglutination test is available and may be of value in selected patients (19). Acute- and convalescent-phase sera should be submitted to CDC through the state health department.

Use of marker systems

Although phage typing of *L. monocytogenes* has not been extensively investigated, it has been used in a presumptive typing system (32), and some studies have indicated that it is potentially useful for epidemiologic and taxonomic investigations (2, 31).

Miscellaneous procedures

(i) Additional carbohydrate fermentation studies may be helpful in characterizing *Listeria* strains (7). In our laboratory, *L. monocytogenes* serotypes lacking the flagellar C factor (1a, 2, 3a, 3c) infrequently ferment melezitose.

(ii) Virulence can be confirmed experimentally by ophthalmic pathogenicity in rabbits (Anton test) (16), intraperitoneal inoculation of mice (18), and inoculation of the chorioallantoic membrane of eggs (25). It is not necessary to determine virulence for routine identification and confirmation of clinical isolates.

(iii) Pathogenic strains of *L. monocytogenes* from the United States generally appear to differ from nonpathogenic strains on the basis of three *in vitro* characteristics: (a) accentuated hemolysis of sheep blood in the presence of *Staphylococcus aureus* β-toxin (modified CAMP phenomenon), (b) fermentation of rhamnose, and (c) failure to ferment xylose (14).

Antimicrobic Susceptibility and Resistance

A number of reports have discussed broth or agar dilution antibiotic susceptibility testing of *L. monocytogenes* strains to a variety of antimicrobial

TABLE 31.2—SUSCEPTIBILITY OF *LISTERIA MONOCYTOGENES* STRAINS TO NINE ANTIBIOTICS[a]

| ANTIBIOTICS | MIC (μG/ML)[b] | | MIC BREAKPOINT (μG/ML) |
	RANGE	MEDIAN	SUSCEPTIBLE
Erythromycin	0.06–0.05	0.125	≤ 2.0
Penicillin	≤0.06–1.0	0.25	≤ 1.5
Ampicillin	0.06–1.0	0.25	≤ 1.5
Tetracycline	≤0.05–2.0	1.0	≤ 4.0
Gentamicin	0.5–8.0	2.0	≤ 6.0
Kanamycin	8.0–32.0	16.0	≤ 6.0
Streptomycin	8.0–64.0	16.0	≤ 6.0
Chloramphenicol	4.0–8.0	4.0	≤12.5
Cephalothin	2.0–8.0	4.0	≤10.0

[a] Modified from Reference 34.
[b] Results of broth microdilution method with Trypticase soy broth.

agents (5, 23, 24). Results of these studies have varied with media and methodology and are greatly influenced by such factors as inoculum size and definition of endpoints. Recent studies (34) with a large number of clinical isolates from the United States (Table 31.2) indicate a homogeneous population of organisms sensitive to the antibiotics most often recommended for treatment (ampicillin, penicillin, erythromycin, and tetracycline). Unlike most other susceptible organisms, the minimal bactericidal concentration (MBC) for ampicillin and penicillin significantly exceeded the minimal inhibitory concentratior. (MIC). The significance of this observation and the possible emergence of resistant strains in clinical failures during treatment with a given antibiotic has not been determined. Antibiotic combinations including a penicillin and an aminoglycoside demonstrate *in vitro* synergism with most isolates and appear to have at least a theoretical advantage as initial therapy for high-risk groups such as neonates and immunosuppressed patients (9, 21, 34).

Evaluation of Laboratory Findings

Prompt diagnosis of infections caused by *L. monocytogenes* requires close cooperation between the clinician and the laboratory. Listeriosis should be suspected if gram-positive bacilli are seen on Gram-stained material or isolated on culture from patients with clinical manifestations compatible with infections caused by this organism. Presumptive biochemical characterization should be undertaken, and a tentative report including antibiotic susceptibilities should be provided for organisms conforming to the characteristics described for *L. monocytogenes*. Definitive serological identification can be made on isolates submitted to CDC through the state health department.

References

1. ALBRITTON WL, WIGGINS GL, and FEELEY JC: Neonatal listeriosis: distribution of serotypes in relation to age at onset of disease. J Pediatr 88:481–483, 1976

2. AUDURIER A, ROCOURT J, and COURTIEU AL: Isolement et caracterisation de bacterio-phages de *Listeria monocytogenes*. Ann Microbiol (Inst Pasteur) 128A:185–198, 1977
3. CHERRY WB and MOODY MD: Fluorescent antibody techniques in diagnostic microbiology. Bacteriol Rev 29:222–250, 1965
4. COOPER RF, DENNIS SM, and McMAHON KJ: Characterization of *Listeria monocytogenes* serotype 5. Am J Vet Res 34:975–978, 1973
5. COURTIEU AL, ESPAZE EP, and DRUGEON H: *In vitro* sensitivity to antibiotics of some *Listeria* strains isolated in France. *In* Problems of Listeriosis. Woodbine M (ed.). Proceedings of the Sixth International Symposium. Leicester Univ Press, Leicester, England, 1975, pp 45–51
6. DINCSOY MY, BOOKER CR, and SCOTT RB: Skin manifestation in listeria infection. J Natl Med Assoc 57:290–296, 1965
7. EMODY L and RALOVICH B: Ability of *Listeria monocytogenes* strains to attack carbohydrates and related compounds. Acta Microbiol Acad Sci Hung 19:287–291, 1972
8. GOMEZ-MAMPASO E, MICHAUX L, DERAFAEL L, CARVAJAL A, and BAQUERO F: Faecal *Listeria monocytogenes* carriers and perinatal mortality. *In* Problems of Listeriosis. Woodbine M (ed.). Proceedings of the Sixth International Symposium. Leicester Univ Press, Leicester, England, 1975, pp 206–213
9. GORDON RC, BARRETT FF, and CLARK DJ: Influence of several antibiotics, singly and in combination, on the growth of *Listeria monocytogenes*. J Pediatr 80:667–670, 1972
10. GRAY ML: A rapid method for the detection of colonies of *Listeria monocytogenes*. Zentralbl Bakteriol Parasitenkd Abt Infektionskr Hyg 1: Orig 169:373–377, 1957
11. GRAY ML and KILLINGER AH: *Listeria monocytogenes* and listeric infections. Bacteriol Rev 30:29–32, 1966
12. GRAY ML, STAFSETH HJ, THORP F JR, SCHOLL LB, and RILEY WF JR: A new technique for isolating *Listerellae* from the bovine brain. J Bacteriol 55:471–476, 1948
13. GREGORIO SB and EVELAND WC: Isolation of *Listeria monocytogenes* from inapparent sources in Michigan. *In* Problems of Listeriosis. Woodbine M (ed.). Proceedings of the Sixth International Symposium. Leicester Univ Press, Leicester, England, 1975, pp 87–93
14. GROVES RD and WELSHIMER HJ: Separation of pathogenic from apathogenic *Listeria monocytogenes* by three *in vitro* reactions. J Clin Microbiol 5:559–563, 1977
15. IWANOW I: Establishment of nonmotile strains of *Listeria monocytogenes* type 5. *In* Problems of Listeriosis. Woodbine M (ed.). Proceedings of the Sixth International Symposium. Leicester Univ Press, Leicester, England, 1975, pp 18–26
16. JULIANELLE LA and MORRIS MD: Pathologic changes in *Listerella* infection. Ann Intern Med 14:608, 1940
17. KAMPELMACHER EH, HUYSINGA WT, and VAN NOORLE JANSEN LM: The presence of *Listeria monocytogenes* in feces of pregnant women and neonates. Zentralbl Bakteriol Parasitenkd Abt Infektionskr Hyg 1: Orig Reihe A 222:258–262, 1972
18. KAUTTER DA, SILVERMAN SJ, ROESSLER WG, and DRAWDY JF: Virulence of *Listeria monocytogenes* for experimental animals. J Infect Dis 112:167–180, 1963
19. LARSEN SA, WIGGINS GL, and ALBRITTON WL: Immune response to *Listeria*. *In* Manual of Clinical Immunology. Rose NR and Friedman H (eds.). American Society for Microbiology, Washington, DC, 1976, pp 318–321
20. MEDOFF G, KUNZ LJ, and WEINBERG AN: Listeriosis in humans: an evaluation. J Infect Dis 123:247–250, 1971
21. MOELLERING RC JR, MEDOFF G, LEECH I, WENNERSTEN C, and KUNA LJ: Antibiotic synergism against *Listeria monocytogenes*. Antimicrob Agents Chemother 1:30–34, 1972
22. MOORE RM and ZEHMER RB: Listeriosis in the United States, 1971. J Infect Dis 127:610–611, 1973
23. NELSON JD, SHELTON S, and PARKS D: Antibiotic susceptibility of *Listeria monocytogenes* and treatment of neonatal listeriosis with ampicillin. Acta Paediatr Scand 56:151–158, 1967
24. NYSTROM KG and KARLSSON KA: Sensitivity of *Listeria monocytogenes in vitro* to different antibiotics and chemotherapeutics. Acta Paediatr 50:113–116, 1961
25. PATERSON JS: Flagellar antigens of organisms of the genus *Listerella*. J Pathol Bacteriol 48:25, 1939

26. RALOVICH B: Selective and enrichment media to isolate *Listeria*. *In* Problems of Listeriosis. Woodbine M (ed.). Proceedings of the Sixth International Symposium. Leicester Univ Press, Leicester, England, 1975, pp 286–294

27. SEELIGER HPR: Listeriosis. S. Karger, Basel-New York, 1961

28. SEELIGER HPR and FINGER H: Analytical serology of *Listeria*. *In* Analytical Serology of Microorganisms. Kwapinski JBG (ed.). John Wiley and Sons, New York, 1969, pp 549–608

29. SEELIGER HPR and FINGER H: Listeriosis. *In* Infectious Diseases of the Fetus and Newborn Infant. Remington JS and Klein JO (eds.). WB Saunders Co, Philadelphia, 1976, pp 333–365

30. STUART SE and WELSHIMER HJ: Taxonomic re-examination of *Listeria* Pirie and transfer of *Listeria grayi* and *Listeria murraya*. Int J Syst Bacteriol 24:177–185. 1974

31. SWORD CP and PICKETT MJ: The isolation and characterization of bacteriophages from *Listeria monocytogenes*. J Gen Microbiol 25:241–248, 1961

32. WATSON BB and EVELAND WC: The application of phage-fluorescent antiphage staining system in specific identification of *Listeria monocytogenes*. I. Species specificity and immunofluorescent sensitivity of *Listeria monocytogenes* phage observed in smear preparations. J Infect Dis 115:363–369, 1965

33. WEIS J and SEELIGER HPR: Incidence of *Listeria monocytogenes* in nature. Appl Microbiol 30:29–32, 1975

34. WIGGINS GL, ALBRITTON WL, and FEELEY JC: Antibiotic susceptibility of clinical isolates of *Listeria monocytogenes*. Antimicrob Agents Chemother 13:854–860, 1978

35. WILKINSON BJ and JONES D: A numerical taxonomic survey of *Listeria* and related bacteria. J Gen Microbiol 98:399–421, 1977

CHAPTER 32

MYCOPLASMA INFECTION

Wallace A. Clyde, Jr.

Introduction

Mycoplasma is the common term used to indicate the unique micro-organisms which constitute Class Mollicutes. At present over 60 mycoplasmas have been given species designations, and they are grouped taxonomically into three families and six genera. These organisms have been linked etiologically with a wide variety of disease processes that affect man and other mammals, birds, insects, and plants. Some species appear to be nonpathogenic, existing as components of the autochthonous microflora or in soil, warm springs, or coal refuse. In view of these ecologic considerations, it can be appreciated that the mycoplasmas are a heterogeneous group. However, as with other microbial classes, members of Class Mollicutes share certain common features.

The cardinal characteristic of mycoplasmas is lack of cell-wall materials of the type seen in bacteria. The organisms are bound by tri-layered unit membranes, a quality that confers absolute insensitivity to the penicillins as well as failure to react with organic dyes used in many staining procedures. Mycoplasmas are considerably smaller than bacteria, in the size range of 0.1–0.3 μm for the largest dimension, and thus easily pass filters which retain larger structures. Accordingly, individual organisms cannot be resolved by standard light microscopy, but they can be seen with well-aligned dark-field and phase-contrast instruments. While lack of rigid cell wall structure suggests that mycoplasmas would be naturally pleomorphic, in fact several species are known to have characteristic shapes—spirals, filaments, ovals—under optimal conditions. Some have differentiated poles or organelles used for attachment to surfaces and are motile.

Another prime feature of mycoplasmas is growth as small colonies (0.05–2 mm diameter) which embed in the interstices of solid media. For this reason special techniques are required for laboratory manipulations such as staining and subculture. Generally these organisms can be considered fastidious, requiring a rich medium containing native protein and supplements including amino acids and peptides. Many substances are inhibitory to mycoplasma growth, which dictates precise quality control of all medium formulations used for the cultivation of these organisms. Since mycoplasmas grow more slowly than bacterial and mycotic organisms, primary isolation must involve selective media. Most mycoplasmas will grow in the presence of penicillin, amphoteri-

cin B, and thallium acetate, which are often used to inhibit other forms in impure inocula. Medium composition, pH, atmosphere, and incubation temperature all must be tailored to the particular mycoplasmal species being cultured.

The focus of this chapter is on mycoplasmas indigenous to man, although
others will be mentioned if there is public health significance or when matters
concern diagnostic accuracy. Table 32.1 lists species that have been isolated
from man, anatomic sites in which they are usually found, and their known
disease associations. The species include one pathogen (*M. pneumoniae*), two
which can best be considered as opportunistic pathogens (*M. hominis, U. urealyticum*), and several which are found among the normal microbial flora.

Mycoplasmas Causing Disease in Man

Mycoplasma pneumoniae

Mycoplasma pneumoniae is a minute filament (0.1 × 2.0 μm) having the
capacity for gliding motility. A differentiated terminal organelle attaches the
organism to host cell membranes with a neuraminic acid receptor mechanism.
Growth on solid medium requires the presence of serum and heat stable components from aqueous extracts of baker's yeast. With incubation at 35–37 C,
colonies measuring 10–100 μm in diameter can be seen in 7–10 days. Generally colonies are spherical and slightly granular, with a faint lemon-yellow
color, but features vary depending on medium composition and degree of
crowding on the agar. In broth medium growth produces no gross turbidity,

TABLE 32.1—MYCOPLASMA SPECIES INDIGENOUS TO MAN*

SPECIES	HABITAT	PATHOBIOLOGY	DISTINCTIVE FEATURES
M. pneumoniae	Respiratory tract	Tracheo-bronchitis pneumonia	Slow-growing; ferments carbohydrates; β-hemolysis of sheep erythrocytes.
M. orale	Pharynx	Normal flora	Hydrolyzes arginine; colony resembles *M. pneumoniae*.
M. buccale	Oropharynx	Normal flora	Isolated rarely.
M. faucium	Oropharynx	Normal flora	Isolated rarely.
M. salivarium	Gingiva, oropharynx	Normal flora	Hydrolyzes arginine; large fried-egg colony.
M. fermentans	Genital tract, rarely pharynx	Normal flora	Ferments carbohydrates; hydrolyzes arginine.
M. hominis	Genital tract, oropharynx occasionally	Normal flora, salpingitis, postpartum sepsis, neonatal abscesses	Hydrolyzes arginine; large fried-egg colony; grows rapidly.
U. urealyticum	Genital tract, oropharynx occasionally	Normal flora, urethritis, congenital pneumonia, amnionitis	Tiny colonies grow rapidly; acid pH optimum for growth; produces urease.

* Other species which have been isolated include *M. lipophilum, M. primatum,* and *A. laidlawii.*

but when viewed microscopically (100×), refractile "spherules" are seen attached to the culture vessel surfaces. Many carbohydrates are fermented by the organisms, and the pH reduction accompanying acid metabolite production is a convenient reflection of growth in liquid medium containing suitable substrate and indicator dye. Production of peroxide is another metabolic feature useful in identification of the species. Although various phenotypic strain variations have been described, only one serotype of *M. pneumoniae* is recognized (24).

Mycoplasma hominis

Mycoplasma hominis is generally a spherical organism or short filament in the size range of 0.2 μm. Growth requirements are less stringent than for *M. pneumoniae*, although serum must be present as a source of sterol. Solid media incubated at 35–37 C yield colonies measuring 0.1–1.0 mm in diameter within 2–4 days. If well-separated the colonies show the classical "fried egg" morphology of mycoplasmas, produced by a central portion that is more deeply embedded in the agar than is the peripheral zone. In older colonies the periphery takes on a vacuolated appearance due to production of large, probably degenerative forms. In liquid media growth results in a faint homogeneous turbidity best visualized with oblique fluorescent illumination. Carbohydrates are not fermented, but arginine deaminase activity results in production of ammonia with a consequent pH rise accompanying growth. There is evidence that there are multiple serotypes of *M. hominis* (23).

Ureaplasma urealyticum

Ureaplasma urealyticum is a small spherical organism which, like *M. pneumoniae,* has the ability to attach to host cells. Members of this genus were formerly called "T" (for tiny) strains because of small colony size (5–25 μm) on solid media. This may represent medium deficiency rather than a fixed characteristic, since larger colonies can be grown with special buffering systems. Anaerobic conditions have been used widely for propagation, but recent information suggests that the presence of CO_2 (5%–10%) may be more important than the reduction of oxygen. After incubation for 24–48 hr at 35–37 C, colonies are seen as thin, rather granular, fried-egg forms on solid media. Organisms grow with similar rapidity in liquid media, but no turbidity is evident. As the species name implies, these organisms produce a urease which is a unique metabolic feature among the mycoplasmas. Cleavage of urea with production of ammonia raises medium pH rapidly and constitutes a visible reflection of growth in the presence of appropriate indicators. At present 8 distinct serotypes of *U. urealyticum* have been designated (3).

Clinical Manifestations

The expression of *M. pneumoniae* infections ranges from entirely subclinical disease through tracheobronchitis to pneumonia. This mycoplasma was identified originally as the causative agent of so-called primary atypical pneumonia and has been characterized most completely in this syndrome. After a 2- to 4-week incubation period, symptoms begin insidiously with dry throat, fever, and malaise. This influenza-like illness continues with development of persistent dry cough followed by productive cough and headache. Physical examination may be unremarkable initially, but as cough becomes productive, fine rales sometimes associated with localized wheezing may be heard. Chest X ray usually reveals a patchy bronchopneumonia involving one of the lower lobes, but a wide spectrum of changes including segmental atelectasis and lobar consolidation have been described. Unusual manifestations include frank hemoptysis, pleuritic pain, pleural effusion, and various nonrespiratory findings such as nondescript rashes, erythema multiforme, hemolytic anemia, arthritis, and several neurologic syndromes. Disease is usually mild and self-limited, running its course in 2–4 weeks. Resolution of symptoms and signs is accelerated with appropriate antibiotic therapy.

The manifestations of *M. hominis* infection are less well-defined, since the organism is found frequently as a component of the normal pharyngeal and genital tract flora. It has been isolated somewhat more frequently from subjects with respiratory illnesses including pharyngitis, but there are no pathognomonic findings. Pharyngitis was produced experimentally in adult volunteers inoculated with this organism (27). Instances of postpartum fever have been associated with *M. hominis* sepsis, presumably resulting from opportunistic invasion of the compromised female genital tract; this is a self-limited process without known complications or sequelae (26). The frequency of this cause of postpartum fever is unknown, but is important to establish from the standpoint of differential diagnosis and for therapeutic considerations. Isolated cases of "sterile" scalp abscesses yielding only *M. hominis* on culture have been described in newborn infants (22). Minor scalp wounds are a likely portal of entry for these infections, and the increasing use of obstetrical instrumentation including intrauterine monitoring devices raises the potential for problems of this type.

Ureaplasma urealyticum is another common inhabitant of the genital tracts of both sexes. Venereal transmission is suggested by the observation that colonization frequency is directly proportional to degree of sexual activity (26). A relationship has been established between *U. urealyticum* and nongonococcal urethritis in the male, but the etiologic association between organisms and disease is a matter of unresolved controversy. *Ureaplasma* species have also been linked to instances of amnionitis, fetal wastage, and congenital or neonatal pneumonia (5, 21, 31). Appropriate studies have not yet been done to assess the true importance of ureaplasmas in these situations.

Epidemiology

Respiratory disease caused by *M. pneumoniae* occurs both endemically and in irregular, protracted epidemics. Although the disease may occur in any season, it has been observed frequently in the fall when tracheobronchitis and pneumonia from other causes are less common. Transmission is presumed to occur by a person-to-person droplet route. As evidenced by studies in families, communicability seems to be of high order, although not all infected individuals manifest overt clinical disease (17). Pneumonia caused by *M. pneumoniae* has its peak incidence in late childhood and adolescence. Disease is uncommon below age 5, although some such infections do occur (16). In studies of college populations, this organism has accounted for up to 50% of all cases of pneumonia; as a corollary, the incidence of pneumonia is low in years when *M. pneumoniae* is less prevalent. Many outbreaks have been described in institutional settings and among the Armed Forces. In a metropolitan study the yearly incidence of *M. pneumoniae* pneumonia was estimated to be as high as 3.2/1000 population; depending upon age grouping concerned, this represented the cause of 6%–28% of all pneumonia cases observed (1). Prospective studies have shown that infections, including those associated with pneumonia, can recur within 2–4 years suggesting that re-infections are not unusual.

The epidemiology of *M. hominis* and *U. urealyticum* is less clearly defined since, unlike *M. pneumoniae,* they can be found as normal mucosal flora in many individuals. Surveillance studies have shown a low incidence in children and among nuns and a high incidence among adults with multiple consorts, suggesting that genital colonization is by venereal transmission (26). The fact that sexually transmitted diseases of all kinds follow this same pattern has complicated assessment of the disease relationship of *U. urealyticum* in epidemiologic studies. Transmission of mycoplasmas from mother to newborn infant has been demonstrated, but generally there has been no associated morbidity except for a trend toward lower birth weight (22).

Public Health Significance

As indicated above, *M. pneumoniae* is a major contributor to the lower respiratory disease of adolescents and young adults, thereby constituting a significant health problem among students, the work force, and military personnel. Since the disease is rarely fatal, the impact is measured more in terms of lost school and work days as well as in health care effort and cost. If the controversies concerning the etiologic role of ureaplasmas are resolved, they could become another important venereal disease or cause of fetal wastage.

Mycoplasmas have other implications for public health in addition to their role in human disease. It is now known that various diseases affecting the quality and yield of grains and citrus fruits are caused by *Spiroplasma* species transmitted via insect vectors. The many mycoplasma diseases of avian, bovine, ovine, and porcine species can influence the production of these important protein sources if not successfully controlled. The prototypic mycoplasmal disease—bovine pleuropneumonia caused by *M. mycoides*—is still a problem among cattle in underdeveloped areas of the world today, although it has been controlled by quarantine measures in more advanced countries. Less progress has been made in control of swine pneumonias (*M. hyorhinis, M. hyopneumoniae*) and in respiratory diseases of poultry (*M. gallisepticum* and others).

The importance of viral diagnosis and surveillance programs to public health represents another point where mycoplasmas exert a more subtle but significant influence. Mycoplasmas persist in tissue cultures in the presence of antimicrobials which inhibit bacteria and fungi, creating a problem for laboratories especially in the maintenance of continuous cell lines. Depending upon species involved the organisms can interfere with either cell or viral growth or can themselves produce confusing cytopathic effects. Formerly cell cultures were often contaminated with human oropharyngeal mycoplasma species. Recognition of this problem with consequent improvement in technique has altered the epidemiology of culture contamination so that currently the main source is serum or other biologic supplements used in media. Problems associated with mycoplasmal contamination of tissue cultures are costly in terms of effort and expense related to the increased quality control measures in the laboratory which are necessitated.

Collection and Processing of Specimens

Specimens and Handling

In the case of *M. pneumoniae* infections, organisms are found throughout the respiratory tract. Thus nasopharyngeal or oropharyngeal swabs, sputum, and tracheal aspirates can be used for culture diagnosis. Tissues are more difficult to process because hemoglobin and other inhibitors (antibodies, lysolecithin, antibiotics) may interfere with successful isolation attempts. The use of "holding" or transport media has not received systematic study relative to *M. pneumoniae,* and no definitive recommendations can be made in this regard. The organisms are relatively stable at 4 to –20 C for several days, but –65 C is required for more extended storage. Ideally, appropriate liquid growth medium should be inoculated on site because the organisms then easily survive transport to the laboratory at ambient temperatures.

Paired serum samples, taken during the acute and convalescent phases of illness, are a useful adjunct to diagnosing *M. pneumoniae* disease. Since the same blood specimens are often used for cold hemagglutinin titration, they should be allowed to clot at 22–37 C before sera are removed. If a growth inhibition serology is to be performed (see below), hemolyzed samples should not be analyzed, and antibiotic administration to the patient should be noted.

Suitable specimens for isolating *M. hominis* include throat swabs, whole blood, urethral discharge, and cervical swabs depending upon the clinical situation involved. For *U. urealyticum* urethral scrapings, voided urine, and fetal membranes or tissues may be used. The direct inoculation of liquid growth medium is again recommended for transport to the laboratory. At present there is little reason to collect serum specimens for diagnostic serology, since the techniques necessary remain in the research phase and are not routinely available.

Time of Collection

Specimens for isolation of *M. pneumoniae* are usually collected during the acute phase of illness. However, longitudinal studies have shown that the organisms persist in the nasopharynx for 4–6 weeks, so that a late specimen may be used to obtain a diagnosis. Because of the long incubation period and insidious onset of clinical disease, serum antibodies may be elevated in acute-phase specimens. A serum sample collected 2–4 weeks later is useful for further diagnostic interpretation.

Microbiologic Procedures

Microscopic Examination

As indicated above, mycoplasmas are too small to visualize with ordinary light microscopy, and they fail to react with organic dyes such as those used in the Gram-staining procedure. Direct diagnosis of *M. pneumoniae* infection has been described in reports of using immunofluorescence for sputum samples (19), the limiting factor being availability of suitable reagents. Sputum cytology may be useful in obtaining a tentative diagnosis and in excluding other possibilities (10). The findings may include few or no bacteria, a mixture of polymorphonuclear leukocytes and macrophages, clumps of ciliated epithelial cells, and desquamated apical tips of ciliated cells (ciliocytophthoria). Occasionally seen are "rosette" configurations, an epithelial cell surrounded by polymorphonuclear cells, which may represent immune phagocytosis.

Inoculation of Primary Media

As in other areas of diagnostic microbiology, various media and cultural conditions would be required to isolate all recognized mycoplasmal species. It is beyond the scope of this chapter to discuss or even review them all. Even for the three mycoplasmas of man discussed above, various isolation techniques have been described. Since adequate comparative study of these methods has not been done, only procedures which have been most widely used will be described in detail with variations the author has found useful. Included are modifications of the media originally described by Hayflick for *M. pneumoniae* (Table 32.2) (18) and by Shepard for *U. urealyticum* (Table 32.3) (33); both formulae support the growth of *M. hominis*. A recent report suggests a superior formula for the primary isolation of *M. pneumoniae* (39).

Both solid and liquid versions of the 2 media may be used for diagnostic work. Agar has the advantages of handling ease and rapid recognition of growth, along with the disadvantage of short shelf life. Broth offers greater isolation sensitivity and storage quality (aliquots can be held frozen if desired) than agar, but subculture to agar is required for demonstration of growth and identification procedures. Choices thus depend upon the aim of study and needs of individual laboratories.

Solid mycoplasma media

Media should be freshly prepared or stored at 4 C less than 2 weeks to avoid drying and loss of antibiotic activity. Plates can be inoculated directly with charged cotton swabs passed over the entire agar surface. It is not necessary to dilute the inoculum by streaking with a bacteriological loop, since relatively few organisms appear on primary clinical cultures, and the soft agar is easily torn or roughened, making subsequent microscopic observation difficult. If a liquid specimen must be spread, use of a sterile glass rod bent in the form of a small hockey stick gives good results. After inoculation plates should be handled carefully to prevent drying. Sealing in a small plastic bag is prudent if there will be a delay in transporting plates to the laboratory for humidified incubation.

TABLE 32.2—MYCOPLASMA MEDIUM*

COMPONENTS	AMOUNT (PER LITER)	COMMENTS
Basic ingredients:		
Mycoplasma broth base	21.0 g	Lots must be pre-tested for ability to support optimum growth of *M. pneumoniae*.
Yeast extract	100.0 ml	Active dry baker's yeast 10% w/v in distilled water, autoclaved at 121 C for 5 min and clarified by filtration and centrifugation. A simpler procedure involves autoclaving a 25% w/v yeast suspension in a dialysis casing, dialyzing against distilled water 2–4 days at 4 C, and using the dialysate. Products should be sterilized by autoclaving and stored at −20 C.
Horse serum	200.0 ml	Lots must be pre-tested for ability to support optimum growth of *M. pneumoniae*. An alternative is IgG-free serum.
Distilled water	700.0 ml	Glass-distilled or high-quality de-ionized water recommended.
Optional supplements:		
Penicillin sodium	1,000,000 U	Usually suffices for respiratory tract flora inhibition.
Thallium(ous) acetate	0.5 g	Helpful in suppressing gram-negative flora; *inhibits ureaplasmas*.
Amphotericin B	0.5 g	Helpful in suppressing fungal growth; avoid use if possible, since product contains sodium deoxycholate as a solubilizer.
Dextrose	20.0 ml	U.S.P. sterile 50% solution (broth medium only).
Arginine HCl	4.0 ml	Filter-sterilized 50% stock solution; store −20 C (broth medium only).
Phenol red (sodium salt)	4.0 ml	Autoclave-sterilized 1% stock solution (broth medium only).
Purified agar	8.5 g	Crude agars often inhibitory; equivalent amounts of agarose or Ionagar give superior results.

* Modified after Hayflick (18) and Chanock, Hayflick, and Barile (7).

No pretreatment of specimens is ordinarily required, since the media are formulated to select for mycoplasma growth. Sputum samples should be homogenized by grinding in a mortar and pestle or by being drawn and expelled several times through a needle and syringe. Enzyme or detergent treatment of samples is deleterious to the organisms and should be avoided.

In the laboratory plates should be placed lid side down in a well-humidified incubator at 35–37 C. Growth of *M. pneumoniae* is improved in an atmosphere containing 5% CO_2. The original descriptions of ureaplasmas specified strict anaerobiosis for growth, but some workers now achieve good results by use of 10% CO_2. No special conditions are required for growth of *M. hominis*.

TABLE 32.3—UREAPLASMA MEDIUM*

COMPONENTS	AMOUNT (PER LITER)	COMMENTS
Basic ingredients:		
Mycoplasma broth base	15.0 g	Dissolve, adjust pH to 5.5 with 2 N HCl, auto-
Distilled water	700.0 ml	clave before adding remaining ingredients.
Horse serum	200.0 ml	Unheated. IgG-free serum is unsatisfactory.
Yeast extract	100.0 ml	See Table 32.2.
Urea	2.0 ml	Filter-sterilized 10% solution; store at −20 C.
L-cysteine HCl	5.0 ml	Filter-sterilized 2% solution; store at −20 C.
Enrichment (co-factors, amino acids, vitamins)	1.0 ml	Commercial product (CVA Enrichment, Gibco Diagnostics, or Iso VitaleX, Baltimore Biological Laboratories).
Optional Supplements:		
Penicillin sodium	1,000,000 U	
Phenol red (sodium salt)	1.0 ml	See Table 32.2. Broth medium only.
Purified agar	8.5 gm	For solid medium, add to broth base.
Manganous chloride		Tested only in Shepard's differential medium formula A-7 (19); urea test reagent offers a simple alternative (urea, 1.0 g; manganous chloride, 0.8 g; water, 100 ml). Colonies ≤48 hr old turn brown immediately after a drop is added to agar.

*Based on formulae described by M.C. Shepard (33) and personal communication.

Liquid mycoplasma media

Screw-capped vials of growth media are convenient to handle in the field. These may be inoculated directly with swabs, curettes, loops, or pipettes, taking customary care to prevent contamination of the vial rim. Since pH of the medium is important to maintain vials should be tightly capped during transportation to the laboratory; they should be held at ambient or body temperature rather than cooled.

Identification Procedures

Mycoplasmas grow relatively slowly; examination of cultures for growth at 2, 7, and 14 days is recommended. Because of their small size, mycoplasma colonies rarely can be seen with the naked eye. Agar plate cultures are conveniently scanned with a dissecting microscope at 15–20×, following which suspect colonies can be examined more closely at 35–100× with a standard microscope. Colonies are nearly transparent and are easier to see by looking through the agar and tilting the microscope mirrors to produce an oblique beam. Typical colonies of several human mycoplasma species are shown in Figure 32.1. Morphology is influenced greatly by medium composition, culture age, colony spacing, and incubation conditions. Microscopic examination of agar media introduces the observer to a variety of artifacts which must be distinguished from mycoplasma colonies. Examples are agar chips, granular debris from supplements, crystals, cells from the inoculum, and so-called pseudocolonies. Pseudocolonies are structures composed of fatty or soapy materials from the media which "grow" by accretion in the manner of crystal formation. Some common morphologic varieties are: flat, granular structures; striated volcano-like cones; and dark objects with spiraling arms that resemble pinwheels. Pseudocolonies are more common in old media incubated for prolonged periods. Considerable experience is required to exclude artifacts and make an educated guess of species identity based on colony morphology. Further steps are indicated for diagnosis.

When liquid primary media are used, growth is difficult to detect unless there has been a change in pH as a result of mycoplasma metabolism (acid for *M. pneumoniae*, alkaline for *M. hominis* and *U. urealyticum*). Cultures which appear frankly turbid are probably contaminated by bacterial or fungal growth. After they are inoculated, tubes should be inspected daily for pH change. If a shift is noted, the broth should be subcultured by transferring a drop to the agar medium of corresponding formulation. Organism viability may be lost under extremes of pH, and it is advisable to store a small aliquot at −65 C for later use rather than to continue incubation. If no color change is detected, a blind subculture can be made at specified intervals, such as 3, 7, and 14–21 days.

Once mycoplasma growth has been established a number of techniques

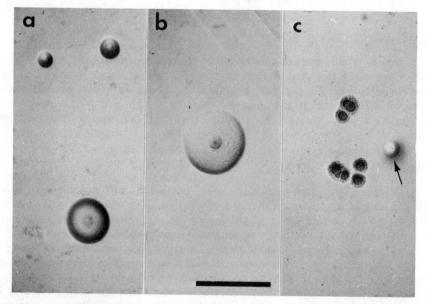

Figure 32.1. Typical colonies of mycoplasmas isolated from human sources: a, *M. pneumoniae*; b, *M. hominis*; c, *U. urealyticum*, serotype VIII. Arrow indicates an artifact (air bubble in agar). Unfixed, unstained. Bar = 0.2 mm.

may be used for speciation of the isolate. The schema depicted in Figure 32.2 is recommended as being widely adaptable to most laboratories but other options will be mentioned.

Growth on agar media

To establish subcultures, a block of agar bearing colonies is cut from the plate with a small sterile spatula. The specimen is dropped into a tube containing 2–4 ml of broth media with indicator and substrates to reflect metabolic activity. The tube is incubated and observed daily for pH shift, which is recorded; this subculture can then be used for the serologic test described below. To the remainder of the primary plate is added a thin layer of melted 5% sheep's blood agar (melted 1% agar in saline cooled to 45 C before erythrocytes are added). This overlay is allowed to solidify after which the plate is reincubated for 24–48 hr and observed grossly for hemolytic zones.

Among the mycoplasma species of man only *M. pneumoniae* produces β hemolysis of sheep's blood (8), this effect being due to elaboration of peroxide by the organisms which diffuses into the surrounding agar (36). The combination of respiratory tract-derived, slow-growing, granular, rounded colonies which are hemolytic under these conditions accordingly identifies *M. pneumoniae.* False-positive results are produced occasionally by incompletely suppressed bacterial colonies, which can be distinguished by noting a dense, dark center in the hemolytic zone viewed with transmitted light (*M. pneumoniae* colonies are nearly transparent). Air bubbles or agar chips in the blood agar overlay can be identified microscopically. At times other mycoplasmal species, especially *M. salivarium,* may discolor or partially lyse overlying blood agar; absence of β hemolysis and the colony morphology allow differentiation from *M. pneumoniae.*

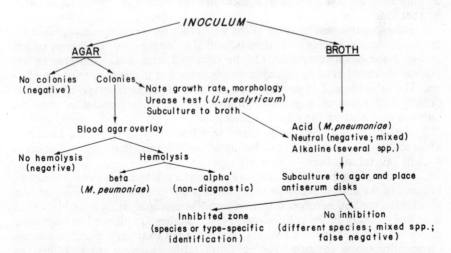

Figure 32.2. Schema for isolation and identification of mycoplasmas from human sources as described in the text.

Ureaplasmas are readily identified on primary agar plate cultures by virtue of their unique urease activity with ammonia production. This is detected by use of manganous sulfate incorporated in the medium (35), or added as a solution (0.8% $MnSO_4$ with 1.0% urea) (34) when colonies appear. The reaction product turns the minute colonies a golden brown color which can be observed microscopically. No further steps are required unless serotyping is to be performed.

Growth in broth media

After presence of organisms is established by pH shift or appearance of typical colonies on agar medium subculture, the primary broth may be used for serologic identification. In the case of mixed mycoplasma species it is necessary to clone organisms by removing single, well-isolated agar colonies to broth for propagation.

Serologic Procedures

Serologic identification of isolates

Advantage is taken of the fact that mycoplasmal growth is inhibited in the presence of specific antiserum (9). A few drops (0.05–0.1 ml) of broth culture containing the unknown organism are placed on a new agar plate and spread evenly with a sterile glass rod bent in the form of a hockey stick. Sterile absorbent paper disks (of the type used for antibiotic sensitivity testing) each are saturated with 0.025–0.05 ml of individual mycoplasma antisera to be used and are applied to the inoculated plate. The plate is incubated to permit colony development, then examined grossly and microscopically for an inhibited zone around a disk as shown schematically in Figure 32.3. Appearance of a definite zone around a given disk identifies the organism species represented by that antiserum.

False-positive results occur if the antiserum used is not monospecific for the mycoplasma species it represents, and if colony growth is uneven or too sparse. False-negative results may be obtained with weak antisera, an inoculum that contained too many mycoplasmas, and if mixed species are present. The inhibition of *Ureasplasma* strains and *M. hominis* is type-specific, requiring either use of a pooled "omniserum" for these species or multiple antisera representing the different serotypes.

Antiserum disks can be prepared in advance by allowing the saturated disks to dry (37). Dried disks can be stored conveniently in sterile containers at 4 C for several months.

Species identification by antiserum growth inhibition is time-consuming because of the subculture steps required to propagate and purify cultures. An alternative method involves direct immunofluorescence using agar blocks cut from the primary or subculture plates (2). Colonies are allowed to react with fluorescein-labeled specific antisera, and are then examined under a fluorescence microscope equipped for epi-illumination. Species are identified by bright, specific fluorescence after reaction with homologous antiserum. This technique has significant advantages in processing time and in permitting recognition of mixed cultures; unfortunately, suitable equipment and reagents are not widely available. The protein composition of mycoplasmas is species and type specific which permits identification by the band patterns produced in high-resolution gel electrophoresis. This method is too complex to be recommended for the usual diagnostic situation.

Patient serology

A wide variety of techniques has been described to measure immune responses to mycoplasmas. Some examples include complement fixation procedures, agglutination and hemagglutination (direct and indirect) methods, various types of inhibition of either mycoplasma growth or metabolism, radio-immuno-precipitation, complement-dependent mycoplasmacidal assays, and indirect immunofluorescence antibody titrations. These tests represent extremes of sensitivity, specificity, and complexity; choices for use will require consideration of study purpose and laboratory capability. Immune responses to *M. pneumoniae* have been studied most extensively, but indications for serologic tests against *M. hominis* and ureaplasmas are less clear and optimal methodology is the subject of on-going research efforts. Accordingly, only tests useful for diagnosis of *M. pneumoniae* infections will be discussed in this context. These include the cold hemagglutination test, complement fixation method, and others to be mentioned briefly.

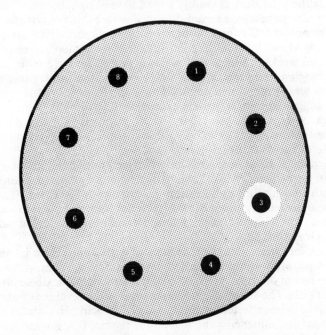

Figure 32.3.   Schematic representation of mycoplasma growth inhibition by antiserum-impregnated paper disks. A clear zone around antiserum number 3 identifies the organism, whereas uninhibited growth is depicted around seven heterologous antisera.

Cold hemagglutination. This procedure was described originally in relation to "primary atypical pneumonia," now known to be caused by *M. pneumoniae* (29). Dilutions of patients' sera are mixed with a suspension of human erythrocytes and incubated at 4 C overnight. Hemagglutination which disappears on warming the test to 37 C constitutes a positive reaction. The phenomenon is based on development of antibodies in the IgM class which react with the I-antigen of the erythrocyte membrane (14). Significant reactions are represented by a fourfold rise (or fall) in titers between paired sera, or single values equal to or greater than a dilution endpoint of 1:128.

Cold hemagglutinins are useful diagnostically, because they rise during the first and second weeks of illness and disappear around the sixth week. However, as they develop in only half of patients proven to be infected with *M. pneumoniae,* their absence by no means excludes the diagnosis. Cold hemagglutinins also have been reported to occur in nonmycoplasma diseases although frequently the titers range less than 128. Continued use of the procedure is justified by simplicity of the test, availability in most serology laboratories, and early appearance of cold hemagglutinins relative to more specific antibodies.

Complement fixation. These procedures for *M. pneumoniae* serology became practicable soon after organism propagation in artificial media was first described (6, 7, 20). Standard methodology used with other test antigens is suitable; thus the procedure is readily added to existing laboratory routines. It has been popular to incubate serum dilutions with 2 units of complement and 4 units of antigen at 4 C overnight before adding the hemolytic system. Antibodies of the IgM and IgG classes contribute to this reaction, developing in the second or third weeks of illness and persisting often for 6–12 months (15). As in other serologic procedures, a fourfold or greater rise in titer measured between paired sera is more meaningful than a single value. Acute relationship to illness is suggested by single titers exceeding 128, or by demonstrating that the titer can be reduced significantly by mercaptoethanol treatment of the serum (since IgM, which is sensitive to this chemical, may predominate early in the course of the disease) (13).

Complement is fixed in the reaction between antibodies and a glycolipid moiety of *M. pneumoniae.* A workable antigen can be prepared by suspending washed organisms in saline and heating the product at 100 C for 10 min to reduce anti-complementary properties. A superior and more specific antigen is obtained using the chloroform-methanol extraction procedure described by Kenny and Grayston (20).

Other serologic tests. Other procedures may be appropriate in certain applications. A growth inhibition method involves adding a known quantity of organisms to serum dilutions in broth medium containing dextrose and phenol red indicator (38). The serum dilution end point is the level preventing organism growth otherwise reflected by production of an acid pH. Careful control of the many variables influencing the reaction is required. A similar test is based on the ability of *M. pneumoniae* to reduce colorless triphenyl-tetrazolium chloride to red formazan, a reaction inhibited by the presence of antiserum (32). These methods are more sensitive than the complement-fixation test, and measure predominantly IgG developing late in convalescence (15). For these reasons they are useful in assessing prior experience with *M. pneumoniae* and for sero-epidemiologic investigations.

Special Methods for Epidemiologic Investigations

Strain variations of *M. pneumoniae* have been described, but they have been produced in the laboratory and are not known to exist under natural disease conditions (24). At present, isolates have identical biologic properties and existence of distinct serotypes has not been described. In contrast, there are eight designated serotypes of *U. urealyticum* (3) and the suggestion of at least three more. Evidence has appeared that multiple serotypes of *M. hominis* exist as well (23), but these have not received official taxonomic status. Epidemiologic studies involving either *M. hominis* or *U. urealyticum* would be facilitated by typing capability in view of the common colonization of asymptomatic individuals and other considerations.

Animal Inoculation

Although isolation of mycoplasmas by inoculation of experimental animals has considerable historical and research significance, this method has been supplanted for clinical diagnosis by availability of improved artificial media and other *in vitro* systems. The initial isolation of *M. pneumoniae* (originally Eaton's agent of atypical pneumonia) was achieved by intranasal inoculation of cotton rats and hamsters (12). Later, the lungs of infected chicken embryos provided the source of antigen for the first practical serologic tool employing indirect immunofluorescence (25). Workers using animals for experimental purposes should recognize that there are mycoplasmas indigenous to these hosts, and due caution must be exercised.

Miscellaneous Procedures

As indicated above, strain variations of *M. pneumoniae* have not been recognized in nature but have been produced in the laboratory. Virulence of strains can be tested by assessing their effects in experimental systems. Histologic changes are produced in the lungs of hamsters inoculated with virulent strains of the organism, while attenuated or avirulent strains produce little or no pathologic change, respectively (24). Virulent strains also produce alteration of ciliary function in tracheal organ cultures, while avirulent strains do not (11).

Antimicrobial Susceptibility

A characteristic feature of mycoplasmas is absolute insensitivity to antibiotics whose mode of action is interference with cell wall synthesis, such as the penicillins and polymyxins. However, most strains are sensitive to members of the tetracycline group. A few species, including *M. pneumoniae* and *U. urealyticum*, are sensitive to the macrolide antibiotics. Although erythromycin has no effect on *M. hominis*, many strains are sensitive to clindamycin (4). Antimicrobial resistance beyond these generalities has not been a notable clinical problem to date, although a major problem in control of tissue culture contaminants is the rapid emergence of mycoplasmas with multiple antibiotic resistance patterns.

In performing susceptibility testing, the relatively slow growth of mycoplasmas and the lability and protein binding of many antibiotics must be considered. No standardized procedures (such as the Kirby-Bauer method) have been described for work with mycoplasmas. Studies have been reported in which modifications of antibiotic disk methods or agar or broth dilution techniques were used. Inhibition of incorporation of radioactive substrates has received only limited attention. In all methods, careful control of inoculum size is important.

Mycoplasmas may be made resistant to some antibiotics in the laboratory by serially passing them in increasingly higher concentrations of the drugs. This has practical importance for serology using the growth inhibition approach, since antibiotics taken by patients may persist in the serum sample. For example, erythromycin is stable for long periods in sera, and use of an erythromycin-resistant strain of *M. pneumoniae* for growth inhibition serology is a useful strategy (28).

Evaluation of Data

Meaningful information from mycoplasma culture services can be obtained only with very careful quality control measures. Appropriate specimens must be transported correctly and processed under conditions favoring growth of the organisms being sought. Generally, the isolation of *M. pneumoniae* in association with a compatible clinical picture is diagnostic; however, it should be remembered that the organism is carried in the upper respiratory tract for 4–6 weeks during convalescence, and that subclinical or asymptomatic infections are frequent. For the reasons stated, it is helpful to have additional evidence of acute infection, such as presence of cold hemagglutinins or the development of specific antibodies between properly timed sera.

Isolation of *M. hominis* and *U. urealyticum* is more difficult to interpret. As previously stated, they are commonly found among the genital tract flora in both sexes, so that their presence does not necessarily imply an etiologic association with intercurrent disease states. Recovery of these mycoplasmas from areas which are normally sterile—blood, unopened abscesses, intact products of conception, internal organs—may be more meaningful. At present means of measuring host-immune responses to the organisms are still being explored; successful technical advances in this area would facilitate our understanding of the pathogenic role of *M. hominis* and *U. urealyticum*.

References

1. ALEXANDER ER, FOY HM, KENNY GE, KRONMAL RA, MCMAHAN R, CLARKE ER, MAC-COLL WA, and GRAYSTON JT: Pneumonia due to *Mycoplasma pneumoniae*. Its incidence in the membership of a cooperative medical group. N Engl J Med 275:131–136, 1966

2. BARILE MF and DELGIUDICE RA: Isolations of mycoplasmas and their rapid identification by plate epi-immunofluorescence. *In* Pathogenic Mycoplasmas. A Ciba Foundation Symposium. Elsevier, Amsterdam, 1972, pp 165–185

3. BLACK FT: Serological methods for classification of human T mycoplasmas. Fifth Int Congr Infect Dis 1:407–411, 1970

4. BRAUN P, KLEIN JO, and KASS EH: Susceptibility of genital mycoplasmas to antimicrobial agents. Appl Microbiol 19:62–70, 1970

5. BRUNELL PA, DISCHE RM, and WALKER MB: *Mycoplasma,* amnionitis, and respiratory distress syndrome. J Am Med Assoc 207:2097–2099, 1969

6. CHANOCK RM, HAYFLICK L, and BARILE MF: Growth on artificial medium of an agent associated with atypical pneumonia and its identification as PPLO. Proc Natl Acad Sci USA 48:41–49, 1962

7. CHANOCK RM, JAMES MD, FOX HH, TURNER HC, MUFSON MA, and HAYFLICK L: Growth of Eaton PPLO in broth and preparation of complement fixing antigen. Proc Soc Exp Biol Med 110:884–889, 1962

8. CLYDE WA JR: Hemolysis in identifying Eaton's pleuropneumonialike organism. Science 139:55, 1963

9. CLYDE WA JR: Mycoplasma species identification based upon growth inhibition by specific antisera. J Immunol 92:958–965, 1964

10. COLLIER AM and CLYDE WA JR: Appearance of *Mycoplasma pneumoniae* in lungs of experimentally infected hamsters and sputum from patients with natural disease. Am Rev Respir Dis 110:765–773, 1974

11. COLLIER AM, CLYDE WA JR, and DENNY FW: Biologic effects of *Mycoplasma pneumoniae* and other mycoplasmas from man on hamster tracheal organ culture. Proc Soc Exp Biol Med 132:1153–1158, 1969

12. EATON MD, MEIKLEJOHN G, and VAN HERICK W: Studies on the etiology of primary atypical pneumonia. I. A filterable agent transmissible to cotton rats, hamsters and chick embryos. J Exp Med 79:649–668, 1944

13. EMMONS J, SCHLUEDERBERG A, and CORDERO L: An aid to the rapid diagnosis of *Mycoplasma pneumoniae* infections. J Infect Dis 119:650–653, 1969

14. FEIZI T and TAYLOR-ROBINSON D: Cold agglutinins, anti-I and *Mycoplasma pneumoniae.* Immunology 13:405–409, 1967

15. FERNALD GW, CLYDE WA JR, and DENNY FW: Nature of the immune response to *Mycoplasma pneumoniae.* J Immunol 98:1028–1038, 1967

16. FERNALD GW, COLLIER AM, and CLYDE WA JR: Respiratory infections due to *Mycoplasma pneumoniae* in infants and children. Pediatrics 55:327–335, 1975

17. FOY HM, GRAYSTON JT, KENNY GE, ALEXANDER ER, and MCMAHAN R: Epidemiology of *Mycoplasma pneumoniae* infection in families. J Am Med Assoc 197:859–866, 1966

18. HAYFLICK L: Tissue cultures and mycoplasmas. Tex Rep Biol Med 23:285–303, 1965

19. HERS JF: Fluorescent antibody technique in respiratory viral diseases. Am Rev Respir Dis 88:316–333, 1963

20. KENNY GE and GRAYSTON JT: Eaton PPLO (*Mycoplasma pneumoniae*) complement fixing antigen: extraction with organic solvents. J Immunol 95:19–25, 1965

21. KUNDSIN RB: The role of mycoplasmas in human reproductive failure. Ann NY Acad Sci 174:794–797, 1970

22. LEE YH, MCCORMACK WM, MARCY SM, and KLEIN JO: The genital mycoplasmas. Their role in disorders of reproduction and in pediatric infections. Pediatr Clin North Am 21:457–466, 1974

23. LIN J-SL, ALPERT S, and RADNAY KM: Combined type-specific antisera in the identification of *Mycoplasma hominis.* J Infect Dis 131:727–730, 1975

24. LIPMAN RP, CLYDE WA JR, and DENNY FW: Characteristics of virulent, attenuated and avirulent *Mycoplasma pneumoniae* strains. J Bacteriol 100:1037–1043, 1969

25. LIU C, EATON MD, and HEYL JT: Studies on primary atypical pneumonia. II. Observations concerning the development and immunological characteristics of antibody in patients. J Exp Med 109:545–556, 1959

26. MCCORMACK WM, BRAUN P, LEE YH, KLEIN JO, and KASS EH: The genital mycoplasmas. N Engl J Med 288:78–89, 1973

27. MUFSON MA, LUDWIG WM, PURCELL RH, CATE TR, TAYLOR-ROBINSON D, and CHAN-

OCK RM: Exudative pharyngitis following experimental *Mycoplasma hominis* type 1 infection. J Am Med Assoc 192:1146–1152, 1965

28. NIITU Y, HASEGAWA S, and KUBOTA H: Usefulness of an erythromycin-resistant strain of *Mycoplasma pneumoniae* for the fermentation-inhibition test. Antimicrob Agents Chemother 5:111–113, 1974

29. PETERSON OL, HAM TH, and FINLAND M: Cold agglutinins (autohemagglutinins) in primary atypical pneumonia. Science 97:167, 1943

30. RAZIN S and ROTTEM S: Identification of mycoplasma and other micro-organisms by polyacrylamide-gel electrophoresis of cell proteins. J Bacteriol 94:1807–1810, 1967

31. ROMANO N, ROMANO F, and CAROLLO F: T-strains of mycoplasma in bronchopneumonic lungs of an aborted fetus. N Engl J Med 285:950–952, 1971

32. SENTERFIT LB and JENSEN KE: Antimetabolic antibodies to *Mycoplasma pneumoniae* measured by tetrazolium reduction inhibition. Proc Soc Exp Biol Med 122:786–790, 1966

33. SHEPARD MC: Cultivation and properties of T-strains of mycoplasma associated with nongonococcal urethritis. Ann NY Acad Sci 143:505–514, 1967

34. SHEPARD MC: Differential methods for identification of T mycoplasmas based on demonstration of urease. J Infect Dis 127:S22–S25, 1973

35. SHEPARD MC and LUNCEFORD CD: Differential agar medium (A7) for identification of *Ureaplasma urealyticum* (human T mycoplasmas) in primary cultures of clinical material. J Clin Microbiol 3:613–625, 1976

36. SOMERSON NL, WALLS BE, and CHANOCK RM: Hemolysin of *M. pneumoniae:* tentative identification as a peroxide. Science 150:226–228, 1965

37. STANBRIDGE E and HAYFLICK L: Growth inhibition test for identification of *Mycoplasma* species utilizing dried antiserum-impregnated paper discs. J Bacteriol 93:1392–1396, 1967

38. TAYLOR-ROBINSON D, PURCELL RH, WONG DC, and CHANOCK RM: A colour test for the measurement of antibody to certain mycoplasma species based upon the inhibition of acid production. J Hyg 64:91–104, 1966

39. TULLY JG, ROSE DL, WHITCOMB RF, and WENZEL RP: Enhanced isolation of *Mycoplasma pneumonia* from throat washings with a newly modified culture medium. J Infect Dis 139:478–482, 1979

CHAPTER 33

NEISSERIAL INFECTIONS

Dieter H. M. Gröschel and Benjamin L. Portnoy

Introduction

Neisserial infections are caused by bacteria of the genus *Neisseria*. In the eighth edition of *Bergey's Manual of Determinative Bacteriology* (8) this genus is listed in the family *Neisseriaceae* together with the genera *Branhamella*, *Moraxella*, and *Acinetobacter* (35). Neisseriae are gram-negative cocci and frequently appear in pairs with adjacent sides flattened, utilize few carbohydrates, and produce catalase and cytochrome-oxidase. They show few or no genetic affinities to *Branhamella* and differ in the guanine-cytosine (G + C) content of their DNA. Characteristics differentiating the species of the genus *Neisseria* are given in Table 33.1. Two species of the genus *Neisseria* cause worldwide endemic and epidemic contagious diseases—gonococcus and meningococcus. Other species have been implicated in human disease. In this chapter we discuss both gonorrhea and meningococcal infection and other neisserial infections.

Gonorrhea

Introduction

Causative organism

The cause of gonorrhea, *Neisseria gonorrhoeae*, commonly called gonococcus, was first described by Albert Neisser in 1879. Like other neisseriae it is an organism with a human reservoir and an affinity to mucous membranes. It is a gram-negative, nonmotile, nonencapsulated diplococcus that may occasionally grow in tetrads and clusters. (A recent report by Richardson and Sadoff indicates that fresh isolates of gonococci may be encapsulated and that this capsule can be induced *in vitro* in the presence of microaerophilic α-hemolytic streptococci (61).) The cocci are small (ca. 0.6×0.8 μm) and grow as small colonies on primary isolation. After repeated subculture, larger colonies with larger bacterial cells (1.2 to 1.5 μm) will develop that are avirulent upon inoculation in male volunteers. The small colony types, T_1 and T_2, consist of piliated virulent cells; the avirulent cells form colony types T_3 and T_4 (43, 45). Optimal growth requires aerobic incubation at 35–37 C in an atmosphere of

TABLE 33.1—CHARACTERISTICS DIFFERENTIATING THE SPECIES OF GENUS *NEISSERIA*

| | CAP-SULES | ACID FROM | | | | | | POLYSAC-CHARIDE FROM 5% SUCROSE | H_2S[1] PROD. | REDUCTION OF | | PIG-MENT[2] | EXTRA CO_2[3] | GROWTH | |
		GLU-COSE	MAL-TOSE	FRUC-TOSE	SU-CROSE	LAC-TOSE + ONPG				NO_3	NO_2			AT 22 C	ON NU-TRIENT AGAR (37 C)
N. gonorrhoeae	−[4]	+	−	−	−	−	NG	−	−	−	−	VI	−	−
N. meningitidis	V	+	+	−	−	−	NG	−	−	d	−	I	−	−
N. lactamica	−	+	+	−	−	+	−	+	−	+	+	d	V	+
N. sicca	V	+	+	+	+	−	+	+	−	+	d	NO	+	+
N. subflava	+	+	+	V	V	−	d	+	−	+	+	NO	+	+
N. flavescens	−	−	−	−	−	−	+	+	−	+	+	NO	+	+
N. mucosa	+	+	+	+	+	−	+	+	+	+	−	NO	+	+

− Most strains negative (≥ 90%)
+ Most strains positive (≥ 90%)
d Some strains positive, some negative
V Character inconstant, may sometimes be positive
NG No growth on 5% sucrose plates

[1] With lead acetate paper
[2] On Loeffler slant
[3] VI Extra CO_2 very important for growth
   I Extra CO_2 important for growth
   NO Extra CO_2 not important for growth
[4] See text description of causative organism of gonorrhea.

increased CO_2 tension on moist, supplemented protein hydrolysate agar media in which toxic fatty acids and trace metals are bound by blood, serum, starch, or charcoal. They will not grow on nutrient agar, eosin-methylene blue, or MacConkey agars. The organisms are sensitive to drying and exposure to sunlight and autolyze easily, especially in the absence of increased CO_2 tension.

Clinical manifestations

Urethritis usually begins 2 to 5 days after the male patient is infected by the gonococcus. Symptoms may vary from a scant watery urethral discharge to dysuria and a copious thick purulent discharge. Up to 40% of men with gonococcal infection of the urethra have no symptoms, and thus serve as an important reservoir of gonorrhea (34).

In women, the columnar epithelium of the cervix is the common site of gonococcal infection. Most patients are asymptomatic, but some are seen initially because of vaginal discharge. The vaginal wall of the postpubertal woman is relatively resistant to gonococcal infection, but the periurethral glands and the Bartholin's glands may be infected by the organisms, and abscesses may form.

Rectal infection by gonococci (48) is usually asymptomatic, but a severe proctitis with an anal discharge and diarrhea may occur. In women, this infection represents either secondary spread of the gonococci by contaminated vaginal discharge or primary introduction during anal intercourse. In men, rectal gonorrhea is a disease of the homosexual patient infected during anal intercourse.

Pharyngeal gonorrhea is acquired by fellatio and possibly cunnilingus with an infected host. Asymptomatic infection is common, but an occasional patient will have a purulent pharyngitis (76).

Gonococcal infection may spread from an infected cervix to the fallopian tubes, ovaries, and pelvic walls. The resulting pelvic inflammatory disease produces lower abdominal pain, fever, and an increased vaginal discharge. Local scarring of the fallopian tube may lead to ectopic pregnancy or infertility, even after a single episode of infection.

Pelvic inflammatory disease is common. However, the etiologic agent in repeated attacks has not been clearly established, and other bacteria may be responsible. Inflammation of the liver capsule, a perihepatitis, may accompany pelvic inflammatory disease. This Fitzhugh-Curtis syndrome probably represents direct spread of gonococci from the pelvic focus, but lymphatic spread also has been suggested.

Disseminated gonococcal infection may accompany simple urogenital gonococcal infection but usually represents hematogenous spread from an asymptomatic urogenital, rectal, or pharyngeal infection. Initially, bacteremia produces fever and chills, and the organism may be cultured from the blood. Papular erythematous skin lesions appear, and these later develop vesicular or pustular centers. Joint symptoms ranging from mild tenosynovitis to polyarthritis appear at the same time as the skin lesions. If untreated, a single joint will often develop purulent arthritis, and gonococci may be found on culture of the joint fluid. A few cases of disseminated gonococcal infection present as endocarditis or meningitis (37).

Ophthalmia neonatorum is still responsible for an occasional infection of the eye in a newborn baby. The gonococcus infects the eye during birth, and symptoms begin within a day or two after delivery. If untreated, blindness may occur. Fortunately, silver nitrate prophylaxis at time of birth has almost eliminated this clinical form of gonorrhea.

Epidemiology

Gonorrhea is by far the most commonly reported infectious disease in the United States. The rate of gonorrhea has steadily increased since 1957; however, between 1975 and 1978 the rate seems to have leveled off at about 470 cases per 100,000 population. The 15- to 29-year-old age group is responsible for most of the reported cases of gonorrhea. In men, ages 20–24, the rate of reported gonorrhea during the 3 years following 1975 has been around 2,500 cases per 100,000 population, or about 2.4% of men in this age group.

Disseminated gonococcal infection has been reported in clusters, suggesting that some strains of the organism have a virulence factor (33). These strains of the organism have a low antibiotic resistance and have distinctive growth requirements.

Gonococci that produce penicillinase have been identified around the world. In the United States, these strains have not become a major clinical problem to date, but the potential for the spread of a totally penicillin-resistant gonococcus exists (12).

Public health significance

Between 1975 and 1979, over one million cases of gonorrhea were reported annually to the Center for Disease Control. This figure certainly represents only part of the actual number of cases. Morbidity from disseminated gonococcal infection, pelvic inflammatory disease, and localized genital infection is obviously significant.

The large number of cases of gonorrhea and the increasing case rate always evoke questions about prevention of gonorrhea. So far, no easy, successful preventive measure has been developed for our society. Venereal disease education beginning in early teen-age years, easy and effective treatment, free venereal disease clinics, and confidentiality in treatment of minors have all been introduced; but no dramatic lowering of the gonorrhea rate has occurred. An effective vaccine for gonorrhea does not seem to be a likely development in the next few years. Epidemiologic tracing of contacts by trained professionals has been an effective tool in preventing syphilis, but the staggering number of gonorrhea cases makes this an unlikely solution to slowing the spread of gonorrhea. The practicing physician or staff of the public venereal disease clinic must remember that a case of gonorrhea involves at least one infected person besides the patient, and vigorous efforts must be made to bring all of them to treatment.

Collection and Processing of Specimens

Type of specimen

Specimens for microscopic and cultural diagnosis of gonococcal infections must be collected from the suspected site and processed without delay to avoid desiccation, overgrowth by other flora, or exposure to detrimental factors. Either cotton-, polyester-, or calcium alginate-tipped swabs are used to obtain the specimen from the mucosal surface. In a hospital or laboratory, the specimen is inoculated immediately on a Thayer-Martin agar plate if contamination by other flora is suspected or on chocolate agar if a pure culture is expected. For a clinic or office without microbiology laboratory facilities, the Lester-Martin transport and growth (Transgrow) medium in a CO_2-containing flask is available.

Urogenital mucosa. In women, the diagnosis of infection usually is made by cultures since the Gram stain alone may be misleading due to the often very low numbers of gonococci and the presence of other bacteria with similar morphology. The specimens are most commonly obtained from the posterior vaginal fornix and the cervix after removal of the cervical mucous plug. Proper exposure of the sites requires a vaginal speculum that should be free of any antimicrobial substance such as bacteriostats in a lubricant and disinfectant or detergent residuals from the cleaning process. If the urethra or Skene's and Bartholin's glands are infected, exudate must be collected by applying pressure on these sites with a swab or a microbiological loop.

In men, a small amount of urethral discharge is either obtained by swab or as a drop on a microscope slide. A smear of the discharge from men will usually contain the organism. If the man is asymptomatic or without discharge at the time of examination, a specimen from within the urethra is obtained either with a calibrated (0.001 ml) new platinum loop or a pediatric nasopharyngeal calcium alginate swab. Since nongonococcal urethritis or a mixed infection may be present, especially in the pretreated or "therapy-resistant" man, in selected cases it may be important to culture the specimen for other bacteria and yeasts as well as chlamydia or mycoplasma. A wet preparation may be examined for the presence of *Trichomonas vaginalis.* If the urethral smear and culture are negative and clinical findings suggest involvement of the prostate and seminal vesicles, an exprimate may be cultured and microscopically examined. Occasionally, culture of centrifuged or uncentrifuged, first-voided urine may yield positive results (25).

Other mucosal membranes. Isolation of neisseriae from mucosal sites other than the genital tract is more difficult to accomplish because of the heavy contamination with normal site flora, often resistant to the antimicrobials used in selective media.

The rectum is frequently infected, occasionally as the only site, in homosexual males as well as in females. The swab specimen should be obtained from the crypts just inside the sphincter ani without contacting feces. The growth medium should contain trimethoprim lactate in addition to the usual vancomycin-colistin-nystatin additives to suppress, especially swarming, enteric bacteria. The same medium is recommended for swab specimens in patients suspected of having gonococcal pharyngitis. Ophthalmia requires the preparation of several slides for Gram stain and possibly fluorescent antibody staining.

Body fluids and needle aspirates. In arthritis or tenosynovitis synovial fluid is obtained, diluted with sterile Trypticase soy broth, and centrifuged. The sediment is used for culture and microscopy (42). Anticoagulants should be avoided as they may interfere with the viability of the gonococcus. Aspirates from tuboovarian abscesses should be obtained anaerobically and cultured for anaerobes as well as gonococci and other bacteria. Cutaneous lesions accompanying arthritis or sepsis may yield growth of gonococci, but here fluorescent antibody staining of smears may be more profitable (75). Blood cultures for the diagnosis of gonococcaemia are best performed in commercially available closed bottle systems with brain heart infusion or Trypticase soy broth under increased CO_2 tension. Kellogg (42) recommends a biphasic medium. The presence of sodium polyanethol sulfonate may inhibit or retard the growth of some gonococcus strains but, on the other hand, will interfere with the more detrimental leukocyte phagocytosis and thus preserve the organism.

Transport

Using the direct inoculation of specimens on transport medium in flasks (Transgrow) has greatly reduced the problems of viability during transportation. If direct media inoculation is not possible, a swab transport system as described by Stuart et al. (68) and Amies and Douglas (1) can be used. Due to the inevitable loss of viability of gonococci, swab transport beyond 6 hr is not recommended. Inoculated selective or nonselective plates may be transported in miniature candle jars or in plastic bags containing a CO_2 atmosphere developed by a CO_2 generating tablet (49, 69).

Number of specimens

Whereas in the heterosexual male a single urethral specimen is usually sufficient, in the female swabs from different vaginal sites (cervix, posterior fornix, urethral), the rectum, and pharynx are recommended. In high-risk groups with negative laboratory results, repeat specimens may be necessary. The same plate may be inoculated if swabs are obtained from cervical and rectal sites of the same patient (14). Depending on the sexual practices of the individual patient, specimens from other body sites should be taken and inoculated on separate plates of selective medium. After treatment, follow-up cultures are recommended; smears alone are not reliable as an indicator of successful treatment since dead gonococci may still be present and will be stained.

Diagnostic Procedures

Microscopic examination

In acute gonococcal urethritis of the male, a Gram-stained smear of urethral exudate usually reveals the typical picture of gonorrhea: many pus cells and intra- and extracellular gram-negative diplococci. However, in very early or late infections, only extracellular diplococci may be found. Direct smears prepared from other mucosal sites are usually unsatisfactory because of the presence of other bacteria resembling gram-negative diplococci.

Preparation and staining. Smears for the microscopic examination should be prepared immediately upon collection of the specimen. The microscopic slide must be clean and free of fingerprints. It is marked with patient identification by either a diamond writer or, on frosted-end slides, with pencil. The pus or exudate sample is applied with a loop or swab and spread over an area of at least 1 cm². Care must be taken not to destroy the pus cells by streaking too vigorously and the film should be thin. After air-drying and heat fixation, the slide is ready for staining or shipment. For shipment, the slides should be separated, preferably in a slide container to avoid loss of the film.

Staining should be performed with the Gram procedure as outlined in the *Manual of Clinical Microbiology* (53), using the modified Hucker's crystal violet. Regular quality control of the staining components and the procedure is required.

Fluorescent antibody (FA) staining techniques have been described in previous editions of *Diagnostic Procedures for Bacterial, Mycotic and Parasitic Infections* (70), but they should be limited to laboratories that have highly specific and sensitive antisera available. For routine examination of direct smears, especially those made from specimens containing normal site flora, they are not recommended (44).

Examination and report. The stained smear is carefully examined with an oil immersion objective at 800–1000× magnification. The presence and amount of polymorphonuclear leukocytes and epithelial cells and the morphology, Gram reaction, and location (intra- or extracellular) of the bacteria are recorded. A useful semiquantitative recording method is given in reference 44. The report of the Gram-stained smear should state all findings and may include the statement that the observed bacteria "morphologically resemble gonococci," if the experienced laboratorian considers the microscopic appearance to be typical for findings in acute gonorrhea in the male.

For body fluids and conjunctival pus as well as for material from skin lesions the Gram stain is recommended, but FA staining has been applied successfully.

Culture procedures

Media. Specimens from the genitourinary tract, rectum, and pharynx should be inoculated at least on the selective Thayer-Martin or similar, enriched medium containing antibiotics. Specimens from other or normally sterile sites (body fluids, pus, conjunctival exudate) are inoculated at least on nonselective chocolate agar. Depending on the goals of culturing other media may be included. All media used for the specific isolation of gonococci must be controlled for their ability to support the growth of small inocula of quality control strains and of recently isolated patient strains. Various new culture detection systems have been described and tested but it is too early to assess their usefulness in the clinical or public health laboratory. Due to their high cost, they may be more applicable for the occasional patient in a physician's office. A recently described medium containing Imferon (iron-dextran complex) claims to increase the speed and rate of isolation of gonococci from clinical specimens (54).

Inoculation. Selective plate or flask media are usually inoculated with a swab by streaking over the entire agar surface and rotating the swab to assure contact of all areas with the agar. Specimens obtained with a loop are also seeded over the entire surface. Nonselective media are inoculated in the usual manner by heavily applying the specimen to a small area and then using the loop dilution technique for obtaining isolated colonies.

Incubation. Inoculated plates are transferred as quickly as possible to an environment of about 70% humidity in ~ 5% CO_2 at 35–37 C. This environment may be obtained in a CO_2 incubator, a sealed container with a CO_2 generating tablet, or in a candle extinction jar. If a candle jar is used, spiced or decorative candles must be avoided due to the antimicrobial activity of most of the perfumes and additives; only white wax (devotional) candles should be used. A quality control of the growth environment is required.

Examination of cultures. Cultures should be inspected after overnight incubation and returned to the CO_2 environment quickly if negative. At least 48 hr of incubation are required before cultures can be considered negative.

Colonies of *N. gonorrhoeae* are usually very small after overnight growth and may be overlooked. Suspect colonies may be tested for oxidase reaction either by dropping the reagent, fresh 1% tetramethyl-para-phenylenediamine-dihydrochloride (53), directly on the plate or by inoculating a part of the colony with a platinum loop onto a filter paper strip impregnated with the reagent. In both cases, neisseriae will turn the reagent to a dark purple within 10 sec. Quality control will assure that oxidase reagent will always perform as expected. The morphology of oxidase-positive colonies must be confirmed by the Gram stain, since other bacteria and yeasts may also produce oxidase. False-negative or slow reactions may occur with old cultures and with the use of acid media (containing glucose, or increased CO_2 atmosphere such as the Transgrow flask). Plates densely overgrown with different colonies may be flooded with the reagent, but any positive colonies must be subcultured immediately to chocolate agar to avoid death of the bacteria. Cultures of urethral pus from males showing growth of oxidase-positive, gram-negative diplococci may be called presumptively positive for gonococci. For definite identification, single suspected colonies are transferred to chocolate agar plates and densely streaked.

Identification of isolates

Identification procedures require good growth of isolated colonies on the primary isolation medium or pure subcultures. In all cases, the purity of the inoculum for biochemical testing must be confirmed with the oxidase reaction and Gram staining.

Most commonly, carbohydrate degradation studies (see Table 33.1) will be performed by growing the gonococci in cystine Trypticase agar (CTA) medium containing 1% reagent grade, filter-sterilized glucose, maltose, sucrose, or lactose. A dense suspension of the organism is prepared in a small volume of saline or peptone water. With a pipette, aliquots are dropped on the surface of the CTA medium and with a needle or loop the inoculum is stabbed into the upper third of the agar column. The tubes are tightly closed. Test results are read after 16–20 hr of incubation at 35 to 37 C and considered to be negative only after 48 hr of total incubation time. Since other enzymes may degrade peptone and produce an alkaline pH, prolonged incubation may give false-negative results (11). Carbohydrates are degraded primarily by an oxidative pathway rather than by fermentation (6); thus acid production is often very low. False-positive results may occur if tubes are incubated in CO_2 incubators or even in regular incubators if the screwcaps are not tightly closed. Occasional *N. gonorrhoeae* strains fail to grow in CTA medium, but supplementing the medium with 1% inactivated rabbit serum may overcome the nutritional deficiency (57). If unsupplemented CTA medium is used, it is necessary to determine whether or not the organisms have grown at all in the tubed media. Uninoculated control tubes for each carbohydrate should be incubated in parallel to observe for spontaneous acid formation. Also, all tubes with positive reactions should be controlled for the absence of contaminating microorganisms by Gram stain.

A nongrowth carbohydrate degradation test was described by Brown (8) and by Yong and Prytula (77) as a modification of Kellogg's and Turner's method (46). (For details see reference 44.) An adaptation of this test to the Minitek system (52) and the radiometric method (60, 67) has been reported recently. In addition, numerous variations and modifications of carbohydrate degradation tests may be found in the world literature. A novel approach to rapid enzymatic profile determination was reported by D'Amato et al. (3). With properly prepared monospecific fluorescent antigonococcal conjugates, culture isolates may also be confirmed. A combination of tests (FA, rapid carbohydrate tests, and penicillinase production) was reported by Young (78). Menck (51) used a slide coagglutination test (Phadebact) to identify isolates.

Presumptive results may be reported based on adequate clinical information, knowledge of the exact source of the specimen, and the findings of typical bacteria on microscopic examination of a direct Gram-stained smear or after the detection of oxidase-positive, gram-negative bacteria with typical colony morphology on culture plates. Isolation of *N. gonorrhoeae* can be reported only after the isolate has been identified by biochemical tests or specific fluorescent antibody procedures.

Serologic procedures

Pure isolates of *N. gonorrhoeae* may be identified with fluorescent dye-conjugated antigonococcal serum or immunoglobulins. These sera need to be tested for specificity and sensitivity, since commercial sera have shown cross-reactions with meningococci, staphylococci, streptococci, and other bacteria. Hen antiserum to gonococcal lipopolysaccharide was found to be a reliable FA reagent (72).

Attempts to serotype gonococci have been reported, but presently this procedure is not useful for the diagnostic laboratory (2, 28). No serologic test can be recommended for the routine diagnosis of gonococcal infections. However, for screening purposes several of the newer test procedures (radioimmunoassay for antibody to gonococcal pili, the latex agglutination test, or the indirect fluorescent antibody test) have shown some promising results. (The reader is referred to reference 17 for discussion of the problem of gonococcal serology.) The study of serotypes and the preparation of well-defined antigens may improve the usefulness of serological tests for both case finding and diagnosis in the absence of positive culture results.

Epidemiologic markers

The most useful markers currently available for epidemiologic studies of gonococcal infections are the colony types (see above) and pili antibodies mentioned above. Auxotypes that correlate with strains of gonococci isolated from disseminated infection have been described, but this potential epidemiologic marker has only recently been reported. The discovery of penicillinase-producing gonococci may add another useful epidemiological marker.

Antimicrobial Susceptibility

Until recently, antibiotic susceptibility studies were not necessary for gonococci and, therefore, no standardized test procedures have been developed. The disk diffusion susceptibility test of Bauer et al. is not reliable. Although a steady increase in penicillin resistance has been noted over the past decades, the usually recommended and regularly adjusted doses of penicillin achieve drug concentrations in body fluids and secretions adequate for bactericidal action. The failure of patients to respond to penicillin therapy led to the discovery of penicillinase-producing gonococci (3, 55). Recent reports indicate that the beta-lactamase production is mediated by a plasmid resembling the R plasmids in *Enterobacteriaceae* and *Haemophilus influenzae* (20, 64) and that resistance can be transferred by conjugation (47). Thus, it may be useful to test penicillin-resistant strains of gonococci for penicillinase production. Cumitech 4 (44) recommends the use of a 10-unit penicillin disk placed on a chocolate agar plate, inoculated according to the National Committee for Clinical Laboratory Standards (NCCLS) standards for disk diffusion susceptibility testing. Zones of inhibition of less than 20 mm suggest penicillinase-producing strains. It is recommended that all gonococci suspected of penicillinase production be forwarded to a reference health department laboratory for confirmation and epidemiologic information.

Evaluation of Laboratory Findings

In urethral exudates of the male with typical clinical signs of gonorrhea, there is a high correlation (up to 90%) between the classical appearance of a Gram-stained smear and the confirmed diagnosis of gonorrhea. Similarly, the absence of gram-negative diplococci correlates well with a failure to culture gonococci (40). In specimens with mixed flora, however, the appearance of intracellular, gram-negative diplococci is not enough to make a presumptive diagnosis. Specimens from patients who are taking small doses of antibiotics, e.g., tetracycline for acne conditions, or who come to the doctor after having received a "cure from a friend" are unsuitable candidates for presumptive diagnosis by Gram-stained smear alone.

False-negative laboratory results may occur if disinfectants, detergents, or antiseptics have interfered with the viability of the bacteria. Toxic materials (inhibitory cotton on homemade swabs, toxic candles in the candle jar), inadequate transport systems, old or deteriorated medium, failure of oxidase reagent, low inoculum size in biochemical tests, and use of impure sugars for fermentation may produce false negatives. A rare strain of gonococcus sensitive to vancomycin (44) may not grow on Thayer-Martin media which contain this antibiotic. False results may also be due to improperly trained laboratory personnel or inadequate procedures.

Meningococcal and Other Neisserial Infections

Introduction

Causative organisms

Although gonorrhea was known as a communicable venereal disease for 700 years, the other major neisserial infection, epidemic cerebrospinal meningitis, was not clearly recognized as a contagious disease until early in the 19th century. Weichselbaum first isolated the causative organism from purulent spinal fluid in 1887. Like the gonococcus, *Neisseria meningitidis* (meningococcus), is a small, gram-negative diplococcus that demonstrates different colony types and piliation. In contrast to *Neisseria gonorrhoeae*, there is no consistent relationship of pili to colony morphology (50). Freshly isolated strains may be encapsulated.

Meningococci are fastidious bacteria requiring enriched media for primary isolation. Their optimal growth temperature is 35 to 37 C in a moist environment. CO_2 concentrations of 2%–8% are stimulating and, for some strains, necessary. Although laboratory strains may grow on simple synthetic media, freshly isolated patient strains will not form colonies on nutrient agar. The diplococci autolyze easily and are sensitive to desiccation and sunlight.

The so-called nonpathogenic neisseriae are part of the normal flora of the pharynx and the female genital tract. They usually grow on nutrient agar at 22 C and are often pigmented. In this chapter, only the species *N. sicca*, *N. subflava*, *N. flavescens*, *N. mucosa*, and *N. lactamica* are discussed, since they are frequently isolated from human specimens, occasionally cause disease, and may be difficult to differentiate from pathogenic species upon primary isolation.

Clinical manifestations

Meningococcal infection typically presents as meningitis and/or bacteremia. Meningococcemia without meningitis begins with sudden high fever, prostration, myalgias, and, in most cases, a petechial eruption. Some cases are dramatically fulminant and lead to shock and death. In those who recover from fulminant meningococcemia, loss of gangrenous skin or digits is common.

Meningococcal meningitis may occur alone or in association with meningococcemia. Symptoms of an upper respiratory infection frequently precede the onset of meningitis. The sudden appearance of high fever, headache, vomiting, and confusion typical of meningococcal meningitis occurs in over half the cases along with the petechial or purpuric rash of meningococcemia.

Rarer manifestations of meningococcal infection account for 5% of cases. Chronic meningococcemia with fever, rash, and arthritis may last weeks or months. Primary meningococcal pneumonia, arthritis, pericarditis, endocarditis, and urethritis have been reported (9, 36, 38).

Epidemiology

Man is the only known reservoir for meningococcus, and transmission of the bacteria is accomplished by inhalation of infected droplets of nasopharyngeal secretions.

Meningococci can be serogrouped, and the most commonly identified groups are A, B, C, and Y. Historically, group A was the most prevalent, but currently group B is the most common and C the next most common.

Since the meningococcus is spread from person to person, close contacts of a case of meningococcal infection are at risk of becoming carriers or of developing disease, p = 3/1000 contacts (13). A choice of chemoprophylaxis agents for contacts is frequently made on the basis of which serogroup is prevalent in the community, since groups B and Y are usually sensitive to sulfonamide while groups A and C are resistant to sulfonamide and require rifampin treatment.

Meningococcal infections reach peak incidence in late winter and early spring, and the lower incidence is in the summer. Infants between 6 months and 1 year of age have the highest attack rate of meningococcal infection of all age groups. Persons under 20 years of age account for 75% of cases.

Public health significance

A case of meningococcal meningitis or meningococcemia rarely fails to strike terror among persons who have had contact with the patient. Health departments or physicians are often able to reduce the panic following such a case by educational means. It is helpful for health departments to have informative brochures available on meningococcal infections, and occasionally a televised interview with a public health official will prevent widespread panic from developing.

Vaccines are available for serogroups A and C meningococcal infection (58). The polysaccharide vaccines have been licensed in this country, and they appear to have only rare serious adverse reactions. The vaccines should be used to control outbreaks of serogroup A or C infection, and they may be used as an adjunctive measure in preventing the spread of infection among household contacts of a case.

Collection and Processing of Specimens

Type of specimen

Specimens for the diagnosis of nongonococcal neisserial infections include cerebrospinal fluid, blood, aspirate from petechial lesions, nasopharyngeal swabs, sputum, aspirates from various effusions, and others. Specimens should be obtained prior to initiation of antimicrobial therapy. Liquid materials are collected in sterile tubes with tightly fitting closures. In most hospitals, disposable plastic containers will be used. If glass tubes are recycled, it is advisable to sterilize these in a dry heat oven in order to incinerate residual microorganisms and avoid confusing findings on smears. Blood is best obtained with a needle and syringe or an evacuated sterile glass tube, or directly transferred in a blood culture container. Petechiae are aspirated with sterile saline solution in a small syringe with a fine needle. For nasopharyngeal specimens, the calcium alginate- or polyester-tipped pediatric swabs are preferred.

Cerebrospinal fluid. The specimen is obtained by lumbar puncture after appropriate antiseptic preparation of the area. Residual antiseptic must be removed to avoid accidental transfer of residuals into the specimen container.

After measuring the opening pressure of the spinal fluid, 2–5 ml aliquots of fluid are obtained in three sterile tubes. The tubes should be sent to the laboratory at once. In addition to microbiological tests, cytologic and chemical studies are requested. Part of the specimen may be used to detect soluble antigens in the spinal fluid by countercurrent immunoelectrophoresis (30). It should be arranged that all specimens are first brought to the Microbiology Laboratory, especially if very small amounts of spinal fluid are available. The supernatant from the microbiology specimen may then be passed on for the chemical determination of protein and glucose concentrations. Bloody specimens may give confusing chemical and cytological results but should always be processed. Very small amounts of spinal fluid are unreliable, especially in the early stages of meningitis. A repeat spinal puncture should be requested. Repeat cultures are suggested if the patient does not respond well to the appropriate antibiotic therapy.

Blood. Most physicians order at least one blood culture in cases of suspected meningitis. Meningococcemia also may occur without meningitis and may result in metastatic lesions. Other *Neisseria* spp. are occasionally isolated from blood cultures (10, 27). Occasionally, intracellular diplococci may be detected in blood smears submitted for differential counts or may be found in specially prepared Gram-stained films from a buffy coat.

Petechiae. These metastatic lesions of the skin often contain viable bacteria. In doubtful cases, their aspiration may allow the microscopic and culture demonstration of meningococci.

Posterior nasopharynx. Swabs from the nasopharynx of untreated cases may assist in the diagnosis of a case of meningococcal infection. The nasopharyngeal swab is most helpful in the screening of suspected carriers or in checking household contacts of a case.

Sputum. Occasionally, meningococcal infection may involve the respiratory tract, either during meningococcemia or as a primary infection (41, 59). Expectorated sputum may be submitted, but specimens obtained by transtracheal aspiration will avoid the confusion of contamination by nasopharyngeal organisms.

Other body fluids. Fluids from pericardial, pleural, joint, or other effusions should be obtained as cerebrospinal fluid is.

Transporting specimens

It is important that any specimen obtained from a patient suspected of a neisserial disease not be exposed to desiccation, chilling, or unfavorable pH. Therefore, rapid transport of all specimens to the laboratory is required. Blood specimens for culture should be inoculated into culture bottles at once. Aspirates and swabs are best inoculated on primary culture media at bedside, but transport media or swabs discussed for gonococci may be used.

Laboratory processing

Since meningococcal meningitis and bacteremia are life-threatening infections, the processing of specimens is one of the few emergency procedures for the clinical microbiology laboratory. Any delay may reduce the viability of organisms and prolong the reporting time unnecessarily. Unless very turbid, fluid such as cerebrospinal fluid should be centrifuged at 2500 rpm for 15 min and the sediment used for both smear and culturing (39). Countercurrent immunoelectrophoresis (30) will rapidly detect groups A and C meningococcal infections in blood or spinal fluid. Specimens for this procedure should be processed without delay so that a firm diagnosis may be reported to the physician as quickly as possible. The laboratory management must train personnel to give preferential treatment to all specimens from patients with meningitis, especially outside of regular working hours.

Diagnostic Procedures

Microscopic examination

Direct microscopic examination is useful for original specimens such as fluids, buffy coat preparations, or petechial aspirates, as well as for monitoring liquid culture media and determining Gram characteristic and morphology of colonies grown on solid media.

Preparation and staining. For all stains, a thin film is spread on a microscope slide, air dried, either heat fixed or fixed in absolute methanol for 10 min to preserve leukocyte morphology (11), and stained by the Gram method (53). Some laboratorians add a smear stained with Loeffler's methylene blue. This staining procedure is quick, and methylene blue-stained diplococci are often better recognized than by the Gram stain. The microscope slides must be absolutely clean to avoid erroneous readings of the stained smears.

If the Gram stain reveals many gram-negative diplococci, one can attempt to detect the encapsulated meningococci of groups A and C by capsular swelling (Quellung) test. Meningococci in body fluids as well as pure culture isolates may be tested with homologous group-specific antisera (4).

Smears prepared from specimens containing organisms of the normal host flora (nasopharyngeal swab, sputum, etc.) are not useful for direct microscopic examination since meningococci cannot be differentiated morphologically from other neisseriae. Due to cross-reactions the fluorescent antibody technique is not recommended.

Examination and report. The stained smear of a cerebrospinal fluid sediment is examined with an oil immersion objective for at least 10 min before it can be called negative. In certain cases, especially in early *Haemophilus influenzae* meningitis, it may take much longer to detect single gram-negative rods. The presence, type, and amount of leukocytes are noted. In a typical case, gram-negative, mainly intracellular coffee bean-shaped cocci in pairs (0.8 × 0.6 μm) will be observed. Often they will be in groups of 2–4. Occasionally, the smear is negative but meningococci are found on the culture plate. In fulminating cases one may find few leukocytes and mostly extracellular diplococci. In patients pretreated with cell wall-active antibiotics, highly pleomorphic, bizarre bacterial forms can be observed. The finding of very faintly stained, not well-defined, extracellular bacteria suggests a secondary contamination but may mislead the inexperienced observer.

Gram-stained preparations from early cultures usually show pleomorphism with formation of tetrads and even, short chains, varying intensity of staining, as well as very small and very large bacterial cells.

Direct smears from buffy coats or petechiae usually show predominantly intracellular gram-negative diplococci.

A report on the reading of direct smears should be communicated immediately to the attending physician or his delegate. The report should give an exact description of the findings. It may include the statement by the experienced microbiologist that organisms observed in cerebrospinal fluid morphologically resemble meningococci. Without knowledge about the patient, the same statement should not be made about the detection of gram-negative diplococci in specimens from buffy coat or skin lesions, since gonococci are indistinguishable.

Group-specific capsular swelling may be considered presumptive identification of *Neisseria meningitidis*. Indirect fluorescent antibody technique has been used on both spinal fluid and young culture preparations. Cross-reactions make the method not very reliable for the diagnostic laboratory.

Culture procedures

Media. All culture media used for the propagation of meningococci should be allowed to warm to 25 C. Agar plates should be fresh and moist but not wet. For body fluids, at least a chocolate or blood agar plate or a similar enriched medium should be inoculated, and a tube of Mueller-Hinton broth, brain heart infusion broth supplemented with 10% to 20% serum or ascitic fluid, or another enriched broth medium added. For specimens obtained from sites with normal flora or suspected of containing other microorganisms, the medium of Thayer and Martin or a similar selective medium should be included. All media used for the isolation of meningococci must have been shown to support the growth of *Neisseria meningitidis*.

For culture of blood and other body fluids and effusions the regularly used commercial blood culture containers with brain heart infusion or Trypticase soy broth and CO_2 atmosphere are most useful. Thiol or thioglycolate broths may retard or interfere with the growth of meningococci. Like gonococci some strains of *Neisseria meningitidis* may be inhibited by sodium polyanethol sulfonate (22), but a recent report indicates that this inhibition may be overcome by the addition of gelatin (21). Sodium amylosulfate does not seem to inhibit growth (62).

Inoculation. Solid culture media are best inoculated with 0.5 to 1 ml of cerebrospinal or other body fluids. All remaining fluid should be added at a ratio of 1:10 to 1:5 to a broth medium.

For blood cultures, 10–15 ml of blood is dispensed to one to three blood bottles, resulting in a 1:10 dilution of the blood. All evacuated bottles must be vented. Blood cultures must be subcultured blindly on chocolate or blood agar even if the radiometric BACTEC method is used. Some microbiologists like to inoculate 0.5–1 ml of patient blood directly on a chocolate agar plate.

A buffy coat prepared for smears can be inoculated in liquid (blood culture) media or on chocolate agar plates.

Swab specimens are directly inoculated on selective (Thayer-Martin) medium by covering the entire surface while turning the swab. Nonselective media are heavily inoculated by the entire swab in one-third of the plate and the inoculum then is spread by a loop in the usual manner to obtain single isolated colonies.

Incubation. Inoculated plates and tubes are incubated at 35 to 37 C in an atmosphere of increased CO_2 tension (2% to 8%) and moisture.

Examination of cultures. Meningococci usually grow to visible colonies after 18 to 20 hr of incubation. Plates without growth should be reincubated. The colonies are round, smooth, glistening, translucent (on Mueller-Hinton agar) and nonpigmented. Some group B strains become yellowish with age. The colonies can be easily emulsified in saline.

Other members of the genus *Neisseria* may initially resemble the pathogenic species, especially *N. lactamica, N. flavescens,* and *N. subflava,* but they develop pigment after continued incubation. Colonies of *N. sicca* are wrinkled or rough, dry, adherent or entirely movable, those of *N. mucosa* are mucoid and often adherent, and colonies of *N. flavescens* are smooth and opaque. *N. sicca, N. subflava,* and *N. flavescens* will usually not grow on Thayer-Martin medium unless heavily inoculated.

The oxidase reaction described above and the Gram stain allow the presumptive identification of neisseriae in young mixed or pure cultures. Subcultures to blood or chocolate agar should be prepared at once.

Identification of isolates

As aerobic bacteria, neisseriae are unable to grow on chocolate agar in a strictly anaerobic environment (11). As a human pathogen, *N. meningitidis,* like *N. gonorrhoeae* and some *N. lactamica* strains, is well adapted to the nutritionally rich environment of the mucosa and to temperatures of 37 C. Other *Neisseria* spp. grow at 22 C on enriched media and can also multiply on a simple beef extract-peptone-water agar at 37 C. Some nonpathogenic neisseriae may not grow on Thayer-Martin medium. These characteristics, in addition to pigment formation, can be used for a preliminary separation of *Neisseria* spp.

Definitive identification of *Neisseria* is accomplished by biochemical tests (see Table 33.1). In the previous edition of this book, Feldman warns about the use of phosphate-buffered saline with meningococci, since phosphate is lethal to these bacteria (24). *Neisseria lactamica* hydrolyzes lactose with the enzyme β-galactosidase. Thus the ONPG test can be used instead of lactose degradation. Some *Neisseria* spp. can be identified by their ability to reduce nitrate or nitrite. (For technique see ref. 11.) According to Diena et al. (18) meningococci form colonies on Dubos oleic acid agar medium whereas gonococci will not. Meningococci can also be confirmed by slide agglutination or by the capsular swelling (only groups A and C) with monospecific antisera.

Presumptive results must be reported on all isolates from life-threatening infections such as meningitis and septicemia. Knowledge about the clinical status and, in the case of meningitis, about the cytology and chemistry results on the cerebrospinal fluid will assist the experienced microbiologist in arriving at a presumptive laboratory diagnosis. However, one must be aware that occasionally neisseriae other than *N. meningitidis* will cause meningitis and bloodstream infections. Also, one should expect meningococci from unusual sites, for example, the vagina (31). Preliminary reports on blood cultures should be sent to the physician in accordance with the usual procedures of the laboratory.

Definitive identification may be delayed in cases with unusual biochemical reactions. In such cases it is better to report "*N. meningitidis* cannot be excluded" than to overlook an atypical pathogen.

Serologic procedures and epidemiologic markers

Isolates of *N. meningitidis* can be grouped into four main (superficial) antigen groups, A, B, C, and D. The most commonly encountered serogroups in the United States are groups B and C. Five additional serogroups are rarely associated with disease production, the Slaterus serogroups X, Y, Z, and Z[1] (65, 66) and the Evans serogroup 135 (23).

Some grouping sera are commercially available. Capsular swelling can be shown with the encapsulated group A and group C strains. Other grouping procedures are slide agglutination (11) or immunofluorescence. Cross-reactions may occur due to common somatic antigens not only with other neisseriae but also with unrelated bacteria (15). Recently, coagglutination with specific antibody-coated Protein A-rich staphylococci was reported (79). For epidemiologic studies *N. meningitidis* of group B and group C can be subdivided into serotypes (26, 29). Bacteriocins produced by certain meningococcal strains have been applied for identification (15). For the detection of soluble antigens of *Neisseria meningitidis* in spinal fluid, blood, and joint fluids countercurrent immunoelectrophoresis with group-specific antisera is used, especially in pediatric hospitals (30, 56).

The detection of antibodies directed against meningococci is mainly of epidemiologic interest. Edwards and Driscoll (19) described a passive hemagglutination test for screening of naval recruits for carrier stage. Wenzel et al. (74) found this passive hemagglutination test to be quite specific, but an indirect immunofluorescence method for testing for antibodies in nasal secretions showed considerable cross-reactions among meningococcal serogroups. For testing serum antibody response to meningococcal polysaccharides, a latex agglutination test similar to the one used for gonorrhea was developed (71).

Antimicrobial Susceptibility

Neisseria meningitidis is susceptible to penicillin. As of now, penicillin resistance has not been reported and for clinical and epidemiological reasons it is hoped that the epidemic strains of meningococci will not acquire the β-lactamase-inducing plasmids.

In cases of true penicillin hypersensitivity, an antimicrobial susceptibility test may be desired by the clinician. The presently used disk diffusion (Bauer-Kirby) test with Mueller-Hinton agar is not standardized for *Neisseria meningitidis* or *Neisseria gonorrhoeae*. Generally recommended is the agar dilution method with Mueller-Hinton agar, GC medium base with supplement, or chocolate agar (73). Bennett et al. described a sulfonamide disk test for meningococci (5). Recently Hammerberg et al. (32) reinvestigated the disk test. The authors found that there exists complete correlation between agar dilution MIC determination and the disk diffusion test for sulfonamides if certain standards are observed. Reproducible results with the agar dilution susceptibility test using Mueller-Hinton agar require an inoculum of 10^6 CFU/ml grown in Mueller-Hinton broth. Correlation between the agar dilution test and a disk diffusion test on Mueller-Hinton agar requires an inoculum of 10^7 CFU/ml. With a 300-μg disk of sulfadiazine or sulfathiazole, it resulted in reproducible zone sizes of less than 20 mm diameter for resistant and 30 mm or more for susceptible strains. Sulfisoxazole disks gave erratic results.

Evaluation of Laboratory Findings

Meningococcal infection often is strongly suspected on the basis of clinical findings but the diagnosis must be confirmed by the isolation and identification of the organism in cerebrospinal fluid, blood, or lesion aspirate. The reader should keep in mind that in the early stages of bacterial meningitis rather vague, flu-like symptoms may occur, and that in the very young, the very old, and in debilitated patients many, if not all, classical signs of infection and meningeal irritation may be absent. The clinician will then rely only on laboratory findings for a diagnosis. Four rapid test procedures are performed in the laboratory that will assist in the management of patients: the Gram stain, the cytological examination of spinal fluid and the chemical determination of its sugar and protein content, and a serological test to detect the presence of meningococcal antigens in blood or spinal fluids.

The Gram stain prepared from the sediment of the spinal fluid specimen, from buffy coat cells, or from lesion aspirates will reveal the type of blood cells, the presence of bacteria, their Gram reaction and morphology, and their intracellular or extracellular location. If the patient has already been treated with antibiotics, rather unusual bacterial forms may be seen which can easily be mistaken for artifacts. Secondary contamination of the specimen either from the skin or from careless handling of the specimen containers, the presence of microbial "ghosts" in specimen tubes, or the use of unclean slides (fingerprints) may result in erroneous interpretation of microscopic findings, especially by an inexperienced observer. A bloody spinal tap may obscure the presence of microorganisms, and the microscopist may fail to examine the smear with the usual care. In the presence of microorganisms on the smear of spinal fluid, the increased white cell count in the spinal fluid with preponderance of polymorphonuclear leukocytes and the decreased spinal fluid sugar level with a concomitant increase in protein support the presumptive diagnosis of meningitis. Yet, the non-microbiological laboratory test results must be reviewed carefully. Patients with meningitis may have normal spinal fluid chemistry and cytology values; a "normal CSF sugar content" in reality may be quite low in a diabetic or in patients receiving intravenous dextrose infusions. Therefore, a serum glucose determination must be performed simultaneously with the spinal fluid analysis.

The results of bacteriological cultures are dependent on appropriate quality control procedures in the laboratory. If a purulent specimen is not cultured within a short period of time after obtaining it, phagocytosis and post-phagocytic killing may continue and the culture may not show growth. The most common reason, however, for the discrepancy of having a positive

Gram-stained smear and a negative culture for meningococci is the prior administration of antibiotics, even in very low dosage. Here the detection of meningococcal antigens by serological means serves to confirm the suspected diagnosis. All culture isolates require definite identification procedures. This is important to recognize infections with unusual neisseriae, to reveal unusual sites of infection, and for public health and infection control reasons.

Uncomplicated cases of meningococcal meningitis or sepsis usually will yield positive spinal fluid or blood cultures if obtained prior to therapy. It is the complicated case that requires special attention by the microbiologist in close cooperation with the attending physician.

References

1. AMIES CR and DOUGLAS JI: Some defects in bacteriological transport media. Can J Public Health 56:27, 1965
2. APICELLA MA: Serogrouping of *Neisseria gonorrhoeae*: identification of four immunologically distinct acidic polysaccharides. J Infect Dis 134:377–383, 1976
3. ASHFORD WA, GOLASH RG, and HEMMING VG: Penicillinase-producing *Neisseria gonorrhoeae*. Lancet 2:657–658, 1976
4. AUSTRIAN R: *Streptococcus pneumoniae* (Pneumococcus). *In* Manual of Clinical Microbiology, 2nd edition. Lennette EH, Spaulding EH, and Truant JP (eds.). American Society for Microbiology, Washington, DC, 1974
5. BENNETT JV, CAMP HM, and EICKHOFF TC: Rapid sulfonamide disc sensitivity test for meningococci. Appl Microbiol 16:1056–1060, 1968
6. BERGER U: Über den Kohlehydratstoffwechsel von *Neisseria* und *Gemella*. Zentralbl Bakteriol Parasitenkd Infektionskr Hyg Abt I: Orig 180:147–149, 1960
7. BROWN WJ: Modification of the rapid fermentation test for *Neisseria gonorrhoeae*. Appl Microbiol 27:1027–1030, 1974
8. BUCHANAN RE and GIBBONS NE (eds.): Bergey's Manual of Determinative Bacteriology, 8th edition. Williams & Wilkins Co, Baltimore, Md, 1974, pp 427–433
9. BYEFF PD and SUSKIEWICA L: Meningococcal arthritis. J Am Med Assoc 235:2572, 1976
10. CARRINGTON GO: Unusual isolates of *Neisseria* from blood. *In* Pathogenic Microorganisms from Atypical Clinical Sources. Von Graevenitz A and Sall T (eds.). M. Dekker, New York, 1975
11. CATLIN BW: *Neisseria meningitidis* (Meningococcus). *In* Manual of Clinical Microbiology, 2nd edition. Lennette EH, Spaulding EH, and Truant JP (eds.). American Society for Microbiology, Washington, DC, 1974
12. CENTER FOR DISEASE CONTROL: Follow-up on antibiotic resistant *Neisseria gonorrhoeae*. Morbid Mortal Weekly Rep 26:29, 1977
13. CENTER FOR DISEASE CONTROL: Meningococcal disease: secondary attack rate and chemoprophylaxis in the United States. J Am Med Assoc 235:261–265, 1974
14. CHAPEL TA, KEANE MB, and GATEWOOD C: Combining cervical and rectal cultures for gonorrhea on a single modified Thayer-Martin plate. Health Lab Sci 13:190–193, 1976
15. COUNTS GW, SEELEY L, and BEATY HN: Identification of an epidemic strain of *Neisseria meningitidis* by bacteriocin typing. J Infect Dis 124:26–32, 1971
16. D'AMATO RF, ERIQUEZ LA, THOMFORDE KM, and SINGERMAN E: Rapid identification of *Neisseria gonorrhoeae* and *Neisseria meningitidis* by using enzymatic profiles. J Clin Microbiol 7:77–81, 1978
17. DANS PE, TOTHENBERG R, and HOLMES KK: Editorial: Gonococcal serology: how soon, how useful and how much. J Infect Dis 135:330–334, 1977
18. DIENA BB, WALLACE R, KENNY CP, and GREENBERG L: Dubos oleic acid agar medium in the differentiation of meningococci and gonococci. Appl Microbiol 19:1025, 1970
19. EDWARDS EA and DRISCOLL WS: Group-specific hemagglutination test for *Neisseria meningitidis* antibodies. Proc Soc Exp Biol Med 126:876–879, 1967

20. ELWELL LP, ROBERTS M, MAYER LW, and FALKOW S: Plasmid-mediated beta-lactamase production in *Neisseria gonorrhoeae*. Antimicrob Agents Chemother 11:528–533, 1977

21. ENG J and HOLTEN E: Gelatin neutralization of the inhibitory effect of sodium polyanethol sulfonate on *Neisseria meningitidis* in blood culture media. J Clin Microbiol 6:1–3, 1977

22. ENG J and IVELAND H: Inhibitory effect in vitro of sodium polyanethol sulfonate on the growth of *Neisseria meningitidis*. J Clin Microbiol 1:444–447, 1975

23. EVANS JR, ARTENSTEIN MS, and HUNTER DH: Prevalence of meningococcal serogroups and description of three new groups. Am J Epidemiol 87:643–646, 1968

24. FELDMAN HA: Neisseria infections other than gonococcal. *In* Diagnostic Procedures for Bacterial, Mycotic and Parasitic Infections, 5th edition. Bodily HL, Updyke EL, and Mason JO (eds.). American Public Health Association, New York, 1970

25. FENG WC, MADEIROS AA, and MURRAY ES: Diagnosis of gonorrhea in male patients by culture of uncentrifuged first-voided urine. J Am Med Assoc 237:896–897, 1977

26. FRASCH CE and CHAPMAN SS: Classification of *Neisseria meningitidis* group B into distinct serotypes. 3. Application of a new bactericidal-inhibition technique to distribution of serotypes among cases and carriers. J Infect Dis 127:149–154, 1973

27. GAY RM and SEVIER RE: *Neisseria sicca* endocarditis: report of a case and review of the literature. J. Clin Microbiol 8:729–732, 1978

28. GEIZER I: Studies on serotyping of *Neisseria gonorrhoeae*. Zentralbl Bakteriol I. Orig A 232:213–220, 1975

29. GOLD R, WINKLEWAKE JL, MARS RS, and ARTENSTEIN MS: Identification of an epidemic strain of group C *Neisseria meningitidis* by bactericidal serotyping. J Infect Dis 124:593–597, 1971

30. GREENWOOD BM, WHITTLE HC, and DOMINIC-RAJKOVIC O: Countercurrent immunoelectrophoresis in the diagnosis of meningococcal infections. Lancet 3:519–521, 1971

31. GREGORY JE and ABRAMSON E: Meningococci in vaginitis. Am J Dis Child 121:423, 1971

32. HAMMERBERG S, MARKS MI, and WEINMASTER G: Re-evaluation of the disc diffusion method for sulfonamide susceptibility testing of *Neisseria meningitidis*. Antimicrob Agents Chemother 10:869–871, 1976

33. HANDSFIELD HH and HOLMES KK: Microepidemic of virulent gonococcal infection. J Am Vener Dis Assoc 1:20–22, 1974

34. HANDSFIELD HH, LIPMAN TO, HARNISCH JP, et al: Asymptomatic gonorrhea in men. N Engl J Med 290:117–123, 1974

35. HENRIKSEN SD: *Moraxella, Neisseria, Branhamella* and *Acinetobacter*. Annu Rev Microbiol 30:63–83, 1976

36. HERMAN RA and RUBINS HA: Meningococcal pericarditis without meningitis presenting as tamponade. N Engl J Med 290:143–144, 1974

37. HOLMES KK, COUNTS GW, and BEATY HN: Disseminated gonococcal infection. Ann Intern Med 74:979–993, 1971

38. IRWIN RS, WOELK WK, and COUDON WL: Primary meningococcal pneumonia. Ann Intern Med 82:493–498, 1975

39. ISENBERG HD, WASHINGTON JA II, BALOWS A, and SONNENWIRTH AC: Collection, handling and processing of specimens. *In* Manual of Clinical Microbiology, 2nd edition. Lennette EH, Spaulding EH, and Truant JP (eds.). American Society for Microbiology, Washington, DC, 1974

40. JACOBS NF and KRAUS SJ: Gonococcal and nongonococcal urethritis in man. Clinical and laboratory differentiation. Ann Intern Med 82:7–12, 1975

41. JACOBS SA and NORDEN CW: Pneumonia caused by *Neisseria meningitidis*. J Am Med Assoc 227:67–78, 1974

42. KELLOGG DS: *Neisseria gonorrhoeae* (Gonoccus). *In* Manual of Clinical Microbiology, 2nd edition. Lennette EH, Spaulding EH, and Truant JP (eds.). American Society for Microbiology, Washington, DC, 1974

43. KELLOGG DS, COHEN IR, NORINS LC, SCHROETER AL, and REISING G: *Neisseria gonorrhoeae*. II. Colonial variation and pathogenicity during 36 months in vitro. J Bacteriol 95:596–605, 1968

44. KELLOGG DS, HOLMES KK, and HILL GA: Cumitech 4: Laboratory Diagnosis of Gonorrhoea. American Society for Microbiology, Washington, DC, 1976

45. KELLOGG DS, PEACOCK WL, DEACON WE, BROWN L, and PIRKLE CI: *Neisseria gonorrhoeae.* I. Virulence genetically linked to clonal variation. J Bacteriol 85:1274–1279, 1963

46. KELLOGG DS and TURNER EM: Rapid fermentation confirmation test of *Neisseria gonorrhoeae.* Appl Microbiol 25:50–52, 1973

47. KIRVEN LA and THORNSBERRY C: Transfer of beta-lactamase genes of *Neisseria gonorrhoeae* by conjugation. Antimicrob Agents Chemother 11:1004–1006, 1977

48. KLEIN EJ, FISHER LW, CHOW AW, et al: Anorectal gonococcal infection. Ann Intern Med 86:340–346, 1977

49. MARTIN JE JR and JACKSON RL: A biological environmental chamber for the culture of *Neisseria gonorrhoeae.* J Am Vener Dis Assoc 2:28–30, 1975

50. MCGEE ZA, DOURMASHKIN RR, GROSS JG, CLARK JB, and TAYLOR-ROBINSON D: Relationship of pili to colonial morphology among pathogenic and nonpathogenic species of *Neisseria.* Infect Immun 15:594–600, 1977

51. MENCK H: Identification of *Neisseria gonorrhoeae* in cultures from tonsillo-pharyngeal specimens by means of a slide co-agglutination test (Phadebact Gonococcus Test). Acta Pathol Microbiol Scand (B) 84:139–144, 1976

52. MORSE SA and BARTENSTEIN L: Adaptation of the Minitek system for rapid identification of *Neisseria gonorrhoeae.* J Clin Microbiol 3:8–13, 1976

53. PAIK G and SUGGS MT: Reagents, stains and miscellaneous test procedures. *In* Manual of Clinical Microbiology, 2nd edition. Lennette EH, Spaulding EH, and Truant JP (eds.). American Society for Microbiology, Washington, DC, 1974, pp 942–943

54. PAYNE SM and FINKELSTEIN RA: Imferon agar: improved medium for isolation of pathogenic *Neisseria.* J Clin Microbiol 6:293–297, 1977

55. PHILLIPS I: Beta-lactamase-producing penicillin-resistant gonococcus. Lancet 3:656–657, 1976

56. PICKERING LK: Chemoprophylaxis against *Neisseria meningitidis.* The role of countercurrent immunoelectrophoresis. J Am Med Assoc 236:1882–1883, 1976

57. POLLOCK HM: Evaluation of methods for the rapid identification of *Neisseria gonorrhoeae* in a routine clinical laboratory. J Clin Microbiol 4:19–21, 1976

58. PUBLIC HEALTH SERVICE ADVISORY COMMITTEE ON IMMUNIZATION PRACTICES: Meningococcal polysaccharide vaccines. Morbid Mortal Weekly Rep 24:381–382, 1975

59. PUTSCH RW, HAMILTON JD, and WOLINSKY E: *Neisseria meningitidis,* a respiratory pathogen? J Infect Dis 121:48–54, 1970

60. RAPACZ S and KASPER J: Comparison of a radiometric method with a carbohydrate fermentation method in the speciation of *Neisseria.* Abstr Annu Meet Am Soc Microbiol, 38:C76, 1976

61. RICHARDSON WP and SADOFF JC: Production of a capsule by *Neisseria gonorrhoeae.* Infect Immun 15:663–664, 1977

62. RINTALA L and POLLOCK HM: Effects of two blood culture anticoagulants on growth of *Neisseria meningitidis.* J Clin Microbiol 7:332–336, 1978

63. ROBBINS JB, MYEROWITZ L, WHISNANT JK, ARGANAN M, SCHNEERSON R, HANDZEL ZT, and GOTSCHLICH EC: Enteric bacteria cross-reactive with *Neisseria meningitidis* groups A and C and *Diplococcus pneumoniae* types 1 and 3. Infect Immun 6:651–656, 1972

64. ROBERTS M and FALKOW S: Conjugal transfer of R plasmids in *Neisseria gonorrhoeae.* Nature (London) 226:630–631, 1977

65. SLATERUS KW: Serological typing of meningococci by means of microprecipitation. Antonie van Leeuwenhoek J Microbiol Serol 27:305–315, 1961

66. SLATERUS KW, RUYS AC, and SIEBERG IG: Types of meningococci isolated from carriers and patients in a nonepidemic period in the Netherlands. Antonie van Leeuwenhoek J Microbiol Serol 29:265–270, 1963

67. STRAUSS RR, HOLDERBACH J, and FRIEDMAN H: Comparison of a radiometric procedure with conventional methods for identification of *Neisseria.* J Clin Microbiol 7:419–422, 1978

68. STUART RD, TOSHACH SR, and PATSULA TM: The problem of transport specimens for culture of gonococci. Can J Public Health 45:73–83, 1954

69. SYMINGTON DA: Improved transport system for *Neisseria gonorrhoeae* specimens. J Clin Microbiol 2:498–503, 1975

70. THAYER JD: Gonorrhea. *In* Diagnostic Procedures for Bacterial, Mycotic and Parasitic Infections, 5th edition. Bodily HL, Updyke EL, and Mason JO (eds.). American Public Health Association, New York, 1970
71. TRAMONT EC and ARTENSTEIN MS: Latex agglutination test for measurement of antibodies to meningococcal polysaccharides. Infect Immun 5:346–351, 1972
72. WALLACE R, ASHTON FE, RYAN A, DIENA BB, MALYSHEFF C, and PERRY MB: The lipopolysaccharide (R-type) as a common antigen of *Neisseria gonorrhoeae*. II. Use of hen antiserum to gonococcal lipopolysaccharide in a rapid slide test for the identification of *N. gonorrhoeae* from isolates and secondary cultures. Can J Microbiol 24:271–275, 1978
73. WASHINGTON JA II and BARRY AL: Dilution test procedures. *In* Manual of Clinical Microbiology, 2nd edition. Lennette EH, Spaulding EH, and Truant JP (eds.). American Society for Microbiology, Washington, DC, 1974
74. WENZEL RP, MITZEL JR, DAVIES JA, and BEAM WE JR: Serum and nasal secretion immune response in meningococcal disease. Infect Immun 5:627–629, 1972
75. WHITE LA and KELLOGG DS: *Neisseria gonorrhoeae* identification in direct smears by a fluorescent antibody-counter stain method. Appl Microbiol 13:171–174, 1965
76. WIESNER PJ, TRONCA E, BONIN P, et al: Clinical spectrum of pharyngeal gonococcal infection. N Engl J Med 228:181–185, 1972
77. YONG DCT and PRYTULA A: Rapid microcarbohydrate test for confirmation of *Neisseria gonorrhoeae*. J Clin Microbiol 8:643–647, 1978
78. YOUNG H: Identification and penicillinase testing of *Neisseria gonorrhoeae* from primary isolation cultures on modified New York City medium. J Clin Microbiol 7:247–250, 1978
79. ZIMMERMAN SE and SMITH JW: Identification and grouping of *Neisseria meningitidis* directly on agar plates by coagglutination with specific antibody-coated Protein A-containing staphylococci. J Clin Microbiol 7:470–473, 1978

CHAPTER 34

PASTEURELLOSES

G. R. Carter

Introduction

Organisms of the genus *Pasteurella* are small gram-negative rods or coccobacilli that grow well on blood- or serum-supplemented solid media either aerobically or anaerobically. Unlike *Yersinia* spp. which were until recently classed as *Pasteurella*, *Pasteurella* spp. grow best at 35 to 37 C, are nonmotile, and are oxidase positive.

Included in the genus *Pasteurella* are the following species: Official—*P. multocida, P. haemolytica, P. pneumotropica,* and *P. ureae*; unofficial—*P. gallinarum, P. anatipestifer,* and *P. aerogenes.* All occur naturally in animals except *P. ureae,* which has only been recovered from humans. All are commensals and potential pathogens in their natural hosts. All but *P. gallinarum* and *P. anatipestifer* have been implicated in human disease.

Pasteurella multocida

P. multocida, the type species of the genus, is considerably heterogeneous and has varieties that differ in colonial characteristics, antigenic nature, and their capacity to produce disease in animals. As more information is obtained on the principal varieties it may be possible to designate distinct biotypes. Recently the author proposed the eventual recognition of five biotypes (8).

General Characteristics

The organism in clinical materials and in freshly recovered cultures consists of gram-negative rods or coccobacilli. They are facultative anaerobes that grow best at 35 to 37 C on solid media supplemented with blood or serum, although growth is also adequate on many nonsupplemented media. After 24 to 48 hr of incubation, colonies resemble in appearance and size colonies of *E. coli, Salmonella,* and other enterobacteria. They are fermentative and nonmotile and do not form spores. They are also non-hemolytic, do not grow on MacConkey agar, produce indole, and reduce nitrate.

Clinical Manifestations

That *P. multocida* can infect human beings has been known for many years; however, only recently have many hospital and public health laboratories learned to recognize this species. In an early review, it was pointed out that the first human infection attributed to *P. multocida* involved a farmer's wife with puerperal fever (29). She was found to have a bacteremia, and the organism was isolated by blood culture.

The different kinds of infections or infectious processes from which *P. multocida* has been isolated are numerous. In general two principal categories of disease are seen. The most common category is infected animal bites. These bites, and in some instances scratches, are most often inflicted by dogs or cats, but other animals including the tiger, opossum, lion, rabbit, and rat have been involved (18, 23). The other category is "internal" infections for which the most likely portal of entry is the respiratory or alimentary tract.

In bite or scratch infections, which most often involve the hands, arms, and legs, a painful, reddened, extensive swelling is usually seen within 24 to 48 hr. There is considerable cellulitis, and a purulent (sometimes sanguineous) discharge will exude from the puncture wounds. On occasions the synovial sheath and periosteum are penetrated, and an osteomyelitis follows. Ordinarily these infections remain localized, and there have been few reports of subsequent bacteremia or septicemia. The possibility of septicemia would seem more likely in the debilitated or compromised patient. It is of interest that the canine and feline strains of *P. multocida*—unlike cultures from cattle, swine, and poultry—rarely cause septicemias or other serious manifestations in natural infections in these species.

Of the so-called internal infections, those involving the respiratory tract are most common, and the respiratory tract is the most likely portal of entry for them. Because there is now a voluminous literature on human infections with this species, only salient points are covered here. Cases and reports of nonbite infections as late as 1965 have been reported on (24). A study of the many reports of internal infections leads to the conclusion that in most instances *P. multocida* is a secondary invader rather than a primary pathogen. Probably the most common internal disease process from which the organism is recovered is bronchiectasis. Of 37 cases of "internal" human pasteurellosis 30 of them were diagnosed as bronchiectasis (35). Other diagnoses involving the respiratory tract have been: chronic bronchitis, empyema, sinusitis, pulmonary cavitation (pulmonary emphysema), infected pulmonary tuberculosis lesions, pleurisy, pneumonia, and pulmonary fibrosis.

The portal of entry for the nonrespiratory internal infections is not known for certain, but it would seem that the most likely routes are wounds and the respiratory or digestive tract. There have been a number of reports of meningitis caused by *P. multocida* (13, 24). Both very young and elderly patients were affected, and in some cases there was a history of accidental or surgical trauma.

There have been a number of reports of septicemia caused by this species (1, 38). In many of these cases, the septicemias were in patients with extensive cirrhosis of the liver. The source of the organism in several of the septicemias was believed to be a dog or cat that had bitten the patient earlier (34, 37).

Among the miscellany of infections reported are the following: puerperal fever leading to septicemia, pyoarthrosis, septic arthritis, appendicular abscess, conjunctivitis, urethritis, brain abscess, otitis, mastoiditis, abdominal abscesses, mouth ulcer, urinary tract infections, acute epiglottitis, infection of mycotic aneurysm, osteomyelitis, endocarditis, corneal ulcer, panophthalmitis, leg ulcer, and infection of compound fractures.

P. multocida has been isolated from a wide range of infected and apparently normal domestic and wild animals. It is a common commensal on the mucous membranes of the upper digestive and respiratory tract. A review of several reports lists carrier rates as follows: cattle, 6%–8%; pig, 26%–51%; sheep, 40%; dogs, 10% (nose) and 54% (tonsils) (41). The organism can be recovered from the gingiva of many cats and from the mouths of many dogs. The organism is inoculated into tissues during the act of biting and the damaged tissues provide a favorable milieu for growth.

P. multocida is carried with impunity and usually only results in infection if there are predisposing influences such as environmental stresses, impaired resistance for various reasons, or primary virus or mycoplasma infections. The fact of the many carriers and the considerable number of infections in domestic animals must result in the release and shedding into the immediate environment of large numbers of *P. multocida*. This shedding is no doubt heaviest in such locations as stables, feedlots, and abattoirs, and consequently it is amongst those individuals working in such locations that most internal infections are seen (35). Another likely source of the organism could be animal and poultry products that could become contaminated in the same way that meat products and carcasses are contaminated with *Salmonella*. *P. multocida* is a not uncommon cause of mastitis in cattle, sheep, and goats, and there is the possibility of human beings becoming infected while milking or as a result of the consumption of unpasteurized milk.

The major diseases of domestic animals caused by *P. multocida* are the following: *Primary disease* (8). Hemorrhagic septicemia of cattle and buffaloes. This important economical disease occurs mainly in tropical and subtropical countries and is caused by two serotypes of *P. multocida*, neither of which has been reported as causing human infections (29). Fowl cholera, an acute to chronic disease primarily of chickens, turkeys, ducks, geese, and wild fowl. The disease is widespread in many countries resulting in great losses particularly in turkeys in the United States (18). Occasional primary pasteurellosis may occur in many animal species. *Secondary disease*. *P. multocida* is a common and important secondary invader of pneumonic lesions in cattle, sheep, swine, and goats particularly, resulting in large numbers of cases of chronic to severe pneumonias. Shipment, transport, and crowding of animals—particularly during inclement weather—predispose to this disease. In addition to these principal diseases *P. multocida* is recovered from a variety of sporadic infections in many animal species.

P. multocida can colonize the upper respiratory tract of apparently normal human beings. There have been several instances in the writer's experience in which the organism has been isolated from the nasal passages and sputum of healthy individuals working in veterinary microbiology laboratories. It was isolated from the throats of two of 71 veterinary students in England (42). There are no reports of person-to-person transmission of *P. multocida*.

Collecting and Processing Specimens

The specimens submitted will depend upon the particular disease manifestation. From the respiratory tract early morning sputa, bronchial washings, nasal swabs, and tracheal aspirates are submitted. From patients with suspected bite or scratch infections, exudate expressed from the wounds is submitted. Other materials submitted include urine, tissues, blood, pleural fluid, and cerebrospinal fluid. If a septicemia or bacteremia is suspected, repeated blood cultures are indicated. Material should always be collected aseptically. When convenient, clinical material is collected on a swab placed in a transport medium before being sent to the laboratory. It is good practice to submit more than one specimen because repeated isolation of *P. multocida* from a particular disease process will help confirm its significance. Specimens and tissues to be shipped should be refrigerated or frozen and surrounded by dry ice.

Ordinarily it is not necessary to submit paired sera for serologic examination. The serologic tests used to detect and measure antibody are sufficiently involved that such procedures are only meaningful if they are carried out in a laboratory with expertise in the serology of this species.

Diagnostic Procedures

In infections caused by *P. multocida*, Gram-stained smears of material taken from the infectious process will show gram-negative rods and coccobacilli. Because this species resembles a number of other gram-negative species morphologically and tinctorially, smears provide only suggestive evidence. In order to confirm a diagnosis, it is necessary to isolate and identify *P. multocida*.

The optimum temperature for growth is 35 to 37 C. Organisms will grow at several degrees warmer, but the amount of growth is diminished as the temperature is lowered to 25 C. The optimum pH for growth is around 7, and cultures grow equally well aerobically or anaerobically.

Isolation and cultivation

Primary isolation should be attempted on blood agar. Any of the standard blood agar formulations are satisfactory. Blood agar is preferred to serum agar, or other unsupplemented media such as tryptose or Trypticase agar because low concentrations of *P. multocida* occasionally fail to grow unless blood is present. The characteristic odor and colonial morphology are also more readily recognized on blood agar. Although strains rarely fail to grow initially on generously inoculated blood agar, it is a good practice to inoculate simultaneously one or several tubes of a nutritious semi-solid medium such as Schaedlers or Brain Heart Infusion broth containing 0.15% agar. If the organism does not grow on blood agar, the broths are plated to blood agar as soon as there is evidence of growth.

It is usually not necessary to triturate tissues prior to culturing. The tissue can be lightly flamed on the outside to remove contaminants, trimmed with sterile scissors, and applied directly as a sectioned surface to the blood agar surface. The inoculum is then streaked over the total plate surface. Inocula can also be taken from incised tissues after searing the surface with a hot spatula.

Small- to moderate-sized dewdrop-like colonies are usually evident after 24 hr incubation. Occasionally it is advisable to reincubate plates for an additional 24 hr. The colonies are round, grayish, nonhemolytic and to the uninitiated eye do not look too unlike species of enterobacteria such as *E. coli* or *Salmonella*. However, with practice one can distinguish the colonies of *P. multocida* from those of the enterobacteria. The characteristic "musty" odor of most cultures gives an indication of its probable identity. The colonial morphology will vary considerably with strains (see Fig 34.1). Cultures from internal infections are more likely to yield large mucoid colonies with flowing margins, whereas those from infected cat and dog bites are usually small. Organisms from the mucoid colonies have large capsules, whereas those from the feline and canine cultures usually have little or no capsules.

Many cultures of *P. multocida* have a great capacity for colonial variation. This is particularly the case with strains from internal infections. Smooth (iri-

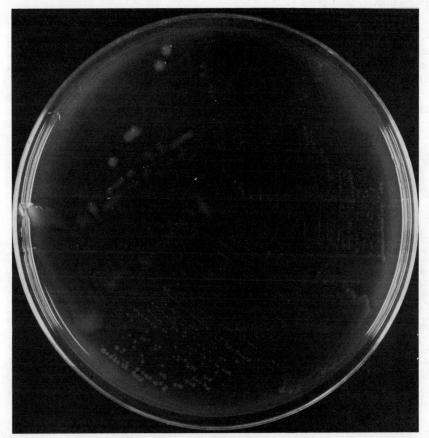

Figure 34.1—Colonies of *Pasteurella multocida* on blood agar. Left: mucoid colonies of a swine culture. Right: small colonies of a canine culture. Center: colonies of a feline culture.

descent), mucoid (iridescent), blue, and rough variants can be identified when cultures on dextrose starch agar (Difco) are examined with oblique light (6).

Animal inoculation. Unless the specimen is heavily contaminated, animals need not be inoculated in order to recover *P. multocida.* Mice are the preferred species, and washings or suspensions of various specimens are inoculated intraperitoneally in several doses ranging from 0.1–0.5 ml. If mice succumb to pasteurella infection, deaths usually occur in 18–96 hr. The organism can be readily recovered from infected mice if the heart's blood, liver, and spleen are inoculated onto blood agar.

It should be kept in mind that the cultures from feline and canine bite infections are frequently of relatively lower pathogenicity for mice. For this reason those mice that do not die should also be necropsied and cultured. Those cultures from internal infections that most likely originated from farm animals are usually more pathogenic for mice.

Identification procedures

P. multocida is a small gram-negative, nonsporeforming, nonmotile rod or coccobacillus which usually occurs singly (see Fig 34.2). When cultures lose their smooth or mucoid colonial character, various filamentous forms are seen. Freshly isolated cultures occasionally have some cell wall-deficient organisms which result in rather bizarre pleomorphism.

Organisms from internal infections will often be capsulated and those which yield large mucoid colonies possess capsules composed largely of hyaluronic acid. The hyaluronic acid capsules can be easily detected with staphylo-

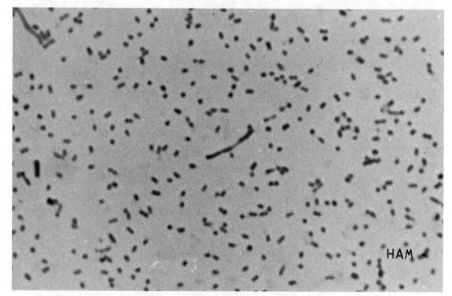

Figure 34.2—*Pasteurella multocida* from a blood agar plate culture. Gram stain, ×3000 (H. A. McAllister). From G. R. Carter, *Diagnostic Procedures in Veterinary Microbiology,* 2nd ed. Charles C. Thomas, 1973.

coccal hyaluronidase (10). Organisms from bite infections usually have little or no capsule.

Although the organism grows best on media supplemented with blood or serum, it also grows well on such solid media as Tryptose and Trypticase soy agar, triple sugar iron agar, and most of the differential media used in studying biochemical characteristics. It does not always grow well in nutrient or peptone water, and heart infusion broth is preferred for indole tests.

The characteristics which lead one to suspect *P. multocida* are: gram-negative rod or coccobacillus, facultative anaerobe, nonhemolytic, nonmotile, reduces nitrate, produces indole (rare exceptions), produces oxidase, and does not grow on MacConkey agar. On triple sugar iron agar, there is an acid slant, an acid butt, no H_2S or gas; however, the color change for acid is not as marked as for some of the enterobacteria. Cultures can then be identified definitively by the additional differential characteristics listed in Table 34.1. Other *Pasteurella* species are listed in this table because, as mentioned later in this chapter, several are capable of causing human infections.

Serologic procedures are not required in identifying this species. Serologic and antigenic features of the organism and the detection and measurement of specific antibody are discussed below.

Although lyophilization is the preferred means of preserving this organism, many strains will survive for weeks or months on Stock Culture agar (Difco) stored at room temperature; they soon die if refrigerated.

Serologic and antigenic nature

As mentioned earlier, *P. multocida* is a very heterogeneous species, with strains probably distinctive enough to be considered biotypes. Characteristics that differ among strains are pathogenicity, host predilection, biochemical activity, colonial morphology, and antigenic nature (8).

Four different capsular types designated A, B, D, and E can be identified with a passive or indirect hemagglutination procedure in which the capsular polysaccharides are adsorbed onto red blood cells (4, 5). As was pointed out

TABLE 34.1—DIFFERENTIAL CHARACTERISTICS OF *PASTEURELLA* SPECIES
(All species are nonmotile, oxidase and catalase positive)

	P. MUL-TOCIDA	*P. PNEUMO-TROPICA*	*P. UREAE*	*P. HAEMO-LYTICA*	*P. AERO-GENES*	*P. GALLI-NARUM*	*P. ANATI-PESTIFER*
Hemolysis	−	−	Green	Beta	−	−	−
Growth on							
MacConkey	(−)[1]	(−)	−	+	+	−	−
Indole	+	+	−	−	−	−	−
Urease	−	+	+	−	+	−	+
Fermentation:							
Glucose	A[2]	A	A	A	AG[3]	A	−
Sucrose	A	A	A	A	AG	A	−
Lactose	(−)	(A)	−	(A)	−	−	−
Mannitol	(A)	−	A	A	−	−	−

[1] ( ) most strains.   [2] A = acid.   [3] AG = acid and gas.

earlier, there is a correlation between capsular type, disease production, and host predilection. Recently, nonserologic procedures were developed for identifying types A and D cultures (10, 11).

Cultures of types A and D have different O or somatic antigens, as shown in an agglutination procedure in which organisms are made agglutinable by acid treatment (33). What are probably the same O antigens have also been identified with an agar gel precipitin test (17), and more than a dozen different O antigens have been identified among type A avian cultures. It has also been shown that the different O or somatic varieties of type A cultures can be readily identified in a slide agglutination procedure in which organisms are first rendered agglutinable by treatment with testicular or staphylococcal hyaluronidase (7, 9).

The serologic and antigenic nature of the feline and canine strains has received little attention, at least partially because they are not important pathogens of these animals. It is also more difficult to use conventional procedures because many strains produce little if any capsule, and suspensions of organisms often have a tendency to autoagglutinate.

It may be beyond the means of most hospital and public health laboratories to do serotyping or detect and measure antibody in a patient's serum. Such considerations as inagglutinability, absence of capsule, and autoagglutination of cultures make detecting antibody difficult. Frequently a patient's serum will not directly agglutinate a suspension of the infecting organism because of the large capsule. In such instances, a culture must be treated with hyaluronidase or plated until an agglutinable variant is obtained. If additional work is required, it is usually advisable to submit the culture or sera to a reference laboratory with expertise in the serology of this species.

Antimicrobial Susceptibility and Resistance

The conventional Kirby-Bauer procedure for testing for antimicrobial susceptibility is recommended. The organism grows well on Mueller-Hinton agar.

Penicillin has been used for many years with good results in treating human infections. However, the need for the susceptibility testing of all cultures is underscored by a recent report of multiple drug resistance in *P. multocida* recovered from cattle and swine (12). Strains tested were most frequently resistant to streptomycin, followed by penicillin and tetracycline.

In the absence of acquired drug resistance, cultures are susceptible to: penicillin, ampicillin, tetracylines, chlortetracycline, novobiocin, streptomycin, erythromycin, neomycin, polymyxin, gentamicin, cephalothin, and sulfonamides. The susceptibility of isolates from humans to several of these drugs was documented in a recent report (40).

Evaluation of Laboratory Findings

P. multocida can be considered the primary infectious agent in animal-bite or -scratch infections if it is recovered in sufficient concentrations after repeated culturing. That *P. multocida* has a causal role in most internal infections is confirmed by the clinical improvement of affected patients after antimicrobial treatment. Treatment should be continued until the elimination of the organism is confirmed by negative culture results.

Pasteurella pneumotropica

P. pneumotropica resembles *P. multocida* but has several different biochemical characteristics and also is less likely to cause disease in animals. It was first found to be a fairly common commensal of rats, mice, and guinea pigs (25), and later of cats (44) and dogs. Human infections caused by this species are uncommon.

General Characteristics

This organism, like the type species *P. multocida*, is a small, nonmotile, fermentative, oxidase positive, gram-negative rod or coccobacillus, which grows aerobically or anaerobically. Its colonial and microscopic morphology strongly resemble that of a nonmucoid *P. multocida*. In the original description of this species it was stated that it had an "indistinct capsule" (25).

Clinical Manifestations

This commensal of the upper respiratory and digestive tracts of mice, rats, guinea pigs, dogs, cats, and some other animals has a low potential for causing disease. When it does cause disease, it is usually mild and involves the respiratory tract—particularly the lungs of rats and mice. It would seem that when associated with pneumonia its role is usually secondary, as it is in chronic murine pneumonia of the rat. Among the diseases of mice in which it has been implicated are conjunctivitis, metritis, urocystitis, abscesses, and dermatitis (3). Various infections have also been reported from a kangaroo rat, dog, hamster, and rat (3).

Only a few human infections have been attributed to this organism. In a comprehensive study of unusual pathogenic gram-negative rods, sources of human strains of *P. pneumotropica* were "one cellulitis following rat bite," "one peritoneal fluid following appendectomy," and one infection of unknown source (28). Several dog-bite infections, one of which was fatal, and one cat-bite infection have been reported (31) and also the association of the organism (originally thought to be *P. multocida*) with rhinitis and tonsilitis in a young boy (19). A fatal septicemia following a dog-bite infection has been reported (32), as has a septicemia in a patient being treated for myeloid leukemia (39).

Collecting and Processing Specimens

Specimens are handled as described for *P. multocida.*

Diagnostic Procedures

The procedures described for *P. multocida* also apply to *P. pneumotropica.* The colonies resemble those of nonmucoid *P. multocida* but have a grayish-yellow cast. Gram-stained smears from colonies disclose small gram-negative rods or coccobacilli indistinguishable from those of *P. multocida.*

The biochemical characteristics of *P. pneumotropica* resemble those of *P. multocida.* The principal difference is the production of urease by the former organism. Like *P. multocida*, it is nonhemolytic, nonmotile, oxidase positive, reduces nitrate, and produces indole. Differential media used for definitive identification are listed in Table 34.1. In a recent report three different biotypes were proposed on the basis of differences in several biochemical reactions (47).

Ordinarily, serologic procedures and animal inoculations are not done. Strains of *P. pneumotropica* are less pathogenic for mice on inoculation than cultures of *P. multocida* from cattle, sheep, swine, and poultry.

Cultures from infected humans should be tested for susceptibility to antimicrobics. The Kirby-Bauer method with Mueller-Hinton agar is quite adequate. There are few reports on the susceptibility of this species. A strain recovered from an infected human was susceptible to tetracycline, chloramphenicol, colistin, sodium cephalothin, nalidixic acid, and streptomycin. It was resistant to ampicillin (36). Another human isolate was reported to be susceptible to penicillin, ampicillin, carbenicillin, oxytetracyline, chloramphenicol, kanamycin, polymyxin, cephalothin, gentamicin, and a sulphamethoxazole/trimethoprim combination (39).

Pasteurella ureae

This organism was originally considered to be a variety of *P. haemolytica*, a species which occurs naturally only in animals (20). The official and widely accepted name at present is *P. ureae*. In contrast to the other *Pasteurella* species, it has only been recovered from human beings.

It resembles *P. multocida* in microscopic and colonial morphology and in oxygen and growth requirements. Like the type species, it is nonmotile, fermentative, oxidase positive, and occurs naturally as a commensal in human beings.

Clinical Manifestations

P. ureae is an uncommon commensal which sometimes acts as an opportunist in compromised individuals and as a secondary invader in traumatized tissue or tissues in which there is already an infectious or pathologic process. It has been recovered most frequently from patients with bronchiectasis and chronic bronchitis (26). Other diseases with which it has been associated are sinusitis and ozaena (20), pneumonia (43), septicemia (15), and meningitis (45).

P. ureae occurs in human beings as a rather uncommon commensal of the upper respiratory and digestive tracts. It is isolated occasionally from human sputa, and one group of authors found it in 1% of their sputum specimens (27). In another study it was recovered from the nasal passages of three individuals and from the upper respiratory tract of seven (20, 21).

Diagnostic Procedures

The diagnostic procedures recommended are essentially similar to those recommended for *P. multocida.* The organism grows well on blood agar, which is recommended for isolation. Mice are not used for isolation. After 24 to 48 hr of incubation, colonies are similar in size and appearance to those of many cultures of *P. multocida*. Greening is seen around colonies with some later partial hemolysis.

This organism differs from *P. multocida* in producing a strong urease reaction but no indole. Like the former species it is oxidase positive, does not grow on MacConkey agar, reduces nitrate, and ferments glucose, sucrose, and some other carbohydrates with the production of acid. The differential tests listed in Table 34.1 should be done for definitive identification.

The very limited information on *in vitro* antimicrobial susceptibility suggests a spectrum of susceptibility that roughly resembles that of *P. multocida* and *P. pneumotropica*.

Additional *Pasteurella* Species

P. haemolytica

This is an important commensal and pathogen of domestic and wild animals. To date only four cultures have been recovered from human beings. One was from blood of a patient injured while dressing a deer, and another was isolated from a gall bladder (28). The third was recovered from a patient with endocarditis (14) and the fourth from "berry bush" lacerations and scratches sustained while hunting (32). A deer which the patient subsequently dressed was thought to be the source of the *P. haemolytica*.

This species resembles *P. multocida* in its colonial and microscopic morphology but differs in being beta-hemolytic, not producing indole, and growing on MacConkey agar. The amount of beta hemolysis depends on the kind of blood used in the blood agar. If sheeps' blood is used, the beta hemolysis may only be evident under a colony which was scraped from the agar. Two very distinct varieties of *P. haemolytica* have been described (2). For definitive identification, the differential characteristics listed in Table 34.1 should be referred to.

Pasteurella new species I "gas" (*multocida?*)

This organism, which resembles *P. multocida* in microscopic appearance, colonial morphology, and in oxygen and growth requirements, was recovered from humans with various types of infections. The sources of 44 isolates were as follows: dog bite, 17; animal, 10; cat bite, 2; cat scratch, 1; wound, 5; blood, 3; throat, 2; lung and pleural effusion, 1; and unknown, 2 (46). The property that readily distinguishes these cultures from typical *P. multocida* is that the former produces gas from glucose.

This variety occurs as a commensal in the upper respiratory and digestive tracts of dogs and cats, as do *P. multocida* and *P. pneumotropica*. It has been suggested that these aerogenic strains are a biotype of *P. pneumotropica*. Except for the production of gas they appear to be identical in their biochemical reactions to one of the three biotypes of *P. pneumotropica* referred to above (47).

P. aerogenes

This aerogenic organism, which has been given the tentative name *P. aerogenes*, occurs as part of the normal flora of the intestine of swine (30). It has only rarely been associated with disease in swine, and there has only been one isolation to date from a human being. This individual had been bitten by a boar.

The principal differential characteristics of this apparently new species are listed in Table 34.1.

P. gallinarum, P. anatipestifer, and Pasteurella-like Organisms

Although there have been no human infections as yet attributed to *P. gallinarum* (16, 22) or *P. anatipestifer* (22), these species are listed in Table 34.1 to aid in their identification should they be recovered from human specimens. Occasionally pasteurella-like organisms recovered from animals do not conform in one or more reactions to species descriptions based on typical biochemical characteristics. These are sometimes referred to as *Pasteurella*-like organisms. An alternative way of reporting them is to state, e.g., that an isolate resembles *P. multocida* or another *Pasteurella* species except for an aberrant reaction (or reactions).

References

1. BEARN AG, JACOBS K, and MCCARTY M: *Pasteurella multocida* septicemia in man. Am J Med 18:167–168, 1955
2. BIBERSTEIN EL and FRANCIS CK: Nucleic acid homologies between the A and T types of *Pasteurella haemolytica*. J Med Microbiol 1:105–108, 1968
3. BRENNAN PC, FRITZ TE, and FLYNN RJ: *Pasteurella pneumotropica*: Cultural and biochemical characteristics and its association with disease in laboratory animals. Lab Anim Care 15:307–312, 1965
4. CARTER GR: Studies on *Pasteurella multocida*. I. A hemagglutination test for the identification of serological types. Am J Vet Res 16:481–484, 1955
5. CARTER GR: A new serological type of *Pasteurella multocida* from Central Africa. Vet Rec 73:1052, 1961
6. CARTER GR: Pasteurellosis: *Pasteurella multocida* and *Pasteurella hemolytica*. In Advances in Veterinary Science, Vol. 11. Academic Press, New York, 1967, pp 321–379
7. CARTER GR: Simplified identification of somatic varieties of *Pasteurella multocida* causing fowl cholera. Avian Dis 16:1109–1114, 1972
8. CARTER GR: A proposal for five biotypes of *Pasteurella multocida*. 19th Annual Proceedings of the American Association of Veterinary Diagnosticians, 1976, pp 189–196
9. CARTER GR, CHENGAPPA MM, and GUPTA AN: A preliminary report on somatic types of type A *Pasteurella multocida* from cattle and swine. 20th Annual Proceedings of the American Association of Diagnosticians, 1977
10. CARTER GR and RUNDELL SW: Identification of type A strains of *Pasteurella multocida* using staphylococcal hyaluronidase. Vet Rec 96:343, 1975
11. CARTER GR and SUBRONTO P: Identification of type D strains of *Pasteurella multocida* with acriflavine. Am J Vet Res 34:293–294, 1972
12. CHANG WH and CARTER GR: Multiple drug resistance in *Pasteurella multocida* and *Pasteurella haemolytica* from cattle and swine. J Am Vet Med Assoc 169:710–712, 1976
13. CONTRONI G and JONES RS: *Pasteurella* meningitis: a review of the literature. Am J Med Tech 33:379–386, 1967
14. DOTY GL, LOOMUS GN, and WOLF PL: *Pasteurella* endocarditis. N Engl J Med 268:830–832, 1963
15. GATTY F, SENYHAEVE V, and WEAVER R: First description of a case of human septicemia due to *Pasteurella ureae*. Annu Soc Belges Trop 48:463–468, 1968
16. HALL WT, HEDDLESTON KL, LEGENHAUSEN DH, and HUGHES RW: Studies on pasteurellosis. I. A new species of *Pasteurella* encountered in chronic fowl cholera. Am J Vet Res 25:598–604, 1955
17. HEDDLESTON KL, GALLAGHER JE, and REBERS PA: Fowl cholera: gel diffusion precipitin test for serotyping *Pasteurella multocida* from avian species. Avian Dis 16:925–936, 1972

18. HENDERSON A: *Pasteurella multocida* infection in man: a review of the literature. Antonie van Leeuwenhoek J Microbiol Serol 29:359–367, 1963

19. HENDRIKSEN SD: Some pasteurella strains from the human respiratory tract. Acta Pathol Microbiol Scand 55:355–356, 1962

20. HENDRIKSEN SD and JYSSUM K: A new variety of *Pasteurella haemolytica* from the human respiratory tract. Acta Pathol Microbiol Scand 50:443, 1960

21. HENDRIKSEN SD and JYSSUM K: A study of some *Pasteurella* strains from the human respiratory tract. Acta Pathol Microbiol Scand 51:354–368, 1961

22. HITCHNER SB, DOMERUTH CH, PURCHASE HG, and WILLIAMS JE (eds.): Isolation and Identification of Avian Pathogens. Arnold Printing Corp, Ithaca, NY, 1975

23. HUBBERT WT and ROSEN MN: I. *Pasteurella multocida* infection due to animal bite. Am J Public Health 60:1103–1117, 1970

24. HUBBERT WT and ROSEN MN: II. *Pasteurella multocida* infection in man unrelated to animal bite. Am J Public Health 69:1109–1117, 1970

25. JAWETZ E: A pneumotropic *Pasteurella* of laboratory animals. I. Bacteriological and serological characteristics of the organism. J Infect Dis 86:172–183, 1950

26. JONES DM: A *Pasteurella*-like organism from the human respiratory tract. J Pathol Bacteriol 83:143–151, 1962

27. JONES DM and O'CONNOR PM: *Pasteurella haemolytica* var. *ureae* from human sputum. J Clin Pathol 15:247–248, 1962

28. KING EO: The identification of unusual pathogenic Gram-negative bacteria. 64th Annual Meeting of the American Society for Microbiology, Washington, DC, 1964

29. LEVY-BRUHL M: Les pasteurelloses humaines. Ann Med 44:408–437, 1938

30. MCALLISTER HA and CARTER GR: An aerogenic *Pasteurella*-like organism recovered from swine. Am J Vet Res 35:917–922, 1974

31. MEDLEY S: A dog bite wound infected with *Pasteurella pneumotropica*. Med J Aust 2:224–225, 1977

32. MILLER JK: Human pasteurellosis in New York State. New York State J Med 66:2527–2531, 1966

33. NAMIOKA S and MURATA M: Serological studies on *P. multocida*. III. O antigenic analysis of cultures isolated from various animals. Cornell Vet 51:522–528, 1961

34. NORMANN B, NILEHN B, RAJS J, and KARLBERG B: A fatal human case of *Pasteurella multocida* septicemia after cat bite. Scand J Infect Dis 3:251–254, 1971

35. OLSEN AM and NEEDHAM GM: *Pasteurella multocida* in suppurative diseases of the respiratory tract. Am J Med Sci 224:77–81, 1952

36. OLSON JR and MEADOWS TR: *Pasteurella pneumotropica* infection resulting from a cat bite. J Clin Pathol 51:709–710, 1969

37. PALUTKE WA, BOYD CB, and CARTER GR: *Pasteurella multocida* septicemia in a patient with cirrhosis. Am J Med Sci 266:305–308, 1973

38. PELTIER M, ARQUIE E, JONCHERE H, and LE BLOUGH G: Septicemie mortella a *Pasteurella*. Bull Soc Pathol Exot 31:475–479, 1938

39. ROGERS BT, ANDERSON JC, PALMER CA, and HENDERSON WG: Septicaemia due to *Pasteurella pneumotropica*. J Clin Pathol 26:396–398, 1973

40. ROSENTHAL SL and FREUNDLICH LF: *In vitro* antibiotic sensitivity of *Pasteurella multocida*. Health Lab Sci 13(4):246–249, 1976

41. SMITH JE: Studies on *Pasteurella septica*. I. The occurrence in the nose [sic] and tonsils of dogs. J Comp Pathol Ther 65:239–245, 1955

42. SMITH JE: Studies on *Pasteurella septica*. III. Strains from human beings. J Comp Pathol 69:231–235, 1959

43. STARKEBAUM GA and PLORDE JJ: *Pasteurella* pneumonia: report of a case and review of the literature. J Clin Microbiol 5:332–335, 1977

44. VAN DORSSEN CA, DE SMIDT AC, and STAM JWE: Over het voorkomen van *Pasteurella pneumotropica* bin katten. Tijdschr Diergeneeskd 89:674–682, 1964

45. WANG WLL and HAIBY G: Meningitis caused by *Pasteurella ureae*. J Clin Pathol 45:562–565, 1966

46. WEAVER RE: Unclassified groups of aerobic Gram-negative bacteria isolated from clinical specimens. Current Topics in Clinical Microbiology Seminar, American Society for Microbiology, Boston, Mass, 1970

47. WINBLAD S: *Pasteurella* taxonomy and nomenclature. *In* Contributions to Microbiology and Immunology, Vol. 2. Karger, Basel, 1973, pp 170–176

CHAPTER 35

PSEUDOMONAS AND MISCELLANEOUS NONFERMENTERS

Peter C. Fuchs

Introduction

General Description

The genus *Pseudomonas* is a rather heterogeneous group of organisms, with few phenotypic characteristics to clearly distinguish it from other genera. Nucleic acid homology studies show significant differences within the currently recognized genus. At least five distinct groups can be distinguished, each of which may ultimately merit separate genus status (65). Members of the genus are aerobic, asporogenous, gram-negative bacilli, which are usually motile with polar flagella. Anaerobic growth may occur with those species (e.g., *P. aeruginosa*) capable of denitrification as a means of anaerobic respiration. They are nonfermentative microbes, but most species utilize carbohydrates by oxidation and are oxidase positive.

Another genus incorporating significant gram-negative nonfermenting bacteria is *Acinetobacter*. Members of this genus may also be oxidizers or non-oxidizers, but are readily differentiated from *Pseudomonas* by being nonmotile and oxidase negative. Microbes of the genera *Alcaligenes* and *Moraxella* are occasionally found in clinical material, and both are oxidase-positive, gram-negative nonfermenters. *Alcaligenes*, though motile, has peritrichous flagella, and *Moraxella* is nonmotile. Table 35.1 shows the characteristics at the genus level for *Pseudomonas* and other commonly found clinical gram-negative non-fermenters. The single characteristic that best differentiates *Pseudomonas* from the others is polar flagellation—though at least one species (*P. mallei*) is non-motile. Several less common isolates collected at the Center for Disease Control (CDC) and as yet unnamed also have polar flagella (e.g., IIK, Va, VE-1, VE-2) (86).

Clinical Manifestations

The disease spectrum of this group of organisms is protean. *P. aeruginosa* and most of the other related species rarely infect immunologically competent individuals. Although *P. aeruginosa* may cause almost any kind of infectious process [urinary tract infection, pneumonia, wound infection, endocarditis (72), meningitis (5), osteomyelitis (56), bacteremia (26), etc.], this organism also produces a number of characteristic clinical syndromes.

Burn patients are unusually susceptible to *P. aeruginosa* infection of the burn wound. Once an infection is established, vascular wall invasion by the organism may cause sepsis and dissemination of infection. Although *Pseudomonas* infections in moderate to moderately severe burns can be prevented or controlled by modern topical antimicrobic preparations, *P. aeruginosa* infection with sepsis remains a common cause of death in severely burned patients (90). The bedside diagnosis of *P. aeruginosa* infections of burns may be made easily by examining the burn under a Wood's light for the characteristic fluorescence (84).

Patients with malignant neoplastic disease, especially those with acute leukemia and those receiving antineoplastic therapy associated with marrow suppression (e.g., radiotherapy and chemotherapy), are particularly susceptible to *P. aeruginosa* infection with sepsis (10, 26, 74). Often such infections respond poorly to antimicrobic therapy. One of the factors in this increased susceptibility and poor therapeutic response is the low neutrophil count of many of these patients (74). Neutrophils are now recognized as a major defense against *P. aeruginosa* infection, and patients with neutrophil counts under 1000/μl of blood often fail to respond to even the best available antimicrobic therapy. This is the rationale for granulocyte transfusions in such patients.

Patients with cystic fibrosis are particularly prone to *P. aeruginosa* infection of the respiratory tract (48). About half these patients have respiratory tract colonization by *P. aeruginosa* (53). Isolates from such infections or colonizations are often mucoid and may exhibit antimicrobic susceptibility patterns different from non-mucoid variants of the same strains (75). Sputa from nearly half of cystic fibrosis patients which contain *P. aeruginosa* will have two or more phenotypically and serotypically distinct strains (75). Antimicrobic susceptibilities often differ significantly among the different strains in the same

TABLE 35.1—DIFFERENTIAL CHARACTERISTICS OF COMMON NONFERMENTING GRAM-NEGATIVE GENERA

GENUS	OXIDASE	GLUCOSE OXIDIZER	FLAGELLA
Pseudomonas	V	V	Polar
Achromobacter	+	+	Peritrichous
Flavobacterium	+	+	−
*Kingella**	+	+	−
Brucella	+	V	−
Alcaligenes	+	−	Peritrichous
Bordetella	V	−	V (Peritrichous)
Moraxella	+	−	−
Acinetobacter	−	V	−

V = varies with species
− = negative
+ = positive
* Formerly named *Moraxella kingii* (45)

patient. Therefore, when antimicrobic susceptibility tests are requested on such specimens, all the different strains of *P. aeruginosa* should be tested.

The prevalence of mucoid strains in such patients is a unique phenomenon. Since mucoid variants are rarely encountered outside the respiratory tracts of cystic fibrosis patients, a biochemical defect involving slime formation in such patients has been postulated. Mucoid strains have been induced *in vitro* by both bacteriophages (57) and the selective pressures of antimicrobics in growth media (37).

Infections of the eyelids and conjunctivitis caused by *P. aeruginosa* are generally not too severe. Corneal ulcers due to *P. aeruginosa*, however, are potentially devastating (2). The collagenase elaborated by this organism may lead to perforation within hours. Therefore, such an infection is a true emergency and requires immediate diagnosis and therapy.

P. aeruginosa and a few other nonfermenters are commonly isolated from the ear canals of patients with otitis externa. The significance of this relationship is not always clear. A rarely seen form of otitis externa, malignant otitis externa, is commonly caused by *P. aeruginosa* and generally occurs in diabetics (16). This infection is progressive and may lead to 7th nerve palsy and ultimately death.

Glanders, a disease caused by *P. mallei* and primarily occurring in horses, may rarely produce disease in humans. However, the disease is virtually nonexistent in the Western Hemisphere today.

Melioidosis, on the other hand, a disease caused by the related organism, *P. pseudomallei*, is more commonly seen in man. Based on serologic studies of endemic populations, it appears that the great majority of infections are asymptomatic (63). Most clinically significant infections are initially apparent as pulmonary infections which, if untreated, may progress to sepsis, dissemination of infection, and death (47, 87). After an infection, *P. pseudomallei* may be latent within the host for years. Reactivated infection may occur many years later during periods of stress without re-exposure to the organism (49).

Many other species of *Pseudomonas* and related genera have been isolated from clinical specimens, though less commonly than *P. aeruginosa*. Often these isolates represent colonization, but true infections with such organisms have been well documented. Some examples of such infections are listed in Table 35.2.

Epidemiology

Pseudomonas and other common "water bug" members of the nonfermenter group are ubiquitous in the environment—commonly isolated from soil, water, or any moist environment. Foods, particularly vegetables, are colonized with such microbes. Ingestion of such foods provides a ready means of colonization of the intestinal tract by *Pseudomonas* (13, 80).

P. aeruginosa may be found as part of the fecal flora of many normal individuals, but is rarely, if ever, a major component of such flora in healthy people (90). Occasionally, *Pseudomonas* may transiently colonize the pharynx, skin, and other areas of a healthy individual's body. Pharyngeal and intestinal colonization, however, is more frequent in seriously ill hospitalized patients (50), and those receiving antibiotics (80).

Table 35.2—Examples of Infections by Less Common Nonfermentative Gram-Negative Bacilli

Organism	Type of Infection	References	Organism	Type of Infection	References
Achromobacter xylosoxidans	Wounds	70	*Pseudomonas cepacia*	Sepsis	27, 34, 67
	Otitis	70		Wounds	6, 27, 34, 67
				Urinary tract	27, 34
Acinetobacter calcoaceticus	Sepsis	36		Respiratory tract	20, 27, 34
	Wounds	36		Endocarditis	42, 64
	Urinary tract	36		Meningitis	21
	Respiratory tract	36			
	Meningitis	39	*Pseudomonas fluorescens/putida*	Wounds	34
	Otitis	19		Urinary tract	34
Acinetobacter lwoffi	Meningitis	14	*Pseudomonas maltophilia*	Sepsis	42, 62
	Otitis	19		Wounds	34, 35
				Urinary tract	34, 35
Alcaligenes faecalis	Respiratory tract	76		Respiratory tract	34
	Meningitis	76		Meningitis	66
Flavobacterium	Meningitis	43	*Pseudomonas putrefaciens*	Sepsis	34, 82
	Respiratory tract	81		Wounds	23, 82
	Endocarditis	88		Otitis	34, 46
Moraxella species	Endocarditis	17, 77	*Pseudomonas stutzeri*	Sepsis	54
	Otitis	19		Wounds	34, 58
				Otitis	34
			Pseudomonas (other species)	Sepsis	4, 34
				Wounds	34
				Urinary tract	34
				Respiratory tract	34
				Meningitis	18

The mechanism of this phenomenon is not well understood. The finding of increased *Pseudomonas* infection rates in intestinal carriers of *P. aeruginosa* (74) and the presence of the same strain in both the intestinal tract and site of infection in many leukemic patients (10, 74) support the intestinal source hypothesis. Colonization of other sites by *P. aeruginosa* appears to originate in the environment, presumably via transient carriage on the hands of persons caring for patients who have burns, tracheotomies, etc. (52). The major source and precursor of infection by *P. aeruginosa*, regardless of the mechanism, is the colonization of the body surfaces of patients.

Many outbreaks of *P. aeruginosa* infections in hospitals have been traced to specific mechanisms and sources. Examples include: nebulizers and humidifiers of respiratory therapy equipment (68); urological surgical instruments (60); resuscitation apparatus (25); faucet aerators (40); and disinfectant solutions. Similar sources and mechanisms have been incriminated for other pseudomonads, especially *P. cepacia* (24, 79) and *A. calcoaceticus* (78) (*Acinetobacter calcoaceticus var. anitratus, Herellea vaginicola*).

Pseudomonas is a significant factor in the epidemiology of nosocomial infections. Among the common microbes producing nosocomial infections in the United States, *P. aeruginosa* ranked 6th in frequency in 1975 (15). *P. aeruginosa* causes infections such as urinary tract infections, wound (including burn) infections, and respiratory tract infections, in decreasing order of frequency. Sepsis occurs in 5%–10% of all patients with *P. aeruginosa* infections. *P. aeruginosa* ranks 4th among all organisms causing secondary nosocomial bacteremias (15).

Like other pseudomonads, *P. pseudomallei* is found in soil and water, but unlike the others it is not geographically ubiquitous. It is primarily endemic in southeast Asia, but has occasionally been isolated in tropical and subtropical parts of the world, such as Central and South America. There is at least one report of indigenous infection by *P. pseudomallei* or a closely related species in the United States (58). Infection is usually acquired through the skin via cuts, abrasions, wounds, etc. Infections via inhalation and ingestion have also been described. Infections in the United States have been seen in returnees from southeast Asia. Person to person transmission does not occur or is extremely rare.

Public Health Significance and Preventive Measures

Since pseudomonads are only opportunistic pathogens and rarely are of significance outside the health care facility environment, they have essentially no public health significance in the usual sense. The one exception to this is *P. pseudomallei*, the etiologic agent of melioidosis. Because of recent military involvement in southeast Asia, veterans returning to the United States from such areas as Vietnam are occasionally found to be infected with this agent. Person to person spread does not seem to occur or at least too rarely to warrant quarantine or isolation measures. Prophylaxis consists of general hygiene and avoidance of endemic areas.

In recent years, vaccines consisting of various serotypes of *P. aeruginosa* have been prepared and used for active immunization of burn patients. Early studies indicate this may effectively reduce the incidence of *P. aeruginosa* infections in such patients (1, 73). In three controlled trials (two in England, one in India) the use of a vaccine prepared from 16 *P. aeruginosa* serotypes resulted in a profound reduction of *P. aeruginosa* infection, bacteremia, and mortality in the Indian hospital, where such infections and mortality are normally high (51); in the British hospital the incidence of *P. aeruginosa* infections and death were too low to be assessed. Preliminary trials with such vaccines in leukemic children appear less promising (41).

Collection and Processing of Specimens

No special procedures or precautions beyond those recommended for other nonfastidious microbes, such as the *Enterobacteriaceae* and staphylococci, are required for specimen collection and processing. In general, the specimen should be sent to the laboratory promptly and processed quickly. Should delay be unavoidable, refrigerate specimens such as urine.

Diagnostic Procedures

Microscopic Examination

There are no intrinsic morphologic features which distinguish *Pseudomonas* from other common gram-negative bacilli on direct Gram-stained smears. Although *P. aeruginosa* is a slender, gram-negative bacillus measuring about 0.5–1.0 μm by 2–3 μm, these dimensions are neither specific for this organism nor all-inclusive. In certain specimens (e.g., corneal ulcer), smears containing gram-negative bacilli should be assumed to contain *P. aeruginosa* until culture results prove otherwise. Members of the genera *Moraxella* and *Acinetobacter* may be coccobacillary and arranged in pairs. In urethral and cervical smears, they may resemble or even be mistaken for gram-negative diplococci.

Microscopic examination of paraffin sections of *P. aeruginosa*-infected tissue characteristically reveals acute vasculitis with invasion of blood vessel walls by gram-negative bacilli. Intravascular thrombosis and extravascular hemorrhages with surrounding hemorrhagic necrosis are commonly associated with this condition (30).

Primary Culture Media

The organisms included in this section grow well on all the usual media used for primary isolation of nonfastidious bacteria.

On such media, well-formed colonies are usually present in 18–24 hr. Colonial morphology varies considerably, not only between species, but also within the same species. *P. pseudomallei* and *P. stutzeri* characteristically produce wrinkled, heaped-up colonies in 48–72 hr. Typically, *P. aeruginosa* produces large (2–4 mm), slightly convex, glistening, grayish colonies. They may smell sweet and grape-like and are often hemolytic on blood agar. Most strains elaborate pyocyanin, a chloroform- and water-soluble bluish, phenazine pigment. Most strains also produce pyoverdin, a pigment which is yellow, fluorescent, water-soluble, and chloroform-insoluble. Pyoverdin can be detected by examining the colonies under ultraviolet light. Other pigments such as pyorubin (red) and pyomelanin (brown-black) are also occasionally produced. Although pyocyanin is specific for *P. aeruginosa*, pyoverdin is also produced by *P. fluorescens* and *P. putida*. These pigments may not show up in a significant proportion of strains and their absence cannot be relied upon to rule out *P. aeruginosa*. Various yellow and tan pigments are produced by other pseudomonads. Special media to increase pyocyanin production (Tech Agar-BBL) and pyoverdin production (Flo Agar-BBL) are available.

Though not recommended for routine culture, selective media such as cetrimide containing media (e.g., Pseudosel Agar-BBL) may be useful when *P. aeruginosa* specifically is sought from a source containing other microbes (e.g., detection of *P. aeruginosa* in the environment, in carriers or infections during epidemics, or for special epidemiologic studies). On such media, growth alone is not specific for *P. aeruginosa*, unless the characteristic bluish pyocyanin pigment is also seen. Other pseudomonads and *Enterobacteriaceae* may also grow on them. Therefore, further identification procedures should be performed.

Identification Procedures

The identification of these organisms is made by determining the appropriate biochemical, physiologic, and morphologic characteristics. Many approaches are now available for the identification of nonfermenters. Some of the better recognized schemata include those of King as modified by Weaver et al. (86), Gilardi (32, 33), Pickett (69), and Henriksen (44). Although each of these schemata is valid, their reliability and validity are largely dependent on utilizing the methods and media described by the author of a particular schema. The most common members of this group are described below, but for the less commonly seen isolates, the reader should refer to the authors listed above.

With a few biochemical and physiological tests, most of the nonfermenters seen in clinical material can be easily identified. Table 35.3 lists the characteristics of the more common nonfermentative clinical isolates which can be identified by tests and media readily available in most clinical microbiology laboratories.

As a group, the nonfermenters are usually recognizable by their inactivity or alkaline reaction on TSI or Kligler's iron agar. They can then be easily broken into subgroups on the basis of three easy-to-perform reactions: glucose oxidation (Hugh and Leifson's OF Basal Medium-BBL); oxidase test (Kovacs); and motility (hanging drop or motility test medium-BBL). The number of additional tests required for species identification can be minimized by concentrating on those reactions yielding maximum differentiation within a particular subgroup (see highlighted reactions in Table 35.3). For the occasional strains giving atypical reaction patterns, additional tests may be needed for identification.

The flagellar stain is a very useful test for differentiating *Pseudomonas* species (polar flagella) from peritrichously flagellated nonfermenters such as

TABLE 35.3—CHARACTERISTICS OF THE MORE COMMON NONFERMENTATIVE CLINICAL ISOLATES

IDENTIFICATION (CHARACTERISTICS*)	NUMBER	POLAR FLAGELLA	PYOCYANIN	ESCULIN HYDROLYSIS	LACTOSE OXIDATION	42 C GROWTH	PHENYLALANINE	CITRATE	UREASE	MALTOSE OXIDATION	XYLOSE OXIDATION	MANNITOL OXIDATION	H_2S IN TSI	GELATINASE	INDOL	GAS FROM NITRATE	FLUORESCENCE	MOTILITY	OXIDASE (KOVACS)	GLUCOSE OXIDATION
Pseudomonas aeruginosa	1-2	+	+ᵛ	−	−	+	−	+	+ᵛ	−	+	+ᵛ	−	+ᵛ	−	+	+ᵛ	+ᵛ	+	+
Pseudomonas fluorescens	>2	+	−	−	v	−	−	+	v	−	+	+ᵛ	−	+	−	−	+ᵛ	+	+	+
Pseudomonas putida	>2	+	−	−	v	−	−	+	v	v	+	−ᵛ	−	−	−	−	+ᵛ	+	+	+
Pseudomonas pseudomallei	>2	+	−	+ᵛ	+	+	−	+	−	+ᵛ	+	+	−	+	−	+	−	+	+ʷ	+
Pseudomonas stutzeri	1-2	+	−	−	−	+	−	+	v	+ᵛ	+	+ᵛ	−	−	−	+	−	+	+	+
Pseudomonas putrefaciens	1-2	+	−	−	v	+	−	−	−ᵛ	v	−	−	+	+	−	−	−	+	+	+
Pseudomonas cepacia	>2	+	−	+ᵛ	+	v	−	+	−ᵛ	+ᵛ	+	+ᵛ	−	+ᵛ	−	−	−	+	+ʷ	+
Achromobacter xylosoxidans	−	−	−	−	−	−ᵛ	−	+	−ᵛ	−	+	−	−	−	−	−	−	+	+	+
Flavobacterium meningosepticum	−	−	−	−	v	−ᵛ	−	−	−ᵛ	+	−	+	−	+	+	−	−	−	+	+
Flavobacterium species	−	−	−	−	−	−ᵛ	−	−	−ᵛ	+	−	−	−	+	+	−	−	−	+	+
Kingella kingii	−	−	−	−	−	−	−	−	−	+	−	−	−	−	−	−	−	−	+	+

	Acinetobacter calcoaceticus	*Pseudomonas mallei*	*Pseudomonas maltophilia*	*Pseudomonas species*	*Alcaligenes species*	*Bordetella bronchiseptica*	*Moraxella phenylpyruvica*	*Moraxella osloensis*	*Mima polymorpha var. oxidans*	*Acinetobacter lwoffi*
			>2	v						
	−	−	+	+	−	−	−	−	−	−
	−	−	−	−	−	−	−	−	−	−
	−	−	+ᵛ	−	−	−	−	−	−	−
	+	−	v	−	−	−	−	−	−	−
	−ᵛ	−ᵛ	+ᵛ	−	−	−	−ᵛ	−ᵛ	−ᵛ	−
	−	−	−	−	−	−	+	−	−	−
	v	−	v	+	+	+	−	−	+	−
	v	−	v	−	+	+ˢ	−	−	−	−
	−	−	+	−	−	−	−	−	−	−
	+	−	−	−	−	−	−	−	−	−
	−	−	−	−	−	−	−	−	−	−
	−	−	−	−	−	−	−	−	−	−
	v	−	+	v	−	−	−	−	−	−
	−	−	−	−	−	−	−	−	−	−
	−	−	−	v	−	−	−	−	−	−
	−	−	−	−	−	−	−	−	−	−
	−	−	+	+	+	+	−	−	−	−
	−	−	−	+	+	+	+	+	+	−
	+	+	+ᵛ	−	−	−	−	−	−	+

* Boldfaced reactions = strong differential reactions
+ = > 95% positive
+ᵛ = 75%–95% positive
s = very strong
− = > 95% negative
−ᵛ = 75%–95% negative
v = variable
w = weak

A. xylosoxidans. Leifson beautifully illustrates the art of the flagella stain (55). The standard tannic acid method for flagella staining requires meticulous care and expertise, but a simplified silver plating technique has been recently described (89) which provides staining of comparable quality.

Gas-liquid chromatographic analysis of metabolic products has been successfully utilized in the speciation of pseudomonads (61, 83), but is not widely used for this purpose.

Serologic Procedures

With one exception, serologic tests have little or no practical value in the diagnosis of infections by this group of organisms. The exception is serological testing for melioidosis. The complement-fixation or passive hemagglutination (*P. pseudomallei* polysaccharide adsorbed onto ovine erythrocytes) tests are most useful (47). Because this disease is rare in the United States, the maintenance of reagents for this test is not justifiable in most clinical microbiology laboratories.

Typing

Because *P. aeruginosa* accounts for over 75% of gram-negative nonfermentative isolates from clinical material, and because of its importance in nosocomial infections, strain identification by various typing methods is most useful for epidemiologic studies of this species. At least six typing methods have been used in *P. aeruginosa* strain identification: serologic typing, two forms of pyocin typing, bacteriophage typing, antibiogram typing, and biotyping.

Serologic typing

This is performed through an agglutination test based on the reactivity of somatic O antigens of intact cells with specific antisera. Despite some cross-reactivity, clear differentiation between O types is usually possible (9, 11). Commercial antisera (Difco) are now available, and the simplicity of the slide agglutination test should make this method of typing practical. Despite 10%–11% cross-reactivity, the method has been very effective in epidemiologic studies (11).

Pyocin typing

Pyocins refer to *P. aeruginosa*-specific bacteriocins (antimicrobic substances produced by organisms which inhibit other strains of the same species). Two methods of typing are possible (9, 28, 29): pyocin production (active typing) and pyocin susceptibility (passive typing).

In pyocin production typing, a set of indicator strains of *P. aeruginosa* is tested for its susceptibility to the pyocin produced by the strains to be typed. Based on the pattern of resistance and susceptibility of the indicator strains to the test strains, specific pyocin types can be identified.

In pyocin susceptibility typing, the strains to be typed are tested for their susceptibility to a set of different pyocin-producing indicator strains of *P. aeruginosa.* Again, based on the patterns of resistance and susceptibility of the test organisms to the pyocin-producing indicator strains, specific types can be identified. Pyocin production has been shown to be a more stable and reproducible feature of *P. aeruginosa* strains than pyocin susceptibility (28) and has become a useful tool for typing this organism in epidemiologic studies (9).

Bacteriophage typing

Because lysogenic *P. aeruginosa* are common, methods of phage typing have been developed which determine the susceptibility of test organisms to a series of different bacteriophages (38). Because of its slightly greater complexity and its poorer reproducibility (8, 29), phage typing has not been as popular as the first two methods of *P. aeruginosa* strain identification.

Antibiogram

Most strains of *P. aeruginosa* have a fairly standard antimicrobic susceptibility pattern (Table 35.4). However, occasional strains have a different pattern, such as resistance to gentamicin and/or carbenicillin. These changes are often plasmid mediated (12) and thus may be passed to other strains or lost spontaneously. Consequently, this characteristic cannot be used alone to identify a strain. Nevertheless, variant antibiogram patterns are useful in the early detection of problems in the hospital setting and are epidemiologically valuable (22).

Biotyping

Typing can be done easily by determining the patterns of biochemical, physiologic, and morphologic properties, but if there is no outstanding characteristic present to identify an outbreak strain, the value of biotyping is limited. Many strains of *P. aeruginosa* have identical patterns of biochemical reactivity. On the other hand, some properties appear to vary within the same strain. For example, in one study multiple biotypes based on a small number of phenotypic characteristics (pigment production, fluorescein production, hemolysis, etc.) were found in an outbreak caused by a single strain (single pyocin type and serotype) of *P. aeruginosa* (9).

Many of these different systems for typing *P. aeruginosa* have been combined (7, 9, 29) in attempts to more accurately "fingerprint"strains in epidemiologic investigations. From such studies, it appears that serologic or pyocin typing, used separately or together, provide the most discriminating, reproducible, and practical solution to the problem.

Antibiotic Susceptibility

Many pseudomonads are typically resistant to commonly used antimicrobics, a feature of great clinical significance. The antimicrobic susceptibility pattern of many species of *Pseudomonas* and other nonfermenters is quite characteristic for each particular species (3, 31, 59) (Table 35.4). In many instances, the pattern of susceptibility to certain antimicrobics is sufficiently characteristic to warrant the use of antibiograms as a quality control check on species identification.

The susceptibility of *P. aeruginosa* to aminoglycosides and polymyxins is

TABLE 35.4—ANTIBIOGRAMS FOR PSEUDOMONADS AND RELATED SPECIES

Organism	Penicillin G	Cephalothin	Nitrofurantoin	Ampicillin	Erythromycin	Tetracycline	Carbenicillin	Gentamicin	Polymyxins	Chloramphenicol	Kanamycin	Streptomycin	Neomycin	Novobiocin	Nalidixic Acid
Pseudomonas cepacia	R	R	R	R	R^v	R^v	R^v	R^v	R^v	S^v	R^v	R^v	R^v	R^v	V
Pseudomonas aeruginosa	R	R	R	R	R	R^v	S^v	S^v	S	R^v	R^v	R^v	S^v	R	R^v
Pseudomonas putida	R	R	R	R	R	V	R	S^v	V	S	R	V	S	R	
Pseudomonas fluorescens	R	R	R	R	R^v	S	R^v	S	S	V	S^v	V	S	R	R^v
Pseudomonas pseudomallei	R	R	R	S^v	R	S	S^v	R	R	S^v	S	R	S^v	S^v	S^v
Pseudomonas maltophilia	R^v	R^v	R	R^v	R^v	R	S^v	V	S	S^v	V	R^v	V	R	S^v
Pseudomonas stutzeri	R	R	S^v	S^v	V	S^v	S	S	S	V	S^v	S^v	S^v	R	S
Pseudomonas putrefaciens	R	V	R	V	V	V	V	S	S	S	S	S	S	R	S
Acinetobacter calcoaceticus	R^v	R	R^v	V	V	R	S	S	S	R^v	S	S^v	S	R^v	S
Acinetobacter lwoffi	R	V	R^v	R^v	V	R^v	R	S	R	V	S	R^v	S	V	S
Flavobacterium meningosepticum	V	R	R^v	V	S	R	S	R^v	S	S^v	R	R^v	V	S	S^v
Alcaligenes sp.	V	S	V	R	V	R^v	S	S	S	V	V	R^v	V	R^v	V
Moraxella sp.	S	S	S^v	S	S	S	S	S	S	S^v	S^v	S^v	S	S^v	S

S = > 95% susceptible
S^v = 75%–95% susceptible
R = > 95% resistant
R^v = 75%–95% resistant
V = 75%–95% variable

markedly influenced by the concentration of cations (71, 85) such as calcium and magnesium in the test medium—MIC's are increased with increasing concentrations of cations. Mueller-Hinton media containing 20–35 mg of Mg^{++} and 50–100 mg Ca^{++} per liter should be utilized for both dilution (broth and agar) and disk diffusion susceptibility tests. Most batches of Mueller-Hinton agar contain such concentrations of cations, but Mueller-Hinton broth usually needs to be supplemented with additional cations.

Evaluation of Laboratory Findings

Because many nonfermenters are everywhere in the environment and in human body surface flora, such organisms are commonly isolated from clinical material. When isolated from blood, cerebrospinal fluid, tissue, urine in counts greater than $10^5/ml$, etc., the clinical significance of such isolates is usually readily apparent. Likewise, if such an organism is the sole or predominant organism isolated from a source with a different normal flora (e.g., sputum), one might assume the organism is significant.

Often this is not the case. *Pseudomonas* and other nonfermenters are frequently isolated in small numbers from the pharynx, sputum, intestinal tract, genito-urinary tract, etc.—particularly in hospitalized patients. Unless such isolates are being identified for epidemiologic purposes, it is best to consult the clinician instead of wasting time, expense and effort on identifying isolates which are probably not clinically significant. The identification of such isolates may be misleading and costly for the patient, especially if he receives inappropriate treatment as a result.

References

1. ALEXANDER JW, FISHER MW, MACMILLAN BG et al: Prevention of invasive *Pseudomonas* infection in burns with a new vaccine. Arch Surg 99:249–256, 1969
2. ALLEN HF: Current status of prevention, diagnosis and management of bacterial corneal ulcers. Ann Ophthalmol 3:235–246, 1971
3. ALTMANN G and BOGOKOVSKY B: *In vitro* sensitivity of *Flavobacterium meningosepticum* to antimicrobial agents. J Med Microbiol 4:296–299, 1971
4. ATKINSON BE, SMITH DL, and LOCKWOOD WR: *Pseudomonas testosteroni* septicemia. Ann Intern Med 83:369–370, 1975
5. AYLIFFE GA, LOWBURY EJL, HAMILTON JG et al: Hospital infection with *Pseudomonas aeruginosa* in neurosurgery. Lancet 2:365–368, 1965
6. BASSETT DCJ, STOKES KJ, and THOMAS WRG: Wound infection with *Pseudomonas multivorans*. A water-borne contaminant of disinfectant solution. Lancet 1:1188–1191, 1970
7. BERGAN T: Epidemiological markers for *Pseudomonas aeruginosa*. 3. Comparison of bacteriophage typing, serogrouping, and pyocine typing on heterogenous clinical material. Acta Pathol Microbiol Scand Sect B 81:91–101, 1973
8. BERGAN T and LYSTAD A: Reproducibility in bacteriophage sensitivity pattern of *Pseudomonas aeruginosa*. Acta Pathol Microbiol Scand Sect B 80:345–350, 1972
9. BOBO RA, NEWTON EJ, JONES LF et al: Nursery outbreak of *Pseudomonas aeruginosa*: epidemiological conclusions from five different typing methods. Appl Microbiol 25:414–420, 1973
10. BODEY GP: Epidemiological studies of *Pseudomonas* species in patients with leukemia. Am J Med Sci 260:82–89, 1970
11. BROKOPP CD, GOMEZ-LUS R, and FARMER JJ III: Serological typing of *Pseudomonas aeruginosa*: use of commercial antisera and live antigens. J Clin Microbiol 5:640–649, 1977

12. BRYAN LE, SHAHRABADI MS, and VAN DEN ELZEN HM: Gentamycin resistance in *Pseudomonas aeruginosa*: R-factor-mediated resistance. Antimicrob Agents Chemother 6:191–199, 1974

13. BUCK AC and COOKE EM: The fate of ingested *Pseudomonas aeruginosa* in normal persons. J Med Microbiol 2:521–525, 1969

14. BURROWS S and KING MJ: Meningitis due to *Mima polymorpha*. Am J Clin Pathol 46:234–238, 1966

15. CENTER FOR DISEASE CONTROL. 1977. National Nosocomial Infection Study Report, Annual Summary, 1975

16. CHANDLER JR: Malignant external otitis and facial paralysis. Otolaryngol Clin North Am 7:375–383, 1974

17. CHRISTENSEN CE and EMMANOUILIDES GC: Bacterial endocarditis due to "Moraxella New Species I." N Engl J Med 277:803–804, 1967

18. COWLISHAW WA, HUGHES ME, and SIMPSON HCR: Meningitis caused by an alkali-producing pseudomonad. J Clin Pathol 29:1088–1090, 1976

19. DADSWELL JV: *Acinetobacter* and similar organisms in ear infections. J Med Microbiol 9:345–353, 1976

20. DAILEY RH and BENNER EJ: Necrotizing pneumonitis due to the pseudomonad "Eugonic oxidizer—group I." N Engl J Med 279:361–362, 1968

21. DARBY CP: Treating *Pseudomonas cepacia* meningitis with trimethoprim-sulfamethoxazole. Am J Dis Child 130:1365–1366, 1976

22. DAYTON SL, BLASI DD, CHIPPS D, and SMITH RF: Epidemiological tracing of *Pseudomonas aeruginosa*: antibiogram and serotyping, Appl Microbiol 27:1167–1169, 1974

23. DEBOIS J, DEGREEF H, VANDEPITTE J, and SPAEPEN J: *Pseudomonas putrefaciens* as a cause of infection in humans. J Clin Pathol 28:993–996, 1975

24. DIXON RE, KASLOW RA, MACKEL DC et al: Aqueous quaternary ammonium antiseptics and disinfectants. Use and misuse. J Am Med Assoc 236:2415–2417, 1976

25. DREWETT SE, PAYNE DJH, TUKE W, and VERDON PE: Eradication of *Pseudomonas aeruginosa* infection from a special care nursery. Lancet 1:946–948, 1972

26. DUPONT HL and SPINK WW: Infections due to gram-negative organisms: an analysis of 860 patients with bacteremia at the University of Minnesota Medical Center. 1958–1960. Medicine 48:307–332, 1969

27. EDERER GM and MATSEN JM: Colonization and infection with *Pseudomonas cepacia*. J Infect Dis 125:613–618, 1972

28. FALKINER FR and KEANE CT: Epidemiological information from active and passive pyocine typing of *Pseudomonas aeruginosa*. J Med Microbiol 10:447–459, 1977

29. FARMER JJ III and HERMAN LG: Epidemiological fingerprinting of *Pseudomonas aeruginosa* by the production of and sensitivity to pyocine and bacteriophage. Appl Microbiol 18:760–765, 1969

30. FORKNER CE JR: *Pseudomonas aeruginosa* Infection. Grune and Stratton, Inc, New York, 1960

31. GILARDI GL: Antimicrobial susceptibility as a diagnostic aid in the identification of nonfermenting gram-negative bacteria. Appl Microbiol 22:821–823, 1971

32. GILARDI GL: Characterization of nonfermentative, nonfastidious gram-negative bacteria encountered in medical bacteriology. J Appl Bacteriol 34:623–644, 1971

33. GILARDI GL: Diagnostic criteria for differentiation of *Pseudomonas* pathogenic to man. Appl Microbiol 16:1497–1502, 1968

34. GILARDI GL: Infrequently encountered *Pseudomonas* species causing infection in humans. Ann Intern Med 77:211–215, 1972

35. GILARDI GL: *Pseudomonas maltophilia* infections in man. Am J Clin Pathol 51:58–61, 1969

36. GLEW RH, MOELLERING RC JR, and KUNZ LJ: Infections with *Acinetobacter calcoaceticus (Herella vaginicola)*: clinical and laboratory studies. Medicine 56:79–97, 1977

37. GOVAN JRW and FYFE JAM: Mucoid *Pseudomonas aeruginosa* and cystic fibrosis: resistance of the mucoid form to carbenicillin, flucloxicillin and tobramycin and the isolation of mucoid variants *in vitro*. J Antimicrob Chemother 4:233–240, 1978

38. GRABER CD, LATTA L, VOGEL EH, and BRAME R: Bacteriophage grouping of *Pseudomonas aeruginosa*, with special emphasis on lysotypes occurring in infected burns. Am J Clin Pathol 37:54, 1962

39. GREEN D: *Bacterium anitratum* meningitis. Arch Intern Med 106:870–873, 1960

40. GROSS DF, BENCHIMOL A, and DIMOND EG: The faucet aerator—a source of *Pseudomonas* infection. N. Engl J Med 274:1430–1431, 1966
41. HAGHBIN M, ARMSTRONG D, and MURPHY ML: Controlled prospective trial of *Pseudomonas aeruginosa* vaccine in children with acute leukemia. Cancer 32:761–766, 1973
42. HAMILTON J, BURCH W, GRIMMETT G et al: Successful treatment of *Pseudomonas cepacia* endocarditis with trimethoprim-sulfamethoxazole. Antimicrob Agents Chemother 4:551–554, 1973
43. HAZUKA BT, DAJANI AS, TALBOT K, and KEEN B: Two outbreaks of *Flavobacterium meningosepticum* type E in a neonatal intensive care unit. J Clin Microbiol 7:450–455, 1977
44. HENRIKSEN SD: *Moraxella, Acinetobacter,* and the *Mimeae.* Bacteriol Rev 37:522–561, 1973
45. HENRIKSEN SD and BØVRE K: Transfer of *Moraxella kingae* Henriksen and Bøvre to the genus *Kingella* gen. nov. in the family *Neisseriaceae.* Int J Syst Bacteriol 26:447–450, 1976
46. HOLMES B, LAPAGE SP, and MALNICK H: Strains of *Pseudomonas putrefaciens* from clinical material. J Clin Pathol 28:149–155, 1975
47. HOWE C, SAMPATH A, and SPOTNITZ M: The *Pseudomallei* group: a review. J Infect Dis 124:598–606, 1971
48. IACOCCA VF, SIBINGA MS, and BARBERO GJ: Respiratory tract bacteriology in cystic fibrosis. Am J Dis Child 106:315–324, 1963
49. JACKSON AE, MOORE WL JR, and SANFORD JP: Recrudescent melioidosis associated with diabetic ketoacidosis. Arch Intern Med 130:268–271, 1972
50. JOHANSON WG, PIERCE AK, and SANFORD JP: Changing pharyngeal flora of hospitalized patients. Emergence of gram-negative bacilli. N Engl J Med 281:1137–1140, 1969
51. JONES RJ, ROE EA, and GUPTA JL: Controlled trials of a polyvalent pseudomonas vaccine in burns. Lancet 1:977–983, 1979
52. KOMINOS SD, COPELAND CE, and GROSIAK B: Mode of transmission of *Pseudomonas aeruginosa* in a burn unit and an intensive care unit in a general hospital. Appl Microbiol 23:309–312, 1972
53. KULCZYCKI LL, MURPHY TM, and BELLANTI JA: *Pseudomonas* colonizaion in cystic fibrosis. A study of 110 patients. J Am Med Assoc 240:30–34, 1978
54. LAPAGE SP, HILL LR, and REEVE JE: *Pseudomonas stutzeri* in pathological material. J. Med Microbiol 1:195–202, 1968
55. LEIFSON E: Atlas of Bacterial Flagellation. Academic Press, New York and London, 1960
56. LEWIS R, GORBACH S, ALTNER P: Spinal *Pseudomonas* chondro-osteomyelitis in heroin users. N Engl J Med 286:1303, 1972
57. MARTIN DR: Mucoid variation in *Pseudomonas aeruginosa* induced by the action of phage. J Med Microbiol 6:111–118, 1973
58. MCCORMICK JB, WEAVER RE, HAYES PS et al: Wound infection by an indigenous *Pseudomonas pseudomallei*-like organism isolated from the soil: case report and epidemiologic study. J Infect Dis 135:103–107, 1977
59. MOODY MR, YOUNG VM, and KENTON DM: *In vitro* antibiotic susceptibility of pseudomonads other than *Pseudomonas aeruginosa* recovered from cancer patients. Antimicrob Agents Chemother 2:344–349, 1972
60. MOORE B and FORMAN A: An outbreak of urinary *Pseudomonas aeruginosa* infection acquired during urological operations. Lancet 2:929–931, 1966
61. MOSS CW and SAMUELS SB: Short-chain acids of *Pseudomonas* species encountered in clinical specimens. Appl Microbiol 27:570–574, 1974
62. NARASIMHAN SL, GOPAUL DL, and HATCH LA: *Pseudomonas maltophilia* bacteremia associated with a prolapsed mitral valve. Am J Clin Pathol 68:304–306, 1977
63. NIGG C: Serologic studies on subclinical melioidosis. J Immunol 91:18–28, 1963
64. NORIEGA ER, RUBENSTEIN E, SIMBERKOFF MS, and RALAL JJ JR: Subacute and acute endocarditis due to *Pseudomonas cepacia* in heroin addicts. Am J Med 59:29–36, 1975
65. PALLERONI NJ, KUNISAWA R, CONTOPOULOU R, and DOUDOROFF M: Nucleic acid homologies in the genus *Pseudomonas.* Int J Syst Bacteriol 23:333–339, 1973
66. PATRICK S, HINDMARCH JM, HAGUE RV, and HARRIS DM: Meningitis caused by *Pseudomonas maltophilia.* J Clin Pathol 28:741–743, 1975
67. PHILLIPS I, EYKYN S, CURTIS MA, and SNELL: JJS: *Pseudomonas cepacia* (multivorans) septicaemia in an intensive care unit. Lancet 1:375–377, 1971
68. PHILLIPS I and SPENCER G: *Pseudomonas aeruginosa* cross-infection due to contaminated respiratory apparatus. Lancet 2:1325–1327, 1965

69. PICKETT MJ and PEDERSEN MM: Nonfermentative bacilli associated with man. II. Detection and identification. Am J Clin Pathol 54:164–177, 1970
70. PIEN FD and HIGA HY: *Achromobacter xylosoxidans* isolates in Hawaii. J Clin Microbiol 7:239–241, 1978
71. RELLER LB, SCHOENKNECHT FD, KENNY MA, and SHERRIS JC: Antibiotic susceptibility testing of *Pseudomonas aeruginosa*: selection of a control strain and criteria for magnesium and calcium content in media. J Infect Dis 130:454–463, 1974
72. REYES MP, PALUTKE WA, WYLIN RF et al: *Pseudomonas* endocarditis in the Detroit Medical Center 1969-1972. Medicine 52:173–194, 1973
73. SACHS A: Active immunoprophylaxis in burns with a new multivalent vaccine. Lancet 2:959–961, 1970
74. SCHIMPFF SC, MOODY M, and YOUNG VM: Relationship of of colonization with *Pseudomonas aeruginosa* to development of *Pseudomonas* bacteremia in cancer patients. Antimicrob Agents Chemother—1970, 240–244, 1971
75. SEALE TW, THIRKILL H, TARPAY M, FLUX M, and RENNERT OM: Serotypes and antibiotic susceptibilities of *Pseudomonas aeruginosa* isolates from single sputa of cystic fibrosis patients. J Clin Microbiol 9:72–78, 1979
76. SHERMAN JD, INGALL D, WIENER J, and PRYLES CV: *Alcaligenes faecalis* infection in the newborn. Am J Dis Child 100:212–215, 1960
77. SILBERFARB PM and LAWE JE: Endocarditis due to *Moraxella liquefaciens*. Arch Intern Med 122:512–513, 1968
78. SMITH PW and MASSANARI RM: Room humidifiers as the source of *Acinetobacter* infections. J Am Med Assoc 237:795–797, 1977
79. SPELLER DCE, STEPHENS ME, and VIANT AC: Hospital infection by *Pseudomonas cepacia*. Lancet 1:798–799, 1971
80. STOODLEY BJ and THOM BT: Observations on the intestinal carriage of *Pseudomonas aeruginosa*. J Med Microbiol 3:367–375, 1970
81. TERES D: ICU-acquired pneumonia due to *Flavobacterium meningosepticum*. J Am Med Assoc 228:732, 1974
82. VANDEPITTE J and DEBOIS J: *Pseudomonas putrefaciens* as a cause of bacteremia in humans. J Clin Microbiol 7:70–72, 1978
83. WADE TJ and MANDLE RJ: Chromatographic characterization procedure: preliminary studies on some *Pseudomonas* species. Appl Microbiol 27:303–311, 1974
84. WARD CG, CLARKSON JG, TAPLIN D, and POLK HC JR: Wood's light fluorescence and *Pseudomonas* burn wound infection. J Am Med Assoc 202:1039–1040, 1967
85. WASHINGTON JA II, SNYDER RJ, KOHNER PC et al: Effect of cation content of agar on the activity of gentamicin, tobramycin, and amikacin against *Pseudomonas aeruginosa*. J Infect Dis 137:103–111, 1978
86. WEAVER RE, TATUM HW, and HOLLIS DC: The Identification of Unusual Pathologic Gram-negative Bacteria (Elizabeth O. King). Center for Disease Control, Atlanta, Ga, 1972
87. WEBER DR, DOUGLASS LE, BRUNDAGE WG, and STALLKAMP TC: Acute varieties of melioidosis occurring in U.S. soldiers in Vietnam. Am J Med 46:234–244, 1969
88. WERTHAMER S and WEINER M: Subacute bacterial endocarditis due to *Flavobacterium meningosepticum*. Am J Clin Pathol 57:410–412, 1972
89. WEST M, BURDASH NM, and FREIMUTH F: Simplified silverplating stain for flagella. J Clin Microbiol 6:414–419, 1977
90. YOUNG LS and ARMSTRONG D: *Pseudomonas aeruginosa* infections. CRC Crit Rev Clin Lab Sci 3:291–347, 1972

CHAPTER 36

RAT-BITE FEVER

William J. Martone and Charlotte M. Patton

Two etiologic agents can cause rat-bite fever: spirillary rat-bite fever, or Sodoku, is caused by *Spirillum minus,* whereas streptobacillary rat-bite fever is caused by *Streptobacillus moniliformis.* Although infection most commonly follows the bite of a rat, other animals have also been implicated in transmission of the disease, particularly that caused by *St. moniliformis* (1).

Spirillum minus

Sp. minus is a rigid, spiral-shaped organism, 3–5 μm in length, with single or, occasionally, multiple bipolar flagella. The most outstanding feature of the organism, the characteristic darting-to-and-fro motility and rotation about the long axis, is best observed with dark-field microscopy. Speculation that *Sp. minus* and *Campylobacter* spp. are closely related is partially based on their close morphologic resemblance and their similar motilities (9).

Clinical manifestations of infection with *Sp. minus* and *St. moniliformis* are similar; in many instances differentiation on clinical grounds alone may not be possible. The incubation period for spirillary rat-bite fever is variable but is usually longer than 10 days, whereas for streptobacillary rat-bite fever it is usually shorter than 10 days (14). Although the site of the original bite may heal initially, an inflammatory recrudescence characterized by swelling, erythema, induration, pain, and even ulceration may coincide with the development of other symptoms. Fever, which tends to be relapsing, may be accompanied by headache, nausea, vomiting, myalgia, regional lymphadenopathy, rash, and leukocytosis. Although arthralgia may occur, arthritis is unusual, being more characteristic of *St. moniliformis* than of *Sp. minus* infection. A false-positive serologic test for syphilis is said to occur more commonly with *Sp. minus* infections.

Recovery from spirillary rat-bite fever is usually complete after penicillin therapy; tetracycline may be used as an alternative drug for penicillin-sensitive individuals. In the absence of specific antimicrobial therapy, the disease may run a chronic course, frequently taking months to resolve (13).

Confirmatory laboratory evidence of *Sp. minus* infection must rely on animal inoculation because no artificial growth medium has been developed. Sporadic reports claiming successful cultivation of *Sp. minus* have not been substantiated; further work on the development of an artificial medium is clearly needed.

Although organisms occasionally may be discovered by direct dark-field microscopy of patient's blood or lesion scrapings, care must be taken to exclude the possibility of artifacts or other spiral organisms. When rat-bite fever is suspected, mice should be inoculated intraperitoneally with 0.5–1 ml of patient's blood or lesion scrapings suspended in saline. The infection in mice is usually inapparent clinically and must be documented microscopically. Peritoneal exudate and/or blood should be examined by dark-field microscopy weekly for 4 weeks. Alternatively, blood, peritoneal exudate, or cardiac impressions may be stained with Giemsa stain and examined by light microscopy (6). The inoculation of four mice has generally been suggested; however, the optimal number of animals required has not been adequately studied. Some authors have recommended that guinea pigs be inoculated in addition to mice (1)

Since *Sp. minus* infection is said to occur in a variable percentage of uninoculated laboratory rodents, care must be taken to exclude prior infection by preexamination or the use of controls.

A reliable serologic test for spirillary rat-bite fever is not available.

Streptobacillus moniliformis

Streptobacillus moniliformis is a gram-negative, non-acid-fast, nonmotile, pleomorphic rod 0.3–0.7 μm in width and 1–5 μm in length. Filaments are common and often have spherical or oval swellings. Chains of bacilli and coccobacilli are frequently observed and account for the descriptive name given to the organism. An L-phase variant occurs commonly on solid media 2–4 days after the development of the bacterial colony.

St. moniliformis infection may follow the bite of a rat or, more uncommonly, bites of other animals. Sporadic and epidemic disease may also occur with no history of rat bite, the most notable example being the Haverhill, Massachusetts, epidemic of 1928. Illness in this outbreak, referred to as "Haverhill fever," or "erythema arthriticum epidemicum," is thought to have been caused by drinking contaminated unpasteurized milk (12). Today, the term "Haverhill fever" is still applied to cases of human infection for which no history of rat bite can be found.

The incubation period for *St. moniliformis* infection is variable but is usually less than 10 days. If a rat bite has occurred, healing is usually uneventful, although swelling and tenderness may be present initially. Fever, chills, headache, vomiting, and leukocytosis are common but do not necessarily distinguish *St. moniliformis* from *Sp. minus* infection. The fever with *Sp. minus* infection, however, may have a greater tendency for a relapsing pattern than that with *St. moniliformis* infection. The rash in streptobacillary disease, which may be macular, maculopapular, petechial, or pustular, is more pronounced on the extremities, frequently affecting the palms and soles.

Polyarthritis, involving mainly the elbows, wrists, knees, and/or ankles, is one of the hallmarks of infection with *St. moniliformis*. Arthritis reportedly occurs in over 70% of the cases and is one of the features that distinguish *St. moniliformis* from *Sp. minus* infection (14).

Patients usually recover completely from *St. moniliformis* infection after penicillin therapy. Untreated, the disease may run a chronic course and take weeks to months to resolve. Superimposed complications such as endocarditis have resulted in fatalities but should be prevented by prompt antimicrobial therapy (13).

Rodents appear to be the most important natural reservoirs of *St. moniliformis*. Carriage of the organism in the upper respiratory passages of laboratory and wild rats is common. Mice are apparently more susceptible than rats to severe *St. moniliformis* infection, with epizootic disease having been reported in the former (4, 15). Humans are a dead-end host for infection.

Infection is confirmed in the laboratory by recovering the organism from blood, joint fluid, or abscess aspirates. Agglutination of *St. moniliformis* antigen by patient's serum may also be demonstrated, but obtaining an isolate of the organism is the preferred method of laboratory diagnosis.

Collection and Handling of Specimens

One outstanding growth characteristic of *St. moniliformis* is its requirement for serum, ascitic fluid, or blood in artificial media. This property must be considered when laboratory specimens are being collected and handled. To minimize destruction of the organism, specimens should be inoculated onto culture media as soon as possible after collection.

Blood

A 10- to 15-ml sample of citrated blood should be collected, with 1 ml of each sample being used as inoculum for several tubes containing 5–6 ml of broth enriched with 20% ascitic fluid or 10%–30% horse or rabbit serum. Trypticase soy, tryptose phosphate, and veal infusion broth with a final pH of 7.3–7.6 have been used satisfactorily as basal media. Thioglycolate medium (10 ml) has also been used successfully for primary isolation. If serum- or ascitic fluid-enriched media are not available for primary isolation, routine blood culture media can be used, but the volume of patient's blood should be increased to 20% (11). Neither Trypticase soy broth nor thioglycolate medium should contain Liquoid (sodium polyanethol sulfonate), as this substance has been shown to be inhibitory to *St. moniliformis* (10).

A satisfactory solid medium can be prepared by adding 1.5% agar to the basal broths. Freshly prepared agar plates can be inoculated with the sediment from a citrated blood specimen after the specimen is centrifuged for 30 min (1).

Both liquid and solid media should be incubated at 35–37 C in a moist, reduced-oxygen atmosphere obtained either in a candle jar or a humidified CO_2 incubator with 5%–10% CO_2.

Joint Fluid

Joint fluid should be citrated to prevent clotting. Direct smears of joint fluid stained by the Gram, Wayson, or Giemsa method and examined microscopically may provide a presumptive identification of *St. moniliformis.* Tubes containing enriched broth or enriched thioglycolate medium should be inoculated with 1–2 ml of the joint fluid. The surface of freshly prepared, moist agar should also be inoculated with 0.1 ml of the material. The broth and solid media should be incubated as indicated for blood cultures.

Pus or Exudate from Abscess

Adequate amounts of specimen should be aspirated with a sterile syringe, transferred to a tube, and processed as for joint fluids. If only a small amount of material is available, it can be collected on a swab and used to inoculate solid and liquid media.

Identification Procedures

In *Bergey's Manual, St. moniliformis* is identified as a gram-negative, facultatively anaerobic rod with uncertain generic affiliation (2). The cellular morphology and cultural characteristics appear to be more helpful than conventional biochemical characteristics in identifying the organism.

Microscopic Examination

The morphologic characteristics of *St. moniliformis* are variable, with cell size and arrangement being influenced by the conditions of culture, including culture age. The bacteria may appear small and uniform in stained smears of pus or joint fluid. Stains of growth from broth cultures or solid media usually demonstrate the characteristic tangled, pleomorphic filamentous forms, with oval or elongated swellings. The swellings, which are often beaded or granular, stain more intensely than the filaments. Chains of bacilli or coccobacilli may also be observed. Giemsa and Wayson stains are usually more satisfactory than the Gram stain for demonstrating cellular detail. Wet-mount preparations of 3- to 4-day-old cultures, examined by dark-field microscopy, may reveal masses of spherules or bubbles.

Culture Procedures

Broth. Growth in broth appears as whitish granules often referred to as "fluff balls" or bread crumbs. The growth usually appears at the bottom of the tube as discrete particles suspended in the broth or on the surface of sedimented red blood cells in blood cultures. The culture medium remains clear except for areas of particulate bacterial growth.

Blind transfers from the original culture to both solid media and broth are suggested if *St. moniliformis* is suspected, but no growth is observed in 2–3 days. A 0.5- to 1.0-ml inoculum should be used for the successive transfers.

Once growth has been obtained, daily subculture is usually required to maintain viability of the organism. A rapid decrease in the pH of the broth, considered lethal to the organism, is one possible explanation for loss of viability (1).

Young broth cultures and/or stock strains, suspended in defibrinated blood, may be quick frozen and stored at −25 to −70 C. Culture viability has been demonstrated for several years using this method (2).

Solid media. Growth of *St. moniliformis* on solid media is often slower than growth in broth. Initial growth of primary isolates may take 1–2 weeks. A high atmospheric moisture content should be maintained as the organisms are susceptible to drying. Although subcultures may grow well aerobically and anaerobically, increased concentrations of CO_2 are generally required for primary isolates and some laboratory strains. On solid media, organisms maintain viability for 3–7 days, requiring less frequent subculture than those maintained in broth. Although *St. moniliformis* has been successfully subcultured on media with starch, glycogen, and dextrin replacing the serum component, it is uncertain whether these components will consistently support growth for primary isolates (3).

Bacterial colonies and L-phase (L_1) colonies can be seen on serum-enriched media. After 2–3 days of growth, the primary or bacterial colonies are 1–3 mm in diameter and tend to be smooth, white, glistening, and butyrous in consistency. Surface colonies on sheep blood agar are similar in appearance and are nonhemolytic.

L_1 colonies may appear spontaneously several days after the primary bacterial colonies and may be found within, adjacent to, or beneath the primary colony. On microscopic examination, they have the characteristic dense central core or "fried egg" appearance. Transfers of L_1 colonies are best accomplished by the agar "cut out" technique of Kleinberger, since they are usually embedded in the media (7, 8).

The L_1 forms are felt to contribute little to the pathogenicity of *St. moniliformis.* Artificially induced L_1 murine infection has been described, but infection was apparently the result of *in vivo* reversion to the filamentous bacterial form (5).

Biochemical characteristics. *St. moniliformis* is catalase-, oxidase-, urease-, and indole-negative; will not reduce nitrate; and will not grow on MacConkey, *Salmonella-Shigella,* citrate, or cetrimide agars. The production of H_2S can frequently be detected only by the lead acetate filter paper method.

Biochemical fermentation reactions have been reported to occur with various basal media enriched with horse serum, rabbit serum, or ascitic fluid. Variable biochemical reactions may thus be caused by strain variation and/or differences in growth conditions. The most consistently reported reactions are as follows: 1) acid but no gas from glucose, maltose, dextrin, glycogen, and starch, and 2) no acid from mannitol, glycerol, dulcitol, rhamnose, sorbitol, inositol, or inulin. Other carbohydrates may be variably fermented.

Serologic Tests

Commercially prepared antigen and antiserum are not available for detecting antibodies to *St. moniliformis,* but both antigen and antiserum can be prepared as needed (1). Difficulty in the preparation of a smooth antigen, which occurs because of the organism's tendency to grow in clumps, may be overcome by adding 3% glycerol to the broth medium.

A serum agglutinating titer of 1:80 is considered positive for *St. moniliformis*. Low titers may persist for several years, and the demonstration of a rising titer between acute-phase and convalescent-phase sera is valuable for the diagnosis of recent infection.

Animal Inoculation

Animal inoculation is not usually necessary for the isolation of *St. moniliformis* from clinical specimens. However, clinical distinction of *Sp. minus* from *St. moniliformis* infection may not be possible, and mouse inoculation is advisable when rat-bite fever is suspected. The mice, which can be inoculated intraperitoneally with 0.5–1.0 ml citrated patient's blood, may have either acute infection with septicemia and early death or chronic infection with arthritis and conjunctivitis. As indicated with *Sp. minus*, laboratory mice should be shown to be free of prior *St. moniliformis* infection.

References

1. BROWN TMcP and NUNEMAKER JC: Rat-bite fever: A review of the American cases with reevaluation of etiology; report of cases. Bull Johns Hopkins Hosp 70:201–328, 1942
2. BUCHANAN RE and GIBBONS NE (eds.): Bergey's Manual of Determinative Bacteriology, Williams & Wilkins Co, Baltimore, Md, 1974
3. DUMOFF M and DUFFY CE: The substitution of starch, glycogen, and dextrin for natural body fluids in the cultivation of *Streptobacillus moniliformis*. J Bacteriol 61:535–539, 1951
4. FREUNDT EA: *Streptobacillus moniliformis* infection in mice. Acta Pathol Microbiol Scand 38:231–245, 1956
5. FREUNDT EA: Experimental investigations into the pathogenicity of the L-phase variant of *Streptobacillus moniliformis*. Acta Pathol Microbiol Scand 38:246–258, 1956
6. JELLISON WL, ENEBOE PL, PARKER RR, and HUGHES LE: Rat-bite fever in Montana. Public Health Rep 64:1661–1665, 1949
7. KLEINBERGER E: The colonial development of the organisms of pleuropneumonia and agalactia on serum agar and variations of the morphology under different conditions of growth. J Pathol Bacteriol 39:409–420, 1934
8. KLEINBERGER E: The natural occurrence of pleuropneumonia-like organisms in apparent symbiosis with *Streptobacillus moniliformis* and other bacteria. J Pathol Bacteriol 40:93–105, 1935
9. KRIEG NR: Biology of the chemoheterotropic spirilla. Bacteriol Rev 40:55–115, 1976
10. LAMBE DW, McPHEDRAN AM, MERTZ JA, and STEWART P: *Streptobacillus moniliformis* isolated from a case of Haverhill fever: biochemical characterization and inhibitory effect of sodium polyanethol sulfonate. Am J Clin Pathol 60:854–860, 1973
11. MORTON HE: *Streptobacillus moniliformis*. *In* Bacterial and Mycotic Infections of Man. Dubos RJ and Hirsch JG (eds.) J. B. Lippincott Co, Philadephia, 1965
12. PLACE EH and SUTTON LE: Erythema arthriticum epidemicum (Haverhill fever). Arch Intern Med 54:659–684, 1934
13. ROUGHGARDEN JW: Antimicrobial therapy of ratbite fever. Arch Intern Med 116:39–54, 1965
14. WATKINS CG: Ratbite fever. J Pediatr 28:429–448, 1946
15. WILLAMS S: An outbreak of infection due to *Streptobacillus moniliformis* among wild mice. Med J Aust 1:357–359, 1941

CHAPTER 37

STAPHYLOCOCCAL INFECTIONS

Peter Byrd Smith

Introduction

Causative Organism

The staphylococci are spherical cells arranged in irregular grapelike clusters. The grouping is particularly characteristic in a stained preparation from an agar culture. In broth, the clusters are usually small, and many of the cocci grow singly, in pairs, or in short chains; they never form long chains. The average diameter of the cocci is about 0.8 to 1 μm, and in any one culture they tend to be fairly uniform in size and appearance. (Many micrococci also grow in irregular clusters; however, the clusters often appear to be aggregations of single or paired cocci and the individual cells tend to be somewhat larger and less uniform in size than the staphylococci.)

Staphylococci stain well with the usual basic and acid dyes and are grampositive; cultures more than 48 hr old may vary, and occasionally gram-negative cocci are present. Staphylococci are not motile and do not form spores. Staphylococci seen in the clinical laboratory do not usually possess capsules, although strains which appear to be truly encapsulated are occasionally isolated from human sources.

The staphylococci are aerobic and facultatively anaerobic. They grow best at 35 C, but also grow between 15 and 42 C. Staphylococci grow readily on almost all commonly used noninhibitory culture media.

Colonies grown on agar are round, raised, opaque, smooth, and glistening, and characteristically appear deep gold to cream or white. Color develops only in cultures grown aerobically and is most definite on solid media containing blood or a carbohydrate. Although color is generally distinct after cultures are incubated at 35 C, it often intensifies when they are held at room temperature for another day or two. Cultures in broth are nonpigmented and usually are uniformly turbid, with an amorphous sediment.

On blood agar, colonies of most freshly isolated strains of pathogenic staphylococci are surrounded by a zone of hemolysis; a few strains are nonhemolytic. Pathogenic staphylococci produce three antigenically distinct hemolysins designated alpha, beta, and delta. The three differ in their ability to lyse erythrocytes of various animal species and produce distinctive zones of hemolysis on blood agar. Alpha hemolysin lyses sheep and rabbit red blood cells but has little or no effect on human cells. It produces a wide, clear zone of hemolysis with an ill-defined outer margin. Beta hemolysin lyses sheep cells but not rabbit or human cells. On sheep blood agar after incubation at 35 C for 24 hr, beta hemolysin produces a wide zone of what is best described as incomplete or partial hemolysis. However, when the blood agar plate is held overnight at room temperature or in the refrigerator, the zone of partial hemolysis becomes clear and complete. Delta hemolysin lyses human, sheep, and rabbit red blood cells and produces a narrow zone of complete hemolysis with a well-defined border. Many strains pathogenic for man produce both alpha and delta hemolysins, some produce one of the hemolysins, and a few produce all three. Beta hemolysin is usually found in strains that are pathogenic for animals; a number of these same strains also produce alpha or delta hemolysin and some produce both.

Staphylococci are catalase positive and ferment a number of carbohydrates, including glucose, lactose, maltose, mannitol, sucrose, and glycerol. The ability to ferment mannitol (anaerobically) is generally accepted as a characteristic of pathogenic staphylococci. This carbohydrate is sometimes incorporated into agar media used for their primary isolation.

Staphylococci normally inhabit mucous membranes and the skin, either transiently or as part of the resident bacterial flora. Potentially pathogenic staphylococci can be isolated from the nasopharynx of about 50% of all individuals and from the skin of about 20%. These staphylococci are also often found in the air, dust, fomites, and the environment in general, which contributes substantially to the complexity of control and epidemiology of staphylococcal infections. Nonpathogenic staphylococci are found even more frequently, because they constitute a substantial proportion of the resident flora of body surfaces, water, air, and soil. It is therefore important to differentiate potentially pathogenic from nonpathogenic staphylococci.

The staphylococci are a genus in the family *Micrococcaceae* and have undergone a varied taxonomic history. In earlier classifications several species were identified on the basis of their pigmentation: *Staphylococcus aureus* (golden), *S. citreus* (lemon yellow), and *S. albus* (white, nonpigmented). The most recent edition of *Bergey's Manual of Determinative Bacteriology* recognizes three species: *Staphylococcus aureus*, *S. epidermidis*, and *S. saprophyticus* (2). *S. aureus* is coagulase positive, ferments mannitol anaerobically, produces thermostable nuclease, and usually produces an orange-yellow pigment. *S. epidermidis* is coagulase negative, does not ferment mannitol anaerobically, does not produce thermostable nuclease, and is usually white. *S. saprophyticus* is rarely found and represents a taxonomic compromise. Staphylococci can be distinguished from micrococci because the former can produce acid from glucose anaerobically in a tryptone-yeast extract medium containing bromcresol purple as an indicator (7).

Clinical Forms of Staphylococcal Disease

S. aureus is responsible for various human clinical diseases which are characterized by inflammation, necrosis of the tissues, and abscess formations. The infections vary in severity from mild, localized suppurations of the skin to pyemia or a sometimes fatal septicemia. Certain acute infections, notably osteomyelitis and furunculosis, often become chronic or recur over long periods. *S. aureus* is the usual cause of furunculosis, carbunculosis, and osteomyelitis, and is commonly associated with infections of wounds or burns as the primary pathogen or in combination with other microorganisms. It can also cause pneumonia, meningitis, bacteremia, endocarditis, pyrathrosis, conjunctivitis, renal abscess, and impetigo. *S. aureus* is apparently the most common cause of bacterial food poisoning.

Nosocomial staphylococcal infections caused by antibiotic-resistant strains have assumed major importance in recent years, particularly those appearing as breast abscesses in nursing mothers or as epidemics among newborn infants. Antibiotic-resistant staphylococci also have been incriminated as a cause of enterocolitis following massive oral doses of broad-spectrum antibiotics, which reduce or eliminate the normal intestinal flora. Although coagulase-negative staphylococci generally are regarded as nonpathogenic, they have caused some cases of subacute endocarditis, postcardiotomy endocarditis, and bacteremia following ventriculovenous cerebrospinal fluid shunt operations (6). The incidence of such cases has apparently increased in recent years, either in fact or because of more effective surveillance. Many *S. epidermidis* strains isolated from patients with such infections are antibiotic resistant, particularly to methicillin.

Epidemiology

Man is continually exposed to potentially pathogenic staphylococci. As indicated above, many people carry *S. aureus* in the nasopharynx or on the skin (the nasal passages of infants are often colonized by the time they are 24 hr old), and potentially pathogenic staphylococci are sometimes found in the environment. *S. aureus* may be transiently or intermittently carried, although some individuals continue to carry the organisms for many months. The incidence of nasopharyngeal carriers is high among people who are in frequent, close contact with infected patients (e.g., the medical and nursing staffs of hospitals). *S. aureus* found in the hospital must be assumed to have come fairly recently from a human source. It is especially prevalent in the immediate vicinity of heavily infected patients.

The presence of antibiotic-resistant staphylococci in hospitals is well documented. The "hospital strains," carried by personnel or living in the environment, are often readily disseminated and are always a potential source of cross-infection. Hospitalized patients are always at risk of being infected by these ubiquitous staphylococci, both because of their exposure to carriers and because of their condition when hospitalized (e.g., a metabolic or nutritional disturbance, a blood dyscrasia, or a lengthy, complex surgical procedure). Staphylococci can easily enter and colonize patients during the venipunctures and skin punctures required for some laboratory tests and therapeutic procedures or through any other break in the skin.

Staphylococcal food poisoning results from ingesting enterotoxin formed as staphylococci grew in the food. The usual source of such staphylococci is the food handler who harbors the organisms in the nasopharynx or on the skin or has a superficial staphylococcal skin lesion. This toxin can form in food which is inadequately refrigerated or left too long at room temperature. Foods such as custard-filled bakery goods, meat and meat products, puddings, salads, and dairy products have all been incriminated in staphylococcal food poisoning.

Public Health Significance

Most staphylococcal infections occur as sporadic, unrelated cases and not as epidemics, in the usual sense of that term. However, staphylococcal food poisoning and impetigo often cause outbreaks involving groups of people. If such an outbreak occurs, the public health laboratory can be asked to assist in isolating and identifying the causative organism and tracing its source and mode of transmission. An outbreak of food poisoning may be confined to a small family group or may involve participants in a banquet or some other communal meal. Outbreaks of impetigo often occur among groups of children in school or camp.

Outbreaks of nosocomial staphylococcal infections can usually be treated as within-institution problems by the hospital's medical and laboratory staffs. The local or state public health laboratory can assist in identifying the causative strain, either by phage-typing the cultures isolated or by submitting the cultures to a reference laboratory for typing. Nosocomial staphylococcal infections can be prevented with rigidly applied good housekeeping and sanitary practices. Inadequate cleanliness of personnel and equipment is one of the most important factors in staphylococcal infection outbreaks. Nosocomial infections can become a limited "community" problem, because patients who become infected in the hospital may still carry the causative organisms after they are discharged and may transmit them to family members or other contacts.

Collection and Processing of Specimens

Kinds of Specimens and Times of Collection

Because most tissues and organs of the body are subject to infection with staphylococci, numerous types of specimens can be submitted for laboratory examination, including pus from wounds, abscesses, or fistulas; blood; urine; feces; sputum; cerebrospinal fluid; and serous exudates. In epidemiologic investigations of staphylococcal outbreaks, specimens examined should include material from lesions and swabs taken from the nasopharynx and skin of patients and suspected carriers. In outbreaks of staphylococcal food poisoning, cultures should be made of specimens of feces and vomitus of affected persons, samples of suspected foods, nasopharyngeal and skin swabs from food handlers and overt lesions, if found on food handlers.

If antimicrobial therapy is planned for a patient, at least one such specimen should be taken for culture (or blood for a culture when indicated) before therapy is started. Results of testing *S. aureus* isolates for sensitivity to antimicrobial agents provide both a guide for the clinician in planning therapy and reference data should later cultures yield staphylococci of a markedly different susceptibility (which may suggest the presence of a new strain of staphylococcus) or reveal the presence of other bacterial species. Again, it should be emphasized that the original specimen should be obtained as early in the course of disease as possible.

After the first specimen has been obtained, the bacteriologic diagnosis established, and susceptibility of the organism to antimicrobial agents determined, the number of subsequent specimens that must be tested largely depends on the patient's clinical progress. The clinician should not continue to order specimens for culture indiscriminately, but should examine only those that will provide informative data on the efficacy of the therapeutic agent or that will explain untoward developments.

Methods of Collecting Specimens

Micrococci and coagulase-negative staphylococci are commonly present on the human skin and mucous membranes; pathogenic staphylococci are also sometimes present, as are diphtheroid bacilli, *Escherichia coli,* yeasts, and occasionally other microorganisms. Special care must be taken to eliminate or reduce the number of these organisms when specimen collection involves direct contact with the skin.

Although staphylococci are relatively hardy, specimens should be delivered to the laboratory promptly. If a delay in culturing is anticipated, specimens should be refrigerated if only to prevent overgrowth of fortuitous organisms.

Blood culture

With a sterile sponge, clean the skin over the selected vein with 70% alcohol and paint the area with tincture of iodine. When the iodine is dry, remove with alcohol. This procedure must be done carefully and thoroughly. Collect 10 ml of blood in a sterile syringe, and transfer the specimen aseptically to a sterile tube containing an anticoagulant or directly to culture medium as described below. Because it may not be practical to obtain 10 ml of blood from infants, collect whatever amount is practical and proceed as below under "Processing of Specimens," making proportional adjustments in volumes of materials used.

Aspirated fluids (cerebrospinal, pleural, pericardial, peritoneal, and synovial fluids)

Prepare the skin as directed for blood culture, collect the fluid in a sterile syringe, and transfer the material to a sterile screw-capped tube for transport to the laboratory.

Pus

In superficial lesions, remove surface debris and pick up the exudate with a sterile swab; if the lesion is dry, moisten the swab first with sterile saline or broth.

When sampling furuncles, carbuncles, or subcutaneous abscesses, clean the surface of the lesion and the adjacent skin with 70% alcohol to minimize the chance of contamination by the skin flora. Incise the lesion (this must be done by the physician), remove the first pus that exudes, and collect the specimen from the deeper part of the lesion with a sterile swab. Pustules in the region of the nose and mouth must never be squeezed to express pus, because the highly vascular nature of this area renders it especially vulnerable to extension of the infection or even to invasion of the bloodstream.

Draining sinus or fistula

Cleanse the adjacent skin surface and collect the specimen on a sterile swab inserted deep into the sinus, taking care not to touch the surrounding skin.

Wounds

Remove any surface pus or scar and collect pus or exudate from within the wound on a sterile swab.

Sputum

Collect the specimen in a sterile wide-mouthed glass or plastic container. Specimens of saliva are not acceptable. The patient should be instructed to cough deeply to bring up sputum from the lungs.

Urine

For both male and female patients, cleanse the genitalia thoroughly and collect a midstream specimen in a sterile widemouthed glass or plastic container. Specimens can be collected by catheter when this procedure is indicated. However, many authorities feel that catheterizing to obtain a routine urine specimen is inherently dangerous because the procedure itself may lead to a urinary tract infection. When catheterization is necessary, strict aseptic precautions should be observed.

Feces

Collect the specimen in a container of a type approved by the laboratory performing the bacteriologic examination. When it is not feasible to collect a stool specimen, fecal material can be obtained with a rectal swab.

Nasopharynx

Moisten a thin sterile swab in sterile saline or broth, drain excess fluid, and insert deep in both nares with a gentle rotary motion; do not force insertion if an obstruction is encountered. Throat cultures are not usually considered necessary in attempts to detect carriers of staphylococci because the organisms are far more often found in the nasopharynx than in the throat.

Skin

Moisten a large sterile swab in sterile saline or broth and rub it thoroughly over the selected area of the skin; when culturing the hand, rub the swab over the surfaces of the hand and between the fingers. Collect a specimen from the umbilicus of newborn infants by rubbing a moist sterile swab over the cord, the cord end, and the cord clamp.

Serum

It is not necessary to obtain serum from patients with suspected staphylococcal infections because no diagnostically reliable serologic tests are presently available for detecting active infection. Recent developments in detecting teichoic acid antigens of staphylococci may be useful for serologic detection of staphylococcal endocarditis, but these techniques are not yet fully developed.

Processing of Specimens

Treat all specimens (except feces, blood, and specimens from the nasopharynx and skin surfaces) as follows:

1. Make a direct smear and do a Gram stain;
2. Inoculate material on a blood agar plate. Place a heavy inoculum on a small area near one edge of the plate. Starting from this area and using an inoculating loop, streak the inoculum over the surface of the plate, cross-hatching carefully to obtain well-isolated colonies. Incubate at 35 C. If the direct smear shows many gram-negative rods, inoculate a selective agar plate in the same manner.

Do not make a direct smear of fecal specimens, except in food poisoning or enterocolitis. In these cases, if large numbers of gram-positive cocci in clusters are seen in the smear, make a preliminary report of this fact and proceed with the culture, inoculating both blood agar and selective agar plates. Inoculate other specimens of feces or rectal swabs heavily on the selective agar, cross-hatching carefully, and incubate at 35 C for 24 to 48 hr.

Do not make direct smears of specimens from the nasopharynx or skin. Streak these specimens carefully on blood agar and incubate at 35 C. Streak specimens from the perineum on both blood agar and selective agar plates.

For blood cultures, two procedures are available:

1. Draw the blood under strict conditions as described above and inoculate at the bedside directly into an appropriate culture medium, which can be one prepared in the laboratory or obtained commercially. Many laboratories now favor using specially designed kits, also available commercially, with which the blood is transferred in a closed system under partial vacuum directly from the vein into the blood culture bottle; this procedure eliminates the need to use a syringe and reduces the chance of contamination.
2. Draw 10 ml of blood and transfer aseptically at the bedside to a sterile tube containing enough anticoagulant to prevent clotting. Mix the blood and anticoagulant immediately by gently rotating the tube. In the laboratory:
   a) Pipette 4 ml into a flask containing 50 ml of broth.
   b) Pipette 6 ml into a flask containing 50 ml of blood agar base or some other suitable agar medium which has been melted and cooled to about 45 C (comfortably warm to the skin of the wrist).
   c) Mix the blood and agar by rotating the flask, and pour approximately equal amounts into each of three sterile petri dishes. This makes possible a rough estimate of the number of colonies per milliliter, on the basis of about 2 ml of blood per plate. When only a small amount of blood can be obtained, transfer it to anticoagulant solution, add to 15 ml of melted, cooled agar in a tube, and pour into a single petri dish.

Diagnostic Procedures

Microscopic Examination

Direct examination of Gram-stained smears of certain specimens provides information about the kinds of organisms present and is often a useful guide in selecting appropriate culture media for their isolation. Make smears and do a Gram stain on all the following specimens:

Pus

Pus can be obtained from abscesses, wounds, sinuses, and sputum.

Cerebrospinal fluid

If the fluid is turbid, make a smear directly from the specimen; if clear, make a smear of the sediment after centrifugation.

Serous exudates (pleural, pericardial, peritoneal, and synovial fluids)

Make a direct smear from the uncentrifuged specimen.

Urine

When a smear is required, spread a loopful of the fresh, uncentrifuged specimen on the slide. The value of a direct smear for the detection of staphylococci is debatable since the presence of only a few cocci is of little significance, for these organisms may be present fortuitously. However, the presence of several cocci in every microscopic field is more significant and is suggestive of active infection.

Feces

Do not make direct Gram-stained smears, except in cases of enterocolitis following oral administration of antibiotics or in cases of food poisoning. In such instances, the presence of very large numbers of staphylococci strongly suggests that they may be the cause of the condition.

In direct Gram-stained smears of clinical specimens, staphylococci are usually grouped in small clusters or in pairs but also occur singly; in fluid specimens, short chains of three or four cocci may also be seen occasionally. Care must be taken not to confuse them with other gram-positive cocci such as pneumococci, streptococci, or poorly decolorized gram-negative cocci. Direct Gram-stained smears supply only presumptive evidence of the presence of staphylococci; their identification must be confirmed biochemically. Other staining or microscopic techniques are of little value in identifying staphylococci.

Culture Procedures

Primary isolation

All specimens of clinical material should be cultured on appropriate media, following the routine practice of the individual laboratory for the isolation of miscellaneous pathogens.

For primary isolation of *S. aureus* from clinical specimens, blood agar and a selective agar are adequate. Staphylococci grown on blood agar are quite typical in appearance, and colonies are easily recognized. A selective agar may be used in addition to blood agar, when it is expected that heavy contamination by other microorganisms is likely, as might occur in cultures of wounds or feces.

Sheep blood agar is preferred because the growth and hemolytic action of *S. aureus* are particularly characteristic on this medium. To prepare the medium, add sterile defibrinated sheep blood, available commercially, in a final concentration of 5% to any good base medium, such as blood agar base, or to Trypticase soy, tryptose, or brain-heart infusion agar. Because of its ready availability, outdated human blood from blood banks is used in some laboratories. Although the colonial appearance of *S. aureus* on human blood agar is characteristic, hemolysis is less likely to be observed, and the medium may occasionally be inhibitory because of the presence of antibiotics.

If human blood-bank blood is used, every batch must first be tested as follows: Prepare a few blood agar plates with the selected blood and streak them with a group A beta-hemolytic streptococcus. If there is any inhibition of growth of the streptococcus, do not use that batch of blood in culture media.

The high content of sodium chloride (7.5%) in mannitol salt agar inhibits the growth of coagulase-negative staphylococci, micrococci, and most gram-negative rods, but permits the growth of *S. aureus* (3). The colonies usually are pigmented and surrounded by a yellow zone indicative of acid production from mannitol. Incubation for 48 hr at 35 C is often necessary to obtain good growth.

Several other culture media have been devised for the selective or differential isolation of staphylococci. Among them, phenylethyl alcohol agar (5) sometimes has been substituted for mannitol salt agar for culturing specimens likely to contain large numbers of gram-negative bacilli. It is prepared as blood agar by adding 5% defibrinated blood to it. Hemolysis on this medium may be atypical. Columbia colistin nalidixic acid agar (CNA) is also used for selective isolation, because it inhibits gram-negative bacilli but is slightly less inhibitory for gram-positive cocci than phenylethyl alcohol agar is (4). On CNA with blood, *S. aureus* is typically pigmented, hemolytic, and about 1–2 mm in size after 24 hr of incubation at 37 C. Tellurite glycine agar is a selective medium on which *S. aureus* appears typically as black colonies after incubation for 24 hr at 35 C (8). The selective agents potassium tellurite, glycine, and lithium chloride completely or partially inhibit coagulase-negative staphylococci, micrococci and gram-negative bacilli. If these organisms grow, they do so poorly and slowly. The medium must be very carefully prepared, and the inhibiting concentration of the selective agents is critical.

Any or all of these media can be used for primary isolation of staphylococci from foods, clinical specimens, or the environment. However, tellurite glycine agar is most often used in attempts to detect *S. aureus* in foods, either for quality control purposes or in investigations of staphylococcal food poisoning. In this connection, it should be noted that although *S. aureus* is isolated from foods, this does not prove that it was the organism responsible for food poisoning. The presence of large populations of *S. aureus* provides presumptive evidence, but it is confirmed only by demonstrating the presence of staphylococcal enterotoxin or by demonstrating that the organisms cultured are capable of producing enterotoxin. Food poisoning outbreaks have been traced to foods containing staphylococcal enterotoxin but having low levels of viable *S. aureus* cells (1).

Examination of cultures

Identification of staphylococci is based on gross appearance of the colonies, microscopical appearance of a Gram-stained smear of the culture, and coagulase test results. After incubation for 18 to 24 hr at 35 C, typical colonies of *S. aureus* on blood agar usually are pigmented and are surrounded by a zone of hemolysis. The color may range from deep gold to pale cream or white, and rare strains may be nonhemolytic. Colonies of *S. epidermidis* on blood agar are usually porcelain-white and nonhemolytic.

Examine a Gram-stained smear from an isolated, pigmented, hemolytic colony or from a staphylococcus-like colony when no typical colonies are seen. If the smear contains gram-positive cocci of typical morphology and grouping, they can be regarded as staphylococci. *S. aureus* and *S. epidermidis* can be differentiated with the coagulase test (see below), which should be performed on every culture exhibiting growth which has the characteristic cultural and morphologic appearance of staphylococci.

Transfer the selected colony to (a) a 1:5 saline dilution of plasma or to plasma broth for the coagulase test; (b) broth for testing susceptibility to antimicrobial agents; and (c) an agar slant, for future study as indicated. If growth on the original plate is poor, reincubate it overnight. When no isolated colonies are present but the plate shows massive growth of gram-positive cocci in clusters, set up a coagulase test for preliminary information and streak the growth onto a second blood agar plate to determine purity of the culture. Repeat the coagulase test on an isolated colony from the second plate and subculture to broth for testing susceptibility to antimicrobial agents.

On mannitol salt agar, colonies of *S. aureus* are usually pigmented and are surrounded by a yellow zone, indicating acid production from mannitol. The porcelain-white colonies of *S. epidermidis* generally show no yellow zone. Inspect the plate after incubation for 24 hr at 35 C. Select a pigmented, acid-producing colony and proceed as with a blood agar plate. If growth is poor and coagulase-positive staphylococci were not isolated from a blood agar plate made from the same specimen, reincubate it overnight and proceed with the examination of any staphylococcus-like colonies present. It is sometimes necessary to incubate mannitol salt agar plates for 48 hr before characteristic staphylococcal growth develops.

It must be remembered that *Streptococcus faecalis* grows readily on mannitol salt agar, sometimes clots blood plasma (due to utilization of citrate), and often is not readily distinguishable from staphylococci in Gram-stained smears. It is important to perform a catalase test on any colonies on mannitol salt agar that are suspected of being staphylococci, because this test effectively differentiates *S. faecalis* (catalase negative) from the staphylococci (catalase positive). This differentiation is especially necessary when examining mannitol salt agar plates inoculated with fecal specimens.

Coagulase test. The ability to clot blood plasma is generally accepted as the most reliable laboratory criterion for the identification of *S. aureus*. Some strains of *E. coli, Pseudomonas aeruginosa,* and *S. faecalis* also clot plasma; the gram-negative bacilli can be distinguished readily from staphylococci in a Gram-stained smear, and *S. faecalis* is catalase negative.

For the coagulase test, either rabbit or human blood plasma can be used. Although fresh plasma is preferred, both rabbit and human plasma are available commercially in lyophilized form and are satisfactory if they are sterile. Because of its ready availability, outdated human plasma from the blood bank is sometimes used. Individual samples of human blood-bank plasma vary considerably in their suitability for the coagulase test; every batch must be checked before use by setting up coagulase tests with several known coagulase-positive and coagulase-negative cultures of staphylococci; the coagulase-positive cultures should include both strong and weak reactors. It may be necessary to dilute human plasma slightly (1:5) to obtain a positive test.

The two methods available are the tube test and the slide test. Although referred to here and in the original article by the originators of the procedure as a "slide test," it is not a true coagulase test but rather a reaction in which the staphylococci clump in the presence of blood plasma.

If time permits, the tube test should be performed with an overnight culture of *S. aureus* in brain-heart infusion broth or any other good general purpose broth. To 0.5 ml of diluted plasma, add 0.05 to 1.0 ml of culture, and incubate the mixture at 37 C, preferably in a water bath. Classically, any degree of clotting which occurs within 4 hr is read as a positive reaction. If sterile plasma was used, tubes which contain no clot after 4 hr can be re-incubated overnight. Some commercially available coagulase plasmas are not sterile, however, so one must be certain of the product used before prolonging incubation.

Alternatively, a large colony typical of *S. aureus* may be picked directly from an isolation plate, emulsified in 0.5 ml of plasma, and incubated as above. However, this procedure may lead to selection of a weak or poor coagulase-producing colony.

Controls must be included in coagulase tests and should consist of strong, weak, and negative coagulase-producing strains. It should be emphasized that a positive reaction consists of clot formation; reactions in which a flocculent precipitate forms or in which there are "stringy" formations should be considered negative.

For the slide test, emulsify a portion of the colony in a drop of water on a microscope slide to give a distinctly milky suspension. A suspension that clumps spontaneously is unsatisfactory. The test cannot be performed with material taken directly from agar containing high salt concentrations. Add a drop of undiluted plasma to the suspension and mix by continuous stirring for 10 sec with a loop needle. Alternatively, the slide can be rocked gently, but active mixing with a loop is usually better. A positive slide test is one in which easily visible clumps appear in the suspension within 10 sec. A uniformly turbid suspension with no visible clumping in 10 sec represents a negative slide test. Late clumping (after 10 sec) is not significant. If the slide test is negative and the smear from the colony contains gram-positive cocci of typical morphology and grouping, set up a tube test.

The slide test is useful as a screening procedure for examining a large number of cultures or many colonies on a single plate. Skill is required to perform and read the test; but this can be acquired by performing several series of slide tests with known coagulase-positive and coagulase-negative cultures in parallel with tube tests.

Serologic procedures

At present there are no definitive serologic procedures readily available either for identifying staphylococci or for detecting antibodies in sera. Although much work to devise such methods has been done, those which have been developed are either performed in only a few reference laboratories (serologic typing) or have not yet proven to be of diagnostic value (antibody detection).

Serologic procedures have been applied successfully in detecting staphylococcal enterotoxins. Oudin and Ouchterlony diffusion techniques have been used, as well as hemagglutination and fluorescent antibody procedures. However, few laboratories have the expertise and equipment required to extract enterotoxins from foods and to perform the serologic tests subsequently required. These techniques are not recommended for the clinical laboratory, but assistance in performing the tests can be obtained from Food and Drug Administration laboratories or state public health laboratories.

Marker Systems of Epidemiologic Value

Several marker systems have been used for epidemiologic investigations of staphylococcal infections, but the only three which are widely used are biotyping, antibiograms, and bacteriophage typing. The first two of these can be and often are used in any bacteriology laboratory. The third system is occasionally used in larger institutions and in state or national reference laboratories.

Biotyping is the process of typing or grouping cultures on the basis of similarities (or differences) in their metabolic activities. It usually requires more biochemical tests than may be required for identification, especially in the case of staphylococci. This disadvantage is offset by the ready availability of media and substrates and by the familiarity of most microbiologists with the methods used. The microbiologist can examine records of biochemical reactions and data on organisms isolated from clinical specimens to detect trends or patterns of reactions which may be somewhat unusual or unexpected. This may signal the emergence and spread of a particular strain within a hospital, thus permitting more rapid control of infections and detection of the source of the problem. The major problem with biotyping is that of biological variation. Bacterial cultures usually consist of a nonhomogeneous population of cells, within certain limits, so a single colony may or may not be representative of the majority of the population.

Antibiograms can also be used as markers in epidemiologic investigations. The resistance patterns found among strains of staphylococci within a particular hospital or from a particular patient population are often quite similar. Thus, the appearance of a new resistance pattern in several cultures within a limited time frame may signal the emergence of a new staphylococcal strain. Obviously, for such a trend to be detected, accurate and detailed records must be regularly maintained in the laboratory. It must also be recognized that patterns of resistance to antimicrobics may change, depending on the usage of drugs within a hospital or community and on the ability of the microorganisms to develop resistance to these drugs. It is very important that the laboratory be aware of changes in drug usage, so that intelligent analysis of resistance patterns can be made and the drugs tested can be changed when necessary.

Because microbiologists are probably more familiar with the two systems mentioned above than with bacteriophage typing, it will be discussed in slightly more detail. Bacteriophage typing is based on the susceptibility of *S. aureus* cultures to a collection of bacteriophages. The bacteriophages and the procedures for their use have been highly standardized to improve reproducibility. Thus, this typing procedure yields results which can be compared among different laboratories and indeed among different countries.

Only coagulase-positive staphylococci, i.e., *S. aureus*, should be phage typed, and cultures should be selected in sets which appear to be epidemiologically related. Phage typing yields no information of diagnostic or therapeutic value, so it is not recommended as a routine laboratory procedure. Cultures to be typed should be accompanied by all available epidemiologic data, since it is the *combination* of phage typing and epidemiologic information which allows an accurate assessment of the relationships among cultures.

Bacteriophage typing is performed with a set of internationally standardized phages, which are used at dilutions established by titration of each phage on its homologous propagating strain. The composition of the typing set changes occasionally as new nontypable strains of *S. aureus* appear. In 1980, the basic typing set was composed of these phages:

group I: 29, 52, 52A, 79, 80
group II: 3A, 3C, 55, 71
group III: 6, 42E, 47, 53, 54, 75, 77, 83A, 84, 85
Misc: 81, 94, 95, 96.

One drop of each of the phages is placed on a lawn of young cells of *S. aureus* on an agar plate. After the drops have dried, the plate is incubated overnight (preferably at 30 C), and the plate is inspected for lysis of the culture by any of the phages. Most cultures, if sensitive, are lysed by more than one of the phages, so patterns are recorded. Most laboratories should not attempt to establish their own phage typing service because the procedures of maintenance and standardization of the phages and propagating strains are expensive in terms of time and personnel required. In addition, considerable experience is required to prepare and use the phages properly and to interpret the lytic reactions correctly. Many large hospitals do provide this service, however, as do some state public health laboratories. A national reference center at the Center for Disease Control in Atlanta can assist in this activity.

Coagulase-negative staphylococci from epidemic situations can be typed with any of the 3 systems mentioned above, but little has been accomplished that is of practical value for most laboratories at present.

Testing for Susceptibility to Antimicrobial Agents

The procedures for testing susceptibility of bacteria to antimicrobial agents are elsewhere in this book.

Many of the strains of *S. aureus* responsible for disease in man are resistant to one or more of the antimicrobial agents now in common use. Therefore, before therapy is initiated, susceptibility tests must be performed on all cultures of coagulase-positive staphylococci isolated from patients with pathologic conditions. Susceptibility tests need not be done on coagulase-positive staphylococci from the presumably healthy nasopharynx or skin. Possible exceptions are cultures of *S. aureus* isolated from suspected carriers in a given epidemiologic situation. While comparison of the antibiograms of such cultures with those of cultures obtained from lesions may lead to correct identification of the responsible staphylococcus, it must be remembered that an antibiogram does not supply as definitive an identification as does phage typing.

Two points deserve special mention. First, determining the susceptibility of an organism to methicillin may require procedures somewhat different from those normally used. Second, it is not usually necessary to test the susceptibility of coagulase-negative staphylococci because normally they are not pathogenic. However, a completely different situation exists with *S. epidermidis* cultures from patients with endocarditis, artificial valves, or prostheses. When bacteriologic and clinical evidence indicates that *S. epidermidis* is the causative agent in such infections, susceptibility tests must be performed. A high proportion of *S. epidermidis* strains isolated from such patients are multiply resistant to antimicrobics and may have extremely high levels of resistance.

Evaluation of Laboratory Findings

Report the results of clinical specimens according to the routine practice of the individual laboratory, describing all organisms found in the cultures.

Report as *S. aureus* cultures of gram-positive cocci with typical morphology and grouping which are coagulase positive, regardless of pigmentation or hemolytic activity. Most freshly isolated cultures possess these last two characteristics, but they are influenced by conditions of growth (culture medium, type of blood, aerobiosis, etc). An acceptable alternative to a report of *S. aureus* is "coagulase-positive staphylococci."

Report as *S. epidermidis* or "coagulase-negative staphylococci" gram-positive cocci with typical morphology and grouping, which are white and coagulase-negative on microscopic examination.

Reports based exclusively on Gram stains and microscopic morphology or on colony appearance and coagulase test results can be considered only presumptive and must be confirmed by additional tests. It must be re-emphasized that enterococci can resemble staphylococci microscopically and that several other bacterial groups can coagulate plasma.

References

1. ARMIJO R, HENDERSON DA, TIMOTHEE R, and ROBINSON HB: Food poisoning outbreaks associated with spray-dried milk—an epidemiologic study. Am J Public Health 47:1093–1100, 1957

2. BUCHANAN RE and GIBBONS NE (eds.): Bergey's Manual of Determinative Bacteriology, 8th edition. Williams & Wilkins Co, Baltimore, 1974

3. CHAPMAN GH: The significance of sodium chloride in studies on staphylococci. J Bacteriol 50:201–203, 1945

4. ELLNER PD, STOESSEL CJ, DRAKEFORD E, and VASI F: A new culture medium for medical bacteriology. Tech Bull Regist Med Technol 36:58–60, 1966

5. LILLEY BD and BREWER JH: The selective antibacterial action of phenylethyl alcohol. J Am Pharm Assoc 42:6–8, 1953

6. QUINN EL, COX F, and FISHER M: The problem of associating coagulase-negative staphylococci with disease. Ann NY Acad Sci 128:428–442, 1965

7. SUBCOMMITTEE ON TAXONOMY OF STAPHYLOCOCCI AND MICROCOCCI: Recommendations. Int Bull Bacteriol Nomencl Taxon 15:109–110, 1965

8. ZEBOWITZ E, EVANS JB, and NIVEN CF JR: Tellurite glycine agar: a selective plating medium for the quantitative isolation of coagulase-positive staphylococci. J Bacteriol 70:686–690, 1955

General References

Recent Advances in Staphylococcal Research. Yotis WW (ed.). Ann NY Acad Sci, 1974, Vol 236

The Staphylococci. Cohen JO (ed.). John Wiley & Sons, Inc, New York, 1972

Compendium of Methods for Microbiological Examination of Foods. Speck MD (ed.). APHA, Washington, DC, 1976

CHAPTER 38

STREPTOCOCCAL INFECTIONS

Lawrence J. Kunz and Robert C. Moellering, Jr.

Introduction

The streptococci are a heterogeneous group of organisms constituting a genus that includes some 20 species of bacteria. Although the members of the genus share a significant number of morphologic and physiologic characteristics, they differ widely among themselves in certain biological properties, especially in their capacity to produce disease in man and other animals.

The Etiologic Agents

Streptococci are gram-positive spherical-to-ovoid cells less than 2 μm in diameter. Cell division occurs in parallel planes in adjacent cells, resulting in pairs and chains and not in tetrads, packets, or clusters. Chain formation is promoted by growth in broth (rather than on solid media) and is dependent to some extent on species.

Members of the genus *Streptococcus* are facultative anaerobes. (Strictly anaerobic streptococci belong to the genus *Peptostreptococcus.*) They are fermentative, catalase negative, and generally active metabolically. With rare exception, they have complex nutritional requirements that call for enriched media for their isolation and study; some variants require further supplementation of ordinary enriched media to sustain their growth.

Streptococci may be grossly differentiated for operational purposes on the basis of the type of reaction produced around colonies on blood agar, the so-called "hemolytic reactions." Alpha (greening), beta (hemolysis), and gamma (no change) reactions are loosely associated with certain species or groups of streptococci, but such relationships are tenuous and are strongly influenced by the composition and pH of the media, species of blood used, and gaseous atmosphere of cultivation. Many of the streptococci elaborate polysaccharide antigens either within the cell wall or between the cell wall and cytoplasmic membrane. These antigens, which are easily extractable by a variety of methods, serve as grouping antigens, segregating various clusters of similar organisms into serogroups designated by capital letters. The organisms in most serogroups contain additional antigens that differentiate serotypes within the respective group; these typing antigens may be either polysaccharide or protein in nature. To some extent, typing antigens interfere with precise sero-grouping through cross-reactions with antisera employed for grouping individual strains. Serotyping has been particularly useful in the epidemiology of infections involving streptococci of serogroups A and B and the pneumo-coccus, *S. pneumoniae*.

Strains that are not amenable to serologic identification because they lack demonstrable grouping antigens can be differentiated and identified through physiologic characterization. In summary, some of the streptococci are identi-fied by serologic means, others by biochemical and physiologic characteristics, and still others by a combination of methods.

The nomenclature of streptococci isolated in the clinical laboratory in-cludes serologic designations, classical binomials, and informal descriptive terms. Many of the binomials historically recall the influence of dairy and vet-erinary bacteriology on streptococcal research. This may be noted in Table 38.1, which lists serologic equivalents of some of these terms. Other medically important streptococcal species, usually listed among the so-called "viridans" group, include *S. salivarius, S. mitis, S. milleri*, etc. The group A streptococcus (*S. pyogenes*) produces a number of extracellular, biologically active products such as streptolysin O, deoxyribonuclease B, and hyaluronidase. Tests for the presence of antibodies to these substances are performed on the sera of pa-tients for evidence of recent infection. These serologic tests are useful in diag-nostic procedures dealing with the complications of infections due to *S. pyo-genes*.

Clinical Manifestations of Streptococcal Infections

The clinical manifestations of streptococcal infections are well known. In-deed, such infections are among the commonest encountered in clinical medi-cine. Streptococci are associated with a wide spectrum of disease that encom-passes virtually all of the major clinical manifestations produced by bacterial

TABLE 38.1—RELATIONSHIP OF LANCEFIELD SEROLOGIC GROUPS TO CERTAIN NAMED
STREPTOCOCCAL SPECIES

SEROLOGIC GROUP	STREPTOCOCCAL SPECIES
A	*S. pyogenes*
B	*S. agalactiae*
C	*S. equi, S. zooepidemicus, S. equisimilis, S. dysgalactiae*
D	*S. faecalis, S. faecium, S. bovis, S. equinus*
E	*S. infrequens, (S. uberis?)*
F	*S. anginosus (S. milleri?)*
G	*S. anginosus**
H	*S. sanguis*
K	*S. salivarius*
N	*S. lactis, S. cremoris*

* Applies only to type I, group G.

pathogens. In general, illness caused by the beta-hemolytic strains is more acute and more likely to be associated with suppurative lesions, while illness resulting from the alpha- and gamma-reacting organisms is usually subacute and rarely associated with abscess formation. Exceptions occur, however, as will be noted subsequently.

Traditionally, infections due to *S. pyogenes* have been accorded the greatest amount of emphasis in discussions of streptococcal disease (excluding that caused by *S. pneumoniae*). This is understandable since the clinical illness produced by these organisms is often dramatic, occurs throughout the world, and may be accompanied by serious sequelae such as rheumatic fever or glomerulonephritis.

The group A streptococci are capable of producing many different types of infections, including pharyngitis, tonsillitis, pyoderma, impetigo, cellulitis, necrotizing fasciitis, erysipelas, surgical or other wound infections, septicemia, otitis media, sinusitis, mastoiditis, pneumonia, osteomyelitis, endocarditis, and meningitis (66). Pharyngitis and pyoderma are the commonest manifestations of infections due to group A streptococci. The pharyngitis is usually characterized by fever and severe sore throat, although it is becoming increasingly clear that asymptomatic pharyngeal colonization also occurs in a large number of patients (3). Complications may develop during either the acute or convalescent stage of the illness and include both suppurative and nonsuppurative sequelae. The former result from contiguous spread of the infection resulting in peritonsillar, intratonsillar, or parapharyngeal space abscesses, sinusitis, otitis media, mastoiditis, lateral sinus thrombophlebitis, brain abscess, meningitis, and bacteremia, which sometimes results in metastatic abscess formation. Strains producing erythrogenic toxin cause scarlet fever in patients who do not possess antibodies to the toxin. Late nonsuppurative sequelae of group A streptococcal pharyngitis include rheumatic fever and glomerulonephritis. Glomerulonephritis, but not rheumatic fever, can also result from streptococcal pyoderma. Infections due to the group A streptococci result in the production of antibodies directed against a number of extracellular products produced by these organisms. Detection of serum antibodies to these products, e.g., anti-streptolysin O (ASO), anti-deoxyribonuclease-B (ADN-B), anti-hyaluronidase (AH), provides presumptive evidence of prior infection with group A streptococci. These antibodies are useful epidemiologic tools and may also be helpful when one is dealing with patients who appear to have rheumatic fever or glomerulonephritis in the absence of a prior streptococcal infection.

Pneumonia due to group A streptococci often begins as an interstitial process and is usually accompanied by a rapidly developing pleural effusion and/or empyema. It is remarkable that bacteremia due to group A streptococci is less frequent than that due to group D or nongroupable streptococci and has become less common in the United States in the past 40 years (23). It most frequently arises from a traumatic or surgical skin wound and may be associated with disseminated intravascular coagulation and symmetrical peripheral gangrene of the digits.

Diseases caused by the group B streptococci have become a subject of considerable interest and discussion in recent years (54). This organism is now recognized as a major cause of neonatal septicemia and congenital pneumonia and as a cause of meningitis in both neonates and young infants (4, 54). Otitis media, septic arthritis, osteomyelitis, adenitis, and cellulitis can also be caused by group B streptococci in young children. During the past decade it has likewise become clear that group B streptococci can also cause infections in adults, with urinary tract infections predominating (7, 29). Pneumonia, cellulitis, endometritis, septic arthritis, endocarditis, meningitis, pharyngitis, and peritonitis have also been described (7, 15, 29). Diabetics and other patients with impaired host defense mechanisms, such as cirrhotics and patients who are immunosuppressed, seem to be the victims of a disproportionate number of such infections.

Infections due to group C streptococci in man are uncommon. The most frequently described syndrome is a pharyngitis, similar to that caused by group A streptococci (8, 23). Skin and wound infections, puerpural sepsis, pulmonary infections, and endocarditis have also been described (23). Glomerulonephritis may complicate group C streptococci infections (22), but rheumatic fever has not been described as a nonsuppurative complication.

Both enterococcal and non-enterococcal group D streptococci cause serious infection in man. Differentiation of enterococcal from non-enterococcal strains is important because of the markedly differing antibiotic susceptibilities of these organisms (48). Enterococci are common causes of urinary tract infections. They are also isolated frequently (usually in combination with other fecal flora) from intraabdominal abscesses and peritonitis. Enterococci account for approximately 10% of the cases of bacterial endocarditis presently seen in the United States. Bacteremia (most commonly from an intraabdominal or genitourinary source) is much more frequent than endocarditis. Metastatic suppurative complications almost never occur. Enterococci occasionally cause burn wound infections, especially in the presence of porcine heterografts. Meningitis and pulmonary infections due to enterococci have been described but are quite uncommon.

The clinical importance of distinguishing enterococci from the non-enterococcal *S. bovis* has only recently been appreciated (48, 58). Most clinically significant *S. bovis* isolates have been described as causes of bacteremia and endocarditis (where they occur almost as frequently as enterococci). It is likely that other sites of infection will emerge as these organisms are more frequently recognized by microbiologists and clinicians.

The clinical significance of group F streptococci has yet to be clearly defined. These organisms are most commonly isolated from the respiratory tract (6), where they appear to be nonpathogenic. They have been documented as causative agents of dental abscesses, and reports of bacteremia, sinusitis, empyema, brain abscess, meningitis, puerpural sepsis, and wound infections have occurred (23). Present experience is insufficient to enable one to determine whether the paucity of clinical data concerning these organisms is due to lack of routine identification or to their rarity as causes of clinical disease. It is probable that many cultures of *S. milleri* are included among the medically important streptococci that react with group F antisera.

Group G streptococci appear to be capable of causing pharyngitis that is clinically indistinguishable from that caused by group A streptococci (34).

Along with infections due to groups A and C streptococci, infections caused by group G streptococci also may result in a rise in serum ASO titers (34). Despite this, nonsuppurative sequelae (acute rheumatic fever, acute glomerulonephritis) have not been documented following infections with group G streptococci, except for a single case of acute rheumatic fever reported by Duma et al. (23). In addition to pharyngitis, group G streptococci have also been documented as causes of bacteremia, endocarditis, puerpural sepsis, empyema, and skin or wound infections (23).

The clinical presentations of the diseases produced by the remaining groupable streptococci (H, K–T) and the nongroupable streptococci have so many features in common that they will be considered together. Human isolates of groups P–T are so uncommon that their clinical significance is difficult to assess (13). The remaining organisms are part of the normal upper-respiratory-tract flora and can be implicated (often with other organisms) in dental infections, aspiration pneumonia, and empyema, as well as occasional cases of wound or skin infections and meningitis. These organisms (especially group H and nongroupable streptococci) are the most frequent etiologic agents of subacute bacterial endocarditis. Two species of nongroupable streptococci merit special notice. *S. mutans* has been implicated as a major cause of dental caries in man and experimental animals (32). *S. milleri* has been reported to be a frequent cause of suppurative lesions (53), a property that distinguishes it from most of the other alpha- and gamma-reacting streptococci, which rarely cause abscess formation.

S. pneumoniae is widely recognized as the most frequent cause of bacterial pneumonia in persons of all ages. Classically this agent produces lobar consolidation with a high prevalence of associated bacteremia. Pleural effusion and empyema may also complicate pneumococcal pneumonia. Although pneumonia clearly accounts for the majority of the serious infections caused by the pneumococci, these organisms can also cause meningitis (especially in older persons), otitis media, sinusitis, mastoiditis, arthritis, osteomyelitis, cellulitis, peritonitis, pericarditis, and endocarditis.

Epidemiology

The epidemiology of streptococcal infections is diverse and complicated. Many of the streptococci are part of the normal oropharyngeal, skin, and fecal flora of man. In the case of organisms which are not part of the normal flora, such as the group A streptococci, there is often a high rate of asymptomatic pharyngeal infection or colonization, making it difficult to equate isolation of the organism with clinical disease. Although most streptococcal groups have been isolated from animals, little evidence exists that animals serve as significant vectors for transmission of streptococcal disease to man. In most instances infections result either from acquisition of pathogenic organisms via contact with persons who are infected or who are asymptomatic carriers or from contact with materials contaminated by man, or they result from a breakdown in local or general host defense mechanisms, allowing infection to occur with organisms that are part of the normal flora. Thus, group A streptococci causing pharyngitis are most commonly spread by droplets expelled from the nose and throat of infected persons (66). As a result, overcrowding, depressed living conditions, increasing urbanization, and poor health standards are associated with the occurrence of streptococcal pharyngitis and with increased incidences of rheumatic fever. Explosive outbreaks of streptococcal pharyngitis have occurred when food such as unpasteurized milk, ice cream, or egg salad has been contaminated with streptococci of groups A, C, or G (22, 34, 66). Group A streptococcal skin infections are most likely spread by direct contact with persons who have preexisting streptococcal skin infections. In this setting pharyngeal colonization appears to be secondary to skin colonization and infection (20). The possibility that fomites or insect vectors may play a role in the transmission has been raised but is unproven (20). Group A streptococci can survive passage through the gastrointestinal tract to establish an anal carriage state. Persistent anal carriers have occasionally been implicated as vectors in the spread of streptococcal infection, especially in postoperative wounds. A number of studies suggest that group A streptococci of certain M or T serotypes (especially M-49 and M-52 through M-61) show a predilection for causing skin infections (20). A different series of M types, not all of which cause skin infection, has been associated with the development of poststreptococcal glomerulonephritis. These have been called "nephritogenic strains." Whether or not certain strains are more likely to cause pharyngitis and tonsillitis is less clear. Moreover, although it appears that there may be "rheumatogenic strains," these are not well characterized (60). Studies in Memphis, Tennessee, give particular credence to such concepts (60). In this area group A streptococcal infections are quite common, but there is a striking seasonal separation of the occurrence of pyoderma-nephritis on the one hand and acute rheumatic fever on the other. In the summer, when streptococcal pyoderma is prevalent, large numbers of cases of acute nephritis appear, whereas acute rheumatic fever is virtually absent. In the fall, when school begins, pyoderma and acute nephritis decline rapidly and acute rheumatic fever appears within a month or two thereafter.

The incidence of acute rheumatic fever has declined strikingly in North America and Europe in recent years. The reasons for this are not entirely clear, but it may be related to improved living conditions and to the widespread (and sometimes promiscuous) use of penicillin among members of these populations. It is also possible that there has been a decline in the rheumatogenic potential of the strains currently associated with group A streptococcal pharyngitis (9).

A number of studies [summarized by Patterson and Hafeez (54)] suggest that although variable from area to area, the incidence of group B streptococcal infections in infants has increased in different parts of the United States during the past decade. Group B streptococci find their primary reservoir in the female genital tract, with carriage rates of 2.3%–29.8% in adult females. Although there may be venereal spread of the organisms, it is also possible that fecal colonization leads to vaginal colonization in many instances (54). Infants are infected in one of two ways. Those who develop congenital pneumonia, neonatal sepsis, or neonatal meningitis (early-onset disease) are almost certainly infected during passage through the birth canal (or possibly *in utero* if the membranes rupture prematurely). In the case of infections in older infants (late-onset disease), infections are usually nosocomial (54).

Group D streptococci are found as normal constituents of the fecal flora in man. This accounts for the propensity of enterococci to cause intra-abdominal and urinary tract infections. Enterococcal bacteremia and endocarditis are often related to abdominal surgery, genitourinary instrumentation, and processes involving manipulation of the birth canal. Recent studies suggest that there may be an association between bacteremia and endocarditis due to *S. bovis* and the presence of neoplastic processes involving the gastrointestinal tract (40). Whether this association is simply a manifestation of the fact that a process that interrupts the integrity of the gastrointestinal mucosa may predispose to bacteremia with bowel flora including *S. bovis,* or whether this association is so specific that all patients with *S. bovis* bacteremia should have an extensive gastrointestinal evaluation remains to be proven by further studies. The observation that patients with carcinoma of the bowel may have an increased fecal carriage rate of *S. bovis,* however, raises the strong possibility that the association may be significant (40).

Streptococci of groups F, H, K, L, M, N, and O and the non-groupable streptococci are all found as constituents of the normal oropharyngeal flora in man. As a result, bacteremia or endocarditis due to these organisms strongly suggests an oropharyngeal portal of entry and should alert the clinician to the possibility that the patient with such a process might have significant oral or dental pathology.

S. pneumoniae may be cultured from the pharynx of as many as 50% of normal persons. Recent studies suggest that colonization rates are highest in young children and in adults with children at home (33). It appears that infection with indigenous pneumococci occurs when events take place that abridge the normal respiratory tract defense mechanisms. These include aspiration of oropharyngeal secretions, antecedent viral respiratory infections, exposure to noxious gases and various environmental pollutants, anesthesia, cardiac failure, and trauma. Although over 80 serotypes of *S. pneumoniae* can be identified, only a relatively few (serotypes 1, 3, 4, 5, 8, 9, 12) are implicated as the cause of the majority of serious pneumococcal infections in man (51).

Public Health Significance

Streptococci cause a wider variety of clinical infections than any other genus of bacteria. Infections due to these organisms occur worldwide. Unfortunately, adequate provisions for reporting streptococcal illness do not exist in the United States or the rest of the world. Thus, it is impossible to derive accurate data concerning the true incidence of streptococcal infections.

However, it has been estimated that in 1971 there were 1,662,000 cases of pneumonia resulting in 34,689,000 days of restricted activity in the United States alone (35). At least half of these cases of pneumonia were caused by bacteria, the majority of which were *S. pneumoniae* (61). Pneumonia accounts for about 10% of admissions to acute medical hospital wards and ranks fifth (with influenza) among the 10 leading causes of death in the United States

(35). At present there are no proven methods for prevention of pneumococcal infections, although long-term penicillin prophylaxis may be effective in some patients with specific host defense abnormalities such as asplenia, and pneumococcal polysaccharide vaccine has shown promising results in early clinical trials.

Pharyngitis and pyoderma due to the group A streptococci are probably the commonest infections caused by the streptococci and undoubtedly result in much time lost from the work force in the United States and elsewhere. In a pediatric practice in New York, approximately 10% of office visits were related to streptococcal disease in 1966 (12). It has been estimated that the annual incidence of poststreptococcal rheumatic fever in the United States is between 100,000 and 200,000 cases annually and that at least 50,000 new cases of rheumatic heart disease develop each year. Poststreptococcal glomerulonephritis likewise may result in chronic renal impairment in at least some of its victims, adding significantly to the public health costs of these diseases. Since chronic antibiotic prophylaxis can prevent recurrence of rheumatic fever in patients with rheumatic heart disease, and since acute administration of intramuscular benzathine penicillin has been shown to reduce the number of new cases of pyoderma in epidemics (55), it seems prudent to continue efforts at antibiotic prophylaxis for patients at high risk of developing poststreptococcal complications. More data concerning the epidemiology and pathogenesis of group A streptococcal disease are needed, however, before totally effective programs of prophylaxis can be designed.

Accurate data concerning the incidence of disease caused by non-group A streptococci in the United States and elsewhere simply do not exist. Nonetheless, these infections clearly occur with a high enough frequency to add significantly to the burden of public health costs, particularly since endocarditis due to these organisms commonly requires at least 2 and usually 4–8 weeks of hospitalization. Moreover, streptococcal bacterial endocarditis often results in valvular destruction sufficient to necessitate surgical replacement of the damaged valve. At present, the hospital costs associated with such surgery in the United States are in the vicinity of $12,000–$20,000 per patient.

For patients with known valvular heart disease who are at high risk of developing bacterial endocarditis, antibiotic prophylaxis seems clearly indicated whenever they are exposed to procedures, such as dental or genitourinary manipulations, likely to result in significant bacteremia. The efficacy of such prophylaxis has not been proven, however, and considerable debate remains concerning the most effective antibiotic regimen to use for prophylaxis (38).

Collection and Processing of Specimens

Bacteriologic diagnosis of streptococcal diseases, as with other types of infectious processes, depends on judicious selection, collection, and processing of specimens. In the absence of appropriate clinical material, the necessary diagnostic procedures either cannot be applied or are applied ineffectively. Not only must proper techniques be employed in the collection of specimens for culture, but because streptococci comprise a large part of the normal flora of several areas of the human body, bacteriology laboratory personnel must utilize knowledge and discretion in examining cultures and in selecting colonies for study and identification. Following are guidelines for collection of specimens and for examination of cultures of clinical specimens.

Throat Cultures

Cultures of tonsils and posterior pharynx are necessary to obtain bacterial confirmation of the diagnosis in patients with suspected streptococcal pharyngitis. A tongue depressor should be used to expose the posterior pharynx. A sterile swab is then rubbed firmly over the tonsils (if present) and posterior pharynx, touching any exudate present. It is important to avoid contact of the swab with the tongue, gingiva, or buccal mucosa to prevent gross contamination with normal flora. The swab should then be returned to its sterile container for transportation to the laboratory. Streptococci are quite resistant to drying. Therefore, if transportation is delayed more than a few hours, the swab can be placed in sterile tube or aluminum foil packet containing a drying agent or it can be rubbed onto a piece of sterile filter paper, which is then air dried, placed in a sterile envelope, and mailed to the laboratory.

The swab or filter paper should be streaked onto blood agar plates (see below) and the plates incubated in 3%–5% CO_2 at 37 C.

As already noted, the normal oropharynx is heavily colonized with harmless streptococci. The only organism that ought routinely be sought in patients with pharyngitis is the group A beta-hemolytic streptococcus. Occasionally, a nonhemolytic group A strain may be involved (37); rarely, an epidemic of group G organisms may be encountered (34); group B streptococci have been reported in certain instances (15); most infrequently an atypical strain may be the etiologic agent (46). None of these possibilities should require that every throat culture be examined so thoroughly as to detect the rare presence of 1 of these aberrant strains. The astute observer, however, should be intellectually prepared to expect or recognize their possible involvement, at least when large numbers of cases are prevalent (37).

Nasal/Nasopharyngeal Cultures

For young children whose lack of cooperation makes it impossible to obtain an adequate throat culture, nasopharyngeal cultures may occasionally yield interpretable diagnostic information. With this exception, and except for determining the etiology of discrete lesions, cultures of the nose or nasopharynx should be requested only for determining carriers (of streptococci or *other* microorganisms) for definite epidemiologic purposes. Nasal cultures may be obtained by swabbing the anterior nares at a depth of 1–2 cm with a cotton-tipped wire. Nasopharyngeal cultures may be obtained by advancing a wire swab along the floor of the nasal cavity and under the medial turbinate until the pharyngeal wall is reached. Specimens should be handled as described for throat cultures.

The organism sought should be clearly specified in order to facilitate the study through the use of appropriate media selected for the particular organism. The presence of irrelevant commensal organisms in the cultures can then be rationally and economically ignored. The use of an enrichment medium for detection of small numbers of group A streptococci is indicated only in a survey for asymptomatic carriers of *S. pyogenes.*

Sputum Cultures

Sputum cultures may be useful in the diagnosis of lower respiratory tract infections due to pneumococci and other streptococci. Unfortunately, the majority of expectorated sputum specimens are heavily contaminated with oropharyngeal flora, which may make isolation or interpretation of true pathogens difficult. Specimens obtained by nasotracheal aspiration should contain fewer "contaminants." Transtracheal aspiration obviates this problem; thus, specimens obtained via this method are much more reliable. By whatever method the specimen is obtained, it should be transferred immediately to a sterile container for transportation to the laboratory.

The sputum specimen should be streaked on blood agar plates as well as on a medium, such as MacConkey agar, that is selective for gram-negative bacilli.

Use of selective media is recommended for pneumococci or for *S. pyogenes* in the presence of other organisms, especially gram-negative rods. Pneumonia due to *S. pyogenes* is a distinctive, rapidly progressing respiratory infection that demands early consideration and recognition for successful therapy. Although suspicion of the etiology from microscopic examination of sputum may be delayed because of confusion with pneumococci, isolation of beta-hemolytic streptococci from sputum of a rapidly deteriorating patient with pneumonia should suggest the precise etiologic diagnosis.

Blood Cultures

Blood cultures should be obtained from all patients with possible bacteremia or endocarditis. Bacteremia in settings other than intravascular infections such as endocarditis is usually discontinuous. Cultures are more likely to be positive under these circumstances if obtained during a rigor or just prior to the patient's fever spike. For obvious reasons this may be difficult to accomplish. In patients with endocarditis or endarteritis, the bacteremia is continuous although the number of organisms present varies from moment to moment. The exact timing of blood cultures in this setting is less important, except as it relates to the rapidity with which the patient is being evaluated. Among patients with infective endocarditis who eventually have positive blood cultures, the first culture will be positive in 80%–90% of cases, and a positive result is obtained in approximately 99% after three cultures (63). In view of this, three blood cultures should be adequate to confirm the diagnosis in most patients with bacterial endocarditis. Exceptions include patients who have recently received antibiotics and patients with prosthetic valve endocarditis; additional cultures may occasionally be necessary for these persons. Arterial cultures have no advantage over venous cultures.

The skin at the venipuncture site should be cleansed with 70% alcohol, followed by an application of 1%–2% iodine solution. Alternatively, povidone-iodine (Betadine) may be used. The iodine should be removed with alcohol after the venipuncture. If blood culture flasks with rubber diaphragm stoppers are used, the alcohol or iodine preparation should also be used to cleanse the diaphragm, and the disinfecting agent allowed to act for approximately 1 min before use. With sterile technique approximately 10 ml of blood should be drawn into a syringe. Then, 5 ml of blood is inoculated into each of two flasks containing 50–100 ml of culture media. One flask should contain a standard nutrient medium such as Trypticase soy broth, brain heart infusion broth, or dextrose phosphate broth and, after being vented, should be incubated aerobically. The second should contain a medium such as fluid thioglycollate broth that will support the growth of anaerobic organisms. It is most important to obtain the proper volume of blood for culture. If too little is obtained, the number of microorganisms (which may be present in as low a concentration as one or less organism per ml) contained therein will be too small to permit isolation. On the other hand, if too large a quantity of blood is obtained, the concentration of natural inhibiting substances, including leukocytes, antibodies, and complement, may be great enough to inhibit growth of many organisms. To prevent this action, the blood should be diluted 1:10–1:20 in the culture medium. The addition of 0.05% sodium polyanethol sulfonate (SPS) to the aerobic flask may increase the yield of positive cultures since it is anticomplementary, precipitates immunoglobulins, and inactivates leukocytes. In addition, it has some ability to antagonize the effects of polymyxin and the aminoglycoside antibiotics. Adding penicillinase to the blood culture flasks from patients who have recently received penicillin may improve the yield of positive cultures (21). If penicillinase is added, however, a portion of the reagent should be cultured separately as a sterility check since contaminated penicillinase can produce pseudobacteremia.

Cultures of blood containing streptococci present few problems in recognition. An occasional strain of *Peptostreptococcus* may be inhibited by SPS (for this reason it is considered prudent to include SPS in routine aerobic blood culture medium and to omit it from anaerobic broth medium). To prevent "self-sterilization" of blood cultures containing acid-sensitive bacteria such as pneumococci, routine aerobic blood culture media should be provided with some buffering mechanism for avoiding acid loading. The growth of bizarre, biochemically aberrant streptococci (46), including capnophilic pneumococci (2), usually is supported in an already enriched basic broth medium that is automatically supplemented by the inoculum of patient's blood. The problem of both capnophilic and other biochemically aberrant strains of streptococci is thus reduced to the matter of subculturing them to solid media, of recognizing their metabolic deficit, and ultimately, of identifying them. Though academically challenging, the problem of predicting on the basis of microscopic morphology the presence of pneumococci rather than of other streptococci in broth cultures is fortunately one that is not often of critical importance to the patient because of the nearly uniform susceptibility of species to penicillin. However, the recent emergence of multiresistant strains of pneumococci in South Africa and elsewhere may necessitate revision of that concept.

Urine Cultures

Proper collection and handling of urine specimens is of utmost importance if the results of cultures are to be of value. Straight catheterization or suprapubic aspiration under sterile technique provides the best method of obtaining valid specimens. However, since these methods (especially catheterization) carry a risk of introducing organisms into the noninfected urinary tract, they should be used only when it is impossible to obtain adequate voided specimens. For the latter the genitalia should be thoroughly cleansed and a midstream specimen of urine collected in a sterile, wide-mouth receptacle. The urine should then be transferred aseptically to a sterile screw-capped container for immediate transportation to the laboratory. Delay in transport, especially if the specimen is not refrigerated, may result in the overgrowth of contaminating organisms in the urine.

Urine specimens should be plated on an enriched, general-purpose medium and, because of the frequency with which enteric gram-negative bacilli are isolated, on an enteric differential medium as well. Methods of culturing should be employed so that quantitative or, at least, semiquantitative estimates can be made of the bacterial content of the specimen for interpretation of etiologic significance of the isolated bacteria.

While the streptococcal etiology of urinary tract infection may be inferred from the finding of streptococci in a Gram-stained smear of the specimen, the probability of predicting a specific agent is somewhat uncertain. Although the enterococcus is more frequently involved in urinary tract infections than other streptococci, this fact should not preclude consideration of the less frequent but not unlikely group B streptococcus. Confirmatory cultures in the case of streptococcal urinary tract pathogens are necessary because of the need to select effective antibacterial agents for treating enterococci less susceptible to antibiotics than group B organisms.

Skin Cultures

Direct cultures of the intact skin are generally useful only for determining carriage rates in epidemiologic studies. To perform such cultures, rub a swab moistened with sterile saline (without perservative) or broth over the selected skin area, and then place it in a sterile container for transportation to the laboratory.

For patients with skin infections, attempts should be made to obtain pus or tissue fluid for culture. If there are crusted areas, the top of a lesion should be removed with a sterile needle and the underlying pus or tissue fluid removed with a sterile swab for culture. If furuncles or subcutaneous abscesses are present, the overlying skin should be cleansed with 70% alcohol and iodine, the lesion incised with a sterile scalpel blade, and the pus removed with a sterile swab. For patients with cellulitis, the skin should be cleansed with alcohol and iodine, and a small sterile needle introduced into the advancing margin of the lesion. If no fluid can be aspirated, 0.5–1.0 ml of sterile saline (without preservative) can be injected and then aspirated for culture. If the amount of fluid aspirated is large enough, it can be expelled onto a sterile swab for transport to the laboratory. Otherwise, the syringe and needle can be transported to the laboratory, and the fluid in the needle expelled directly onto culture medium. An anaerobic broth medium might be used in addition to enriched blood agar medium to provide for the chance occurrence of an unexpected anaerobic pathogen.

Early preliminary evidence of the etiology of certain skin conditions may be obtained by examining Gram-stained smears of the specimen; rational culture methods and therapy may occasionally be suggested as well. Similarly, early examination of cultures of specimens of skin infections can serve as guides to rational therapy. Selection of skin sites to be sampled is of no little importance.

Fluid, Exudate Cultures (Cerebrospinal Fluid; Pleural, Pericardial, Peritoneal, Synovial Fluids; Abscess Contents)

These materials, especially if obtained under sterile conditions from patients not receiving antimicrobial therapy are most likely to yield a positive diagnosis because the number of infecting organisms is great and there is no "normal flora" present to obscure cultures. The skin should be prepared as described for blood cultures, and the fluid collected with a sterile syringe. It should be transferred immediately to a sterile, screw-capped tube for transportation to the laboratory.

A standard procedure for culturing materials such as these should be followed. Provision should be made for the possible presence of anaerobic bacteria or of eugonic gram-negative rods, which may complicate the bacteriologic examination of the culture. A Gram-stained smear of the specimen, carefully examined and interpreted, may serve as a useful guide for setting up initial cultures. The finding of gram-positive cocci in pairs or chains in specimens of cerebrospinal fluid either in smear or in culture is, on a statistical basis, good evidence that the pneumococcus is the etiologic agent of meningitis. Nevertheless, the need to confirm the etiology by subsequent bacteriologic examination of cultures of the CSF is not to be neglected. Confirmation of microscopic observations, identification of presumptively identified species, and presence of additional, unrelated organisms in cultures of other specimens all require that careful, complete bacteriologic determinations be performed on cultures involving streptococci, no less than those containing other genera or species. Selective media should be employed when the presence of other organisms, especially gram-negative enteric rods, is suspected in order to facilitate the isolation of streptococcal species.

Diagnostic Procedures

Microscopic Examination of Specimens

As already stated, the presence of infection involving streptococci can frequently be determined both quickly and easily by microscopic examination of Gram-stained smears of certain types of specimens. Because of the large numbers of streptococci normally colonizing the mouth and pharynx, examination of smears of the throat for evidence of infection by *S. pyogenes* is almost always inconclusive and may be misleading. Similarly, smears of vaginal secretions may contain indigenous streptococcal flora. On the contrary, Gram-stained smears of pus, exudates, and normally sterile body fluids are usually helpful.

Accordingly, appropriately prepared smears are examined from pus from wounds, abscesses, and sinuses; from sputum and exudates from body spaces and cavities; from cerebrospinal fluid; from urine; and from skin lesions.

The same precautions apply to collecting, processing, examining, and interpreting smears for streptococci as for other microorganisms. For example, cerebrospinal fluid should be centrifuged if direct examination proves negative, and the sediment examined for inflammatory cells and bacteria; in the case of urine specimens the correlation between "positive" smears and "significant" colony counts is approximately 80%; the detection of microorganisms with various morphologies may serve as a useful guide in selecting media to ensure isolation of all of the organisms observed. Caution must be observed in the interpretation of smears containing organisms resembling streptococci. Occasionally, it may be difficult to determine whether the gram-positive cocci represent staphylococci or streptococci; rarely the paired, short rods of *Listeria monocytogenes* may be mistaken for streptococci resembling, in particular, *S. pneumoniae*. Although pneumococci are often said to be recognized by the "lancet-shape" of the diplococci, the conferring of species designation on gram-positive cocci in pairs or chains, long or short, is presumptive and may be hazardous. Finally, it must be emphasized that aging organisms occasionally lose their capacity to retain gram-positivity, especially in cultures, and may then resemble gram-negative bacteria.

Culture of Specimens

Since bacteriologic culture media for primary isolation usually include one highly enriched medium, the nutritional requirements of all but the most bizarre streptococci will usually be satisfied by routine initial culturing. Brucella agar, Trypticase soy agar, or Columbia agar, for example, supplemented with blood, is adequate for growth of all but the exceptional strains. In this country sheep blood is the most recommended and the widely used animal blood supplement. It has generally superseded horse blood because it does not support the growth of *Haemophilus hemolyticus*, which produces beta-hemolytic zones on horse blood agar (41). It otherwise offers no significant benefit over horse blood.

When blood agar plates are streaked with specimens expected to contain streptococci, e.g., throat swabs, the inoculating loop should be used to stab into the agar once or twice in each sector of streaking. Occasional nonhemolytic strains of *S. pyogenes* may produce hemolytic colonies within the depths of the stabs.

If mixed cultures are anticipated or suggested by the nature of the infection or by microscopic observations of the Gram-stained smear, the primary culture procedures should include selective and differential media designed for isolation of the types of organisms suspected. Selective media for *S. pyogenes* include media containing 1 or more antibiotics such as gentamicin, colistin, and nalidixic acid; broth containing nalidixic acid and gentamicin for group B streptococci (5); blood agar containing gentamicin for *S. pneumoniae* (10); Pfizer Selective Enterococcus (PSE) agar for enterococci and *S. bovis*; and Colistin Nalidixic Acid (CNA) agar (25) and phenylethyl alcohol agar (PEA) for both streptococci and staphylococci. The limitations of each medium selective for streptococci should be questioned; inhibition of some strains should be expected.

Broth media for blood culture and for preparing cell crops for extracting antigens for serogrouping are discussed elsewhere. Because at least one streptococcal species, *S. pneumoniae*, autolyzes when pH of culture media is lowered by fermentation of added glucose, it is necessary either to limit glucose content of the medium or to buffer the medium adequately. Brucella broth with added phosphate (dextrose phosphate broth) is an example of such a medium in which the phosphate tends to sustain the viability of pneumococci in aging acid cultures.

Cultures should be incubated in an atmosphere of 3%–5% CO_2 in air to satisfy the need of *S. pneumoniae* for increased CO_2 tension to initiate growth (2) and to promote the rapid growth of minute colony-forming strains of *S. anginosus* (43). There is little evidence for the frequently stated need for anaerobic incubation of blood agar cultures of facultatively anaerobic streptococci in order to demonstrate beta hemolysis. On the contrary, evidence suggests that strains which require anaerobic incubation for hemolysis are relatively rare (52). The occurrence of strains lacking streptolysin S does not appear to be widespread except, of course, during an epidemic such as that described by James et al. (37). Alternatively, the submerged colonies in pour plates will reveal hemolysis due to oxygen labile streptolysin O in strains lacking streptolysin S, as will submerged growth in the recommended stab in the agar of a surface-streaked blood agar plate.

Isolation and Recognition of Streptococci

Colonies of streptococci vary from barely visible, pinpoint colonies of groups F and G (*"Streptococcus anginosus"*) to eugonic colonial forms of some of the group D strains that may grow as large as 1–1.5 mm in 18–24 hr. Colonies may range from transparent to opaque, generally being grayish-white in appearance. Under appropriate conditions group B strains (and rarely other varieties) may form colored pigment.

Depending on the resources of the laboratory, the requirements imposed on it, and the circumstances of the specimen and culture, streptococci can be isolated and identified at several levels of speed and sophistication. Initial recognition of colonies as streptococci may be facilitated with the aid of the Gram stain; the catalase test aids in differentiating streptococci from staphylococci. Colonies can be tentatively identified as members of the more familiar and more commonly occurring groups or species of streptococci if the microbiologist is sufficiently familiar with the gross appearance of the respective groups. In such cases presumptive or definitive identification may be expedited by early performance of appropriate tests. A guide to relative frequency of occurrence of some of the more common streptococci can be found in Table 38.2, in which the groups and species isolated in a large general hospital in a given year are listed. A schema for identifying presumptively certain of these organisms is shown in Table 38.3.

Individual species may be identified with one of several methods. For example, suspected group A streptococci can be identified presumptively with a positive bacitracin test, pneumococcus by a positive optochin test, group B streptococcus by hydrolysis of hippurate, etc. As with other groups or genera of bacteria, the isolates can be more definitively identified by evaluating the pattern of acceptable reactions obtained with a series of tests rather than the results of any single test.

Identification at a second level, somewhat more comprehensive and less presumptive, can be achieved by substituting serologic grouping for the less-specific bacitracin and hippurate tests.

A few serogroups can be definitively identified serologically by using specific fluorescein-conjugated antisera for recognizing grouping antigens. This test has been widely applied to group A organisms in young broth cultures (50)

TABLE 38.2—FREQUENCY OF OCCURRENCE OF CERTAIN STREPTOCOCCI IN CULTURES OF CLINICAL SPECIMENS*

GROUP OR SPECIES			NUMBER OF ISOLATES
Serogroup A			1,012
B			1,114
C			516
D†	Enterococci	6239	6,353
	S. bovis	114	
	S. equinus	0	
E			0
F			442
G			575
H			33
K			16
L			8
M			7
N			2
O			9
N G‡			493
S. pneumoniae			809
Others (unnamed or incompletely identified)			4,004
TOTAL			15,393

* Bacteriology Laboratory, The Massachusetts General Hospital, Boston, August 1976–July 1977. Isolates from throat cultures were tested with sera of groups A–G only; isolates from all other specimens were tested routinely only with sera of groups A–O, because of rarity of occurrence of streptococci of groups P–T in our earlier experience (13).

† Usually not identified by serogrouping.

‡ Could not be grouped serologically.

TABLE 38.3—PRESUMPTIVE IDENTIFICATION OF CERTAIN FREQUENTLY OCCURRING MEDICALLY IMPORTANT STREPTOCOCCI*

PRESUMPTIVE IDENTIFICATION	REACTION ON BLOOD AGAR	BACITRACIN SENSITIVITY	OPTOCHIN SENSITIVITY	HIPPURATE HYDROLYSIS	TOLERANCE TO 6.5% NaCl	BILE-ESCULIN†
Group A	β	+	-(+)‡	-	-	-
Group B	β	-(+)	-(+)	+	±§	-
Enterococcus	α β γ	-	-	-(+)	+	+
S. bovis	α	-	-	-	-	+
Pneumococcus	α	±	+	-	-	-
Not groups A, B, D	β	-(+)	-(+)	-	-	-
Viridans	α	-	-	-(+)	-	-(+)

* Adapted from Facklam (28).
† Growth and esculin hydrolysis on bile-esculin agar.
‡ (+) = Occasional strains positive.
§± = May be positive or negative.

and, in more recent years, to group B streptococci (59). Because of the sensitivity of the method, carefully prepared specific antisera must be used to avoid ambiguous cross-reaction with organisms containing related antigens (64).

Serogrouping is also performed by the microprecipitin test on extracts of Lancefield grouping antigens with specific streptococcal grouping antisera. The extracts can be prepared according to any of several methods described later. The system of using serogrouping combined with speciating of group D organisms can be used for definitive identification of most medically important streptococci, except for the viridans organisms.

Being able to differentiate the species of group D organisms is medically important because of the relative antibiotic resistance of the enterococci relative to that of the susceptible nonenterococcal *S. bovis*. The latter can be relatively easily recognized as a nonenterococcal species by its inability to grow in broth containing 6.5% NaCl or to hydrolyze arginine and by its ability to hydrolyze starch.

The viridans streptococci include a dozen or so species and clusters of more or less related organisms for which no widely accepted, comprehensive schema for identification exists. Lack of agreement on taxonomy or nomenclature (or both) accounts to a great degree for the lack of a satisfactory identification system. This is illustrated in the recent report on a comprehensive system (27), in which the author draws particular attention to the discrepancies in taxonomy and nomenclature among several of the major works in this area of streptococcal identification (14, 17, 27). An abstract of the extensive contribution of Facklam (27) is shown in Table 38.4. To be noted particularly is the

TABLE 38.4—REACTIONS OF CERTAIN MORE FREQUENTLY OCCURRING VIRIDANS STREPTOCOCCI*

	S. MU-TANS (152)†	*S. SAN-GUIS* I (202)	*S. SALI-VARIUS* (81)	*S. MG-*‡ *INTER-MEDIUS* (231)	*S. SAN-GUIS* II (231)	*S. MITIS* (177)	*S. ANGI-NOSUS-CONSTEL-LATUS*§ (55)
Alpha	59 ‖	94	10	45	95	92	40
Gamma	29	6	90	55	5	8	60
Arginine	1	64	0	26	21	16	24
Esculin	90	77	91	100	0	0	73
Mannitol	100	0	0	0	0	0	0
Lactose	99	94	89	100	100	100	0
Inulin	99	100	100	0	0	0	0
Raffinose	85	45	95	18	100	0	9
Gel-sucrose broth	88	72	0	10	43	10	0
Gel-sucrose agar	96	84	66	13	49	13	0

* Adapted from Facklam (27).
† Number in parentheses indicates number of strains tested.
‡ Includes lactose+ *S. milleri*.
§ Includes lactose− *S. milleri*.
‖ Percentage of strains positive.

omission of *S. milleri* from the nomenclature in this listing, as well as in the principal taxonomic authority in this country (19).

Although there is no generally agreed-upon system for differentiating viridans streptococci, one comparable to that extracted from Facklam's study (Table 38.4) can be tentatively used for identification of the principal viridans species.

Special Biochemical and Physiologic Diagnostic Tests

Bacitracin sensitivity test. Sensitivity of group A streptococci to low concentrations of bacitracin can be used in identifying beta-hemolytic streptococci as *S. pyogenes.* Differential disks should be used rather than susceptibility test disks, because the latter are too potent.

1. Select a colony from the culture to be tested; streak it evenly over the surface of half a blood agar plate.
2. Place a bacitracin disk in the center of the area streaked.
3. Incubate overnight.
4. A zone of inhibition of any size indicates sensitivity and presumptive identification of the culture as *S. pyogenes.*

The test yields practically no false-negative results; false-positive tests occur, particularly with group B, C, and G strains, at different frequencies depending on the occurrence of the various groups among prevalent streptococcal species being tested.

Optochin sensitivity test. *S. pneumoniae* can be differentiated from non-pneumococcal alpha-reacting streptococci by its sensitivity to optochin (ethyl hydrocupreine hydrochloride) (11).

1. Streak half the surface of a blood agar plate with a colony from the strain to be examined.
2. Place an optochin disk in the center of the streaked area.
3. Incubate overnight in the absence of increased CO_2 (56).
4. Zones of inhibition of at least 15 mm represent highly presumptive evidence of the presence of pneumococci.

Hippurate hydrolysis. Of the beta-hemolytic streptococci, *S. agalactiae* (serogroup B) is unique in being able to hydrolyze sodium hippurate. A rapid test (36) has been adapted from one recommended by Facklam for presumptive identification of commonly found streptococci (28).

1. Transfer a large loopful of the organism to be tested from a blood agar (TSA with 5% sheep blood) plate to a tube containing 0.4 ml of 1% aqueous sodium hippurate.
2. Incubate at 32 C for 2 hr.
3. Add 0.2 ml of ninhydrin solution to detect glycine end product (3.5 g ninhydrin in 100 ml 1:1 mixture of acetone and butanol). Do not mix.
4. Incubate reaction mixture at 37 C for 10 min.
5. Hydrolysis of hippurate is indicated by deep purple color; negative reactions are colorless or are occasionally faintly tinged with purple.

Other streptococci may hydrolyse hippurate; usually, these strains are enterococci and are not hemolytic.

Starch hydrolysis. S. bovis can be differentiated from enterococci with several tests, including starch hydrolysis.

1. Streak brain heart infusion agar containing 2% soluble starch with the colony to be tested.
2. Incubate 48 hr.
3. Test for absence of starch by flooding area of heavy growth with Gram's iodine.
4. Hydrolysis of starch is noted by absence of characteristic blue-black color of the starch iodine complex.

Anaerobic incubation and presence of fermentable carbohydrate, e.g., glucose, may interfere with the usefulness of the test (24).

Tolerance to 6.5% NaCl. Failure to be inhibited by 6.5% NaCl in otherwise satisfactory broth culture medium is one of the several characteristics that differentiate enterococci from antibiotic-sensitive group D streptococci, particularly *S. bovis.*

1. Inoculate heart infusion broth or Todd-Hewitt broth supplemented with NaCl to 6.5% concentration with a colony of the organism to be tested.
2. Incubate for 48 hr.
3. Observe broth culture for turbidity, acid production from glucose (if any), or other evidence of growth.

Streptococci other than enterococci may be salt-tolerant; accordingly, multiple criteria should be used to identify enterococci, as has been appropriately emphasized (26).

CAMP test. Group B streptococci can be presumptively identified in the CAMP reaction (16, 18). A known β-toxin–producing strain of staphylococcus must be used.

1. Streak the β-toxin–producing staphylococcus across the center of a sheep-blood agar plate.
2. Streak the streptococci to be tested at right angles to the testing *Staphylococcus* from the edge of streak across the uninoculated portion of the plate. If several unknown strains are to be tested, place the parallel streaks at least 2 cm apart.
3. Incubate aerobically 18 hr. Positive reactions can be observed within 5–6 hr.
4. A positive CAMP reaction is indicated by an arrowhead-shaped zone of hemolysis around the test organism where it abuts the *Staphylococcus.*

Although the CAMP reaction occurs with group B streptococci under both aerobic and anaerobic conditions, it must be emphasized that group A strains react only under anaerobic conditions.

Serologic Grouping and Typing

The fluorescent-antibody (FA) technique for serogrouping. Many of the commonly occurring, medically important streptococci can be identified by determining the presence of the group-specific, cell-wall carbohydrate. FA techniques can be used if group-specific antisera are available. Identification of streptococci with FA testing is limited almost exclusively to groups A and B (50, 59), for which appropriate sera are available. The test is most often performed on throat specimens; tests of young broth cultures of throat swabs have proven to be superior to direct tests of uncultured swabs.

1. Incubate throat swabs in 1 ml of broth for 2–5 hr.
2. After removing the swab (to be subsequently cultured for confirmatory testing), centrifuge the cells to be tested, and wash them once in buffered saline.
3. Prepare smears; air dry them, and fix them with 95% ethanol before staining them with fluorescein-conjugated antisera of known potency and specificity. Specific reactions must be unequivocal; staining of unsatisfactory intensity should be considered negative or ambiguous, and the specimen should be subjected to repeated testing or to other confirmatory identification procedures.

Extraction of antigens for serogrouping by precipitin technique. The Lancefield precipitin technique for detecting serogrouping antigens of streptococci (42) has wider application than the FA technique for identifying medically important members of the genus. The grouping antigen can be extracted with one of several techniques [the more complicated method of Fuller (31), using hot formamide, will not be described].

The hot-HCl extraction method of Lancefield involves treating the cell crop from a Todd-Hewitt broth culture of the unknown organism with 0.2 N hydrochloric acid in a boiling water bath. Supplement the broth with 0.8% glucose, which is required for the production of group D antigen. Extraction proceeds for 10 min. Neutralize the harvested extract after centrifugation with 0.2 N NaOH and clarify it by recentrifugation. It is then ready for testing by the precipitin reaction.

The autoclave extraction method of Rantz and Randall (57), a simplified method for extracting C polysaccharide from streptococci, has enjoyed wide usage. After overnight broth cultures (40 ml) are centrifuged, resuspend cell crops in 0.5 ml of isotonic solution of NaCl, and autoclave at 15 psi for 15 min. Test the supernatant fluid for the presence of serogrouping antigens. This extraction method is by far the simplest of the several procedures available.

The Maxted method for extracting C polysaccharide involves using a filtrate of cultures of *Streptomyces albus* as the extractant (45). This technique is also a simplified procedure but fails to produce suitable antigen preparations from group D streptococci and from some of the streptococcal serological groups after G (65).

Analysis of these procedures led to the development of a technique by Watson et al. (65) for extracting group-specific antigens from all medically important groupable streptococci. With it, a mixture of enzymes including lysozyme, active against group D streptococci, in combination with the *S. albus* extract of Maxted is used. With only moderately large cell crops harvested from the surface of primary isolation media and, more particularly, from cell crops from overnight cultures, extracts can be relatively easily prepared by this method. Its utility as a diagnostic procedure must be further documented.

The precipitin technique for serogrouping. The antigen-antibody reactions by which serogroup antigens in extracts of unknown cultures are detected and identified by known grouping sera are performed in glass capillary tubes that require only economic amounts of reagents. A 1-cm column of antiserum is allowed to flow by capillary action into a tube, followed by a similar column of extract without an intervening bubble of air. The capillary tube is then inserted into clay or similar material, mounted in an upright position, and observed for the formation of a grayish-white precipitate at the interface of the antiserum and extract. Strong reactions may occur within a few minutes; weaker specific reactions or specific cross-reactions with common antisera may occur more slowly and require as much as 10 to 30 min of observation. Rapid, clear-cut, specific reactions are recorded as such; ambiguous reactions or reactions of extracts with multiple antisera must be carefully interpreted, and the specificity of the antisera of the serogroups must be reevaluated.

Streptococcal serotyping. Streptococcal infections, particularly those involving *S. pyogenes, S. agalactiae,* and *S. pneumoniae,* have been better understood as a result of studies of the various serotypes. Many strains of *S. pyogenes* can be serotyped in the precipitin technique on the basis of M protein surface antigen (some 60 serotypes), or that of T antigen agglutination, or a combination of both. Because of the limited availability of type-specific sera, group A streptococci are usually serotyped at a reference laboratory.

When typing sera for group B streptococci are available, serotyping (types Ia, Ib, Ic, II, and III) can be done with antigens obtained by the hot hydrochloric acid method of extraction. Cultures of *S. pneumoniae* are differentiated by capsular polysaccharide antigens in the Quellung reaction. More than 80 serotypes have been designated, and specific antisera can be purchased from the Statens Seruminstitut, Copenhagen, Denmark. Some of the typing antisera are available to certain laboratories by special request from CDC, Atlanta, Georgia (1).

Antigen recognition (miscellaneous). Bacterial antigens can also be detected and identified with other serologic methods such as counter-immunoelectrophoresis (CIE) and coagglutination. The latter method depends on the reaction of antigen (either in solution or on the intact cell) with antibody that has been adsorbed to protein A on the surface of staphylococcal cells. Latex particles are also used as carrier of antibody molecules. At this time, the cross-reactions between streptococcal group antigens and the causes of such cross-reactions reported for the coagglutination method must be further evaluated.

CIE is an especially sensitive method for detecting antigen. Its usefulness for grouping and typing streptococci requires evaluation for sensitivity and specificity, and for economy of time, effort, and cost.

Detection of Antistreptococcal Antibodies

The late appearance of sequelae of group A streptococcal infections made necessary the development of serologic tests for infection, because *S. pyogenes* was frequently not isolated in cultures when there was evidence of rheumatic fever or acute glomerulonephritis. Tests for antibodies to streptolysin O (ASO) and deoxyribonuclease B (ADN-B) have been found to be most useful. ASO tests are usually positive (~80%–85%) in acute rheumatic fever; the ADN-B test is the test of choice for streptococcal pyoderma and its complications. Reagents for both tests are available commercially.

The ASO test depends on the neutralization of the hemolytic action of streptolysin O reagent on erythrocytes by antibodies in the patient's serum. Since the hemolysin is oxygen labile, the test must be performed under conditions which prevent inactivation. Constant volumes of streptolysin O are added to dilutions of the patient's serum. After incubation to permit neutralization, standard volumes of erythrocytes are added to the reaction mixtures, which are again incubated. The end point of the test is the highest dilution of patient's serum that inhibits hemolysis. When the streptolysin reagent used has been measured against a standard (Todd) reference, the end point or titer of serum is the reciprocal of the serum dilution expressed in Todd units (i.e., 1/ 166 = 166 Todd units). The upper limit of "normal" varies geographically and by age and is ~ 150 Todd units.

The ADN-B test is, like the ASO test, a neutralization test in which the streptococcal enzyme deoxyribonuclease B (DNaseB) is used as the antigen. Constant volumes of DNaseB are added to dilutions of the patient's serum. After incubation to allow any antibody to combine with the antigen, a constant volume of deoxyribonucleic acid (DNA) is added to the reaction mixture, which is then reincubated. The tubes are then tested for depolymerization of the DNA, which occurs in the absence of ADN-B. Polymerized DNA is detected with one of several reagents, depending on the system used. As with the ASO test, the upper limits of normal vary with age and geography, the average being somewhere around 150 units.

For a review of tests for antibodies to streptococci, the reader is referred to Klein (39).

Antimicrobial Susceptibility Testing

With the exception of the group D enterococci (and a few strains of *S. pneumoniae*), all of the streptococci are susceptible to ampicillin and penicillin G (30, 44). Thus, it is not necessary to determine routinely the susceptibility of nonenterococcal streptococci to penicillin G and related antibiotics. However, the recent emergence in New Guinea, South Africa, and elsewhere of strains of *S. pneumoniae* which are relatively penicillin resistant may change this policy—at least as far as the pneumococci are concerned. Some authorities feel that it is reasonable to subject streptococcal isolates from cerebrospinal fluid and blood cultures to penicillin susceptibility testing since occasional strains of nongroup A streptococci (especially group B and some nongroupable strains) may be found for which the minimal inhibitory concentrations (MICs) of penicillin range up to 1 μg/ml. However, there are no data to demonstrate that penicillin G is clinically ineffective against these strains. The cephalosporins and semisynthetic, penicillinase-resistant penicillins are effective against most streptococci except enterococci, although the MICs of these agents are often higher than those of penicillin or ampicillin. Enterococci are generally more resistant to penicillin G, with concentrations of 1–8 μg/ml being required to inhibit the growth of most of these strains (62). The susceptibility pattern of enterococci to penicillin is so predictable that these strains probably need not be routinely tested. Despite this fact, susceptibility testing is generally performed for enterococci in most clinical laboratories. Endocarditis and other serious infections caused by enterococci are usually treated with combinations of penicillin and an aminoglycoside such as streptomycin or gentamicin, because such combinations may exhibit synergistic antimicrobial activity against enterococci. However, not all combinations are synergistic. The presence or absence of synergism may be predicted by screening for high-level resistance (MIC > 2000 μg/ml) to the aminoglycoside. Strains of *S. faecalis* that are highly resistant are not synergistically killed by combinations of penicillin with the aminoglycoside to which they are highly resistant (49). In the absence of high-level resistance, synergism almost invariably occurs, except with amikacin.

S. *faecium* is resistant to synergism when penicillin is combined with kanamycin, tobramycin, netilmicin, or sisomicin, irrespective of the presence or absence of high-level resistance to the aminoglycosides (47).

Some streptococcal isolates, including some of those of *S. pneumoniae*, are resistant to the tetracyclines, the sulfonamides, erythromycin, lincomycin, and clindamycin. Therefore, susceptibility testing should be performed if these drugs are to be used in the treatment of streptococcal infections. Most streptococci are resistant to clinically achievable concentrations of the aminoglycosides and the polymyxins. These agents need not be included among the battery of antimicrobial agents selected for routine testing against streptococci.

Special Test Procedures

Although Mueller-Hinton agar and broth are the media recommended by the World Health Organization International Collaborative Study on Antibiotic Susceptibility Testing, these media do not consistently support the growth of streptococci. Thus, the media must be supplemented. For agar-dilution and agar-diffusion testing, the addition of 5% defibrinated sheep blood is recommended (44). Supplementation of broth with blood makes it difficult to assess turbidity end points. Thus, for broth dilution studies, horse serum can be added to Mueller-Hinton broth to enhance growth (44). Alternatively, a medium such as dextrose phosphate broth, which readily supports streptococcal growth, can be used. (See Chapter 44.)

The method of testing for high-level aminoglycoside resistance (for synergism determination in enterococci) is as follows.

1. Susceptibility testing plates used in this determination contain either no antibiotics (control), or streptomycin, kanamycin, or gentamicin (or other aminoglycoside) in a concentration of 2000 μg/ml.
2. Prepare stock solutions containing 500 mg/ml of antibiotic in sterile distilled water. Dissolve dextrose phosphate broth powder (Pfizer-Albimi), 15.5 g, in 500 ml of distilled water, and add Bacto-agar (Difco), 5 g (1%); autoclave the mixture.
3. Cool the liquid medium to 45–50 C in a water bath; add 2 ml of antibiotic solution; after they are mixed, pour the 15–20 ml aliquots of the solution into each of a series of 100-mm sterile petri dishes, and allow to harden at room temperature. (Mueller-Hinton agar with 5% defibrinated sheep blood can be substituted for dextrose phosphate agar.)
4. Select a representative enterococcal colony from an overnight culture on

semisolid medium. With a platinum loop, streak half of the colony onto the test plate and half on a control plate without antibiotics.

5. After they are incubated overnight at 37 C, examine plates for growth. Confluent growth (or the presence of multiple isolated colonies) on the antibiotic-containing test plate denotes high-level resistance.

Reporting and Evaluation of Laboratory Findings

The results of testing cultures of clinical specimens that are intended, either explicitly or implicitly, to provide evidence for the presence or absence of streptococci must be reported in precise, medically useful terms. Reporting of group A, B, C, etc, streptococci should be based on positive serologic identification of the serogroup. Presumptive identification should be reported as such when, for example, group A streptococci are identified in the bacitracin test or group B streptococci by hippurate hydrolysis, etc.

Group D streptococci should be further differentiated as enterococci or nonenterococcal streptococci on the basis of several tests because of the important implications of susceptibility to antibiotics for these organisms. Recent evidence suggests that it may be useful to differentiate *S. faecium* from *S. faecalis* because of differences among these species in susceptibility to antimicrobial agents alone and in combination (26, 47).

Named species should be established on the basis of as substantial a series of reactions as the intellectual and physical resources of the laboratory will permit. The degree of certainty of the designation should be included in the wording of the report, with terms such as "presumptive," "probable," and the like being used when indicated; their absence should denote the degree of certainty with which the organism was identified. For example, unidentifiable streptococci can be described as "alpha, beta, or gamma streptococci" (their otherwise namelessness being presumed) or "serologically ungroupable" (if serogrouping was actually unsuccessfully attempted), or they may be characterized in some other agreed-upon manner (e.g., capnophilic, fastidious, satelliting, etc). In the interests of economy, relevance, and perspective, it should be appreciated that rare or few colonies of nonhemolytic streptococci found in mixed cultures which contain many other potentially pathogenic organisms usually do not need to be fully characterized for general medical purposes.

Whether clinically relevant streptococcal groups or species need to be subjected to infrasubspecific differentiation such as serotyping depends on the individual clinical situation.

Finally, the question of using serologic tests to provide indirect evidence of prior streptococcal infection should be addressed. The more popular ASO test of patients' sera for antibodies to streptococci is not the most sensitive test for this purpose; the ADN-B test or a combination of the two should be substituted for it. For the physician it must be emphasized that so-called "normal ranges" vary both with age of subject and prevalence of infection—the latter determined by season and geography. An important concern of the physician and public health worker is understanding the variation in antibody responses of the patient to pharyngitis and pyoderma and the significance of the responses in relation to the two important sequelae of streptococcal infections.

References

1. AUSTRIAN R: *Streptococcus pneumoniae* (Pneumococcus). *In* Manual of Clinical Microbiology, 2nd edition. Lennette EH, Spaulding EH, and Truant JP (eds.). American Society for Microbiology, Washington, DC, 1974, pp 109–115
2. AUSTRIAN R and COLLINS P: Importance of carbon dioxide in the isolation of pneumococci. J Bacteriol 92:1281–1284, 1966
3. AYOUB EM, ANTHONY BF, MAUCERI AA, and SANDERS WE JR: Asymptomatic epidemic acquisition of group A streptococcus: Antibody response to extracellular and type-specific antigens. J Infect Dis 132:20–27, 1975
4. BAKER CJ and BARRETT F: Group B streptococcal infections in infants. The importance of the various serotypes. J Am Med Assoc 230:1158–1160, 1974
5. BAKER CJ, CLARK DJ, and BARRETT FF: Selective broth medium for isolation of group B streptococci. Appl Microbiol 26:884–885, 1973
6. BANNATYNE RM and RANDALL C: Ecology of 350 isolates of group F streptococcus. Am J Clin Pathol 67:184–186, 1977
7. BAYER AS, CHOW AW, ANTHONY BF, and GUZE LB: Serious infections in adults due to group B streptococci. Clinical and serotypic characterization. Am J Med 61:498–503, 1976
8. BENJAMIN JT and PERRIELLO VA JR: Pharyngitis due to group C hemolytic streptococci in children. J Pediatr 89:254–256, 1976
9. BISNO AL, PEARCE IA, and STOLLERMAN GH: Streptococcal infections that fail to cause recurrences of rheumatic fever. J Infect Dis 136:278–285, 1977
10. BLACK WA and VAN BUSKIRK F: Gentamicin blood agar used as a general purpose selective medium. Appl Microbiol 25:905–907, 1973
11. BOWEN MK, THIELE LC, STEARMAN BD, and SCHAUB IG: The optochin sensitivity test: A reliable method for identification of pneumococci. J Lab Clin Med 49:641–642, 1957
12. BREESE BB, DISNEY FA, and TALPEY W: The nature of a small pediatric group practice. II. The incidence of beta streptococcal illness in a private pediatric practice. Pediatrics 38:277–285, 1966
13. BROOME CV, MOELLERING RC JR, and WATSON BK: Clinical significance of Lancefield groups L-T streptococci isolated from blood and cerebrospinal fluid. J Infect Dis 133:382–392, 1976
14. CARLSSON J: A numerical taxonomic study of human oral streptococci. Odontol Revy 19:137–160, 1968
15. CHRETIEN JH, MCGINNISS CG, THOMPSON J, DELAHA E, and GARAGUSI VF: Group B beta-hemolytic streptococci causing pharyngitis. J Clin Microbiol 10:263–266, 1979
16. CHRISTIE R, ATKINS NE, and MUNCH-PETERSEN E: A note on a lytic phenomenon shown by group B streptococci. Aust J Exp Biol Med Sci 22:197–200, 1949
17. COLMAN G and WILLIAMS REO: Taxonomy of some human *Viridans streptococci*. *In* Streptococci and Streptococcal Diseases. Wannamaker LW and Matsen JM (eds.). Academic Press, New York, 1972, pp 281–299
18. DARLING CL: Standardization and evaluation of the CAMP reaction for the prompt presumptive identification of *Streptococcus agalactiae* (Lancefield group B) in clinical material. J Clin Microbiol 1:171–174, 1975
19. DEIBEL RH and SEELEY HW JR: Family II. Streptococcaceae. *In* Bergey's Manual of Determinative Bacteriology. Buchanan RE and Gibbons NE (eds.). Williams & Wilkins Co, Baltimore, 1974, pp 490–509
20. DILLON HC: Streptococcal infections of the skin and their complications: Impetigo and nephritis. *In* Streptococci and Streptococcal Diseases. Wannamaker LW and Matsen JM (ed.). Academic Press, New York and London, 1972, pp 571–587
21. DOWLING HF and HIRSH HL: The use of penicillinase in cultures of body fluids obtained from patients under treatment with penicillin. Am J Med Sci 210:756–762, 1945
22. DUCA E, TEODOROVICI G, RADU C, VITA A, TALASMAN-NICULESCU P, BERNESCU E, FELDI C, and ROSCA V: A new nephritogenic *Streptococcus*. J Hyg 67:691–698, 1969
23. DUMA RJ, WEINBERG AN, MEDREK TF, and KUNZ LJ: Streptococcal infections. A bacteriologic and clinical study of streptococcal bacteremia. Medicine 48:87–127, 1969
24. DUNICAN LK and SEELEY HW: Starch hydrolysis by *Streptococcus equinus*. J Bacteriol 83:264–269, 1962

25. ELLNER PD, STOESSEL CJ, DRAKEFORD E, and VASI F: A new culture medium for medical bacteriology. Am J Clin Pathol 45:502–504, 1966

26. FACKLAM RR: Recognition of group D streptococcal species of human origin by biochemical and physiological tests. Appl. Microbiol 23:1131–1139, 1972

27. FACKLAM RR: Physiological differentiation of Viridans streptococci. J Clin Microbiol 5:184–201, 1977

28. FACKLAM RR, PADULA JF, THACKER LG, WORTHAM EC, and SCONYERS BJ: Presumptive identification of group A, B, and D streptococci. Appl Microbiol 27:107–113, 1974

29. FEINGOLD DS, STAGG NL, and KUNZ LJ: Extrarespiratory streptococcal infections. Importance of the various serological groups. N Engl J Med 275:356–361, 1966

30. FINLAND M, GARNER C, WILCOX C, and SABATH LD: Susceptibility of beta-hemolytic streptococci to 65 antibacterial agents. Antimicrob Agents Chemother 9:11–19, 1976

31. FULLER AT: The formamide method for the extraction of polysaccharides from hemolytic streptococci. Br J Exp Pathol 19:130–139, 1938

32. GIBBONS RJ and VAN HOUTE J: Dental caries. Annu Rev Med 26:121–136, 1975

33. HENDLEY JO, SANDE MA, STEWART PM, and GWALTNEY JM JR: Spread of *Streptococcus pneumoniae* in families. I. Carriage rates and distribution of types. J Infect Dis 132:55–61, 1975

34. HILL HR, CALDWELL GG, WILSON E, HAGER D, and ZIMMERMAN RA: Epidemic of pharyngitis due to streptococci of Lancefield group G. Lancet 2:371–374, 1969

35. HOEPRICH PD: Bacterial pneumonias. *In* Infectious Diseases. Hoeprich PD (ed.). Harper and Row, Hagerstown, Md, 1972, pp 311–324

36. HWANG M and EDERER GM: Rapid hippurate hydrolysis method for presumptive identification of group B streptococci. J Clin Microbiol 1:114–115, 1975

37. JAMES L and MCFARLAND RB: An epidemic of pharyngitis due to a nonhemolytic group A streptococcus at Lowry Airforce Base. N Engl J Med 284:750–752, 1971

38. KAYE D: Prophylaxis against bacterial endocarditis: a dilemma. *In* Infective Endocarditis. Kaplan EL and Taranta AV (eds.). Am Heart Assoc Monogr No. 52. Dallas, Tex, 1977, pp 67–69

39. KLEIN GC: Immune response to streptococcal infection. *In* Manual of Clinical Immunology. Rose NR and Friedman H (eds.). Am Soc Microbiol, Washington, DC, 1976, pp 264–273

40. KLEIN RS, RECCO RA, CATALANO MT, EDBERG SC, CASEY JI, and STEIGBIGEL NH: Association of *Streptococcus bovis* with carcinoma of the colon. N Engl J Med 297:800–802, 1977

41. KRUMWIEDE E and KUTTNER AG: A growth inhibitory substance for the influenza group of organisms in the blood of various animal species. J Exp Med 67:429–441, 1938

42. LANCEFIELD RC: A serological differentiation of human and other groups of hemolytic streptococci. J Exp Med 57:571–595, 1933

43. LIU P: Carbon dioxide requirement of group F and minute colony G hemolytic streptococci. J Bacteriol 68:282–288, 1954

44. MATSEN JM and COGHLAN CR: Antibiotic testing and susceptibility patterns of streptococci. *In* Streptococci and Streptococcal Diseases. Wannamaker LW and Matsen JM (eds.). Academic Press, New York and London, 1972, pp 189–204

45. MAXTED WR: Preparation of streptococcal extracts for Lancefield grouping. Lancet 2:255–256, 1948

46. MCCARTHY LR, and BOTTONE EJ: Bacteremia and endocarditis caused by satelliting streptococci. Am J Clin Pathol 61:585–591, 1974

47. MOELLERING RC JR, KORZENIOWSKI OM, SANDE MA, and WENNERSTEN CB: Species-specific resistance to antimicrobial synergism in *Streptococcus faecium* and *Streptococcus faecalis*. J Infect Dis 140:203–208, 1979

48. MOELLERING RC JR, WATSON BK, and KUNZ LJ: Endocarditis due to group D streptococci. Comparison of disease caused by *Streptococcus bovis* with that produced by the enterococci. Am J Med 57:239–250, 1974

49. MOELLERING RC JR, WENNERSTEN C, MEDREK T, and WEINBERG AN: Prevalence of high-level resistance to aminoglycosides in clinical isolates of enterococci. Antimicrob Agents Chemother—1970: 335–340, 1971

50. MOODY MD, SIEGEL AC, PITTMAN B, and WINTER CC: Fluorescent antibody identification of group A steptococci from throat swabs. Am J Public Health 53:1083–1092, 1963

51. MUFSON MA, KRUSS DM, WASIL RE, and METZGER WI: Capsular types and outcome of bacteremic pneumococcal disease in the antibiotic era. Arch Intern Med 134:505–510, 1974
52. MURRAY PR, WOLD AD, SCHRECK CA, and WASHINGTON JA II: Effects of selective media and atmosphere of incubation on the isolation of group A streptococci. J Clin Microbiol 4:54–56, 1976
53. PARKER MT and BALL LC: Streptococci and aerococci associated with systemic infection in man. J Med Microbiol 9:275–302, 1976
54. PATTERSON EJ and HAFEEZ AEB: Group B streptococci in human disease. Bacteriol Rev 40:774–792, 1976
55. PETER G and SMITH AL: Group A streptococcal infections of the skin and pharynx. N Engl J Med 297:311–317 and 365–370, 1977
56. RAGSDALE AR and SANFORD JP: Interfering effect of incubation in carbon dioxide on the identification of pneumococci by optochin discs. Appl Microbiol 22:854–855, 1971
57. RANTZ LA and RANDALL E: Use of autoclaved extracts of hemolytic streptococci for serological grouping. Stanford Med Bull 13:290–291, 1955
58. RAVERBY WD, BOTTONE EJ and KEUSCH GT: Group D streptococcal bacteremia, especially infections due to *Streptococcus bovis*. N Engl J Med 289:1400–1403, 1973
59. ROMERO R and WILKINSON HW: Identification of group B streptococci by immuno-fluorescence staining. Appl Microbiol 28:199–204, 1974
60. STOLLERMAN GH: Nephritogenic and rheumatogenic group A streptococci. J Infect Dis 120:258–263, 1969
61. SULLIVAN RJ JR, DOWDLE WR, MARINE WM, and HIERHOLZER JC: Adult pneumonia in a general hospital. Arch Intern Med 129:935–942, 1972
62. TOALA P, MCDONALD A, WILCOX C, and FINLAND M: Susceptibility of group D streptococcus (enterococcus) to 21 antibiotics *in vitro*, with special reference to species differences. Am J Med Sci 258:416–430, 1969
63. WASHINGTON JA II: Blood cultures. Mayo Clin Proc 50:91–98, 1975
64. WATSON BK, KUNZ LJ, and MOELLERING RC JR: Identification of streptococci: serogrouping by immunofluorescence. J Clin Microbiol 1:268–273, 1975
65. WATSON BK, MOELLERING RC JR, and KUNZ LJ: Identification of streptococci: use of lysozyme and *Streptomyces albus* filtrate in the preparation of extracts for Lancefield grouping. J Clin Microbiol 1:274–278, 1975
66. WOODBURY C: Streptococcal Disease. The Upjohn Co, 1973, pp 51

CHAPTER 39

SYPHILIS

Peter L. Perine, Alwilda L. Wallace, Joseph H. Blount, and Stuart T. Brown

Introduction

Causative Agent

Syphilis or lues is caused by *Treponema pallidum,* a thin, motile spiral organism belonging to the order Spirochaetales and the family *Treponemataceae.* It is approximately 0.2 μm wide and 7–20 μm long, and because of its small mass, it cannot be easily visualized except by the darkfield or phase-contrast microscope. *T. pallidum* cannot be cultured on artificial medium. The organisms used for certain serologic tests are usually obtained from the testicles of experimentally infected rabbits.

Syphilis is one of the treponematoses, a group of chronic diseases caused by closely related treponemes. These include the tropical diseases, yaws and pinta, which are caused by *T. pertenue* and *T. carateum,* respectively. Because these treponemes have a morphology and antigenic structure which is virtually identical to *T. pallidum* they cannot be differentiated except by the character of lesions and the course of infection they produce in man and experimental animals.

The *Treponemataceae* also contain a number of avirulent, cultivatable, members that are part of the normal oral, gastrointestinal and urogenital microbial flora. They commonly cause confusion in the diagnosis of syphilis since their morphology is very similar to that of *T. pallidum* and they may at times become opportunistic pathogens, contaminating genital lesions or infecting syphiliticlike lesions. Moreover, many of these organisms share common antigens with *T. pallidum,* giving rise to cross-reacting antibodies that may react in "specific" treponemal serologic tests. This antigenic relationship has its beneficial aspects, however, because large numbers of certain avirulent treponema, particularly the Reiter biotype of *T. phagendenis,* can be grown, purified, and used as antigen in serologic tests.

Clinical Description of Disease

Syphilis is a chronic granulomatous disease that characteristically progresses by "stages" of clinically apparent infection. Each stage has different manifestations and lesion morphology, and stages are separated by periods of latency or quiescence when the only evidence of infection is a reactive sero-logic test for syphilis. Syphilis can mimic almost any disease and a detailed discussion of its clinical manifestations is beyond the scope of this text.

Except for congenital infection, syphilis is almost always transmitted by sexual exposure. *T. pallidum* breaches the skin or mucous membrane barrier and spreads within hours from the site of invasion to the regional lymphatics and small blood vessels, causing a bacteremia that may continue throughout the course of untreated infection. The majority of the infecting spirochetes re-main and slowly multiply at the site of invasion, however, and after an in-cubation period ranging from 9 days to 90 days (average, 21 days), the primary syphilitic lesion, the chancre, appears. The chancre is most frequently a pain-less, ulcer-like lesion with raised borders and a necrotic base. The serum from the chancre contains *T. pallidum* and is highly infectious. The chancre heals spontaneously without scarring over a period of 2–3 weeks.

The secondary stage of syphilis occurs 6 weeks to 6 months after the chancre heals, although in some cases it may begin before the chancre heals. The secondary stage reflects the bacteremia that began at the onset of infection and virtually every organ and tissue of the body may be involved. As a result, the symptoms and signs of secondary syphilis are legion. In addition to consti-tutional symptoms such as fever, headache and malaise, there may be general-ized lymphadenopathy and a variety of skin rashes, hepatitis, myositis, men-ingitis, neuropathies, glomerulonephritis and nephrosis. Syphilitic nephrosis has been attributed to soluble immune complexes composed of treponemal an-tigen and antibody.

Secondary lesions heal spontaneously over a period of several weeks, and then the disease enters the latent stage. This is arbitrarily divided into early and late latent stages, the former being the 2-year period of time when lesions of secondary syphilis may recur. There are no clinical manifestations in the la-tent stage and the only evidence of infection is a reactive serologic test for syphilis.

Tertiary syphilis represents the destructive stage of the disease. It may be-gin 5 to 20 or more years after the initial infection. Only one-third of untreated patients develop tertiary lesions, which are of three types: 80% are aneurysms of the aortic arch leading to dilation of the aortic valve with regurgitation; 15% involve the central nervous system and produce meningitis, cerebrovascular accidents, neuropathies of the cranial nerve (the classical Argyl-Robinson pu-pil of neurosyphilis which accommodates but does not react to light), epilepsy, general paresis (insanity) or tabes dorsalis; and gumma, the rarest tertiary le-sion, which histologically resembles a tubercle. Gummas are usually "benign" since they seldom cause death or disability, although they are space-occupying lesions and may occur in vital organs.

Congenital syphilis results from the passage of *T. pallidum* across the pla-centa from the mother to the fetus. The risk of transmission decreases with the duration of untreated infection in the mother, i.e., a mother with latent syphilis has a very low chance of transmitting syphilis to her baby during pregnancy. The fetus may be aborted, stillborn or liveborn with or without clinical evi-dence of syphilis. The lesions of early congenital syphilis are of the secondary type and may be present at birth or more often develop 3 weeks to 6 months later. The lesions of early congenital syphilis include skin rashes, pneumonia, ascites, anemia and painful bone lesions. The lesions of late congenital syphilis (untreated disease of more than 2 years' duration) include blindness secondary to optic atrophy, nerve deafness, gummas and deformed bones, which may not appear until puberty.

Epidemiology

Since man is the only natural host for *T. pallidum,* someone with syphilis obviously acquired the infection from another syphilitic. Only primary and secondary syphilis are infectious. For epidemiologic purposes, however, public health personnel, who have been specially trained in the interview-contact referral·process, also find and examine sexual partners of patients with early latent syphilis. This procedure ensures that those infected with syphilis are adequately treated and unable to spread the disease further. Sexual partners of patients with early syphilis who have no clinical or serologic evidence of infection but who might be incubating syphilis are also treated. These control measures, initiated in the late 1930s, have resulted in a dramatic decline in all stages of syphilis over the past three decades. Total syphilis of all stages decreased from 575,593 in 1943 to 64,875 in 1978, down 88.7%, or 510,718, in the last 35 years. Treating large numbers of patients for syphilis has consequently produced a significant reduction in the late damaging sequelae of syphilis (Fig 39.1).

The *incidence* of syphilis is defined as the number of new syphilis infections occurring within a 1-year period. Although syphilis infections are reportable by law in all 50 states, the District of Columbia, Puerto Rico and the Virgin Islands, the reported number may understate actual incidence because infections occur which are not diagnosed, and some diagnosed cases are not reported to the health departments. The Venereal Disease Control Division of the Center for Disease Control estimates that the actual incidence of syphilis was more than 80,000 cases in 1978—about two to three times the reported incidence!

The *prevalence* of syphilis is the number of cases needing treatment at a given time. This large reservoir of untreated cases is composed primarily of those that have progressed to the latent stages of infection and are detectable only by means of blood tests. The prevalence reservoir in 1978 was estimated to number about 300,000. If untreated, syphilis may progress to destructive neurosyphilis, cardiovascular syphilis, and other serious chronic manifestations. The prevalence of syphilis has declined steadily since 1943, primarily because of disease prevention plus the serologic screening programs which detected and treated larger numbers of persons for syphilis.

Certain aspects of syphilis epidemiology are of practical importance. Not all patients with primary syphilis progress through the subsequent stages of infection. Secondary syphilis is usually the first clinical manifestation of syphilis in women and homosexual men since the primary lesion is likely to be hidden. The recent "revolution" in sexual mores and practices has increased the incidence of primary syphilitic lesions at extragenital sites, particularly in the oropharynx and rectum. In certain areas of the country, syphilis is particularly

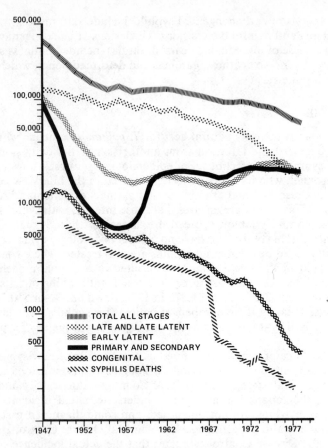

Figure 39.1—Reported cases of syphilis, 1947–1978.

common among homosexual men. Like many communicable diseases, syphilis rates are consistently higher in urban than in rural areas and syphilis is found more frequently among the sexually active population between 15–30 years of age.

Public Health Significance

If social notoriety and the economic consequences of morbidity and mortality are measures of public health significance, then few infectious diseases are the equal of syphilis. Before the introduction of arsenical treatment for syphilis in the early twentieth century, syphilis was one of the leading causes of death in the Western World and it is still a major killer in certain underdeveloped countries of Africa and Asia.

Syphilis first appeared in Europe in the late 15th century, shortly after Columbus returned from the New World. Whether or not it was imported by his crew from the West Indies, where syphilis is alleged to be of long standing, or resulted from a mutation of one of the non-venereal treponemes then existing in Europe is controversial. Perhaps the first recorded syphilis epidemic occurred in the Spring of 1495 when a violent plague, which most contemporary records attribute to syphilis, broke out among the armies participating in the siege of Naples. The malignant nature of the infection in its early stages broke the siege, and the disbanding troops rapidly spread "the great pox" throughout Europe, where it became one of the scourges of the 16th century. Syphilis thereafter evolved slowly to become the less virulent, chronic infection recognized today.

The venereal transmission of syphilis was recognized from its inception, and perhaps because of this characteristic, efforts to control the disease, including such measures as banishment and incarceration during the infectious stages, were unsuccessful. Moreover, treatment with a variety of ointments, unctions, fumigations, etc., were not only ineffective, but often so toxic as to cause more disability and death than the disease itself. In the absence of an effective cure, a syphilitic faced a lifelong threat of a horrible death from tertiary syphilis, regarded by many nonsyphilitics as just retribution for the sinful acquisition of the infection. Some of these social stigmas and punitive attitudes about syphilis survive today.

The syphilis problem is generally measured by the extent and trend of reported cases and by other types of information such as the results of serologic screening programs and deaths from syphilis. Little is known about these statistics in the United States before 1941 except that syphilis was one of the leading causes of rejection from the armed services in World War I, and despite a modest federal and state VD control program, the incidence of syphilis progressively increased during the 1920s and 1930s. This increase culminated in the passage of the Venereal Disease Control Act by Congress in 1938, which significantly increased federal monetary support to state health departments with the long-range goal of eradicating syphilis.

The impact of the VD control programs, which became effective in 1939, was immediate and massive. The number of clinics providing free diagnosis and treatment increased from 1746 to 2405 within the first year, and the number of new cases of syphilis treated rose from 197,000 to 314,000 (1). The reported incidence of syphilis increased sharply during World War II, partly as a result of better case detection and reporting, and partly because of the social chaos of those times. However, since World War II, the trend of syphilis has been characterized by an initial and rapid decline and then a resurgence in the number of new cases and a progressive decline in the number of latent syphilis cases detected and treated.

With the introduction of penicillin as a simple and highly effective cure, the reported incidence of primary and secondary syphilis dropped from a high of 106,539 cases in 1947 to 6392 in 1956 (4). Many public health authorities believed that syphilis was for all practical purposes eradicated. Consequently, funds for VD control were reduced so that many VD control programs were either dismantled or were in such disarray that they were unable to cope with the resurgence of infectious syphilis in the 1960s.

The reported incidence of primary and secondary syphilis (4) increased almost progressively from 3.9 to 12.1 cases per 100,000 population from 1956 to 1975 (6392 to 25,561 cases). The reasons for this increase are speculative, but many attributed it to an increase in sexual promiscuity and permissiveness. It is generally agreed that this increased incidence did not result from improved case detection and reporting since the degree of underreporting remained fairly constant throughout this period. A revitalized federally assisted syphilis control program begun in 1962 appears to have stemmed the rise in syphilis incidence; reported cases declined more than 15% between 1975 and 1978, or from 25,561 to 21,656 cases. Also, the number of reported early latent syphilis cases continued a decline that started in 1962. This decline suggests that more cases are being prevented or treated in the infectious stages as a result of intensified case detection and prevention activities.

Forty-five states plus the District of Columbia, incorporating 94% of the population of the United States, require notification to the proper health officials of all reactive serologic tests for syphilis. In 1978, 1,466,288 reactors were reported to health departments by laboratories (Table 39.1). Of these, 155,340 required consultation with the patients' physician or investigation of their medical records to determine the cause of reactivity. A total of 49,065 cases of previously unknown syphilis were identified, including 24,638 infectious and early latent cases.

Testing Procedures and Recommendations for Use

Types of Tests

Serologic tests for syphilis are of two general types: the first and oldest are the nontreponemal antigen tests which utilize lipid (cardiolipin) as antigen. The second type are treponemal antigen tests which use pathogenic *T. pallidum* or closely related treponemal antigens to detect "specific" antibodies. Cardiolipin is a normal constituent of mammalian cells and reacts with IgM or IgG immunoglobulins known as "reagin" antibody. Reagin is a historical designation and should not be confused with the IgE class of immunoglobulins. Several tests are available to detect reagin antibody. These do not vary significantly in their sensitivity in syphilis; therefore most public health and clinical laboratories perform only one cardiolipin test, because results from additional non-

TABLE 39.1—ESTIMATED VOLUME OF SEROLOGIC TESTING FOR SYPHILIS IN THE UNITED STATES AND OUTLYING AREAS (1978)*

TYPE OF LABORATORY	NO. OF LABORATORIES	NO. OF SPECIMENS PROCESSED	NO. OF REACTIVE SPECIMENS	% REACTIVE
Private	7400	30,560,846	635,942	2.1
Public	1570	13,813,111	795,031	5.8
Federal	273	1,236,373	35,315	2.9
Total	9243	45,610,330	1,466,288	3.2

* Excludes Upstate New York.

treponemal tests offer little or no help to the clinician. Treponemal antigen tests are available at an increasing number of local and state laboratories.

Nontreponemal Antigen Tests

Nontreponemal antigen tests comprise the majority of all syphilis serologic tests performed in hospital, private, and public health laboratories. The standard nontreponemal antigen tests discussed in this chapter are the Venereal Disease Research Laboratory (VDRL) slide test, the Unheated Serum Reagin (USR) test, and the Rapid Plasma Reagin (RPR) (18-mm circle) Card test on serum. Automated Reagin Test (ART) systems are commercially available with standardized reagents and methods (27) for laboratories that test large numbers of specimens.

The VDRL slide test, the oldest and most widely used of these tests, is practical, inexpensive and reproducible. The quantitative VDRL slide test is easily performed on specimens having reactivity in a qualitative test. Techniques for the qualitative and quantitative VDRL slide tests on spinal fluid are simple, requiring only a small amount of fluid. VDRL slide tests use a standard antigen that is an alcoholic solution of cardiolipin, purified lecithin, and cholesterol in optimal proportions.

The USR and RPR (18-mm circle) card tests are known as rapid reagin tests; these tests use a modified VDRL antigen suspension containing choline chloride, making heat inactivation of serum unnecessary and apparently enhancing test reactivity. The RPR card test antigen suspension contains specially prepared carbon particles as a visualization agent. The antigen suspensions used in these tests are stable for specified periods of time under controlled conditions. The use of the rapid reagin tests is rapidly increasing since they are simple to perform and require little specialized equipment; also most of this equipment is disposable, so glassware cleaning is eliminated. Additional rapid reagin tests are in various stages of development and evaluation, but appear to offer few advantages in performance or availability over those now available.

Treponemal Antigen Tests

Treponemal antigen tests use pathogenic *T. pallidum* as antigen to detect specific treponemal antibodies. Although these are more specific for syphilis than the nontreponemal antigen tests, they are also more expensive and technically more difficult to perform. There is no advantage in quantitating the treponemal antibody detected by these tests since this has no diagnostic or therapeutic value at present.

The standard treponemal test is the fluorescent treponemal antibody-absorption (FTA-ABS) test; the microhemagglutination assay for antibodies to *T. pallidum* (MHA-TP) has provisional test status and is used by an increasing number of laboratories. The *T. pallidum* immobilization (TPI) test developed by Nelson and Mayer in 1949 uses viable *T. pallidum* extracted from infected rabbit testicular tissue (17). Its technical complexity is such that it is no longer routinely available in clinical laboratories in the United States.

The FTA-ABS test is an indirect fluorescent antibody test, which is a modification of the original FTA test published by Deacon et al. (5). The antigen is a suspension of dead *T. pallidum*, Nichols' strain, extracted from rabbit testicular tissue. The conjugate (reaction indicator) is a fluorescein-labeled antihuman globulin. The test is performed by first diluting the test serum 1:5 in "Sorbent," a standardized product prepared from cultures of Reiter treponemes. The diluted serum is added to antigen previously fixed on a glass slide, incubated, and then washed to remove excess serum and sorbent. Conjugate is then added, the slide is incubated and washed as before, and the test is read microscopically with an ultraviolet light source. The FTA-ABS test is more sensitive than the TPI test and appears to have comparable specificity.

The MHA-TP test (3) is a modification of a hemagglutination procedure reported by Rathlev in 1965 (22) and by Tomizawa and Kasamatsu in 1966 (26). The antigen is a suspension of formalinized, tanned sheep erythrocytes which have been sensitized with sonicated *T. pallidum*, Nichols' strain. The patient's serum, first treated with an absorbing diluent to increase specificity, is tested by a qualitative microhemagglutination method; test results are read macroscopically. The MHA-TP test is less sensitive than the FTA-ABS test in primary syphilis but gives essentially the same results in the later stages of disease (14). Available data indicate that the specificity of the MHA-TP test in populations known to be at high risk for false-positive nontreponemal tests may be somewhat less than the FTA-ABS test. Further studies are needed before the MHA-TP is given the status of a standard test.

Recommendation for Test Use

Tests with serum specimens

In selecting serologic tests for use in public health and clinical laboratories, consideration must be given to a number of factors: The volume of tests, number and caliber of technical personnel, physical facilities, cost, and availability of reference services. It is recommended that all blood specimens submitted for diagnostic purposes be examined by means of a standard cardiolipin antigen test such as the VDRL slide test or a rapid reagin test. On specimens that are nonreactive to the standard test, additional tests are unnecessary unless specifically requested and justified. Specimens having any degree of reactivity with the standard test should be rechecked and titered to an end point by a standard quantitative test like the VDRL slide quantitative test. Quantitative test results provide additional information to the clinician by establishing a base line for following the serologic response to treatment.

The treponemal tests are not intended for routine use, but are reserved for diagnostic problem cases at the special request of the clinician. Their greatest value is in distinguishing syphilitic reactions from false-positive (FP) reactions in the non-treponemal antigen tests and in aiding in the establishment of a diagnosis of syphilis in a patient with clinical evidence of tertiary syphilis but with nonreactive cardiolipin test results.

Most hospital and clinical laboratories perform only the qualitative and quantitative nontreponemal antigen tests, the one in most common use being the VDRL slide test. Most state public health laboratories and some local public health and clinical laboratories are equipped to perform the FTA-ABS or MHA-TP test on diagnostic problem cases. State public health laboratories may have established criteria for the acceptance of specimens on which a treponemal test is requested.

Tests with cerebrospinal fluid specimens

Neurosyphilis may exist in the presence of normal spinal fluid, but not frequently. A reactive reagin test on the spinal fluid indicates central nervous system involvement; however, a nonreactive test does not rule out central nervous system syphilis, especially tabes dorsalis. Furthermore, the spinal fluid is abnormal in 33% or more patients in the late primary or early secondary stage of syphilis.

In the case of a reactive reagin test on the spinal fluid, the presence of WBC cells (more than four cells per mm³) and/or an increased total protein indicate active disease of the central nervous system. The cell count on the spinal fluid is the most sensitive indicator of activity. After adequate treatment the cell count is the first test to return to normal, usually within 6 months. The reactive reagin test is generally the last test to become normal, sometimes taking months or years to do so.

The spinal fluid should be examined macroscopically; spinal fluid grossly contaminated with blood or bacteria is not considered satisfactory for examination. The cell count should be performed as soon as possible. The tests for total protein and reagin do not require that the spinal fluid be fresh.

The VDRL method for the quantitative determination of spinal fluid protein is discussed here because of its reproducibility and simplicity, but any reliable method for spinal fluid protein determination can be used. The technique described for detecting reagin is the VDRL Slide Spinal Fluid test. Limited studies on the use of treponemal tests with spinal fluid have been done; their use cannot be recommended at this time. In addition, reactive treponemal antigen tests on spinal fluid appear to offer no assistance to the clinician in evaluating patients (14).

Interpretation of Test Results

The diagnosis of syphilis depends on a combination of clinical, laboratory, and epidemiologic information. The combination of results needed to confirm the diagnosis varies with the stage of the disease.

The most specific diagnostic test for infectious syphilis is a positive darkfield microscopic examination of exudate from a clinically suspicious lesion. The diagnosis of syphilis is supported but not established by reactive serologic tests for syphilis. As previously mentioned, the serologic evidence for syphilis consists of both nonspecific reaginic and specific treponemal antibodies. The former are believed to be produced in response to lipid antigens released from host cells as a result of the treponeme-induced host immune response. The titer of reagin, therefore, is a measure of the degree of cellular injury or syphilis activity. Reaginic antibody is also produced by immunization and in a number of infectious and autoimmune diseases, such as malaria, rheumatoid arthritis and systemic lupus erythematosus. A reactive reagin test in the absence of syphilis is considered a false-positive (FP) reaction, referred to in the past as a biologic false-positive reaction (BFP). Therefore, to support the diagnosis of syphilis, other evidence such as a positive darkfield examination, clinical evidence of syphilis or a reactive treponemal antigen test must be obtained. Patients with a reactive non-treponemal antigen test but with no other serologic or clinical evidence of syphilis should be evaluated further to determine, if possible, the cause of this reactivity.

Treponemal antibody is produced not only in response to infection by *T. pallidum* and the other pathogenic treponemes but as the result of colonization and/or opportunistic infection by the avirulent treponemes of the normal microbial flora. Avirulent treponemal antibodies are thought to be removed by absorbing test serum with protein factions (sorbent), derived from Reiter treponeme cultures, before FTA and MHA-TP tests. This immunologic action of sorbent is questionable, however, since treatment of test serum with some hyperosmolar solutions has a similar effect. For unknown reasons, both the FTA-ABS and MHA-TP tests may occasionally be reactive in patients who do not have syphilis, most commonly in those with auto-immune diseases.

The various serologic tests become reactive at different times in different patients (Table 39.2). In general, all of the tests are reactive in secondary syphilis and those reactive with treponemal antigens remain so thereafter in untreated syphilis with the exception of the TPI. Reaginic antibody usually decreases in quantity with the duration of untreated disease. Approximately one-third of patients with late latent syphilis have nonreactive reaginic tests, which may reflect "spontaneous" cure of the infection. Rarely, the treponemal antigen tests will also become nonreactive in these cases.

Adequate treatment should decrease the titer of reaginic antibody in all but the late stages of infection. In seropositive primary, secondary and early latent syphilis the majority of patients with a reactive test will become nonreactive within 2 years after treatment (Table 39.3) (24). Untreated patients who remained reactive until late latent, tertiary, or late congenital syphilis seldom become seronegative after treatment. Reactive CSF reagin tests usually revert to nonreactive with adequate therapy.

A significant increase in reagin titer (an increase of two doubling dilutions or more) may indicate treatment failure or reinfection in early syphilis. Rein-

TABLE 39.2—REACTIVITY OF SERODIAGNOSTIC TESTS IN UNTREATED SYPHILIS*

| | STAGE OF DISEASE | | | |
TEST	PRIMARY	SECONDARY	LATENT	TERTIARY
VDRL	72%	100%	73%	77%
FTA-ABS	91%	100%	97%	100%
TPI	46%	98%	95%	95%
MHA-TP	69%	100%	98%	100%

* Data compiled by the Center for Disease Control. Percentage figures provided should not be interpreted as absolute values because there are small numbers in certain categories and test results vary from study to study.

fection is likely if the increase in reagin titer follows an initial decline; this may occur in the absence of clinical signs of reinfection and is an indication for retreatment. Patients with latent and tertiary syphilis may continue to be seropositive (serofast) with stable, low reagin titers after two years of observation. This persistent seropositivity does not indicate treatment failure or reinfection and these patients are likely to remain seropositive for their lifetimes, even if retreated.

Treponemal antigen tests are less likely to become nonreactive than the reagin tests. The earlier treatment is begun, the greater the chances that the treponemal test will become nonreactive; about 10% of reactive FTA-ABS primary syphilis patients treated early in their infection are nonreactive two years after treatment (24).

Collection and Submission of Specimens

Blood specimens for the VDRL Slide, USR, RPR (18-mm circle) Card, Fluorescent Treponemal Antibody-Absorption (FTA-ABS), and MHA-TP tests

1. Collection tubes should be clean, dry, and sterile to prevent contamination and hemolysis of the specimen. Vacuum tubes or tubes with paraffin-coated corks can be used.

2. At least 5–8 ml of blood should be drawn, placed in the tube aseptically, and allowed to clot at room temperature. Store the tube in refrigerator until sent to the laboratory. Specimens should not be placed in the mail over long weekends or holidays, when delivery may be delayed. NOTE: Hemolysis may be caused by wet or dirty syringes, needles, or tubes; chemicals; freezing; or extreme heat.

3. If serum is submitted to the laboratory, indicate whether it has been heated (time and temperature) and whether preservatives have been added.

Spinal fluid specimens for nontreponemal antigen tests and total protein determinations

1. Collection tubes should be clean and sterile. Merthiolated tubes may be prepared for the collection of specimens: Prepare a 1% aqueous solution of Merthiolate; place 0.1 ml in a clean sterile tube and dry in a desiccator over $CaCl_2$. This compound inhibits bacterial growth without affecting the nontreponemal antigen tests for syphilis or affecting the results obtained with the turbidimetric methods for determining total proteins in spinal fluids. Stopper with paraffin-coated corks.

2. Collect 2–8 ml of spinal fluid aseptically.

TABLE 39 3—EFFECT OF TREATMENT ON REACTIVE REAGIN TESTS FOR EARLY SYPHILIS

| STAGE OF DISEASE | TIME FOR SEROCONVERSION TO NONREACTIVE STATUS | | |
	3 MOS	12 MOS	24 MOS
Primary	21%*	76%	97%
Secondary	1%	42%	76%

* Percent of patients.

3. If the specimen is centrifuged before transmittal to the laboratory, note the original condition or appearance of the specimen on the request slip. NOTE: Specimens grossly contaminated with blood or bacteria are unsatisfactory for testing.

General Information

Preparation and use of control sera (10, 27)

Control sera of graded reactivity should be included in each serologic test. For the nontreponemal flocculation tests with serum and spinal fluid, the antigen suspension to be used each day is first examined with control sera. The results obtained with the controls should reproduce the established reactivity pattern. If the results are not acceptable, routine testing should be delayed until optimal reactivity has been established (by preparing another antigen suspension, correcting room temperature, adjusting equipment, etc). For the FTA-ABS and MHA-TP tests the control sera are included in the test run. If the pattern of reactivity is not acceptable, results of the tests on individual specimens are considered invalid and are not reported.

Control sera of graded reactivity for nontreponemal and treponemal test procedures are available from commercial sources or they may be prepared from individual sera or from sera pooled after testing (27). Reactive serum of high titer may be used to prepare spinal fluid controls. A pattern of reactivity should be established for each new lot of control serum prepared in the laboratory, or confirmed for each new lot of control serum obtained from a commercial source, by comparing the new control serum with a standard control serum.

Use of safety pipetting devices for syphilis serology

In keeping with the recommendation to eliminate mouth pipetting of possibly infectious sera, studies to determine the efficacy of substitutes for pipettes have been made by CDC. The following are recommendations for measuring sera for qualitative and quantitative tests:

1. Plastic Dispenstirs that deliver approximately 0.05 ml of serum per drop when held in a vertical position can be used for the RPR (18-mm circle) Card, USR, and VDRL qualitative tests.

2. Safety pipetting devices with disposable plastic tips that deliver 0.05 ml (50 lambda) can be used for preparing serial 2-fold dilutions of serum for the RPR (18-mm circle) Card and VDRL quantitative tests.

3. Each laboratory should determine the type of safety pipetting device it prefers on the basis of accuracy of measurement, reproducibility, ease of use, and cost.

Nontreponemal Antigen Tests

Rapid Plasma Reagin (RPR) (18-mm Circle) Card Test on Serum (18, 19, 27)

Equipment, glassware, and reagents

All equipment and supplies necessary to perform the RPR (18-mm circle) card test are contained in a kit (Hynson, Westcott and Dunning, Baltimore,

Md.) with the exception of serum controls, the rotating machine, and the cover.

The test kits contain

1. RPR card test antigen—This antigen suspension is similar to that prepared for the USR test. It also contains a suspension of specially prepared charcoal particles. Store antigen suspension in ampules or in the plastic dispensing bottle at 2–8 C. An unopened ampule has a shelf life of at least 12 months from the date of manufacture; antigen suspension in the plastic dispensing bottle (refrigerated) usually remains satisfactory for approximately 3 months. Do not use antigen suspension beyond the expiration date shown on the ampule. A new lot of antigen suspension should be compared with an antigen suspension of known reactivity before being placed in routine use (27).

20-gauge needle without bevel

Plastic dispensing bottle

Plastic-coated cards, each with ten 18-mm circle spots

Dispenstirs, 0.05 ml per drop,

or

Capillary pipettes, 0.05-ml capacity

Rubber bulbs

Stirrers

2. Rotating machine—Fixed-speed, or adjustable to 100 rpm, and circumscribing a ¾-inch diameter circle on a horizontal plane.

3. Humidifier cover—Any convenient cover containing a moistened blotter may be used to cover the cards during rotation.

Testing accuracy of delivery needles

1. It is of primary importance that the proper amount of reagents be used. For this reason, the needles used should be checked each day.

2. For the RPR (18-mm circle) Card test, dispense antigen suspension from a plastic dispensing bottle with a 20-gauge disposable needle without bevel. These needles should deliver 60 ± 2 drops of antigen suspension per ml when held in a vertical position. Practice will allow rapid delivery of antigen suspension, but care should be exercised to obtain drops of uniform size.

3. To check accuracy of the needle, place needle on a 2-ml syringe or on a 1-ml pipette. Fill the syringe or pipette with the antigen suspension and, holding in a vertical position, count the number of drops delivered from 0.5 ml. The needle is considered to be satisfactory if 30 ± 1 drops are obtained from 0.5 ml of suspension.

4. A needle not meeting this specification should be replaced with another needle that does meet this specification.

Preliminary testing of antigen suspension

1. Attach needle hub to tapered fitting on plastic dispensing bottle. Shake antigen ampule to resuspend antigen particles, snap ampule neck at breakline, and withdraw all the RPR card antigen suspension into the dispensing bottle by suction, collapsing the bottle and using it as a bulb. Shake dispenser gently before each series of antigen drops is delivered.

2. Test control sera (Hynson, Westcott & Dunning, Inc, Baltimore, Md)

of graded reactivity each day as described under "Rapid Plasma Reagin (18-mm circle) Card test with serum."

3. Use only those suspensions that have given the designated reactions with the controls.

Preparation of sera

1. Centrifuge blood specimens at room temperature and at a force sufficient to separate the serum from the cells. Generally, 1500–2000 rpm for 5 min is satisfactory.

2. Specimens may be retained in the original collection tube.

NOTE: Sera are tested without heating and should be at 73 F–85 F (23 C–29 C) at the time of testing.

RPR 18-mm (circle) card test on serum

NOTE: Slide flocculation tests for syphilis are affected by room temperature. For reliable and reproducible results, the controls, RPR card antigen suspension, and test specimens should be at room temperature, 73 F–85 F (23 C–29 C) when tests are performed.

1. Place 0.05 ml of unheated serum onto an 18-mm circle of the test card, using a Dispenstir or a 0.05-ml capillary pipette with attached rubber bulb.

2. Spread serum with inverted Dispenstir (closed end) or a stirrer (broad end) to fill the entire circle.

3. Add exactly 1 drop (1/60 ml) of RPR card test antigen suspension to each test area containing serum. Do not stir.

4. Place card on rotator, and cover with humidifier cover.

5. Rotate 8 min at 100 rpm on mechanical rotating machine.

6. Read tests without magnification immediately after rotation. A brief rotating and tilting of the card by hand should be used to aid in differentiating nonreactive from minimally reactive results.

7. Report results as follows:

Reading	Report
Small to large clumps	Reactive (R)
No clumping or very slight roughness	Nonreactive (N)

NOTE: Specimens which clump to any degree should be subjected to further serologic study, including quantitation.

8. Quantitative tests are performed according to directions included in the kit. (Serum dilutions for the quantitative test may be prepared directly on cards in the same manner as described for the VDRL Slide Quantitative Test on Serum.)

9. Upon completion of the daily tests, remove needle, rinse in water, and air dry. (Avoid wiping needle, as this removes silicone coating.) Recap dispensing bottle and store in refrigerator.

Unheated Serum Reagin (USR) Test on Serum (20,21,27)

Equipment

1. Centrifuge (Ivan Sorvall, Inc, Norwalk, Conn), angle-head, Servall SS-1, Type "XL" or equivalent, and tachometer.

2. Tubes, stainless-steel, 50-ml capacity, without flange.
3. Cotton gauze.
4. Rotating machine, adjustable to 180 rpm, circumscribing a circle of ¾-inch diameter on a horizontal plane.
5. Ringmaker, to make paraffin rings approximately 14 mm in diameter.
6. Slide holder, for 2 × 3 in microscope slides.
7. Hypodermic needle, 18-gauge, without bevel.

Glassware

1. Slides, 2 × 3 inch, with paraffin rings approximately 14 mm in diameter. (Glass slides with ceramic rings may be used with the following precautions: The rings must be high enough to prevent spillage when slides are rotated at prescribed speeds. Slides must be cleaned so that serum will spread to the inner surface of the ceramic rings. This type of slide should be discarded if or when the ceramic rings begin to flake off.)
2. Syringe, Luer-Type, 1- or 2-ml.
3. Bottle, 30-ml, round, glass-stoppered, narrow-mouth, approximately 35-mm in diameter, with flat innerbottom surface.
NOTE: *Some of the bottles now available are unsatisfactory for preparing antigen suspension because of the convex innerbottom surface which causes the saline to be distributed only at the periphery.*

Reagents

1. VDRL antigen.
2. VDRL buffered saline.
3. Phosphate (0.02 M), Merthiolate (0.2%) solution.
Dissolve 1.42 g Na_2HPO_4, 1.36 g KH_2PO_4, 1.00 g Merthiolate in distilled water to a final volume of 500 ml. The pH of this solution should be 6.9. Store in dark at room temperature. May be used for a period of 3 months.
4. Choline chloride solution (40%)
   a. Because of its hygroscopic nature, the entire contents of a previously unopened bottle may be used in preparing the solution.
   Example: Dissolve the entire contents of a 250-g bottle of choline chloride in distilled water to a final volume of 625 ml.
   b. Filter and store at room temperature. May be used for 1 year. Refilter if visible particles form.
5. EDTA (0.1 M)
Dissolve 3.72 g EDTA [(ethylenedinitrilo) tetraacetic acid disodium salt] to a volume of 100 ml in distilled water. Can be used for 1 year.
6. Resuspending solution. To prepare 10 ml of resuspending solution, combine the following:

EDTA (0.1 M)..1.25 ml
Choline chloride (40%)..2.5 ml
Phosphate (0.02 M), Merthiolate (0.2%) ....5.0 ml
Distilled water...1.25 ml

Prepare solution each time antigen suspensions are made.

Preparation of antigen suspension (available commercially)

1. Prepare antigen suspension as for the VDRL slide tests.
NOTE: Bulk batches of 100 ml of VDRL antigen suspension may be prepared

for the USR antigen suspension in a 250-ml, glass-stoppered pyrex bottle (or equivalent) with appropriate amounts of antigen and buffered saline. Add the antigen rapidly with a 10-ml pipette directly onto the buffered saline while continuously rotating the bottle. Times and speeds of rotation and shaking after addition of the antigen are the same as for VDRL antigen suspension preparation.

2. Centrifuge measured amounts of the antigen suspension in stainless steel tubes in an angle centrifuge at room temperature at a relative centrifugal force of approximately 2000 g for 15 min. Start timing when centrifuge reaches desired speed. Centrifuge from 5 to 30 ml in a single centrifuge tube.

3. Locate the sediment, and decant supernatant fluid by inverting tube away from the side containing the sediment. While holding tube in an inverted position, wipe the inside with cotton gauze without disturbing the sediment.

4. Resuspend in a volume of resuspending solution equal to that of the original volume of antigen suspension that was centrifuged.

5. If more than one centrifuge tube is used, combine all suspensions in a bottle, stopper tightly, and shake gently for a few seconds to obtain an even suspension. This is the completed antigen suspension.

6. Before being placed in routine use, a new lot of antigen suspension should be compared with an antigen suspension of known reactivity (27).

7. Store antigen suspension at 3 C–10 C. Antigen suspension stored in this manner has been found to give satisfactory results for at least 6 months. However, do not use the antigen suspension if, at any time, the expected results are not obtained with control sera of graded reactivity.

Testing accuracy of delivery needles

1. It is of primary importance that the proper amounts of reagents be used, and for this reason, the needles used should be checked each day. Practice will allow rapid delivery of antigen suspension, but care should be exercised to obtain drops of uniform size.

2. For the USR test, dispense antigen suspension from a syringe fitted with an 18-gauge needle without bevel which will deliver 45 ± 1 drops of antigen suspension per ml when checked with a 1- or 2-ml syringe held vertically.

3. Adjust needles not meeting these specifications to deliver the correct volume before using (27).

Preliminary testing of antigen suspension

1. For daily use, withdraw sufficient antigen suspension from the stock bottle for one day's testing and return the stock bottle to the refrigerator. Keep the antigen suspension at room temperature for not less than 30 min before it is to be used.

2. Test control sera of graded reactivity each day as described under "Unheated Serum Reagin (USR) test on serum."

3. Reactions with control sera should reproduce the established reactivity pattern. The nonreactive serum should show complete dispersion of antigen particles.

4. Do not use an unsatisfactory antigen suspension.

Preparation of sera

1. Centrifuge blood specimens at room temperature at a force sufficient to separate the serum from the cellular elements. Generally, 1500–2000 rpm for 5 min is adequate.

2. Sera can be retained in the original collection tube.

NOTE: The sera are tested without heating and should be at 73 F–85 F (23 C–29 C) at time of testing.

USR test on serum

NOTE: Slide flocculation tests for syphilis are affected by room temperature. For reliable and reproducible results, control sera, USR antigen suspension, and test specimens should be at room temperature, 73 F–85 F (23 C–29 C), when tests are performed.

1. Place 0.05 ml of unheated serum from the original collecting tube into one ring of a paraffin-ringed glass slide.

2. Add 1 drop (1/45 ml) of antigen suspension onto each serum.

3. Rotate slide on rotating machine for 4 min at 180 rpm.

4. Read test microscopically with a 10× ocular and a 10× objective immediately after rotation.

5. Report the results as follows:

Reading	Report
Medium and large clumps	Reactive (R)
Small clumps	Weakly Reactive (W)
No clumping, or very slight roughness	Nonreactive (N)

NOTE: Specimens giving any degree of clumping should be subjected to further serologic study, including quantitation.

Venereal Disease Research Laboratory (VDRL) Slide Tests (13,18,24)

Equipment

1. Rotating machine, adjustable to 180 rpm, circumscribing a circle ¾ inch in diameter on a horizontal plane.

2. Ringmaker, to make paraffin rings approximately 14 mm in diameter.

3. Slide holder, for 2 × 3 in microscope slides.

4. Hypodermic needles, without bevels.
   a. For serum test: 18 gauge.
   b. For spinal fluid test: 21- or 22-gauge.

Glassware

1. Slides, 2 × 3 in, with 12 paraffin or ceramic rings approximately 14 mm in diameter, for serum test. (Glass slides with ceramic rings may also be used with the following precautions: The rings must be high enough to prevent spillage when slides are rotated at prescribed speeds. Slides must be cleaned so that serum will spread to the inner surfaces of the ceramic rings. This type of slide should be discarded if or when the ceramic rings begin to flake off.)

2. Slides, agglutination, approximately 2 × 3 in, with concavities measuring 16 mm in diameter and 1.75 mm in depth, for spinal fluid test.

3. Syringe, Luer-type, 1- or 2-ml.

4. Bottles, 30-ml, round, glass-stoppered, narrow-mouthed, approximately 35 mm in diameter, with flat innerbottom surfaces.

NOTE: *Some of the bottles now available are unsatisfactory for preparing antigen suspension because of the convex innerbottom surface which causes the saline to be distributed only at the periphery.*

Reagents

1. VDRL antigen:

a. Antigen for this test is a colorless, alcoholic solution containing 0.03% cardiolipin, 0.9% cholesterol, and sufficient purified lecithin to produce standard reactivity. During recent years, this amount of lecithin has been 0.21% ± 0.01%. Each lot of antigen must be serologically standardized by proper comparision with an antigen of known reactivity.

b. Antigen is dispensed in screw-capped (Vinylite liners) bottles or hermetically sealed glass ampules and should be stored in the dark at either refrigerator (6 C–10 C) or room temperature. The components of this antigen remain in solution at these temperatures, so that any precipitate noted will indicate changes resulting from factors such as evaporation or additive materials contributed by pipettes. Antigen that contains precipitate should be discarded.

c. A new lot of antigen should be compared with a standard antigen before being accepted for routine use. Testing should be performed on more than one testing day with control sera, individual sera of graded reactivity, and nonreactive sera. Reportable test results on individual specimens in qualitative and quantitative tests should be comparable with results obtained with the standard reagent (27).

2. VDRL buffered saline containing 1% sodium chloride, pH 6.0 ± 0.1:
Formaldehyde, neutral (A.C.S.) ....0.5 ml
Secondary sodium phosphate, anhydrous (A.C.S.) (Na_2HPO_4)..0.037 g
Primary potassium phosphate (A.C.S.) (KH_2PO_4).......................0.170 g
Sodium chloride (A.C.S.)..10.0 g
Distilled water ....1000.0 ml
Check pH of solution and store in screw-capped or glass-stoppered bottles.
NOTE: When an unexplained change in test reactivity occurs, check the pH of the VDRL buffered saline to determine if this is a contributing factor. Saline outside the range of pH 6.0 ± 0.1 should be discarded.

3. 0.9% saline:
Add 900 mg of dry sodium chloride (A.C.S.) to each 100 ml of distilled water.

4. 10% saline:
Add 10 g of dry sodium chloride (A.C.S.) to each 100 ml of distilled water.

VDRL Slide Test on Serum

Preparation of antigen suspension

NOTE: Temperature of buffered saline and antigen should be in the range 73–85 F (23–29 C) at the time antigen suspension is prepared.

1. Pipette 0.4 ml of buffered saline to the bottom of a 30-ml round glass-stoppered bottle.

2. Add 0.5 ml of antigen (from the lower half of a 1.0-ml pipette graduated to the tip) directly onto the saline while continuously but gently rotating the bottle on a flat surface.

NOTE: Antigen is added drop by drop, but rapidly, so that approximately 6 sec are allowed each 0.5 ml of antigen. Pipette tip should remain in upper third of bottle and rotation should not be vigorous enough to splash saline onto pipette. Proper speed of rotation is obtained when the center of the bottle circumscribes a circle 2 inch in diameter approximately three times per sec.

3. Blow last drop of antigen from pipette without touching pipette to saline.

4. Continue rotation of bottle for 10 sec.

5. Add 4.1 ml of buffered saline from 5-ml pipette.

6. Place top on bottle and shake from bottom to top and back approximately 30 times in 10 sec.

7. Antigen suspension is ready for use and may be used during one day.

8. A double volume of antigen suspension may be prepared at one time by using doubled quantities of antigen and saline. A 10-ml pipette should be used for delivering the 8.2-ml volume of saline. If larger quantities are required, more than one antigen suspension should be prepared. Test these suspensions with control sera, pool the ones with satisfactory reactivity, and test the pool with control sera.

9. Mix antigen suspension gently each time it is used. Do not mix suspension by forcing back and forth through the syringe and needle, since this may cause breakdown of particles and loss of reactivity.

Testing accuracy of delivery needles

1. It is of primary importance that the proper amounts of reagents be used, and for this reason the needles used each day should be checked. Practice will allow rapid delivery of antigen suspension and saline, but care should be exercised to obtain drops of uniform size.

2. For the slide tests on serum, dispense antigen suspension from a syringe fitted with an 18-gauge needle without bevel which will deliver 60 drops ± 2 drops of antigen suspension per ml when syringe and needle are held vertically.

3. Adjust needles not meeting these specifications to deliver the correct volumes before their use (27).

Preliminary testing of antigen suspension

1. Test the control sera of graded reactivity as described under "VDRL slide qualitative test on serum."

2. Reactions with control sera should reproduce the established reactivity pattern. The nonreactive serum should show complete dispersion of antigen particles.

3. Do not use an unsatisfactory antigen suspension or pool of antigen suspensions.

NOTE: Control sera of graded reactivity (Reactive, Weakly Reactive, and

Nonreactive) are always included during a testing period to insure proper reactivity of antigen suspension at the time tests are performed.

Preparation of serum

1. Heat clear serum, obtained from centrifuged, clotted blood, in 56 C water bath for 30 min before testing.
2. Examine all sera when removed from the water bath and recentrifuge those found to contain particulate debris.
3. Reheat at 56 C for 10 min those sera to be tested more than 4 hr after the original heating period.
4. When tested, the sera must be at room temperature.

VDRL Slide Qualitative Test on Serum

NOTE: Slide flocculation tests for syphilis are affected by room temperature. For reliable and reproducible results, tests should be performed within the temperature range 73 F–85 F (23 C–29 C). At lower temperatures, test reactivity is decreased; at higher temperatures, test reactivity is increased.

1. Place 0.05 ml of heated serum into one ring of a paraffin-ringed or ceramic-ringed slide.

NOTE: Glass slides with concavities, wells or glass rings are not recommended for this test.

2. Place 1 drop (1/60 ml) of antigen suspension onto each serum with an 18-gauge needle and a syringe.
3. Rotate slides for 4 min. (Mechanical rotators that circumscribe a circle 3/4 inch in diameter should be set at 180 rpm.)

NOTE: When tests are performed in a dry climate, slides may be covered with a box lid containing a moistened blotter during rotation to prevent excessive evaporation.

4. Read tests microscopically with a 10× ocular and a 10× objective immediately after rotation.
5. Report the results as follows:

Reading	Report
Medium and large clumps	Reactive (R)
Small clumps	Weakly reactive (W)
No clumping or very slight roughness	Nonreactive (N)

6. A prozone reaction is encountered occasionally. This type of reaction is demonstrated when complete or partial inhibition of reactivity occurs with undiluted serum and maximum reactivity is obtained only with diluted serum. This prozone phenomenon may be so pronounced that only a Weakly Reactive or "rough" Nonreactive result is produced in the qualitative test by a serum which will be strongly Reactive when diluted. *It is therefore recommended that all sera producing Weakly Reactive or "rough" Nonreactive results in the qualitative test be retested by using the quantitative procedure before a report of the VDRL Slide test is submitted.* When a Reactive result is obtained on some dilution of a serum that produced only a Weakly Reactive or "rough" Nonreactive result before dilution, report the test as Reactive and include the quantitative titer (see examples, step 9, "VDRL Slide Quantitative Test on Serum").

VDRL Slide Quantitative Test on Serum

Test quantitatively, *to an end-point titer,* all sera that produce Reactive, Weakly Reactive, or "rough" Nonreactive results in the qualitative VDRL slide test. The dilutions of the serum to be tested are: undiluted (1:1), 1:2, 1:4, etc. Three serum quantitative tests through 1:8 dilution (see Table 39.4, below) or two serum quantitative tests through 1:32 dilution may be performed on one slide.

1. Select tubes of serum for quantitation and place in a rack.

2. Measure 0.05 ml of 0.9 percent saline onto the second, third, and fourth paraffin rings in a row on the slide. Do not spread saline. Saline may be delivered from an 18-gauge needle without point (0.025 ml per drop—use 2 drops), or a large needle or calibrated dropper that delivers 0.05 ml in a single drop; these should be checked daily for accuracy of delivery.

3. Using a safety pipettor with disposable tip (that delivers 0.05 ml or 50 lambda), measure 0.05 ml of serum to the first and second rings. Avoid contamination of the instrument with serum.

4. Use the same pipettor and tip to prepare serial 2-fold dilutions by drawing the serum/saline mixture up and down in the tip five or six times. Avoid excess bubbles. (Use a clean plastic tip for each serum tested.)

5. Mix the serum and saline in ring #2 (1:2 dil); transfer 0.05 ml of the 1:2 dilution to ring #3, and mix (1:4 dil); transfer 0.05 ml of the 1:4 dilution to ring #4, mix (1:8 dil), and discard 0.05 ml. Additional serial dilutions may be set up for strongly reactive sera. (If the 0.05 ml of serum dilution has not spread within the entire area of a paraffin ring, spread this with the pipettor tip before proceeding to the next ring.)

6. Add 1 drop (1/60 ml) of VDRL antigen suspension to each ring with an 18-gauge needle and syringe (used for antigen suspension in the qualitative test).

7. Rotate slides for 4 min. (Mechanical rotators that circumscribe a 3/4-inch diameter circle should be set at 180 rpm.)

TABLE 39.4

UNDILUTED SERUM (1:1)	SERUM DILUTIONS					Report
	1:2	1:4	1:8	1:16	1:32	
R	W	N	N	N	N	Reactive, undiluted only, or 1 dil
R	R	W	N	N	N	Reactive, 1:2 dilution, or 2 dils
R	R	R	W	N	N	Reactive, 1:4 dilution, or 4 dils
W	W	R	R	W	N	Reactive, 1:8 dilution, or 8 dils
N (rough)	W	R	R	R	N	Reactive, 1:16 dilution, or 16 dils
W	N	N	N	N	N	Weakly Reactive, undiluted only, or 0 dils

NOTE: When tests are performed in a dry climate, slides may be covered with a moisture chamber during rotation to prevent excessive evaporation.

8. Read tests microscopically with a 10× ocular and a 10× objective, immediately after rotation. Record the reading for each dilution tested.

9. Report titer in terms of the greatest serum dilution that produces a Reactive (not Weakly Reactive) result, in accordance with the examples in Table 39.4.

VDRL Slide Test on Spinal Fluid

Preparation of the sensitized antigen suspension.

1. Prepare antigen suspension as described for the VDRL slide tests on serum (see "Preparation of antigen suspension," this Section).

2. Add 1 part of 10% saline to 1 part of VDRL slide test suspension.

3. Mix by gently rotating the bottle or inverting the tube and allow to stand at least 5 min but not more than 2 hr before use.

Testing accuracy of delivery needles.

1. It is of primary importance that the proper amount of reagent be used, and for this reason needles used each day should be checked. Practice will allow rapid delivery of antigen suspension, but care should be exercised to obtain drops of uniform size.

2. For the slide qualitative and quantitative tests on spinal fluid, dispense sensitized antigen suspension from a syringe fitted with a 21- or 22-gauge needle which will deliver 100 drops ± 2 drops of sensitized antigen suspension per ml when syringe and needle are held vertically.

3. Adjust needles not meeting these specifications to deliver the correct volume before using (27).

Preliminary testing of sensitized antigen suspension.

1. Satisfactory control sera for the spinal fluid test are conveniently prepared by diluting strongly reactive serum in 0.9% saline (27).

2. For daily use, remove one tube of the reactive control serum from the freezer, thaw, and mix thoroughly. Prepare the designated serum dilutions in 0.9% saline. The controls are tested without preliminary heating in the slide test.

3. Test the control serum dilutions as described under "VDRL slide qualitative test on spinal fluid."

4. Reactions on the control serum dilutions should reproduce the established reactivity pattern and the nonreactive dilution should show complete dispersion of antigen particles.

5. Do not use an unsatisfactory sensitized antigen suspension.

NOTE: Control serum dilutions of graded reactivity (reactive, minimally reactive, and nonreactive) are always included during a testing period to insure proper reactivity of the sensitized antigen suspension at the time tests are performed.

Preparation of spinal fluid.

Centrifuge and decant each spinal fluid. The spinal fluid is tested without preliminary heating. Spinal fluids which are visibly contaminated or contain gross blood are unsatisfactory for testing.

VDRL Slide Qualitative Test on Spinal Fluid

NOTE: Slide flocculation tests for syphilis are affected by room temperature. For reliable and reproducible results, tests should be performed within the temperature range 73 F–85 F (23 C–29 C). At lower temperatures, test reactivity is decreased; at higher temperatures, test reactivity is increased.

　　1. Place 0.05 ml of spinal fluid into one concavity of an agglutination slide.

　　2. Add 1 drop (0.01 ml) of sensitized antigen suspension to each spinal fluid with a 21- or 22-gauge needle.

　　3. Rotate slides for 8 min on a mechanical rotator at 180 rpm.

NOTE: When tests are performed in a dry climate, the slides may be covered with a box lid containing a moistened blotter during rotation to prevent evaporation.

　　4. Read tests microscopically, with a 10× ocular and a 10× objective, immediately after rotation.

　　5. Report the results as follows:

Reading	Report
Definite clumping	Reactive (R)
No clumping or very slight roughness	Nonreactive (N)

VDRL Slide Quantitative Test on Spinal Fluid

Quantitative tests are performed on all spinal fluids found to be reactive in the qualitative tests. These tests may be performed in the same manner as the quantitative tests on serum.

Treponemal Antigen Tests

Fluorescent Treponemal Antibody Absorption (FTA-ABS) Test on Serum (6, 7, 11–13, 15, 19–21, 25, 27)

Equipment and supplies

　　1. Incubator, adjustable to 35 C–37 C
　　2. Darkfield fluorescence microscope assembly
　　3. Bibulous paper
　　4. Diamond-point pencil (optional)
　　5. Template, used as a guide for cutting circles 1.0 cm in diameter on glass slides (optional)
　　6. Slide board or holder
　　7. Moist chamber (Place moistened paper inside a convenient cover fitting the slide board.)
　　8. Loop, bacteriological, standard 2-mm, 26-gauge platinum
　　9. Oil, immersion, low-fluorescence, nondrying

Glassware

　　1. Microscope slides, 1 × 3 in, frosted end, approximately 1 mm thick
　　2. Cover slips, No. 1, 22 mm sq
　　3. Dish, staining, glass or plastic, with removable slide carriers
　　4. Glass rods, approximately 100 × 4 mm, both ends fire-polished

Reagents

1. *T. pallidum* antigen

a) The antigen for the FTA-ABS test is a suspension of *T. pallidum* (Nichols strain) extracted from rabbit testicular tissue. The extract should contain a minimum of 30 organisms per high dry field. The antigen may be stored at 6 C–10 C or processed by lyophilization.

b) Store lyophilized antigen at 6 C–10 C and rehydrate for use according to the accompanying directions.

c) Discard antigen suspension if it becomes bacterially contaminated or does not demonstrate the proper reactivity with control sera.

2. FTA-ABS test sorbent

a) Sorbent is a standardized product prepared from cultures of Reiter treponemes. This may be purchased in lyophilized or liquid state.

b) Store lyophilized antigen at 6 C–10 C and rehydrate for use accordpanying directions.

3. Fluorescein-labeled antihuman globulin (conjugate)

a) The conjugate should be of proven quality for the FTA-ABS test. Test each new lot of conjugate to determine its working titer and to verify that it meets the criteria for nonspecific staining and standard reactivity.

b) Store lyophilized conjugate at 6 C–10 C. Dispense rehydrated conjugate in not less than 0.3-ml quantities and store at −20 C or lower. For practical purposes, a conjugate with a working titer of 1:400 or higher can be diluted 1:10 with sterile phosphate-buffered saline (containing Merthiolate in a concentration of 1:5000) before storage.

c) When conjugate is thawed for use, do not refreeze, but store at 6 C–10 C. It may be used as long as satisfactory reactivity is obtained with test controls.

d) If a change in FTA-ABS test reactivity is noted in routine laboratory testing, the conjugate should be retitered to determine whether or not it is the contributing factor.

4. Phosphate-buffered saline (PBS), pH 7.2 ± 0.1

Formula per L:

NaCl..7.65 g

Na_2HPO_4 ....0.724 g

KH_2PO_4 ....0.21 g

Several liters may be prepared and stored in a large Pyrex (or equivalent) or polyethylene bottle. Determine the pH of each lot of PBS prepared for the FTA-ABS test. PBS outside the range of pH 7.2 ± 0.1 should be discarded.

5. Tween 80

To prepare PBS containing 2% Tween 80, heat the two reagents in a 56 C water bath. To 98 ml of PBS, add 2 ml of Tween 80 by measuring from the bottom of a pipette, and rinse out the pipette. The 2% Tween 80 solution should be pH 7.0–7.2. Check the pH periodically, as the solution may become acid. This solution keeps well at refrigerator temperature; discard if a precipitate develops or if the pH changes.

6. Mounting medium

The mounting medium consists of 1 part PBS at pH 7.2, plus 9 parts glycerine of reagent quality.

7. Acetone (A.C.S.)

Check-testing new lots of reagents (27)

NOTE: Each new lot of reagents should be tested in parallel with a standard reagent before being placed in routine use.

1. *T. pallidum* antigen

a) A new lot of antigen should be compared with a standard antigen before being placed in routine use. Testing should be performed on more than one testing day with control sera, individual sera of graded reactivity, and nonreactive sera.

b) A sufficient number of organisms should remain on the slide after staining so that tests may be read without difficulty.

c) The antigen should not contain background material which stains to the extent that it interferes with the reading of the tests.

d) The antigen should not stain nonspecifically with a standard conjugate at its working titer.

e) Reportable test results on controls and individual sera should be comparable with those obtained with the standard antigen.

2. FTA-ABS test sorbent

a) A new lot of sorbent should be compared with a standard sorbent before being placed in routine use. Testing should be performed on more than one testing day with control sera, individual sera of graded reactivity, and nonsyphilitic sera demonstrating nonspecific reactivity.

b) The new sorbent should remove nonspecific reactivity of the nonspecific serum control.

c) The new sorbent should not reduce intensity of fluorescence of the reactive (4+) control serum to less than 3+.

d) The nonspecific staining control with the new sorbent should be nonreactive.

e) Reportable test results on controls and individual sera should be comparable with those obtained with standard sorbent.

f) The sorbent should be usable when rehydrated to the indicated volume on the label or according to accompanying directions.

3. Fluorescein-labeled antihuman globulin (conjugate)

a) A satisfactory conjugate should not stain a standard antigen nonspecifically at three doubling dilutions below the working titer of the conjugate.

b) Reportable test results on controls and individual sera should be comparable with those obtained with the standard conjugate.

NOTE: Most manufacturers designate on the label the working titer of the conjugate which was determined under the testing conditions and with the equipment in their laboratories. Since conditions and equipment vary from one laboratory to another, it is necessary to titer and to check-test a new lot of conjugate with the fluorescence microscope assembly available.

Titration

1. Prepare serial doubling dilutions of the new conjugate in PBS containing 2% Tween 80 to include the titer indicated by the manufacturer. Examples—(a) 1:2.5, 1:5, 1:10, 1:20, 1:40, 1:80, 1:160
(b) 1:12.5, 1:25, 1:50, 1:100, 1:200, 1:400, 1:800
Prepare higher dilutions if necessary.

2. Test each conjugate dilution with the Reactive (4+) control serum diluted 1:5 in PBS in accordance with the FTA-ABS technique.

3. Include a nonspecific staining control with each conjugate dilution.

4. A standard conjugate, at its titer, is set up at the same time with a Reactive (4+) control serum, a Minimally Reactive (1+) control serum, and a Nonspecific staining control with PBS for the purpose of controlling reagents and test conditions. An example of the titration of new conjugate is shown in Table 39.5.

5. Read slides in the following order: (a) Examine the three control slides to insure that reagents and testing conditions are satisfactory. (b) Examine the slides with new conjugate; start with the lowest dilution of conjugate. Record readings in plusses.

6. The end point titer is the highest dilution giving maximum (4+) fluorescence. The working titer of the new conjugate is one doubling dilution below the end point. In the example, the dilution selected for the working titer is 1:200.

7. The new conjugate should not stain nonspecifically at three doubling dilutions below the working titer of the conjugate. In the example, the conjugate would meet this criterion, since there is no nonspecific staining with the 1:25 dilution.

8. Dispense conjugate in not less than 0.3-ml quantities and store at −20 C or lower. (For practical purposes, a conjugate with a working titer of 1:400 or higher may be diluted 1:10 with sterile PBS containing Merthiolate in a concentration 1:5000 before storage in the freezer.)

9. Verify titer of the conjugate after at least 3 days' storage in the freezer.

Check-testing conjugate

If the criterion of acceptability for the nonspecific staining has been met and a working titer has been determined, the new conjugate should be check-tested in parallel with a standard conjugate before being placed into routine use.

TABLE 39.5

CONJUGATES	NONSPECIFIC STAINING CONTROL (PBS)	REACTIVE (4+) CONTROL SERUM (1:5 IN PBS)	REACTIVE (1+) CONTROL SERUM
Standard conjugate, titer 1:400	−	4+	1+
New conjugate dilution:			
1:12.5	<1+	4+	
1:25	−	4+	
1:50	−	4+	
1:100	−	4+	
1:200	−	4+	
1:400	−	4+	
1:800	−	3+	

1. Each new lot of conjugate should be tested in parallel with a standard conjugate before being placed in routine use. Testing should be performed on more than one testing day with control sera, individual sera of graded reactivity, and nonreactive sera.

2. Individual sera tested in parallel with a standard and a new conjugate are read against the minimally reactive (1+) controls set up with the respective conjugates.

3. A new conjugate is considered to be satisfactory when comparable test results are obtained with both conjugates.

Preparation of T. pallidum antigen smears

1. Mix antigen suspension well with a disposable pipette and rubber bulb by drawing the suspension into and expelling it from the pipette at least 10 times to break the treponemal clumps and insure an even distribution of treponemes. Determine by darkfield examination that treponemes are adequately dispersed before making slides for FTA test. Additional mixing may be required.

2. On clean slides, cut two circles 1 cm in diameter with a diamond-point pencil. Wipe slides with clean gauze to remove loose glass particles. Slides with pre-etched circles may be used.

3. Smear one-half to one loopful of *T. pallidum* antigen evenly within each circle by using a standard 2-mm, 26-gauge platinum wire loop. Experience with individual lots of antigen may indicate that a smaller or larger quantity should be spread in each circle. Allow to air dry at least 15 min.

4. Fix smears in acetone for 10 min and allow to air dry thoroughly; not more than 60 slides should be fixed with 200 ml of acetone. Store acetone-fixed smears at −20 C or lower. Fixed, frozen smears are usable indefinitely, provided that satisfactory results are obtained with the controls. Do not thaw and refreeze antigen smears. [Smears may be fixed for 20 sec in a solution of 10% methyl alcohol in distilled water. (Not more than 20 slides should be fixed with 200 ml of 10% methyl alcohol; this solution should be prepared on the day of use.) Antigen smears to be fixed by this method should be prepared on the day of test.]

Preparation of sera

Note: Bacterial contamination or excessive hemolysis may render specimens unsatisfactory for testing.

1. Heat the test and control sera at 56 C for 30 min before testing.

2. Reheat previously heated test sera for 10 min at 56 C on the day of testing.

Controls

Store and use control sera from commercial sources according to the accompanying directions.

1. *Reactive (4+) control*—This consists of a reactive serum or a dilution of reactive serum demonstrating strong (4+) fluorescence when diluted 1:5 in PBS and only slightly reduced fluorescence when diluted 1:5 in sorbent. (A reduction of no more than 1+ fluorescence, i.e., 4+ changing to 3+.)

a) Using a 0.2-ml pipette and measuring from the bottom, add 0.05 ml of reactive control serum into a tube containing 0.2 ml of PBS. Mix well, at least eight times.

b) Using a 0.2-ml pipette measuring from the bottom, add 0.05 ml of reactive control serum to a tube containing 0.2 ml of sorbent. Mix well, at least eight times.

2. *Minimally reactive (1+) control* consists of a dilution of reactive serum demonstrating the minimal degree of fluorescence reported as "reactive" for use as a reading standard. The reactive (4+) control serum may be used for this control when diluted in PBS according to directions.

3. *Nonspecific serum control* consists of a nonsyphilitic serum known to demonstrate at least 2+ nonspecific reactivity in the FTA test at a dilution in PBS of 1:5 or higher.

a) Using a 0.2-ml pipette and measuring from the bottom, add 0.05 ml of nonspecific control serum into a tube containing 0.2 ml of PBS. Mix well, at least eight times.

b) Using another 0.2-ml pipette and measuring from the bottom, add 0.05 ml of nonspecific control serum into a tube containing 0.2 ml of sorbent. Mix well, at least eight times.

4. *Nonspecific staining controls* consist of (a) antigen smear treated with 0.03 ml of PBS and (b) antigen smear treated with 0.03 ml of sorbent.

Note: Controls #1, #3, and #4 are included for the purpose of controlling reagents and test conditions. Control #2 [minimally reactive (1+) control serum] is included as the reading standard.

CONTROL PATTERN ILLUSTRATION:

Control	Reaction
Reactive control	
a. 1:5 PBS dilution	R4+
b. 1:5 sorbent dilution	R(4+–3+)
Minimally reactive (1+) control	R1+
Nonspecific serum controls	
a. 1:5 PBS dilution	R(2+–4+)
b. 1:5 sorbent dilution	N
Nonspecific staining controls	
a. Antigen, PBS, and conjugate	N
b. Antigen, sorbent, and conjugate	N

Test runs in which these control results are not obtained are considered unsatisfactory and should not be reported.

FTA-ABS test on serum

1. Identify previously prepared slides by numbering the frosted end with a lead pencil (see "Preparation of *T. pallidum* antigen smears").

2. Number the tubes to correspond to the sera and control sera being tested and place in racks.

3. Prepare Reactive (4+), Minimally Reactive (1+), and Nonspecific control serum dilutions in sorbent and/or PBS according to the directions in "Controls."

4. Pipette 0.2 ml of sorbent into a test tube for each test serum.

5. Using a 0.2-ml pipette and measuring from the bottom, add 0.05 ml of the heated test serum into the appropriate tube and mix eight times.

6. Cover the appropriate antigen smears with 0.03 ml of the Reactive (4+), Minimally Reactive (1+), and Nonspecific control serum dilutions.

7. Cover the appropriate antigen smears with 0.03 ml of the PBS and 0.03 ml of the sorbent for "Nonspecific staining controls (a) and (b)," respectively.

8. Cover the appropriate antigen smears with 0.03 ml of the test serum dilutions.

9. Prevent evaporation by placing slides within a moist chamber.

10. Place slides in an incubator at 35 C–37 C for 30 min.

11. Rinsing procedure:

a) Place slides in slide carriers and rinse slides with running PBS for approximately 5 sec.

b) Place slides in staining dish containing PBS for 5 min.

c) Agitate slides by dipping them in and out of the PBS at least 10 times.

d) Using fresh PBS, repeat steps b and c.

e) Rinse slides in running distilled water for approximately 5 sec.

12. *Gently* blot slides with bibulous paper to remove all water drops.

13. Dilute conjugate to its working titer in PBS containing 2% Tween 80.

14. Place approximately 0.03 ml of diluted conjugate on each smear. Spread uniformly with a glass rod to cover entire smear.

15. Repeat steps 9, 10, 11, and 12.

16. Mount slides immediately by placing a small drop of mounting medium on each smear and applying a cover slip.

17. Examine slides as soon as possible. If a delay in reading is necessary, place slides in a darkened room and read within 4 hr.

18. Study smears microscopically by using an ultraviolet light source and a high-power dry objective. A combination of BG 12 exciting filter, not more than 3 mm in thickness, and OG 1 barrier filter (or their equivalents)* has been found to be satisfactory for routine use.

19. Check nonreactive smears by using illumination from a tungsten light source in order to verify the presence of treponemes.

20. Using the minimally reactive (1+) control slide as the reading standard, record the intensity of fluorescence of the treponemes according to the tabulation in Tables 39.6, and 39.7

Microhemagglutination Assay for *Treponema pallidum* antibodies (MHA-TP) (provisional technique) (3)

Equipment and supplies

1. Microdiluters (0.025 ml) (Cooke Engineering Co, 900 Slaters Lane, Alexandria, VA).

---

* Filter equivalents — Exciting filters: BG 12 = o = AO 702
  Barrier filters: OG 1   = o = AO 724 or 1124
  = o = B & L Y-8
  = o = Zeiss 50/– (II/O)

TABLE 39.6

READING	INTENSITY OF FLUORESCENCE	REPORT
2+ to 4+	Moderate to strong	Reactive (R)
1+	Equivalent to Minimally Reactive (1+) control	Reactive (R)‡
<1+	Weak, but definite, less than minimally reactive (1+) control	Borderline (B)‡
−	None, or vaguely visible	Nonreactive (N)

‡ Retest all specimens with intensity of fluorescence of 1+ or less. When a specimen initially read as 1+ is retested and is subsequently read as 1+ or greater, the test is reported as "reactive." All other results on retest are reported as "borderline." It is not necessary to retest nonfluorescent (nonreactive) specimens.

2. Pipette droppers calibrated to deliver 0.025 ml (Cooke Engineering Co).

3. Go no-go delivery testers for 0.025 ml (blotters) (Cooke Engineering Co).

4. Tray viewer (Ames Company, Division of Miles Laboratories, Inc, Elkhart, IN).

5. Disposable, clear plastic trays with eight rows of 15 cups each (Ames Co). The round-bottomed (U-shaped) cups should be smooth and free from dust and lint.

6. 12- × 75-mm test tubes.

7. 1.0-ml serologic pipettes graduated in 1/100 ml.

8. 0.1-ml or 0.2-ml serologic pipettes graduated in 1/100 ml. To avoid mouth pipetting of serum, use push-button automatic pipettes with disposable tips calibrated to deliver 0.025 ml (25 μl) and 0.020 ml (20 μl).

Reagents

Rehydrate the lyophilized reagents (prepared by Fuji Zoki Pharmaceutical Co, Tokyo, Japan; distributed by Ames Co) with sterile distilled water according to the manufacturer's instructions. Store lyophilized and rehydrated reagents at 2 C–8 C. These reagents should be discarded if they become contaminated or do not demonstrate the proper reactivity with control sera.

1. Absorbing diluent (liquid). This consists of sonicated cell membranes from sheep and ox erythrocytes, normal rabbit testicular extract, sonicated Reiter treponemes, normal rabbit serum, Tween 80 and acacia powder in phosphate buffered saline (PBS), pH 7.2. This reagent is used to preabsorb and dilute sera, and to prepare the working dilutions of the sensitized and unsensitized cell suspensions.

2. Antigen. *Treponema pallidum* sensitized sheep cells (lyophilized).

a) The rehydrated antigen is a 2.5 percent suspension of formalinized, tanned sheep erythrocytes which have been sensitized with sonicated *T. pallidum* (Nichols strain). Reconstituted reagents should be used within 5 days.

b) Prepare the working dilution of antigen *for one test day* by adding one part of the rehydrated suspension to 5.5 parts of absorbing diluent (1:6.5 dilution). The quantity of working dilution needed is 0.075 ml for each serum dilution tested plus a slight excess.

3. Unsensitized sheep cells (lyophilized).

a) When rehydrated, this is a 2.5 percent suspension of formalinized, tanned sheep erythrocytes (*not* sensitized with *T. pallidum* antigen). Reconstituted reagents should be used within 5 days.

b) Prepare the working dilution (1:6.5) for one test day, allowing 0.075 ml for each serum tested plus a slight excess.

4. Sterile distilled water.

5. 0.85 percent saline.

Controls

1. Control sera (lyophilized) (prepared by Fuji Zoki Pharmaceutical Co, Tokyo, Japan; distributed by Ames Co). Store lyophilized control sera at 2 C–8 C. When rehydrated, the control sera may be stored at −20 C. These sera are supplied unabsorbed.

a) The reactive control serum should not vary more than plus or minus one doubling dilution from the end-point titer established for that serum. (The dilutions are expressed in terms of the *final serum dilution* obtained after the addition of all reagents.)

b. The nonreactive control serum should be nonreactive at the 1:80 serum dilution.

2. Unsensitized erythrocyte-serum control. Each test and control serum tested with sensitized sheep erythrocytes (antigen) is also tested at its lowest dilution with unsensitized erythrocytes. This serum control should be nonreactive.

TABLE 39.7—FTA-ABS REPORTING SCHEME:

TEST READING	REPEAT	REPORT
4+		R
3+		R
2+		R
	1+ or greater	R
1+	<1+ or N	B
<1+	1+, <1+, or −	B
−		N

Suggested attachment to reports of "Borderline" test results:

The borderline report of the FTA-ABS test performed in our laboratory on the specimen obtained from (patient's name) means that the results cannot be interpreted as either Reactive or Nonreactive.

If this is the first specimen you have submitted for FTA-ABS testing on this patient, another specimen should be submitted for FTA-ABS testing.

If this is a second specimen from this patient on which an FTA-ABS test has been made and the report is again "Borderline," it is impossible to state definitely that the patient does or does not have serologic evidence of syphilitic infection. A careful review of the patient's history and physical findings is suggested, and diagnosis will necessarily rest upon the clinical evidence in view of the Borderline serologic findings.

3. Reagents controls. Both sensitized erythrocytes (antigen) and unsensitized erythrocytes mixed with absorbing diluent should give nonreactive test results.

Preparation of sera for testing

1. Add 0.02 ml of unheated test and control sera to 0.38 ml of absorbing diluent in test tubes (1:20 dilutions).
2. Mix at least eight times and incubate at room temperature (25 C ± 5) for 30 min.
3. The absorbed test and control sera (1:20 dilutions) are now ready to be tested. The residual of the absorbed sera may be stored at 2−8 C and can be retested on the same day. Absorbed sera should be at room temperature when tested.

Preparation of microdiluting equipment

1. Microdiluter preparation
a) Rotate microdiluters in distilled water to clean.
b) Flame microdiluters to incandescence over a Bunsen burner; quench in distilled water to cool; and blot to expel liquid.
2. Go no-go delivery test. (The delivery test and prewetting are accomplished in the same operation.)
a) Fill each microdiluter by touching it to the surface of 0.85% saline. Do not wet canopy (top) of the loop.
b) Touch the microdiluter to the marked center of one of the circles on the go no-go delivery tester (blotter), and observe the dampened area within the circle.
c) A properly prepared microdiluter will deliver all contained fluid which will be sufficient to *immediately* dampen the area within the circle. The solution from an improperly prepared microdiluter will not be sufficient to dampen the entire area within the circle.
3. The calibrated pipette dropper must be clean. To assure proper delivery of fluid, gently blot excess solution from the outside of the pipette dropper with a cleansing tissue after filling. Hold the dropper in a vertical position when adding fluid to the tray cups.

Qualitative assay on serum (see Table 39.8)

1. Record the controls and serum numbers on the daily worksheets to correspond to their respective tray and cup numbers.
2. Place 0.025 ml of each absorbed test serum (1:20 dilution) into two adjacent cups in the tray; e.g., cup no. 1 in rows A and B; cup no. 2 in rows A and B, etc.
3. Using a pipette dropper calibrated to deliver 0.025 ml, add 0.075 ml (3 drops) of the working dilution of sensitized cells (antigen) to each cup in rows A, C, E, and G (absorbed serum Test).
4. Add 0.075 ml (3 drops) of the working dilution of unsensitized cells to each cup in rows B, D, F, and H (absorbed serum Control).
5. The *final serum dilution* in each test and control cup is 1:80.
6. Set up Reactive and Nonreactive control sera (see Table 39.8).

a) Prepare 2-fold dilutions of the absorbed reactive control serum (1:20 dilution) in absorbing diluent to exceed the end-point titer (final serum dilution) established for this serum; e.g., 1:80, 1:160, 1:320, 1:640, etc. (Dilutions may be prepared in 0.025-ml quantities in the tray cups with microtiter equipment; or these may be prepared in test tubes and 0.025 ml transferred to the cups.) Measure 0.025 ml of the absorbed reactive control serum (1:20 dilution) into another cup for the unsensitized erythrocyte-serum control.

b) Measure 0.025 ml of the absorbed nonreactive control serum (1:20 dilution) into each of two adjacent cups (test and serum control).

TABLE 39.8—OUTLINE OF MHA-TP QUALITATIVE TEST

	DILUTED (1:6.5) UNSENSITIZED CELLS, ML	DILUTED (1:6.5) SENSITIZED CELLS, ML	FINAL SERUM DILUTION
ABSORBED TEST SERA (1:20) ML			
Serum Test (Rows A,C,E,G)...............................0.025	—	0.075	1:80
Serum Control (Rows B,D,F,H) 0.025	0.075	—	1:80

ABSORBED CONTROL SERA (1:20)					
CUP No.	REACTIVE CONTROL + SERUM, ml	ABSORB-ING DILUENT, ml	= CONTROL SERUM DILUTION		
1	0.025 (1:20)	—	1:20	—	0.075	1:80
2	0.025 (1:20)	0.025	1:40	—	0.075	1:160
3	0.025 (1:40)	0.025	1:80	—	0.075	1:320
4	0.025 (1:80)	0.025	1:160	—	0.075	1:640
5	0.025 (1:160)	0.025	1:320	—	0.075	1:1280
6	0.025 (1:320)	0.025	1:640	—	0.075	1:2560
7	0.025 (1:640)	0.025	1:1280	—	0.075	1:5120
8	0.025 (1:1280)	0.025	1:2560	—	0.075	1:10240
9	0.025 (1:2560)	0.025	1:5120	—	0.075	1:20480
10	0.025 (1:5120)	0.025	1:10240	—	0.075	1:40960
11	0.025 (1:20)	—	1:20 C*	0.075	—	1:80

NONREACTIVE CONTROL SERUM, ML					
1	0.025 (1:20)	—	1:20	—	0.075	1:80
2	0.025 (1:20)	—	1:20 C*	0.075	—	1:80

REAGENTS CONTROLS					
1	—	0.025	—	—	0.075	—
2	—	0.025	—	0.075	—	—

* C = Control.

c) Add 0.075 ml of the unsensitized cells to each cup for the reactive and nonreactive unsensitized erythrocyte-serum controls.

d) Add 0.075 ml of the sensitized cells to all other cups containing reactive control serum dilutions and the Nonreactive control serum dilution.

7. Set up reagent controls.

a) Add 0.075 ml sensitized erythrocytes to 0.025 ml absorbing diluent in one cup.

b) Add 0.075 ml unsensitized erythrocytes to 0.025 ml absorbing diluent in another cup.

NOTE: Other methods of adding the 0.075-ml quantities of sensitized cells and unsensitized cells may be used if delivery is checked for accuracy.

8. Shake the trays gently, stack, and cover with an empty tray.

9. Incubate the trays at room temperature (25 C ± 5 C) for at least 4 hr. The incubation period may be extended to overnight.

10. Read the settling patterns of the red blood cells with an angled mirror (tray viewer) to visualize the patterns from below.

11. Readings are scored on a scale of − to 4+, and the degree of hemagglutination is judged according to the criteria in Table 39.9.

12. The results of the controls included for each test day should conform to the criteria outlined in the "Controls" section.

13. Reporting scheme for qualitative test

a. Report as "Reactive" a serum showing hemagglutination of 1+ or higher with sensitized cells (antigen), provided there is no hemagglutination with unsensitized cells.

b. Report as "Nonreactive" a serum showing no hemagglutination (− or ±) with sensitized cells and unsensitized cells.

14. If nonspecific hemagglutination occurs with the unsensitized cells (serum control), retest the serum and report results as described under "Quantitative assay on serum," step 10.

Quantitative assay on serum

Presently available data suggest that no additional valuable diagnostic information is obtained with the quantitative test. The following technique is in-

TABLE 39.9

DEGREE OF HEMAGGLUTINATION	READING	INTERPRETATION
Smooth mat of cells covering entire bottom of cup, edges sometimes folded	4+	Reactive
Smooth mat of cells covering less area of cup	3+	Reactive
Smooth mat of cells surrounded by red circle	2+	Reactive
Smooth mat of cells surrounded by smaller red circle with agglutination outside circle	1+	Reactive
Button of cells having small "hole" in center	±	Nonreactive
Definite compact button in center of cup or may have a very small "hole" in the center	−	Nonreactive

cluded, however, because it is needed for control purposes in the qualitative test.

1. Place 0.025 ml of the absorbing diluent in each cup required for dilutions, leaving the cups in the first and last rows empty.

2. Add 0.050 ml of the absorbed test and control sera (1:20 dilution) to appropriate cups in the first row; add 0.025 ml of each to the last row of cups (serum controls).

3. Prepare serial dilutions of serum with microdiluters. Place 0.025-ml microdiluters in cups containing 0.050 ml of absorbed serum. Rotate 4 sec to fill microdiluter. Remove microdiluters, place in next cups of same row, and rotate. Prepare further dilutions of serum by transferring 0.025 ml from one cup to the next, discarding the excess from the last cup by checking delivery on the blotter.

4. After completing the dilutions in each tray, clean the microdiluters by rotating in distilled water, blotting, dipping in 0.85 percent saline, and blotting to check delivery.

5. Add 0.075 ml unsensitized cells to cups in the last row (serum controls).

6. Add 0.075 ml sensitized cells (antigen) to all other cups containing absorbed serum dilutions.

7. Set up reagent controls.

8. Complete tests and read in the manner described for the qualitative microhemagglutination assay.

9. Quantitative tests showing nonreactive results in the control cup are reported in terms of the highest dilution giving a Reactive result (1+, 2+, 3+, or 4+) as illustrated in Table 39.10.

10. If nonspecific hemagglutination occurs with the unsensitized erythrocytes (serum control), retest the serum in the following manner:

a) Prepare dilutions of the absorbed serum in two rows of cups.

b) Add 0.075 ml of sensitized cells to each cup in one row.

c) Add 0.075 ml of unsensitized cells to the other row.

d) Report as "Reactive," without reference to titer, if:

(1) The hemagglutination with sensitized cells is at least two doubling dilutions greater than with unsensitized cells.

AND

(2) The first dilution showing no hemagglutination with unsensitized cells has a 3+ or 4+ reaction with sensitized cells.

TABLE 39.10—FINAL SERUM DILUTION

1:80	1:160	1:320	1:640	1:1280	1:2560	REPORT
4+	4+	3+	1+	±	−	R 1:640
3+	2+	1+	−	−	−	R 1:320
1+	−	−	−	−	−	R 1:80
±	−	−	−	−	−	N
−	−	−	−	−	−	N
2+	4+	4+	4+	2+	±	R 1:1280

e) Report as "inconclusive, nonspecific hemagglutination in serum control," if:

(1) The hemagglutination with sensitized cells is only one doubling dilution greater than with unsensitized cells;

OR

(2) The hemagglutination with sensitized cells is at the same dilution as with unsensitized cells.

ILLUSTRATION: see Table 39.11.

Miscellaneous Tests

Total protein determination on spinal fluid specimens (2, 9, 27)

Equipment

1. Spectrophotometer
2. Semilogarithmic graph paper

Glassware

1. Test tubes, 13 × 100 mm outside dimensions
2. Spectrophotometer cuvettes

Reagents

1. 10% trichloroacetic acid solution

Dissolve 10 g of trichloroacetic acid (CP) in 100 ml of distilled water. Store at room temperature in a glass-stoppered flask.

2. 0.9% saline

Add 900 mg of dry sodium chloride to each 100 ml of distilled water.

3. Standard serum

Select fresh, clear human serum, free from bacteria and hemolysis. Filter serum through a Seitz filter with a sterilizing pad. Measure serum and add 1 mg of powdered Merthiolate for each milliliter of serum. Determine total protein content by Kjeldahl analysis. Bottle aseptically and store in the refrigerator.

TABLE 39.11—FINAL SERUM DILUTION

SERUM	1:80	1:160	1:320	1:640	1:1280	REPORT
1 (Sensitized cells	4+	4+	4+	3+	1+)	Reactive
(Unsensitized cells	4+	4+	2+	−	−)	
2 (Sensitized cells	4+	3+	2+	−	−)	Inconclusive,
(Unsensitized cells	4+	2+	−	−	−)	nonspecific
3 (Sensitized cells	4+	−	−	−	−)	Hemagglutination
(Unsensitized cells	4+	−	−	−	−)	in serum control

Calibration curve and conversion table

1. Prepare a 60-mg% protein standard solution in triplicate by diluting standard serum with 0.9% saline.

EXAMPLE: If protein content of serum (Kjeldahl) is 7325 mg%, find dilution factor for 60-mg% standard by dividing 60 into 7325.

$$\frac{7325}{60} = 122, \text{ or dilution factor}$$

Therefore, 1 part of serum is diluted with 121 parts of 0.9% saline to make 60-mg% standard solution.

2. Prepare 10, 20, 30, 40, and 50-mg% protein solutions from each of the 60-mg% protein solutions as in Table 39.12.

3. Test the triplicate protein standard solutions in the same manner as described for spinal fluid (see "Performance of the test" below).

4. Average the triplicate percent transmittance values for each protein concentration and plot on semilogarithmic paper.

5. Draw a straight line fitting these points on the graph, and the point of 100% transmittance at 0 concentration.

6. Prepare a conversion chart from the graph by listing every percent transmittance value with its corresponding milligram-percent protein concentration.

7. Periodically test fresh 10, 20, 30, 40, 50 and 60-mg% protein solutions to check on the accuracy of the spectrophotometer and reagents.

Preparation of spinal fluid

Centrifuge and decant spinal fluid. Spinal fluids containing visible contamination or blood, or which are xanthochromic, are unsatisfactory for testing.

Performance of the test

1. Pipette 1.0 ml of spinal fluid into a 13- × 100-mm test tube. (Depending on the size of the spectrophotometer cuvettes, smaller or larger amounts of spinal fluid and trichloroacetic acid may be tested in the same proportions.)

Note—*Protein solutions of known concentration (20, 40, and 60 mg%) should be included as controls each time tests are performed.*

TABLE 39.12

MG% CONCENTRATION	60 MG% SOLUTION (ml)	0.9% SALINE (ml)
10	0.5	2.5
20	1.0	2.0
30	1.5	1.5
40	2.0	1.0
50	2.5	0.5

2. Add 1.0 ml of 10% trichloroacetic acid solution to each spinal fluid and control.

3. Invert the tube twice to mix contents. Avoid foaming.

4. Place tubes in a 37 C water bath for 10 min.

5. Adjust spectrophotometer by setting the wave length to 420 nm.

6. Adjust the spectrophotometer to 100% transmittance with a water blank.

7. Immediately before each reading, invert the tube containing the control or unknown and pour into the cuvette. Avoid foaming.

8. Read the percent transmittance of the controls and the unknowns.

9. Convert percent transmittance of unknowns and controls to milligram-percent total protein by reference to the calibration chart.

Note—*If spinal fluids contain concentrations of protein greater than 60 mg%, they should be appropriately diluted with 0.9% saline and retested. Values obtained from the calibration chart are then multiplied by the dilution factor.*

Cell count on CSF specimens (28)

Equipment and reagents

1. Fuchs-Rosenthal counting chamber slide. This chamber has a ruled area of 16 mm^2 and, with the cover glass on, it has a depth of 0.2 mm, giving the chamber a capacity of slightly more than 3 mm^3.

2. White blood cell pipette

3. Diluting fluid:

crystal violet ....0.1 g
glacial acetic acid ....1.0 ml
distilled water ....50.0 ml
few drops of 5% solution of phenol

4. Wright's stain

Total cell count procedure

1. Draw diluting fluid up to the 1 mark of the white blood cell pipette.

2. Then draw spinal fluid, which has been well shaken, up to the 11 mark.

3. Mix well, discard 2 to 3 drops, and fill counting chamber.

4. Count number of cells in entire ruled area and divide by 3 to give the number of cells per mm^3. The calculations compensate for the dilution factor.

Differential cell count procedure

1. Centrifuge specimen, and make a thin smear of the sediment on microscope slides.

2. Air dry.

3. Stain with Wright's stain as for a blood smear.

4. Count and tabulate cells.

Darkfield microscopy examination for *T. pallidum* (16, 23, 27)

The diagnosis of syphilis can be made by demonstrating *T. pallidum* in material from suspected lesions and/or aspirates from lymph nodes. To demonstrate a spiral organism with the characteristic morphology and motility of *T. pallidum* requires proper equipment, adequately trained personnel, and perseverance. A positive darkfield result constitutes an *absolute* diagnosis of primary, secondary, early congenital, or infectious relapse syphilis. In primary syphilis it may be possible to identify the etiologic agent and make a diagnosis before the appearance of measurable treponemal antibodies or reagin. Every genital lesion should be considered syphilitic unless proved otherwise, and each lesion should be subjected to a darkfield examination. In addition, other lesions of the skin or mucous membranes should be examined if there is the slightest suspicion of syphilis.

1. Collection of specimens

The objective in collecting a specimen for darkfield examination is to obtain serous fluid that is rich in treponemes and as free as possible of red blood cells, inasmuch as such cells may tend to obscure the treponemes. Thorough cleansing of the lesion is required to remove tissue debris and superficial spirochetal flora.

Rubber gloves should be used and other necessary precautions taken to avoid accidental infection. If the lesion is covered with a scab or crust, remove it. Cleanse the lesion with a gauze sponge wet with tap water or physiological saline. The use of antiseptics or soap should be avoided because of their potential antitreponemal effects. After drying the area, abrade the lesion with a dry sponge to provoke slight bleeding and exudation of serum. As oozing occurs, wipe away the first few drops and await the appearance of relatively clear serum. It is sometimes necessary to apply pressure at the base of the lesion or to apply a suction cup over the lesion to promote the appearance of serum. It is more desirable to obtain the serum from the depths of the lesion rather than from its surface because of the greater likelihood of finding motile treponemes. For direct examination, apply several clean cover slips or slides to the oozing lesion, or use a bacteriological loop to transfer the serum from the lesion to glass slides. Flatten the cover slip evenly on the slide with the blunt end of an applicator stick in such a manner as to remove air bubbles.

Lesions of early syphilis which are not manifest but suspected call for special comment. In the female, lesions of the cervix and vaginal vault present special problems for the collection of satisfactory material for darkfield microscopy. With visualization by bivalve speculum, remove all cervical or vaginal discharge of an interfering nature. Then cleanse the lesion with physiological saline, dry it, and abrade it as before (in this instance by rubbing with a gauze square held by a Kelly clamp). As bleeding stops and serum exudes, obtain material with a bacteriological loop.

In either sex, lesions of the skin in even a fading stage can be sampled, by (1) making multiple small linear incisions; (2) scraping with a sharp scalpel (or the side of the bevel of a hypodermic needle, using it as a knife edge); or (3) aspiration of the base of the lesion with a small-caliber hypodermic needle and syringe.

Mucous membrane lesions (patches) usually present little problem except in the mouth, where other treponemes (such as *Treponema denticola (microdentium), Treponema macrodentium*) and spiral organisms are frequently a part of the indigenous flora. In the oral cavity, with care and proper cleansing, drying and isolation, material may be collected so long as it is not at or near the edge of the gingival margin. *T. denticola,* which can be confused with *T. pallidum,* can normally be found in this area.

It may be difficult or impossible to find treponemes when local therapy has been applied to any syphilitic lesion. If, after examining several specimens, it is not possible to demonstrate the organism from the lesion, obtain a sample from a regional lymph node, particularly if it is palpable. To accomplish this, either wash out or introduce about 0.5 ml of sterile physiological saline into a small (2-ml) sterile syringe to which is attached a small hypodermic needle. Sterilize the skin overlying the node by painting with iodine and alcohol or some other suitable agent. Hold the node firmly and insert the needle well into it. The ability to manipulate the node freely is a good indication that its capsule has been pierced. Inject the physiological saline and gently manipulate the needle in various directions to macerate the tissue, aspirating as much fluid as possible. Discharge the aspirated material on slides for immediate examination.

Ideally, the darkfield procedure should be accomplished immediately, either by bringing the patient to the microscope or the microscope to the patient. If this is not possible, measures should be taken to facilitate the prompt delivery of specimens to the examining laboratory. Any appreciable delay in transit may result in questionable findings caused by reduced or complete loss of motility of the treponemes.

2. Examination

Using a properly adjusted darkfield microscope, examine the specimen for organisms of characteristic morphology and motility. Make careful and exhaustive search before rendering a negative report. Although a detailed review of darkfield microscopy is not possible here, a summary of the more frequent sources of error in the use of this technique may be helpful as a checklist:

a) *Preparation error*
  (1) Inclusion of too many refractile elements (red blood cells, air bubbles, tissue fragments, etc.)
  (2) Dirty or defective glassware (fine scratches on slides and cover slips)
  (3) Slides too thick or too thin (proper slide thickness is engraved on the top of the condenser)
  (4) Cover slips too thick (usually No. 1 size cover slip is satisfactory)
  (5) Excessive fluid between glass slide and cover slip with too rapid a flow of liquid across field of vision and too much depth to scan
  (6) Too little fluid between glass slide and cover slip with evaporation effects accentuated
  (7) Forgetting to place oil between condenser and the slide, as well as between oil-immersion objective and cover slip
  (8) Use of the concave side of the mirror

b) *Condenser error*
  (1) Not properly centered
  (2) Not properly focused, too high or too low
  (3) Oil and dust on the subsurface or reflecting area of the condenser

c) *Objective error*
   (1) Too high numerical aperture used
   (2) Failure to compensate high numerical aperture with funnel stop or iris diaphragm
   (3) Oil on 10× or 45× objectives
d. *Inadequate light source*

Definitive differentiation of *T. pallidum* from other treponemes and spiral organisms depends on size and other morphologic characteristics and upon characteristic motility. *T. pallidum* is a small spirilliform (corkscrew-shaped) organisms with 8 to 14 regular rigid spirals. The length is usually 6–14 μm, with an average of 10 μm. This average length is slightly larger than the average red blood cell (8 μm), and an occasional red blood cell in the preparation can be used as the practical criterion of length. The thickness seldom varies from 0.25 to 0.30 μm. The spiral amplitude appears to be 1 μm, and the spiral depth varies from 0.5 to 1.0 μm. The coiled appearance is maintained despite active motility.

Characteristic motions are (1) movements slowly forward and backward (translation); (2) rotation about the long axis like a corkscrew; and (3) slight bending, twisting or undulation from side to side. There is no waving or flattening as can be noted in larger saprophytic spiral organisms. The most common bending is in the middle and is as stiffly executed as the bending of a coil spring that comes back in place when released.

T. refringens-like organisms may be found in oral and genital lesions. These may be differentiated from *T. pallidum* by the variability in the length of the organism and in the number of spirals (from three to 20), the coarseness of the spirals, the rapid movement back and forth across the field with a writhing motion, and their extreme flexibility, manifested in part by relaxation of the spirals. It should be remembered that *T. denticola*, which can be confused with *T. pallidum*, can normally be found at or near the gingival margin.

A practical criterion for differentiating *T. pallidum* from nonpathogenic spiral organisms found commonly in the mouth and upon the genitalia is that organisms observed in microscopic fields of the slide which are quite uniform in size, shape and motility (as described) will usually be *T. pallidum*. On the other hand, *T. refringens*-like organisms, as previously described, are usually quite mixed, so that any one preparation will contain spiral forms of various sizes, shapes and motility. It must be remembered, of course, that some lesions will contain mixed flora and *T. pallidum*. When in doubt under such circumstances, the aspirate of the enlarged regional lymph node draining the site of the lesion will be found to contain only *T. pallidum* (if present) and no *T. refringens*-like forms.

Caution should be exercised in interpreting results on slides that contain numerous artifacts or refractile objects. The untrained and the unwary may be deceived by miscellaneous pieces of cellular debris, cotton strands, flagella, cilia, motile bacteria and fine scratches on glass slides. These and forms made of spiral fibrin filaments that have an appearance similar to treponemes can, with Brownian movement, be quite deceptive.

In summary, *T. pallidum* is a thin, *tightly wound*, rigid spiral organism, exhibiting little flexion, that does not move rapidly from place to place.

Any *loosely wound* spiral organism exhibiting great flexion that moves rapidly from place to place is *not T. pallidum.*

3. Interpretation of findings

The earliest and empirically the most specific means of diagnosing syphilis is by darkfield microscopy. The demonstration of treponemes of characteristic morphology and motility constitutes a positive diagnosis of syphilis in either primary, secondary, early congenital, or infectious relapse stages, regardless of the outcome of serologic testing. In primary syphilis, it may be possible to identify the etiologic agent and to diagnose the disease before the serologic tests become reactive. Serologic followup of untreated, darkfield-positive, seronegative primary syphilis cases may show a development of reactivity within several days to several weeks of treatment. Other stages of early, darkfield-positive syphilis should be routinely seroreactive.

Again, every genital lesion should be considered syphilitic until proved otherwise. Those extragenital lesions characterized by indolence, induration and regional lymphadenopathy should be regarded as probably syphilitic. Failure to find the organism does not exclude a diagnosis of syphilis. Negative results obtained in darkfield examination may mean that organisms were not found in sufficient numbers in the specimen to be observed, that the patient received antitreponemal drugs locally or systemically, that the lesion is "fading" or approaching natural resolution or disappearance, that the lesion is one of late syphilis, or finally that the lesion is not syphilitic. The darkfield examination should be repeated at least three times and serologic followup should be continued for about 4 months—at weekly intervals for the first month and biweekly intervals thereafter—before the probability of syphilis is excluded.

References

1. ANDERSON OW: Syphilis and Society, Health Information Foundation, Research Ser 22, 1965, pp 10–16
2. BOSSAK HN and ROSENBERG AA: A quantitative turbidimetric method for the determination of spinal fluid protein. J Vener Dis Inf 30:100–103, 1949
3. CENTER FOR DISEASE CONTROL: Micro-hemagglutination assay for *T. pallidum* antibodies (MHA-TP), provisional technique. CDC, HEW, Atlanta, Ga. Revised, Jan, 1977.
4. CENTER FOR DISEASE CONTROL: STD Fact Sheet, Edition Thirty-Four, Center for Disease Control, Public Health Service, HEW, Atlanta, Ga
5. DEACON WE, FALCONE VH, and HARRIS A: A fluorescent test for treponemal antibodies. Proc Soc Exp Biol Med 96:477–480, 1957
6. DEACON WE, LUCAS JB, and PRICE EV: Fluorescent treponemal antibody-absorption (FTA-ABS) test for syphilis. J Am Med Assoc 198:624–628, 1966
7. DUNCAN WP, BOSSAK HN, and HARRIS A: VDRL slide spinal fluid test. Am J Clin Pathol 35:93–95, 1961
8. FALCONE VH, STOUT GW, and MOORE MB JR: Evaluation of rapid plasma reagin (circle) card test. Public Health Rep. 79:491–495, 1964
9. HARDING VL and HARRIS A: The effect of temperature variants on quantitative turbidimetric determinations of spinal fluid protein, using trichloracetic acid. J Vener Dis Inf 30:325–327, 1949
10. HARRIS A, HARDING VL, and BOSSAK HN: Serum standards for serologic tests for syphilis. J Vener Dis Inf 32:310–318, 1951
11. HARRIS A, ROSENBERG AA, and DEL VECCHIO ER: The VDRL slide flocculation test for syphilis. II. A supplementary report. J Vener Dis Inf 29:72–75, 1948

12. HARRIS A, ROSENBERG AA, and RIEDEL LM: A microflocculation test for syphilis using cardiolipin antigen. Preliminary report. J Vener Dis Inf 27:169–174, 1946

13. HUNTER EF, DEACON WE, and MEYER PE: An improved FTA test for syphilis, the absorption procedure (FTA-ABS). Public Health Rep 79:410–412, 1964

14. JAFFE HJ, LARSEN SA, JONES OG, and DANS PE: Hemagglutination tests for syphilis antibody. Am J Clin Pathol (in press), 1978

15. NATIONAL COMMUNICABLE DISEASE CENTER, VENEREAL DISEASE RESEARCH LABORATORY: Technique for the fluorescent treponemal antibody-absorption (FTA-ABS) test. Health Lab Sci 5:23–30, 1968

16. NEEDHAM GH: The Practical Use of the Microscope. Charles C. Thomas, Springfield, Ill, 1958

17. NELSON RA JR and MAYER MM: Immobilization of *Treponema pallidum in vitro* by antibody produced in syphilitic infection. J Exp Med 89:369–393, 1949

18. PORTNOY J: Modifications of the rapid plasma reagin (RPR) card test for syphilis, for use in large scale testing. Am J Clin Pathol 40:473–479, 1963

19. PORTNOY J: A note on the performance of modifications of the rapid plasma reagin (RPR) card test for syphilis, for use in large scale testing. Public Health Lab 23:43, 1965

20. PORTNOY J, BOSSAK HN, FALCONE VH, and HARRIS A: Rapid reagin test with unheated serum and new improved antigen suspension. Public Health Rep 76:933–935, 1961

21. PORTNOY J and GARSON W: New and improved antigen suspension for rapid reagin tests for syphilis. Public Health Rep 75:985–988, 1960

22. RATHLEV T: Hemagglutination tests utilizing antigen from pathogenic and apathogenic *T. pallidum*, WHO/VDT/RES 77.65:1–5, 1965

23. REYNOLDS FW and HESBACHER EN: Darkfield microscopy: Some principles and applications. J Vener Dis Inf 31:17–23, 1950

24. SCHROETER AL, LUCAS JB, PRICE EV, and FALCONE VH: Treatment for early syphilis and reactivity of serologic test. J Am Med Assoc 221:471–476, 1972

25. STOUT GW, KELLOGG DS JR, FALCONE VH, MCGREW BE, and LEWIS JS: Preparation and standardization of the sorbent used in the fluorescent treponemal antibody-absorption (FTA-ABS) test. Health Lab Sci 4:5–8, 1967

26. TOMIZAWA T and KASAMATSU S: Hemagglutination tests for diagnosis of syphilis: A preliminary report. Jpn J Med Sci Biol 19:305–308, 1966

27. US DEPT HEALTH, EDUCATION AND WELFARE: Manual of Tests for Syphilis, 1969 Rev. U.S. Dept of Health, Education, and Welfare, PHS Pub. No. 411. US Govt Printing Office, Washington, DC 1969

28. WELLS BB: Exudates, transudates, and cerebrospinal fluid. *In* Todd-Sanford, Clinical Diagnosis by Laboratory Methods, 13th edition. Davidsohn I and Wells BB (eds.). W. B. Saunders, Philadelphia, 1963, pp 915–926

CHAPTER 40

TUBERCULOSIS AND OTHER MYCOBACTERIOSES

Robert C. Good, Vella Silcox, and James O. Kilburn

Introduction

Until 1954 discussions of *Mycobacteriaceae* of medical importance were limited to *Mycobacterium tuberculosis, M. bovis,* and *M. leprae.* Even though isolated reports had intimated that other mycobacteria might be associated with human disease, it remained for Timpe and Runyon (48) to carry out a complete study relating isolates to disease and characterizing the involved mycobacterial species. *M. bovis* infections have been controlled through pasteurizing milk and tuberculin testing of dairy herds. *M. tuberculosis* infections have been controlled through improved living standards and, particularly, through adequate chemotherapy. However, as the incidence of tuberculosis declines, the relative percentage of mycobacterioses caused by other species rises. The etiologic agents have been referred to as "unclassified" or "atypical," but both terms have now lost their usefulness and should not be perpetuated. Timpe and Runyon (48) placed the organisms into three groups which were later expanded to four by Runyon (39) on the basis of cultural characteristics. The groupings are a convenient method of indicating organisms with certain broad characteristics, but they are not taxonomically valid.

Etiologic Agents

Members of the genus *Mycobacterium* are nonmotile, nonsporeforming, slightly curved or straight rods, 0.2–0.6 by 1.0–10.0 μm, which resist staining with basic dyes as a result of their high cell-wall lipid content. For this reason, cells do not stain well by Gram's method and usually appear to be weakly gram-positive. If special methods are used to promote uptake of dye (see below), the bacilli cannot be readily decolorized, even in acidified solutions of organic solvents. Therefore, mycobacteria are described as acid fast. Stain may be taken up uniformly, but usually cells appear beaded or granular, with heavily stained areas separated by unstained spaces. During growth on culture media, cells may lose their acid fastness, and less than 10% of the cells of some species may retain the dye. This often leads to confusion with some species of *Rhodococcus Nocardia* and *Corynebacterium,* which may also appear to be weakly acid fast.

Mycobacteria grow slowly, with colonies from dilute inocula developing

675

on culture media after 2 days to 8 weeks of incubation. Some species requre special nutritional agents, and *M. leprae* has not been successfully cultivated *in vitro*. Optimal temperatures for growth vary from approximately 28 C to 40 C. Since permissible growth temperatures are often in narrow limits, primary cultures of a specimen must often be incubated at more than one temperature. Most of the pathogenic species grow well on complex media such as those containing egg yolk or specific accessory growth factors. Colonies vary from rough, heaped, coiled masses to smooth, rounded groupings which appear off-white, buff to yellow, or orange. Mycobacteria are aerobic and grow as pellicles on liquid media unless a surface-active agent such as polysorbate 80 is added to promote dispersed growth.

Many species of mycobacteria are saprophytic and are commonly found in soil and water; others are obligate parasites. The strictly saprophytic species must be clearly differentiated to avoid useless or inadequate therapy. Therefore, tests to identify pathogenic species are well-defined and must be performed with precision to characterize disease-causing agents adequately.

Clinical Manifestations and Epidemiology

Ten mycobacterial species or complexes are recognized as causes of human disease (40). These are *M. leprae, M. ulcerans, M. tuberculosis* complex (includes *M. bovis* and *M. africanum*), *M. avium-scrofulaceum* complex (often abbreviated as MAIS group since it also includes *M. intracellulare*), *M. kansasii, M. marinum, M. simiae, M. szulgai, M. xenopi,* and *M. fortuitum* complex (includes *M. chelonei*). Three species have been recognized recently: *M. asiaticum, M. malmoense* and *M. haemophilum* (see reference 41). *M. tuberculosis* causes approximately 95% of human mycobacterioses in the United States today—admittedly an estimate, because tuberculosis is the only reportable mycobacteriosis. The organisms may attack any organ, but the primary site of infection is usually the lungs. Tubercle bacilli are aerosolized by infected individuals when coughing or sneezing or by other mechanisms which force air rapidly over infected tissue to form droplet nuclei which measure 1–5 μm. Due to their small size, infective droplet nuclei remain suspended in the air for long periods. When inhaled, they are small enough to be carried into the alveoli without being expelled.

In nonimmune individuals, bacilli induce the formation of a nodule (tubercle) in the lung parenchyma. When such bacilli multiply, they may migrate through the draining lymphatics to a mediastinal lymph node where similar lesions may develop. Lesions in both areas can stabilize for long periods. At this point, the individual is considered to be infected, but not diseased, since clinical signs of illness are not evident. However, delayed-type hypersensitivity develops in infected individuals in 4–8 weeks, so that infection can be recognized by the cutaneous reaction resulting from the injection of tuberculin, a cell-free reagent prepared from liquid medium after pellicle growth has been removed.

When primary lesions in the lung expand, bacilli tend to be most numerous at the periphery, whereas the central area undergoes necrosis. Necrotic areas remain semisolid, resembling cheese—hence, caseous necrosis. When the area of caseous necrosis softens or liquefies, it is expelled, leaving a cavity with irregular edges. Expelled necrotic tissue rich in bacilli is the source of infective droplet nuclei.

The tuberculosis case rate continues to decline steadily in the United States. In 1979, 27,817 cases were reported, for an overall case rate of 12.6 per 100,000 (provisional data). Approximately twice as many males as females are diseased, and most cases are among the 45- to 64-year-old group. The highest case rate is among people 65 and older. The appearance of new cases in these older groups indicates reactivation of primary lesions after many years of dormancy rather than newly acquired infections. Sensitivity to tuberculin in younger age groups has also declined, so that the uninfected population is growing larger.

Other acid-fast bacilli cause diseases which may simulate tuberculosis or may produce chronic, granulomatous, subcutaneous abscesses or lymph node infections. There is little information regarding the epidemiology of these infections, but there have been no reports of person-to-person transmission. Host factors such as trauma, metabolic disease, or immunologic deficiency probably promote susceptibility to infection; however, the infecting species must be identified since prognosis and therapeutic management differ for the infections caused by each.

Public Health Significance

The role of public health departments in the management of tuberculosis patients has changed in the last few years. In the past, major efforts were focused on case finding, and patients with active disease were then placed in sanatoria for therapy. Shortly after effective therapeutic treatment is begun, patients cease shedding viable organisms so that hospitalization may not be necessary or may be required for only brief periods. Public health department personnel must now be fully cognizant of problems associated with chemotherapy so that they can follow the course of the ambulatory patient whose disease remains active.

Case finding is now limited to thorough follow-up of case contacts with tuberculin testing, roentgenography, or both. The public health department must also be responsible for administering preventive therapy to new converters.

Bacteriologic tests to monitor patients having therapy require greater participation by the public health laboratory than was necessary when specialized laboratories were available in sanatoria. Proficiency must be maintained and standard methods used in order to provide accurate diagnosis of cases and drug susceptibility data which are essential in determining case ratios and therapeutic efficacy for all mycobacterioses.

Levels of Laboratory Service

The scarcity of specialized laboratories to isolate and identify mycobacteria poses a problem for general clinical laboratories, which must now assume this responsibility. As case loads decline, fewer positive specimens are seen, but test procedures have become more complex in order to allow identification of a wider range of species. In recognition of this problem the Council of the American Thoracic Society adopted an official statement recommending levels of basic tuberculosis bacteriology which would require degrees of proficiency (12, 24). Specimens or cultures should be referred to a laboratory performing at a higher level if additional examinations are required.

Level I laboratories are those which prepare smears from specimens directly or after they are concentrated, stain, and examine for acid-fast bacilli. Laboratories for individual or groups of physicians and many general clinical or hospital laboratories and outpatient clinics may choose to offer this level of service.

Level II laboratories inoculate specimens to primary isolation media, perform preliminary identification tests, and determine susceptibility of isolates to the primary antituberculosis drugs (isoniazid, rifampin, ethambutol, streptomycin, and para-aminosalicylic acid). Selected laboratories which perform at this level should be available in central locations. They are generally state, city, or county public health laboratories, private clinical laboratories, and laboratories in hospitals in which tuberculosis patients are being treated.

Level III laboratories are public or private laboratories which maintain proficiency in performing a large battery of tests for identifying mycobacterial species and for determining susceptibility to both primary and secondary antituberculosis drugs.

The value of establishing levels of performance has been recognized by several public and private proficiency testing programs which grade responses on the basis of stated level of performance. However, it is the responsibility of individual laboratories to assure that trained personnel are available to perform tests. Because of the time involved in isolating and identifying mycobacteria, laboratory personnel should not rotate more frequently than every 6 months in Level II and Level III laboratories. Rotation at shorter intervals does not permit development of the necessary skills for identification and susceptibility testing.

Safety Procedures in the Mycobacteriology Laboratory

Procedures must be established in the mycobacteriology laboratory to insure that infectious materials are confined. Isolation rooms in a suite set aside for work with mycobacteria are required. The safety measures discussed elsewhere in this volume must be applied. Specifically, the laboratory must: be maintained under negative pressure; be equipped with adequate biologic safety cabinets; have restricted-admission isolation rooms; and be provided with discard pans pretested for leaks. Personnel must maintain clean, uncluttered work areas; autoclave all discard materials as they leave the isolation area; use disinfectant solution to decontaminate other materials taken from the isolation room; and work on towels soaked in disinfectant solution. Ultraviolet (UV) lights emitting rays primarily at wavelength 2537 Å, the bactericidal range, will decontaminate room air and hoods; however, lamps should be turned off before workers enter the laboratory. UV lamps should be cleaned every 2 weeks with an ethanol-moistened cloth because they lose efficiency rapidly as dust accumulates.

Because the primary danger of infection is through inhaling infectious aerosols, procedures which lead to the production of droplet nuclei should not be used. All procedures involving open tubes or plates must be carried out in the biologic safety cabinets. As an added precaution, personnel should wear masks with characteristics at least consistent with a high-quality surgical mask (filtration efficiency >95% for droplets 1–2 μm). Because of their high lipid content, mycobacteria on inoculation loops splatter when heated. Before they are flamed, loops or spades should be cleaned of excess organisms by being dipped in a 250- to 500-ml wide-mouth Erlenmeyer flask containing washed sea sand and 95% ethanol to prevent splatter.

Street clothes should never be worn in isolation rooms. Protective clothing which can be autoclaved after use should always be worn. Protective shoe coverings provide protection against spills. As an alternative, canvas shoes can be worn and then placed under a UV light at the room exit.

Well-equipped laboratories with all appropriate safety features may be available, but safety is ultimately the responsibility of the individual technician. Therefore, personnel must be fully trained to use safe working procedures. In addition, each individual should have a tuberculin skin test and a chest roentgenogram before working in the laboratory. If the results are negative, tuberculin tests can be repeated at 6- to 12-month intervals to monitor exposure to tubercle bacilli. If roentgenograms are deemed necessary (e.g., for tuberculin-positive individuals), they can be repeated at 12-month intervals. If there are no tuberculin conversions in a laboratory, personnel need be examined only once a year; in the event of conversions, examinations should be made more often. If conversion from tuberculin negative to tuberculin positive occurs, refer the employee to a physician for examination and treatment, examine laboratory procedures for safety, test laboratory equipment to assure that air flow is correct, and review laboratory safety procedures with all personnel.

Collection and Processing of Specimens

Successful detection and identification of mycobacteria are dependent on the quality of the specimen submitted. In all cases, procedures which assure minimal contamination with other microorganisms must be used. Specimens must be collected in clean, sterile containers and delivered to the laboratory promptly. If delivery is delayed, specimens should be refrigerated to inhibit the growth of contaminating microorganisms.

Specimens

Sputum. An adequate sputum specimen consists of 5–10 ml of material coughed from the bronchial tree. Patients should be instructed on the value of a sputum specimen rather than saliva or nasopharyngeal exudate. Sputum specimens should be collected in the early morning, and a series of three to six separate specimens should be collected on consecutive days and processed. Collecting sputa in sterile, 50-ml, conical, screw-capped centrifuge tubes is convenient, since specimens will not have to be transferred to other containers for processing in the laboratory. Reusable tubes must be pretreated with acid cleaning solution. One-use, disposable, screw-capped, 50-ml centrifuge tubes are excellent receptacles.

Induced sputum. Patients who do not produce sputum readily can be induced to cough by having them inhale warm, sterile, 10% sodium chloride aerosol. The specimens are more liquid than sputum and may be mistaken for saliva if not properly labeled. However, a better specimen is usually obtained by this method than by gastric lavage, which results in greater contamination.

Gastric lavage. Specimens from patients who cannot produce sputum can be obtained by gastric lavage. In order to obtain adequate material for processing, specimens should be taken at least 8 hr after ingestion of food or water, preferably in the early morning. Swallowed sputum which has not been highly diluted can then be recovered by passing 20–50 ml of sterile water through a sterile tube to the stomach and withdrawing the specimen in a sterile, 50-ml disposable syringe. Specimens should be processed promptly or preserved with 100 mg of powdered sodium carbonate if held for more than 4 hr.

Urine. Multiple midstream specimens collected in the early morning are preferred to a 24-hr pooled specimen; however, the entire voided specimen may provide better results. The collected specimen should be refrigerated until processed.

Tissue. Tissue specimens must be collected aseptically and delivered to the laboratory promptly. Large specimens should be examined to identify areas presumed most likely to contain numbers of bacilli. These areas selected for processing can be transported to the laboratory in sterile distilled water or neutral buffered saline. If tissues cannot be delivered to the laboratory rapidly, they should be frozen immediately and transmitted without being thawed.

Miscellaneous specimens. Other specimens such as pleural fluid, exudates or aspirates from lesions, spinal fluid, bronchial washings, joint fluid, and laryngeal swabs should be collected aseptically and placed in sterile containers for immediate delivery to the laboratory. The volume of some specimens may be very small, and the material must be handled carefully to prevent loss.

Processing

Since specimens containing mycobacteria are usually contaminated with other microorganisms, they must be decontaminated to provide an adequate sample for culture. Decontamination procedures rely on the resistance of mycobacteria to the action of harsh chemicals which will kill most contaminants, but even the mildest agents will reduce the number of recoverable mycobacteria. Directions for digestion and decontamination must be followed carefully to prevent overexposure of specimens to the action of decontaminating agents. The most successful decontamination procedures include digestion with a mucolytic agent to yield a homogeneous specimen. Methods currently used in the United States include treatment with N-acetyl-L-cysteine-sodium hydroxide, Zephiran-trisodium phosphate, sodium hydroxide alone, or oxalic acid.

N-acetyl-L-cysteine-sodium hydroxide procedure (23). This procedure is adaptable for most specimens but was designed primarily for treatment of sputum specimens.

1. *Sputum.* To a 5- to 10-ml sputum specimen in a 50-ml, conical, glass or plastic, screw-capped centrifuge tube, add an equal volume of NALC-NaOH reagent (see Chapter 46 for preparation). Mix on a test-tube mixer until specimen is liquefied (5–30 sec). Do not allow the specimens to froth, because the mucolytic properties of the NALC solution will be inactivated. After the specimen stands for 15 min at room temperature to complete decontamination, fill the tube to 50 ml with M/15 phosphate buffer (pH 6.8), close securely, mix contents of the tube, and centrifuge at 3000 rpm (2000–2400 × g) for 15 min. *Tubes should be enclosed in sealed centrifuge cups* to prevent generating an aerosol should the tube break or leak.

After centrifuging, decant the supernatant liquid into a discard receptacle containing disinfectant solution, taking care to avoid splashing or otherwise generating an aerosol. Flame the lip of the tube to prevent contamination of the exterior surface. Carefully remove part of the sediment with a sterile 3-mm bacteriologic loop or applicator stick, and prepare a 1- × 2-cm smear on a new glass slide. (If little sediment is obtained, resuspend before preparing smears.) Resuspend the remaining sediment in 1 ml of 0.2% bovine albumin solution (see Chapter 46 for preparation). Proceed with staining and examining smears, and then inoculate primary isolation media.

2. *Other specimens.* Laryngeal swabs or body fluids not taken aseptically can be handled in a manner similar to that described for sputum. Place laryngeal swabs in sterile centrifuge tubes with 2 ml of distilled water or saline and 2 ml of NALC-NaOH. After the contents of the tubes have been thoroughly mixed, allow to digest 15 min, remove swab, and process liquid in tube as previously described. Fluid specimens (such as pleural fluid and spinal fluid) of less than 10 ml should be processed as described for sputum.

Because they are larger, specimens such as those obtained by gastric lavage are processed in a modified manner. If the specimen is mucoid, mix 50–100 mg of NALC powder with the specimen to liquefy it. Centrifuge the specimen for 30 min, discard the supernatant fluid, and resuspend the sediment in 2–5 ml sterile water or buffer. After an equal volume of NALC-NaOH solution is added, processing proceeds as directed above. If the specimen is not mucoid, it is centrifuged and the sediment resuspended in 2–5 ml of water or buffer before processing as above.

Tissues taken aseptically are homogenized in 3 ml of 0.2% bovine albumin with a glass or Teflon tissue homogenizer, diluted, and inoculated directly to primary isolation media. As a precaution, 1 ml of homogenized specimen can be mixed with 1 ml of penicillin solution (1000 units/ml), incubated at 37 C for 30 min, centrifuged, and resuspended in 0.2% albumin. Grossly contaminated tissues should be homogenized and treated as described for gastric lavage.

Zephiran-trisodium phosphate procedure (61). Add an equal quantity of Zephiran-trisodium phosphate reagent (see Chapter 46) to sputum in a screw-capped container, and agitate vigorously for 30 min on a mechanical shaker. Allow the mixture to stand undisturbed for 30 min, transfer it to a 50-ml centrifuge tube, and centrifuge at 3000 rpm (2000 to 2400 × g) for 20 min. Carefully decant the supernatant liquid as described above and resuspend the sediment in 20 ml of Neutralizing Buffer (Difco Laboratories, Detroit, Michigan). Since traces of benzalkonium chloride may inhibit the growth of mycobacteria on some media, use a buffer containing phospholipid to assure neutralization. Centrifuge the suspension in buffer again as above for 20 min. Discard the supernatant fluid, and mix the sediment in the small amount of residual fluid in the tube. Proceed to inoculation of primary isolation media.

Other specimens can also be processed in this manner after initial preparation as described for the NALC-NaOH procedure.

Sodium hydroxide procedure. The procedure for digestion and decontamination with sodium hydroxide is the same as that described for NALC-NaOH. A maximum concentration of 4% NaOH (2% final concentration) is tolerated by mycobacteria, but a 2% NaOH solution (1% final concentration) is preferred. If too many cultures are contaminated, increase the concentration of NaOH to 3% or 4% rather than increasing the time of decontamination. However, better results are routinely obtained with the NALC-NaOH procedure, since the mycolytic agent permits a lower concentration of NaOH to be used.

Oxalic acid procedure (7). Specimens containing pseudomonads are often difficult to decontaminate, but treatment with oxalic acid may be effective. Mix an equal volume of 5% oxalic acid (50 g of oxalic acid dissolved in 950 ml of distilled water and sterilized by heating to 121 C for 15 min) with the specimen. After 30-min reaction time, dilute with 0.85% sodium chloride solution, and centrifuge as described above. After decanting the supernatant fluid, add an indicator to the sediment, and neutralize with 4% NaOH. Proceed with inoculation of primary culture media.

Cetylpyridinium chloride procedure (46). Sputum specimens which must be transported for as long as 24 hr can be decontaminated during shipment with cetylpyridinium chloride (CPC). This method is not intended to replace the NALC-NaOH procedure, since CPC decontaminates more slowly, and the residual quaternary ammonium compound may inhibit mycobacterial growth on other than egg-based media. Growth inhibition may not result if the residual CPC is inactivated with Neutralizing Buffer (Difco), but this has not been investigated.

Mix freshly collected sputum in a 50-ml screw-capped centrifuge tube with an equal portion of CPC-NaCl solution. (Dissolve 1% CPC and 2% NaCl in distilled water. The solution is stable in tightly stoppered bottles shielded from excessive light and heat; however, crystals may form below 22 C.) Shake the specimen until it is liquefied, and place it in appropriate mailing containers for shipment to the processing laboratory. Reaction time should be at least 24 hr. When they are received in the processing laboratory, specimens are diluted to 50 ml with sterile distilled water (or Neutralizing Buffer) and then centrifuged and resuspended as described in the NALC-NaOH procedure.

Diagnostic Procedures

Staining and Microscopy

The acid-fast staining characteristic of mycobacteria provides the basis for making a presumptive laboratory diagnosis of disease. All specimens from patients with suspected mycobacterial infection should be examined for acid-fast bacilli. The results are often used in conjunction with clinical findings to establish a tentative diagnosis, to monitor the efficacy of a therapeutic regimen, or to confirm that tuberculosis patients can be discharged. Therefore, smears must be prepared and stained by standardized and controlled procedures, and microscopic evaluations must be made with care. If the standard Ziehl-Neelsen (Z-N) procedure is used, red-staining bacilli may be masked by the blue staining background in thick smears. Artifacts are commonly seen when smears are stained by the fluorochrome procedure. In both instances, differentiation is possible only by careful examination of the entire smear.

The acid-fast characteristic of mycobacteria is detected with both the Z-N and fluorochrome procedures, because the ability of bacilli to retain dye when exposed to acid alcohol is being determined. However, results of microscopy and culture may not always agree because too few organisms are present to be detected with microscopy, staining procedures are inadequate, bacilli are dead as a result of chemotherapy or too harsh decontamination procedures, or culture media do not support the growth of the isolate. Even though microscopic evaluation is helpful and often reliable, it can provide only presumptive information.

Preparation of smears (45)

Glass slides used to prepare smears for acid-fast staining must be new and clean, since used slides may still have bacilli on their surfaces. With a 3-mm inoculating loop or an applicator stick, transfer a portion of the specimen to a clearly labeled slide and smear evenly over a 2 cm^2 area. Material for smears can be the sediment from a concentrated specimen or a direct preparation of pus, caseum, tissue impression, or caseous clumps carefully selected from the sputum specimen. A properly prepared smear should be thin enough so that newsprint can be read through it at a distance of 5–10 cm. After smears are prepared, air dry and heat fix them on an electric slide warmer at 65–75 C for 2 hr, or pass them through a flame until the slide is just hot enough to cause slight pain when touched to the back of the hand.

If the specimen is not to be used for culture (as in Level I laboratories), it can be treated with sodium hypochlorite solution to kill all viable bacilli. Household bleach containing 5%–6% sodium hypochlorite is adequate for this purpose. Mix the specimen with an equal volume of sodium hypochlorite solution in a 50-ml centrifuge tube, and shake it. Allow the mixture to sit for at least 10 min, but not longer than 30 min, to kill tubercle bacilli and other microorganisms. Add water to fill the tube, mix, and centrifuge at 2000 × g for 15 min. Decant supernatant fluid, resuspend sediment in a few drops of water, and prepare smear as directed above.

Bright-field microscopy (45)

Detecting acid-fast bacilli with bright-field microscopy depends on selectively staining bacilli which contrast with the non-acid-fast staining background. Two staining procedures in routine use are the Ziehl-Neelsen and Kinyoun methods described below.

Ziehl-Neelsen procedure.

1. Cover heat-fixed smear with absorbent paper. Add enough (4–5 drops) Ziehl-Neelsen carbol-fuchsin (see Chapter 46) to saturate paper.

2. Gently heat the bottom of the slide until the stain begins to steam. Continue heating for 5 min, but do not allow the stain to boil or dry. Add more carbol-fuchsin if necessary.

3. Carefully lift paper from slide with forceps.

4. Rinse smear with tap water.

5. Flood smear with acid alcohol (3 ml of concentrated hydrochloric acid to 97 ml of 95% ethanol) for 2 min.

6. Rinse smear with tap water.

7. Flood slide with aqueous methylene blue (0.3 g methylene blue chloride in 100 ml distilled water) for 1–2 min.

8. Rinse in tap water, drain, and dry.

Kinyoun acid-fast procedure.

1. Cover heat-fixed smear with absorbent paper, and add sufficient (4–5 drops) Kinyoun carbol-fuchsin reagent (see Chapter 46) to saturate paper. Allow the stain to remain in contact for 5 min. Do not heat.

2. Carefully lift off paper with forceps.

3. Wash smear with tap water and drain.

4. Flood smear with acid alcohol (3 ml of concentrated hydrochloric acid in 97 ml of 95% ethanol), and destain for 2 min.

5. Rinse with tap water and drain.

6. Flood smear with aqueous methylene blue (0.3 g of methylene blue hydrochloride in 100 ml of distilled water), and stain for 1–2 min.

7. Rinse with tap water, drain, and air dry.

With both of the above methods, acid-fast mycobacteria stain red on a blue background. Other counterstains such as malachite green, brilliant green, or picric acid can be used if there are problems with red-blue differentiation.

Fluorescence microscopy (45)

Acid-fast bacilli stained with a fluorochrome such as auramine O retain the dye following exposure to acid alcohol. These acid-fast staining procedures are gaining wide acceptance because of the ease and accuracy with which they allow brightly fluorescing bacilli to be distinguished on a dark background. Currently used procedures include the Blair, Smithwick, and Truant methods described below.

Blair fluorescence staining procedure.

1. Flood heat-fixed smear with auramine O-phenol reagent (see Chapter 46), and stain for 15 min.

2. Rinse with chlorine-free water, and drain.

3. Flood with acid-alcohol reagent (0.5 ml of concentrated hydrochloric acid to 100 ml of 70% ethanol) for 2 min.

4. Rinse with water.

5. Flood smear with potassium permanganate reagent (0.5 g of potassium permanganate, $KMnO_4$, dissolved in 100 ml of distilled water) for 2 min.

6. Rinse, drain, and air dry.

Smithwick fluorescence staining procedure.

1. Flood heat-fixed smear with auramine O-phenol reagent (see Chapter 46), and stain for 15 min.

2. Rinse with chlorine-free water, and drain.

3. Flood with acid alcohol (0.5 ml of concentrated hydrochloric acid in 100 ml of 70% ethanol) for 2 min.

4. Rinse with water, and drain.

5. Flood smear with acridine orange reagent (see Chapter 46), and stain for 2 min.

6. Rinse with water, drain, and air dry.

Truant fluorescence staining procedure.

1. Flood heat-fixed smear with auramine O-rhodamine B-phenol reagent (see Chapter 46) and allow to react for 15 min.

2. Rinse with chlorine-free water and drain.

3. Flood with acid alcohol reagent (0.5 ml concentrated hydrochloric acid in 100 ml 70% ethanol) for 2 min.

4. Rinse and drain.

5. Cover slide with potassium permanganate solution (0.5 g potassium permanganate, $KMnO_4$, in 100 ml distilled water) and let stand for 2 min.

6. Flush slide with water, then drain and let air dry.

Observation of acid-fast stained smears

Carbol-fuchsin-stained smears are examined with the oil immersion lens at 900–1000× magnification. Mycobacteria appear as red-stained organisms (coccobacilli, long bacilli, filamentous or banded forms) against a blue background.

Fluorochrome-stained smears are examined with the high dry lens at 250–400× magnification. Mycobacteria stained with auramine O-phenol fluoresce yellow to yellow-green on a black background; those stained with auramine O-rhodamine B-phenol fluoresce yellow-orange. Background material fluoresces weakly orange or red if counterstained with acridine orange. A microscope used to detect fluorescence must have a lamp which emits light in the blue visible or UV range. Barrier filters which select for specific wave lengths transmit light which excites the dye to fluoresce. The Zeiss BG-12 and Corning 5113 excitation filters and the Corning OG-1 barrier filter are satisfactory for these purposes. In fluorescence microscopy, a dark-field condenser with a drop of nonfluorescing immersion oil on the top surface is usually used; however, dry dark-field condensers which permit a broader field of vision are available. A method for blue-light fluorescence microscopy in which a low-voltage, high-amperage concentrated filament type lamp is used in combination with selective filters has been described by Richards and Miller (38). The original article should be consulted for instructions for assembling the light source to use with a standard medical microscope. Pollock and Wieman (36) recently reported using blue-light microscopy successfully in detecting acid-fast bacilli in clinical specimens.

Since detecting acid-fast bacilli in stained preparations is of primary importance in diagnosis and patient discharge, smears must be examined carefully and the results reported in a uniform manner. As shown in Table 40.1, the number of fields that must be examined for acid-fast bacilli varies with the magnification used. Therefore, one of the advantages of fluorochrome staining procedures is that less time is needed for observation.

The American Thoracic Society of the American Lung Association rec-

TABLE 40.1—RECOMMENDED MINIMUM NUMBER OF FIELDS TO SEARCH AT SELECTED
MAGNIFICATIONS BEFORE REPORTING AN ACID-FAST STAINED SMEAR AS NEGATIVE FOR AFB[a]

MAGNIFICATION[b]	NUMBER OF FIELDS
250X	30
400X	55
450X	70
630X	130
1000X	300

[a] Reproduced with permission of R. W. Smithwick (45).

[b] This final magnification represents the objective lens magnification multiplied by the eye-piece magnification.

ommends that mycobacteria observed microscopically be reported as rare, few, or numerous (1). However, the reporting procedure described by Smithwick (45) is better quantitated:

Number of Organisms Seen	Report
0	Negative for AFB (−)
1–2/300 fields	Number seen (±)
1–9/100 fields	Number/100 fields (1+)
1–9/10 fields	Number/10 fields (2+)
1–9/field	Number/field (3+)
>9/field	>9/field (4+)

This method of reporting is based on examinations made at magnifications of 800–1000×. Fewer than three acid-fast bacilli per slide (300 fields) is not considered positive but indicates that additional specimens should be examined. Reports at the lower magnifications used with fluorochrome staining should be corrected appropriately: at magnification of 650×, divide the count by 2; of 450×, divide the count by 4; and of 250×, divide the count by 10. The resulting number will be approximately the same as that found at 1000× (45).

Primary Isolation

Mycobacteria, especially *M. tuberculosis,* are resistant to the harsh chemicals used for digesting and decontaminating specimens, but surviving cells may be injured or the total population may be reduced. Therefore, multiple enriched isolation media are used to favor the growth of bacilli. Egg-based media such as Lowenstein-Jensen (L-J) medium (13) or American Trudeau Society (ATS) medium (2) are always included for primary isolation. Slants or bottles of L-J and ATS media are available from a number of commercial suppliers; among these are Difco Laboratories, Inc., Detroit, Mich.; BBL, Cockeysville, Md; Gibco Diagnostics, Madison, Wis.; and REML, Lenexa, Kan. For preparation from basic ingredients, consult original references or see the manual by Vestal (51). Specimens are also inoculated onto Middlebrook 7H10 (30) or 7H11 agars (6) or Dubos oleic agar (9) for quantitation and determination of colonial morphology. Dehydrated bases for preparing Middlebrook 7H10 and 7H11 agars and Dubos oleic agar and Middlebrook 7H9 liquid medium are available commercially, e.g., from Difco Laboratories, Inc., Detroit, Mich.; BBL, Cockeysville, Md; Gibco Diagnostics, Madison, Wis.; and

REML, Lenexa, Kan. For preparation from basic ingredients, consult original references or see the manual by Vestal (51). The last three media were formulated to neutralize any toxic substances in specimens or to promote the growth of nutritionally dependent strains such as those which are isoniazid resistant. A liquid medium such as Middlebrook 7H9 broth (30) may also be included.

Even with adequate decontamination of specimens, as many as 6% of all cultures may be contaminated. In an attempt to prevent the loss of mycobacteria as a result of contamination, Mitchison et al. (31, 32) added antibacterial drugs to Middlebrook 7H11 agar when isolating *M. tuberculosis* and *M. bovis*. Since some species did not grow well on the medium, McClatchy et al. (28) reduced the concentration of carbenicillin but used specimens decontaminated by the NALC-NaOH procedure. The final drug concentrations per ml of medium were: polymyxin B, 200 μg; amphotericin B, 10 μg; trimethoprim lactate, 20 μg; and carbenicillin, 50 μg. Overall results were favorable in that contamination was reduced on drug-containing medium, but some strains of *M. kansasii, M. intracellulare,* and *M. gordonae* did not grow well. Including the selective medium along with other primary isolation media improves the chances for successful culture of mycobacteria.

To prepare inoculum for primary isolation media, dilute sediment from the processed specimen 1:10 in sterile distilled water. Inoculate half of the agar-based medium in an I plate with 0.1 ml of undiluted specimen and the other half with 0.1 ml of the 1:10 dilution. Spread inoculum over the surface of agar media with a bent glass rod which has been sterilized by dipping in an alcohol flask and then flaming. Inoculation with diluted specimen is necessary to obtain isolated colonies for determining culture purity and colonial morphology and to dilute out potentially toxic substances which would inhibit growth. After inoculated plates have been allowed to dry (overnight incubation at room temperature is acceptable), they are placed inverted into CO_2-permeable plastic bags which are then sealed.

Inoculate slants of egg-based medium with 0.1 ml of undiluted and 0.1 ml of diluted specimen, and spread over the surface with an inoculating needle. Incubate tubes with loosened caps in a horizontal position until excess moisture evaporates or absorbs (overnight to 1 week in the incubator). Inoculate at least two tubes of egg-based medium and two plates or tubes of agar-based medium with each specimen. Only by using multiple specimens inoculated to different types of media and more gentle decontamination procedures can we eliminate routine guinea pig inoculation.

Place inoculated plates and tubes in an incubator at 36 C $\pm$ 1 C in an atmosphere of 5%-10% CO_2 in air. Incubate cultures of skin lesions or environmental specimens at $\leq$33 C to promote the growth of *M. marinum, M. ulcerans,* or the rapid growers which do not grow well at higher temperatures.

Incubate primary cultures for 6-8 weeks before discarding them as negative. During this period, observe tubes each week with a hand lens and plates each week with a dissecting microscope. At the first reading, caps on tubes containing egg-based medium are tightly closed, after which the tubes can be transferred to an incubator without CO_2. The basic four cultures on primary isolation media are observed for simple characteristics which allow a preliminary subdivision into species.

Growth rate. Slowly growing mycobacteria usually require more than 10 days to develop on solid media inoculated with a diluted 7- to 10-day broth culture, whereas rapidly growing species develop mature colonies in less than 7 days particularly at 28 C. On primary isolation media, rapid growers may develop more slowly, but generally the rate of growth can be determined from the primary culture.

Growth temperature. M. *tuberculosis* and other mycobacteria recovered from pulmonary lesions or similar deep tissues grow well at 35 C, but mycobacteria which infect cutaneous sites, such as M. *marinum,* do not grow well above 33 C. Rapid growers may require 14–21 days to develop at 35 C, but colonies will reach maturity in 2–4 days at 24 C–28 C. If definitive information is needed for species identification, inoculate slants of egg-based medium with a 100-fold dilution of a barely turbid suspension and incubate at 24 C, 32 C, 37 C, and 42–45 C.

Colonial morphology. Observe characteristic colonial morphology on Middlebrook 7H10 agar or Dubos oleic agar with the low-power objective on a standard microscope or with a dissecting microscope. Rough colonies (R) appear when bacilli arrange into cords or strands. Smooth colonies (S) contain an even distribution of cells and appear more homogeneous. Graduations between rough and smooth also occur. Additional terms helpful in specifying morphology are found in the manual by Vestal (51).

Pigmentation. Many mycobacterial species produce colonies which are cream to light buff, but others are yellow to red due to synthesis of carotenoid pigments. Scotochromogenic species produce pigment in the dark, as well as in the light, but color may intensify with prolonged exposure to light. Photochromogenic species are not pigmented if grown in the dark but produce pigment after exposure to light for ≥1 hr. Caps on tubes must be loosened to permit entrance of oxygen, so that pigment can be synthesized by both scotochromogens and photochromogens.

When nonpigmented colonies are first observed, place tubes with caps loosened or plates near a light source for ≥1 hr before returning them to the incubator. For best results, expose young, actively growing cultures to light, since other cultures do not consistently respond. Colonies of photochromogenic species become pigmented 6–12 hr after exposure. When grown in continuous light for 2–3 weeks, M. *kansasii* and M. *marinum* produce crystals of pigment which are visible with 100× magnification.

M. *fortuitim* colonies may turn green when grown on media containing malachite green. Coloration does not result from synthesis of pigment but from incorporation of dye into the colony.

Identification Procedures

Mycobacterial species can be identified with a series of biochemical tests which are easily performed and widely acceptable. Many of the tests are highly reproducible (58, 59), but controls with known strains must be included to assure reliable results. Many additional tests are used in taxonomic studies of the genus, but only those of differential value to the diagnostic laboratory have been included in the following section.

Growth on primary isolation media is inoculated to a tube of 7H9 broth to prepare inocula for many of the following test media. In some cases, tests can be performed directly on growth from the primary isolation media. If liquid medium is used, sufficient growth for inoculation is obtained after 7–10 days of incubation. On the basis of preliminary observations of colony morphology, growth rate, optimum growth temperature, and pigmentation, differential tests can be selected to identify isolates.

The following tests are listed alphabetically for convenience rather than in order of importance.

Arylsulfatase, 3-day and 14-day. The 3-day arylsulfatase test is primarily for differentiating potential pathogens from other rapid growers which are not usually positive until 14 days. Also, *M. marinum, M. xenopi,* and M. triviale may be positive in 3 days. The 14-day test is useful in identifying *M. marinum, M. szulgai, M. xenopi, M. triviale,* and *M. flavescens.*

Two techniques are used for detecting phenolphthalein enzymatically split from tripotassium phenolphthalein sulfate: the Center for Disease Control's (CDC's) method, which utilizes a liquid medium, and the Wayne method, which utilizes an agar medium. When the test is performed, uninoculated medium and medium inoculated with *M. fortuitum* should be included as controls.

CDC's method (15). Inoculate tubes of arylsulfatase medium-CDC (see Chapter 46) with 0.1 ml of a 7-day liquid culture or a spadeful of growth from solid medium. Incubate cultures at 36 C. After 3 days of incubation, test the tube of medium containing 0.001 M substrate for free phenolphthalein by adding not more than 6 drops of 2 N sodium carbonate solution (10.6 g of anhydrous Na_2CO_3 made to 100 ml with distilled water). After 2 weeks of incubation, test the tube containing 0.003 M substrate in the same way. Appearance of a pink coloration indicates a positive test. Compare color with a set of standards so that intensity can be reproducibly recorded on a scale of − to 5+ (see reference 15 for preparing standards).

Wayne method (54). Prepare a barely turbid suspension of the test culture in sterile water, and inoculate 1 drop to arylsulfatase medium-Wayne (see Chapter 46; commercially available as Wayne sulfatase agar, BBL, Cockeysville, Md; Arylsulfatase Agar, Butt, Remel, Lenexa, Kan.). Incubate at 37 C for 3 days. Add 1 ml of 1.0 M sodium carbonate solution. Pink or red appearing on the surface of the medium indicates a positive reaction.

Catalase. Except for some isoniazid-resistant strains of *M. tuberculosis,* all mycobacterial isolates produce various quantities of catalase. Presence of the enzyme can be detected quickly by adding 1–2 drops of a freshly prepared solution of hydrogen peroxide solution (a mixture of equal portions of 30% hydrogen peroxide, Superoxol: Merck & Co., Rahway, N.J., and a 10% solution of Tween 80) to cultures on a plate or slant. Bubbles of oxygen released within 5 min around colonies indicate catalase activity. This reaction may be rapid or slow, representing high or low catalase activity. More information is obtained by performing the semiquantitative test and determining the stability of the enzyme at 68 C.

Heat-stable catalase (26). M. tuberculosis, M. bovis, M. gastri, and occasional strains of *M. marinum, M. kansasii, M. avium* complex, *M. malmoense,* and *M. fortuitum* complex do not produce heat-stable catalase. To perform the test, suspend several colonies in 0.5 ml of 0.067 M phosphate buffer, pH 7 (see Chapter 46), in a 16- × 125-mm screw-capped tube, and heat in a water bath at 68 C for 20 min. Cool the suspension to room temperature, and add 0.5 ml of the hydrogen peroxide solution prepared as above. Bubbles of oxygen will be released by positive cultures. Hold tubes for 20 min before discarding as negative. Controls should include *M. tuberculosis* (negative) and *M. gordonae* or *M. fortuitum* (positive).

Semiquantitative catalase (25). Results of the semiquantitative catalase test are more standardized than those of the basic test described above; therefore, test results are more reliable for differentiating species. Prepare L-J butt tubes by inspissation in an upright position of 5 ml medium contained in 20- × 150-mm tubes (also available from Difco Laboratories, Inc., Detroit, Mich; and Remel, Lenexa, Kan.). Inoculate the butt with 0.1 ml of well-grown, 7-day-old liquid culture, and incubate 2 weeks at 36 C ± 1 C with loosened caps. Add 1 ml of the peroxide solution described above, and hold tubes in an upright position. After 5 min at room temperature, measure the column of bubbles in mm and record as <45 mm (weak positive), >45 mm (strong positive), or negative. Include appropriate controls in the test.

Iron uptake (49). Except for *M. chelonei,* only rapidly growing mycobacteria are positive for iron uptake. Inoculate slants of L-J medium prepared with 1.5% ferric ammonium citrate with 1 drop of a barely turbid aqueous suspension of cells. More consistent results are obtained if the final concentration is 2.5% ferric ammonium citrate. Incubate for 21 days at 28 C. If positive, colonies are rusty-brown, and the medium is light tan. Controls should include *M. fortuitum* (+) and *M. chelonei* (−).

As an alternative procedure (56), inoculate slants of plain L-J as above, and incubate them until definite growth is observed. Add 1 drop of 20% aqueous ferric ammonium citrate for each 1 ml of L-J medium, e.g., if L-J slant is prepared with 8 ml of medium, add 8 drops of reagent. Resume incubation for a maximum of 21 days, and record reaction as indicated above.

Growth on MacConkey agar (18). This test differentiates two groups of rapid growers. The potentially pathogenic species, *M. fortuitum* and *M. chelonei,* show growth within 5 days, whereas most other species do not. Inoculate plates of MacConkey agar without crystal violet (BBL, Cockeysville, Md., and Difco Laboratories, Inc., Detroit, Mich.) with a 7-day liquid culture. Streak plates according to instructions for isolating individual colonies. Incubate plates at 28 C ± 2 C and examine for growth after 5 and 11 days. Only strains of *M. fortuitum* and *M. chelonei* grow throughout the streak, whereas other species grow only where the inoculum is very heavy. Include *M. fortuitum* and *M. phlei* as positive and negative controls, respectively.

Niacin production (42, 59). The test for niacin is one of the most commonly used procedures for identifying *M. tuberculosis.* When growing on egg-based media or in agar media supplemented with 0.25% L-asparagine or 0.1% potassium aspartate, *M. tuberculosis* releases large quantities of niacin into the medium. Only *M. simiae,* which can readily be differentiated from *M. tuberculosis,* produces as much as or more of the compound. Rarely, niacin-negative strains of *M. tuberculosis* are found, but if other characteristics indicate that the isolate is of this species, the test should be repeated with a culture showing luxuriant growth, i.e., after up to 6 weeks of growth.

Add 1 ml of sterile water to a 3- to 4-week-old culture on L-J or ATS medium, and hold the tube so that the water covers the medium around the colonies. If growth is confluent, puncture the surface to allow niacin to be extracted from the medium. After 15 min, remove 0.5 ml of the liquid containing extracted niacin, and transfer it to a clean, screw-capped tube. Add 0.5 ml of 4% aniline solution and 0.5 ml of 10% cyanogen bromide (see Chapter 46 for preparation of solutions). If yellow appears immediately, niacin is present. Discard into germicide made alkaline with NaOH to prevent hydrolysis of reagent to hydrocyanic acid.

A paper-strip method for detecting niacin has been developed (20, 63) and is widely accepted because it is reproducible, easily performed, and does not involve handling toxic chemicals. Tests must be performed according to instructions supplied by the manufacturer (PathoTec Niacin from General Diagnostics Division, Warner-Lambert Co., Morris Plains, N.J.; Niacin Test Strips, TB from Difco Laboratories, Detroit, Mich.).

Nitrate reduction (53). *M. tuberculosis, M. kansasii, M. szulgai,* and some strains of *M. terrae* complex reduce nitrate to nitrite, whereas other slowly growing species do not. With the notable exception of *M. chelonei,* rapidly growing mycobacteria also reduce nitrate. Tests must be performed with growth from well-grown cultures (3–4 weeks for slow growers, 2–4 weeks for rapid growers). Emulsify a heavy loop of growth in 3–4 drops of sterile distilled water in a 16- × 125-mm screw-capped tube. Add 2 ml of nitrate reductase substrate (see Chapter 46), shake to obtain an even suspension, and incubate in a 37 C water bath for 2 hr. Add 1 drop of a 1:2 dilution of concentrated HCl, and gently mix. Add 2 drops of 0.2% aqueous solution of sulfanilamide and 2 drops of 0.1% aqueous N-(1-naphthyl)ethylenediamine dihydrochloride. Observe for the immediate development of a definite red color. Compare with a reagent control and a positive control test set up with *M. kansasii* or *M. tuberculosis.* Add a pinch of zinc dust to all negative tubes to reduce nitrate. If red develops, the test was indeed negative. If color does not develop after zinc dust is added, reaction has proceeded beyond nitrite and can be recorded as positive if a second test reacts the same way. Positive reactions can be quantitated by comparing against a set of color standards. If needed, prepare them as directed by Vestal (51).

Enzyme activity is increased by adding electron donors to the reaction mixture (5). If neutralized solutions of Tween 80, lactic acid, propionic acid, or pyruvic acid are added to a final concentration of 0.5%, enzymatic activity of positive strains increases, but the reactions of strains which do not produce nitrate reductase are not altered.

Pyrazinamidase test (55). This test for detecting free pyrazinoic acid is based on the rate of enzyme degradation of pyrazinamide. *M. marinum* is positive in 4 days, and *M. kansasii* is negative in 4 days, but many strains may become positive in 7 days. *M. bovis* is negative at 4 days and usually at 7 days, but *M. avium, M. intracellulare,* and *M. tuberculosis* are positive in 4 days.

Prepare pyrazinamidase test agar by dissolving 6.5 g of commercially available Dubos broth base with Tween in a liter of distilled water. Add 100 mg of pyrazinamide, 2 g of sodium pyruvate, and 15 g of agar, and heat the mixture to melt the agar. Dispense the solution in 5-ml amounts into 16- × 125-mm screw-capped tubes, and autoclave them at 121 C for 15 min. Allow agar to solidify with the tubes in an upright position. Inoculate the surface of the agar butt heavily with growth from an L-J slant. Prepare two tubes for each culture being tested. After incubating the cultures for 4 days at 35 C–37 C, add 1 ml of freshly prepared aqueous 1% ferrous ammonium sulfate solution. Place tubes at 4 C for 4 hr. Hold tubes against a white background, and examine for a pink band which develops in the agar. After 7 days of incubation, test the second tube in a similar manner. Include a tube of uninoculated medium as the negative control, and inoculate one tube with *M. avium* or *M. intracellulare* as the positive control.

Sodium chloride tolerance (19). Except for *M. chelonei,* ssp. *chelonei,* most rapidly growing mycobacteria will grow on medium containing 5% NaCl. All slow growers are inhibited except *M. triviale* and some strains of *M. flavescens.* To perform the test, prepare L-J or ATS medium in slants with a final concentration of 5% sodium chloride (tubed media are commercially available). Inoculate slants of media prepared with and without sodium chloride with 0.1 ml of a barely turbid suspension prepared by diluting liquid culture or emulsifying growth from a slant in sterile water. Incubate slowly growing strains at 35 C and rapidly growing strains at 28 C with caps loosened until moisture evaporates. Tighten caps, and continue incubating cultures for no longer than 4 weeks. After growth is observed on control medium, examine the NaCl medium each week for 3 weeks. If >50 colonies are seen on the NaCl-containing medium, the culture is tolerant, but if <50 colonies are seen, it is sensitive. Confluent or heavy growth should develop on control medium during the period of incubation.

Tellurite reduction (22). Rapid growers and organisms in the *M. avium-intracellulare* complex reduce tellurite salt to metallic tellurium in 3–4 days. Heavily inoculated cultures to be tested are grown in 5 ml of Middlebrook 7H9 liquid medium with Tween 80 (with no glycerol added) contained in 20- × 150-mm screw-capped tubes at 35 C for 7 days. Add 2 drops of sterile 0.2% aqueous potassium tellurite solution (0.1 g potassium tellurite dissolved in 50 ml of distilled water and sterilized by autoclaving) to the heavily turbid broth culture. Continue incubation for 3 additional days before examining tubes for a precipitate of the black metallic tellurium. To avoid errors, inoculate heavily to obtain turbid suspensions at 7 days. Do not use cultures incubated > 7 days, but prepare fresh cultures if growth is not heavy enough. Include uninoculated medium and a culture of *M. avium* complex as controls.

Thiophene-2-carboxylic acid hydrazide (TCH) susceptibility (4, 52). This test is used primarily to differentiate *M. bovis* from *M. tuberculosis,* although it can be used to differentiate *M. bovis* from other nonchromogenic mycobacteria. *M. bovis* strains are usually susceptible to low concentrations of the drug, but resistant variants may be found because of cross-resistance with isoniazid. As the test is performed in this country (51), dilute a 7- to 10-day-old culture in 7H9 liquid medium 1:10 and 1:1000 in sterile saline or distilled water. Deliver 3 drops of each suspension from a sterile capillary pipette to the surface of 7H10 or Dubos Middlebrook agar containing 10 μg of TCH (Aldrich Chemical Co., Milwaukee, Wis.) per ml of medium. Prepare the medium as slants in screw-capped tubes (4 ml medium per tube) or in sectioned petri dishes (5 ml per quadrant). Inoculate cultures to media prepared with and without TCH. Organisms are susceptible if growth in TCH medium is less than 1% of growth on control media without drug. Culture the two dilutions separately in order to estimate the number of colonies resistant to the drug.

In the test as originally described (4), susceptibility to 1 μg of TCH per ml was used to differentiate *M. bovis*, but response to this low level has not always been reliable. Wayne et al. (59) found in a collaborative study that tests in which 1 μg of TCH per ml of either L-J or 7H10 medium was used were very reproducible (96.9% consensus) with laboratory-adapted cultures. Tests in which 10 μg per ml were used were also very reproducible, but occasional strains of *M. tuberculosis* were inhibited. Test results must be interpreted in conjunction with other taxonomic criteria to assure correct identification of clinical isolates.

Tween hydrolysis (57). Clinically significant scotochromogens and non-photochromogens usually cannot enzymatically hydrolyze Tween 80 (poly-oxyethylene sorbitan monooleate). Therefore, this test is useful in differentiating clinically significant species from saprophytic species of these groups. Since *M. kansasii* rapidly hydrolyzes Tween 80, it should be used as a positive control. Prepare the substrate by dissolving, in order, 500 mg of Tween 80 and 2.0 mg of neutral red in 100 ml of 0.067 M phosphate buffer, pH 7.0. (Caution: Dye weight is based on 100% neutral red; if less than 100%, calculate the quantity that will yield 2.0 mg.) Dispense this solution into 16- × 125-mm screw-capped test tubes in 2-ml amounts, and autoclave it for 15 min at 121 C. Final medium should be amber. When tubes are cool, suspend in the substrate a large loop of growth from an actively growing culture on solid medium. Incubate the suspension in substrate at 35 C, and examine it daily for conversion from amber to pink. Cells may turn pink, but unless the fluid changes color the test is negative. A color change can be detected most easily by comparing the test specimen with an uninoculated tube of medium held against a white background. This test has been reported to be highly reproducible in interlaboratory studies (58).

The Tween 80 substrate described above should be freshly prepared or stored for no longer than 2 weeks in the dark at 4 C to prevent deterioration. A concentrated substrate stable for up to 6 months has been described by Kilburn et al. (21) and is available commercially (Difco Laboratories, Inc., Detroit, Mich. Remel, Lenexa, Kan.). If commercial substrate is used, manufacturer's instructions must be followed to obtain reliable test results.

Urease. The ability of some species to hydrolyze urea is a useful differential characteristic, particularly for separating urease-positive *M. scrofulaceum* from pigmented, urease-negative strains of the *M. avium* complex. Other species such as *M. xenopi* and *M. gordonae* are negative, whereas *M. bovis* and *M. tuberculosis* are positive.

Several methods of performing the test have been proposed (33, 50, 55, 58), but the following simple method has been used in the CDC laboratory for 18 months with great success. Add 3 ml of sterile distilled water to Bacto-Urea R Broth Vials (Difco Laboratories, Inc., Detroit, Mich.) to rehydrate the contents immediately before use. Inoculate the vial heavily with a spade of growth from a well-grown culture. Incubate the inoculated substrate at 35 C in air for 72 hr. A positive test is indicated by a color change to bright red. Include a culture of *M. scrofulaceum, M. fortuitum,* or *M. gastri* as a positive control and uninoculated medium as a negative control.

A reliable test which is currently in use in our laboratory was described by Steadham (47) in 1979. To perform the test, inoculate 1.5 ml of Steadham urea broth (see Chapter 46) in 13 × 100 mm tubes with a spade of growth from an actively growing culture on an L-J slant. Inoculum must be heavy enough to impart a definite tubidity to the broth. Incubate for 3 days at 35–37 C and observe for the development of a pink to red color. Compare with positive and negative controls. Steadham (47) recommends incubation for 7 days before making final readings. Results may be quantitated using standards prepared for the nitrate reduction test (51), but a positive reaction must develop color equivalent to or greater than the 2+ standard.

A rapid test which involves detection of radio-labeled carbon dioxide has recently been described (8). The test is complete in 30 min with both rapid and slow growers, but reproducibility with large numbers of strains has not been determined.

Identification of Isolates

Reactions used for primary separation of mycobacterial species are growth rate, colony morphology, pigmentation, and optimal growth temperature. Flow charts which incorporate these initial reactions have been designed (27, 35, 51), but procedures differ after primary observations have been made.

Reactions useful for identifying rapid growers are shown in Table 40.2. *M. fortuitum* and *M. chelonei* have often been identified as causes of disease (ulcers on lower extremities, eye infections, pulmonary disease, infection following cardiac surgery), and identification to species is helpful in epidemiologic studies. The species in this group are rapid growers at 25–28 C, but they may appear as slow growers at 35–37 C. Rare isolates reverse this pattern and grow slowly at 28 C and rapidly at 35 C. Although not listed in the table, niacin-positive strains of *M. chelonei* are not uncommon.

Characteristics of slowly growing mycobacteria are shown in Table 40.3. The primary pathogen responsible for most mycobacterial disease is *M. tuberculosis*, which can be differentiated from other species on the basis of the niacin test, TCH resistance, nitrate reductase, and catalase activity. Since all mycobacteria except certain isoniazid-resistant strains produce catalase, a column of foam > or < 45 mm is used as the differential characteristic. Other pathogenic species have been isolated with greater frequency as the number of *M. tuberculosis* isolates declines. Nonpathogenic species must be differentiated in order to prevent needless therapy, and pathogenic species must be identified so that appropriate therapy can be given. Since *M. africanum* has not yet been isolated in this hemisphere, its differential characteristics are not shown in the table. Additional aids in identifying species can be found in the references (41, 43, 51).

Serologic Procedures

The use of serologic procedures to aid in identifying *Mycobacterium* spp. has not been uniformly successful because of the complex antigenic relationships among members of the genus. The most successful procedure is the agglutination reaction described by Schaefer (44), but cross-reactions and autoagglutination are common. An acceptable scheme for numbering serologic

TABLE 40.2—CHARACTERISTICS FOR IDENTIFICATION OF RAPIDLY GROWING MYCOBACTERIA

SPECIES	PIGMENT	GROWTH ON MAC-CONKEY AGAR	NITRATE REDUC-TION	NACL TOLERANCE	IRON UPTAKE	ARYLSUL-FATASE 3-DAY	TWEEN HYDROLYSIS 5-DAY	CATALASE >45mm	CATALASE 68 C
M. fortuitum	None	+	+	+	+	+	+/−[b]	+	+
M. chelonei	None	+	−	Variable[a]	−	+	−/+[c]	+	+
M. smegmatis	None	−	+	+	+	−	+	+	+
M. phlei	Orange/Yellow	−	+			−	+	+	+
Other Rapid Growers	Variable	−		Variable	Variable				

a M. chelonei subsp. abscessus = positive; M. chelonei subsp. chelonei = negative.
b 55% of strains positive.
c 30% of M. chelonei subsp. abscessus are positive; M. chelonei subsp. chelonei is negative (43).

TABLE 40.3—CHARACTERISTICS FOR IDENTIFICATION OF SLOWLY GROWING MYCOBACTERIA

Species	Colony Morphology[a]	Pigment[b]	Niacin	Growth on TCH	Nitrate Reduction	Catalase >45 mm	Catalase 68C	Tween Hydrolysis 10 Days	Tellurite Reduction 3 Days	Pyrazinamidase 4 Days	Pyrazinamidase 7 Days	Urease	NaCl (5%) Tolerance	Arylsulfatase 2 Weeks
M. tuberculosis	Rg	N	+	+	+	−	−	−/+[c]	−/+	+	+	+	−	−
M. bovis	Rg	N	−	+	−	−	−	−	−	−	−	+	−	−
M. ulcerans	Rg	N	−	+	−	+	+	+	−(?)	−	Unk.	+	−	−/+
M. kansasii	Sm/Rg	P	−	+	+	+	+	+	−	+/−	+/−	+	−	−
M. simiae	Sm	P	+	+	−	+	+	−	−	+	−	−[f]	−	++
M. marinum[d]	Sm	P	−/+	+	−	−	+	+	−	+/−	+	+	−	−
M. scrofulaceum	Sm	S	−	+	−	+	+	−	−	−	−	+	−	+
M. szulgai	Sm/Rg	S/P[e]	−	+	+	+	+	+/−	−	−/+	+/−	+	−	±
M. gordonae	Sm	S	−	+	−	+	+	+	−	+/−	+/−	−	−	++
M. xenopi	Sm/Rg	S	−	+	−	−	+/−[h]	−	+	+/−	+/−	−	−	−/+
M. avium complex	Sm/Rg	N	−	+	−	−	+/−	−	+	Unk	Unk	−	−	−
M. malmoense	Sm	N	−	+	−	−	+/−	+	−	Unk	−/+	+	−	−
M. gastri	Sm	N	−	+	−	−	−	+	−	−/+	+	+	−	−
M. terrae complex	Sm/Rg	N	−	+	+/−	+	+	+	−	−/+	+	−	−[g]	Variable
M. flavescens	Sm/Rg	S	−	+	+/−	+	+	+	−	+	+	+	+/−	+/++

a Rg = rough; Sm = smooth.

b N = none; P = photoinducible; S = scotochromogenic.

c −/+ indicates majority of strains negative; +/− indicates majority of strains positive; ± = weak reaction; Unk = unknown.

d If grown at 28 C–33 C, M. marinum colonies develop in < 7 days.

e M. szulgai is photochromogenic at 25 C and scotochromogenic at 35 C.

f When test is performed as directed in text (47), M. simiae is positive; however, if other procedures are used, isolates may be negative.

g M. triviale in the M. terrae complex will grow in the presence of 5% NaCl.

h Negative 68 C catalase may be seen with poorly growing strains.

variants in the *M. avium* complex (*M. avium, M. intracellulare,* and *M. scrofulaceum*) has been proposed (62). In this scheme, *M. avium* strains are serovars 1–3; *M. intracellulare* strains are serovars 4–20 (currently up to serovar 28), with additional numbers left open; *M. scrofulaceum* strains are serovars 41–43. Other species contain only one or two serovars, but species identification is possible for *M. malmoense, M. szulgai, M. kansasii, M. simiae, M. gastri, M. fortuitum,* and *M. chelonei*. Additional serovars have been identified for *M. scrofulaceum, M. gordonae, M. xenopi,* and *M. marinum* (10).

M. avium complex serovars have been grouped to form the basis of an epidemiologic study in Germany (29). The authors concluded that serovars 1–3 (*M. avium*) are an important source of human infection which arises from the natural host and that the remaining serovars are associated with environmental sources.

Typing sera for identifying mycobacteria are not commercially available; only limited supplies have been produced in special reference laboratories. Problems with cross-reactivity and autoagglutination must be taken into account when interpreting results. Some laboratories are experimenting with fluorescent-antibody procedures in order to circumvent some of the problems with the agglutination reactions. A study with the enzyme-linked immunosorbent assay indicated that this procedure may be valuable for diagnosing tuberculosis (34). However, additional tests with serum from diseased and infected individuals are required to evaluate the procedure fully.

Mycobacteriophage Typing

A general review of mycobacteriophages has been included in the excellent overall review of *Mycobacterium* by Barksdale and Kim (3). As pointed out by these authors, mycobacteriophages are essentially similar to other phages, and a satisfactory phage-typing scheme can be developed. Problems associated with developing a reproducible typing scheme have centered around the propagation of phages on the appropriate host strain and around variations in techniques for determining susceptibility of isolates. Cooperative studies to establish standard techniques (37) have led to the recognition of four major phage types of *M. tuberculosis* (A_x, A_2, B, and C) by using 11 mycobacteriophages. With a similar technique, Grange et al. (11) identified three phage types in isolates from British and Asian patients and compared the results with those from previous studies. Of strains from British patients, 50%–60% were type A, 30%–45% were type B, and the remaining strains were intermediate between the two. Of strains from Asian patients, 54%–66% were type A, 2%–6% were type B, and 28%–43% were intermediate between the two. Addition of more selective phages will allow further separation of types for epidemiologic studies.

Jones and Greenberg (16) described a phage which further divides the existing types of *M. tuberculosis* into two subtypes. The phage was modified by propagating it on an alternate host strain so that its ability to lyse mycobacteria was selectively altered. Jones (14) also successfully used a mycobacteriophage to differentiate BCG strains from *M. bovis* and *M. tuberculosis*. The ability to differentiate these isolates is of practical importance because BCG is widely used in cancer immunotherapy.

At present, phage typing procedures are still in the experimental phase. However, as efforts continue to simplify and standardize procedures (17), a reliable typing scheme for mycobacteria will evolve. Until it is developed, phage typing of mycobacteria must remain a specialized technique for exploratory studies.

Antimycobacterial Drug Susceptibility Testing

Drug susceptibility tests of mycobacterial cultures are not performed or interpreted in the same way as the conventional diffusion techniques commonly used in clinical microbiology. However, the responsiveness of isolates to specific antimycobacterial drugs is helpful to the clinician in selecting the most effective therapeutic regimen. In practice, newly diagnosed, previously untreated patients with tuberculosis are started on therapy before results of drug susceptibility tests are known, and therapy is altered as needed after reports are available. Results of susceptibility tests are necessary for assessing therapy for patients who have been treated before and are thus more likely to have developed resistance.

It is difficult to standardize mycobacterial drug susceptibility tests because of variations in stability of the drugs which are inactivated at different rates by sterilization, binding or inactivation of drugs in different media, concentration or destruction of drugs during medium storage, inoculum and numbers of organisms per volume of drug-containing medium, and distribution of susceptible and resistant populations in the inoculum. Therefore, each phase of the drug susceptibility test must be standardized and finally controlled with known cultures to assure valid results.

Drug tests can be performed with either the disk or conventional methods. The disk method of Wayne and Krasnow (60) is more convenient for Level II laboratories to use to determine susceptibility to first-line drugs (isoniazid, streptomycin, ethambutol, rifampin, and p-aminosalicylic acid). The conventional method (51) is used in determining susceptibility to the second-line drugs (kanamycin, ethionamide, cycloserine, pyrazinamide, and capreomycin). The disk method is described below, and Vestal (51) should be consulted for performing conventional tests. Since comparable results are obtained with both methods on first-line drugs, reliable results can be obtained with commercially available disks even though drug concentrations may vary from 68%–135% of the potency stated on the disks.

Direct test. Susceptibility to antimycobacterial drugs is always tested with dilutions of the clinical specimen (direct test) unless no acid-fast bacilli are observed by microscopic examination. If smear results are negative or if direct test plates are contaminated, the indirect test may be the only way to determine susceptibility. However, the indirect test is subject to variation because of inoculum selection from the primary culture.

Preparation of medium. Complete 7H10 medium is carefully prepared so that 5-ml quantities are available for each test quadrant. Drug-containing disks (available from BBL) to be used in the test (24) are listed in Table 40.4. Place each disk in the center of a section of a quadrant Petri dish, and hold it in place with a drop of 7H10 medium. Dispense 5 ml of complete 7H10 agar at 45–48 C into all quadrants, including control quadrants which do not contain disks. For each determination, prepare nine quadrants with disks (Table 40.4); a tenth quadrant serves as the control for a total of three plates. Two quadrants are not used (or may be used as control quadrants on each plate). Prepare plates in duplicate to test two dilutions of inoculum. After the medium hardens, incubate it overnight to allow the drugs to diffuse and to allow detection of contamination. Use plates immediately, or store at 4 C for up to 4 weeks. While they are stored, protect the medium from dehydration which would cause an increase in drug concentrations.

Inoculum preparation, incubation, and reading. When acid-fast bacilli are seen in smears of sputa or of other specimens, use the direct method of inoculation. Dilutions to be tested are based on the number of acid-fast bacilli and are adjusted as follows:

Acid-Fast Bacilli Observed	Dilution of Inoculum
<1 per field	Undiluted and 10^{-2}
1–10 per field	10^{-1} and 10^{-3}
>10 per field	10^{-2} and 10^{-4}

Adjust inocula so that the number of colonies can be counted, both for drug-containing and control quadrants, since cultures with at least 1% of control growth on drug-containing media are considered resistant. From experience, populations which contain 1% resistant cells do not respond to therapy, because the resistant cells rapidly predominate.

Add 3 drops of the inoculum dilution from a capillary pipette (approximately 0.1 ml) to each quadrant of drug and control media. Inoculate one set of plates with the higher dilution selected on the basis of microscopic examination of specimen, and inoculate a second set of plates with the lower dilution. Seal plates in individual polyethylene bags. When the inoculated surface no

TABLE 40.4—DRUG POTENCIES OF DISKS USED FOR MYCOBACTERIAL SUSCEPTIBILITY TESTS

DRUG	POTENCY (μg/disk)	FINAL DRUG CONCENTRATION (μg/ml)*
Isoniazid	1	0.2
Isoniazid	5	1.0
Rifampin	5	1.0
Streptomycin	10	2.0
Streptomycin	50	10.0
Ethambutol	25	5.0
Ethambutol	50	10.0
p-Aminosalicylic Acid	10	2.0
p-Aminosalicylic Acid	50	10.0

* Concentration in μg/ml when 5 ml of medium are added to quadrant containing disk of stated concentration.

longer contains free liquid, invert plates and incubate in air containing 5%–10% carbon dioxide at 35–37 C.

Read plates each week for 3 weeks. Most slowly growing mycobacteria will not produce visible colonies until after 14 days. After 3 weeks of incubation, record the results. Record bacterial colony development on control and drug-containing medium as follows: confluent colonies, 4+; nearly confluent, 3+; 100–200 colonies, 2+; 50–100 colonies, +; and <50, actual count.

When the results from both dilutions of inoculum are complete, estimate the number of resistant colonies on drug-containing media. (For example, if the number of colonies on drug quadrants inoculated with the lower dilution [10^{-1}] exceeds the number of colonies which developed on the control quadrant inoculated with the higher dilution [10^{-3}], the culture contains more than 1% resistant cells.)

Indirect test. As stated above, always use the direct test when acid-fast bacilli are seen in microscopic examination of the specimen. If it is necessary to determine susceptibility from a previously grown culture, be careful to test a representative population. Inoculum can be prepared from young cultures on solid medium by scraping colonies from all parts of the surface and suspending the cells in a medium containing Tween. Clumping can be reduced by adding 4–5 small glass beads to the tube and placing it on a Vortex mixer for about 1 min. Allow heavy clumps to settle for 15 min, and use the upper portion of the suspension to prepare a barely turbid suspension in another tube of Tween-containing broth. Use this suspension to prepare 10^{-2} and 10^{-4} dilutions, and inoculate them to plates as described above. All other procedures are identical to those described for the direct test.

If the cultures for drug susceptibility testing are old, suspend growth from the primary culture in Tween-containing medium, and use it to inoculate a second tube of broth. Sufficient growth should be available for test after 7–10 days of incubation at 35–37 C. Prepare dilutions, and inoculate plates as directed above. Although this step is often necessary in reference laboratories, it should be avoided if possible because it can cause an alteration in resistant cells in the population.

Evaluation of Laboratory Findings

The presence of *M. tuberculosis, M. bovis, M. kansasii,* and/or other slowly growing pathogenic species is significant because they are etiologic agents of human disease. Other species such as *M. gordonae, M. flavescens,* and members of the *M. terrae* complex are only rarely pathogenic and may be present in various environmental sites including food and water. Rapidly growing species, *M. fortuitum* and *M. chelonei,* which also occur widely, are potential pathogens which can cause disease, particularly in the compromised host.

Since many mycobacteria are found in a number of environmental sites as well as in bronchial secretions and the oral cavity of humans, diagnosis of disease caused by mycobacteria other than *M. tuberculosis* is based on rigid standards defined in a statement of the American Thoracic Society (1). Definite diagnosis requires evidence of a disease (such as infiltrate visible on a chest roentgenogram) for which a cause has not been determined by careful clinical and laboratory studies; and either (a) isolation of the same mycobacterial species repeatedly, usually in the absence of any other pathogen, or (b) isolation of mycobacteria from a closed lesion. In the latter instance, the specimen must be collected and handled under sterile conditions. In the laboratory, aqueous solutions have sometimes been contaminated with mycobacteria. Therefore, a series of cultures containing organisms such as *M. gordonae* or *M. terrae* should alert the laboratorian to possible contamination.

All cultures should be held for at least 1 month, and preferably longer, after identification and drug susceptibility reports have been sent out. This holding period allows the attending physician to request additional tests, particularly drug susceptibilities, or to have identification confirmed in a reference laboratory. If strains of *M. tuberculosis* resistant to multiple drugs are found, it is particularly important to have further tests done in a reference laboratory.

In order to assure accuracy in test procedures, every laboratory must participate in a governmental or commercial proficiency testing program. Information regarding proper selection of the appropriate program can be obtained from state laboratory directors.

References

1. AMERICAN THORACIC SOCIETY: Diagnostic Standards and Classification of Tuberculosis and Other Mycobacterial Diseases. American Lung Association, New York, NY, 1974
2. AMERICAN TRUDEAU SOCIETY: Report of the committee on evaluation of laboratory procedures. Am Rev Tuberc 54:428–432, 1946
3. BARKSDALE L and KIM K-S: *Mycobacterium.* Bacteriol Rev 41:217–372, 1977
4. BONICKE R: Die Differenzierung humaner und boviner Tuberkelbakterin mit Hilfe von Thiophen-2-carbonsauer-hydrazid. Naturwissenschaften 46:392, 1958
5. BONICKE R, JUHASZ SE, and DIEMER U: Studies on the nitrate reductase activity of mycobacteria in the presence of fatty acids and related compounds. Am Rev Respir Dis 102:507–515, 1970
6. COHN ML, WAGGONER RF, and MCCLATCHY JK: The 7H11 medium for the cultivation of mycobacteria. Am Rev Respir Dis 98:295–296, 1968
7. CORPER HJ and UYEI N: Oxalic acid as a reagent for isolating tubercle bacilli and a study of the growth of acid fast non-pathogens on different mediums with their reactions to chemical reagents. J Lab Clin Med 15:348–369, 1930
8. COX FR, COX ME, and MARTIN JR: Rapid urease test for mycobacteria: preliminary observations. J Clin Microbiol 5:656–657, 1977
9. DUBOS RJ and MIDDLEBROOK G: Media for tubercle bacilli. Am Rev Tuberc 56:334–345, 1947
10. GOSLEE S, RYNEARSON TK, and WOLINSKY E: Additional serotypes of *Mycobacterium scrofulaceum, Mycobacterium gordonae, Mycobacterium marinum,* and *Mycobacterium xenopi* determined by agglutination. Int J Syst Bacteriol 26:136–142, 1976
11. GRANGE JM, ABER VR, ALLEN BW, MITCHISON DA, MIKHAIL JR, McSWIGGAN DW, and COLLINS CH: Comparison of strains of *Mycobacterium tuberculosis* from British, Ugandan and Asian patients: a study in bacteriophage typing, susceptibility to hydrogen peroxide and sensitivity to thiophen-2-carbonic acid hydrazide. Tubercle 58:207–215, 1977
12. HAWKINS JE, KARLSON AG, WAYNE LG, and WOLINSKY E: Quality of laboratory services for mycobacterial diseases. Am Rev Respir Dis 110:376–377, 1974
13. JENSEN KA: Reinzuchtung und Typenbestimmung von Tuberkelbazillenstammen. Eine Vereinfachung der Methoden fur die Praxis. Zentralbl Bakteriol Parasitenkd Infektionskr Hyg Abt 1 125:222–239, 1932
14. JONES WD JR: Differentiation of known strains of BCG from isolates of *Mycobacterium bovis*

and *Mycobacterium tuberculosis* by using mycobacteriophage 33D. J Clin Microbiol 1:391–392, 1975

15. JONES WD JR, ABBOTT VD, VESTAL AL, and KUBICA GP: A hitherto undescribed group of nonchromogenic mycobacteria. Am Rev Respir Dis 94:790–795, 1966

16. JONES WD JR and GREENBERG J: Use of phage F-φWJ-1 of *Mycobacterium fortuitum* to discern more phage types of *Mycobacterium tuberculosis*. J Clin Microbiol 3:324–326, 1976

17. JONES WD JR and GREENBERG J: Modification of methods used in bacteriophage typing of *Mycobacterium tuberculosis* isolates. J Clin Microbiol 7:467–469, 1978

18. JONES WD JR and KUBICA GP: The use of MacConkey's agar for the differential typing of *Mycobacterium fortuitum*. Am J Med Technol 30:187–190, 1964

19. KESTLE DG, ABBOTT VD, and KUBICA GP: Differential identification of mycobacteria. II. Subgroups of Groups II and III (Runyon) with different clinical significance. Am Rev Respir Dis 95:1041–1052, 1967

20. KILBURN JO and KUBICA GP: Reagent impregnated paper strips for detection of niacin. Am J Clin Pathol 50:530–532, 1968

21. KILBURN JO, O'DONNELL KF, SILCOX VA, and DAVID HL: Preparation of a stable mycobacterial Tween hydrolysis test substrate. Appl Microbiol 26:826, 1973

22. KILBURN JO, SILCOX VA, and KUBICA GP: Differential identification of mycobacteria. V. The tellurite reduction test. Am Rev Respir Dis 99:94–100, 1969

23. KUBICA GP, DYE WE, COHN ML, and MIDDLEBROOK G: Sputum digestion and decontamination with N-acetyl-L-cysteine-sodium hydroxide for culture of mycobacteria. Am Rev Respir Dis 87:775–779, 1963

24. KUBICA GP, GROSS WM, HAWKINS JE, SOMMERS HM, VESTAL AL, and WAYNE LG: Laboratory services for mycobacterial diseases. Am Rev Respir Dis 112:773–787, 1975

25. KUBICA GP, JONES WD JR, ABBOTT VD, BEAM RE, KILBURN JO, and CATER JC JR: Differential identification of mycobacteria. I. Tests on catalase activity. Am Rev Respir Dis 94:400–405, 1966

26. KUBICA GP and POOL GL: Studies on the catalase activity of acid-fast bacilli. I. An attempt to subgroup these organisms on the basis of their catalase activities at different temperatures and pH. Am Rev Respir Dis 81:387–391, 1960

27. MARKS J: A new practical classification of the mycobacteria. J Med Microbiol 9:253–262, 1976

28. McCLATCHY JK, WAGGONER RF, KANES W, CERNICH MS, and BOLTON TL: Isolation of mycobacteria from clinical specimens by use of selective 7H11 medium. Am J Clin Pathol 65:412–415, 1976

29. MEISSNER G and ANZ W: Sources of *Mycobacterium avium* complex infection resulting in human disease. Am Rev Respir Dis 116:1057–1064, 1977

30. MIDDLEBROOK G and COHN ML: Bacteriology of tuberculosis: laboratory methods. Am J Public Health 48:844–853, 1958

31. MITCHISON DA, ALLEN BW, CARROL L, DICKINSON JM, and ABER VR: A selective oleic acid albumin agar medium for tubercle bacilli. J Med Microbiol 5:165–175, 1972

32. MITCHISON DA, ALLEN BW, and LAMBERT RA: Selective media in the isolation of tubercle bacilli from tissues. J Clin Pathol 26:250–252, 1973

33. MURPHY DB and HAWKINS JE: Use of urease test disks in the identification of mycobacteria. J Clin Microbiol 1:465–468, 1975

34. NASSAU E, PARSONS ER, and JOHNSON GD: The detection of antibodies to *Mycobacterium tuberculosis* by microplate enzyme-linked immunosorbent assay (ELISA). Tubercle 57:67–70, 1976

35. PATTYN SR and PORTAELS F: Identification and clinical significance of mycobacteria. Zentralbl Bakteriol Parasitenkd Infektionskr Hyg Abt I 219:114–140, 1972

36. POLLOCK HM and WIEMAN EJ: Smear results in the diagnosis of mycobacterioses using blue-light fluorescence microscopy. J Clin Microbiol 5:329–331, 1977

37. RADO TA, BATES JH, ENGLE HWB, MANKIEWICZ E, MUROHASHI T, MIZUGUCHI Y, and SULA L: World Health Organization Studies on bacteriophage typing of mycobacteria. Subdivision of the species *Mycobacterium tuberculosis*. Am Rev Respir Dis 111:459–468, 1975

38. RICHARDS OW and MILLER DK: An efficient method for the identification of *M. tuberculosis* with a simple fluorescence microscope. Am J Clin Pathol 11 (Tech Sec 5): 1–8, 1941

39. RUNYON EH: Anonymous mycobacteria in human disease. Med Clin North Am 43:273–290, 1959

40. RUNYON EH: Ten mycobacterial pathogens. Tubercle 55:235–240, 1974
41. RUNYON EH, KARLSON AG, KUBICA GP, and WAYNE LG (revised by Sommers HM and McClatchy JK): Mycobacterium. *In* Manual of Clinical Microbiology 3rd edition. Lennette EH, Balows A, Hausler WJ Jr, and Truant JP (eds.). American Society for Microbiology, Washington, DC 1980, pp 150–179.
42. RUNYON EH, SELIN MJ, and HARRIS HW: Distinguishing mycobacteria by the niacin test. Am Rev Tuberc 79:663–665, 1959
43. SAITO H, GORDON RE, JUHLIN I, et al: Cooperative numerical analysis of rapidly growing mycobacteria: the second report. Int J Syst Bacteriol 27:75–85, 1977
44. SCHAEFER WB: Serologic identification and classification of the atypical mycobacteria by their agglutination. Am Rev Respir Dis 92:85–93, 1965
45. SMITHWICK RW: Laboratory Manual for Acid-Fast Microscopy, 2nd edition. US Dept of Health, Education, and Welfare, Center for Disease Control, Atlanta, Ga, 1976
46. SMITHWICK RW, STRATIGOS CB, and DAVID HL: Use of cetylpyridinium chloride and sodium chloride for the decontamination of sputum specimens that are transported to the laboratory for the isolation of *Mycobacterium tuberculosis.* J Clin Microbiol 1:411–413, 1975
47. STEADHAM JE: Reliable urease test for identification of mycobacteria. J Clin Microbiol 10:134–137, 1979
48. TIMPE A and RUNYON EH: The relationship of atypical acid-fast bacteria to human disease. J Lab Clin Med 44:202–209, 1954
49. TISON F, TACQUET A, and DEVULDER B: Un test simple d'étude des mycobacteries: La transformation du citrate de fer ammoniacal. Ann Inst Pasteur 106:797–801, 1964
50. TODA T, HAGIHARA Y, and TAKEYA K: A simple urease test for the classification of mycobacteria. Am Rev Respir Dis 83:757–761, 1961
51. VESTAL AL: Procedures for the Isolation and Identification of Mycobacteria. HEW Pub No (CDC) 77-8230, 1975
52. VESTAL AL and KUBICA GP: Differential identification of mycobacteria. III. Use of thiacetazone, thiophen-2-carboxylic acid hydrazide and triphenyltetrazolium chloride. Scand J Respir Dis 48:142–148, 1967
53. VIRTANEN S: A study of nitrate reduction by mycobacteria. Acta Tuberc Scand Suppl 48:1–119, 1960
54. WAYNE LG: Recognition of *Mycobacterium fortuitum* by means of the 3-day phenolphthalein sulfatase test. Am J Clin Pathol 36:185–197, 1961
55. WAYNE LG: Simple pyrazinamidase and urease tests for routine identification of mycobacteria. Am Rev Respir Dis 109:147–151, 1974
56. WAYNE LG and DOUBEK JR: Diagnostic key to mycobacteria encountered in clinical laboratories. Appl Microbiol 16:925–931, 1968
57. WAYNE LG, DOUBEK JR, and RUSSELL RL: Classification and identification of mycobacteria. I. Tests employing Tween 80 as substrate. Am Rev Respir Dis 90:588–597, 1964
58. WAYNE LG, ENGBAEK HC, ENGEL HWB, et al: Highly reproducible techniques for use in systematic bacteriology in the Genus *Mycobacterium:* Tests for pigment, urease, resistance to sodium chloride, hydrolysis of Tween 80, and β-galactosidase. Int J Syst Bacteriol 24:412–419, 1974
59. WAYNE LG, ENGEL HWB, GRASSI C, et al: Highly reproducible techniques for use in systematic bacteriology in the Genus *Mycobacterium:* Tests for niacin and catalase and for resistance to isoniazid, thiophene-2-carboxylic acid hydrazide, hydroxylamine, and p-nitrobenzoate. Int J Syst Bacteriol 26:311–318, 1976
60. WAYNE LG and KRASNOW I: Preparation of tuberculosis susceptibility testing mediums by means of impregnated disks. Am J Clin Pathol 45:769–771, 1966
61. WAYNE LG, KRASNOW I, and KIDD GC: Finding the "hidden positive" in tuberculosis eradication programs. The role of sensitive trisodium phosphate-benzalkonium (zephiran) culture technique. Am Rev Respir Dis 86:537–541, 1962
62. WOLINSKY E and SCHAEFER WB: Proposed numbering scheme for mycobacterial serotypes by agglutination. Int J Syst Bacteriol 23:182–183, 1973
63. YOUNG WD JR, MASLANSKY A, LEFAR MS, and KRONISH DP: Development of a paper strip test for detection of niacin produced by mycobacteria. Appl Microbiol 20:939–945, 1970

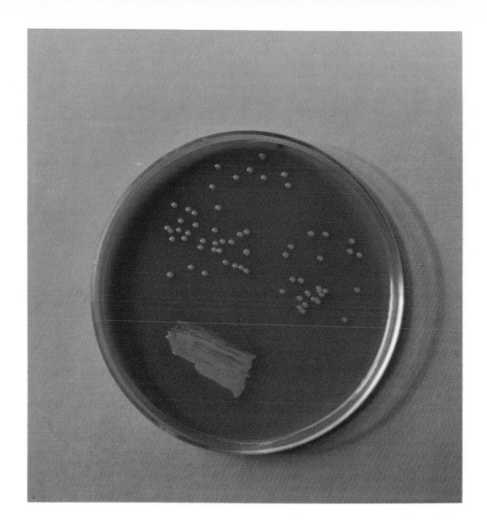

Figure 41.1.—Cystine-glucose-blood agar plate inoculated with *Francisella tularensis.* The colonies are of 96-hr growth. The large growth mass arose in 24 hr from a smear of an infected mouse spleen.

Introduction

Tularemia is an infectious disease caused by *Francisella tularensis.* Clinical symptoms can vary, and the disease has been called various colloquial names including "rabbit fever," "deerfly fever," and "plague-like disease of rodents" (21). Over the years, the causative organism has been thought to belong to the genus *Bacterium,* followed by *Pasteurella* and *Brucella,* and now to *Francisella,* order Eubacteriales. *Bergey's Manual of Determinative Bacteriology* (16) lists *Francisella* under "Genera of uncertain affiliation in the Gram-negative aerobic rods and cocci."

Causative Organism

The organism has been described as a very small coccoid to ellipsoid pleomorphic rod, nonmotile, and gram-negative. Rod and coccal forms with dimensions of 0.2 μm by 0.2 μm to 0.7 μm are common, whereas bizarre forms such as ribbons, buds, balloon, and filamentous cells have been described (22). The organisms occur singly; capsules are rare or absent. It is a strict aerobe and requires an enriched medium for propagation. It is not strongly resistant to physical or chemical disinfection; however, it is extremely infectious, and suspected specimens should be handled with great care. The organism will remain viable for long periods at low temperatures in suitable substrates such as water, soil, and animal tissues.

On suitable bacteriological media, colonies are round, with entire edges and smooth, shiny surfaces. They are gray to blue-white with a creamy or buttery consistency and adhere to the surface of the medium. Their growth sticks to the oese when touched and is easily disrupted to form a smooth suspension in an aqueous solution. On cystine-glucose-blood agar (CGBA) a small zone of partial hemolysis usually surrounds the colonies. A colony mass from a large inoculum can be seen at 24 hr of incubation, but single colonies often require 2–4 days to reach a diameter of 1 mm (Fig 41.1). Smooth and nonsmooth variants occur; the latter are believed to be of attenuated virulence (17). However, this concept has not been totally accepted.

Clinical Manifestations

Tularemia in humans is highly variable depending upon route of infection, the infecting dose, and the subspecies of the organism involved.

The ulceroglandular form is the most common (constituting about 80% of the reported cases), with a slowly healing ulcer at the site of entry and regional lymph node involvement. This infection often results from injury while handling infected animal carcasses or from the bite of an infected blood-sucking arthropod such as a tick or fly. Sometimes no ulcer can be found, possibly because it is obscured by body hair or absent, as *F. tularensis* has been shown to penetrate the intact skin (20).

Oculoglandular tularemia can result from rubbing contaminated materials into the eyes (8). Conjunctivitis occurs, and regional lymph nodes may enlarge and suppurate.

The pulmonary or pneumonic form of tularemia can result from inhaling infectious aerosol or dust. Pneumonia and pleuritis which sometimes accompany severe tularemia (regardless of the source) indicate a poor prognosis.

Typhoidal, gastrointestinal, and oropharyngeal infections leading to "penicillin resistant tonsillopharyngitis" (7), pseudomembranous ulcerative colitis (4), and other unique syndromes can be caused by ingesting the organism, e.g., as in laboratory accidents.

The incubation period, which averages about 3 days, is followed by sudden onset of flu-like symptoms. Often vomiting and diarrhea accompany the headache, fever, prostration, and generalized aching. The primary ulcer, if present and untreated, is slow to heal and becomes punched-out in appearance; the regional lymph nodes enlarge and become tender. Exanthem, infrequently present, occurs on the upper body, neck, face, and limbs. It usually appears during the first or second week and persists for 2–3 weeks.

Chronic tularemia, i.e., purulent adenitis, was common before the era of antibiotics and still occurs when patients are inadequately treated with tetracyclines (1).

Rarely, an infection caused by ingesting insufficiently cooked infected meat (such as wild rabbit) or inhaling a large number of type A organisms produces a fulminating, fatal disease (9). With such infections—human or animal and regardless of the route of infection—all exudates, excreta, and secreta contain numerous bacilli and are extremely infectious. However, person-to-person transmission is very rare (13).

Epidemiology

Tularemia is primarily a disease of wild animals. It is a plague-like disease of rodents and lagomorphs, perpetuated among the host animals by their ectoparasites, cannibalism, or contaminated habitat. Early names such as "rabbit fever" and "glandular type of tick fever" reveal the most common sources of human infection. However, many mammals, birds, and blood-sucking arthropods have also been infected with *F. tularensis*. Man is only incidentally involved; persons engaged in outdoor activities which expose them to infected ticks, animals, or their habitat risk contracting tularemia.

There are two generally recognized subspecies, *Francisella tularensis tularensis* (type A) and *Francisella tularensis palaearctica* (type B). Subspecies differ in degree of virulence for domestic rabbits (*Oryctolagus cuniculi*), in the kinds of animals involved in the natural cycles, and in certain metabolic characteristics. There is a current effort to designate other subspecies that produce characteristic diseases peculiar to geographic location. Antigenically, the two subspecies are indistinguishable.

F. tularensis tularensis (type A) is the more virulent of the two subspecies. It is referred to as the tick-deerfly-rabbit-sheep type and occurs naturally only in North America. Rabbits will succumb to one to 10 viable organisms inoculated parenterally. The organism produces an even more serious disease in humans, accounting for most reported cases in North America. The fatality rate among patients untreated with antibiotics is 5%–7%. *F. tularensis tularensis* utilizes glycerol and possesses the enzyme citrullineureidase (14).

F. tularensis palaearctica (type B) is referred to as the beaver-muskrat-water type and is found in most countries of the Northern Hemisphere. It is the less virulent of the two subspecies; rabbits will survive parenteral inoculation with very large numbers of organisms (2). It produces a mild, often subclinical, disease in humans, possibly accounting for the discrepancy between the number of seroreactors and reported cases. Beavers, muskrats, and voles succumb in large numbers during epizootics, releasing the organisms into the soil and water of their habitat. Chronic shedding nephritis among voles has been demonstrated (3). Type B organisms have frequently been isolated from natural running water (18).

These animal associations are not rigid, and epidemiologic findings can only provide a basis for presumptive identification of the subspecies involved. Many other mammals, birds, reptiles, and arthropods have been found infected.

Public Health Significance

In the Soviet Union, where large epidemics of tularemia have occurred among agricultural workers, mass vaccination with an attenuated strain of live *F. tularensis* type B has apparently been very successful (15, 25). A live vaccine is available in the United States on a strictly controlled basis for occupationally exposed individuals. Beaver and muskrat trappers, rabbit hunters, butchers, sheepherders, and laboratory and veterinary workers are considered to be occupationally exposed. Except among the last two groups, however, many infections are inapparent or are misdiagnosed. For example, of the members of a large group of trappers who were skin-tested and bled for serologic tests, 78% of the reactors had no history of or recollection of a tularemia-like illness (19).

Laboratory infections are common; tularemia has been a leading laboratory-acquired infection since its general recognition in the 1920s. Unvaccinated laboratory personnel should be extremely careful when handling infectious material. However, protective clothing, mask- and face-shielding, and proper bacteriologic techniques minimize the risk of laboratory infection, and qualified individuals should not be discouraged from attempting isolations.

In the western United States, specific diagnosis differentiating tularemia from plague is especially important (23). Pneumonic plague can be transmitted from person to person and can be a serious problem in a hospital. Early treatment with antibiotics has greatly reduced reported morbidity and mortality from tularemia. Because of wide use of antibiotics and rapid recovery from disease, the source of the infection is often overlooked. This could be an important reason for the fairly rapid decline in the number of reported cases of tularemia since streptomycin was introduced in 1946.

F. tularensis is quite susceptible to disinfection. It can be killed with heating to 56 C for 10 min. As little as 0.4 ppm chlorine in water (5) or a minute amount of detergent will also kill it.

Collection and Processing of Specimens

Blood specimens for serologic tests should be taken according to the fundamental principles for measuring antibody titers; an acute-phase specimen should be taken as soon as the infection is suspected or the patient begins treatment, and a convalescent-phase specimen should be obtained not less than 2 nor optimally more than 3 weeks after onset.

Blood is usually not a good source of isolates, because the organism is present in the bloodstream only during acute septicemia. Sputum or scrapings from the walls of abscessed nodes or ulcers or conjunctiva (if there is ocular involvement) should be taken before antibiotics are given. Additional specimens should be taken if there are signs of complications such as rapid enlargement of liver and spleen or intermittent or continuous high fever.

Suspected material to which the patient has been exposed, such as domestic and wild animal carcasses, untreated water, and biting arthropods (ticks) can readily be tested. Animal carcasses must be handled very carefully, because they can contain numerous organisms.

Since *F. tularensis* is resistant to penicillin, this antibiotic has been used to reduce the number of contaminating penicillin-susceptible organisms in a specimen. This practice should be followed only when the specimen is known to be heavily contaminated and only for that portion of the specimen to be used for isolating *F. tularensis,* because the specimen might then be unsuitable for isolating other pathogens.

Diagnostic Procedures

Microscopic Examination

Conventional microscopic examination of suspected material is of little diagnostic value except for demonstrating that the organism is gram-negative. The organism is extremely small and is not easily differentiated against the background staining of most tissue preparations. Polychromatic stains such as

Giemsa or hematoxylin-eosin show that the organisms occur singly or in clumps both intracellularly and extracellularly and that they have a hint of bipolar staining. Stained preparations of exudates or tissues of infected laboratory animals may contain enormous numbers of organisms.

Direct fluorescent antibody tests can be quickly and reliably performed with smears of biopsy material or exudates (10). Specific fluorescein-conjugated antiserum or a complete diagnostic reagent kit for fluorescent antibody test with associated technical information is available commercially.

Selection and Inoculation of Specimens

Primary isolation from a specimen may be difficult, even though it may contain large numbers of *F. tularensis;* contaminating organisms can easily overgrow cultures or produce enough acid to prevent growth of *F. tularensis* on the enriched media needed for isolation.

Solid coagulated egg yolk medium described by Francis (6), liquid medium described by Snyder et al. (24), and thioglycolate medium support growth of *F. tularensis* but usually require large inocula. Cystine glucose blood agar (CGBA) is the medium of choice. It is available commercially or can be prepared in the laboratory (see Media).

Isolates can be obtained readily by the subcutaneous inoculation of specimens into mice, hamsters, or cavies. If the material is grossly contaminated, inoculation by scarification is preferred. The animals usually succumb in 5–8 days if 1 to 10 viable organisms are inoculated. The experimental host can be sacrificed at 2–3 days, and pure cultures can be obtained from the spleen by subinoculation onto suitable bacteriological media.

Animals should be inoculated only under proper isolation conditions, because the entire environment can become infectious. All secreta and excreta can be infectious, contaminating the bedding, food, water, etc., and there is the accompanying risk of aerosol.

Necropsy of animals with fatal tularemia reveals a typically enlarged liver and spleen, sometimes with white necrotic foci of infection. Lungs are often consolidated and associated with a frothy fluid. Sometimes there is an excess amber serous peritoneal exudate. All of the above tissues and fluids are highly infectious and should be good source material for further testing by animal inoculation, direct culture, modified Ascoli (11), and direct fluorescent antibody techniques.

Identification Procedures

The blue-gray colonies which appear on CGBA in 24–96 hr at 37 C (Fig 41.1) are suggestive of *F. tularensis.* Poor or no growth on blood-containing media without cystine and complete lack of growth on ordinary media are useful guides for bacteriologic diagnosis. A closely related organism, *Francisella novicida,* is similar to *F. tularensis* in many ways, but it will grow well on blood agar without cystine. The pathogenicity of *F. novicida* for man is unknown, and the organism is so infrequently found in nature that it is not likely to be confused with *F. tularensis* (16).

Biochemical reactions are of little value in diagnosing tularemia. The organism may utilize dextrose, glycerol, maltose, mannitol, and fructose, and produces acid but no gas. If the possible source of infection is of epidemiologic interest, the test for utilization of glycerol would differentiate types A and B. The medium used is cystine-heart agar without blood but with 1% glycerol and enough bromthymol-blue indicator to give a distinct green color. Utilization is shown by a color change to yellow (acid) and indicates that the isolate is the more virulent type A. Type B isolates usually turn the medium dark blue (alkaline) or sometimes cause no change.

Serologic Procedures

Many serologic tests have been used in studying tularemia. Tube agglutination is the most useful procedure for demonstrating the presence of or rise in antibody titer. Slide agglutination is often used for measuring antibody titer or for identifying a culture. The precipitin test can be used to measure antibody titer and demonstrate the presence of antigen. Hemagglutination and complement-fixation tests have been described but have limited use. Skin tests have been used experimentally for determining prevalence of past infection in large populations.

Identifying an Isolate

The slide agglutination test is the most rapid method of identification. Kits and reagents are available commercially. A glass slide divided in half by a wax pencil mark will keep the anti-*tularensis* serum and the normal serum separated. A drop of an emulsified suspected colony is placed on each side of the wax line and mixed with the respective sera, with care being taken to keep them separate. The slide is tilted to and fro over a narrow light source. Flocculation in the antiserum suspension and homogeneity in the control indicate a positive test. By diluting an unknown serum and using a known antigen, the titer of the former can be determined. However, the tube agglutination test described later is preferred for this function.

The precipitin test is useful for grossly contaminated, even decayed specimens, such as spleens and livers of naturally infected field-collected animals. The specimen is ground in a mortar with sand and 2–3 volumes of saline. A modified Ascoli antigen (11) is extracted by boiling the suspension gently for 5 min. It is then centrifuged for 30 min at 6000 × g or filtered through paper (Whatman No. 4), and the clear fluid is retained. The test is performed by drawing known anti-*tularensis* serum up to about a third the length of a capillary tube. The tube is wiped with gauze. A similar amount of antigen is drawn into the tube, the tube is inverted, and the end is inserted into plasticine. The top of the tube is capped with a pledget of plasticine. Tubes are incubated at 37 C for 2 hr and refrigerated overnight. The bottoms of columns should be checked for the presence of precipitate. Twofold dilutions of serum or antigen can be made in saline, depending upon which component is to be tested. This test is specific, and no cross-reactions with other agents have been reported.

Patients' Sera

The tube agglutination test is the standard procedure used in most diagnostic laboratories for determining antibody titer. The antigen can be obtained commercially or can be prepared in the laboratory (see Antigen). When possible acute- and convalescent-phase sera should be tested simultaneously. A known positive and a known negative serum should be included as controls. Six agglutination tubes are placed in a rack for each sample. In tube 1, 0.9 ml of saline is placed; 0.5 ml is placed in each of the others. The test serum (0.1 ml) is added to tube 1 and mixed thoroughly; 0.5 ml is transferred in a clean pipette from tube 1 to tube 2 and mixed. This procedure is continued, tube by tube, through tube 6, with 0.5 ml of the mixture finally being discarded from tube 6. Sometimes a 7th tube is used, and this 0.5 ml of mixture is held, without added antigen, for further dilution if no end point is obtained. The standardized antigen (0.5 ml) is added to each tube and shaken thoroughly. The final serum dilutions are now 1:20, 1:40 . . . 1:640. The tubes are incubated in a 56 C water bath for 2 hr and refrigerated overnight. Results of each tube are read as 4+ to 1+ agglutination or negative.

4+ = water clear supernatant and compact sediment.

3+ = slightly turbid supernatant and compact sediment.

2+ = turbid supernatant and dispersible floccular sediment.

1+ = floccular turbidity only.

Negative = as homogeneous as the known negative serum.

Only 2+ to 4+ results are reported as positive, and the end point is the highest dilution of serum causing such agglutination.

A microagglutination test has been described (12) that promises to save time and material.

Interpretation of Results

A titer of <20 is considered negative. Titers of 20 to 80 are maintained for years by people with no history of the disease. A 4-fold rise in titer from acute to convalescent phase of illness or a convalescent titer of at least 160 is diagnostic for tularemia. Titers of 320 or 640 are common, and even patients who were treated with streptomycin often attain titers of 10,240 or higher.

The diagnostician should be aware that organisms of the genus *Brucella* sometimes cross-react with anti-*F. tularensis* serum and vice versa, but at a much lower titer (20–40). Cross-reacting antibodies usually do not show as high a titer as the specific tularemia titer during an active infection.

Serologic diagnosis is of limited value in determining the course of therapy because of the delay in appearance of agglutinating antibodies (usually 10 days to 2 weeks after onset of illness).

Antibiotic Susceptibility

Streptomycin is the drug of choice, and if used properly, can result in prompt and complete recovery. However, streptomycin-resistant variants have been found. Tetracyclines are quite effective, but relapses and chronic infections have been associated with their use. Chloramphenicol and kanamycin are effective but because of their potential toxicity are not used except in special circumstances. Penicillin and sulfonamides have no effect on the disease.

Bacteriologically, confusion of *F. tularensis* with any other pathogen or incidental bacterium is very unlikely. An organism that fits the morphologic and cultural description and reacts with specific anti-*F. tularensis* serum should be reported as *F. tularensis*. Repeated negative cultures do not exclude tularemia, because the organism can be very elusive. Specific diagnosis is usually based on demonstrating an antibody response. This author believes that many patients are treated and cured by serendipity, without their disease ever being correctly diagnosed.

Most reported tularemia infections are diagnosed by the inordinately few physicians who are aware of the disease and are looking for it.

Antigen for Tube Agglutination Test

The attentuated strain *F. tularensis,* Jap, is used. A 48-hr culture on CGBA (usually several Blake bottles) is harvested and washed several times in saline containing 0.5% formalin, centrifuging each time for 1 hr at 35,000 × g. Finally, the pellet of bacterial cells is suspended in twice its volume of the formol-saline for storage. It should be tested for sterility at this point. This stock antigen can be stored for years at 4 C. It is diluted 1:300 when used for tube agglutination antigen.

Media

At the Rocky Mountain Laboratory, cystine-glucose-blood agar is prepared from dehydrated cystine-heart-agar with glucose. After it is rehydrated, the medium is autoclaved and placed in a 60 C water bath until the temperature has equalized. Defibrinated rabbit blood (5%) is added, and the mixture is held at 60 C for 1 hr with occasional shaking before it is dispensed. The medium should be incubated for several days at 37 C to insure sterility and to remove excess moisture. The final medium should be a light-milk-chocolate-color (Fig 41.1). Variations from this color can indicate an inferior medium which will support less luxuriant growth of *F. tularensis*. The source of rabbit blood should be carefully examined, as commercial rabbit feed often contains antibiotics inhibitory to *F. tularensis*, and breeders rely heavily on medicated feed to maintain healthy rabbit colonies.

Addendum in Proof

Two recent articles dealing with the diagnosis of tularemia have come to my attention:

BERDAL B and SØDERLUND E: Brief reports: Cultivation and isolation of *Francisella tularensis* on selective chocolate agar as used routinely for the isolation of gonococci. Acta Pathol Microbiol Scand Sect B 85:108–109, 1977

CUNHA B and QUINTILIANI R: The atypical pneumonias. Postgrad Med, Vol 66, No. 3, September 1979

Berdal and Søderland observed luxuriant growth of *F. tularensis* after 10 repeated passes on Thayer-Martin derivative CLNT-agar (chocolate agar with colistin, 7.5 µg/ml, nystatin, 12.5 µg/ml, lincomycin, 0.5 µg/ml, and trimethoprim lactate, 5 µg/ml, added). *F. tularensis* was introduced into 10 different cultures of mixed flora from human throat subcultures. *Streptococcus* sp., *Micrococcus* sp., and diphtheroids were prominent in the mixture. *F. tularensis* could be reisolated from 6 of the 10 mixtures. Use of this medium, especially if it is already on hand for the isolation of gonococci, could be of great value in isolating *F. tularensis* from its associated contaminants.

Cunha and Quintiliani reported that the roentgenographic features of pleuropulmonary tularemia are variable; however, the presence of bilateral hilar adenopathy is characteristic only of this organism. But due to the potential severity of atypical pneumonia early treatment is essential and other elusive etiologic agents must be considered. See chapters on *Legionella, Mycoplasma,* Q fever, and psittacosis (as apply), or the excellent review by Cunha and Quintiliani comparing features of pleuropulmonary tularemia and other atypical pneumonias (with proper referrals).

References

1. BELL JF: Tularemia. *In* Steele JH (ed). CRC Handbook Series in Zoonoses. CRC Press, Inc., Boca Raton, 2:161–193, 1980
2. BELL JF, OWEN CR, and LARSON CL: Virulence of *Bacterium tularense*. I. A study of virulence of *Bacterium tularense* in mice, guinea pigs, and rabbits. J Infect Dis 97:162–166, 1955
3. BELL JF and STEWART SJ: Chronic shedding tularemia nephritis in rodents: Possible relation to occurrence of *Francisella tularensis* in lotic waters. J Wildl Dis 11:421–430, 1975
4. EMMONS RW, RUSKIN J, BISSETT MJ, UYEDA DA, WOOD RM, and LEAR CL: Tularemia in a mule deer. J Wildl Dis 12:459–463, 1976
5. FOOTE HB, JELLISON WL, STEINHAUSE EA, and KOHLS GM: Effect of chlorination on *Pasteurella tularensis* in aqueous suspension. J Am Water Works Assoc 35 (7):902–910, 1943
6. FRANCIS E: Cultivation of *Bacterium tularense* on mediums new to this organism. Hyg Lab Bull #130, March, 1922
7. FULGINITI VA and HOYLE C: Oropharyngeal tularemia. Rocky Mount Med J 63 (2):41–42, 67, 1966
8. GUERRANT RL, HUMPHRIES MK, BUTLER JE, and JACKSON RS: Tickborne ocularglandular tularemia. Arch Intern Med 136:811–813
9. JELLISON WJ: Tularemia in North America. University of Montana, Missoula, 1974
10. KARLSSON KA, DAHLSTRAND S, HANKO E, and SÖDERLIND O: Demonstration of *Francisella tularensis* (syn. *Pasteurella tularensis*) in sylvan animals with the aid of fluorescent antibodies. Acta Pathol Microbiol Scand Section B 78:647–651, 1970
11. LARSON CL: Studies on thermostable antigens extracted from *Bacterium tularense* and from tissues of animals dead of tularemia. J Immunol 66:249, 1951
12. MASSEY ED and MANGIAFICO JA: Microagglutination test for detecting and measuring serum agglutinins of *Francisella tularensis*. Appl Microbiol 27:25–27, 1974
13. MCCRUMB FR JR: Aerosol infection of man with *Pasteurella tularensis*. Bacteriol Rev 25:262–267, 1961
14. MILLER LG: Further studies on tularemia in Alaska: Virulence and biochemical characteristics of indigenous strains. Can J Microbiol 20:1585–1590, 1974
15. OGARKOV IP, BELYAEV PA, AL'MYASEV KKH, and BOL'SHAKOV VN: Notes from practice.

Features of outbreaks of tularemia in the Urals and the Ural Region in 1957. Zh Mikrobiol Epidemiol Immunobiol 31(9):131–134, 1960

16. OWEN CR: *In* Bergey's Manual of Determinative Bacteriology, 8th edition. Buchanan RE and Gibbons NE (eds.). Williams & Wilkins Co, Baltimore, 1974, p 283

17. OWEN CR, BELL JF, LARSON CL, and ORMSBEE RA: Virulence of *Bacterium tularense*. II. Evaluation of criteria of virulence of *Bacterium tularense*. J Infect Dis 97:167–176, 1955

18. PARKER RR, STEINHAUS EA, KOHLS GM, and JELLISON WL: Contamination of natural waters and mud with *Pasteurella tularensis* and tularemia in beavers and muskrats in the northwestern United States. Natl Inst Health Bull No. 193, 1951

19. PHILIP RN, CASPER EA, and LACKMAN DP: The skin test in epidemiologic study of tularemia in Montana trappers. J Infect Dis 117(5):393–403, 1967

20. QUAN SF, MCMANUS AG, and VON FINTEL H: Infectivity of tularemia applied to intact skin and ingested in drinking water. Science 123:942–943, 1956

21. REILLY JR: Tularemia. *In* Infectious Diseases of Wild Mammals. Davis JW, Karstad LH, and Trainer DO (eds.). Iowa State University Press, Ames, 1970, p 175

22. RIBI E and SHEPPARD C: Morphology of *Bacterium tularense* during its growth cycle in liquid medium as revealed by the electron microscope. Exp Cell Res 8:474–487, 1955

23. SITES VR, POLAND JD, and HUDSON BW: Bubonic plague misdiagnosed as tularemia. J Am Med Assoc 222(13):1642–1643, 1972

24. SNYDER TL, PENFIELD RA, ENGLEY FB, and CREASY JC: Cultivation of *Bacterium tularense* in peptone media. Proc Soc Exp Biol Med 63:26–30, 1946

25. UGLOVOI GP: Epidemiological features of a winter outbreak of tularemia and an attempt to terminate it. Zh Mikrobiol Epidemiol Immunobiol 31(9):139–140, 1960

CHAPTER 42

VIBRIO INFECTIONS

Harry L. Smith, Jr.

Cholera

Although cholera is rarely seen in the United States, travelers can acquire the infection abroad and the disease at home. An awareness of this possibility is important for the physician and the laboratory analyst who deal with diarrheal disease. A second point is that the diagnosis of cholera does not require special skills, media, etc. Only one reagent—cholera diagnostic serum—is not found in most laboratories. In this chapter, the materials at hand will be emphasized, and specialized media will be given second place.

Recently taxonomists (11) have helped clarify the strict taxonomic classification of vibrios. Clinicians and others may still be confused on the characteristics of *Vibrio cholerae* and whether it causes cholera. On the basis of orthodox and numerical classifications and results of DNA studies (18), most vibrios are designated *Vibrio cholerae* whether they are isolated from feces, water, or other sources. The organisms are then serotyped on the basis of somatic antigens. Those which react with O group 1 serum would correspond to cholera vibrios. Organisms which do not agglutinate in this serum but do so in the other sera included in this set would be designated *V. cholerae* serotype 2, 3, or 4, etc. In the past they were designated as nonagglutinable (NAG), noncholera vibrios (NCVs), cholera-like vibrios, etc.

The author prefers to follow the old schema, in which *V. cholerae* is used to designate organisms which fit the basic criteria for *Vibrio* and are agglutinated by cholera polyvalent (group) serum. The other vibrios, which are discussed later, will be designated "noncholera vibrios (NCVs)."

Description of Causative Agent

Vibrio cholerae is a facultative, gram-negative rod, with varying degrees of curvature. Its definitive characteristics are listed in Tables 42.1 and 42.2; it is agglutinated by cholera polyvalent antiserum.

Clinical Description of Disease

Cholera, in its most severe form, is characterized by sudden onset of an intestinal flux, with large losses of fluid and electrolytes. The resulting hypovo-

TABLE 42.1—MINIMAL NUMBER OF CHARACTERISTICS USED FOR IDENTIFYING *VIBRIO* SPECIES

Indophenol oxidase	+
Glucose fermented gas	+
L-lysine decarboxylase	+
L-ornithine decarboxylase	+
Gram-negative asporogenous rod	
Polar, monotrichous	

lemia leads to shock and death if untreated. Fever or tenesmus is not seen. The stool, described as "rice water," has no fecal odor.

The colonization of the gut lumen by cholera vibrios may produce disease ranging from the acute form just described to an asymptomatic carrier condiiton.

Epidemiology

In recent years cholera has spread in all directions from Bengal. The Western Hemisphere appears to be spared, but other areas which the disease has reached have become seeded with the organisms. Travelers to these areas may acquire infections there and develop symptoms when they return home.

Public Health Significance

Any *V. cholerae* isolate from a person or an environmental sample has marked public health significance. Case reports are universally required by the International Health Regulations. Methods for control are outlined in the *Control of Communicable Diseases in Man,* 12th Edition (4).

If the laboratory uses the taxonomist's designation of *V. cholerae,* its re-

TABLE 42.2—ADDITIONAL BIOCHEMICAL TESTS FOR CHARACTERIZING *V. CHOLERAE*

TEST	REACTION
"String" test	+
Sucrose	+
Arabinose	−
Mannose	+
Inositol	−
Gelatin	+
Indole	+
Nitrite from nitrate	+
MR	±
VP	±
Urea	−
Vibriocin inhibition (0/129)	+
H_2S in TSI	−
Growth in 6% NaCl broth	−

port should stress whether the isolate is a vibrio which causes or is likely to cause cholera.

Collection of Specimens

Stool samples are preferred. They should be obtained with sterile rectal catheters rather than in receptacles which could contain residual disinfectants. Rectal swabs can be used for patients with acute cases but are of little value for convalescent patients or persons suspected of being carriers. The swab must be rectal and not perianal.

If the specimen cannot be cultured immediately, it should be placed in transport medium. Sterile 1% gelatin-1% NaCl (pH 7.2) in a screw-capped tube has worked well in field and laboratory experiments. The transport medium of Monsur (15) or the commercially available Cary and Blair medium can be used.

Specimens must not be refrigerated. Vibrios are very sensitive to cold.

Bacteriological Procedures

Direct microscopic examination

Smears of the rice-water stool of patients with acute cholera may show actively motile organisms in wet mounts and gram-negative rods, vibrios, and spirillar organisms when stained. The organisms cannot be definitively identified as *V. cholerae* solely on this basis. However, Benenson et al. (5) have observed a portion of the rice-water stool under darkfield and then added specific anticholera serum and directly observed the cessation of motility and clumping. The organisms can be identified and serotyped rapidly if reagents are available.

Cultural procedures

A generalized scheme for the isolation of vibrios is shown in Figure 42.1. The critical factor in the success of this procedure is that the physician and/or laboratory analyst suspect the presence of *V. cholerae*. If the stool specimen is inoculated on what might be called "routine" enteric media (MacConkey, EMB, SS, etc.), vibrios are less likely to be isolated. With these media, the number of CFU's seen will be only about 25% of that seen with the nonselective media described below.

Vibrio cholerae does not have exotic requirements for its growth. Strains grow quite well on nonselective media. Gelatin-agar (23) is used in our laboratory because it is easy to prepare from materials in the laboratory (1% Trypticase, 1% NaCl, 3% Bacto-gelatin, 1.8% agar). *V. cholerae* rapidly degrades gelatin and forms a turbid zone around colony within 24 hr. TCBS (thiosulfate-citrate-bile salts-sucrose) agar is commercially available, does not have to be heated to 121 C for 15 min to be sterilized, and produces yellow colonies as indication of sucrose utilization. However, Gangarosa et al. (8) and Balows et al. (2) noted that this selective medium is not a suitable direct source of organisms for slide agglutination tests (*vide infra*).

Suspected colonies can be presumptively identified as *V. cholerae* quickly.

A portion the the colony being tested is rubbed on a microscope slide, and a loopful of 0.5% sodium deoxycholate is added. The analyst attempts to suspend the cells in the fluid. If the organisms produce an even turbidity which persists for at least 1 min, the test is negative. If the organisms lyse so that little if any turbidity develops and the fluid becomes mucoid such that a "string" is seen when the loop is slowly raised, the "string" test is positive (22). The selected colony(ies) is then tested for agglutinability in polyvalent (group) cholera serum, if available. Positive clumping of the organisms provides an adequate basis for designating the organisms *V. cholerae.*

Confirmatory tests are based upon characteristics selected from the minimal list (see Table 42.1) accepted by the International Committee on Systematic Bacteriology (11). The biochemical tests listed in Table 42.2 are used for further characterization and differentiation.

Serological procedures

Cholera can be diagnosed retrospectively. The simplest procedure is to document agglutinins to live cholera vibrios. A fourfold rise in titer between acute-phase serum and that collected 10 to 14 days later is considered diagnostic (9).

Nobechi (16) described three serotypes of *V. cholerae*—Ogawa, Inaba, and Hikojima. Kauffmann (12) listed the antigenic formulae as follows:

Ogawa   = AB
Inaba   = AC
Hikojima = ABC

Absorbed sera must be used in serotyping cholera cultures. Although this procedure adds little to the laboratory or clinical aspects of the disease, it does give the epidemiologist the finer distinction among strains which they may need in epidemiologic tracing.

Antimicrobic Susceptibility and Resistance

As indicated by Carpenter et al. (6), adequate amounts of fluids allow most patients to recover from cholera rapidly. Tetracycline given in four equal portions of 40–50 mg/kg body weight each day for 2 days reduces the duration and volume of the diarrhea and rapidly removes the organisms from the stool.

Noncholera Vibrios and *V. parahaemolyticus*

Description of Causative Agents

The organisms are classified as vibrios according to the characteristics shown in Table 42.1. Not included are the organisms previously known as *Vibrio fetus* and now designated as *Campylobacter fetus.* The name "noncholera vibrios (NCVs)" rather than "nonagglutinable (NAG)" is used for the vibrios because, although not agglutinated by cholera polyvalent serum (O group 1), these organisms can be clumped by sera prepared against them and used for serotyping.

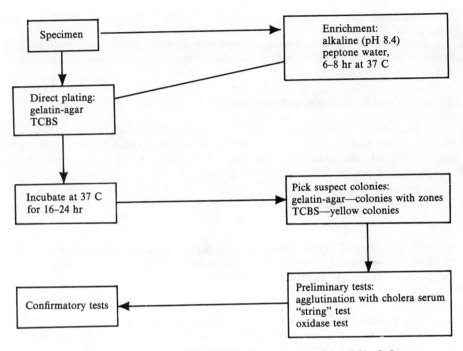

Figure 42.1—Scheme for the isolation and identification of *V. cholerae.*

Vibrio parahaemolyticus is included in this discussion, although there is some question as to whether it is actually a vibrio (3). It has been described as "halophilic" (17), i.e., able to grow in the presence of 6% NaCl.

Clinical Description of Diseases

A broad range of human diseases is associated with these organisms. Intestinal infections mimic the spectrum seen with cholera vibrios, from severe "cholera-like" diarrheas to no symptoms of illness. Both NCV's (1, 13) and *V. parahaemolyticus* (17) have been incriminated.

When the histories of cultures received by our laboratory from workers throughout the world were reviewed, there was evidence that noncholera vibrios are associated with bacteremia, otitis media, and wound infections.

Epidemiology

The epidemiology of human infections caused by noncholera vibrios is an area which needs much work. Study of the ecology of these organisms may indicate the possible sources of human infection. Water is often incriminated as the source of infection. Such things as salinity of water, time of year, depth, etc., are factors which influence the distribution of vibrios (7). One must also question whether the natural habitat is water and the animals in it.

Public Health Significance

Because many laboratories in this country do not consider vibrios during isolation procedures, the significance of these organisms in public health matters is largely unknown.

Collection and Processing of Specimens

The procedures described in the preceding section on *V. cholerae* are applicable when dealing with fecal samples. Specimens taken from materials such as wounds and exudates should be obtained by usual techniques. The sample should not be chilled or allowed to dry.

Bacteriological Procedures

Direct microscopic examination

The presence of highly motile rods in wet-mount preparations of specimens or gram-negative curved rods in stained smears should suggest the need for medium which will support the growth of vibrios.

Cultural procedures

Primary isolation procedures described in the preceding section for vibrios are suitable for NCV's and *V. parahaemolyticus*. The halophilic nature of the latter is not of sufficient magnitude to require that NaCl be added to isolation media. One note of caution if TCBS is used: *V. parahaemolyticus* and some NCV's do not utilize sucrose and will therefore produce green colonies rather than yellow as described for *V. cholerae*.

Biochemical procedures

This group of vibrios can be tested for the characters listed in Table 42.1 of the preceding section. The tests listed in Table 42.2 of that section often give results which can be used to divide them into several groups.

Growth in 6% NaCl broth. V. parahaemolyticus grow, NCV's do not.

Heiberg fermentation pattern. Heiberg (10) reported that cholera and cholera-like vibrios could be classified into six groups depending upon the fermentation of sucrose, arabinose, and mannose. Smith and Goodner (24) proposed two new groups. The combined groupings are presented in Table 42.3.

Other characteristics. Variable results have been observed with other tests listed. The possible permutations are many and can become overly confusing. Our laboratory uses gelatin, indole, and nitrate-to-nitrite as additional characteristics for classification (10).

Serologic procedures

A serologic classification scheme for *V. parahaemolyticus* introduced by Sakazaki et al. (19) is based upon O (somatic) and K (capsular) antigens.

Currently two separate systems are being used to serotype NCV's (12, 24), but efforts are being made to combine them. The sera are not yet available for general use. However, both laboratories have been serotyping cultures sent to them.

TABLE 42.3—HEIBERG FERMENTATION GROUPS

GROUP	SUCROSE	ARABINOSE	MANNOSE
I	+*	−	+
II	+	−	−
III	+	+	+
IV	+	+	−
V	−	−	+
VI	−	−	−
VII	−	+	+
VIII	−	+	−

* + = ferments; − = no fermentation.

One area which could yield valuable information is that of serodiagnosis. McIntyre et al. (14) showed a rise in patients' antibody titers to the homologous strain of NCV during the course of their diseases. Whether this holds true for all NCV infections is not yet known.

Marker systems for epidemiologic investigations

From a public health viewpoint, there is a definite need to separate cholera from noncholera vibrios. The serologic separation, while not acceptable along the lines of strict taxonomy, is useful for the laboratory and the physician. The separation of the NCV's into various groups based upon salt tolerance and biochemical results is not sufficiently refined to serve as markers for epidemiologic purposes. However, combining physiologic characteristics with serotyping has helped (10) in identifying these organisms.

Antimicrobic Susceptibility and Resistance

In vitro studies with 111 strains of *V. parahaemolyticus* and 79 strains of noncholera vibrios (21) indicate general susceptibility to streptomycin, tetracycline, chloramphenicol, and neomycin. More work is needed here.

References

1. ALDOVA E: Isolation of nonagglutinable vibrios from an enteritis outbreak in Czechoslovakia. J Infect Dis 118:25–31, 1968
2. BALOWS A, HERMAN GJ, and DEWITT WE: The isolation and identification of *Vibrio cholerae* - a review. Health Lab Sci 8:167–175, 1971
3. BAUMANN P, BAUMANN L, and MANDEL M: Taxonomy of marine bacteria: the genus *Beneckea*. J Bacteriol 107:268–294, 1971
4. BENENSON AS (ed.): Control of Communicable Diseases in Man, 12th edition. American Public Health Association, Washington, DC, 1975
5. BENENSON AS, ISLAM MR, and GREENOUGH WB III: Rapid identification of *Vibrio cholerae* by darkfield microscopy. Bull WHO 30:827–831, 1964
6. CARPENTER CCJ JR, MAHMOUND AAF, and WARREN KS: Algorithms in the diagnosis and management of exotic diseases. XXVI. Cholera. J Infect Dis 136:461–464, 1977
7. COLWELL RR and KAPER J: *Vibrio cholerae, Vibrio parahaemolyticus,* and other vibrios: occurrence and distribution in Chesapeake Bay. Science 198:394–396, 1977
8. GANGAROSA EJ, DEWITT WE, HUQ I, and ZARIFI A: Laboratory methods in cholera: isolation of *Vibrio cholerae* (El Tor and classical) on TCBS medium in minimally equipped laboratories. Trans Royal Soc Trop Med Hyg 62:693–699, 1968

9. GOODNER K, SMITH HL JR, and STEMPEN H: Serologic diagnosis of cholera. J Albert Einstein Med Ctr 8:143–160

10. HEIBERG B: Des reactions de fermantation chez les vibrions. CR Soc Biol 115:984–986, 1934

11. HUGH R and FEELEY JC: Report (1966–1970) of the Subcommittee on Taxonomy of Vibrios to the International Committee on Nomenclature of Bacteria. Int J Syst Bacteriol 22:123, 1972

12. KAUFFMANN F: On the serology of the cholera vibrio. Acta Pathol Microbiol Scand 27:283–299, 1950

13. MCINTYRE OR and FEELEY JC: Characteristics of noncholera vibrios isolated from cases of human diarrhea. Bull WHO 32:627–632, 1965

14. MCINTYRE OR, FEELEY JC, GREENOUGH WB III, BENENSON AS, HASAN SI, and SAAD A: Diarrhea caused by noncholera vibrios. Am J Trop Med Hyg 14:412–418, 1965

15. MONSUR KA: Bacteriological diagnosis of cholera under field conditions. Bull WHO 28:387–389, 1963

16. NOBECHI K: Contributions to the knowledge of V. cholerae. 3. Immunological studies upon the types of V. cholerae. Sci Repr Govt Inst Infect Dis 2:43–87, 1923

17. SAKAZAKI R: Vibrio parahaemolyticus, a noncholeragenic enteropathogenic vibrio. Proceedings of the Cholera Research Symposium, Honolulu, 1965, pp 30–36

18. SAKAZAKI R, GOMEZ CZ, and SEBALD M: Taxonomical studies on the so-called NAG vibrios. Jpn J Med Sci Biol 20:265–280, 1967

19. SAKAZAKI R, TAMURA K, GOMEZ CZ, and SEN R: Serological studies on the cholera group of vibrios. Jpn J Med Sci Biol 23:13–20, 1970

20. SANYAL SC, GHOSH M, CHOWDHURY M, SEN PC, and SINGH H: Sensitivity of Vibro parahaemolyticus to antibacterial agents. Indian J Med Res 61:324–329, 1973

21. SIL J, SANYAL SC, and MUKHERJEE S: Antibiotic sensitivity of Vibrio cholerae other than O serotype 1 (so-called NAG vibrios). Indian J Med Res 62:491–496, 1974

22. SMITH HL JR: A presumptive test for vibrios: the "string" test. Bull WHO 42:817–818, 1970

23. SMITH HL JR and GOODNER K: Detection of bacterial gelatinases by gelatin-agar plate methods. J Bacteriol 76:662–665, 1958

24. SMITH HL JR and GOODNER K: On the classification of vibrios. Proceedings of the Cholera Research Symposium, Honolulu, 1965, pp 4–8

CHAPTER 43

YERSINIOSES

Thomas J. Quan, Allan M. Barnes, and Jack D. Poland

Introduction

The genus *Yersinia* is comprised of three currently recognized species (formerly placed in the genus *Pasteurella*), *Y. pestis, Y. pseudotuberculosis,* and *Y. enterocolitica,* all of which cause disease in man and various animal species. *Y. pestis* is the etiologic agent of plague, a disease primarily of rodents that can be transmitted to man by the bite of infective fleas or by direct contact with the tissues or carcasses of infected animals. Other humans can be infected by inhaling droplets coughed or expectorated by a patient with plague pneumonia.

Y. pseudotuberculosis and *Y. enterocolitica* cause various human diseases, primarily of an enteric nature—most commonly enterocolitis, terminal ileitis, or mesenteric adenitis often mimicking acute appendicitis, or in older persons, septicemia. Less frequently, these agents cause erythema nodosum, septic arthritis, and rarely meningitis or panophthalmitis. Human infection caused by a *Yersinia* sp. other than *Y. pestis* is referred to as a yersiniosis (plural: yersinioses) to distinguish these syndromes from various forms of plague.

The yersiniae are gram-negative, coccobacillary to bacillary bacteria ranging in size from 0.5–1.0 µm by 1–2 µm. All are nonmotile at 37 C. *Y. pseudotuberculosis* and *Y. enterocolitica* may be motile at temperatures below 30 C, and when motile have peritrichous flagella. On initial isolation, *Y. pseudotuberculosis,* especially, may be nonmotile, but motility can usually be restored by serial passage in semisolid agar media or use of special U tube (27). *Y. pestis* and *Y. pseudotuberculosis,* when stained by polychromatic stains such as Wayson or Giemsa, usually have a bipolar or "closed safety pin" appearance.

All three species are aerobic, facultatively anaerobic, and grow well but slowly on most of the routine selective media for enteric organisms and on enriched media such as blood agar. *Y. pestis* grows from pinpoint-sized colonies (<0.1–0.5 mm) at 24 hr to 1–1.5 mm colonies by 48 hr. Usually within 48 hr the colonies have a characteristic rough, "hammered copper" or cauliflower appearance. *Y. pseudotuberculosis* and *Y. enterocolitica* form slightly larger, usually smooth, entire, transparent to translucent colonies. At least 2 days of incubation at 28 C to 37 C are usually required for all three species to form visible colonies.

Yersinia pestis

Plague is endemic in many parts of the world with temperate climates including Asia, Africa, and North and South America. In the United States, plague poses a recurrent public health threat in states west of the 100th meridian—especially New Mexico, Arizona, and California. Since 1970, human infections have also occurred in Oregon, Colorado, Nevada, Wyoming, and Utah. Plague epizootics have occurred in roughly 5-year cycles among rodent populations—especially rock squirrels, prairie dogs, and other ground squirrels in large areas throughout these and other western states, with serologic evidence of expansion eastward to the 96th meridian in Texas (9). Goldenberg et al. (17) suggested that more human infections would occur in the United States as a result of increased exposure to plague-infected animals concomitant with increased use of the West for recreational purposes and for housing an expanding population. Indeed, between 1970 and 1979, there were 105 confirmed human plague infections (or a yearly average of 10.5) in contrast to 72 confirmed human plague infections from 1925 to 1969 (or a yearly average of only 1.6). Since 1925, all but one of the human plague infections have come from nonurban sources, and no person-to-person pneumonic spread has been documented in the United States. Humans are usually infected by the bite of infective rodent fleas or by direct contact with the carcasses of infected animals. Rodents or their fleas are the most common direct source of infection, but human plague has been acquired from wild or domestic carnivores: specifically, bobcat (39), coyote (46), and house cats (8, 10, 26).

Clinical Manifestations

Plague occurs in three principal clinical forms: bubonic, septicemic, and pneumonic. Bubonic plague is the common form resulting from the percutaneous inoculation of *Y. pestis* by the bite of an infective flea or in skin lesions (such as cuts or abrasions) which are exposed to infected animal tissues. The incubation period is 2 to 7 days after exposure, rarely longer. The disease is characterized by sudden onset of fever, shaking chills, headache, myalgia, prostration, and pain in the area of involved lymph nodes. Untreated, bubonic plague can result in coma and death. Gastrointestinal symptoms of nausea, vomiting, diarrhea (occasionally bloody), and abdominal pain are frequently seen. Possible complications arising from hematogenous dissemination of *Y. pestis* include meningitis; pneumonitis (discussed later); or focal metastatic infections of the eye (endophthalmitis), skin (pustules), liver, or spleen. Gram-negative endotoxemia may result in cardiovascular collapse, consumptive coagulopathy (i.e., DIC), or cardiac failure. This latter event, although rare, may occur without warning when the patient seems almost well enough to be discharged from the hospital.

Classic bubonic plague entails an inflammatory response in the regional lymph nodes which, when enlarged, is referred to as a bubo. Primary buboes occur most commonly in the inguinal, axillary, or cervical areas but may occur in other regions such as epitrochlear, mediastinal, popliteal, supraclavicular, or intra-abdominal areas. Untreated bubonic plague may become septicemic plague. Multiple areas of lymphadenopathy may rarely occur as a result of hematogenous dissemination of *Y. pestis* during intermittent bacteremia or septicemia. Unless clinically detectable lymphadenitis is present, plague septicemia is designated "primary septicemic plague."

Virtually 100% of the *untreated* septicemic plague infections are followed by pulmonary involvement and death. However, functionally transmissible pneumonic infection is estimated to occur with only 5% of such infections because the patients die before alveolar pneumonitis develops or before respiratory spread occurs (38). A chain of human-to-human infections may result, however, when respiratory or pneumonic infection supersedes, since the agent is no longer dependent on the natural animal-flea-animal/human complex. Since 1974, of 91 plague infections 20 (22%) developed pneumonia, seven of which were fatal. None of the contacts of these patients acquired the disease, at least partly because effective prophylactic measures were taken. The incubation period of primary pneumonic plague infections is 2 to 3 days. The disease is characterized by sudden onset of fever, cough, production of bloody sputum, headache, shaking chills, and prostration. The infection is fulminant, and the patient soon dies if not treated. Chances of recovery are markedly reduced if specific therapy is not initiated within 18 hr after onset of symptoms.

Plague is an internationally reportable disease, and when suspected, Federal, state, and local public health authorities must be notified (25). Confirmed infections are reported to the World Health Organization. Epidemiological and epizootiological investigations should be undertaken to ascertain the source of infection for a human, the extent of the plague involvement in reservoir animal species, and the potential for occurrence of additional human infections; and to determine whether there is a hazard to international travel and transport, and whether suitable animal and ectoparasite control measures are indicated. Risk to humans can be reduced or, in certain situations, eliminated by careful application of environmental health principles, animal population management practices, and selective insecticidal measures.

Collection and Processing of Specimens

Although bubonic plague is not transmissible from person to person, reasonable and appropriate precautions must be taken by all personnel attending the patient to minimize the possibility of spreading the disease should secondary pneumonia or draining lesions develop. Face masks, gloves, and gowns worn when in contact with the patient, especially if he has pneumonia, are generally adequate precautions. Two to 3 days after specific antimicrobial therapy is initiated, continued isolation of uncomplicated bubonic plague patients is unnecessary. Vaccination is generally recommended for laboratory and field personnel who are exposed to the plague organism or to infected mammals or ectoparasites. The only vaccine available in the United States is an inactivated plague vaccine, U.S.P., produced by Cutter Laboratories, Berkeley, Calif.; other vaccines have been produced by various institutes in other countries (31). Vaccination is not necessary if stringent laboratory safety procedures are followed and specimens and cultures are handled aseptically.

This conclusion is borne out by years of experience at the Fort Collins laboratory where it is felt that repeated vaccinations produce undesirable side effects.

Specimens of choice for etiological diagnosis are fluid aspirated from the bubo, sputum, or citrated or heparinized blood. Since early bubo formation is seldom purulent or necrotic and is exquisitely painful, lesions can be aspirated under local anesthesia by injecting a small volume of sterile physiologic saline or broth with a syringe and a 20- to 22-gauge needle. The needle and syringe are then thoroughly flushed with additional small volumes of sterile saline or broth. The combined washings and fluid aspirated are used for laboratory study. Blood for at least four cultures should be obtained, since intermittent bacteremia is easily missed when fewer cultures are collected. The four blood samples can be taken within a few minutes of each other and can easily be completed within 1 to 1 1/2 hr, thus not inordinately delaying the initiation of specific therapy. Tissues obtained during necropsy suitable for laboratory examination include excised lymph nodes (buboes), and pieces of liver, spleen, lung, and bone marrow. Of course, if the agent is to be isolated, the tissues should be obtained without preservatives or fixatives (i.e., formalin) and before embalming procedures.

Microscopic Slide Examination

Impression smears of each tissue should be made on each of three microscope slides, one of which should be of acceptable quality for fluorescent antibody testing (see below). After it is air dried, one smear should be fixed with absolute methanol for 2 to 5 min or by light heating; this smear is stained with a polychromatic stain (Wayson or Giemsa) to be examined for bipolar staining rods. The second slide is heat fixed and stained by Gram's method to be examined for gram-negative rods. The third slide, also heat fixed, is used for fluorescent antibody staining techniques which are discussed below. Tissues from rodents or other mammals can be examined for evidence of infection in the same manner as described for those from humans.

Serum Specimens

Paired or serial serum specimens should be taken during the acute phase of the disease and at least 3 weeks later. Sera should be kept sterile and frozen at −20 C or colder until they are processed.

Packaging and Mailing Specimens

When plague is suspected, the nearest public health official must be notified and can be consulted about the proper handling and disposition of suitable specimens. If specimens must be mailed or air freighted to distant laboratories, special precautions must be taken to prevent leakage and contamination of packaging materials and to protect the specimen. Specimens are enclosed in heavy glass or plastic vials sealed with screw caps and tape to prevent leakage. Vials are placed in double mailing containers packed with sufficient absorbent material to retain liquid portions in the event of breakage and are shipped by the fastest method available. Cary Blair transport medium (R) or similar media are suitable for transporting and maintaining plague-infected tissues. If no commercial medium is available, Broquet's fluid can be substituted. Broquet's fluid is prepared by dissolving 20 ml of glycerol (C.P.), 1.11 g anhydrous disodium phosphate, and 0.02 g citric acid in 100 ml distilled water. The solution is steamed at 100 C for 10 min and dispensed into and stored in sterile vials.

Cultures of organisms presumptively identified as *Y. pestis* also can be shipped to a reference laboratory on agar slants (e.g., TSA, blood agar, nutrient agar) if similarly packaged in double containers and appropriately labelled with biologic hazard stickers.

Serum specimens drawn during acute and convalescent periods should be sent frozen on dry ice, especially if transit time is expected to be prolonged or if the weather during transit is hot.

Rodent or other mammal specimens, whole or in parts, can be packed in dry ice and sent by air express if properly wrapped and labelled (18).

Flea Specimens

During epidemiological or research studies, fleas can be collected from animals, nests, or burrows. Although the procedures used are not complex, they should be done by experienced field workers. Active fleas are difficult specimens with which to work, so they are generally killed or anesthetized. Generally, fleas are removed from a dead or anesthetized animal by combing them (we use a modified toothbrush) into a white enamel pan 8–10 inches deep. The outer rows of bristles of the brush are removed, leaving a single, central row of bristles in place. The animal is held over the pan by the tail (small mammals), and the fur is combed vigorously. Fleas are picked up from the pan and placed in vials of 2% sodium chloride solution containing 0.001% Tween 80. (The fleas drown in the Tween 80; the pan is deep enough to contain fleas which recover quickly from anesthesia.) As anesthesia, ether is preferable to chloroform because the latter is toxic to *Y. pestis* (17). Vials containing fleas are refrigerated but not frozen and should not be stored for more than 2 weeks before they are processed.

Laboratory Examination of Fleas

Once collected, fleas are sent to a reference laboratory to be checked for *Y. pestis* infection. Data accompanying such shipments must include date and location of collection and a list of the host species from which fleas were obtained. Genus and species of fleas are identified by an entomologist trained in flea taxonomy. If held for prolonged periods in saline prior to trituration, fleas should be washed with hydrogen peroxide (0.6% in sterile physiologic saline), rinsed, and resuspended in fresh, sterile saline (17, 18). To recover *Y. pestis,* up to 25 fleas can be pooled by host species and location of collection and triturated in a mortar with a pestle or in a small tissue homogenizer containing a small amount of physiologic saline. Small aliquots (0.1–0.5 ml) of the triturate are then inoculated subcutaneously into mice or a guinea pig. Inoculated animals are held and observed for morbidity and mortality up to 3 weeks. Animals which die after inoculation are necropsied, and portions of liver and spleen are excised for bacterial isolation procedures.

Although *Y. pestis* theoretically should be recoverable by direct culture of the flea, experience has shown that such cultures are overgrown by other microbes, notably fungi. However, should direct cultures be needed, Quan et al. (40) have described effective procedures to obtain them. Fluorescent antibody staining techniques can also be used on fleas after they have been subjected to special procedures (23).

Diagnostic Procedures

Laboratory diagnosis of *Y. pestis* infection is based on isolating and identifying the organism from patients' specimens (blood or tissue) or by demonstrating a significant increase of specific humoral antibodies within 3 to 5 weeks after the onset of illness.

When plague is suspected, specimens should be taken for laboratory analysis, and the patient should be given adequate (but not excessive) therapy immediately (38). Examination of bubo aspirate by stained slides or by fluorescent antibody must be done immediately to differentiate gram-positive coccal from gram-negative rod etiologies of the lymphadenitis. Proper therapy can be initiated when this examination is completed, if it is done immediately; however, therapy should not await laboratory confirmation or even early culture results when *Y. pestis* infection is seriously suspected.

In addition to the symptoms listed above, clinical laboratory findings for plague infections may include a polymorphonuclear leukocytosis (20,000 to 25,000/mm^3), lowered platelet counts, and occurrence of fibrin split products. Although intermittent bacteremia is commonly recognized even during the first 2 or 3 days of illness, an early progressive bacteremia is usually present only in patients with septicemic plague or during terminal stages of fatal infections. With bubonic plague, large numbers of organisms are localized in the inflamed, enlarged lymph nodes. Numerous organisms are usually present in sputa from pneumonic plague patients. In either circumstance, dye stains can provide supportive (but not presumptive) evidence of *Y. pestis*, and fluorescent antibody test results can provide presumptive evidence of *Y. pestis*.

Identification of Y. pestis

Identification of *Y. pestis* is dependent on isolating it from clinical, animal, or flea specimens in pure cultures and subjecting it to biochemical and biological characterization tests.

Cultivation. One-half to one milliliter of the fluid specimen (blood, bubo aspirate, CSF) is inoculated into each of several tubes of sterile broth (infusion broth, brain heart infusion broth, Trypticase soy broth, or similar media). The specimen (0.25–0.5 ml) is spread on three or four blood agar base or extract agar slants or plates. The inoculated media are incubated at 28 C to 37 C and examined for growth daily for at least 7–10 days. If no growth appears after that time, the specimen can be classified as negative and discarded.

Tissue specimens of human or animal origin are triturated with a small volume of sterile saline or broth, and the resulting suspension is processed in the same manner as fluid specimens.

Growth characteristics. Aerobic and facultatively anaerobic, *Y. pestis* can grow at temperatures of −2 C to 45 C, with its optimal range being 25 C to 30 C. Best growth occurs within a pH range of 7.2 to 7.6, with tolerance limits of pH 5.0 to 9.6.

A nonfastidious organism, *Y. pestis* can grow on a wide variety of routinely used, commercially available media, e.g., brain heart infusion, Trypticase soy broth or agar, nutrient broth or agar, and common blood agar bases (with or without blood added). More enriched media are also suitable although not required for isolation or maintenance purposes at the clinical laboratory (e.g., cystine Trypticase blood agar).

In stationary, pure, fluid cultures, *Y. pestis* exhibits a flocculent growth after 24 hr of incubation at 28 C or 35 C. Turbid growth is never produced in broth; rather a "stalactite"-type pattern of growth is seen, with floccules which adhere to one side of the tube and settle to the bottom when the tube is jarred.

Although *Y. pestis* grows well on or in these media, it grows more slowly than do most other bacteria. Even after massive inoculation on agar plates, growth after 24 hr of incubation consists of pinpoint, thin, transparent colonies, individual representatives of which can be detected only with magnification. Often the only visible manifestation of growth on blood agar is a slight darkening of the medium. After an additional 24 hr of incubation, colonies reach 1–1.5 mm in diameter and are gray to grayish-white. Under stereoscopic magnification, the colonies have a hammered copper appearance with undulated edges. After 37 C incubation, the colonies—especially those of fully virulent strains—are sticky (an indication that they have produced envelope substance). If the incubation period is extended beyond 2 days, isolated colonies may reach diameters of 4 to 7 mm by the 10th day; crowded colonies seldom exceed 2 or 3 mm.

Microscopically, the plague organism is nonflagellated and nonsporulating. Organisms grown at 37 C on blood agar or in tissue-smear preparations usually have definite envelopes but are not truly encapsulated. Envelopes of organisms grown in culture can be seen after treatment with standard India ink preparation.

On Gram staining, *Y. pestis* appears as a gram-negative rod or coccobacillus. The bipolar character is not marked by Gram staining but is best demonstrated with Wayson stain or another suitable polychromatic stain such as Giemsa. With Wayson stain, *Y. pestis* cells are characteristically light blue to reddish with dark blue polar bodies; they appear swollen, barrel-shaped, or like "closed safety pins." Microscopic pleomorphism is not uncommon and is determined in part by physiological and/or environmental factors such as oxygen tension, drugs, chemicals, age, and pH. In young agar cultures, the organisms are short (mostly single rods), with occasional chains or pairs. In young broth cultures cells are longer and broader, occurring in chains of 4 to 16 or so with rare single cells. Bizarre, involuted forms and the more common pleomorphic forms are seen in cultures older than 3–5 days. Broth cultures begin to autolyze after about 72 hr of incubation at 37 C and somewhat later at 28 C.

Biochemical reactions are not used extensively in identifying *Y. pestis*. Characteristic reactions of *Y. pestis* to routine tests are listed in Tables 43.1, 43.2, and 43.3 along with those of the other *Yersinia* species.

New commercial miniaturized biochemical test systems (e.g., API, Mini-

TABLE 43.1—DEFINITIVE CHARACTERISTICS OF THE GENUS *YERSINIA*[a]

Gram stain: Gram-negative coccobacilli-bacilli, 0.5–1.0 by 1–2 μm.
Growth temperature tolerances: −2 C to 45 C.
Capsule: Not present.

β-Galactosidase:	Positive	Acid from lactose:	Negative*
Oxidase:	Negative	Lysine decarboxylase:	Negative
Malonate:	Not used	Tetrathionate:	Not reduced
Methyl red:	Positive	Arginine dihydrolase:	Negative
Citrate utilization:	Negative*	Phenylalanine deaminase:	Negative
Nitrate reduction:	Positive**	Gelatin hydrolysis:	Negative
Acid without gas from:		Acid from:	
Fructose	Positive	Dulcitol	Negative
Glucose	Positive	Erythritol	Negative
Glycerol	Positive**	Fucose	Negative
Maltose	Positive	Glycogen	Negative
Mannitol	Positive	Inositol	Negative
Mannose	Positive	Melezitose	Negative
Trehalose	Positive	Raffinose	Negative*

Voges Proskauer 37 C ⎱ Variable (*Y. pestis* and *Y. pseudotuberculosis* negative;
Indol 37 C ⎰ *Y. enterocolitica* sometimes positive)
Motility 37 C   Negative
22 C   *Y. pestis* negative; *Y. pseudotuberculosis* and *Y. enterocolitica* positive

[a] Adapted from Mollaret and Thal (33).
* Some strains of *Y. enterocolitica* may be positive.
** One variety of *Y. pestis* negative.

tek, Enterotube) can be used in tentatively but not conclusively identifying *Y. pestis*, although not all of these systems include *Y. pestis* in their numerical taxonomic keys. If *Y. pestis* keys are included, only the most common numerical codes found for stains are listed. It should be noted that if the miniaturized systems are used, because *Y. pestis* grows slowly, more than one colony may be required to prepare the inoculum and more than 24 hr of incubation may be required to achieve correct results.

Strains of *Y. pestis* give remarkably uniform biochemical test results, although there is some variation in fermentation patterns for a few carbohydrates (e.g., salicin, xylose, amygdalin). There are three named varieties of *Y. pestis* on the basis of different patterns of glycerol fermentation and nitrate reduction: var. *orientalis* is glycerol negative and reduces nitrate; var. *mediaevalis* is glycerol positive and does not reduce nitrate; var. *antigua* is glycerol positive and reduces nitrate. Each variety seems to occur in geographically unique niches with occasional overlap in certain areas (e.g., Africa, Asia) (15). Only *orientalis* has been found in the United States.

The Plague Branch of the Center for Disease Control (CDC) uses the following tests to confirm identification of *Y. pestis*: macroscopic and microscopic appearance of the cultures both on agar and in broth, sensitivity to specific bacteriophage, production of F1 (Fraction 1, an envelope antigen) as demon-

TABLE 43.2—DIFFERENTIAL CHARACTERISTICS OF THE GENUS *YERSINIA*[a]

TEST	*Y. PESTIS*	*Y. PSEUDOTUBERCULOSIS*	*Y. ENTEROCOLITICA*
*Motility 22 C	−	+	+
37 C	−	−	−
*Urea hydrolysis	−	+	+
Esculin hydrolysis	+	+	−(d)
Rhamnose	−(d)	+	−(d)
Salicin	d	+	−(d)
*Sucrose	−	−	+
*Ornithine decarboxylase	−	−	+
Citrate utilization	−	−	−(d)
Indol	−	−	d
Raffinose	−	−	−(d)
Melibiose	d	+	−(d)
Adonitol	−	+	−
*Amygdalin	(+)	−	−
Arabinose	+	+	d
*Cellobiose	−	−	+
Galactose	(+)	+	+
Sorbitol	d	−	+
Starch	w	+	d
Xylose	+(d)	−	d
Growth in KCN	−	−	d
d-tartrate	+	−	−

+, positive; (+), delayed positive; w, weak; −, negative; d, strains differ. (d) A few strains differ from sign given.

[a] Adapted from Mollaret and Thal (21).

* Important tests for differentiating the species.

strated by specific immunofluorescence tests, and pathogenicity for laboratory mice (or guinea pigs).

Tests for other virulence factors are also available but are best left for reference or research laboratories equipped to do them routinely. These include tests for production of V and W antigens, fibrinolysin, coagulase, pigmentation on media containing hemin or Congo red dye, and those for the production of or sensitivity to the bacteriocins, pesticin I and pesticin II (44).

Clinical or public health laboratories in plague areas may rely more heavily on biochemical test pattern produced, morphological appearance of the culture, and lysis by specific bacteriophage.* A bacteriophage suspension is applied to filter paper strips, lyophilized, and sealed in glass ampules, which may retain activity for several years. When needed, the ampule is opened and a paper strip removed and placed across streaks from the test culture and control cultures of known *Y. pestis* and *Y. pseudotuberculosis* type IA and/or other enteric organisms. The phage test is performed on duplicate plates, one of

*Samples of bacteriophage-impregnated paper strips are available to states and local public health laboratories from Plague Branch, Vector-Borne Diseases Division, CDC, P.O. Box 2087, Ft Collins, CO 80522.

TABLE 43.3—ADDITIONAL CHARACTERIZATION TESTS FOR *YERSINIA*

TEST	*Y. PESTIS*	*Y. PSEUDO-TUBERCULOSIS*	*Y. ENTERO-COLITICA*
Sensitivity to:			
Y. pestis bacteriophage 37 C	+	d	−
Y. pestis bacteriophage 22 C	+	−	−
Pesticin 1	−/d	+	d
Toxin production	+	d	d
Bacteriophage types	NA	NA	9
Production of VW antigens[a]	+	+	−
Production of coagulase[a]	+	−	−
Pigmentation on hemin or Congo red agar[a]	+	−	−
Production of fibrinolysin[a]	+	−	−
Pathogenicity for:			
Laboratory mice	+	+	−(d)
Laboratory rats	+	−	−(d)
Guinea pigs	+	+	−(d)
Gerbils	+	+	−(d)
Hamsters	−	−	−

[a] Tests with virulent strains.

+, positive; −, negative; d, strains differ.

(d) A few strains differ from sign given; NA not applicable.

which is incubated at 37 C and one at either room temperature or preferably at 20 C. *Y. pestis* streaks will show definite zones of lysis near the paper strip after incubation at either temperature. *Y. pseudotuberculosis* and some other *Enterobacteriaceae* lyse at 37 C but not at 20 C.

Animal inoculation is an efficient way of rapidly obtaining virulent plague organisms, often in pure culture. Also, this technique allows excellent recovery of *Y. pestis* from grossly contaminated specimens such as carcasses of long dead rodents or other mammals, sputa, or mixed cultures. A small volume (0.1–0.2 ml) of the fluid specimen or of a saline suspension of a triturated solid tissue is inoculated subcutaneously into several laboratory mice or a guinea pig. Percutaneous inoculation, which may be necessary for heavily contaminated specimens or mixed cultures, is done by scarifying the back of the animal with a dull knife blade or roughly plucking the fur and applying a small volume of the inoculum onto the abraded skin. Inoculated animals are observed daily for signs of morbidity or mortality. Dead (or dying) animals are (sacrificed and) necropsied, and pieces of spleen and liver are removed for bacterial isolation as described above. When pure cultures or uncontaminated specimens are processed, intraperitoneal inoculation can be done to obtain faster results. Virulent organisms can be recovered from peritoneal fluid aspirated with a syringe and needle from experimental animals in as little as 18–24 hr after inoculation; if no growth is evident, aspiration can be repeated at about 48 hr.

Because mice are very susceptible to the murine toxin of the plague organism and generally die before gross pathological changes occur, guinea pigs better demonstrate the pathological changes associated with plague.

Fluid suspensions of known or suspected plague organisms are inoculated subcutaneously in the inguinal region. After about the second day, a palpable inguinal bubo develops if the inoculum contained virulent plague organisms. Aseptic aspiration of this bubo should yield a pure culture of *Y. pestis*. Animals allowed to succumb to infection with virulent *Y. pestis* also have: an ulcerated inoculation site, usually abscessed, and surrounded with a gelatinous, sometimes hemorrhagic edema; enlarged and inflamed regional lymph nodes, sometimes partly necrotic, and surrounded with edematous, hemorrhagic tissue. The liver is pale and fatty and, if the animal dies more than 5 days after challenge, numerous yellowish pinpoint or larger nodules are present on its surface and on cut sections. The spleen is rounded, friable, enlarged (often three to four times normal size), dusky red, and congested. Large, 0.5–3.0 mm, white or yellowish nodules may be present throughout and are seen on the surface. Lungs appear congested, and guinea pigs which survive plague infection more than 5 days after inoculation may have pinpoint to 5- or 6-mm nodules in the lungs surrounded by large hemorrhagic zones or by areas of consolidation.

Smears of most tissues of animals which died of plague contain numerous plague organisms. Presumably because they often die within 5 days of infection with *Y. pestis,* wild rodents do not usually have the gross tissue lesions described for guinea pigs, although the organism can be readily isolated from the tissues of the former.

Grossly contaminated specimens suspected of also containing *Y. pestis* can be handled in either of two ways. A suspension of the specimen (e.g., sputum, putrified tissue, or triturated fleas) is mixed with a solution of penicillin (10,000 international units/ml). Each laboratory mouse is inoculated either intraperitoneally or subcutaneously with 1000 units of penicillin. Because penicillin kills *Y. pestis* under *in vitro* conditions, specimens should not be stored even briefly in suspensions containing it. Alternately, the specimen can be percutaneously inoculated.

Disposition of Specimens and Cultures

Unused portions of clinical specimens or cultures are stored at 4 C until the final diagnosis is reached. *Y. pestis* remains viable for years on agar slants at 4 C. Lyophilizing and sealing *Y. pestis* under vacuum is the best means of preserving it and maintaining its native antigenic composition, with Hornibrooks's lactose salt solution being an excellent menstruum for this purpose (21).

Y. pestis is a fragile organism. It is very susceptible to drying and is readily killed by short-term exposures to several commonly used disinfectants (e.g., saponified cresol, sodium hypochlorite, iodophors), although the time it takes to kill the organism varies with density of bacterial suspension, nature of the suspending menstruum, and size of the bacterial clumps. Autoclaving or ethylene oxide treatment are excellent means of sterilizing materials contaminated with *Y. pestis*. Materials which are not expendable and will not tolerate autoclaving or ethylene oxide treatment should be thoroughly soaked and scrubbed with strong bleach (sodium hypochlorite) or iodophor solution.

Serologic Tests

Standard whole-cell agglutination tests of suspected *Y. pestis* cultures can be done with commercially available antiplague serum. If antiplague serum is not commercially available, it should be available from plague research laboratories in various parts of the world.

To serologically identify organisms suspected of causing plague, formalin is added to a concentration of 0.5%–1.0% to a suspension of the organisms and allowed to stand overnight at room temperature. (The suspension can be tested after an hour's formalin treatment if quick results are imperative, but it must be treated as a viable suspension.) The formalin-bacteria suspension is centrifuged, and the bacterial pellet is washed twice with physiologic saline and resuspended to a #4 McFarland standard in fresh physiologic saline. For a quick reading, a drop of bacterial suspension is added to a drop of a 1/150 dilution of high-titered antiplague serum, mixed gently, and checked for agglutination in 10–15 min.

For serodiagnostic tests of a patient's serum, a formalinized suspension of known *Y. pestis* cells is prepared as described above. One to nine dilutions of the patient's serum are prepared in tubes, and an equal volume of the antigen suspension is added to and mixed with each dilution and to a control tube containing only a volume of the diluent. At this point, a drop or two of the serum-antigen mixture can be placed in the wells of an agglutination microscope slide (e.g., Boerner test slide). The slide is shaken gently for 15–30 min and examined for agglutination under low magnification. The tube series is incubated for 2 hr at 35 C–37 C and stored at room temperature for about 18 hr. Agglutination is seen best with the aid of a hand lens. A 100× stock suspension of known *Y. pestis* antigen prepared in this manner should be a satisfactory reagent for bacterial agglutination for at least 3 months if stored in a refrigerator. The stock suspension must be agitated before it is used to ensure thorough dispersion of bacterial cells, and a 1:100 dilution is prepared for use in the agglutination test.

Although procedures for other serologic tests (complement fixation, hemagglutination, precipitation, mouse protection index) have been described (12, 13, 22, 32, 52), since suitable reagents are not commercially available, specimens should be sent to regional plague or reference laboratories which can perform these specialized tests. Unless large numbers of tests are planned, the cost of antigen preparation in terms of time and labor does not justify the benefits gained.

Fluorescent Antibody Examination

Smears of bubo aspirate, sputum, or impression smears of tissues obtained either by needle biopsy or at autopsy from human patients or from animals suspected of having died of plague can also be examined with the rapid specific fluorescent antibody test. Blood films can also be examined, but septicemia severe enough to be evident on such slides is rare except in very advanced infections. Presumptive results of fluorescent antibody tests can be obtained in as little as 1 hr after the specimen is received.

Winter and Moody (51) and Moody and Winter (34) describe the fluorescent antibody test fully. Smears are prepared in duplicate on a glass microscope slide of suitable quality for fluorescent microscopy. The smears are dried in air, lightly heat fixed, and ringed with a wax pencil. (A clinical laboratory not equipped to perform this test can ship slides thus prepared to a regional or reference laboratory for examination.) To one smear is added a drop of *Y. pestis* fluorescein-isothiocyanate-labelled antiserum, and to the second smear is added a drop of the same preparation to which a predetermined volume of unlabelled *Y. pestis* antiserum has been added. The slide is incubated in a moist chamber at room temperature for 30 min and washed twice in PBS for 10 min. The slide is covered with a cover slip mounted in glycerol-PBS mounting medium and is examined by standard fluorescent microscopy techniques. The first smear is the test smear, and any *Y. pestis* present should brightly fluoresce as apple green-colored hollow rods. If the specimen is positive, *Y. pestis* cells in the second smear should fluoresce less brilliantly (fluorescence inhibition test).

The fluorescent antibody technique is most specific when performed on tissue specimens from humans or animals. If *in vitro* cultures are used, they should be incubated at 37 C for at least 24 hr, especially if the immunofluorescence reagents have been prepared with the Fraction 1 (envelope) antigen of *Y. pestis*. Immunofluorescence reagents made with whole-cell *Y. pestis* antigen are considerably less specific than those prepared with Fl antigen, and they can cross-react strongly, because antigens common to other enteric organisms are present. We are unaware of commercially available immunofluorescence reagents for *Y. pestis*. Small volumes of these reagents are available to state and local public health laboratories for diagnostic purposes on request from CDC, Plague Branch, Fort Collins, Colo; from CDC, Atlanta, Ga; and from plague reference laboratories in other parts of the world.

Antimicrobial Sensitivity Testing

Sensitivity tests on isolates of *Y. pestis* as routinely performed in a clinical diagnostic laboratory are notoriously unreliable because *in vitro* results commonly differ significantly from *in vivo* efficacy. For example, slight to wide zones of inhibition of *Y. pestis* growth may occur in the Kirby Bauer disk diffusion method with penicillin, although penicillin has no *in vivo* activity against *Y. pestis*. Patients diagnosed as having or suspected of having plague infections should be treated with tetracycline, streptomycin, or chloramphenicol (2). Certain sulfonamides (e.g., sulfadiazine, trimethoprim-sulfamethoxazole) (1) are also effective and are used successfully when the more effective antibiotics are not available.

Evaluation of Laboratory Findings

Because of the seriousness of plague, with its high ($\geq$ 60%) fatality rate if untreated, and because it can be pneumonically spread, specific therapy should be initiated as soon as plague is suspected on the basis of medical history and clinical examination findings. However, specimens for laboratory diagnosis should be taken before antimicrobials are administered.

Presumptive laboratory diagnosis can be based on: (a) a positive fluorescent antibody test coupled with a good fluorescent inhibition test on tissue smear or culture or (b) isolation of an organism with microscopic and macroscopic characteristics compatible with *Y. pestis* (gram-negative rods, which also show bipolar staining with Wayson or Giemsa stains; hammered-copper appearance, slow-growing colonies, stalactite-type growth in broth). A presumptive diagnosis should not be based solely on Gram stain or Wayson stain preparations, but results of these tests provide supportive evidence when coupled with a compatible epidemiologic history and clinical picture.

A confirmed diagnosis of plague is made when *Y. pestis* has been isolated and identified, on the basis of at least the following characteristics:

1. Microscopic—gram-negative rods, showing bipolar staining with Giemsa or Wayson stain; positive fluorescent antibody test.
2. Macroscopic—slow-growing, hammered-copper colonies, stalactite-type growth in broth.
   -Sensitivity to *Y. pestis* specific bacteriophage at 22 C and 37 C.
   -Biochemical test results consistent with *Y. pestis*.
3. Pathogenic for laboratory mice.

Firm diagnoses can also be made retrospectively when serological tests indicate a rising titer to *Y. pestis* antigen in sera drawn during the acute and convalescent phases of the infection, 3 to 5 weeks apart. A titer of 10 or greater is considered significant in patients who have not been vaccinated against plague.

When plague is seriously suspected, local and state public health authorities must be notified immediately by telephone so that they can promptly investigate to determine the source of infection and institute needed control measures.

Because clinical diseases caused by *Y. pestis* and by *Francisella tularensis* (the tularemia agent) are similar, specimens should be cultured on media that will support growth and recovery of the latter agent as well (see Chapter 41).

Also, when specimens from wild animals are examined, one should remember that agents other than *Y. pestis* could be responsible for the morbidity/mortality. Procedures outlined above should allow some of these agents to be isolated, e.g., *Pasteurella multocida*, *Salmonella* spp.; others may require special procedures, e.g., *Leptospira*, *Listeria*, fungal, rickettsial, or viral agents. The reader is referred to appropriate chapters for the necessary techniques to isolate and identify these agents.

Yersinia enterocolitica and Y. pseudotuberculosis

Y. enterocolitica and *Y. pseudotuberculosis* are both discussed in this section since they cause similar diseases in man and have similar morphological and biochemical properties. Both agents are aerobic, anaerogenic, gram-negative rods, although small amounts of gas may be produced in glucose by an occasional strain of *Y. enterocolitica*. When they are virulent, their cellular morphology is coccobacillary; avirulent strains or those repeatedly passed on artificial media are distinctly bacillary. Both species grow in a wide temperature range (−1 C to 45 C), but prolonged incubation at temperatures higher than 30 C–32 C results in loss of flagella and of antigenic characteristics. As does *Y. pestis*, both species grow well but slowly on many of the usual selective media used in isolating common enteric pathogens. Stationary broth cultures of both agents are uniformly turbid in 18–24 hr, achieving concentrations of about (sometimes exceeding) 2×10^9 cells/ml. In contrast, *Y. pestis* never produces a turbid suspension and seldom produces more than 1×10^8 cells/ml after 24 hr of incubation.

Biochemical reactions which allow differentiation of the two species from each other and from *Y. pestis* are shown in Tables 43.1, 43.2, and 43.3.

Clinical Manifestations

Commonly, both agents cause infections (yersinioses) which appear as enteric disorders, e.g., diarrhea, enteritis, terminal ileitis, mesenteric adenitis, or colitis. These gastrointestinal disorders cannot be clinically distinguished from those caused by other enteric pathogens such as *Salmonella, Shigella,* or enteropathogenic *E. coli*. Infections in young children (≤ 10 years) usually appear as enteritis, often with diarrhea as the only symptom, but sometimes with diffuse abdominal pain and/or fever. In older children and young adults, infection commonly causes terminal ileitis and mesenteric adenitis mimicking acute appendicitis. Older patients usually have severe enteritis, colitis, or septicemia. Occasionally, either agent may cause erythema nodosum, pyuria, skin lesions, ophthalmitis, meningitis, or polyarthritis. *Y. pseudotuberculosis* has been implicated as the etiologic agent of Far East scarlet fever syndrome. Since these organisms are rarely detected in nature or as human pathogens unless aggressively searched for, our knowledge of the spectrum of disease states they produce is likely incomplete (3).

Epidemiology

As Wetzler indicated, *Y. enterocolitica* and *Y. pseudotuberculosis* have been isolated from a wide variety of vertebrate and invertebrate animal hosts and from man (49). As more investigators become interested in and adept at isolating these organisms, the list of their hosts grows. The principal reservoirs of *Y. pseudotuberculosis* are believed to be wild rodents and birds, and the organism is spread by fecal or urine contamination of foodstuffs. In North America, no principal animal reservoir has been defined for *Y. enterocolitica,* although swine seem to act in this capacity in Europe and other areas where serotype 0:3 *Y. enterocolitica* infection occurs most frequently in man (16). Episodes of *Y. enterocolitica* infection in North America have been epidemiologically associated with milk products (11), with contaminated water (7), and with dogs (19) (personal communication, J. Feeley, CDC, Atlanta, Ga.).

Although it may occur, no human-to-human transmission has been documented for either agent. The agents may be transmitted by bites of infective arthropods (e.g., flea, tick), because they have been found in these vectors (42,

49), but this route does not appear to play a major role in human infection (48). The most probable route of human infection still appears to be that of ingesting foods or water contaminated with feces or urine.

Public Health Significance

With a few major exceptions (where common sources have been implicated) no large-scale epidemics caused by either agent have been reported, nor has man-to-man transmission been documented. Individual cases must be diagnosed and treated promptly to prevent development of potentially severe sequelae and to prevent possible inappropriate surgery for "appendicitis." We strongly urge that epidemiological investigations be carried out when individual infections are diagnosed so as to define possible sources of the infection, to uncover additional existing human infections, and to assess the potential of occurrence of new cases. While reporting of these infectious diseases is not required, it is obviously desirable if the epidemiological and clinical features are to be fully elucidated.

Collection and Processing of Specimens

Clinical specimens from which *Y. enterocolitica* can be isolated include stool, blood, excised mesenteric nodes, or appendices obtained during surgery. The organism also has been recovered from sputum, urine, abscess, skin ulcer, spleen, liver, cerebrospinal fluid, and conjunctival washings. *Y. pseudotuberculosis* has not been easily recovered from stool specimens, but otherwise has been readily isolated from the above sources.

Techniques for culturing the agents have been described by Wetzler (34), Wauters (47), Nilehn (37), Toma (45), and others. Other procedures outlined by Saari and Jansen (43), Hanna et al. (20), Botzler et al. (4), and Lee (42) are especially useful for recovering *Y. enterocolitica* from environmental specimens (water, food, or animals).

The only specimens which pose a laboratory diagnostic problem are those which normally contain a mixture of organisms (e.g., stool, sputum, water, or other environmental specimens). Cultures of blood or mesenteric nodes, for example, should be either sterile or contain pure cultures of the etiologic agent.

Both *Y. enterocolitica* and *Y. pseudotuberculosis* grow well but slowly on media commonly used in recovering enteric pathogens, although as Bottone noted (3) several serotypes of *Y. enterocolitica* found in North America are markedly inhibited on SS and Hektoen enteric agars. As reported by Wetzler (48) and Bottone (3), strains of *Y. enterocolitica* which do grow well on some selective media may closely resemble *E. coli*, presumably because sucrose fermentation in the media may be confused with lactose fermentation. Data from the Plague Branch, CDC, Fort Collins, Col., indicate that MacConkey agar or eosin methylene blue agar best support the growth of most serotypes of *Y. enterocolitica* found in the United States (6).

If blood or mesenteric lymph node specimens are directly plated on various enteric media (including blood agar) and incubated at 25 C–37 C for 24 hr, either agent should grow and can best be visualized on agar plates under low power (3–10×) magnification as pinpoint to 0.1 mm, transparent to translucent, smooth colonies of morphologically variable gram-negative bacilli. For well-defined, larger colonies (0.5 to 2 mm) additional incubation at 25 C is recommended.

For specimens that are grossly contaminated (such as feces and water), cold enrichment techniques are recommended. Specimens are inoculated into buffered saline (pH 7.4 to 7.6) and stored for up to 6 weeks at 4 C–7 C. Both *Y. enterocolitica* and *Y. pseudotuberculosis* tolerate and even grow at these reduced temperatures, whereas other organisms present in the specimen gradually die.

Periodic samples of the cold enriched suspensions are taken by plating them on several of the enteric agars and blood agar. Plates are incubated at either 37 C or 25 C for a day and examined for presence of tiny colonies, again using magnification. Because the colonies are small when initially recovered, they must be incubated for at least 48 hr at 25 C, since prolonged incubation above 30 C (i.e., beyond the first 24-hr period) results in loss of serotyping characteristics of the isolated strain.

Special care is required because both agents are pathogenic to man, and the same reasonable precautions that would be taken for other bacterial pathogens must be applied in the laboratory to prevent laboratory-acquired infections.

Serological Methods

The six major recognized somatic serotypes of *Y. pseudotuberculosis* and their subgroups are: I (A & B), II (A & B), III, IV (A & B), V and VI. Human infections with serotypes I, II, and III have been reported from North America, Europe, and Asia; with serotypes IV and V, from Europe and Japan; and a few infections with serotype VI have been reported only from Japan.

Serotyping factors are not shared by the serotypes of *Y. pseudotuberculosis,* but several serofactors of *Y. pseudotuberculosis* are identical to those of *Salmonella* groups as outlined by Wetzler (48) and originally discussed by Knapp (28). For somatic O antigenic analyses or serodiagnostic tests, either whole-cell agglutination tests with killed antigen preparation or hemagglutination tests (14) are useful. Antigens for agglutination tests can be obtained by growing serotyping strains of *Y. pseudotuberculosis* or unknown strains for 48 to 72 hr at 22 C–25 C, harvesting in 0.5% sodium chloride, and either (a) mixing the suspension with an equal volume of 1% formalin in 0.5% saline and allowing the mixture to stand at room temperature overnight or (b) heating the suspension by boiling for several hours or autoclaving at 121 C for 15 min.

For hemagglutination tests, the supernatant fluid from heat-killed or autoclaved cell suspensions is adsorbed onto untanned sheep red blood cells for 30–60 min at 37 C, washed several times, and resuspended to a final concentration of 0.5% to 2% in phosphate buffered saline, pH 7.0. A 2% concentration of sensitized sheep erythrocytes is used in standard tube hemagglutination tests, whereas for microtitration tests the 0.5% concentration is practical. Dilutions of typing antisera or the patient's serum are made, and equal amounts of the antigen suspension are added. For best results, the serum-antigen suspensions are incubated at 37 C for about 2 hr and then placed in the refrigerator (4 C–7 C) overnight before results are observed and recorded.

The disagreement as to diagnostic significance of antibody titers to *Y. pseudotuberculosis* mentioned by Wetzler in 1970 (48) still prevails. Unless cross-reacting common antigens have been removed by adsorption with cells of other enteric agents, results may not be definitive. Also, titers against *Y. pseudotuberculosis* are highest during the acute phase of infection (i.e., within the first week after onset of illness), so the identity of the pathogen is often confirmed by a significant drop of antibody titer rather than a fourfold rise in titer as is common with other disease agents. For diagnostic purposes, a serum agglutination titer of at least 128 can be called positive, and lower titers are not considered to be diagnostic unless the agent has been isolated from the patient.

Serodiagnosis of infection with *Y. enterocolitica* is more difficult in the absence of a bacteriologically confirmed isolate. To date, more then 50 serotypes of this agent have been identified, infections with some of which do not seem to be accompanied by circulating (humoral) antibody production. Somatic serotypes 3 and 9 are most commonly responsible for human infections on a worldwide basis, but are rarely found in the United States where serotype 0:8 is most common. Various other somatic serotypes (0:17; 14; 16; 5; 4,32; 4,33), and a large number of isolates which are nontypeable by methods available (37) have been isolated from clinical specimens.

Serotyping and serodiagnostic tests are generally performed using formalin-killed, whole-cell antigen preparations of cultures grown at 25 C for 48–72 hr as outlined above. For serodiagnostic tests, antigens from all known serotypes must be used. Since these antigens and antisera are not commercially available, cultures and sera should be sent to reference laboratories for serological tests (e.g., CDC; National Center for *Yersinia* in Canada; the Pasteur Institute, Paris, France; or other laboratories of investigators studying these organisms).

Results of serotyping tests on cultures of *Y. enterocolitica* are usually clear-cut and easy to interpret. Serodiagnostic tests on serum specimens from patients for whom no bacteriological isolate is available, however, are quite difficult to interpret except for those patients infected by serotype 0:3. Cross-reactions occur among other serotypes of this agent and among this species and other bacterial groups (e.g., serotype 0:9 with *Brucella*; other serotypes with other enteric bacteria) (5, 35). Arbitrarily, most laboratories performing serodiagnostic tests for *Y. enterocolitica* do not consider titers of less than 128 or 160 to be diagnostically significant in the absence of a confirmed bacterial isolate from the patient.

Use of Marker Systems

Bacteriophages have been isolated from strains of *Y. enterocolitica* whose lytic activity can be used to classify strains of *Y. enterocolitica* into nine major phage types. Strains which cannot be classified into one of these types are designated type X (34). Bacteriophage typing appears to have some epidemiologic significance because specific types occur among isolates from specific geographic areas; for example, Type IX occurs in Europe, Type IXa occurs only in South Africa and Hungary, and Type IXb occurs only in Canada. It is hoped that as more strains of diverse animal and/or environmental origin are examined, a complete pattern of geographic and, perhaps, host distribution and their relationship to human infection will emerge. We are aware of only two laboratories equipped to perform bacteriophage typing, i.e., the Canadian National Reference Center for *Yersinia*, and the Institute Pasteur in Paris, France.

Biotyping

On the basis of results of various biochemical tests, several biotyping patterns have been suggested by Nilehn (37), Wauters (47), Knapp and Thal (29) and are summarized in Table 43.4. Additionally, recent isolates from both human and environmental sources have been reported which do not conform readily to any of the proposed biotyping schemata. The diversity of the *Y. enterocolitica* biochemical test patterns strongly suggests that the species is in fact composed of several closely related species. This premise is supported by results of DNA homology and recombination studies of Moore and Brubaker (35) and of Brenner et al. (5). The study by Brenner and his colleagues showed that there are at least four different groups on the basis of DNA relatedness among the 57 strains of *Y. enterocolitica* examined. Using slightly different techniques, the two groups of researchers also indicated that *Y. enterocolitica* strains are rather distantly related to other members of *Enterobacteriaceae*. Further work in the area of taxonomic relatedness and groupings is needed for full clarification of the status of *Y. enterocolitica*.

Other Tests

Fluorescent antibody tests. Immunofluorescence tests are not routinely used in the laboratory diagnosis of infections with *Y. enterocolitica* or *Y. pseudotuberculosis.*

Animal pathogenicity studies. Y. pseudotuberculosis and recently certain strains of *Y. enterocolitica* have been shown to produce disease and/or death in laboratory animals. Many of the same lesions seen in humans with naturally acquired infection with either agent can be reproduced in the laboratory with appropriate animal models and appropriate doses and routes of inoculation.

Experimental animals of choice for pathogenicity tests include mice, guinea pigs, rabbits, and gerbils. Hamsters are refractory to infection by either agent. Laboratory rats are refractory to *Y. pseudotuberculosis* and resistant to *Y. enterocolitica,* although some lesions such as septic arthritis may be produced (52).

Antimicrobial sensitivity tests. Numerous publications attest to the *in vivo* efficacy of the following antimicrobial drugs in the treatment of *Y. enterocolitica* infections: streptomycin, chloramphenicol, tetracycline, colistin, and trimethoprim-sulfamethoxazole, among others. The organism is usually resistant to penicillin and ampicillin, although some strains recently received by the Plague Branch, CDC, are sensitive *in vitro* to ampicillin.

TABLE 43.4—BIOTYPING SCHEMATA FOR *YERSINIA ENTEROCOLITICA*

SCHEMA OF:	NILEHN (37)					WAUTERS (47)					KNAPP AND THAL (29)			
TEST BIOTYPE →	1	2	3	4	5	1	2	3	4	5	1	2	3	4
Salicin	+	−/x	−/x	−/x	−/x	ND	ND	ND	ND	ND	−	−	+	d
Esculin	+	−/x	−/x	−	−	ND	ND	ND	ND	ND	−	−	+	d
Indole	+	+/(+)	−	−	−	+	(+)	−	−	−	−	+	+	d
Lactose O-F medium	+O	+O	+O	−/x	x	+	+	+	−	−	ND	ND	ND	ND
Xylose/25 C	+	+	+	−/x	−/x	+	+	+	−	−	d	+	+	d
Nitrate reduction	+	+	+	+	−	+	+	+	+	−	ND	ND	ND	ND
Trehalose	+	+	+	+	−	ND	ND	ND	ND	ND	ND	ND	ND	ND
Sorbitol	+	+	+	+	−	+	+	+	+	−	ND	ND	ND	ND
Ornithine decarboxylase/25 C	+	+	+	+	−	ND	ND	ND	ND	−	ND	ND	ND	ND
Acetylmethylcarbinol/25 C	+	+	+	+	−	+	+	+	+	ND	ND	ND	ND	ND
β-galactosidase/25 C	+	+	+	+	−	+	+	+	+	−	ND	ND	ND	ND
Sucrose/25 C	+	+	+	+	d	ND	ND	ND	ND	ND	ND	ND	ND	ND
L-sorbose	+	+	+	+	d	ND	ND	ND	ND	ND	ND	ND	ND	ND
Lecithinase	ND	ND	ND	ND	ND	+	−	−	−	−	ND	ND	ND	ND

+, Positive 1–2 days; −, negative; x, irregularly or delayed positive.
(+), delayed positive (>2 days); ND, not done; d, strains vary.
O, oxidative metabolism.

Y. *pseudotuberculosis* has similar antimicrobial sensitivities to those of Y. *pestis* and Y. *enterocolitica*. Streptomycin, tetracycline, and chloramphenicol are effective in treating human infections caused by it. Again, penicillin and ampicillin are usually ineffective *in vivo*.

Sensitivity to various antimicrobials should be determined in the laboratory with standard techniques such as, e.g., the Kirby-Bauer or minimal inhibitory concentration methods. Caution is urged in equating *in vitro* findings and *in vivo* activity.

Interpretation of Laboratory Findings

Definitive diagnosis of Y. *enterocolitica* and Y. *pseudotuberculosis* is dependent on the isolation and identification of the agent from appropriate specimens. Presumptive diagnosis of infection with either agent can be based on clinical and/or surgical findings in conjunction with a compatible medical history, although if the disease is enteric in nature, other enteric bacterial agents cannot be dismissed as possible causes.

Results of specific serological tests for Y. *pseudotuberculosis* antibody which indicate a high titer during the acute phase of illness and significant drop in titer during the convalescent phase support the diagnosis retrospectively. Similarly, positive serological tests for Y. *enterocolitica* antibody which usually show significantly increasing titers during convalescence can be used to support the diagnosis, although again it must be stressed that serological test results on many serotypes of Y. *enterocolitica* found in the United States must be interpreted cautiously unless a confirmed bacterial isolate is obtained.

References

1. AI NV, HANH ND, DIEM PV and LE NV: Co-trimoxazole in bubonic plague. Br Med J 4:108–109, 1973
2. BAHMANYAR M and CAVANAUGH DC: Plague manual. World Health Organization, Geneva, 1976
3. BOTTONE EJ: *Yersinia enterocolitica*: A. Panoramic view of a charismatic organism. *In* CRC Critical Reviews in Microbiology. CRC Press, Cleveland, Ohio, 1977, pp 211–241
4. BOTZLER RG, WETZLER TF, and COWAN AB: *Yersinia enterocolitica* and *Yersinia*-like organisms isolated from frogs and snails. Bull Wildlife Dis Assoc 4:110–115, 1968
5. BRENNER DJ, STEIGERWALT AG, FALCAO DP, WEAVER RE, and FANNING GR: Characterization of *Yersinia enterocolitica* and *Yersinia pseudotuberculosis* by deoxyribonucleic acid hybridization and by biochemical reactions. Int J Syst Bacteriol 26:180–194, 1976
6. CENTER FOR DISEASE CONTROL: Annual Report of the Vector-Borne Diseases Division, CDC, Fort Collins, Colo, 1975
7. CENTER FOR DISEASE CONTROL: Gastro-intestinal illness, Montana. Morbid Mortal Weekly Rep 24(16):142–143, 1975
8. CENTER FOR DISEASE CONTROL: Plague—Arizona, Colorado, New Mexico. Morbid Mortal Weekly Rep 26(26):215, 1977
9. CENTER FOR DISEASE CONTROL: Plague—United States, 1976. Morbid Mortal Weekly Rep 26(19):159, 1977
10. CENTER FOR DISEASE CONTROL: Plague—United States. Morbid Mortal Weekly Rep 26(41):337, 1977
11. CENTER FOR DISEASE CONTROL: *Yersinia enterocolitica* outbreak in New York. Morbid Mortal Weekly Rep 26(7):53–54, 1977

12. CHEN TH and MEYER KF: Studies on immunization against plague. X. Specific precipitation of *Pasteurella pestis* antigen and antibodies in gels. J Immunol 74:501–507, 1955
13. CHEN TH, QUAN SF, and MEYER KF: Studies on immunization of plague. II. The complement fixation test. J Immunol 68:147–158, 1952
14. CURRIE JA, MARSHALL JD JR, and CROZIER D: Rapid hemagglutination test for the detection of *Pasteurella pseudotuberculosis* antibodies. J Infect Dis 116:117–122, 1966
15. DEVIGNAT R: Varietes de l'espece *Pasteurella pestis*: nouvelle hypothese. Bull WHO 4:247–263, 1951
16. ESSEVELD H and GOUDZWAARD C: On the epidemiology of *Yersinia enterocolitica* infections: pigs as the source of infections in man. *In* Yersinia, Pasteurella, and Francisella. Vol. 2. Contributions to Microbiology and Immunology. Winblad S (ed.). Karger, Basel, Switzerland, 1973, pp 146–149
17. GOLDENBERG MI, HUDSON BN, and KARTMAN L: *Pasteurella* Infections. I. *Pasteurella pestis*. *In* Diagnostic Procedures for Bacterial, Mycotic and Parasitic Infections. Bodily HL, Updyke EL, and Mason JO (eds.). American Public Health Association, Inc, New York, NY, 1970, pp 422–439
18. GOLDENBERG MI, QUAN SF, and PRINCE FM: The survival of *Pasteurella pestis* in materials preserved by solid carbon dioxide (dry ice). Bull WHO 30:741–746, 1964
19. GUTMAN LT, OTTESEN EA, QUAN TJ, NOCE PS, and KATZ SL: An inter-familial outbreak of *Yersinia enterocolitica* enteritis. N Engl J Med 288:1372–1377, 1973
20. HANNA MD, ZINK DL, CARPENTER ZL, and VANDERZANT C: *Yersinia enterocolitica*-like organisms from vacuum packaged beef and lamb. J Food Sci 41:1254–1256, 1976
21. HORNIBROOK JW: A useful menstruum for drying organisms and viruses. J Lab Clin Med 35:788–792, 1950
22. HUDSON BW and KARTMAN L: The use of the passive hemagglutination test in epidemiologic investigations of sylvatic plague in the United States. Bull Wildlife Dis Assoc 3:50–59, 1967
23. HUDSON BW, KARTMAN L, and PRINCE FM: *Pasteurella pestis* detection in fleas by fluorescent antibody staining. Bull WHO 34:709–714, 1966
24. HURVELL B and LINDBERG AA: Immunochemical studies on the cross reactions between *Brucella* species and *Yersinia enterocolitica* type 9. *In* Yersinia, Pasteurella, and Francisella. Vol. 2. Contributions to Microbiology and Immunology. Winblad S (ed.). Karger, Basel, Switzerland, 1973, pp 159–168
25. INTERNATIONAL HEALTH REGULATIONS: WHO, Geneva, Switzerland, 1969
26. ISAACSON M, LEVY D, PIENAAR B, BUBB HD, LOUW JA, and GENIS DK: Unusual cases of human plague in Southern Africa. S Afr Med J 4:2109–2113, 1973
27. KNAPP W: Ein Beitrag zur Beweglichkeit von *Pasteurella pseudotuberculosis*. Z Hyg 142:219, 1956
28. KNAPP W: Über weitere antigene Beziehunger zwischen *Pasteurella pseudotuberculosis* und der *Salmonella* Gruppe. Z Hyg 146:315–317, 1960
29. KNAPP W and THAL E: Differentiation of *Yersinia enterocolitica* by biochemical reactions. *In* Yersinia, Pasteurella, and Francisella. Vol. 2. Contributions to Microbiology and Immunology. Winblad S (ed.). Karger, Basel, Switzerland, 1973, pp 10–16
30. LEE WH: Two plating media modified with Tween 80 for isolating *Yersinia enterocolitica*. Appl Environ Microbiol 33:215–216, 1977
31. MEYER KF, CAVANAUGH DC, BARTONELLI PJ, and MARSHALL JD JR: Plague immunization. I. Past and present trends. J Infect Dis 129(Suppl):S13–S18, 1974
32. MEYER KF and FOSTER LE: Measurement of protective serum antibodies in human volunteers inoculated with plague prophylactics. Stanford Med Bull 6:75–79, 1948
33. MOLLARET HH and THAL E: Yersinia. *In* Bergey's Manual of Determinative Bacteriology, 8th edition. Buchanan RE and Gibbons NE (eds.). Williams & Wilkins Co, Baltimore, 1974, pp 330–332
34. MOODY MD and WINTER CC: Rapid identification of *Pasteurella pestis* with fluorescent antibody. III. Staining *Pasteurella pestis* in tissue impression smears. J Infect Dis 104:288–294, 1959
35. MOORE RL and BRUBAKER RR: Hybridization of deoxyribonucleotide sequences of *Yersinia enterocolitica* and other selected members of *Enterobacteriacea*. Int J Syst Bacteriol 25:336–339, 1975

36. NICOLLE P, MOLLARET HH, and BRAULT J: Recherches sur la lysogenie, la lysosensibilite, la lysotypie et la serologie de *Yersinia enterocolitica*. *In* Yersinia, Pasteurella and Francisella. Vol. 2. Contributions to Microbiology and Immunology. Winblad S (ed.). Karger, Basel, Switzerland, 1973, pp 54–58

37. NILEHN B: Studies on *Yersinia enterocolitica* with special reference to bacterial diagnosis and occurrence in human acute enteric disease. Acta Pathol Microbiol Scand Suppl 206:1–48, 1969

38. POLAND JD: Plague. *In* Infectious Diseases, 2nd edition. Hoeprich PD (ed.). Harper and Row, Hagerstown, Md, 1977

39. POLAND JD, BARNES AM, and HERMAN JJ: Human bubonic plague from exposure to a naturally infected wild carnivore. Am J Epidemiol 97:332–337, 1973

40. QUAN SF, VON FINTEL H, and MCMANUS AG: Ecological studies of wild rodent plague in the San Francisco Bay Area of California. II. Efficiency of bacterial culture compared to animal inoculation as method for detecting *Pasteurella pestis* in wild rodent fleas. Am J Trop Med Hyg 7:411–415, 1958

41. QUAN TJ: Biotypic and serotypic profiles of 359 *Yersinia enterocolitica* cultures of human and environmental origin in the United States. Contrib Microbiol Immunol, 5:83–87, 1979

42. QUAN TJ, MEEK JL, TSUCHIYA KR, HUDSON BW and BARNES AM: Experimental pathogenicity of recent North American isolates of *Yersinia enterocolitica*. J Infect Dis 129:341–343, 1974

43. SAARI TN and JANSEN GP: Waterborne and human *Yersinia enterocolitica* in the Midwest United States. Contrib Microbiol Immunol 5:185–196, 1979

44. SURGALLA MJ, BEESLEY ED, and ALBIZO JM: Practical application of new laboratory methods for plague investigations. Bull WHO 42:993–997, 1970

45. TOMA S, LIOR H, QUINN-HILL M, SHER N, and WALKER WA: *Yersinia enterocolitica* infection: report of two cases. Can J Public Health 63:433–436, 1972

46. VON REYN CF, BARNES AM, WEBER NS, QUAN TJ, and DEAN WJ: Bubonic plague from direct exposure to a naturally infected wild coyote. Am J Trop Med Hyg 25:626–629, 1976

47. WAUTERS G: Contribution à l'étude de *Yersinia enterocolitica*. Doctoral dissertation, Vander, Louvain, Belgium, 1970

48. WETZLER TF: Pseudotuberculosis. *In* Diagnostic Procedures for Bacterial, Mycotic and Parasitic Infections, 5th edition. Bodily HL, Updyke EL, and Mason JO (eds.). American Public Health Association, Inc, New York, NY, 1970, pp 449–468

49. WETZLER TF: Pseudotuberculosis. *In* Infectious Diseases of Wild Mammals. Davis JW, Karstad LH, and Trainer DO (eds.). Iowa State Univ Press, Ames, Iowa, 1970, pp 224–235

50. WINBLAD S: Studies on the O-antigen factors of *Yersinia enterocolitica*. *In* International Symp. on Pseudotuberculosis, Symp. Series on Immunobiol. Standardization, Vol. 9. Regamey E (ed.). Karger, Basel, Switzerland, 1968, pp 27–37

51. WINTER CC and MOODY MD: A rapid identification of Pasteurella pestis with fluorescent antibody. I. Production of specific antiserum with whole cell *Pasteurella pestis* antigen. J Infect Dis 104:274–280; and II. Specific identification of *Pasteurella pestis* in dried smears. Ibid. 281–287, 1959

52. WORLD HEALTH ORGANIZATION COMMITTEE ON PLAGUE: Passive hemagglutination test. WHO Tech Rep Series 447:23–25, 1970

CHAPTER 44

ANTIMICROBIAL SUSCEPTIBILITY TESTS FOR BACTERIA

Clyde Thornsberry and Carolyn N. Baker

Introduction

One of the major roles of the clinical microbiology laboratory is isolating pathogens from appropriate clinical material and assisting the clinician in choosing appropriate antimicrobial therapy. The microbiologist must use appropriate antimicrobial susceptibility methods and perform them in a standardized manner in order to obtain as much useful clinical and epidemiological information as possible.

Antimicrobial susceptibility methods as we know them in the antibiotic era probably began with the report of Rammelkamp and Maxon, who described a broth dilution method for measuring the activity of penicillin on *Staphylococcus aureus* (23). Soon afterward, there were reports of similar methods involving paper disks (17, 35). In 1947, Bondi et al. described a routine paper disk method for performing antimicrobial susceptibility tests (7). Of the many disk tests that evolved during the next 20 years, some involved using various concentrations of drugs and disks. However, beginning in the early 1950's, Kirby and his colleagues began to develop and recommend a method in which they used single high-content disks, and from which categories of clinical susceptibility (i.e., susceptible, intermediate, or resistant) were derived. These interpretations were based on zone diameters from data developed through a statistical study of the correlation of zone diameters and minimal inhibitory concentrations (MICs) and a study of the distribution of zone diameters obtained with organisms whose levels of susceptibility to an antimicrobial agent vary. Their work on the development of this standardized disk method of antimicrobial susceptibility testing culminated in the classic publication of Bauer, Kirby, Sherris, and Turck in 1966 (4). This method has been adopted in most U.S. clinical microbiology laboratories for routine susceptibility testing.

Other factors have contributed to the remarkable acceptance of this method in the United States. A 1968 Supreme Court decision affirmed the right of the Food and Drug Administration (FDA) to certify the commercial disks (40). Furthermore, in 1972 the FDA adopted the standardized Kirby-Bauer method as the procedure to be described in the insert included in each package of disks (10). The National Committee for Clinical Laboratory Standards (NCCLS) also adopted the method and published a standard for it in 1975 (18) and revised it in 1979 (19).

Other susceptibility testing methods have also evolved. The broth dilution method has basically become a microdilution procedure in which volumes of 0.05 or 0.1 ml per well are placed in trays containing 80 or more wells. These trays can be prepared in the laboratory with automated or mechanized systems now available commercially. Two frozen and three dried microdilution MIC systems have been FDA-certified, and can be purchased (3, 13). Other systems of prefilled trays are now being studied.

Agar dilution MICs have been performed routinely for years at the Mayo Clinic (36) with a Steers replicating device (26). Some other large laboratories also now use this method routinely, but most microbiologists find the method inconvenient, even though they recognize that its accuracy and reproducibility are very satisfactory.

Recently, the NCCLS has published a standard for performing dilution susceptibility tests.

Simultaneous identification and susceptibility testing are being studied in both the broth microdilution and agar dilution systems. Because of space limitations, the concentrations of antimicrobial agents tested are necessarily limited. If only one concentration is tested, a category result is obtained, i.e., sensitive or resistant. If two or three concentrations are tested, an MIC can be reported.

Automation has also been applied to susceptibility tests. The Autobac system (Pfizer) (31), the *Escherichia coli* card used in the AMS system (Vitek), the MS-2 system (Abbott) (27), and the API system have been approved by FDA. Other automated or mechanized systems are currently being studied.

Several factors can affect the results of antimicrobial susceptibility tests (28). These may include specific characteristics of the individual organism and drug being tested but also include several methodological factors—i.e., culture medium (components, ionic content, pH), stability of the drug, size of inoculum, time and temperature of incubation, atmosphere of incubation, and variation in end-point determinations.

Mueller-Hinton broth or agar adjusted to a pH of 7.3 ± 0.2 must be used as the medium for the Kirby-Bauer disk method. The cation content should be approximately that of human serum; this is particularly important for tests with aminoglycosides and *Pseudomonas aeruginosa*. Where possible, Mueller-Hinton broth or agar has also been used with tests for MICs. Mueller-Hinton broth, which generally contains negligible cations, can be adjusted by adding 50 mg of calcium and 25 mg of magnesium per liter. Mueller-Hinton agar, however, cannot usually be adjusted to yield predictable results. Therefore, a new lot of Mueller-Hinton agar should be performance tested with an aminoglycoside disk (e.g., gentamicin) and the reference strain *Pseudomonas aeruginosa* ATCC 27853 in a Kirby-Bauer test. The zone of inhibition should fall within the range specified by the NCCLS (19, 30). Blood or blood products can be added to Meuller-Hinton agar, even for the Kirby-Bauer test. In the MIC test, other media can be substituted for Mueller-Hinton if necessary for growth. (It should be emphasized again that other media cannot be substituted in the Kirby-Bauer method.)

The incubation temperature should be 35 C. Higher temperatures may prevent the recognition of methicillin-resistant *Staphylococcus aureus* (29). The time of incubation should not exceed 24 hr unless otherwise specified in the description of the method. Atmospheres of CO_2 and/or anaerobiosis should not be used for the Kirby-Bauer test but can be used for MIC tests if required for growth.

Antimicrobial disks certified by the FDA do not generally cause problems, but they must be kept dry and cold to insure the stability of some drugs. The same is true for the antimicrobial powders used in MIC tests. This stability can be maintained by putting the disks or drugs in a container with a desiccant (preferably with a moisture indicator) and storing them in a freezer.

End-point determination which involves human judgment is subjective for any susceptibility test. In the disk diffusion test, some zones have feathery edges which contribute to subjectivity, and MIC end points may be influenced by the inoculum. However, if end points are read as described for the methods, acceptable accuracy and reproducibility are not difficult to attain.

Routine susceptibility testing in a microbiology laboratory can be done with either the Kirby-Bauer disk diffusion procedure or with an acceptable MIC procedure because sufficiently accurate and reproducible methods have been developed for both. As mentioned previously, most laboratorians in the United States use the Kirby-Bauer method, but a number prefer the broth microdilution and the agar dilution methods. Therefore the choice of method must be based upon each laboratory's needs. If the decision is made to use MICs routinely, an education program for the clinical staff must be initiated. Several laboratories also use automated systems routinely.

The method adopted must always be performed in a standard manner, and a quality control program must be initiated. The heart of the quality control program is the use of standard reference strains (19–21). Recommended strains are listed for each method.

In the remainder of this chapter, we describe in detail the procedures for routinely performed susceptibility tests.

Agar Disk Diffusion Susceptibility Testing (4, 19)

This standardized disk susceptibility test is a modification of the test described by Bauer, Kirby, Sherris, and Turck (4). The test is practical, accurate, and reproducible for detecting the susceptibility of rapidly growing pathogens to antimicrobial agents. The agar overlay method (2) yields equivalent results and has been approved by the FDA (10).

Reagents and Materials

1. Mueller-Hinton agar.
2. Mueller-Hinton broth or Trypticase soy broth.
3. FDA-certified, high-content antimicrobic paper disks specified for the Kirby-Bauer method.
4. Petri plates, 150 × 15 mm.

Medium

Prepare Mueller-Hinton agar as directed by manufacturer; autoclave and cool to 48–50 C. Dispense 60 ml into a 150- × 15-mm petri plate. Let the medium harden. If the plates are to be stored for later use, seal in plastic and place in a refrigerator at 4–8 C. Generally, no more than a week's supply should be prepared; if necessary, plates can be stored more than 1 week if they have been properly sealed and no evaporation has occurred. The pH of the agar should be 7.3 ± 0.2 when checked at room temperature. Commercially prepared plates can also be used.

Before it is used, the surface of the agar should be dry, and no water droplets should be on the petri plate cover.

Performance of the Test

Select four or five similar, well-isolated colonies of the organism to be tested from an 18- to 24-hr pure culture or from the primary isolation plate. Touch the top of each colony successively with the same wire loop, and transfer the bacteria to a tube containing 3 to 5 ml of Mueller-Hinton or Trypticase soy broth. Incubate the tube at 35 C long enough (2 to 8 hr) to produce an organism suspension with slight to moderate cloudiness. Dilute the broth culture with sterile saline or broth *to obtain a turbidity equivalent to that of a 0.5 McFarland turbidity standard.* (To prepare the standard, add 0.5 ml of 1.175% $BaCl_2 \cdot 2H_2O$ solution to 99.5 ml of 1% H_2SO_4. Dispense 3–5 ml of the standard into a tube. Seal the tube to prevent evaporation. When not in use, it can be stored in the dark at room temperature for 6 months or more. The standard must be thoroughly mixed just before use, preferably on a vortex mixer.)

Dip a sterile cotton swab into the adjusted inoculum, lift the swab above the fluid level, and rotate it against the inside of the tube to remove as much excess inoculum as possible. Streak the entire agar surface with the swab evenly in three directions. Let the inoculum dry for 3–5 min with the plate closed. Place disks on the agar with a dispenser or sterile forceps with up to nine disks in the outer circle and two or three in the middle. To avoid overlapping zones, do not place disks likely to produce large zones next to each other, e.g., penicillins and cephalosporins. Also, do not place disks next to each other that contain drugs that are likely to be antagonistic, e.g., erythromycin and clindamycin. Place disks likely to yield small zones, e.g., colistin, in the center area of the plate. Press disks down gently on the agar with sterile forceps to insure even contact. Incubate plates immediately or within 30 min in air at 35 C. Do not use higher temperatures because some methicillin-resistant staphylococci may be missed. Do not incubate in a candle extinction jar or in a CO_2 incubator.

Read plates after 16–24 hr of incubation.

Reading Results

Measure the zone size around each disk against a dark background under reflected light using a light source set at a 45 degree angle. Measure zone diameters (including the 6-mm disk) with a ruler on the undersurface (back) of the petri dish without removing the cover. Carefully prepared templates can also be used to categorize zones. (A reading of 6 mm indicates *no zone*.) If blood agar is used, measure the zones from the surface with the cover off the plate. The end point is complete inhibition of growth as judged by the naked eye, except for sulfonamides and swarming *Proteus* species. With sulfonamides, slight growth (20% or less growth, i.e., 80% or more inhibition of growth) may occur throughout the zone of inhibition, because some Mueller-Hinton agar has components (principally thymidine) which inhibit sulfonamide activity. Strains of *Proteus mirabilis* and *Proteus vulgaris* may swarm back into areas of inhibited growth around certain antimicrobics. The zones of inhibition are usually clearly outlined, and this veil of swarming growth should be ignored. Interpret the zone sizes as shown in Table 44.1.

Control Strains

Each time tests are performed, use one or more appropriate control strains. The following strains are recommended:

Escherichia coli ....ATCC 25922
Pseudomonas aeruginosa..ATCC 27853
Staphylococcus aureus...ATCC 25923

The allowable ranges of zone diameters for each antimicrobic are listed in Table 44.2. When zones for control strains fall outside those limits, the reason should be determined and appropriate remedial action taken. In order to utilize the quality control program fully, zone diameters for the reference strains must be measured, recorded, and compared with previous results.

P. aeruginosa ATCC 27853 may develop carbenicillin-resistant mutants during passage on laboratory media. If this occurs, get a new subculture from lyophilized or frozen stocks.

For more detailed information on quality control of disk susceptibility tests, see references 19 and 30.

Comments

1. Refrigerate individual containers of susceptibility disks at 4–5 C, or store at −20 C or below until needed. Disks containing drugs belonging to the penicillin or cephalosporin families are most susceptible to degradation and should always be kept frozen, except for a small working supply which can be refrigerated for at least 1 week. Allow new containers of susceptibility disks to reach room temperature before opening them. Store dispensers containing susceptibility disks with a desiccant in the refrigerator, but allow them to warm to room temperature before they are used. Discard any leftover disks on the manufacturer's stated expiration date. Disks *must* be kept dry until they are used.

2. Inocula adjusted as described in this method will contain approximately 10^8 colony forming units per ml. Adjustments can be made by other methods, e.g., spectrophotometrically, if the correct inoculum size is obtained. Do not use overnight cultures.

3. Diffusion techniques have been standardized with rapidly growing

Table 44.1—Zone Diameter Interpretive Standards and Approximate Minimal Inhibitory Concentration (MIC) Correlates

Antimicrobial Agent	Disk Content	Zone Diameter, Nearest Whole MM			Approximate MIC Correlates	
		Resistant	Intermediate	Susceptible	Resistant	Susceptible
Amikacin[a]	30 µg	≤14	15-16	≥17	≥32 µg/ml	≤16 µg/ml
Ampicillin when testing gram-negative enteric organisms and enterococci[b]	10 µg	≤11	12-13	≥14	≥32 µg/ml	≤8 µg/ml
Ampicillin[b] when testing staphylococci[c] and penicillin G-susceptible microorganisms	10 µg	≤20	21-28	≥29	β-lactamase[c]	≤0.2 µg/ml
Ampicillin when testing Haemophilus species[d]	10 µg	≤19	—	≥20	>2.0 µg/ml	≤2.0 µg/ml
Bacitracin	10 units	≤8	9-12	≥13	—	—
Carbenicillin when testing Proteus species and Escherichia coli	100 µg	≤17	18-22	≥23	—	≤16 µg/ml
Carbenicillin when testing Pseudomonas aeruginosa	100 µg	≤13	14-16	≥17	≥250 µg/ml	≤125 µg/ml
Cefamandole[e]	30 µg	≤14	15-17	≥18	≥32 µg/ml	≤10 µg/ml
Cefoxitin[e]	30 µg	≤14	15-17	≥18	≥32 µg/ml	≤10 µg/ml
Cephalothin[f]	30 µg	≤14	15-17	≥18	≥32 µg/ml	≤10 µg/ml
Chloramphenicol	30 µg	≤12	13-17	≥18	≥25 µg/ml	≤12.5 µg/ml
Clindamycin[g]	2 µg	≤14	15-16	≥17	≥2 µg/ml	≤1 µg/ml
Colistin[h]	10 µg	≤8	9-10	≥11	≥4 µg/ml	—
Erythromycin	15 µg	≤13	14-17	≥18	≥8 µg/ml	≤2 µg/ml
Gentamicin[a]	10 µg	≤12	13-14	≥15	≥8 µg/ml	≤8 µg/ml
Kanamycin	30 µg	≤13	14-17	≥18	≥25 µg/ml	≤6 µg/ml
Methicillin when testing staphylococci[i]	5 µg	≤9	10-13	≥14	—	≤3 µg/ml
Nalidixic acid[j]	30 µg	≤13	14-18	≥19	≥32 µg/ml	≤12 µg/ml
Neomycin	30 µg	≤12	13-16	≥17	—	—
Nitrofurantoin[j]	300 µg	≤14	15-16	≥17	≥100 µg/ml	≤25 µg/ml
Penicillin G when testing staphylococci[k]	10 units	≤20	21-28	≥29	β-lactamase[c]	≤0.1 µg/ml
Penicillin G when testing other microorganisms[l]	10 units	≤11	12-21	≥22	≥32 µg/ml	≤1.5 µg/ml
Polymyxin B[h]	300 units	≤8	9-11	≥12	≥50 units/ml	—
Streptomycin	10 µg	≤11	12-14	≥15	—	—
Sulfonamides[j,m]	250 or 300 µg	≤12	13-16	≥17	≥350 µg/ml	≤100 µg/ml
Tetracycline[n]	30 µg	≤14	15-18	≥19	≥12 µg/ml	≤4 µg/ml

Trimethoprim-sulfamethoxazole[a]	1.25 μg, 23.75 μg	≤ 10	11–15	≥ 16	≥ 8/152 μg/ml	≤ 2/38 μg/ml
Tobramycin[a]	10 μg	≤ 12	13–14	≥ 15	≥ 8 μg/ml	≤ 8 μg/ml
Vancomycin	30 μg	≤ 9	10–11	≥ 12	—	≤ 5 μg/ml

[a] The zone sizes obtained with aminoglycosides, particularly when testing *Pseudomonas aeruginosa*, are very medium dependent because of variations in cation content. The zone size interpretive standards for amikacin, gentamicin, and tobramycin shown in Table 44.1 are tentative standards recently agreed upon by a subcommittee of the NCCLS (19). These interpretive standards are to be used only with Mueller-Hinton medium that has yielded zone sizes within the correct range shown in Table 44.2 when performance tests were done with *P. aeruginosa* ATCC 27853. In addition, the amikacin disk must be 30 μg rather than the 10-μg disk used previously. Organisms in the intermediate category may be either susceptible or resistant when MICs are performed on them and should therefore more properly be classified as "indeterminate" in their susceptibility to aminoglycosides.

[b] Class disk for ampicillin, hetacillin, and amoxicillin.

[c] Resistant strains of *S. aureus* produce β-lactamase.

[d] For testing *Haemophilus*, use Mueller-Hinton agar supplemented with 1% hemoglobin and 1% IsoVitaleX (BBL) or equivalent. Adjust pH to 7.2. Prepare the inoculum by suspending growth from a 24-hr chocolate agar plate in Mueller-Hinton broth to the density of a 0.5 McFarland standard. The vast majority of ampicillin-resistant strains of *Haemophilus* produce β-lactamase. See text on *Haemophilus* testing.

[e] Cefamandole and cefoxitin were recently approved by the FDA. They have a wider spectrum of activity on gram-negative bacilli than do other approved cephalosporins. Therefore, cephalothin disks cannot be used as the class disk for these two drugs.

[f] The cephalothin disk is used for testing susceptibility to cephalothin, cephaloridine, cephalexin, cefazolin, cephacetrile, cephradine, cephapirin, and cefaclor. Cefamandole and cefoxitin must be tested separately. *Staphylococcus aureus* exhibiting resistance to methicillin disks should be reported as resistant to cephalosporin-type antibiotics, regardless of zone size, because in most cases infections caused by these organisms are clinically resistant to cephalosporins (1, 29). A recent report indicates that methicillin-resistant *S. epidermidis* infections may not respond to cephalosporins (15), but this issue is still unsettled.

[g] The clindamycin disk is used for testing susceptibility to both clindamycin and lincomycin.

[h] Colistin and polymyxin B diffuse poorly in agar, and the diffusion method is thus less accurate than with other antibiotics. Resistance is always significant, but when treatment of systemic infections caused by susceptible strains is being considered, results of a diffusion test should be confirmed with those of a dilution method. MIC correlates cannot be calculated reliably from regression analysis.

[i] Of the staphylococcal β-lactamase-resistant penicillins, methicillin is the class disk, and results also apply to cloxacillin, dicloxacillin, oxacillin, and nafcillin. Oxacillin and nafcillin are, however, more resistant to degradation in storage (30). Cloxacillin disks should not be used because they may not detect methicillin-resistant *S. aureus* (29).

[j] Susceptibility data for nalidixic acid, nitrofurantoin, and sulfonamides (other than trimethoprim-sulfamethoxazole) apply only to organisms isolated from urinary-tract infections.

[k] Penicillin G is used to test the susceptibility of all penicillinase-sensitive penicillins, except ampicillin, amoxicillin, hetacillin, and carbenicillin. Results can be applied to phenoxymethyl penicillin and phenethicillin.

[l] This category includes some organisms such as enterococci and gram-negative bacilli which may cause systemic infections treatable by high doses of penicillin G. Such organisms should be reported susceptible to penicillin G but not to phenoxymethyl penicillin or phenethicillin.

[m] Any of the commercially available 250- or 300-μg sulfonamide disks can be used with the same standards of zone interpretation. Blood-containing media, except media containing lysed horse blood (5, 6), are not satisfactory for testing sulfonamides. The Mueller-Hinton agar should be as thymidine-free as possible for sulfonamide testing.

[n] Tetracycline is the class disk for all tetracyclines, and the results can be applied to chlortetracycline, demeclocycline, doxycycline, methacycline, oxytetracycline, minocycline, and rolitetracycline for most commonly isolated organisms. However, some data show that certain organisms may be more susceptible to doxycycline and minocycline than to tetracycline.

pathogens such as staphylococci, *Pseudomonas aeruginosa*, and *Enterobacteriaceae* and *cannot* be reliably applied to slowly growing organisms because of the much larger zone sizes produced by the latter. However, total resistance (no zone) may be significant. Therefore, susceptibility testing of organisms which are fastidious in their nutritional requirements, which require an anaerobic atmosphere or increased concentration of CO_2 for growth, or which grow unusually slowly should be done with one of the dilution methods, pending development and standardization of suitable diffusion tests. Modifications of the recommended method may be applicable for detecting sulfonamide resistance of *Neisseria meningitidis* (5), and for β-lactamase-producing *N. gonorrhoeae* (6).

4. Use 15- × 150-mm petri plates in the Kirby-Bauer procedure. The proper depth of agar for the test can be obtained by adding 60 ml of agar if the petri plates are flat. However, 15- × 100-mm plates have been used with 25 ml of agar added. In the smaller plates, do not place more than eight disks on the agar surface. In some cases, e.g., β-lactamase-negative staphylococci, eight disks will be too many, because the zone diameters obtained with some of the

TABLE 44.2—SUSCEPTIBILITY OF CONTROL STRAINS

| | | INDIVIDUAL TEST CONTROL LIMITS ZONE DIAMETER OF INHIBITION (MM) | | |
| | DISK | *S. AUREUS* | *E. COLI* | *P. AERUGINOSA* |
ANTIBIOTIC	CONTENT	ATCC 25923	ATCC 25922	ATCC 27853
Amikacin	30 µg	20–26	19–26	18–26
Ampicillin	10 µg	24–35	15–20	—
Bacitracin	10 U	17–22	—	—
Carbenicillin	100 µg	—	24–29	20–24
Cefamandole	30 µg	28–34	24–31	—
Cefoxitin	30 µg	23–28	23–28	—
Cephalothin	30 µg	25–37	18–23	—
Chloramphenicol	30 µg	19–26	21–27	6–12
Clindamycin	2 µg	23–29	—	—
Colistin	10 µg	—	11–15	11–15
Erythromycin	15 µg	23–30	8–14	—
Gentamicin	10 µg	19–27	19–26	16–21
Kanamycin	30 µg	19–26	17–25	—
Methicillin	5 µg	17–22	—	—
Nalidixic acid	30 µg	—	23–28	—
Neomycin	30 µg	18–26	17–23	—
Nitrofurantoin	300 µg	20–24	21–26	—
Penicillin G	10 µg	26–37	—	—
Polymyxin B	300 µg	7–13	12–16	11–16
Streptomycin	10 µg	14–22	12–20	—
Sulfisoxazole	250 or 300 µg	24–34	18–26	—
Tetracycline	30 µg	19–28	18–25	6–14
Trimethoprim—	1.25 µg			
sulfamethoxazole	23.75 µg	24–32	24–32	—
Tobramycin	10 µg	19–29	18–26	19–25
Vancomycin	30 µg	15–19	—	—

antistaphylococcal drugs are very large. Overlapping zones will decrease accuracy and reproducibility. If zones overlap or if a zone is incomplete because the disk is too close to the edge of the plate, too many disks have been used.

5. Disk diffusion susceptibility tests on *Haemophilus* spp. should be performed as follows (19, 30). Use Mueller-Hinton agar supplemented with 1% IsoVitaleX or equivalent (do not use supplement C) and adjust the pH to 7.2. *Adjust the turbidity of the culture to equal the 0.5 McFarland standard or to contain 10^8 CFU/ml.* Inoculate the supplemented Mueller-Hinton agar as described for the Kirby-Bauer method. Allow to dry. Place the disks to be tested onto the surface of the inoculated agar and gently press them onto the agar with sterile forceps. Invert the plates and incubate them at 35 C for 24 hr. A CO_2 atmosphere is not generally necessary. Measure the diameter of zones with a caliper or ruler. A zone of ≥20 mm for ampicillin or penicillin indicates susceptibility; ≤19 mm indicates resistance (and in most cases β-lactamase production). For chloramphenicol and tetracycline we tentatively use the Kirby-Bauer breakpoints (4).

6. We recommend that an oxacillin disk test be used to screen for penicillin resistance (MIC ≥ 2.0 μg/ml) and penicillin-relative resistance (MIC 0.12–1.0 μg/ml) in pneumococci. Perform the test on Mueller-Hinton agar supplemented with 5% sheep blood (we have also used 5% lysed horse blood) and a 1-μg oxacillin disk. Prepare the inoculum by suspending the growth of several colonies in Mueller-Hinton or Trypticase soy broth and adjusting the turbidity to equal the 0.5 McFarland standard. Inoculate the agar as in the Kirby-Bauer test. Incubate either in ambient air or in CO_2 at 35 C. Measure the zones of inhibition after 18–24 hr of incubation. A zone of ≥ 20 mm indicates penicillin susceptibility, and ≤ 12 mm indicates either penicillin resistance or relative resistance (in most cases these zones are 6 or 7 mm). Occasionally, zones of 13–19 mm are obtained; their MICs were either 0.06 or 0.12 μg/ml.

Determining Minimal Inhibitory Concentration (MIC) by Agar Dilution (21)

Reagents and Materials

1. Mueller-Hinton agar.
2. Mueller-Hinton broth or Trypticase soy broth.
3. Antimicrobic powders suitable for susceptibility testing.
4. Steers or other replicator apparatus or 0.001-ml loop.
5. Petri plates, 90-mm square or 100-mm round.

Medium

The 90-mm square petri plate requires 30 ml of agar, whereas a 100-mm round petri plate requires 25 ml of agar. Prepare the amount of agar needed based on these figures. Cool the agar to 48–50 C. Before antimicrobial solutions are added, dispense the agar in appropriate volumes (see section on preparing plates) into bottles or flasks and hold in a 48–50 C water bath. If needed, add 5% defibrinated sheep, rabbit, or horse blood. Chocolatize if desired, but cool the medium to 48–50 C before adding antimicrobics.

Preparing Antimicrobic Solutions

Obtain antimicrobic powders suitable for susceptibility testing from individual pharmaceutical companies. It is necessary to know the potency of the powders; activity should be expressed in μg (or units) of pure substance. Store antimicrobic powders under desiccation at −20 C or less. Prepare stock solutions by putting the antimicrobics into solution in the appropriate diluent as outlined in the ASM *Manual of Clinical Microbiology*, 2nd edition (37) or the NCCLS dilution test standard (21). If a solvent other than the diluent is required initially, use only enough to get the material into solution, and make further dilutions with the appropriate diluent. Stock solutions may be sterilized by membrane filtration (0.22 μm). Distribute the stock solutions into vials or ampoules, seal tightly, and store at −20 C or less. Remove a vial(s) from storage as needed; use within a day or discard. The solution should never be refrozen for later use. Frozen antimicrobic solutions are usually stable for at least 6 months (21).

Preparing Plates

In this test, 1 part of antimicrobic solution is added to 9 parts of agar. Therefore, it is necessary to use the stock solution to prepare intermediate dilutions that are 10 times the desired final concentration. For example, if a final concentration of 128 μg/ml is desired, add 10 ml of a solution containing 1280 μg/ml antimicrobic to 90 ml of Mueller-Hinton agar at 48–50 C, mix by gentle inversion, and pour into four 90-mm round plates. Each plate will contain agar with 128 μg of antimicrobic per ml of medium. Repeat this process for each concentration of each antimicrobic. In each set of tests, always include control agar plates prepared without antimicrobic. Allow the agar to harden at room temperature. For routine use, plates can be stored for 4 weeks at 4 C if they are sealed in plastic bags (a simple heat-sealing device works well). Allow the plates to dry before they are inoculated.

Performing the Test

Inoculate Mueller-Hinton or Trypticase soy broth with four to five similar colonies from a 24-hr primary isolation plate. Incubate at 35 C until the logarithmic or early stationary phase of growth is reached (usually 2–8 hr). Dilute the culture to contain 10^7 colony forming units (CFU) per ml of medium. If the McFarland standard is used, adjust the culture to match the standard, and then make a further dilution of 1:10. If a replicating device is used, transfer each adjusted culture to a well of a sterile seed plate. With the Steers device, as many as 36 cultures per plate can be tested. Use the replicator head to "spot inoculate" the cultures onto the dried agar plates. About 10^4 CFU from each culture will be delivered onto the surface of the agar. Prevent the swarming of *Proteus* cultures by pressing a glass cylinder or assay cup into the agar around the inoculum.

Reading Results

The MIC is the lowest concentration of antimicrobic that inhibits growth. Disregard a barely visible haze or a single colony. If several colonies are found extending beyond an obvious end point, check the purity of the culture and repeat the test.

Control Strains

Each time tests are performed, use one or more appropriate control strains. The following strains are recommended:

Escherichia coli ....ATCC 25922
Pseudomonas aeruginosa..ATCC 27853
Staphylococcus aureus...ATCC 29213
Streptococcus faecalis..ATCC 29212

Determining Minimal Inhibitory Concentration (MIC) with Broth Microdilution (21)

Reagents and Materials

1. Mueller-Hinton broth.
2. Cation supplements.
   a. *Magnesium stock solution*
      Dissolve 83.6 mg of $MgCl_2 \cdot 6H_2O$ in 100 ml of deionized distilled water. This solution contains 10 mg of Mg^{++}/ml. Sterilize by filtration and store at 4 C.
   b. *Calcium stock solution*
      Dissolve 36.75 mg of $CaCl_2 \cdot 2H_2O$ in 100 ml of deionized distilled water. This solution contains 10 mg of Ca^{++}/ml. Sterilize by filtration and store at 4 C.
3. Microdilution trays and filling system. The trays can be filled with one of several available systems (16), or prefilled trays can be purchased (3, 13).
4. Antimicrobic powders suitable for susceptibility testing.

Medium

Prepare the Mueller-Hinton broth as directed by the manufacturer, autoclave, and chill overnight at 4 C (or chill in an ice bath if prepared on the same day trays are to be filled). Add 2.5 ml of chilled Mg^{++} stock solution to each liter of cold broth. The concentration of Mg^{++} will be 25 mg/liter. Add 5.0 ml of chilled Ca^{++} stock solution to each liter of cold broth. The concentration of Ca^{++} will be 50 mg/liter. This medium is hereafter called cation supplemented Mueller-Hinton broth (CSMHB) (21, 30).

Preparing Antimicrobic Solutions

Prepare stock dilutions of antimicrobics and store them as outlined for the agar dilution method.

Preparing and Storing Microdilution Trays

Dilute the stock solution of antimicrobic in sterile distilled water to contain 10 times the final desired concentration (e.g., 1280 μg/ml, 640 μg/ml, etc.). For each drug, add 1 ml of 10 times concentrated antimicrobic solution to 9 ml of CSMHB. Add 1 ml of sterile distilled water to 9 ml of CSMHB to serve as a growth control. Dispense 0.1 ml of each antimicrobic solution and the control solution into the wells of the microdilution tray by hand or, more easily and efficiently, with an automated commercial dispenser. Seal the prepared trays in plastic bags. Immediately place the bags of trays in a freezer at −20 C or less and store until needed. (The frozen trays usually remain stable for at least 4 weeks before any of the antimicrobic agents begin to deteriorate.) Do not store trays in a *self-defrosting freezer.*

Performing the Test

Select three to four well-isolated, similar colonies from an overnight primary isolation plate. Touch each colony with a loop and transfer the growth to a tube of Mueller-Hinton or Trypticase soy broth. Incubate the broth at 35 C for 2–4 hr or until the turbidity is equivalent to that of a McFarland standard (4). If the turbidity is greater than the standard, dilute with broth to equal the standard. The inoculum will then be approximately 10^8 CFU/ml. Dilute in broth or water so that after final inoculation each well contains approximately 10^5 CFU/ml. The amount of diluent will vary according to the volume of inoculum.

With the adjusted inoculum, inoculate each well of the thawed antimicrobic tray with calibrated dropping pipettes or with automated or mechanized inoculators. If the latter are used, all the wells in a plate are inoculated at the same time. Seal the inoculated trays inside plastic bags, or with plastic tape. Incubate at 35 C for 16 to 20 hr in a *forced air incubator.*

Read and record results. (Readers with mirrors are available if desired.) The minimal inhibitory concentration (MIC) is read as the lowest concentration of antimicrobic which completely inhibits growth of the organism as detected with the unaided eye.

Control Strains

Before a new set of plates is accepted for routine use, perform tests with the control organisms. The MICs obtained should be within acceptable limits (21).

Each time tests are performed, use one or more appropriate control strains. The following strains are recommended:

Escherichia coli..ATCC 25922
Pseudomonas aeruginosa...ATCC 27853
Staphylococcus aureus...ATCC 29213
Streptococcus faecalis..ATCC 29212

Susceptibility Tests for Anaerobes (20, 33)

Antimicrobial susceptibility testing of anaerobes can be done with either agar dilution or broth dilution tests if the appropriate atmosphere is used (30, 33). An atmosphere of 85% nitrogen, 10% hydrogen, and 5% carbon dioxide or the atmosphere of the GasPak is very efficacious for this purpose (25). Wilkins-Chalgren agar or broth is a good medium to use in performing MICs on anaerobes (12, 38).

For laboratories that do not perform MICs but wish to do susceptibility testing of anaerobes, the broth-disk methods are recommended as routine procedures. In the Wilkins-Thiel method, a single concentration of antimicrobic is delivered to broth in a commercially available disk (i.e., one used in the Kirby-Bauer test) (39). If the test organism grows in the broth, it is resistant to the drug; if it fails to grow, it is susceptible. In the Kurzynski modification of this method, thioglycollate broth is substituted for brain heart infusion broth so that the test can be done in air (14). In the category method used in our laboratory, two or three clinically important concentrations of each drug are tested (33). Disk diffusion methods are not recommended for anaerobic bacteria.

The antimicrobics to be tested with anaerobic bacteria should generally be limited to drugs known to be effective against anaerobic infections and those that are generally used for this purpose in the institution where the tests are being performed. The basic list should include penicillin G, tetracycline, chloramphenicol, and clindamycin. Erythromycin, carbenicillin, cefoxitin, and metronidazole may be added if used clinically or if requested.

Wilkins-Thiel Broth-Disk Method (30, 33, 39)

For the inoculum, grow the test organism overnight in prereduced chopped-meat broth. The medium to use for the tests is brain heart infusion broth supplemented with 0.0005% hemin, 0.002% menadione, and 0.5% yeast extract. Dispense the medium into tubes in 5-ml volumes, and close with rubber stoppers. To add the antimicrobics, insert a cannula carrying oxygen-free CO_2 into a tube to prevent entry of air, and add the necessary disks (shown in Table 44.3). Inoculate each tube of broth by adding a drop of turbid inoculum

TABLE 44.3—PREPARATION OF ANTIBIOTIC BROTH TUBES FOR THE WILKINS-THIEL METHOD

ANTIBIOTIC	DISK CONTENT	DISK(S) PER TUBE	FINAL CONC/ML*
Penicillin G	10 U	1	2 U
Tetracycline	30 µg	1	6 µg
Clindamycin	2 µg	8	3.2 µg
Chloramphenicol	30 µg	2	12 µg
Erythromycin	15 µg	1	3 µg
Control	0	0	0

* Tubes contain 5 ml of broth.

with a Pasteur pipette, again using the stream of oxygen-free CO_2. Include a growth control broth that contains no antimicrobic. Reseal the tube. Since no oxygen has entered the tubes, each tube can serve as its own anaerobic chamber, but they can also be placed in an anaerobic chamber or jar as a precaution. Incubate for 18–24 hr at 35 C. Compare the turbidity of each antimicrobic tube with the growth control. A 50% reduction in the amount of growth indicates that the organism is susceptible to the drug; if the reduction in growth is less than 50%, the organism is resistant to the drug. In most cases, there is either no growth (susceptible) or equal growth (resistant). Report the results as either susceptible or resistant.

Kurzynski Broth-Disk Method (14, 30, 33)

This method is a modification of the Wilkins-Thiel test. Thioglycollate broth is substituted for brain heart infusion broth so that the test can be performed aerobically. The inoculum is grown in chopped meat glucose broth. Add the appropriate number of disks to the tubes of broth (shown in Table 44.3). Let the tubes stand for 2 hr to complete elution of the antimicrobics. This extended elution time is required because the thioglycollate broth contains 0.07% agar. Inoculate the thioglycollate broth with two drops of turbid inoculum, tighten the cap, and invert twice. Perform the remainder of the test according to the instructions for the Wilkins-Thiel method (39).

The Category Susceptibility Test for Anaerobes (24, 30, 33)

In this method, use two or three clinically important concentrations of each antimicrobic as shown in Table 44.4. A result can be reported as an MIC (based on an expanded scale in contrast to usual MICs that are based on serial twofold dilutions), or it can be reported as one of the four categories shown in Table 44.5.

For the test use Schaedler broth supplemented with 5 µg/ml hemin and 0.1 µg/ml vitamin K. Dispense the medium into sterile 13- × 100-mm screw-capped tubes in 2.7-ml volumes if the antimicrobic is to be added from a solution or in 3.0-ml volumes if the antimicrobic is to be added by disks. Prereduce the medium before using it. If the antimicrobics are to be added in solution, prepare stock solutions containing 1280 µg/ml (5120 µg/ml for carbenicillin).

TABLE 44.4—SUGGESTED ANTIBIOTIC CONCENTRATIONS FOR THE CATEGORY METHOD

ANTIMICROBIAL AGENT	TEST CONCENTRATION (μg/ml)
Penicillin G	0.25, 16, 128
Tetracycline	2, 8, 32
Clindamycin	2, 8, 64
Erythromycin	2, 4, 64
Chloramphenicol	1, 12
Carbenicillin	16, 128, 512
Cefoxitin	4, 16, 64
Metronidazole	4, 32, 128

Dispense into tubes, seal, and store at −70 C. For use, thaw a stock solution, and dilute to 10 times the final desired concentration. Add 0.3 ml of the 10× antimicrobic solution to 2.7 ml of the prereduced medium to obtain the final 1:10 dilution of the drug (33).

The antimicrobics can also be added in disks which contain the appropriate amount of drug (33). Prepare these disks as follows:

a. Make all stock solutions of drugs at 40 times the desired final concentrations per ml, e.g., 40× for 1 ml of broth, 80× for 2 ml of broth, 120× for 3 ml of broth, etc. If the desired concentration is 1 μg/ml in 3 ml of broth, prepare a stock solution of 120 μg/ml.

b. Spread 6-mm blank filter-paper disks on a sterile surface.

c. Drop 0.025 ml of stock solution on each disk.

d. Dry the disks in a laminar flow hood or in an incubator.

e. Place the disks with a desiccant in a container that can be sealed tightly. Store at −20 C or lower.

Add the appropriate disks to tubes containing 3 ml of Schaedler broth shortly before tests are run (it takes only a few minutes for the antimicrobic to elute into the broth).

Prepare the inoculum by removing several similar colonies from an agar plate that has been incubated overnight and suspending them in Schaedler

TABLE 44.5—INTERPRETATION OF CATEGORY SUSCEPTIBILITY TEST RESULTS

	GROWTH IN THE FOUR TUBES			
Category	Control	Low	Medium	High
I	+	−	−	−
II	+	+	−	−
III	+	+	+	−
IV	+	+	+	+

Category I. Very susceptible. Readily inhibited by levels of antibiotic attained in the blood on usual dosage.

Category II. Moderately susceptible. Inhibited by blood levels achieved on high dosage.

Category III. Moderately resistant. Inhibited by levels achieved where drug is concentrated, e.g., in urine.

Category IV. Very resistant. Resistant to usually achievable levels.

broth. Adjust the suspension to equal the turbidity of a 0.5 McFarland standard. An overnight broth culture can also be adjusted to the turbidity of the standard.

To perform the test, add 0.025 ml (disposable droppers are very convenient for this step) of the adjusted inoculum to each tube containing antimicrobics and to a growth control broth containing no antimicrobic. Incubate the tubes in an anaerobic chamber or GasPak jar for 18–24 hr at 35 C. Read the end point as the absence of macroscopic growth. The growth control must show adequate growth. Report the results as MICs or in terms of the categories of susceptibility shown in Table 44.5.

Other variations of category methods have been reported by Fass et al. (9), who used a broth test, and by Hauser et al. (11), who used an agar dilution method.

A standard reference method has been developed by a subcommittee of the NCCLS. It is an agar dilution method in which Wilkins-Chalgren agar is used (20). A set of standard reference strains were recommended by this committee. These reference strains should be used in a quality control program for these tests. The reference strains are:

Bacteroides fragilis...ATCC 25285
Clostridium perfringens..ATCC 13124
Bacteroides thetaiotaomicron ....ATCC 27941

Rapid β-Lactamase Methods (30)

The rapid iodometric, acidometric, and chromogenic cephalosporin techniques are specific tests for the presence of β-lactamase in a bacterial culture. The detection of resistance to penicillin with the disk diffusion test correlates with the production of β-lactamase by *H. influenzae, N. gonorrhoeae, S. aureus,* and *S. epidermidis.* With these tests, positive results are generally obtained quite rapidly with *H. influenzae* and *N. gonorrhoeae* but may take longer with staphylococci. However, staphylococci may produce positive results sooner if they are preinduced (use growth near a methicillin or oxacillin disk, e.g., from the edge of a zone), because many staphylococcal β-lactamases are inducible. The β-lactamases of *H. influenzae* and *N. gonorrhoeae* are not inducible.

These β-lactamase tests should be performed on pure cultures of bacteria, and should not be used for direct tests on body secretions. Control strains known to be β-lactamase positive and β-lactamase negative should be tested simultaneously with the test strains.

The three β-lactamase tests described here work equally well for determining β-lactamase in staphylococci, *H. influenzae,* and *N. gonorrhoeae,* but for many gram-negative bacteria the chromogenic cephalosporin test is more sensitive and the iodometric method the least sensitive. Each method has certain advantages and disadvantages, but we recommend the chromogenic cephalosporin test because of the stability of the reagent and the ease with which the test is performed.

For clinical use we recommend that β-lactamase tests be performed only on *Haemophilus* sp., *Neisseria* sp., and *Staphylococcus* sp.

The Rapid Iodometric Method for β-Lactamase (8, 30)

Prepare the substrate by adding sodium or potassium penicillin G powder to freshly prepared phosphate buffer, pH 6.0, to obtain a solution with a concentration of 6000 μg/ml. Dispense small aliquots of the penicillin solution into vials that can be tightly sealed and frozen in *non-frost-free freezers*. Frost-free freezers are unsuitable because repeated thawing cycles destroy the penicillin. Properly stored aliquots can be thawed and used for up to 1 week or as long as correct results are obtained with control cultures of known reactivity.

To prepare the starch solution, add 1.0 g of soluble starch to 100 ml of distilled water. Place in a boiling water bath until the starch goes into solution. Prepare fresh or store in refrigerator for no more than 1 week. Smaller volumes of this 1% solution can be made, because 10 ml is enough for over 100 tests. Starch designated for use in iodometric tests is commercially available.

The iodine reagent contains 2.03 g of iodine and 53.2 g of potassium iodide dissolved in 100 ml of distilled water. Store at room temperature in a brown glass bottle. Prepare fresh when the solution develops excessive precipitate (usually several months).

To perform the test, dispense 0.1 ml of penicillin solution into a well of a microdilution plate or a small test tube. Remove several similar colonies of an overnight culture with a loop and make a *heavy* turbid suspension in the penicillin solution in the well. An adequate amount of inoculum should produce a cloudy suspension. Stir for 30 sec and let the mixture stand for 1 hr at room temperature to allow time for the β-lactamase to break down the penicillin to penicilloic acid. *H. influenzae* and *N. gonorrhoeae* usually do not require an hour of incubation, but staphylococci may. Add 1 drop of iodine reagent with a Pasteur pipette. Add 2 drops of starch solution. *Stir the mixture for 1 min.* Rapid decolorization indicates the production of β-lactamase. If the solution remains blue for longer than 10 min, the culture did not produce the enzyme.

The Rapid Acidometric Method for β-Lactamase (30,32)

Prepare 0.5% phenol red solution by dissolving 1.0 g of indicator in 30 ml of 0.1 N NaOH and adding distilled water to a volume of 200 ml. Add 2.0 ml of 0.5% phenol red solution to 16.6 ml of sterile, distilled water. Add this solution to a vial containing 20 million units of potassium penicillin G. *Buffering is necessary;* many penicillin preparations contain citrate buffer which is adequate for the test. Add NaOH (1 N) drop by drop until the pH is 8.5. The solution will turn dark red. Since different individuals see colors differently, the pH should be determined with a pH meter. This penicillin substrate can be used immediately or divided into portions in screw-capped tubes and frozen in *non-frost-free freezers*. Frost-free freezers are unsuitable because repeated thawing cycles destroy the penicillin. If the frozen or thawed test solution turns yellow, discard it.

To perform the test, add 0.05 to 0.1 ml of penicillin substrate to a well of a microdilution plate or to a small tube. Remove several similar colonies with a loop and make a heavy turbid suspension in the substrate.

If the culture produced β-lactamase, the solution will turn yellow. In most cases with *H. influenzae* and *N. gonorrhoeae,* the color change occurs within 1 min. β-Lactamase-producing staphylococci should produce the color change within 1 hr if preinduced. If the culture did not produce β-lactamase, the test solution remains dark red.

Chromogenic Cephalosporin Method for β-Lactamase (22, 30)

Dissolve 10 mg of cephalosporin 87/312 (nitrocefin, Glaxo, Inc.) in 1 ml of dimethylsulfoxide (DMSO). Dilute with phosphate buffer, pH 7.0, to a concentration of 500 μg/ml. This solution is yellow when viewed in a microdilution plate or small tube but may appear more orange in larger volumes. However, the red color of a positive test is easily discerned. This solution is stable at 4–10 C for many weeks.

To perform the test, add 0.05 ml of cephalosporin substrate to a well of a microdilution plate or to a small tube. With a loop, remove several colonies of the test organism, and make a heavy turbid suspension in the cephalosporin solution. Mix for 1 min. Observe for color immediately, after 10 min, and after 1 hr.

If the culture produced β-lactamase, the color of the substrate will change from yellow to red. β-Lactamase-producing *H. influenzae* or *N. gonorrhoeae* usually turn the solution red in less than 10 min, but staphylococci may take an hour. Use preinduced staphylococci in the test.

The test can also be performed directly on an agar plate in tests with *H. influenzae* and *N. gonorrhoeae*. The agar plate should contain the organism in pure culture. Place a drop (approximately 0.05 ml) of the cephalosporin reagent on an area of bacterial growth. Tilt the plate slightly to permit the drop to spread across the plate.

If the organism produced β-lactamase, the reagent will turn red along the streak, but if it is β-lactamase negative, the reagent will be yellow along the streak. Usually, the positive test can be read immediately, but a negative result should be confirmed by a second reading after 10 min. Although the red color is less readily seen than when the test is done in the microdilution well, it is generally easy to see. If on rare occasions there is uncertainty, repeat the test in a microdilution well or small tube.

References

1. ACAR JF, COURVALIN P, and CHABBERT YA: Methicillin-resistant staphylococcemia: bacteriological failure of treatment with cephalosporins. Antimicrob Agents Chemother 1970:280–285, 1971
2. BARRY AL, GARCIA F, and THRUPP LD: An improved single-disc method for testing the antibiotic susceptibility of rapidly growing pathogens. Am J Clin Pathol 53:149–158, 1970
3. BARRY AL, JONES RN, and GAVAN TL: Evaluation of the Micro-Media System for quantitative antimicrobial drug susceptibility testing: a collaborative study. Antimicrob Agents Chemother 13:61–69, 1978
4. BAUER AW, KIRBY WMM, SHERRIS JC, and TURCK M: Antibiotic susceptibility testing by a standardized single disc method. Am J Clin Pathol 45:493–496, 1966
5. BENNETT JV, CAMP HM, and EICKHOFF TC: Rapid sulfonamide disc sensitivity test for meningococci. Appl Microbiol 16:1056–1060, 1968
6. BIDDLE JW, SWENSON JM, and THORNSBERRY C: Disc agar antimicrobial susceptibility tests with β-lactamase producing *Neisseria gonorrhoeae*. J Antibiot 31:352–358, 1978

7. BONDI AS, SPAULDING EH, SMITH DE, and DIETZ CC: A routine method for the rapid determination of susceptibility to penicillin and other antibiotics. Am J Med Sci 213:221–225, 1947

8. CATLIN BW: Iodometric detection of *Haemophilus influenzae* beta-lactamase: rapid presumptive test for ampicillin resistance. Antimicrob Agents Chemother 7:265–270, 1975

9. FASS RJ, PRIOR RB, and ROTILIE CA: Simplified method for antimicrobial susceptibility testing of anaerobic bacteria. Antimicrob Agents Chemother 8:444–452, 1975

10. FEDERAL REGISTER. Antibiotic susceptibility discs. 37:20525–20529, 1972

11. HAUSER KJ, JOHNSTON JA, and ZABRANSKY RJ: Economical agar dilution technique for susceptibility testing of anaerobes. Antimicrob Agents Chemother 7:712–714, 1975

12. JONES RN, FUCHS PC, THORNSBERRY C, and RHODES N: Antimicrobial susceptibility tests for anaerobic bacteria. Comparison of Wilkins-Chalgren agar reference method and a microdilution method, and determination of stability of antimicrobics frozen in broth. Current Microbiol 1:81–83, 1978

13. JONES RN, GAVAN TL, and BARRY AL: The evaluation of the Sensititre microdilution antibiotic susceptibility system against recent clinical isolates: a three laboratory collaborative study. J Clin Microbiol 11:426–429, 1980

14. KURZYNSKI TA, YRIOS JW, HELSTAD AG, and FIELD CR: Aerobically incubated thioglycollate broth disc method for antibiotic susceptibility testing of anaerobes. Antimicrob Agents Chemother 10:727–732, 1976

15. LAVERDIERE M, PETERSON PK, VERHOEF J, WILLIAMS DN, and SABATH LD: In vitro activity of cephalosporins against methicillin-resistant, coagulase negative staphylococci. J Infect Dis 137:245–250, 1978

16. MERTENS BF and GERLACH EH: Simultaneous Bacterial Identification and Antimicrobial Susceptibility Testing. Am Soc Clin Pathol Commission on Continuing Education, 1978

17. MORLEY DC: A simple method of testing the sensitivity of wound bacteria to penicillin and sulphathiazole by use of impregnated blotting paper discs. J Pathol Bacteriol 57:379–382, 1945

18. NATIONAL COMMITTEE FOR CLINICAL LABORATORY STANDARDS. Performance Standards for Antimicrobial Disc Susceptibility Tests. Approved Standard ASM-2. Villanova, Pa, 1975

19. NATIONAL COMMITTEE FOR CLINICAL LABORATORY STANDARDS: Performance standards for antimicrobic disc susceptibility tests, 2nd edition. Approved Standard ASM-2. Villanova, Pa, 1979

20. NATIONAL COMMITTEE FOR CLINICAL LABORATORY STANDARDS: Proposed reference dilution procedure for antimicrobic susceptibility testing of anaerobic bacteria. Proposed Standard PSM-11. Villanova, Pa, 1979

21. NATIONAL COMMITTEE FOR CLINICAL LABORATORY STANDARDS: Standard methods for dilution antimicrobial susceptibility tests for bacteria which grow aerobically. Proposed Standard PSM-7. Villanova, Pa, 1980

22. O'CALLAGHAN CH, MORRIS A, KIRBY SM, and SHINGLER AH: Novel method for detection of β-lactamase by using a chromogenic cephalosporin substrate. Antimicrob Agents Chemother 1:283–288, 1972

23. RAMMELKAMP CH and MAXON T: Resistance of *Staphylococcus aureus* to the action of penicillin. Proc Soc Exp Biol Med 51:386–389, 1942

24. STALONS DR and THORNSBERRY C: Broth-dilution method for determining the antibiotic susceptibility of anaerobic bacteria. Antimicrob Agents Chemother 7:15–21, 1975

25. STALONS DR, THORNSBERRY C, and DOWELL VR JR: The effect of culture medium and carbon dioxide concentration on the growth of anaerobic bacteria from clinical specimens. Appl Microbiol 27:1098–1104, 1974

26. STEERS E, FOLTZ E, GRAVES BS, and RIDEN J: An inocula replicating apparatus for routine testing of bacterial susceptibility to antibiotics. Antibiot Chemother 9:307–311, 1959

27. THORNSBERRY C, ANHALT JP, WASHINGTON JA II, MCCARTHY LR, SCHOENKNECHT, FD, SHERRIS JC, and SPENCER HJ: Clinical Laboratory evaluation of the Abbott MS-2 automated antimicrobial susceptibility testing system: report of a collaborative study. J Clin Microbiol, 12:375–390, 1980

28. THORNSBERRY C and BAKER CN: The agar diffusion antimicrobial susceptibility test. *In* Current Techniques for Antibiotic Susceptibility Testing. Balows A (ed.). Charles C. Thomas, Springfield, Ill, 1973, pp 3–8

29. THORNSBERRY C, CARUTHERS JQ, and BAKER CN: Effect of temperature on the in vitro susceptibility of *Staphylococcus aureus* to penicillinase-resistant penicillins. Antimicrob Agents Chemother 4:263–269, 1973

30. THORNSBERRY C, GAVAN TL, and GERLACH EH: Cumitech 6. New Developments in Antimicrobial Agent Susceptibility Testing. Sherris JC (coordinating ed.). American Society for Microbiology, Washington, DC, 1977

31. THORNSBERRY C, GAVAN TL, SHERRIS JC, BALOWS A, MATSEN JM, SABATH LD, SCHOENKNECHT F, THRUPP LD, and WASHINGTON JA II: Laboratory evaluation of a rapid, automated susceptibility testing system: report of a collaborative study. Antimicrob Agents Chemother 7:466–480, 1975

32. THORNSBERRY C and KIRVEN LA: Ampicillin resistance in *Haemophilus influenzae* as determined by a rapid test for beta-lactamase production. Antimicrob Agents Chemother 6:653–654, 1974

33. THORNSBERRY C and SWENSON JM: Antimicrobial susceptibility testing of anaerobes. Lab Med 9:43–48, 1978

34. THORNSBERRY C and SWENSON JM: Antimicrobial susceptibility tests for *Streptococcus pneumoniae*. Lab Med 11:83–86, 1980

35. VINCENT JC and VINCENT HW: Filter paper disc modification of the Oxford cup penicillin determination. Proc Soc Exp Biol Med 55:162–164, 1944

36. WASHINGTON JA: The agar dilution technique. *In* Current Techniques for Antibiotic Susceptibility Testing. Balows A (ed.). Charles C. Thomas, Springfield, Ill, 1974, pp 54–62

37. WASHINGTON JA and BARRY AL: Dilution test procedures. *In* Manual of Clinical Microbiology, 2nd edition. Lennette EH, Spaulding EH, and Truant JP (eds.). American Society for Microbiology, Washington, DC, 1974, pp 410–417

38. WILKINS TD and CHALGREN S: Medium for use in antibiotic susceptibility testing of anaerobic bacteria. Antimicrob Agents Chemother 10:926–928, 1976

39. WILKINS TD and THIEL T: Modified broth-disk method for testing the antibiotic susceptibility of anaerobic bacteria. Antimicrob Agents Chemother 3:350–356, 1973

40. WRIGHT WW: FDA actions on antibiotic susceptibility discs. *In* Current Techniques for Antibiotic Susceptibility Testing. Balows A (ed.). Charles C. Thomas, Springfield, Ill, 1974, pp 26–46

CHAPTER 45

IMMUNODIAGNOSTIC TECHNIQUES FOR BACTERIAL INFECTIONS

Earl A. Edwards, Michael W. Rytel, and Richard L. Hilderbrand

Introduction

Immunodiagnostic techniques for detecting antigen or antibody immediately suggest a variety of applications of immunological and immunochemical methods in diagnosing microbial diseases. Immunodiagnosis lends itself to the study of human diseases because of the sensitivity and specificity that specific immune sera (the immune response) provide. Initially, immunologic diagnosis involved demonstrating circulating antibodies to disease-producing microbial agents. This was done both directly (Widal test) and by showing a rise in titer between serum samples taken in the acute phase compared with those taken during convalescence. The data from such testing and their reliability in diagnosis of various microbial diseases have formed a solid cornerstone from which a much broader and more sophisticated technology has developed.

The initial application of precipitin reaction in the diagnosis of infectious diseases goes back to 1909, when Vincent and Bellot detected meningococcal antigen in cerebrospinal fluids of patients with meningitis (49). Dochez and Avery in 1917 were the first to identify pneumococcal antigen in serum and urine of patients with lobar pneumonia (13).

However, the data collected over the past 2 decades have shown that specific antigen-antibody complexing can be a powerful tool in identifying either antigen or antibody. A thorough description of this reaction was made by Heidelberger and Kendall in the mid 1930s. Landsteiner and Pauling also played a major role in our understanding of the precipitin reaction in the late 1930s and early 1940s. That the precipitin reactions could occur and be visualized in gels was described by Ouchterlony and by Oudin in the late 1940s.

The technique described by Ouchterlony has been widely used to identify multiple antigen and antibody systems. The method also allows one to show the immunologic relationship between two antigens by the line confluence when two antigen preparations are used. The Ouchterlony technique has been extensively used to determine antigen or antibody purity, detect antigen in biological secretions, and to quantitate either antigen or antibody when necessary. Elik was one of the first to use the gel/precipitin reaction as a diagnostic tool to identify pathogenic strains of diphtheria.

This chapter will deal with several of the techniques that have been developed and have proven useful in identifying either antigen or antibody during the past decade. It will give more emphasis to identifying antigens because of the urgency of early identification of microbial agents for proper chemotherapy. In addition, the sensitivity of these techniques allows identification of picogram amounts of antigen, the levels that are frequently found in biological secretions during acute illnesses. Techniques to be described include the double-diffusion test (Ouchterlony), counterimmunoelectrophoresis (CIE), rocket immunoelectrophoresis (Laurell), specifically sensitized Protein A-containing *Staphylococcus aureus* (Kronvall), and enzyme-linked immunosorbent assay (ELISA) (Engvall).

Double-Diffusion or Ouchterlony Test

The double-diffusion test described by Ouchterlony takes advantage of the phenomenon that soluble antigens and their antibodies will precipitate in a gel and the precipitate is permeable to all other antigens and antibodies that have no points of antigenic similarity with the precipitating pair. Thus, identical antigens or antibodies diffusing from two or more wells will form a precipitating band with an angle with one another that will fuse (lines of identity). By the same reasoning, antigens of different specificities will form an angle with one another that will cross (non-identity) or will partly cross and partly fuse (partial identity) (Fig 45.1).

The Ouchterlony test has been used to study microbial antigens and to detect antibodies. The test is relatively insensitive compared with other tests available and has not had broad clinical application but has proven very useful in research. It also suffers from the fact that it takes at least 24–48 hr for the results to become available. However, since the test has been used for presumptive diagnosis, a methodology for the macro double-diffusion test is described.

Materials

1. Agarose
2. 0.15 M sodium chloride (saline)
3. Microscope slide (cleaned with Baboo and then with 95% ethanol; towel dry)
4. Well-punch set (#51450 Gelman or individual well cutters 3.0 mm in diameter)
5. Pasteur pipettes or capillary tubes
6. Moist chamber

Method

1. Prepare 1% agarose in saline, bring to boil to dissolve agarose, and overlay 2–2.5 ml onto a clean microscope slide.
2. Allow agarose to solidify (1 hr in moist chamber).
3. Punch desired number of wells in desired pattern. The distance between wells ranges from 2 to 5 mm. A circular pattern around a central well lends itself to many testing requirements.
4. Carefully remove punched plugs by suction.
5. Fill the central well with immune serum and the surrounding wells with test material (spinal fluid, serum, sputum, etc.).

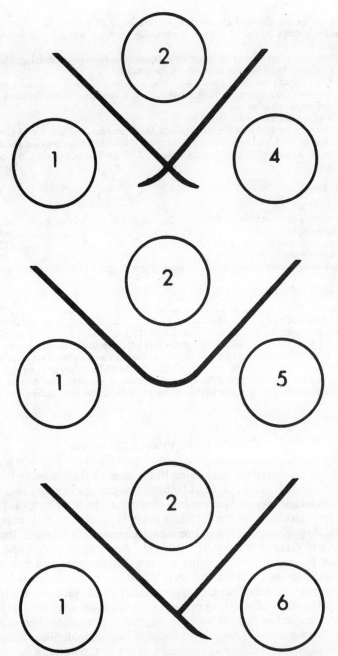

Figure 45.1—A graphic preservation of patterns of precipitation that may be seen using the Ouchterlony technique to identify or compare antigens. Well #2 represents antiserum; wells 1, 4, 5, and 6 represent antigen preparations. Top: reaction of non-identity; middle: reaction of identity; bottom: reaction of partial identity.

6. Place in a moist chamber at room temperature for 24–72 hr.
7. Read the slides by use of oblique illumination. A hand lens 3–7× is highly recommended.
8. The precipitin bands may be easier to interpret after appropriate staining. Should this be necessary, the following steps are recommended:
   a. Rinse or soak the slides (step 7 above) in a saline solution at room temperature for 2–3 days, changing the saline bath daily. This procedure removes the excess antigen and serum proteins.
   b. Soak in distilled water for 1–2 hr.
   c. Place the washed slides in either amido black or coomassie blue for 30 min.
   d. Destain until precipitin bands are readily differentiated from the background.
   e. As an alternative to step c, place slides at 37 C until completely dry. Proceed with step c.

Staining solution

Amido black or
Coomassie brilliant blue R-250...5 g
Ethanol 95% ....450 ml
Glacial acetic acid..100 ml
Distilled water..450 ml
Dissolve stain in acid-ethanol-water solution. Allow to stand 24 hr, filter, and use.

Destaining solution

Ethanol 95% ....450 ml
Glacial acetic acid..100 ml
Distilled water..450 ml
Caution: Unless the glass surface of the slides is carefully cleaned, the agarose may float off the slide during step 8a. It is advisable to precoat the clean slides with a thin layer of a 0.2% agarose, allow them to air dry, and further super dry the slides for several days in a jar with $CaCl_2$. This provides a bonding for the fresh agarose layer applied for double-diffusion testing and reduces the chance of having the agarose float off the glass surface during washing.

Counterimmunoelectrophoresis

Tiselius pioneered the separation of proteins by their moving boundaries, which he carried out in a liquid-phase system; however, the zone electrophoresis technology of Tiselius and Flodein in the early 1950s set the stage for the immunoelectrophoresis techniques which were to follow in the late 1950s and throughout the 1960s. Immunoelectrophoresis was first described by Williams and Grabar in the mid 1950s (52). Application of this technique allowed one to separate and identify mixtures of antigens and was especially used to study serum proteins and their mobilities in an electrical field. It became customary to carry out electrophoresis of serum proteins at pH 8.6 during this early stage of studying protein separation because most proteins are negatively charged at this pH and will migrate to the anode. The exception to this was the case of the three major classes of immunoglobulins. Immunoglobulins M and A (IgM and IgA) remained either at the point of application or migrated toward the cathode. Immunoglobulin G (IgG), being made up of a heterogeneous group of protein moieties, shows a broader range of movement, moving both anodal and cathodal. This (cathodal movement) was found to be caused by the impurities in the gel (agaropectins), which have a strong negative charge. When in an electrical field, these "fixed" negative charges surround themselves with positive charges from the anode, thus moving the liquid buffer from the anode toward the cathode. This movement of buffer is called *electroosmotic flow* or *endosmosis*, and is affected by agar purity, concentration, thickness, buffer molarity, and pH as well as by the voltage at which the electrophoresis is performed. These aspects will be addressed in greater detail below.

The endosmotic effect carries the relatively neutral charge of the immunoglobulins toward the cathode. This characteristic was used in developing the CIE test as first described by Bussard in 1959 (7). He called the test *l'electrosynerese*. The CIE test developed by Bussard has the advantage of using an electric current (and resulting endosmosis) as a migratory force, which increases the speed and sensitivity of the precipitin reaction. The technique was used sparingly until Gocke and Howe published their paper on its use to detect Australia antigen in 1970 (19) and Edwards reported his work with the CIE test to detect bacterial antigens in 1971 (15). Since then, there has been widespread use of the technique to detect both bacterial, viral, fungal, protozoan, and various protein constituents associated with diseases (1, 10, 14, 16, 20, 36). Current uses of CIE are summarized below:

1. Detecting antigen in body fluids.
2. Detecting antibodies.
3. Making prognoses, i.e., positive correlation between presence and amount of antigen and severity of illness and prognosis.
4. Identifying possible role of antigens in disease pathogenesis.
5. Identifying and typing isolates in clinical microbiology laboratory.

Although CIE is a variation of immunoelectrophoresis and agar gel diffusion, the various parameters involved seem much more critical. An illustration of a simple immunoelectrophoresis chamber is shown in Figure 45.2. Since the test has not been standardized with respect to variation in antigen composition, several features of the technique which influence sensitivity will be brought to the attention of the reader.

One of the critical points is to have the correct current/voltage so that the precipitin band is formed between the two wells (Fig 45.3). A number of factors contribute to this success, i.e., well size, distance between wells, composition of agar, depth of agar, composition of buffer, concentration of antigen and antibody. These factors will eventually be standardized as commercially prepared reagents for CIE testing become available; however, at present, these points, which bear directly on the sensitivity of the test, will be discussed.

Well Size

For the antigens that have so far been successfully detected by CIE, wells 3 mm in diameter separated by 2–4 mm (edge to edge) have proven satisfactory. This size well will hold from 5 to 7 μl of fluid. There are variations that can be substituted for this pattern. If the antibody used to detect antigen is relatively weak, the size of the well containing antibody can be increased to 5–8 mm in diameter, thus allowing a larger quantity of antibody to be used, while the antigen well is kept at 3 mm in diameter and vice versa. Variations in well-

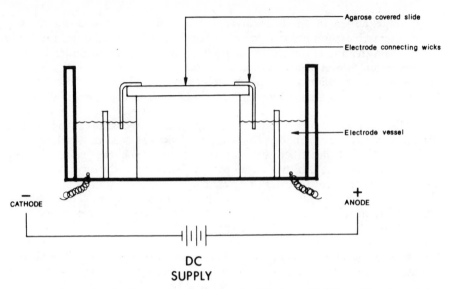

Figure 45.2—A simply designed electrophoresis chamber which is easily adapted to a single microscope slide, multiple slides, or Kodak glass plates.

size patterns should be established with each lot of antiserum to insure the sensitivity needed.

Distance Between Wells

It is recommended that when trying a "new" antigen-antibody system, a series of wells be spaced, starting at 2 mm (edge to edge) and increasing the distance between wells by 2 mm through 5 wells. Such a pattern will reveal an optimal range of distances that will give a precipitin band with the expected antigen concentration.

Composition and Depth of Agar

The less pure the agar, the greater the negative charge and, in turn, the greater the endosmotic flow. This can have catastrophic consequences on the CIE test. Agarose, although the quality varies from company to company and even from batch to batch, appears to give the most consistent results with the antigens so far detected. Each agarose batch should be checked for sensitivity. The depth of the agarose layer over the slide is another variable that has definite influence on the sensitivity of the test. Our experience indicates that agar thicknesses of 3 mm or greater are generally unsatisfactory. Optimal thickness ranges from 1 to 2.5 mm.

Buffer Composition

A wide variety of buffers have been used in CIE; however, barbital buffers seem to be the buffer of choice for most antigens. One exception is the use

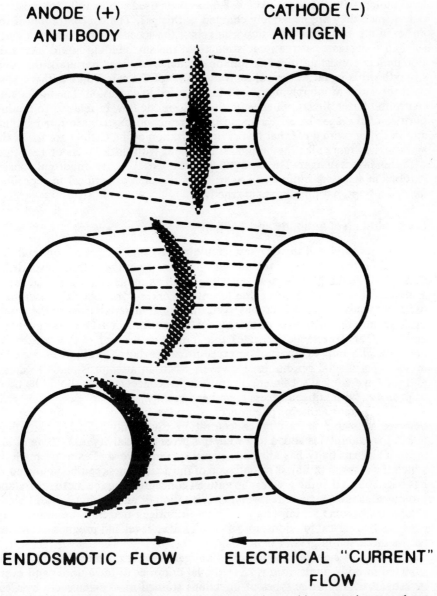

Figure 45.3—Antigen-antibody precipitin patterns observed in counterimmunoelectrophoresis. The upper pattern represents the optimal pattern, not often observed when clinical samples are tested. The lower 2 patterns are frequently seen in clinical samples. The bottom pattern indicates antigen
excess or a support medium with low endosmotic flow.

of a borate buffer when one is testing for pneumococci types 7 and 14 (2). Barbital buffer (0.05–0.1 M) at pH 8.4–8.6 has been used successfully for most antigens since they are negatively charged at this pH. The concentration of the buffer in the agarose layer is important since the speed of migration of a given substance decreases as the ionic strength of the surrounding liquid increases. For buffers consisting of weak monobasic acids (such as barbital), the ionic strength (μ) is equal to the concentration (M) of the salt. Some authors have used the μ and M interchangeably, which has led to confusion. The buffer concentration has a direct influence on the endosmotic flow in relation to the impurities of the agar layer. Endosmosis is greater in less concentrated buffers and in buffers with a pH that favors the ionization of the COOH groups of the agarose, i.e., more alkaline buffers. It is greater with thick layers of agar than with thin layers of agar. These physiochemical variables are important considerations in selecting buffers and agar, both of which are critical to reproducibility and optimal immunologic reactivity.

Concentration of Antibody and Antigen

The sensitivity of the CIE test, assuming all other factors are optimal, depends upon the potency of the antiserum. It has been the authors' experience that this is the limiting factor in detecting small amounts of antigen. The test is also subject to prozone effect due to antigen excess. If a potent antiserum is used, prozones have not been observed in clinical material, even to the extent of 20 μl/ml concentrations of meningococcal antigen in 1 CSF specimen examined. Our experience indicates that potent antiserum is the critical ingredient. The authors have not observed prozones due to antibody excess even under experimental conditions. However, when an attempt is made to detect antibody in a clinical specimen, several antigen concentrations should be tried, as prozones with antigen excess have been seen (2).

With potent antisera, pneumococcal and meningococcal antigen can be detected at from 1 to 2 μg/ml concentration. Since only 5–7 μl of body fluid (CSF, for example) is added to a well, this gives a sensitivity of 5–10 ng of antigen. This sensitivity has allowed several quantitative studies to be made in which the severity of illness or outcome of the acute illness can be predicted. It has been found that the greater the antigen concentration, the more severe and prolonged is the course of recovery. Quantitation of antigen in CSF and blood serum has become an important adjunct to antigen detection because of the consistent empirical relationship between antigen level and prognosis. This aspect is discussed in greater detail below.

Table 45.1 summarizes microbial antigens and antibodies that have been detected in body fluids or *in vitro* in the laboratories of the authors and other investigators. The three types of infections studied most extensively by CIE, besides hepatitis B, are those caused by meningococcus, pneumococcus, and haemophilus (15, 36). Of the various clinical syndromes studied, the highest diagnostic yield was obtained in meningitis caused by these three organisms (over 90% in most studies). The method has been found to be more specific and sensitive than the Gram stain and more rapid than the culture of CSF. It has an additional advantage over the latter in that it may remain positive in partially treated cases. In pneumococcal pneumonia the results have been less satisfactory in that only approximately 50% of bacteremic patients have detect-

TABLE 45.1—DETECTION OF MICROBIAL ANTIGENS AND ANTIBODIES BY CIE IN VARIOUS BODY FLUIDS

ANTIGENS (IN VIVO)	DETECTED IN
Viral:	
Hepatitis B surface antigen	Serum, tears, saliva, urine
Enteroviruses	Cerebrospinal fluid (CSF)
Bacterial:	
Streptococcus pneumoniae	Sputum, serum, urine, CSF, pleural, bullus, joint, peritoneal fluids
Neisseria meningitidis	
A, C, D, X, Y, Z	CSF, serum, joint fluid
Haemophilus influenzae type b	CSF, serum, subdural, joint fluid
Pseudomonas aeruginosa	Serum
Klebsiella pneumoniae	Serum, CSF, urine, pleural fluid
Escherichia coli K1	CSF, serum
Staphylococcus aureus (teichoic acid)	CSF, pericardial fluid
Streptococcus group B	CSF

ANTIBODIES	DETECTED IN
Viral:	
Hepatitis B	Serum
Influenza A_2	Serum
California encephalitis virus	Serum
Cytomegalovirus	Serum
Bacterial:	
Serratia marcescens	Serum
Staphylococcus aureus	Serum
Mycoplasma pneumoniae	Serum
Fungal:	
Candida sp.	Serum
Coccidioides immitis	Serum
Histoplasma capsulatum	Serum
Actinomyces israelii	Serum
Aspergillus fumigatus	Serum
Protozoan:	
Trypanosoma cruzi	Serum
Entamoeba histolytica	Serum
Trichinella spiralis	Serum

ANTIGENS (IN VITRO)	DETECTED IN
Viral:	
Plant viruses	Plant juice, tissue culture fluid
Influenza A_2	Tissue culture, chick chorioallantoic fluid
Cytomegalovirus	Tissue culture fluid
Bacterial:	
Streptococcus pneumoniae	Broth culture extracts
Streptococcus groups A–F	Broth culture extracts
Peptococcus magnus	Broth culture extracts
Klebsiella pneumoniae	Broth culture extracts
Bacteroides fragilis	Broth culture extracts
Enterobacterial common antigen (*E. coli* 014)	Broth culture extracts

able antigen in their serum (36). This figure could be increased to 64% if both serum and urine (concentrated 20-fold by 95% ethanol precipitation at 5 C) were studied. Though CIE appears to be less sensitive (14) than bacterial cultures in identifying cases of pneumococcal pneumonia, it continues to have the advantage of rapidity and, in relation to sputum cultures, specificity. In this regard, current work on this disease focuses on detection by CIE of pneumococcal capsular antigens in sputum (29). The test was reported to be sensitive (100% [8 of 8] sputum specimens from persons with established cases of pneumococcal pneumonia were positive) and specific (saliva of 83 normal individuals was negative).

An additional application of CIE has been in the identification and typing of microbial isolates obtained *in vitro* (16, 43). In general, appropriate dilutions of sonicates of suspensions of bacterial cultures from plates or broth have been employed for study. This approach offers an additional diagnostic dimension in that it may still lead to a more rapid identification of pathogen, which was present in body fluids (blood, CSF, etc.) in insufficient quantity to yield enough antigen for direct detection of CIE.

Finally, one of the most intriguing "spin-offs" of the diagnostic application of CIE has been the demonstration of a direct relationship between the presence and amount of antigen in body fluids and disease morbidity and mortality. This relationship has been reported in a number of infectious diseases (13, 22, 26). Specifically, meningococcal disease patients with antigenemia had a higher incidence of disseminated intravascular coagulation (DIC) and shock and more prolonged duration of coma (22). In patients with pneumococcal infections, there was also a direct relationship between the quantity of circulating antigen and development of DIC, other complications, and mortality rates (12, 37). In both infections antigen levels correlated inversely with antibody response and levels of complement and its components (12, 22). The interpretation of these findings is a matter of speculation, but they may signify formation of toxic immune complexes or impairment of immunologic function, which may have an adverse effect on resistance to the infection. Work is in progress in several laboratories to elucidate this problem.

Materials

1. Variable DC power source with ampere and voltage meters.
2. Chamber with appropriately spaced electrode vessels.
3. Cleaned lantern or microscope slides. Wash with scouring powder, towel dry, then wash in 95% ethanol, and towel dry to remove all residue.
4. Filter paper for electrode wicks (Eaton-Dykman #301 or Gelman S1290 were found to provide superior conductivity).
5. Needles approximately 3 mm in diameter (Gelman well cutters #51466).
6. Agarose (generally 1%). There are several sources that vary in quality from lot to lot. See references 21 and 46.
7. Buffer. A barbital buffer at pH 8.6 has proven satisfactory for many antigen-antibody systems. However, the optimal buffer and pH should be established for each antigen to be identified.

Test Procedure

The technique can briefly be described as follows:
1. A glass slide or lantern slide is covered with 1% agarose in buffer to a depth of 1–2.5 mm (2 ml per microscope slide and 10–14 ml per lantern slide). After the agarose has solid-

ified, two rows of wells are punched in the agarose, the rows being approximately 3 mm apart, edge to edge. The plugs are removed by suction, with use of a Pasteur pipette attached to a faucet aspirator.

2. The prepared plates are then placed in an electrophoresis apparatus for immediate use or stored in a moist chamber in the cold for several (but not more than 4) days until needed. If the slides are not used the same day, a preservative (0.1% sodium azide final concentration) should be added to the agarose to retard bacterial contamination before the agarose is layered over the glass slides.

3. The slides are connected to the electrode vessels by a paper wick. Presoak the filter paper to insure a satisfactory bridge with the agar layer. The sample to be tested (antigen) is placed in the wells on the cathode (−) side of the electrophoresis chamber, and the antibody on the opposite wells (the anode side). The apparatus is connected to a power source and run with use of from 3 to 6 mA per microscope slide or from 12 to 20 mA per lantern slide, as measured at the power source. For diagnostic detection of antibodies, 25 mA has been employed (11).

4. After 1 hr, turn off the power, remove the slides, and look for a precipitin band between the wells by using an oblique lighting effect, holding the slides against a dark background. A hand lens 3–7× is highly recommended. A simple and rapid method of intensifying the precipitin band is to soak the slide in 95% ethanol for 15–20 min or in physiologic saline for several hours. This provides greater contrast so that weak reactions can be more readily observed but does not alter the final results.

Quantitating Antigen (previously identified)

Twofold dilutions of the specimen (1:1–1:128) are run against undiluted type-specific antiserum. Concurrently, for reference quantitation, purified type-specific antigen is also run; the following dilutions are employed: 25, 10, 5, 2.5, 1.0, 0.5, 0.1, 0.05 μg/ml.

Purified lyophilized antigen (for pneumococcus, see reference 25) should be reconstituted at concentrations no less than 5 mg/ml (stock) because of the possibility of polysaccharide adsorbing onto glass or plastic at lower concentrations. The stock solution is stored at −20 C. Any leftover test dilutions below stock concentrations should be discarded.

Table 45.2 shows an example of quantitation of a pneumococcal (PNC)

TABLE 45.2. QUANTITATION OF MENINGOCOCCAL ANTIGEN

CATHODE (−)	DILUTIONS OF SPECIMEN		ANTI-SERA	CONCENTRATION OF PURIFIED PNC (μg/ml)		ANTI-SERA	ANODE (+)
	1:1	0)	0	25.0	0)	0	
	1:2	0)	0	10.0	0)	0	
	1:4	0)	0	5.0	0)	0	
	1:8	0)	0	2.5	0)	0	
	1:16	0)	0	1.0	0)	0	
	1:32	0)	0	0.5	0)	0	
	1:64	0)	0	0.1	0	0	
	1:128	0)	0	0.05	0	0	
	1:256	0)	0				

Results: μg antigen/ml serum = 32 × 0.1 μg/ml = 3.2 μg/ml.
Close parenthesis = antigen/antibody precipitate.

antigen: quantity of antigen (μg/ml) = specimen titer (dilution) $\times$ reference quantitation titer.

Source of Reagents for Diagnostic CIE

Pneumococcal antiserum

Omniserum, pooled antisera (groups A–1), and specific types are available from Statens Seruminstitut, Amager Boulevard 80, DK 2300, Copenhagen S. Denmark. (Instruct them to mark customs slip as follows: "TSUS 437.76/Free Antitoxin.") They are also available from Difco; however, Statens Seruminstitut reagents have been more reliable for the CIE test

Haemophilus influenzae antiserum

This antiserum is supplied by Difco Laboratories, Box 1058A, Detroit, MI 48232; Hyland Labs, 2275 Half Day Rd., Bannockburn, IL, 60015; and Burroughs-Wellcome, P. O. Box 1887, Greenville, NC 27834.

Meningococcal antiserum

Difco and Burroughs-Wellcome (see addresses above) both supply meningococcal antiserum.

Rocket Immunoelectrophoresis

This test has not received wide clinical application. However, it seems to have the potential of being a sensitive method for antigen detection and quantitation. It has the added advantage of allowing several tests to be performed on a single microscope or Kodak slide.

The test is basically a modification of the single-radial-diffusion method of Mancini but uses an electrical current to force diffusion of the antigen in a gel matrix containing antibody. The antigen reacts with antibody in the gel, giving rocket-like zones of precipitation. Not only can antigen be detected but when known concentrations of antigen are added as controls, the rocket heights are proportional to the concentration of the antigen. Thus, by plotting the height of the precipitation formed by the controls on arithmetic graph paper, the values for the unknown samples can be determined by simple extrapolation.

A limited number of different antibody-impregnated agar plates are commercially available. These include IgG, IgA, IgM, C3, haptoglobin, albumin, alpha 1 antitrypsin, and transferrin (ICL Scientific, 18249 Euclid St., Fountain Valley, CA 92708). Because of the technical difficulties in standardizing and preparing the plates with uniform agar layer thickness, it is recommended that no attempt be made (except under experimental conditions) to prepare the plates in-house for diagnostic use.

Coagglutination Tests Using Specifically Sensitized Protein A-Containing S. aureus

The cell walls of most coagulase-positive *S. aureus* strains contain a protein, called protein A, which combines with the gamma globulin of most mammalian species. For many years it was thought that this was a classic antigen-antibody reaction that occurred because of "natural" antibodies stimulated by frequent exposure to this common bacterium. However, Forsgren and Sjöquist found that the reaction was mediated by sites on the Fc part of immunoglobulin IgG and labeled the reaction a "pseudo-immune" reaction. The reaction between the staphylococcal protein A and the Fc part of IgG provides an example that a reaction can be caused by IgG factors other than specific antigen combining sites. All known antibody combining sites are located on the Fab-fragment of the IgG molecule.

Inhibition experiments with isolated heavy and light chains of human IgG showed the protein A activity to be present only in the heavy-chain preparations. When F(ab')₂, Fab, Fc, and F'c fragments were studied, only the Fc fragment preparation gave inhibition of the precipitate formed between a myeloma globulin and protein A. These inhibition studies confirm the original studies of Forsgren and Sjöquist that the reactivity of normal human gamma globulin with staphylococcus protein A resides in the Fc part of the molecule and is analogous to investigations for rheumatoid factor which also reacts with the Fc fragment of the IgG molecule.

This spontaneous "uptake" of IgG by the coagulase-positive *S. aureus* by way of the Fc fraction, leaving the antigen-binding Fab portion of the molecule free to combine with antigen, has many practical applications. Kronvall showed that by sensitizing protein A-containing *S. aureus* with sub-agglutinating amounts of rabbit anti-pneumococcal typing serum, the staphylococcus would take on the specificity of the immune serum and be agglutinated only by the corresponding pneumococcal antigen. The antiserum used must be specific since cross-reactions occur as in any immunologic method. The authors have found the test to be more sensitive than the capillary precipitation test for grouping streptococci but not as sensitive as the CIE test. However, it is a rapid test in that a positive agglutination reaction occurs within 1–3 min.

The sensitized staphylococcus-reagent has been used to group/identify antigens from broth cultures and also to group/identify antigens directly upon the primary isolation plate; thus it is possible to give presumptive identification within hours after having received a test sample compared with 1–4 days with conventional methods. Until further data are gathered on the sensitivity and specificity of the test with use of antisera to a broad range of bacterial species, the test will not replace accepted standard procedures of microbial identification but rather serve to augment these procedures and, if so used, may provide early presumptive identification of an infectious agent.

Materials

1. *S. aureus,* Cowan I Strain, American Type Culture.
2. Trypticase soy broth (TSB) (Baltimore Biological Labs).
3. Clean 500-ml Erlenmeyer flasks and 10-mm × 125-mm test tubes.
4. Polyethylene screw-capped centrifuge tubes (250-ml) or, if a 250-ml centrifuge head is not available, 50-ml polyethylene tubes.

5. Centrifuge with 3–5000 rpm capabilities.
6. Phosphate-buffered saline (PBS) 0.03 M, pH 7.3.

Preparation of S. aureus

1. Check purity of stock culture by culturing for 18 hr at 37 C.
2. Pick a colony of pure S. aureus, and inoculate 2- to 5-ml tubes of TSB.
3. After 6–7 hr of growth (log phase), Gram stain for purity; if pure, pipette (aseptically) 1 ml into a 500-ml Erlenmeyer flask containing 250 ml sterile TSB, and inoculate a blood agar plate to recheck for purity.
4. Incubate flasks and plates at 37 C for 18–24 hr. (An incubator-shaker is preferred; however, static incubation can be used but the yield will be smaller.)
5. As a safety precaution, inactivate the growth either by adding 0.5 ml betapropiolactone, mixing, and allowing to stand at room temperature for 2 hr or by heating at 56 C for 2 hr.
6. Centrifuge to pellet the bacterial cells and wash 3 times with PBS.
7. Make a 10% suspension of the sediment in 0.5% formaldehyde in PBS. Allow to stand at room temperature for 3 hr with occasional shaking.
8. Heat suspension at 80 C in a hot water bath for 1 hr.
9. Wash with PBS three times, and store as a 10% suspension in PBS containing 0.1% sodium azide.

Sensitizing S. aureus

1. Remove 10% stock suspension S. aureus from refrigerator. Mix thoroughly to ensure complete suspension and to break up small clumps that may have developed during storage.
2. Transfer 1 ml (fractions or multiples thereof) of the 10% stock suspension to a clean test tube.
3. Add 0.1 ml of immune serum and mix. (Ratio of immune serum to stock cells should remain at 0.1 to 1.0 ml, respectively.)
4. Allow to "sensitize" for 1–2 hr at room temperature. Shake periodically (every 15 min) to promote optimal sensitization.
5. Pellet staphylococci, wash pellet at least once with PBS, and resuspend to 10 ml with PBS.(This provides a 1% suspension for testing. If a heavier suspension is desired, resuspend washed pellet into a smaller volume.)

Test Procedure to Identify Colony* of Organisms from Primary Isolate

1. Make at least 2 paraffin rings around suspected colonies. A wire ring 12 mm in diameter has been suitable for this purpose. The paraffin has to be hot so that a good seal is made with the agar surface.
2. Add a drop of specifically sensitized staph to 1 paraffin ring and a drop of staph sensitized with normal rabbit serum (negative control) to a paraffin ring around a similar suspected colony.
3. Move the petri dish in a to-and-fro pattern for at least 1 min. Preliminary observations can be made using a dissecting scope. Continue the rotations for 3 min before final reading. Positive aggregates usually form by 1–2 min. The negative (control) should remain negative. (Continued mixing of the staphylococci reagent over the colony is very important for development of visible aggregates).
4. Observe for large aggregates using the dissecting microscope. Other methods of observing aggregation of staphylococcus reagent have not proven satisfactory.
5. Record results.

---

*Group A, B, C, D streptococci; group A, C, Y meningococci; group A, B, C, Cl, D Salmonellae and Shigella sonnei and flexneri; and pneumococcus types 3, 4, 6, 7, 8, 9, 11, 12, 13, 14, 18, 19, and 23 have been shown to give a positive test with polyvalent (omniserum) sensitized staphylococci.

Procedure for Identifying Organisms from a Broth Culture

1. Transfer suspected organisms to 1–5 ml TSB, or in the case of *Salmonella*, inoculate Dulcitol-Selenite enrichment broth and incubate 12–18 hr or until growth is evident.

2. Transfer 1 drop of the growth onto a marked area of a microscope slide, a drop of uninoculated growth medium to another area of the slide, and add 1 drop of specific sensitized staphylococcus reagent to both the test and control test area.

3. Mix thoroughly with an applicator stick. Rotate slide for 1–2 min.

4. Observe for agglutination. The control should remain negative throughout the observation period.

Enzyme-Linked Immunosorbent Assay

In 1971 Engvall and Perlmann (18) and van Weeman and Schuurs (47) independently reported the use of enzymes conjugated to antibodies for the detection and assay of biological molecules. This technique was the outgrowth of the use of enzyme labeled antibodies to detect and localize cellular antigen in light- and electron-microscopy studies (4, 28) and is an alternative to the radioimmunoassay (RIA) method. Enzyme-linked immunosorbent assay (ELISA) has been designated variously as enzyme- or enzymo-immunoassay (EIA) and immunoenzymatic assay. Enzyme-linked immunospecific assay (also ELISA) has been proposed by Engvall as a title with a broader range of application.

The procedures used in enzyme immunoassays are directly analogous to the techniques developed for RIA and are of the same range of sensitivity due to the amplification provided by the enzyme. In comparison with radioimmunoassay, ELISA uses only spectrophotometric or visual detection rather than the expensive instrumentation necessary for quantitation of radioactivity. In addition, with ELISA the need for special training and procedures for handling and disposal of reagents is obviated. RIA and ELISA have been used in similar manners for serodiagnosis (e.g., 45). However, RIA has not been widely applied in diagnostic microbiology although direct and indirect methods for bacterial identification have been developed (44). RIA has also been used for identification of staphylococcal enterotoxins A, B, and C, and for clostridial toxin (6, 31). The principal use of ELISA has been in serology by the use of conjugates directed against a particular antibody.

Several different ELISA procedures have been used to measure antigen and/or antibody. In the "competitive" assay for antigen, labeled antigen and unlabeled antigen compete for a limited quantity of antibody bound to a solid support. The excess antigen is eluted and either the free or bound enzyme is quantitated and related to standard concentrations of antigen.

In the "homogenous" assay an enzyme bound to a hapten is inactivated when an antibody specific for that hapten is present. The addition of free unlabeled hapten, as either a standard or test, will compete for the antibody binding site freeing the hapten and thus the enzyme in proportional quantities. The enzyme can then be quantitated, producing an assay which requires no separation step. This procedure works only for haptens.

For "immunoenzymometric" assay antigen is reacted with excess labeled antibody. Excess solid phase antigen is then added to remove any free labeled antibody and separated. The labeled antibody-antigen complex remaining in solution is then quantitated.

Another method used for quantitating antibody is performed by attaching antigen to a solid support and adding the antibody to be measured. Following incubation an excess of enzyme labeled antibody with specificity for the first antibody is added followed by incubation and quantitation of the bound enzyme.

The method described in this chapter is an example of a "sandwich" assay (see Figure 45.4). The method requires that the antigen (material to be detected) have at least two antibody binding sites.

Summary of Methodology for Sandwich Assay

1. Specific antibody is adsorbed to a solid support (polystyrene or polypropylene) and the support washed.
2. Appropriate antigen in standards or tests is complexed to the specific antibody adsorbed on the solid support and non-bound material removed by washing.
3. The same specific antibody as in 1, which has been chemically conjugated to an enzyme is incubated with the antigen. Non-bound material is again removed by washing.
4. Substrate is added to allow colorimetric quantitation of the bound enzyme. This value is proportional to the quantity of antigen present in standards allowing one to quantitate over the range of standards.

If the second antibody is added unlabeled and a third incubation with excess labeled antibody with specificity for the second antibody is added, the assay is termed a "double sandwich." This last technique has the advantage that one labeled antibody can be used to quantitate a number of specific antibodies from a single species.

Below is a procedural outline for commonly used methods of adsorption, conjugation, and immunoassay. Alternative procedures are included. A master list of required materials has not been presented; however, materials needed will include polystyrene or polypropylene tubes (12 × 75 mm, Sarstedt), Tween 20 (J. T. Baker), glutaraldehyde (Sigma), and either alkaline phosphatase (Sigma Type VII) and p-nitrophenyl phosphate (Sigma) or horseradish peroxidase (Sigma Type VI) and 2.2′-azino-di[3-ethyl-benzthiazoline sulfonate (6)] (ABTS, Boehringer-Mannheim).

Adsorption of specific antibody to solid support

Select 1 of the following 2 methods:

The most frequently used solid support for serodiagnostic methods has been polystyrene (8) in the form of either tubes or plates. The procedure for the adsorption of protein to polystyrene tubes is outlined below.

Dilute specific antibody material to be adsorbed just prior to use with 0.1 M Na_2CO_3 (pH 9.8). For dilution see "Titration of solid phase antibody." Add 1.0 ml of this solution to a polystyrene tube (12 × 75 mm) and allow it to set at 37 C for 3 hr. An additional period (overnight) at 4 C may also be used, but adsorption seems essentially complete within 3 hr. Wash the tubes three times with gentle swirling with 2 ml 0.9% NaCl containing 0.05% Tween 20 (Saline-Tween). The Saline-Tween wash as used throughout this discussion is intended to reduce nonspecific adsorption of antigen or antibody in subsequent

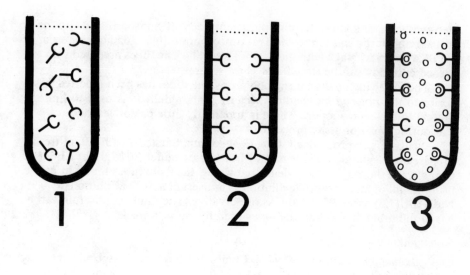

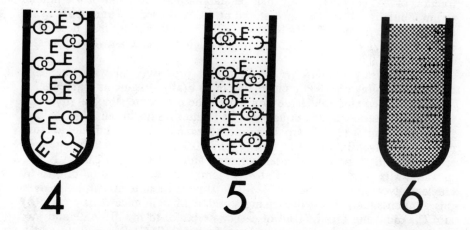

Figure 45.4.—Schematic of "sandwich" ELISA. 1) Specific antibody is added and 2) adsorbed to solid support. 3) Antigen to be measured is added, bound by the specific antibody, and the unbound antigen washed out. 4) Specific antibody conjugated to an enzyme is added and bound to the antigen remaining on solid support antibody, excess labelled antibody is removed by washing. 5) Enzyme substrate is added and 6) the optical density of the products is assayed visually or spectrophotometrically.

steps without removing the solid phase antibody. If nonspecific adsorption is still a problem the wash procedure may incorporate 10% aged human serum or 4% BSA or 0.5 M NaCl with the 0.05% Tween 20. The tubes prepared with adsorbed antibody can be stored at 4 C for several weeks.

The following method using polypropylene tubes has been reported as superior to the polystyrene method because glutaraldehyde is used to link the protein to the solid support. There is apparently little or no "leakage" of protein during wash or assay procedures.

Incubate polypropylene tubes (12 × 75 mm, Sarstedt) with 1.0 ml freshly prepared 0.1% glutaraldehyde in 0.1 M carbonate buffer (pH 9.0) for 3 hr at 56 C and wash thoroughly with deionized water. Incubate tubes for 20 hr at 4 C using 1.0 ml of an appropriate dilution of antiserum in 0.02 M phosphate, 0.9% NaCl (pH 7.2) and 0.02% NaN_3 as preservative. The diluted antiserum can be left in the tubes at 4 C and the tubes used for up to 8 weeks (5).

Conjugation of enzyme-label to antibody

Alkaline phosphatase (AP) (18). Combine 1.0 mg of the specific antibody to be conjugated and 3.0 mg of the AP in 0.2 ml total volume of 0.1 M phosphate buffer (pH 6.8). If either material contains $(NH_4)_2SO_4$ dialyze prior to conjugation procedure. Add 8.0 μl of 6.25% aqueous glutaraldehyde (which has been diluted with phosphate buffer 1:4, v:v) for a final glutaraldehyde concentration of approximately 0.2%. Allow to set for 2 hr at room temperature, dialyze exhaustively at 4 C against 0.05 M tris(hydroxymethyl)aminomethane-hydrochloride (Tris-HCl), pH 8.0, and purify by chromatography on Sephadex G-200 (1.5 × 90 cm) in the same buffer. The conjugate will elute in the void volume and unconjugated material will be retained. The void volume fraction of AP conjugates can then be stabilized by addition of 4% human serum albumin and 0.02% NaN_3 stored at 4 C and used for immunoassay. If necessary, a centrifugation at 10,000 × g for several minutes may be used to remove aggregates. Another procedure for higher specific activity AP is also published (17).

Horseradish peroxidase (HRP) (27). This procedure allows greater efficiency of coupling of HRP to either IgG or to F(ab')₂ fragments than either a one- or two-step glutaraldehyde procedure. The procedure is not as simple as that using glutaraldehyde but has provided better results in our work.

Add 0.1 ml of 1% 1-fluoro-2,4-dinitrobenzene in absolute ethanol to 5 mg of HRP dissolved in 1.0 ml of freshly made 0.3 M sodium bicarbonate (pH 8.1). Mix gently for 1 hr (room temperature) and add 1.0 ml of 0.06 M NaIO₄ in water. Mix gently for 30 min at room temperature. Add 1.0 ml of 0.16 M ethylene glycol in water and mix gently for 1 hr at room temperature. Dialyze this solution against 3 × 1 liter changes of 0.01 M sodium carbonate (pH 9.5) at 4 C. Add 5 mg IgG in 1 ml of carbonate buffer to the dialysate and mix gently for 2–3 hr at room temperature. To the IgG-HRP conjugate add 5 mg NaBH₄ and allow to stand at 4 C overnight. Dialyze this at 4 C against 0.02 M phosphate, and 0.9% NaCl (pH 7.2) (PBS) and remove any precipitate by centrifugation. Purify the conjugate by Sephadex G-200 column (1.5 × 90 cm) chromatography in PBS and take the void volume fraction. HRP conjugate can be stabilized with 1% BSA and stored in aliquots at −20 C without azide.

For either procedure a purified antibody fraction [a 45% $(NH_4)_2SO_4$ fraction, an IgG fragment such as F(ab')$_2$ or an antibody purified by affinity chromatography] can be used for conjugation to improve sensitivity or specificity.

Immunoassay

Alkaline phosphatase.

1. Wash the antibody coated tubes 3 times with 2 ml of Saline-Tween.
2. Dilute standards and serum to be tested with 0.02 M phosphate, 0.9% NaCl, and 0.05% Tween 20 and 0.02% NaN$_3$, pH 7.2 (PBS-Tween). Add 1.0 ml of diluted standard or serum to each tube and incubate at about 30 C with mixing for 3–6 hr. Wash 3 times with Saline-Tween.
3. Dilute enzyme-antibody conjugate to optimal concentration with 0.05 M Tris-HCl, pH 8.0, and add 1 ml of conjugate to each tube. Allow to incubate with gentle mixing at about 30 C for 3–16 hr. Wash 3 times with Saline-Tween.
4. Add 1 ml of 0.05 M sodium carbonate 1 mM MgCl$_2$ buffer (pH 9.8) containing 1 mg/ml p-nitrophenyl phosphate (17).
5. Incubate for a suitable time at room temperature (e.g. 30 min). Add 0.1 ml of 1 N NaOH to stop the reaction and read at 400 nm. Plot increase in absorbance units vs. standards.

Horseradish peroxidase.

1. Wash the antibody coated tubes 3 times with 2 ml Saline-Tween.
2. Dilute standards and serum to be tested with 0.02 M phosphate, 0.9% NaCl, 0.05% Tween 20, pH 7.2 (PBS-Tween). Add 1 ml of diluted standard or serum to each tube and incubate at about 30 C with mixing for 3–6 hr. Wash 3 times with Saline-Tween.
3. Dilute enzyme-antibody conjugate to optimal concentration with PBS-Tween and add 1 ml of conjugate to each tube. Allow to incubate with gentle mixing at about 30 C for 3–16 hr. Wash 3 times with Saline-Tween.
4. Add 1 ml of ABTS reagent. Make this by adding 2 mg of ABTS per 50 ml of 0.03 M citric acid, and 0.04 M phosphate buffer, pH 4.0. Immediately before use add 25 μl of 30% H$_2$O$_2$ per 50 ml of prepared ABTS solution (9).
5. Incubate at 25 C for 10 min. Stop the reaction by addition of 0.05 ml of 0.3% NaN$_3$ or by pouring off of solid phase. Read the optical density at 415 nm.

or alternatively for HRP

4. Add 1 ml of substrate for peroxidase. This is prepared by adding 80 mg of 5-aminosalicylic acid to 100 ml of deionized water at 70 C and cooling to room temperature. Directly prior to use adjust the pH to 6.0 with 1 N NaOH. To 9 ml of 5-aminosalicylic acid add 1 ml of 0.05% hydrogen peroxide (33).
5. Incubate at room temperature for exactly 60 min. Stop the reaction by addition of 0.1 ml of 1 N NaOH and read at 449 nm. Plot the increase in absorbance units vs. standards.

Dilution of reagents

Titration of solid phase antibody. To determine the dilution of antiserum to adsorb to the solid support to give maximal uptake of antigen, take serial 10 fold dilutions of antiserum up to 10,000 fold. Adsorb each dilution to the solid support as described. Then add the highest concentration of antigen which you expect to use in your assay to each dilution. Complete the assay as described above and select the solid phase antibody dilution which gives the greatest enzymatic activity.

Titration of conjugated antibody. To a set of tubes coated with the optimal concentration of specific antibody add the highest concentration of antigen which you expect to use. Incubate, wash, and complete the assay using dilutions (e.g., 1:40, 1:80, 1:160, 1:320, 1:640) of conjugated antiserum. Select the optimal dilution.

Discussion

Developmental work increasing the sensitivity and improving separation methods of ELISA is moving rapidly ahead. In addition, improvements are being made in methods for determination of the end point of the assay and in automation. The application of enzyme kinetic analysis will aid in both automation and quantitation. ELISA faces the limitations which are common to any immunoassay in that the characteristics of the antibody determine sensitivity and specificity of the assay. Also, for initial assays, the components of the assay must be prepared and titrated to maximize the assay. Some technical problems are that the titrations of antibody and conjugated antibody must be completed for each new lot of tubes antiserum and conjugate preparation. Antibody specificity and accuracy in measurement are of utmost importance in quantitation, due to the amplification provided by the enzyme.

In the selection of an enzyme, there are several factors which are of prime consideration.

1. The end product of the enzymatic reaction should be detectable visually if ELISA is to be used for screening purposes, should absorb in either visible or ultraviolet regions for spectrophotometric quantitation, or should be fluorescent for fluorimetric determination.

2. The end product should have a high molar extinction coefficient.

3. The enzyme should have high specific activity.

4. The enzyme should be stable, easily obtainable, and not inhibited by constituents of the material to be tested.

Alkaline phosphatase (AP) meets the enzyme requirements for labeling and has been used frequently. AP is preferable to peroxidase for quantitative ELISA and can be stored at 4 C with 0.02% NaN_3 as preservative for several months. The substrate of choice for AP is p-nitrophenyl phosphate. Since inorganic phosphate is an end product of the enzymatic reaction, one must avoid the use of phosphate buffers in the enzyme substrate solution which could alter the rate of hydrolysis of the substrate.

Another frequently used enzyme with the same range of sensitivity as AP is horseradish peroxidase (HRP). HRP is a smaller molecule than AP and is thus useful in histochemistry because diffusion into tissue is enhanced. For glutaraldehyde conjugation with HRP, one may use a one-step (as described here for conjugation of AP) or two-step procedure (3). HRP has the unusual characteristic of reacting with only one glutaraldehyde molecule which limits self coupling of HRP and allows excess glutaraldehyde to be dialyzed out. The "activated" HRP can be added directly to the IgG which increases coupling efficiency and decreases self coupling of the second protein. Due to simplicity and time, the one-step procedure has been used most frequently. The HRP conjugates can be sterilized by filtration and frozen in small aliquots.

The substrate for HRP is H_2O_2. However, there are a number of chromagens for HRP of which one can be selected for use with the substrate. Diaminobenzidine (DAB) is available as a chromagen but is more useful for histochemistry than for ELISA because the end product forms a ,polymeric compound which is insoluble in aqueous solution. 5-Aminosalicylic acid (5-AS) and O-phenylenediamine (OPD) are good substrates but OPD is difficult to handle because it is somewhat sensitive to light. The chromagen of choice for greatest sensitivity is ABTS.

Beta-galactosidase is a much larger enzyme that is also being used. This enzyme can be used with 4-methylumbelliferone to produce a fluorescent product which has proven to be the most sensitive ELISA assay to date (24).

Application

ELISA has been used to detect antibodies to viral, bacterial, and parasitic antigens and bacterial antigens themselves. The simplicity and speed of the technique has led to an application in veterinary medicine for detecting pathogenic organisms in meat on line at slaughterhouses. Saunders et al. have developed capability for multiple screening of serum antibodies to bacterial pathogens. Initial reports identify *Trichinella spiralis, Brucella abortus* (39) and hog cholera (40) and show good correlation with previous methods and in most cases improved sensitivity. In addition, Saunders has reported the detection of staphylococcal enterotoxin A to a level of 3.2 ng of toxin/ml of prepared food product in 1–3 hr test time (38). Ruitenberg has used ELISA for the identification of *T. spiralis* infection in pigs at the slaughterhouse (34).

A second major application has been in disease screening for infectious disease in humans by field studies in remote areas. The characteristic of the assay that gives a yes or no answer by visual or crude colorimetric methods makes this application possible. Voller et al. (51) have demonstrated the potential of the test in a seroepidemiological study in an area of Columbia where malaria is endemic. Using microtiter trays and visual and spectrophotometric methods, they demonstrated the serological differences in the population of an endemic area and an area where anti-malarial measures have been taken. Voller et al. (50) and Ruitenberg and Buys (32) have applied ELISA micro-techniques to the seroepidemiological studies in African trypanosomiasis.

Other applications have included serodiagnosis of syphilis (48) and schistosomiasis (23), the detection of streptococcal M protein antibodies (35) and detection of hepatitis B surface antigen (54).

Summary

Enzyme-linked immunosorbent assay (ELISA) is a recently developed technology that has sensitivity and accuracy in the range of radioimmunoassay (RIA) technology and has the same specificity. The enzyme label is stable for months and the enzymatic activity can be quantitated spectrophotometrically. The general features for radio- and enzyme-immunoassays are the same. However, in ELISA, separation is usually provided by the use of a polystyrene tube or microtiter tray as a solid support. Alkaline phosphatase (AP) and horseradish peroxidase (HRP) are commonly used enzyme labels and are linked to IgG or antigen by glutaraldehyde or $NaIO_4$. The method can be used visually as a rapid screening device or quantitated by a spectrophotometer. The methodology can be automated and adapted to centrifugal analyzers and can be performed without the need for a separation step in some cases (homogeneous assay technique). Kinetic analysis of enzymatic activity may allow increased accuracy and broader applications.

Two recently written reviews (41, 53) have extensive discussions of principles, methods, and applications.

References

1. AGUILAR-TORRES FG, RYTEL MW, and KAGAN IG: Comparison of counterimmunoelectrophoresis (CIE) with other serologic tests in the detection of antibodies to *Trypanosoma cruzi.* Am J Trop Med Hyg 25:667–670, 1976
2. ANHALT JP and YU PKW: Counterimmunoelectrophoresis of pneumococcal antigens: improved sensitivity for the detection of types VII and XIV. J Clin Microbiol 2:510–515, 1975
3. AVRAMEAS S and TERNYNCK T: Peroxidase labeled antibody and Fab conjugates with enhanced intracellular penetration. Immunochemistry 8:1175–1179, 1971
4. AVRAMEAS S and URIEL J: Méthode de marquage d'antigènes et d'anticorps avec des enzymes et son application en immunodiffusion. C R Acad Sci 262:2543, 1966
5. BOENISCH T: Improved enzyme immunoassay for trace proteins in protides of the biological fluids. 24th colloquium, Peeters H (ed.). Pergamon Press, New York, 1976, pp 743–749
6. BOROFF DA and SHU-CHEN G: Radioimmunoassay for type A toxin of *Clostridium botulinum.* Appl Microbiol 25:545–549, 1973
7. BUSSARD A: Description d'une technique combinant simultanement l'électrophorèse et al précipitation immunologique dans un gel: l'électrosynérèse. Biochim Biophys Acta 34:258–260, 1959
8. CATT K and TREGEAR GW: Solid-phase radioimmunoassay in antibody-coated tubes. Science 158:1570–1573, 1967
9. CAWLEY LP, MINARD BJ, and GILLISSEN JA: Enzyme-linked immunosorb assay (ELISA). Paper presented at the American Society of Clinical Pathologists Workshop on ELISA, September 7–9, 1977, Chicago, Ill
10. DAVIS JS and WINFIELD JB: Serum antibodies to DNA by counterimmunoelectrophoresis (CIE). Clin Immunol Immunopathol 2:510–518, 1974
11. DEE TH and RYTEL MW: Clinical application of counterimmunoelectrophoresis in detection of candida serum precipitins. J Lab Clin Med 85:161–166, 1975
12. DEE TH, SCHIFFMAN G, SOTTILE MI, and RYTEL MW: Immunologic studies in pneumococcal disease. J Lab Clin Med 89:1198–1207, 1977
13. DOCHEZ AR and AVERY DT: The elaboration of specific soluble substance by pneumococcus during growth. J Exp Med 26:477–493, 1917
14. DORFF GJ, COONROD JD, and RYTEL MW: Detection by immunoelectrophoresis of antigen in sera of patients with pneumococcal bacteremia. Lancet 1:578–579, 1971
15. EDWARDS EA: Immunological investigations of meningococcal disease. I. Group-specific *Neisseria meningitidis* antigens in the serum of patients with fulminant meningococcemia. J Immunol 106:314–317, 1971
16. EDWARDS EA and LARSON GL: Serological grouping of hemolytic streptococci by counterimmunoelectrophoresis. Appl Microbiol 26:899–903, 1973
17. ENGVALL E, JONSSON K, and PERLMANN P: Enzyme linked immunosorbent assay. II. Quantitative assay of protein antigen, immunoglobulin G, by means of an enzyme labeled antigen and antibody coated tubes. Biochim Biophys Acta 251:427–434, 1971

18. ENGVALL E and PERLMANN P: Enzyme linked immunosorbent assay (ELISA). Quantitative assay of immunoglobulin G. Immunochemistry 8:871–874, 1971
19. GOCKE DJ and HOWE C: Rapid detection of Australia antigen by counter-immunoelectrophoresis. J Immunol 104:1031–1032, 1970
20. GORDON MA, ALMY RE, GREENE CH, and FENTON JW JR: Diagnostic mycoserology by immunoelectro-osmophoresis: a general, rapid, and sensitive microtechnique. Am J Clin Pathol 56:471–474, 1971
21. HIBRAWI H, GARRISON FD, and SMITH HJ: A comparison of various agarose preparations in a counterimmunoelectrophoresis (CIE) system for assaying urinary myoglobin. J Immunol Methods 14:59–63, 1977
22. HOFFMAN TA and EDWARDS EA: Group-specific polysaccharide antigen and humoral antibody response in disease due to Neisseria meningitidis. J Infect Dis 126:636–644, 1972
23. HULDT G, LAGERQUIST B, PHILLIPS T, DRAPER CC, and VOLLER A: Detection of antibodies in schistosomiasis by enzyme-linked immunosorbent assay (ELISA). Ann Trop Med Parasitol 69:483–488, 1975
24. KATO K, HAMAGUCHI Y, FUKUI H, and ISHIKAWA E: Enzyme-linked immunoassay. Conjugation of rabbit anti(human immunoglobulin G) antibody with β-D-galactosidase from Escherichia coli and its use for immunoglobulin G assay. Eur J Biochem 62:285–290, 1976
25. LUND E: Laboratory diagnosis of pneumococcus infections. Bull WHO 23:5–13, 1960
26. MCCRACKEN GH JR, SARFF LD, GLODE MP, MIZE SG, SCHIFFER MS, ROBBINS JB, GOTSCHLICH EC, ØRSKOV I, and ØRSKOV F: Relation between Escherichia coli K1 capsular polysaccharide antigen and clinical outcome of neonatal meningitis. Lancet ii:246–250, 1974
27. NAKANE PK and KAWAOI A: Peroxidase labeled antibody. A new method of conjugation. J Histochem Cytochem 22:1084–1091, 1974
28. NAKANE PK and PIERCE GB: Enzyme labeled antibodies: preparation and application for the localization of antigens. J Histochem Cytochem 14:929–931, 1967
29. PERLINO CA and SCHULMAN JA: Detection of pneumococcal polysaccharide in the sputum of patients with pneumococcal pneumonia by counterimmunoelectrophoresis. J Lab Clin Med 87:496–502, 1976
30. POLLACK M: Significance of circulating capsular antigen in Klebsiella infections. Infect Immun 13:1543–1548, 1976
31. ROBERN H, DIGHTON M, YANO Y, and DICKIE N: Double antibody radioimmunoassay for staphylococcal enterotoxin C₂. Appl Microbiol 30:525–529, 1975
32. RUITENBERG EJ and BUYS J: Application of the enzyme-linked immunosorbent assay (ELISA) for the serodiagnosis of human African trypanosomiasis (sleeping sickness). Am J Trop Med Hyg 26:31–36, 1977
33. RUITENBERG EJ, STEERENBERG PA, BROSI BJM, and BUYS J: Serodiagnosis of Trichinella spiralis infections in pigs by enzyme-linked immunosorbent assays. Bull WHO 51:108–109, 1974
34. RUITENBERG EJ, STEERENBERG PA, BROSI BJM, and BUYS J: Reliability of the enzyme-linked immunosorbent assay (ELISA) for the serodiagnosis of Trichinella spiralis infections in conventionally raised pigs. J Immunol Methods 10:67–83, 1976
35. RUSSELL H, FACKLAM RR, and EDWARDS LR: Enzyme-linked immunosorbent assay for streptococcal M protein antibodies. J Clin Microbiol 3:501–505, 1976
36. RYTEL MW: Rapid diagnostic methods in infectious diseases. Adv Intern Med 20:37–60, 1975
37. RYTEL MW, DEE TH, FERSTENFELD JE, and HENSLEY GT: Possible pathogenetic role of capsular antigens in fulminant pneumococcal disease with disseminated intravascular coagulation (DIC). Am J Med 57:889–896, 1974
38. SAUNDERS GC and BARTLETT ML: Double antibody solid phase enzyme immunoassay for the detection of staphylococcal enterotoxin A. Appl Environ Microbiol 34:518–522, 1977
39. SAUNDERS GC and CLINARD EH: Rapid micromethod of screening for antibodies to disease agents using the indirect enzyme-labeled antibody test. J Clin Microbiol 3:604–608, 1976
40. SAUNDERS GC and WILDER ME: Disease screening with enzyme-labeled antibodies. J Infect Dis 129:362–364, 1974
41. SCHARPE SL, COOREMAN WM, BLOMME WJ, and LAEKEMAN GM: Quantitative enzyme immunoassay: current status. Clin Chem 22:733–738, 1976

42. SHACKELFORD PG, CAMPBELL J, and FEIGIN RD: Countercurrent immunoelectrophoresis in the evaluation of childhood infections. J Pediatr 85:478–481, 1974

43. SOTTILE MI and RYTEL MW: Application of counterimmunoelectrophoresis in the identification of *Streptococcus pneumoniae* in clinical isolates. J Clin Microbiol 2:173–177, 1975

44. STRANGE RE and HAMBLETON P: An indirect immunoradiometric assay of microbes. J Gen Microbiol 93:401–404, 1976

45. TEW JG, BURMEISTER J, GREENE EJ, PFLAUMER SK, and GOLDSTEIN J: A radioimmunoassay for human antibody specific for microbial antigens. J Immunol Methods 14:231–241, 1977

46. TRIPODI D, KOCHESKY R, LYONS S, and DAVIS O: Immunochemistry of counterimmunoelectrophoresis and the effect of electroendosmotic flow on reactivity. J Immunol Methods 4:1–10, 1974

47. VAN WEEMAN BK and SCHUURS AHWM: Immunoassay using antigen-enzyme conjugates. FEBS Letters 15:232–236, 1971

48. VELDKAMP J and VISSER AM: Application of the enzyme-linked immunosorbent assay (ELISA) in the serodiagnosis of syphilis. Br J Vener Dis 51:227–231, 1975

49. VINCENT MH and BELLOT M: Observations a l'occasion du proces-verbal. Diagnostic de la méningite cérébro-spinale à méningocoques par la "précipito-réaction." Bull Acad Med (Paris) 61:326–332, 1901

50. VOLLER A, BIDWELL DE, and BARTLETT A: A serological study of human *Trypanosoma rhodesiense* infections using a microscale enzyme-linked immunosorbent assay. Tropenmed Parasitol 26:247–251, 1975

51. VOLLER A, BIDWELL D, HULDT G, and ENGVALL E: A microplate method of enzyme-linked immunosorbent assay and its application to malaria. Bull WHO 51:209–211, 1974

52. WILLIAMS CA JR and GRABAR P: Immunoelectrophoretic studies on serum proteins. I. The antigens of human serum. J Immunol 74:158–169, 1955

53. WISDOM GB: Enzyme-immunoassay. Clin Chem 22:1243–1255, 1976

54. WOLTERS G, KUIJPERS L, KACAKI J, and SCHUURS A: Solid phase enzyme-immunoassay for detection of hepatitis B surface antigen. J Clin Pathol 29:873–879, 1976

CHAPTER 46

BIOCHEMICAL TEST PROCEDURES, REAGENTS, STAINS, STAINING METHODS, AND MEDIA

Grace Mary Ederer and Marlys E. Lund

Contents

Biochemical Tests

Reagents

Stains and Staining Methods

Bacteriologic Culture Media

Brucella Selective Agar
Buffered Single Substrate Media (BSS)
Carbohydrate Fermentation Media
Cary and Blair Transport Medium
CDC Anaerobe Blood Agar
CDC Anaerobe Blood Agar with Kanamycin
and Vancomycin
CDC Anaerobe Blood Agar with Phenethyl-
alcohol (PEA)
CDC Stiff Anaerobe Blood Agar
Cetrimide Agar
Charcoal-Yeast Extract (CYE) Agar
Chocolate Agar
Chocolatized Blood Agar
Chopped Meat Glucose (CMG) Medium
Chopped Meat Glucose Starch (CMGS)
Medium
Chopped Meat (CM) Medium
Colistin Nalidixic Acid (CNA) Agar
Coagulated Hen's Egg Yolk
Cooked Meat Medium (CM)
Cystine-Glucose-Blood Agar
Cystine-Tellurite-Blood Agar
Egg Yolk Agars
Enriched Thioglycollate Medium
Erysipelothrix Selective Broth
Feeley-Gorman (F-G) Agar
Fildes Enrichment
Fletcher's Medium
Haemophilus ducreyi Rabbit Blood Agar
Hemin-Vitamin K Solution
Hydrogen Sulfide (H$_2$S) Semi-Solid Medium

Kelly's Medium "A"
Leptospira Medium
Levinthal Broth
Lombard-Dowell (LD) Agar
Lombard-Dowell (LD) Bile Agar
Lombard-Dowell (LD) Egg Yolk Agar
Lombard-Dowell (LD) Esculin Agar
McLeod's Medium, Modified
Milk Media (Lombard-Dowell Base)
Mueller-Hinton Agar Supplemented with
1% Hemoglobin and 1% IsoVitaleX
Neomycin Egg Yolk Agar (NEYA)
Pai Medium, Modified
Peptone-Starch-Dextrose (PSD) Agar
Peptone-Yeast Extract-Glucose (PYG) Broth
P.L.E.T. Selective Agar
Serum-Glucose Agar, Modified
Serum-Peptone Agar
Snyder's Medium
Starch Agar
Steadham Urea Broth
Stuart Leptospira Medium
Thayer-Martin Medium
Transgrow
Tinsdale Medium, Modified
Tryptose-Sulfite-Cycloserine Agar (TSC)
Tetrathionate Broth
Urea Broth
Urea Semi-Solid Medium
Vaginalis Agar
Xylose Lysine Desoxycholate Agar (XLD)

Biochemical Test Procedures

Special biochemical test procedures cited in preceding chapters and commonly used test procedures are described in this section. Following each test procedure are directions for preparing some of the media and reagents. Commercially available media are noted as such, and no instructions for preparing them are included. Media designed for purposes other than biochemical tests of bacteria are described in the last section of this chapter. General references are provided as a supplement to those at the ends of the other chapters.

Acetate Utilization

1. Prepare a saline suspension of the organism. Use a young culture.
2. Using a straight wire, inoculate the acetate medium* with the saline suspension.
3. Incubate the culture at 35 C for 24–48 hr, or a maximum of 7 days.
   Positive: growth and the development of a blue color.
   Negative: no growth, green color.

---

* Media marked with an asterisk are available commercially and should be prepared according to the manufacturer's directions.

Carbohydrate Fermentation

1. Inoculate the appropriate carbohydrates prepared in carbohydrate fermentation medium with inverted insert tubes.
2. Incubate at 35–37 C for 4–5 days, examining daily.
   Positive: dark pink to red color (pH 6.2).
   Gas: bubble comprising at least 3% of volume of insert tube.
   Negative: colorless.

Fermentation broth base: Mix 10 g peptone, 3 g meat extract, 5 g sodium chloride in 1000 ml distilled H_2O. Add 10 ml Andrade's indicator. Adjust pH to 7.1–7.2. Glucose and mannitol can be added to the base in a 1.0% concentration before sterilization. Dulcitol, salicin, adonitol, and inositol can also be added before sterilization, but at a final concentration of 0.5%. Disaccharides such as lactose, sucrose, etc., should be sterilized by filtration and added to previously sterilized medium. (Prepare carbohydrates requiring filter sterilization in a 10% concentration, and dispense the base so that a 1 to 10 dilution can be easily made.) Check the stability of carbohydrates other than those listed to determine whether they should be added before or after sterilizing. Sterilize the fermentation base at 121 C for 15 min.

Andrade's indicator: Dissolve 0.2 g of acid fuchsin in 100 ml of distilled water. Add from 5 to 16 ml of 1.0 N NaOH. After this mixture stands for 24 hr, it should become straw-colored; if not, add an additional 1 or 2 ml of alkali. The amount of alkali will vary somewhat with different lots of dye. Andrade's indicator shows a sharp end point (including easy detection of reversion of acid to alkaline), is not easily reduced, and is inexpensive. Because the indicator improves with age, a quantity which will last several years can be prepared.

Carbohydrate Fermentation Tests

1. Inoculate the appropriate carbohydrates prepared in thioglycollate fermentation base.
2. Incubate aerobically for 1–7 days.
   Positive: acid (purple base changes to yellow).

Thioglycollate fermentation base: Prepare 1 liter of fluid thioglycollate medium without dextrose or indicator (BBL or Difco). Add 2.0 g of glucose-free yeast extract and 2 ml of 1.0% aqueous bromcresol purple. Dispense in 9.0-ml aliquots, and add filter-sterilized carbohydrates to a final concentration of 0.5% to 1.0%. Gas trap vials are not necessary.

Catalase Test

1. Inoculate an agar slant heavily with the organism, and incubate at an optimal temperature for 18–24 hr.
2. Allow 1 ml of 3% hydrogen peroxide to flow over the slant.
   Positive: bubbles of oxygen gas produced.
   Negative: no gas produced.

Points to consider:

a. Red blood cells contain catalase, so the test should not be performed directly on organisms growing on blood-containing medium. Colonies can be picked from blood-containing medium and mixed in a drop of hydrogen peroxide on a glass slide.

b. Cultures of anaerobic bacteria should be exposed to air for half an hour before the catalase test is performed.

Citrate Utilization

Use Simmons citrate medium.* See Acetate Utilization for procedure.

Deaminase, Phenylalanine

1. Inoculate a phenylalanine agar* slant heavily.
2. Incubate the culture at 35 C for 4 hr or 18–24 hr.
3. Dispense 4–5 drops of 10% ferric chloride over the growth on the slant.
    Positive: a dark green color develops on the slant surface and in the fluid.
    Negative: yellowish color of the reagent.

Decarboxylase (Lysine and Ornithine) and Dihydrolase (Arginine)

1. Inoculate a tube of decarboxylase broth base* containing 1.0% of a specific L-amino acid. (If a DL-amino acid is used, raise the concentration to 2.0%.
2. Also inoculate a tube of decarboxylase base without amino acid to serve as a control.
3. Add a 10-mm layer of sterile mineral oil to each tube.
4. Incubate at 35 C, and examine daily until the test becomes positive or for at least 4 days.
    Positive: violet or red-violet color with a yellow color in the control.
    Negative: yellow color in both test and control.

The formulations for decarboxylase broth base of either Moeller or Falkow are available commercially. Dispense 3- to 4-ml amounts in 13- × 100-mm screw-capped tubes. A small amount of floccular precipitate in the ornithine medium does not interfere with its use.

Deoxyribonuclease (DNase Test)

1. Inoculate the organism heavily on one spot of DNase Test Agar with Methyl Green.*

2. Incubate the culture for 18–24 hr at 35 C and observe.
   Positive: a colorless zone is evident around the growth.
   Negative: the green of the medium prevails throughout.

Esculin Hydrolysis

1. Inoculate esculin medium, and incubate for 7 days at 35 C.
2. Add a few drops of 1.0% $FeCl_3$ to the top of the tube.
   Positive: brownish-black color indicates hydrolysis.

Esculin medium: Dissolve 25.0 g of heart infusion broth base (Difco), 1.0 g esculin, and 1.0 g agar in 1 liter of distilled H_2O. Heat to dissolve agar, dispense, and sterilize at 121 C for 15 min.

Gelatin Liquefaction

Tube Method

1. Inoculate gelatin deeps (see below) by stabbing, and incubate them at 20–22 C for up to 30 days.
2. To determine whether liquefaction has occurred, place the tubes in the refrigerator for 30 min. Remove the tubes, and tilt to detect liquefaction. Continue incubation until liquefaction occurs or until the 30-day period is over.
   Positive, strong: liquefaction occurs within 3 days.
   Positive, weak: liquefaction in 4–30 days.

Plate Method

1. Inoculate the center of a plate of gelatin medium (see below), and incubate at 30 C for 3 days.
2. Flood the plate with mercuric chloride solution (12 g of $HgCl_2$, 80 ml distilled H_2O, and 16 ml concentrated HCl) and observe.
   Positive: a clear zone is evident around the growth.

Gelatin medium: Add 120 g gelatin to 1 liter of nutrient broth. Heat to dissolve the gelatin. If deeps are desired for the tube test, dispense accordingly, and autoclave at 121 C for 12 min. Pour plates after sterilization.

Rapid Method

1. Inoculate 0.5 ml of normal saline heavily with the organism.
2. Introduce a strip of exposed, undeveloped x-ray paper (approximately 1 × 1¼ inches) in the suspension.
3. Incubate in a heating block or water bath at 37 C, and observe at hours 2, 4, and 24 for the absence of the green gelatin emulsion on the strip.
   Positive: appearance of the blue transparent support strip.
   Negative: green emulsion remains intact.

Method for Anaerobes

Use Thiogel medium (BBL).

Glucose Fermentation for Staphylococci

1. Inoculate the gram-positive, catalase-positive coccus in question into a special tryptone-yeast-extract agar.
2. Incubate for 24 hr at 35 C.
3. Transfer a heavy inoculum of the organism into properly heated and cooled tryptone-glucose medium, making certain that the inoculum reaches the bottom of the tube.
4. Cover medium with 25 mm or more of sterile paraffin oil.
5. Incubate for 5 days at 35 C, examining daily.
    Purple: glucose not fermented anaerobically.
    Yellow: glucose is fermented anaerobically (acid).

Tryptone-yeast extract agar: Add 1.0 g tryptone, 0.1 g yeast extract, and 1.5 g agar to 100 ml distilled water. (Difco brand of media is recommended.) Adjust the pH to 7.2. Heat to dissolve, autoclave at 121 C for 15 min, cool, and pour plates.

Tryptone-glucose medium: Dissolve 1.0 g tryptone, 0.1 g yeast extract, 1.0 g glucose, 0.004 g bromcresol purple, and 0.2 g agar in 100 ml of distilled water. Heat to dissolve. Adjust pH to 7.0, and dispense into 16- × 120-mm tubes, filling each two-thirds full. Autoclave for 20 min at 115 C.

Note: Before use, steam the medium for 10–15 min to remove any dissolved oxygen. Solidify rapidly by placing the tubes in iced water. Use immediately.

Hippurate Hydrolysis

1. Inoculate hippurate medium with 1–2 drops of an overnight broth culture of streptococci. Prepare a positive (group B streptococci) and a negative (group A streptococci) control in the same manner.
2. Incubate the tubes for 42–66 hr at 35 C.
3. Centrifuge the broth cultures, and remove from each 0.8 ml of the supernate into a 13- × 100-ml tube.
4. To the aliquots of supernate, add 0.4 ml of ferric chloride and shake.
5. Shake occasionally over a 10-min period, and examine.
    Positive: a heavy, cloudy precipitate develops which persists beyond the 10-min observation time.
    Negative: the initial precipitate clears within the 10-min period.

Hippurate medium: Prepare a 1% sodium hippurate solution in heart infusion broth. Dispense in 5-ml amounts into screw-capped tubes. Autoclave at 121 C for 15 min. Since it is important to maintain the volume of this reagent, tighten the screw caps after sterilization.

Ferric chloride reagent: Dissolve 12 g $FeCl_3 \cdot 6H_2O$ in 100 ml of dilute HCl (5.4 ml conc. HCl diluted in 94.6 ml distilled H_2O).

Indole Tests

Kovacs' Method

1. Inoculate a high tryptophane content broth (e.g., 0.1% Tryptone or Trypticase), and incubate at 35 C for 24–48 hr.
2. Add approximately 0.5 ml of Kovacs' reagent.
   Positive: deep pink to red color.
   Negative: yellow color of reagent.

Kovacs' reagent: Dissolve 10 g of p-dimethylaminobenzaldehyde in 150 ml of amyl or isoamyl alcohol by warming the solution in a 56 C water bath. To the mixture slowly add 50 ml of concentrated HCl (A.R.). Dispense into a brown bottle, and store in the refrigerator (4–10 C). The reagent should be a light color.

Ehrlich's Method

1. Add 1 ml of xylene to a 48-hr culture of organisms in a high trypto-phane content broth. (Longer incubation may be required for anaer-obes and nonfermentative gram-negative bacilli.) Shake the xylene-broth mixture well, and allow the xylene to rise to the surface.
2. Carefully add 0.5 ml of Ehrlich's indole reagent down the side of the tube so that it is layered between the medium and the solvent.
   Positive: red ring below the solvent layer.

Ehrlich's indole reagent: Dissolve 1 g of p-dimethylaminobenzaldehyde in 95 ml of absolute alcohol. Carefully add 20 ml of concentrated HCl (A.R.). Mix well, and store in a brown bottle at 4–10 C. Discard if the color darkens.

Tablet Test

1. Pipette 1.0 ml of sterile distilled water into a 13- × 100-mm sterile tube; add one indole tablet (Key Scientific Products Co., Los Angeles, CA), and shake to dissolve it.
2. Inoculate the solution heavily, and incubate at 35 C for 24–48 hr.
3. Proceed as with Kovacs' method.

KCN Test

1. Inoculate a few cells (less than 10^5) into KCN medium* (see below).
2. Flame the lip of the tube, and reinsert the waxed cork. When cooled the wax should provide a firm seal.
3. Incubate tubes at 35 C for 2 days, and observe.
   Positive: visible turbidity.

KCN medium: Prepare 1 liter of KCN broth base according to the manufacturer's directions. Autoclave the base for 15 min at 121 C. Refrigerate the broth base until thoroughly chilled, and add 15 ml of cold 0.5% KCN. Mix, and dispense in 1-ml amounts into 12- × 150-mm or 13-× 100-mm tubes. Stopper quickly with corks soaked in hot melted paraffin. The medium can be stored for 2 weeks at 4 C.

CAUTION: When dispensing KCN, work under a fume hood.

Lecithinase

1. Inoculate an egg yolk agar plate (see formula under Lipase). Streak for isolation, and incubate in an anaerobic jar for 48–72 hr.
2. Remove cover and examine.
   Positive: a cloudy, opaque zone appearing around the colonies.

Lipase

1. Inoculate an egg yolk agar plate. Streak for isolation and incubate in an anaerobic jar for 48–72 hr.
2. Remove cover, and examine under oblique light.
   Positive: an oily, iridescent sheen present over and around the growth.

Egg yolk agar: Combine 20.0 g peptone or Trypticase, 2.5 g Na_2HPO_4, 1.0 g NaCl, 0.1 ml 5% $MgSO_4$, 1 g glucose, 12 g agar, and 500 ml distilled water. Adjust pH to 7.3–7.4, and autoclave at 121 C for 15 min. Cool at 60 C, and add 1 egg yolk. (Decontaminate the eggshell by immersing it in 95% ethyl alcohol for 1 hr before extracting the yolk. Use non-commercial, antibiotic-free eggs.) Mix well and pour plates.

This medium is not pre-reduced and should thus be stored in an anaerobic jar if not used within 4 hr of preparation.

Malonate Utilization

Use malonate broth* and follow the manufacturer's directions. Malonate utilization is indicated by growth and a change of the indicator from green to blue.

Methyl Red Test

1. Inoculate MR-VP medium* with the organism.
2. Incubate the culture at 30 C for 5 days.
3. Add 0.2 ml methyl red reagent per 5 ml of culture.
   Positive: bright red color develops (pH $\leq$ 5.7).
   Negative: yellow or orange color (pH > 5.7)
   Weak positive: red-orange color (pH 5.2–5.7)

Comment: Most *Enterobacteriaceae* can be incubated at 35 C for 48 hr with satisfactory results.

Methyl red reagent: Dissolve 0.1 g methyl red in 300 ml 95% ethanol; add 200 ml distilled water. Store at room temperature to prevent precipitation caused by refrigerating solution.

Motility Test

1. Inoculate a semisolid nutrient medium (0.2% to 0.4% agar) by stabbing 2 cm into the center of the medium.
2. Incubate at 35 C for 1–2 days.
3. If negative, reincubate at 21–25 C for 5 days. (For pseudomonads the temperature should be reduced to 18–20 C.)
   Positive: Diffuse growth migrating from the line of in-
       oculation. Some strains move only slightly; some
       move to the bottom of the tube.
4. Motility of organisms aso can be determined microscopically with a hanging drop preparation or a drop of a broth culture coverslipped.

Motility medium: Dissolve 3 g of beef extract, 10 g of peptone, and 5 g of sodium chloride in 1 liter of distilled water. Add 2, 3, or 4 g of agar. Heat to dissolve agar. Dispense in 8-ml aliquots into 16- × 125-mm tubes, and sterilize at 121 C for 15 min. The medium can also be dispensed into petri dishes after it is sterilized for use in selecting motile strains from a predominantly non-motile stock organism.

Mucate Fermentation

1. Inoculate mucate medium with a 3-mm loopful of an overnight nutrient broth culture of the test organisms.
2. Incubate the tubes at 35 C for 14 days, observing daily.
   Positive: greenish-yellow or yellow (pH $\leq$ 6.5).
   Negative: blue.

Mucate medium: Suspend 10 g of mucic acid in 100 ml distilled water in a 1-liter beaker on a magnetic stirrer. Add 12 ml 0.2% bromthymol blue aqueous solution. Add about 4.6 ml saturated NaOH (careful—this is a strong alkali) gradually until all is added or the indicator remains dark blue. Add 10 g peptone and 883 ml distilled water. Adjust pH to 8.8 (some workers use pH 7.4). Dispense 3 ml into 13- × 100-mm tubes, and autoclave at 121 C for 10 min.

Nitrate Reduction (23)

1. Inoculate a nitrate broth of choice [Indole Nitrite Medium (BBL) is recommended].
2. Incubate at 35 C for 24 hr to 7 days, depending on the organism.
3. Add 5 drops of Solution A (sulfanilic acid) and 5 drops of Solution B (naphthylamine) to the tube.

Positive: a red color develops in 1-2 min.

Negative: no red color. Add a pinch of zinc dust to the tube, because the nitrate may have been reduced to nitrogen gas. If nitrate is still present, the zinc will reduce it to nitrite.

No color development at this point is a positive test. Development of a red color indicates a negative test.

Solution A: Dissolve 8 g of sulfanilic acid to 1000 ml of 5 N acetic acid (1 part glacial acetic acid to 2½ parts distilled water).

Solution B: Add 6 ml of N,N-dimethyl-1-naphthylamine to 1 liter of 5 N acetic acid. Store solution B at room temperature.

Comments: The nitrate reduction test can be performed as a rapid test (2 hr) with a small volume of broth and a heavy inoculum.

Recommendation: The original formula for Solution B included alpha naphthylamine as the reagent. The Occupational Safety and Health Administration (OSHA) determined that alpha naphthylamine was a carcinogen. Because N,N-dimethyl-1-naphthylamine has a similar structural formula (although it is not on the carcinogen list), it would seem wise to handle it with optimal safety precautions. This reagent is available commercially.

Nitrate or Nitrite Reduction

1. Inoculate the suspected *Neisseria* into a Mueller-Hinton broth or heart infusion broth containing 0.1% KNO_3 or KNO_2[†] (or less than 0.1% if growth is impaired).
2. Add 10% sterile serum to improve growth if the organism is fastidious.
3. Incubate at 35 C for up to 5 days, testing periodically by removing a small amount of the culture. See the previous description of the nitrate test for details of testing.

ONPG Test for Beta-Galactosidase

1. Inoculate a 0.5-ml aliquot of ONPG broth with a heavy loopful of growth from a triple sugar iron or Kligler's iron agar slant.
2. Incubate the suspension in a heating block or water bath at 37 C for 1-4 hr.

Positive: a yellow color develops.

Negative: solution remains colorless.

Comment: This test may not be used with yellow-pigmented organisms.

ONPG broth: Dissolve 1 g of peptone and 0.5 g of NaCl in 100 ml distilled H_2O. Autoclave the solution at 121 C for 15 min. Dissolve 0.6 g of O-nitrophenyl-β-D-galactopyranoside (ONPG) in 100 ml of 0.01 M Na_2HPO_4, and

---

[†]Tube the nitrate broth in 10-ml volumes, and the nitrite broth in 15-ml volumes, with inverted Durham tubes to collect nitrogen gas.

sterilize by filtration. Store the sterile ONPG solution at 4–10 C in a dark bottle. Add 25 ml of sterile ONPG solution to 75 ml of the peptone broth. After it is mixed, dispense the ONPG broth aseptically in 0.5-ml aliquots into sterile 13- × 100-mm tubes. The ONPG broth will remain stable for 1 month at 4–10 C, or longer if frozen. ONPG broth SHOULD NOT BE USED IF IT TURNS YELLOW.

Oxidase Test

Kovacs' Method

1. Saturate a filter paper contained in a petri dish with 0.5% tetramethyl-p-phenylenediamine HCl.
2. Pick a portion of the colony to be tested using a *platinum* wire, and rub the colony on the filter paper.
   Positive: a deep purple color appearing in *10 seconds.*
   Comments: The tetramethyl-p-phenylenediamine HCl can be dispensed in small aliquots, corked, and frozen at −20 C. The reagent should be checked daily with a known oxidase-positive organism.
   The reagent can be added directly to the colonies on the plate; the oxidase-positive colonies will turn from pink to purple.
   A 1.0% solution of para-amino-dimethylaniline monohydrochloride can also be used for the oxidase test. The reagent should be allowed to stand for 15 min before being used and discarded after 1–2 hr. When this reagent is added to oxidase-positive colonies, the color will change to pink and darken to black.

Indolphenol Oxidase

1. Inoculate the organism on a nutrient agar slant, and incubate at 35 C for 18–24 hr. Prepare a control slant with a stock strain of a known oxidase-positive organism. DO NOT INCUBATE LONGER THAN 18–24 HR.
2. Add 2–3 drops of Reagent A (1.0% alphanaphthol in 95% ethanol) and 2–3 drops of Reagent B (1.0% aqueous p-amino-dimethylaniline HCl or oxalate) to the growth.
3. Tilt the tube so the reagents mix and pass over the growth.
   Positive: blue color developing in the growth within 2 min.
   Comments: Questionable color reactions or reactions occurring after 2 min should be interpreted as negative.
   The indolphenol oxidase test is less sensitive than the Kovacs' oxidase test.

Oxidative-Fermentative (O-F) Metabolism of Carbohydrates

1. Inoculate 2 tubes of O-F medium* (see below) containing a specific carbohydrate by making 1–2 stabs one-half the depth of the medium.

2. Overlay one tube with sterile, stiff petrolatum or Vaspar. (Sterile mineral oil is not recommended.)
3. Incubate both tubes at 35 C for several days, examining daily.
    Nonoxidizer-nonfermenter: no change in either tube, or alkaline in open tube.
    Oxidizer-nonfermenter: acid (yellow) produced in open tube; no change in closed.
    Fermenter: acid (yellow) produced in both tubes.

Oxidative-fermentative basal medium (Hugh & Leifson) is available commercially. These O-F basal media vary in their performance; it is essential that known oxidative and fermentative organisms be used to test the media before use.

Oxidative-fermentative basal medium (CDC formula): To 100 ml distilled water, add 0.2 g pancreatic digest of casein and 0.2 ml of 1.5% aqueous phenol red. Warm to dissolve peptone, and adjust to pH 7.3. Add 0.3 g agar; dissolve by heating. Dispense 6-ml aliquots into 16- × 125-mm tubes, and autoclave at 121 C for 15 min. While basal medium is melted, add filter-sterilized carbohydrate (dextrose, lactose, etc.) to a final concentration of 1%.

Oxygen Requirements—Special Seals

Special seals for Actinomyces and Arachnia cultures

Tube cultures may be sealed for individual incubation either aerobically with CO_2 or anaerobically with CO_2.

Clip off non-absorbent cotton plug and push the short remaining plug into the tube, leaving a space of ½ to ¾ inch at the top of the tube. Place a small pledget of absorbent cotton on top of the plug. Add reagents to the absorbent cotton as indicated below, and immediately close the tube with a rubber stopper.

Aerobic + CO_2 incubation—Add 5 drops 10% Na_2CO_3 + 5 drops 1 M KH_2PO_4.

Anaerobic + CO_2 incubation—Add 5 drops 10% Na_2CO_3 + 5 drops pyrogallol solution (100 g pyrogallic acid in 150 ml distilled water).

Starch Hydrolysis

1. Inoculate a starch agar plate, and incubate it under the appropriate conditions and for the proper interval (for example, see Chapter 12 for *Actinomyces* and *Arachnia*).
2. Flood the medium with 2–4 ml of Gram's iodine.
    Positive: a colorless area appears around streak indicating starch is hydrolyzed.
    Negative: the entire medium turns blue.

Starch agar (Chapter 12): Suspend 5.0 g soluble starch in 40 ml of cold deionized or distilled H_2O. Add the starch suspension to 1 liter of melted nutrient agar, mix, and sterilize at 121 C for 15 min. Dispense into petri dishes.

Comments: The starch content of the medium may be reduced to 0.2% for aerobic bacteria. Slants can be made instead of plates. The medium also can be prepared as a broth. For nonfermentative gram-negative bacilli, Mueller-Hinton agar can be used for the base of this medium.

Starch agar (*Chapter* 14): Prepare Lombard-Dowell agar (see Media section), adding 5.0 g starch per liter.

Starch Hydrolysis Test

1. Inoculate a plate of Mueller Hinton agar (BBL or Difco) with 1 streak of the test organism. Two or three cultures can be tested on one plate.
2. Incubate for 2 days in 35 C.
3. Flood the plate with a 1:5 dilution of Lugol's iodine solution, and hold plate against a white background.
   Positive: colorless zone around the area of growth.

Lugol's iodine solution: Dissolve 10 g potassium iodine in 100 ml distilled water. Add 5 g iodine crystals slowly, with shaking. Filter and store in a tightly stoppered, brown bottle. Discard after 1 month.

Urease

1. Streak the slant of Christensen's urea medium* with the organism.
2. Incubate at 35 C (or the appropriate temperature for the organism) for 24 hr to 4 days.
   Positive: a bright pink color develops on the slant and may
   extend throughout the medium.
   Negative: no change in color of medium.

Voges-Proskauer Test

Barritt's Method (Coblentz)

1. Inoculate 5 ml MR-VP medium,* and incubate at 35 C for 48 hr.
2. Transfer 1 ml of the culture to a clean tube.
3. Add 0.6 ml of 5% alpha naphthol in absolute ethyl alcohol; mix well.
4. Add 0.2 ml 40% KOH containing 0.5% creatine; shake well.
   Positive: red color in 5 min.

O'Meara's Method

1. Inoculate 1 ml MR-VP broth in a 13- × 100-mm tube, and incubate for 24–48 hr at 35 C.
2. Add 1 ml of 40% KOH containing 0.3% creatine.
   Positive: red-pink color within a few minutes (may be read
   up to 4 hr after the reagent is added before calling
   negative).

Comment: Store the reagent in the refrigerator, and discard after 2 weeks.

Rapid Method

1. Inoculate 0.2 ml of MR-VP broth* heavily from a TSI or KI agar slant, blood agar, chocolate agar, or MacConkey agar. (Do not use EMB.)
2. Incubate at 37 C for 4 hr in a heating block.
3. Add 2–3 drops of each of the Barritt reagents (listed above), shaking between the addition of each reagent.
   Positive: cherry red color within 15 min.
   Negative: any color other than the above.

Reagents

The reagents included in this section are those which were cited in the preceding chapters. For the most part they relate to performing a test described in a specific chapter. Reagents associated with biochemical tests in the preceding section have been included with the description of test performance.

N-Acetyl-L-Cysteine-Sodium Hydroxide Reagent

Dissolve 2.94 g of trisodium citrate dihydrate in 100 ml of distilled water. In a separate container, dissolve 4.0 g of NaOH in 100 ml of distilled water. Mix the 2 solutions, and add 0.5 N-acetyl-L-cysteine powder (Mead Johnson Research Center, Evansville, Ind; Sigma Chemical Co, St. Louis, Mo) immediately before use. The solution is self-sterilizing.

N-acetyl-L-cysteine solutions are unstable and should be used immediately after preparation. If the solution cannot be used immediately, store at 2–4 C in a tightly stoppered container for short periods. Do not use the solution if stored for more than 48 hr.

Sodium citrate and sodium hydroxide solutions can be prepared ahead of time, sterilized, and stored at room temperature. They can be mixed with N-acetyl-L-cysteine in the ratios given above to prepare a 1-day supply of reagent as it is needed.

D-Aminolevulinic Acid (ALA) Reagent

Mix 0.03352 g ALA hydrochloride (Sigma), 0.01972 g $MgSO_4 \cdot 7H_2O$, and 100 ml Sorensen phosphate buffer, 0.1 M, pH 6.9. Dispense 0.5 ml into 13-×100-mm test tubes. Store tubes at −20 C until used.

Andrade Base

See Carbohydrate Fermentation.

Aniline Reagent (For Niacin Test)

Add 4 ml of clear, colorless aniline to 96 ml of 95% ethanol. This 4% solution must be stored in a brown bottle at 2 C to 4 C and protected from bright light. If the solution turns yellow, discard, and prepare fresh.

Bovine Albumin 0.2%

Dissolve 2.0 g of bovine albumin, fraction V (Armour Pharmaceutical Co, Kankakee, Ill; Pentex, Inc, Kankakee, Ill) in 100 ml of 0.85% sodium chloride solution by gentle mixing. A magnetic stirrer can be used to dissolve the albumin, but mixing should be gentle to avoid foaming. Adjust to pH 6.8 with 4% NaOH. Sterilize the solution by passing through a membrane filter (0.45 μm pore size), and aseptically dispense into 18- $\times$ 125-mm screw-capped tubes in 10- to 20-ml amounts. Store this 2% solution at 4 C until needed.

Prepare 0.2% bovine albumin solution by diluting the stock 2% solution 1:10 with sterile distilled water or buffered sodium chloride solution. A convenient procedure is to have sterile diluent in 9- or 18-ml amounts in screw-capped tubes so that 1 or 2 ml of the 2% stock solution can be added as needed.

Cyanogen Bromide Reagent (For Niacin Test)

Caution: Prepare the solution in a fume hood, and wear rubber gloves when handling the chemical.

Dissolve 5 g cyanogen bromide in 50 ml distilled water. Store in a tightly capped brown bottle at 2 to 4 C. If crystals form during storage, they will redissolve when the solution is warmed to room temperature. Since BrCN is volatile, the solution may weaken with prolonged storage. Always discard into dilute solutions of NaOH to prevent formation of hydrocyanic acid.

Nitrate Reductase Substrate

Combine 0.085 g $NaNO_3$, 0.117 g KH_2PO_4, 0.485 g $Na_2HPO_4 \cdot 12H_2O$, and dissolve the mixture in 100 ml of distilled water. The final pH of the solution should be 7.0. Store the substrate at 2–4 C in the dark.

Phosphate Buffer, M/15

Prepare stock solutions A and B.

Solution A: M/15 disodium phosphate—Dissolve 9.47 g anhydrous Na_2HPO_4 in distilled water in a 1000- ml volumetric flask. Add distilled water to volume.

Solution B: M/15 monopotassium phosphate—Dissolve 9.07 g KH_2PO_4 in distilled water in a volumetric flask. Add distilled water to volume.

To prepare buffers with specific pH values, mix volumes of Solutions A and B as follows:

pH	Solution A	Solution B
6.6	37.5 ml	62.5 ml
6.8	50 ml	50 ml
7.0	61.1 ml	38.9 ml

Confirm final values with a pH meter.

Spot Indole Reagent

Concentrated hydrochloric acid ....10 ml
Distilled water...90 ml
Paradimethylaminocinnamaldehyde...1 g

Mix and store at 2–5 C. The solution is stable for at least 6 months when refrigerated.

Zephiran Trisodium Phosphate Reagent

Dissolve 1 kg trisodium phosphate ($Na_3PO_4 \cdot 12H_2O$) in 4 liters of hot distilled water. Add 7.5 ml of Zephiran concentrate (17% benzalkonium chloride, Winthrop Laboratories, New York, NY) and mix well. Store at room temperature in a closed container.

Stains and Staining Methods

Detailed instructions for a number of staining procedures are included in the preceding chapters. When the procedure has been described, only the formula for the stain is included in this section. The staining procedures included here are those cited and referenced in the preceding chapters as well as several other commonly used staining procedures.

Auramine O-Phenol Reagent

Dissolve 0.1 g auramine O in 10 ml 95% ethanol. Dissolve 3 g phenol crystals in 87 ml distilled water. Mix the two solutions, and store a tightly stoppered bottle shielded from light. If crystals form or if the surface appears to be oily, filter the solution prior to use.

Auramine O-Rhodamine B-Phenol Reagent

Mix 75 ml glycerol and 10 ml phenol (heat phenol crystals above melting point, 43 C, cautiously) in 50 ml distilled water. Add 1.5 g auramine O and 0.75 g rhodamine B to the solution, and mix well. After thoroughly mixing, let the solution stand, and then clarify by filtering through glass wool. Store at room temperature in a tightly stoppered bottle shielded from light.

Buffered Diluent with Gelatin, pH 6.4

KH_2PO_4 .... 1.33 g
Na_2HPO_4 .... 0.63 g
NaCl ....12.00 g
Gelatin (bacteriological grade)... 1.0 g
Distilled water.. 1000 ml

Mix and heat to boiling with constant stirring to keep the gelatin from scorching. Store refrigerated at 2–5 C.

Capsule Stain, Modified Leifson's Staining Method

Fix the films suspected to contain anthrax spores in Zenker's fluid for 3 to 5 min; wash in tap water. Flood the slides with Solution A for 10 min. Wash with tap water, and stain with Solution B for 5 to 10 min. Wash with tap water, dry, and examine.

Solution A:
$NH_4Al(SO_4)_2 \cdot 12H_2O$ (saturated aqueous solution) ....20 ml
Tannic acid (20% aqueous solution)..10 ml
Distilled water..10 ml
Ethyl alcohol (95%)..15 ml
Basic fuchsin (saturated solution in 95% ethyl alcohol)..................................3 ml

This solution deteriorates after a week and should be freshly prepared.

Solution B:
Methylene blue...0.1 g
Borax..1.0 g
Distilled water..100 ml

Anthrax bacilli stained by this method appear as dark blue bacilli surrounded by pale blue capsules. The background, including erythrocytes, stains red.

Flagellar Stain

Prepare a suspension of organisms by removing a small amount of growth from 18- to 24-hr-old culture growing on agar. Emulsify the organisms in 1 ml of distilled water. The suspension should be only slightly cloudy. Flame a slide to remove any grease, and label it. Using a capillary pipette, place 1 drop of the organism suspension at the top of a slide tilted at a 45 degree angle. Allow the drop to run to the end. Dry the smear in the slanted position. Place the slide on a staining rack with access to a Bunsen burner. Cover the smear with mordant solution for 4 min. Rinse the slide gently with distilled water. Cover the slide with silver stain, and heat by passing a Bunsen burner flame under the slide until steam is emitted. Let the stain remain on the slide for 4 min, and then rinse carefully with distilled water and slant for air drying.

Mordant solution. Mix together 25 ml of saturated aqueous aluminum potassium sulfate stock solution, 50 ml of *freshly prepared* 10% tannic acid solution, and 5 ml of 5% ferric chloride stock solution. Store the mixture in a dark bottle. The solution can be kept at room temperature for several months.

Silver stain. Prepare fresh (do not make a stock solution) 100 ml of 5% silver nitrate solution. To 90 ml of the freshly prepared silver nitrate solution add

2–5 ml of concentrated ammonium hydroxide drop by drop. First a brown precipitate will form. As more alkali is added, the precipitate will dissolve. Stop adding alkali just as the solution clears. At this point reverse the procedure, adding silver nitrate until the solution becomes faintly cloudy. The 100 ml volume of silver nitrate should be sufficient for the total procedure. Store the solution in a dark bottle at room temperature. The solution is stable for several months.

Giemsa Stain

Prepare a thin film of blood, and let it dry. Fix the film by flooding with absolute methanol, draining, and permitting the film to dry. Flood slide with dilute Giemsa stain (1 part stain to 50 parts phosphate buffer at pH 6.4), and stain for 30–60 min. Wash the stain off the slide using large quantities of phosphate buffer. Dry the smear and examine.

Giemsa stain stock solution: Dissolve 0.75 g Giemsa stain, powdered (certified), in 65.0 ml of pure absolute methanol. Add 35 ml of pure glycerol, and mix well by shaking the mixture with glass beads. Keep tightly stoppered at all times. Filter if necessary.

Phosphate buffer, pH 6.4: Prepare by combining 6.63 g anhydrous monobasic potassium phosphate (KH_2PO_4) and 2.56 g of anhydrous dibasic sodium phosphate (Na_2HPO_4) and diluting the mixture to 1 liter.

Gram Stain (Kopeloff Modification)

Flood a heat-fixed slide with crystal violet (10 g crystal violet in 1000 ml distilled water). Immediately add 5 drops of $NaHCO_3$ solution (50 g $NaHCO_3$ in 1000 ml distilled water). Wash the stain from the slide, and add iodine solution. (Dissolve 4 g NaOH in 25 ml distilled water. Add 20 g iodine and 1 g KI, and mix to dissolve the iodine. Slowly add 975 ml distilled water with mixing between each addition.) Wash the slide and decolorize with acetone-alcohol. (Combine 300 ml acetone with 700 ml 95% ethyl alcohol.) Wash. Counterstain with safranin. (Add sufficient 95% ethyl alcohol to 20 g of safranin to dissolve the dye. Bring the solution to a liter with distilled water.)

Kinyoun's Stain, Modified

Fix smears with gentle heat by passing the slide through à Bunsen burner flame. Flood the slides with Kinyoun carbolfuchsin stain for 3 min; wash in tap water. Decolorize with 1.0% sulfuric acid until the film is a faint pink; wash in tap water. Counterstain with Loeffler's methylene blue stain for 30 sec. Wash and blot dry.

Kinyoun's carbolfuchsin: Dissolve 4.0 g of basic fuchsin (certified) in 20 ml of 95% ethyl alcohol. While shaking the dissolved dye solution, slowly add 100 ml distilled water. Finally add 8.0 ml of liquefied phenol (melt in a 56 C bath). Mix and store.

Methylene blue counterstain: Dissolve 2.5 g of methylene blue in 100 ml of 95% ethyl alcohol.

Krojian-Erskine "20-Minute" Rapid Staining Method for Treponemataceae

Fix tissue in 10% Formalin for 10 min at 67 C. Prepare frozen sections 7–10 μm thick; wash in distilled water. (If paraffin sections are used, double the staining times.) Warm the uranium nitrate and the developer solutions in small Stender dishes in a paraffin oven at 60 C. Dispense distilled water into three Stender dishes. Also dispense 5–10 ml 95% ethanol and 5 ml ethanol with a few drops of gum mastix solution into separate Stender dishes. In a 250 ml beaker, dilute 10 ml of the stock silver nitrate solution with 90 ml distilled water. Place the washed tissue section in the uranium solution; put the dish in the paraffin oven at 60 C for 5 min. Remove the section to one of the Stender dishes with distilled water; the section should open and float. Pass the section rapidly three times through the ethanol solution with added gum mastix. Rinse the section in distilled water; the section should spread out. Transfer the section to the beaker with dilute silver nitrate solution; heat the contents of the beaker to 70–73 C for 2 min while exposing it to the light of a 60 W bulb at a distance of 4 ft. Remove the section, and dip it into warm developer solution six to eight times. The section should spread out at each dipping and finally appear brown. Remove excess gum mastix by transferring the section to 95% ethanol. Place the section in distilled water. It should unfold; if not, repeat the alcohol treatment. Check to make sure the silver nitrate solution has cooled, and place the section in it for another 10–20 sec while exposing it to light. Transfer the section to a large dish of distilled water and then to a glass slide. Dehydrate the section by gently adding isopropanol to the slide; let it remain for 30 sec and gently blow dry. Blot with several thicknesses of Whatman No. 1 filter paper and repeat application of isopropanol, this time for 1 min. Dry and blot. Dip the slide into thin celloidin solution (histological formula). Remove the slide, and dry the bottom surface; dry the upper surface by gentle blowing. Dehydrate the section once more with isopropanol for 1 min. Take the slide through two changes of xylene for several minutes. Mechanically remove excess celloidin from around the tissue, and mount preferably with gum damar. Examine, looking for black Treponemataceae against a yellow to brown background.

Uranium nitrate: Dissolve 1 g uranium nitrate, C.P., in a solution containing 10 ml 95% ethanol, 10 ml of acetone, C.P., 5 ml glycerol, C.P., and 3 ml formic acid, C.P.

Silver nitrate: Dissolve 10 g silver nitrate, C.P., in 100 ml of distilled water. Store this stock solution in a brown bottle. The "working solution" of silver nitrate should be prepared on the day of use by diluting 10 ml of stock silver nitrate solution with 90 ml of distilled water. The "working solution" of silver nitrate should not be used more than three times.

Gum mastix: Add 25 ml of gum mastix to 35 ml absolute ethanol, and let the mixture stand in a brown bottle for 3–5 days at room temperature. Shake the bottle occasionally during this time. The supernate should be used in the staining procedure.

Developer solution: Combine 2.5 ml of 40% formaldehyde, C.P., and 2.5 ml of acetone, C.P. In the order listed add to this solution 0.31 g hydroquinone, 0.1 g sodium sulfite, anhydrous, 2.5 ml pyridine, 2.5 ml gum mastix solution, and 15 ml distilled water. Mix and store in a brown bottle at room temperature. The developer solution should be replaced every 1–2 weeks or at any time a sediment forms.

Methylene Blue Stain

Fix smear in heat and flood slide with methylene blue* stain for 1 min. Wash in tap water, blot dry, and examine.

Methylene blue stain: Dissolve 0.3 g methylene blue in 30.0 ml 95% ethyl alcohol. When the dye is dissolved, add 100 ml of distilled water. The original formulation of Loeffler methylene blue stain required that alkali be added to this formula. The present-day commercial preparations of methylene blue do not require alkalinization.

Wayson's Stain

Fix smear with light heat or by flooding the slide with absolute methanol for 2–5 min. Flood the slide with Wayson's stain for 10–20 sec. Wash with water, and blot dry. Examine, looking for bipolar staining.

Wayson's stain: Dissolve 0.20 g basic fuchsin and 0.75 g methylene blue (each with a 90% dye content) in 20 ml of 95% ethyl alcohol. Filter, and pour the dissolved dye mixture slowly into 200 ml of 5% phenol. Store in a dark glass bottle.

Wright's Stain

Air dry smears, and cover each with 2–3 ml of Wright's stain. Stain for 2 min. Add 2–3 ml phosphate buffer, pH 6.4 (see Giemsa stain for formula of buffer), to the stain, blowing to mix stain and buffer. Rinse with buffer until all the purple stain is removed. Air dry, and examine.

*Wright's stain: The complete formulation contains 3.0 g of Wright's stain (certified, powder form), 30.0 ml glycerol (C.P.), and 970.0 ml absolute methanol (acetone-free). To prepare, place the 3.0 g of Wright's stain in a large mortar. Add about 5 ml of glycerol and about 30 ml of methanol, and grind to dissolve. Continue adding the glycerol and the methanol, with grinding until the dye is completely dissolved and all the glycerol and methanol have been used. Store in dark, tightly stoppered bottle, and allow to mature for approximately 2 weeks. Filter before use.

Zenker's Fluid

Mix 2.5 g potassium bichromate, 8.0 g mercuric chloride, and make up to 100 ml with distilled water.

Not all the mercuric chloride will dissolve; the amount specified will maintain a saturated solution. Smears containing the spores of anthrax bacilli are inactivated within 3 to 5 min when submerged in this fluid. Smears fixed in this fluid must be stained longer with hematoxylin.

Ziehl-Neelsen Carbolfuchsin Reagent

Dissolve 0.3 g basic fuchsin in 10 ml of 95% ethanol, and add the dye solution to 90 ml of a 5% aqueous solution of phenol. Store the reagent in stoppered bottles to prevent evaporation. If crystals form during storage, the reagent should be filtered before being used.

Bacteriologic Culture Media

Microbiology has come a long way from the days when the microbiologist stood in his media kitchen decocting infusions from ground-up heart, brains, liver, and the like. The trend has been toward using more defined media components, with extracts and peptones taking the place of infusions, to the creation of completely chemically defined media. Nevertheless, media preparation remains an art best left when possible to skilled manufacturers.

Blending ingredients commonly used in media for the diagnostic laboratory is no mean task. Even peptones, the most uniform of the chemically undefined media components, made by the same digestive process from the same raw protein source are not necessarily equivalent. For example, Difco Laboratories manufactures two peptones which meet the USP standards for pancreatic digest of casein, namely Casitone and Tryptone. However, these peptones are not interchangeable. Equivalence of peptones can only be determined by trial and error. Furthermore, each lot of peptone, extract, or infusion varies somewhat. When these components are incorporated into a more complex medium, they must be carefully balanced with the other components to assure a satisfactory product. The commercial manufacturer is in a much better position to do this than is the clinical microbiologist.

Commercially available dehydrated media mentioned in various chapters of this book without reference to availability and for which the authors suggest no modification are listed in Table 46.1. They should be prepared strictly according to the manufacturer's directions. Unless a carefully controlled source of deionized water is available, distilled water should be used in preparing all media.

Many media mentioned by the various authors must have enrichment added to a basal medium. Those which must be added to a cooled basal medium include defibrinated blood, ascitic fluid, serum, hemin-vitamin K solu-

TABLE 46.1—RECOMMENDED MEDIA WHICH SHOULD BE PREPARED FROM COMMERCIALLY AVAILABLE DEHYDRATED PRODUCTS*

Bismuth-sulfite agar	MacConkey agar
Brilliant green agar	Mannitol-salt agar
Desoxycholate agar	SS (*Salmonella-Shigella*) agar
Desoxycholate citrate agar	Selenite broth
EMB (eosin-methylene blue agar)	TCBS (thiosulfate-citrate-bile
GN (gram-negative) broth	salts) agar
Hektoen enteric agar	Tellurite-glycine agar
Loeffler's medium	Tergitol 7 agar

* This list does not include basic agars and broths that all practicing microbiologists should know, nor does it include media indicated to be commercially available by authors of the various chapters.

tion, cysteine, dithiothreitol, dithioerythritol, and sodium formaldehyde sulfoxalate. Follow each author's recommendations regarding the percentage of enrichment to be added. If it contains agar, the basal medium should be cooled to 50 C before an enrichment is added. Broth media should be allowed to cool to room temperature before being enriched.

Similarly, inhibitory compounds should be added according to individual recommendations. Antibiotics such as colistin, chloramphenicol, the aminoglycosides, and nalidixic acid are heat stable and can be added to the basal medium before autoclaving. When in doubt, antibiotics should be added after the basal medium is autoclaved and cooled.

Specific formulations are given for recommended modifications of standard media; for simple, basic media which can be compounded from standard agar or broth bases; and for media for which there is no convenient commercially available form. Formulations involve the most complete dehydrated base available. Because the comparability of different manufacturers' peptones is not readily apparent, brand names of peptones appear in the formulations submitted by the various authors. For convenience, sources of brand name peptones are presented in Table 46.2, even though other peptones may be equally suitable. Reagents used in preparing culture media should be of analytical quality. Sugars should be bacteriologically pure. The *Manual of Clinical Microbiology,* Second Edition, provides a more detailed description of most of the media currently used in diagnostic work (15).

TABLE 46.2—SOURCES OF PEPTONES* CALLED FOR IN MEDIA FORMULATIONS

PEPTONE	SUPPLIER
Biosate	BBL
Gelysate	BBL
Peptone*	Difco
Proteose peptone #2	Difco
Proteose peptone #3	Difco
Trypticase	BBL
Tryptose	Difco

* The designation "peptone" is assumed to be used in the generic sense unless the author has designated the manufacturer.

Alkaline Peptone Water

Peptone or gelysate...10 g
Sodium chloride ....5 g
Distilled water...1000 ml

Dissolve completely and adjust to pH 8.4 with 1 N NaOH. Dispense in desired amount into test tubes (0.5–1 ml for transport media). Autoclave at 121 C for 15 min.

Arylsulfatase Medium, Center for Disease Control (CDC)

Solution A

Tripotassium phenolphthalein disulfate...2.6 g
Distilled water...50 ml

Mix thoroughly and filter sterilize through a 0.20 μm membrane filter. Check the solution for free phenolphthalein by adding 6 drops of 1 M sodium carbonate to 2 ml of solution. If the solution turns pink, discard it.

Three-day test medium:

Dubos broth or Middlebrook 7H9 ....200 ml
Solution A ....2.5 ml

Fourteen-day test medium

Dubos broth or Middlebrook 7H9 ....200 ml
Solution A ....7.5 ml

Dispense into sterile 16- × 125-mm screw-capped tubes.

Arylsulfatase Medium, Wayne*

Dubos oleic agar base...100 ml
Glycerol..1.0 ml
Tripotassium phenolphthalein disulfate...65 mg

Heat to dissolve completely. Dispense 2-ml amounts into 16- × 125-mm screw-capped tubes. Autoclave at 121 C for 15 min. Allow to harden in an upright position.

Bordet-Gengou Agar, Modified*

Potato infusion:

Washed, peeled, sliced potatoes...500 g
Glycerol..40 ml
Distilled water..1000 ml

Boil potatoes in the solution of glycerol and water until very soft. Strain through several layers of gauze and restore to volume. Pour infusion into tall cylinders, and allow to stand until clear supernatant can be filtered off. If not used immediately, the infusion should be sterilized.

*Complete basal medium commercially available in dehydrated form. Asterisks throughout this section denote such availability.

Basal medium:

Potato infusion	500 ml
Sodium chloride	11.25 g
Agar	50 g
Distilled water	1500 ml

Dissolve salt, and thoroughly wet the agar with some of the water. Add the rest of the water, and dissolve the agar with heat. Add the potato infusion, and dispense as desired. No adjustment of reaction is necessary. Autoclave at 121 C for 15 min.

Complete medium:

Basal medium	100 ml
Defibrinated sheep blood	20 ml
Penicillin (optional)	60 units

Melt the base agar, and cool to 50 C. For each 100 ml of basal medium, aseptically add 20 ml of fresh (less than 72 hr old) defibrinated sheep blood and 60 units of penicillin. Dispense the medium into sterile petri plates or tubes, and incubate overnight at 35 C to check sterility.

Bovine Albumin—Polysorbate 80 Medium[†] (6)

25x buffer

Na_2HPO_4	16.6 g
KH_2PO_4	2.17 g

Dilute to 1 liter with distilled water.

20x salts

NaCl	38.5 g
NH_4Cl	5.35 g
$MgCl_2 \cdot 6H_2O$	3.81 g

Dilute to 1 liter with distilled water.

Vitamin B_{12} solutions

Vitamin B_{12}	10 g
Dilute to 100 ml with distilled water	

Working solution: 1:10 dilution in distilled water of above stock solution.

1% polysorbate 80

Polysorbate 80	10 ml
Distilled water heated to 60 C	70 ml

Mix gently. Dilute to 1000 ml with distilled water. Store at −60 C.

Buffered albumin

Bovine albumin fraction V	5 g
Single strength buffer	100 ml

[†] Commercially available from Difco Laboratories (dehydrated basal medium and separate enrichment), Phoenix Laboratories, Inc., 1614 North 74 Street, Omaha, NB 68114 (supplied as 5× concentrated modified liquid medium), Reheis Chemical Co, Armour Pharmaceutical Co, Greyhound Tower, Phoenix, AZ 85077 (supplied as 5× concentrated medium; sterile 30% nonpreserved albumin also available).

Add albumin slowly to buffer, stirring gently. Dissolve completely. Filter sterilize through 0.8, 0.45, and 0.20–0.22 μm membrane filters, respectively.

Basal medium

25× buffer	40 ml
20× salts	50 ml
0.03% $CuSO_4·5H_2O$	1 ml
0.04% $ZnSO_4·7H_2O$	10 ml
0.25% $FeSO_4·7H_2O$	20 ml
Distilled water	700 ml

Combine and stir for 30 min. Add 200 mg L-cystine; stir an additional 30 min. Filter through triple thickness of Whatman No. 1 filter paper (40 cm diameter) to obtain a clear filtrate. To the filtrate add 20 ml of working Vitamin B_{12} solution, 0.1 ml of 0.2% thiamine hydrochloride, and 120 ml of 1% polysorbate solution (stored at −60 C). Adjust to 1000 ml.

For semi-solid medium, add 2.5 g agar to 1000 ml basal medium. Boil to dissolve agar, dispense, and autoclave. Cool to 56 C. Add 2 ml of sterile albumin solution which has been prewarmed to 37 C. Swirl tubes to mix. Store at 25 C.

For solid medium, add 12.5 g agar to 1000 ml medium. Boil to dissolve agar and autoclave. Cool to 56 C. To 800 ml cooled basal medium add 200 ml sterile albumin solution which has been prewarmed to 37 C. Swirl to mix ingredients completely, and pour 30 ml per petri plate. Store at 5 C.

Complete medium

Dispense 8.0-ml amounts of basal medium into 19- × 150-mm glass tubes containing an additional 0.5 ml distilled water. Cap with steel closures, and autoclave at 121 C for 15 min. Cool to room temperature, and add 2.0 ml of sterile, buffered albumin solution. Seal with parafilm to prevent evaporation. Store at 25 C.

Notes

1. Use only glass distilled water in all components.
2. Concentrated polysorbate 80 should be stored at 5 to 10 C; the 1% solution must be stored at −60 C.

Bovine Albumin-Polysorbate 80 Medium, Modified (12)

Basal Medium

10% Na_2HPO_4	10 ml
3% KH_2PO_4	10 ml
10% NaCl	10 ml
25% NH_4Cl	1 ml
0.5% thiamine	1 ml
10% w/v glycerol (8% v/v)	1 ml
Distilled water	940 ml

Mix thoroughly. Autoclave at 121 C for 15 min (pH when cooled is 7.15).

Albumin Enrichment

Bovine albumin fraction V	20 g
Sterile distilled water	100 ml

```
1.0% CaCl₂.....................................................................................................2 ml
1.0% MgCl₂·6H₂O........................................................................................2 ml
0.400% ZnSO₄·7H₂O ...................................................................................2 ml
0.300% CuSO₄·5H₂O ...................................................................................2 ml
0.500% FeSO₄·7H₂O ...................................................................................20 ml
0.020% Vitamin B₁₂....................................................................................2 ml
10% Tween 80 (see note) .........................................................................25 ml
```

Add the albumin slowly to the distilled water, stirring gently to avoid foaming. After the albumin is completely dissolved, slowly add the remaining components. Mix continuously. Add 1.6 ml 1 N NaOH, and adjust to a total volume of 200 ml. Filter sterilize.

Note: The medium as referenced contains approximately 1250 mg/liter of Tween 80 in the complete medium. The necessary concentration (% v/v) of the stock Tween 80 must be determined experimentally. Prewarm Tween 80 to 37 C, and place 10 ml into a tared beaker. The number of milliliters of Tween 80 required to make 100 ml of stock 10% w/v solution can be determined with the following formula:

$$x = 1.250 \text{ g} \times \frac{10 \text{ ml}}{\text{g Tween 80}} \times 100 \text{ ml} \times \frac{1}{25 \text{ ml}} \times 2$$

or
$$x \text{ ml} = \frac{100}{\text{g of Tween 80 in 10 ml aliquot}}$$

Complete medium (pH 7.2)

```
Sterile basal medium (pH 7.15).............................................................900 ml
Sterile albumin enrichment (pH 7.4).......................................................100 ml
```

Brucella Selective Agar (4)

```
Heart infusion agar ...............................................................................40 g
Gelatin ....................................................................................................1 g
Glucose ..................................................................................................2.5 g
Distilled water.......................................................................................1000 ml
```

Mix and heat to dissolve ingredients completely. Dispense 190 ml per bottle. Autoclave at 121 C for 15 min. Cool to 50 C.

Aseptically add to each bottle:
```
0.5% (w/v) actidione (Upjohn)................................................................1.0 ml
0.5% (w/v) bacitracin (Upjohn)...............................................................1.0 ml
1.0% (w/v) circulin (Upjohn)..................................................................0.3 ml
0.1% (w/v) polymyxin B (Burroughs Wellcome) ....................................1.2 ml
Defibrinated sheep blood.......................................................................10 ml
```

Mix and pour into petri plates.

Buffered Single Substrate Media (BSS) (10)

Base

```
K₂HPO₄ ...................................................................................................0.087 g
1% phenol red.........................................................................................0.2 ml
Distilled water.........................................................................................100 ml
```

Dissolve completely. Store at room temperature over an excess of chloroform.

Substrates

1. Glucose ....2 g
   Distilled water..10 ml
2. Maltose..2 g
   Distilled water..10 ml
3. Soluble starch ....0.5 g
   Distilled water..10 ml
   Adjust starch solution to pH 8.2.

All substrates should be stored at room temperature over an excess of chloroform.

Carbohydrate Fermentation Media (4)

Suspend 26 g of Difco (0841) dehydrated carbohydrate medium base in 1000 ml of distilled water. Heat to boiling for 1–2 min to dissolve ingredients. Autoclave at 121 C for 15 min.

To 900 ml of sterile basal medium cooled to 45–50 C, aseptically add 100 ml of sterile aqueous carbohydrate stock solution (Table 46.3). Mix well, and dispense aseptically in 7-ml quantities into 15- × 90-mm screwcapped tubes. (Final pH of the medium should be 7.0 ± 0.1 at 25 C). With the caps loose, pass the tubes of medium into an anaerobic glove box so that an atmosphere of approximately 85% N_2, 10% H_2, and 5% CO_2 replaces the air in the tubes. Fasten the caps securely so that they are airtight, and remove tubes from the glove box. Store in a refrigerator at 4 C or at ambient temperature.

Cary and Blair Transport Medium* (3)

NaCl...5.0 g
Na_2HPO_4 ....1.1 g
Sodium thioglycollate ....1.5 g
Agar...5.0 g

TABLE 46.3

CARBOHYDRATE	CONCENTRATION OF STOCK SOLUTION*
D-Glucose	6.0%
D-Maltose	6.0%
D-Mannitol	6.0%
D-Mannose	6.0%
D-Xylose	6.0%
Glycerol	6.0%
Lactose	6.0%
L-Arabinose	6.0%
Rhamnose	6.0%
Salicin	6.0%
Starch	2.5%
Sucrose	6.0%
Trehalose	6.0%

* Sterile aqueous carbohydrate solution sterilized by filtration

Mix thoroughly with heat and continued stirring until solution just clears. Do not overheat. Cool to 50 C, and add 9 ml of 1% $CaCl_2$ solution. Adjust to pH 8.4. Dispense in 7-ml amounts into rinsed, sterilized, screw-capped tubes (9-ml capacity). Steam for 15 min. Cool, and tighten caps.

Note: Use chemically clean glassware which has been rinsed with Sørensen's 0.067 M phosphate buffer, pH 8.1.

CDC Anaerobe Blood Agar (4)

```
Trypticase soy agar (BBL).......................................................................................40.0 g
Agar (additional)...................................................................................................5.0 g
Yeast extract (Difco).............................................................................................5.0 g
Hemin†.................................................................................................................5.0 mg
L-cystine†..........................................................................................................400.0 mg
Vitamin K₁ (3 phytylmenadione)‡.......................................................................10.0 mg
Distilled water................................................................................................1000.0 ml
```

Heat to dissolve completely. Adjust pH to 7.5, and autoclave at 121 C for 15 min. Cool to 48–50 C in a water bath. Add 50 ml of sterile, defibrinated sheep blood. Mix and pour in 20-ml quantities into sterile 15- × 100-mm petri dishes.

After the medium hardens, place the plates in cellophane bags, seal tightly, and store at 4 C.

CDC Anaerobe Blood Agar with Kanamycin (4) and Vancomycin (KVA)

Prepare CDC anaerobe blood agar. At the time of adding the sheep blood, also add 100 mg (base activity) of kanamycin and 7.5 mg (base activity) of vancomycin per liter of medium.

CDC Anaerobe Blood Agar with Phenethylalcohol (PEA) (4)

Prepare CDC anaerobe blood agar, and add 2.5 g phenethylalcohol per liter of medium before autoclaving.

CDC Stiff Anaerobe Blood Agar (4)

Prepare CDC anaerobe blood agar, and add 25.0 g additional agar per liter rather than 5.0 g.

---

† In a small beaker, dissolve the hemin and the L-cystine in 5 ml of 1 N NaOH before adding them to the other ingredients.

‡ Add the vitamin K₁ from a stock alcoholic solution containing 1 g of 3 phytylmenadione (ICN, Clevelend, Ohio), plus 99 ml of absolute ethanol.

Cetrimide Agar (23)

For miscellaneous gram-negative rods

Heart infusion agar ....40.0 g
Cetrimide (hexadecyltrimethylammonium bromide) ....0.9 g
Distilled water ....1000 ml

Mix thoroughly, and mix to dissolve completely. Dispense 5-ml amounts in 15- × 125-ml tubes. Continue mixing media as it is dispensed to insure even distribution of sediment. Autoclave at 121 C for 15 min; then slant the medium.

Note: Cetrimide varies from lot to lot, and the actual amount needed must be determined with known cultures.

For enterics

Same as above except contains 0.5% cetrimide.

For pseudomonads

Use Pseudosel agar.

Charcoal Yeast Extract (CYE) Agar

Yeast extract (Difco) ....10.0 g
Activated charcoal (Norit A) ....1.5 g
Agar (Difco) ....17.0 g
Distilled water ....980 ml

Mix and dissolve by boiling. Autoclave at 121 C for 15 min; cool to 50 C in a water bath.

Prepare fresh solutions of L-cysteine HCl (0.40 g in 10 ml of distilled water) and soluble ferric pyrophosphate[†] or $FeNO_3 \cdot 9H_2O$ (0.25 g in 10 ml of distilled water). Membrane filter-sterilize each solution separately. Add L-cysteine HC1 to basal medium first.

Adjust the complete medium to pH 6.90 at 50 C by adding 4.0 to 4.5 ml of 1.0 N NaOH. The pH of this medium is critical.

Pour 20-ml quantities of media into sterile petri dishes (15 × 100 mm). Swirl the medium between pouring plates to keep charcoal particles suspended.

Precaution: Soluble ferric pyrophosphate must be kept dry and stored in the dark; it is no longer usable if it turns from green to yellow or brown. A freshly mixed solution of the compound is required each time it is needed in preparing media. Do not heat to higher than 60 C to dissolve. The mixture can be readily dissolved by placing it in a 50 C water bath.

Chocolate Agar

Base

GC agar base (BBL) ....7.2 g
Distilled water ....100 ml

[†]Available on request from Center for Disease Control, Biological Products Division, Atlanta, GA 30333.

Mix and boil for 1 min. Autoclave at 121 C for 15 min. Cool to 50 C.

Hemoglobin solution

Hemoglobin ....2 g
Distilled water ....100 ml

Mix the hemoglobin with 2–3 ml of the distilled water to form a smooth paste. Continue mixing and gradually add the balance of the water. Autoclave at 121 C for 15 min. Cool to 50 C.

Complete Medium

Aseptically combine cooled base and hemoglobin solution. Then add 2 ml of IsoVitaleX (BBL). Mix and pour 20–25 ml per petri plate.

Supplements

Thayer-Martin Agar, modified (16): Add 1 ml VCN inhibitor containing 300 µg/ml of vancomycin, 750 µg/ml of colistin, and 1250 units/ml of nystatin to cooled, complete medium.

Transgrow (17): Add 2.0 g agar and 0.3 g glucose per 100 ml double-strength GC agar base (see above) before autoclaving. Add 1 ml VCN inhibitor to cooled, complete medium. Dispense into sterile bottles, and gas with 20% CO_2 in air. Tighten caps securely.

Trimethoprim lactate can be added to either Thayer-Martin agar or Transgrow at a final concentration of 5 µg/ml.

Chocolatized Blood Agar

Prepare the appropriate agar base. Autoclave at 121 C for 15 min, and cool to 50 C. Add blood to a concentration of 5% to 10%. Slowly heat the preparation to 80 C, and hold at that temperature, mixing occasionally, until the mixture turns chocolate brown.

Chopped Meat Glucose (CMG) Medium (4)

Prepare chopped meat medium, and add 3.0 g D-glucose per liter of medium.

Chopped Meat Glucose Starch (CMGS) Medium (4)

Lean beef ....500.0 g
Distilled water ....1000.0 ml
Sodium hydroxide (1 N solution) ....25.0 ml
Trypticase (BBL) ....30.0 g
Yeast extract (Difco) ....5.0 g
K_2HPO_4 ....5.0 g
D-glucose ....3.0 g
Soluble starch ....2.0 g

Obtain fresh lean beef. Remove excess fat and connective tissue and grind in a meat grinder (fine grind). Mix 500 g of the ground beef with 100 ml of distilled water and 25 ml of 1 N NaOH. Heat to boiling while stirring to mix. After the mixture has cooled, refrigerate overnight at 4 C. After refrigeration skim remaining fat off surface of mixture. Filter the mixture through two layers of gauze. Retain the meat particles and the liquid filtrate. Add enough distilled water to the filtrate to give a final volume of 1000 ml.

Add remaining ingredients to the filtrate. Heat until ingredients are dissolved. Adjust the pH of the broth to 7.4.

Add the following to 15- × 143-mm screwcapped tubes:
a) a pinch of iron filings,
b) approximately ¾ inch of meat particles,
c) approximately 2.5 inches (7 ml) of the broth filtrate.

Autoclave at 121 C for 15 min. After the tubes cool and with the caps loose, pass them into an anaerobic glove box so that an atmosphere of approximately 85% N_2, 10% H_2, and 5% CO_2 replaces the air in tubes. After the caps are tightened securely, remove the tubes from the glove box. Store the CMGS tubes in a refrigerator at 4 C or at ambient temperature if necessary.

Chopped Meat (CM) Medium (4)

Lean ground beef	500.0 g
Distilled water	1000.0 ml
Sodium hydroxide (1 N solution)	25.0 ml
Trypticase (BBL)	30.0 g
Yeast extract (Difco)	5.0 g
K_2HPO_4	5.0 g
L-cysteine	0.5 g
Hemin (1% solution)[†]	0.5 ml
Vitamin K_1 (1% alcoholic solution)[‡]	0.1 ml

Obtain fresh, lean beef. Remove excess fat and connective tissue and grind in meat grinder (fine grind). Mix 500 g of the meat with 1000 ml of distilled water and 25 ml of 1 N NaOH. Heat to boiling while stirring. After mixture has cooled, refrigerate overnight at 4 C. After refrigeration skim remaining fat off surface of mixture. Filter the mixture through two layers of gauze. Retain the meat particles and the liquid filtrate. Add enough distilled water to the filtrate to give a final volume of 1000 ml.

Add remaining ingredients to the liquid except the L-cysteine. Heat until the ingredients dissolve completely. Cool to less than 50 C and add the L-cysteine. Mix to dissolve it completely. Adjust the pH of the broth to 7.4.

Wash the meat particles several times with distilled water to remove excess NaOH and spread thinly on a clean towel to partially dry. Dispense about 0.5 g of the meat particles with a small scoop into each 15- × 90-mm screwcapped tube. Add 7 ml of the enriched broth filtrate to each tube. Autoclave the tubes at 121 C for 15 min. After the tubes cool and with the caps loose,

---

[†] The 1% hemin solution is prepared by dissolving 1 g of hemin in 5 ml of 1 N NaOH and diluting to 100 ml with distilled water.

[‡] The 1% alcoholic vitamin K_1 solution is prepared by dissolving 1 g of vitamin K_1 (3 phytyl-menadione, ICN, Cleveland, Ohio) in 99 ml of absolute ethanol.

pass them into an anaerobic glove box so that an atmosphere of approximately 85% N_2, 10% H_2, and 5% CO_2 replaces the air in the tubes. After the caps are tightened securely, remove the tubes from the glove box. Store the CM tubes in a refrigerator at 4 C or at ambient temperature.

Colistin Nalidixic Acid (CNA) Agar* (7)

Columbia agar base	42.5 g
Distilled water	1000 ml

Mix thoroughly and heat to boiling to dissolve completely. Autoclave at 121 C for 15 min. Cool to 50 C, and add 50 ml sterile defibrinated sheep blood and 5 ml of a solution containing 0.3% nalidixic acid and 0.2% colistin. Pour into petri plates.

Note: Columbia CNA agar was originally designed for isolating streptococci, which do grow luxuriantly on this medium. However, colonial morphology and hemolysis may not be "typical." Furthermore, the medium as formulated is somewhat inhibitory to many strains of staphylococci, particularly strains of *Staphylococcus epidermidis*. A modification of this medium has been used at the University of Minnesota for a number of years. This medium contains 40 g per liter of casein-soy agar, 5% sterile defibrinated sheep blood, and colistin and nalidixic acid both at a final concentration of 10 μg/ml.

Coagulated Hen's Egg Yolk (9)

Egg yolks	6 parts
Sterile, normal saline (0.9%)	4 parts

Scrub antibiotic-free hens' eggs, and soak them in 95% ethanol for 1 hr. Separate the yolks aseptically and place into a sterile graduate. Add sterile, normal saline and mix thoroughly. Dispense into sterile tubes, cap, and slant. Tubes should have at least 0.5 inch space between them. Heat for 0.5 hr at 70 C and for an additional 0.5 hr at 72 C in a moist chamber. Uniform temperatures must be maintained. Remove from chamber and replace caps with sterile, paraffined cork stoppers. The medium should be soft with an unglazed surface. Store refrigerated, protected from light.

Note: This medium may be sterilized by other appropriate means (see Pai medium). The original method is given here because the method of preparation applies a much gentler heat, but it requires meticulous aseptic techniques.

Cooked Meat Medium (CM)

Ground beef	500 g
Distilled water	1000 ml
1 N NaOH	25 ml

Trim all fat and connective tissue from meat before grinding. Mix and heat to boiling with stirring. Cool, and skim fat from surface. Filter, saving both meat particles and filtrate. Reconstitute the filtrate to 1000 ml with distilled water and add the following ingredients:

Trypticase or peptone ....30 g
Yeast extract ....5 g
K₂HPO₄ ....5 g
0.025% Resazurin solution ....4 ml

Bring to boil; cool, and add 0.5 g cysteine. Adjust to pH 7.8. Dispense meat particles and filtrate into tubes (1 part meat to about 5 parts fluid). Autoclave at 121 C for 15 min. Store at room temperature.

Cooked Meat Glucose* (CMG): Supplement with 0.5% glucose.

Cystine-Glucose-Blood Agar

Cystine heart agar ....15 g
Distilled water..1000 ml

Mix thoroughly, and heat to boiling to dissolve completely. Autoclave at 121 C for 15 min. Place in a 60 C water bath, and allow temperature to equilibrate. Add 50 ml of sterile defibrinated rabbit blood and hold at 60 C for 1 hr with occasional shaking. Pour into sterile petri plates.

Note: A suitable modification can be prepared by combining sterilized, cooled double-strength cystine heart agar with sterilized and cooled 2% hemoglobin. (See Chocolate Agar for details of preparation.)

Cystine-Tellurite-Blood Agar

Heart infusion agar ....20 g
Bacto-agar (Difco)..2.5 g
Distilled water..500 ml

Adjust to pH 7.4. Autoclave at 121 C for 15 min. Cool to 50 C. Add 25 ml sterile defibrinated rabbit blood, 75 ml of 0.3% (w/v) sterile potassium tellurite solution, and 22 mg of L-cystine. Mix well, and continue to mix as necessary to keep cystine in suspension while pouring plates. Store at 5 C for no more than 1 month.

Egg Yolk Agars

McClung and Toabe

50% egg yolk emulsion: Scrub an antibiotic-free hen's egg, and soak it in 95% ethanol for 1 hr. Aseptically separate the yolk, and emulsify it in an equal volume of saline.

Proteose peptone #2 ....40.0 g
Na₂HPO₄ ....5.0 g
K₂HPO₄ ....1.0 g
NaCl..2.0 g
MgSO₄ · 7H₂O...0.1 g
Glucose ....2.0 g
Agar..20.0 g
Distilled water..1000 ml

Mix thoroughly to obtain a uniform suspension, then adjust to pH 7.6. Heat with frequent mixing, and boil 1 to 2 min. Autoclave at 121 C for 15 min. Cool at 50 C. Add 10 ml egg yolk emulsion to every 90 ml of medium. Pour into sterile petri plates.

McClung and Toabe, modified (11)

Peptone or Trypticase	20.0 g
Na_2HPO_4	2.5 g
NaCl	1.0 g
5% $MgSO_4 \cdot 7H_2O$	0.1 ml
Glucose	1.0 g
Agar	12.5 g
Distilled water	500 ml

Adjust to pH 7.3–7.4. Autoclave at 121 C for 15 min. Cool to 50 C. Add 1 egg yolk from an antibiotic-free hen's egg. Mix thoroughly, and pour into petri plates. Store in an anaerobic jar.

Enriched Thioglycollate Medium

Weigh out 30 g of thioglycollate medium without indicator (BBL 0135C), and suspend in 1000 ml of distilled water. Add 0.5 ml of 1% hemin solution[†] and 0.1 ml of the 1% vitamin K_1 solution.[†] Heat to dissolve ingredients completely. Boil for at least 1–2 min. Dispense in 7-ml quantities into 15- × 90-mm screwcapped tubes. Autoclave at 121 C for 15 min.

After the tubes cool and with caps loose, pass them into an anaerobic glove box so that the atmosphere of approximately 85% N_2, 10% H_2, and 5% CO_2 replaces air in tubes. Fasten caps securely so that they are airtight, and remove the tubes from the glove box. Store the enriched THIO tubes in a refrigerator at 4 C or at ambient temperature if necessary.

Erysipelothrix Selective Broth (23)

Na_2HPO_4	12.02 g
KH_2PO_4	2.09 g
Beef extract	3.00 g
Tryptose or Biosate	15.00 g
NaCl	5.00 g
Distilled water	1000 ml

Filter through Whatman #1 filter paper and autoclave at 121 C for 15 min. Cool to 50 C. Aseptically add: 15 ml mammalian (nonhuman) serum, 400 mg of kanamycin, 50 mg of neomycin, and 25 mg of vancomycin. Dispense aseptically. Store at 4–5 C no longer than 2 weeks.

[†]The hemin solution is prepared by dissolving 1 g of hemin in 5 ml of 1 N NaOH and diluting to 100 ml with distilled water. The vitamin K_1 solution is prepared by dissolving 1 g of vitamin K_1 (3 phytylmenadione, ICN, Cleveland, Ohio) in 99 ml of absolute ethanol.

Feeley-Gorman (F-G) Agar

Casein (acid hydrolysate)	17.5 g
Beef extract	3.0 g
Starch	1.5 g
Agar	17.0 g
Distilled water	980 ml

Mix and dissolve by boiling; autoclave at 121 C for 15 min. Cool to 50 C in a water bath.

Prepare fresh solutions of L-cysteine HCl (0.4 g in 10 ml distilled water) and soluble ferric pyrophosphate[†] or $FeNO_3 \cdot 9H_2O$[‡] (0.25 g in 10 ml distilled water). Filter sterilize each separately. Add the L-cysteine HCl to the basal medium first and then the ferric pyrophosphate (or $FeNO_3 \cdot 9H_2O$). Pour in 20-ml quantities into 15- × 100-mm sterile petri dishes (pH of cool agar should be 6.9).

Precaution: Soluble ferric pyrophosphate must be kept dry and stored in the dark; it is no longer usable if it turns from green to yellow or brown. A freshly mixed solution of the compound must be made each time it is needed in preparing media. Do not heat to higher than 60 C to dissolve. The mixture can be readily dissolved by placing it in a 50 C water bath.

Fildes Enrichment*

Pepsin, granular	1 g
Defibrinated sheep blood	50 ml
Sodium chloride, 0.85%	150 ml
Concentrated hydrochloric acid	6 ml

Mix ingredients in a glass-stoppered bottle by shaking thoroughly. Place bottle in a 56 C water bath for 4 hr. Shake occasionally. Remove from water bath and add about 6 ml of 5 N sodium hydroxide to neutralize. The pH should be 7.0 or slightly lower. Add 1–3 ml of chloroform to mixture, mix, and store at 4 C. Activity is retained for at least 6 months. For completed agar medium, add 10 ml of this enrichment to 200 ml of sterile heart infusion agar melted and cooled to 56 C. Pour approximately 20–25 ml per plate.

Fletcher's Medium* (8)

Peptone	0.3 g
Beef extract	0.2 g
NaCl	0.5 g
Agar	1.5 g
Distilled water	920 ml

[†] Available on request from Center for Disease Control, Biological Products Division, Atlanta, GA 30333.

[‡] The use of $FeNO_3 \cdot 9H_2O$ in F-G agar will support growth but the production of the soluble pigment is diminished considerably.

Heat to boiling to dissolve agar completely. Mix thoroughly. Dispense in desired amounts into 20- × 125-mm screw-capped tubes, and autoclave at 121 C for 15 min. Cool to 56 C, then add sterile rabbit serum to a final concentration of 8% (0.8 ml rabbit serum to every 9.2 ml base).

Haemophilus ducreyi Rabbit Blood Agar

Heart infusion agar (Difco) ....2.0 g
Bacto-agar (Difco)...0.75g
Distilled water...50 ml

Mix thoroughly; boil for 1 min. Autoclave at 121 C for 15 min. Cool to 56 C. Add 10 ml sterile defibrinated rabbit blood. Mix and pour 20–25 ml per plate.

Hemin-Vitamin K Solution (11)

Vitamin K (menadione) solution

Menadione ....0.100 g
95% ethanol ....20 ml

Filter sterilize through 0.20-μm membrane filter.

Hemin solution

Hemin ....50 mg
1 N NaOH ....1 ml

Dissolve hemin in 1 N NaOH, and dilute to 100 ml with distilled water. Autoclave at 121C for 15 min.

Working Solution

Hemin solution ....100 ml
Vitamin K solution...1 ml

Add 1 ml working solution to 100 ml of the medium being enriched.

Hydrogen Sulfide (H₂S) Semi-Solid Medium (4)

Trypticase (BBL)..10.0 g
Yeast extract (Difco)..5.0 g
Lead acetate (10% aqueous solution) ....2.0 ml
Agar..2.0 g
D-glucose ....5.0 g
Distilled water..1000.0 ml

Mix and heat to dissolve. Allow to boil for 1 to 2 min. Adjust pH to 7.2. Dispense in 7-ml quantities into 15- × 90-mm screwcapped tubes. Autoclave at 121 C for 15 min. After the tubes cool and with caps loose, pass them into an anaerobic glove box so that an atmosphere of approximately 85% N_2, 10% H_2, and 5% CO_2 replaces the air in the tubes. Fasten caps securely and remove the tubes from the glove box. Store in a refrigerator at 4 C or at ambient temperature if necessary. The medium may be used to detect both H_2S (blackening) and motility. Inoculate by stabbing.

Kelly's Medium "A"(13)

Solution #1

$Na_2HPO_4 \cdot 7H_2O$	26.52 g
$NaH_2PO_4 \cdot H_2O$	1.03 g
NaCl	1.20 g
KCl	0.85 g
$MgCl_2 \cdot 6H_2O$	0.68 g
Glucose	12.75 g
Proteose peptone #2	5.95 g
Tryptone	2.55 g
Sodium pyruvate	1.06 g
Sodium citrate dihydrate	0.47 g
N-acetylglucosamide	0.53 g
Distilled water	1000 ml

Filter sterilize through 0.20-μm membrane filter. Store at −20 C.

Solution #2

Bovine albumin fraction V	10 g
Distilled water	100 ml

Add albumin fraction V slowly to the water with gentle mixing to avoid foaming. When completely dissolved adjust the pH to 7.8 using 0.1 N sodium hydroxide. Store at −20 C.

Solution #3

Sodium bicarbonate	4.5 g
Distilled water	100 ml

Must be prepared fresh.

Solution #4

Gelatin	7 g
Distilled water	100 ml

Dissolve by gentle heating. Autoclave at 121 C for 15 min. Store at 2–4 C.

Solution #5

Phenol red, certified	0.5 g
Distilled water	100 ml

Store at 2–4 C.

Complete medium

Mix in order:

Solution #1	80 ml
Solution #2	34 ml
Solution #3	4 ml
Solution #5	0.7 ml
Distilled water	1.3 ml

Mix thoroughly and filter-sterilize through a 0.20-μm membrane filter. Dispense in 6-ml amounts into 13- × 100-ml sterile, borosilicate, screw-capped tubes with Teflon liners. Liquefy solution #4 in warm water, and add 2 ml to each tube. Then add 0.5 ml sterile, pooled negative rabbit serum to each tube. Store at room temperature for no longer than 4 weeks.

Leptospira Medium (19)

Basal medium

```
NaCl ..............................................................................................................7.2 g
Nutrient agar ...............................................................................................2.0 g
Distilled water..........................................................................................900 ml
```

Mix thoroughly and heat to dissolve. Tube in 9-ml amounts. Autoclave at 121 C. Cool to 50 C.

Laked rabbit blood

```
Defibrinated rabbit blood ...........................................................................5 ml
Sterile, distilled water...............................................................................15 ml
```

Complete medium

To the sterilized, cooled basal medium add 1 ml of fresh, sterile rabbit serum and 0.1 to 0.2 ml of laked rabbit blood.

Levinthal Broth

```
Brain heart infusion (Difco)......................................................................3.7 g
Distilled water..........................................................................................100 ml
```

Heat to boiling. Add 10 ml of defibrinated horse blood. Filter through Whatman filter paper No. 12. Filter-sterilize through a 0.45-μm membrane filter.

Lombard-Dowell (LD) Agar (4)

```
Trypticase (BBL)........................................................................................5.0 g
Yeast extract (Difco)..................................................................................5.0 g
Sodium chloride .........................................................................................2.5 g
Sodium sulfite............................................................................................0.1 g
L-tryptophan .............................................................................................0.2 g
L-cystine†..................................................................................................0.4 g
Hemin†.......................................................................................................10.0 mg
Vitamin K₁ (3 phytylmenadione)‡..............................................................10.0 mg
Agar............................................................................................................20.0 g
Distilled water..........................................................................................1000.0 ml
```

Heat to dissolve completely. Adjust pH to 7.5, and autoclave at 121 C for 15 min. Cool to 48 C–50 C in a water bath. Pour in 5-ml quantities into one quadrant of a sterile petri dish (Presumpto Plate).

Lombard-Dowell (LD) Bile Agar (4)

Prepare Lombard-Dowell Agar, and add 1.0 g glucose and 20.0 g Oxgall (Difco) per liter, before autoclaving. After cooling, pour 5 ml into one quadrant of a sterile petri dish (Presumpto Plate).

---

† In a small beaker, dissolve the hemin and L-cystine in 5 ml of 1 N NaOH before adding them to the other ingredients.

‡ Add the vitamin K₁ from a stock solution containing 1 g of vitamin K₁ (3 phytylmenadione, ICN, Cleveland, Ohio) plus 99 ml of absolute ethanol.

Lombard-Dowell (LD) Egg Yolk Agar (4)

Trypticase (BBL)	5.0 g
Yeast extract (Difco)	5.0 g
Sodium chloride	2.5 g
Sodium sulfite	0.1 g
L-tryptophan	0.2 g
L-cystine[†]	0.4 g
Hemin[†]	10.0 mg
Vitamin K_1 (3 phytylmenadione)[‡]	10.0 mg
D-glucose	2.0 g
Na_2HPO_4	5.0 g
$MgSO_4$ (5% aqueous solution)	0.2 ml
Agar	20.0 g
Distilled water	900.0 ml

Heat to dissolve completely. Adjust pH to 7.4, and autoclave at 121 C for 15 min. Cool to 55–60 C in a water bath. Add 100 ml of warm (55–60 C) egg yolk suspension (Difco), and mix. Pour in 5-ml quantities into one quadrant of a sterile petri dish (or in 20-ml quantities into 15- × 100-mm petri dishes).

Lombard-Dowell (LD) Esculin Agar (4)

Prepare Lombard-Dowell Agar, adding 1.0 g esculin and 0.5 g ferric citrate per liter, before autoclaving. After cooling, pour 5 ml into one quadrant of a sterile petri dish (Presumpto Plate).

McLeod's Medium, Modified

Heart infusion agar	20.0 g
Bacto-agar (Difco)	2.5 g
Distilled water	500 ml

Adjust to pH 7.8. Autoclave at 121 C for 15 min. Cool to 50 C. Add 25 ml sterile defibrinated rabbit blood. Heat to 70 C, and hold at that temperature until blood is chocolatized. Cool to 50 C. Aseptically add 75 ml of sterile 0.3% (w/v) potassium tellurite solution. Pour into petri plates. Store at 5 C for no more than 1 month.

Milk Media (Lombard-Dowell Base)

Trypticase (BBL)	5.0 g
Yeast extract (Difco)	5.0 g
Sodium chloride	2.5 g
Sodium sulfite	0.1 g
L-tryptophan	0.2 g
Vitamin K_1 (3 phytylmenadione)	10.0 mg

[†]In a small beaker, dissolve the hemin and L-cystine in 5 ml of 1 N NaOH before adding them to the other ingredients.

[‡]Add the vitamin K_1 from a stock solution containing 1 g of vitamin K_1 (3 phytylmenadione, ICN, Cleveland, Ohio) plus 99 ml of absolute ethanol.

```
Agar..................................................................................................................20.0 g
Distilled water................................................................................1000.0 ml
L-cystine...........................................................................................0.4 g
Hemin ..............................................................................................10.0 mg
Skim-milk, powdered...................................................................50.0 g
```

Mix all ingredients except the hemin and L-cystine. Dissolve the hemin and L-cystine in 5 ml of 1 N NaOH before adding to the other ingredients. Add the vitamin K_1 from a stock solution containing 1 g of 3 phytylmenadione plus 99 ml of absolute ethanol, 0.1 ml per 100 ml of medium. After the ingredients are dissolved, adjust the pH of the medium to 7.5. Autoclave the medium at 121 C for 15 min. Allow the medium to cool to 48 C, and dispense 20 ml into plastic 15- × 100-mm petri dishes. If quadrant petri dishes are used, dispense 5 ml of medium per quadrant. Place plates of the solidified medium in cellophane bags, and store in a refrigerator at 4 C.

Streak the medium with 1–2 drops of a cell suspension or broth culture. Incubate at 35 C anaerobically for 48 hr. Digestion of the milk proteins is indicated by a clear zone around the growth of the organism. The medium remains cloudy if the milk is not digested.

Mueller-Hinton Agar Supplemented with 1% Hemoglobin and 1% IsoVitaleX

Component A
```
Mueller-Hinton agar.........................................................................38 g
Distilled water..................................................................................490 ml
```

Component B
```
Hemoglobin powder .........................................................................10 g
Distilled water..................................................................................490 ml
```

Component C
```
IsoVitaleX .........................................................................................20 ml
```

Prepare Components A and B separately, and autoclave at 120 C for 15 min; cool to 50 C, mix together, and hold at 50 C in a water bath. Prepare Component C by adding 10 ml of sterile distilled water to each of two 10-ml vials of IsoVitaleX. Add the contents of both vials to the A-B mixture. Check the pH of the medium, and adjust as needed to a final cold pH of 6.9. Pour 20-ml quantities into sterile plastic petri dishes (15 × 100 mm).

Neomycin Egg Yolk Agar (NEYA) (4)

Prepare Lombard-Dowell egg yolk agar. After adding egg yolk suspension, add 100 mg neomycin sulfate per liter. Pour 20-ml quantities into sterile 15- × 100-mm petri dishes. After the mixture hardens, wrap tightly in cellophane, and store at 4 C.

Pai Medium, Modified (2)

Whole fresh eggs...666 ml
Distilled water...333 ml
Glycerin...80 ml

Beat eggs and water; filter through two layers of gauze. Add glycerin, and mix well. Tube in 3-ml amounts in 13- × 100-mm tubes; place in slanted position. Autoclave as follows: close all valves, open steam inlet, and raise temperature to 100 C. Hold for 1 hr. After 1 hr, turn off steam, and allow pressure to drop slowly to zero.

Peptone-Starch-Dextrose (PSD) Agar (5)

Proteose Peptone #3 ....20 g
Soluble starch ....10 g
Glucose ....2 g
Na_2HPO_4 ....1 g
$NaH_2PO_4 \cdot H_2O$...1 g
Agar..15 g
Distilled water...1000 ml

Add starch to 100 ml of cold water, and mix. Add cold water to 400 ml of boiling water, then add the remaining water (500 ml) and ingredients. Adjust to pH 6.8. Autoclave at 121 C for 15 min. Cool to approximately 50 C, and pour 20–25 ml per plate.

Peptone-Yeast Extract-Glucose (PYG) Broth (4)

Peptone (Difco) ....20.0 g
Yeast extract ....10.0 g
Cysteine-HCl ....0.5 g
Resazurin solution[†]...4.0 ml
Salt solution[‡] ....40.0 ml
D-Glucose..10.0 g
Distilled H_2O..1000.0 ml

Mix the above ingredients in water. Adjust pH to 7.2. Dispense in 7-ml quantities into 15- × 90-mm screwcapped tubes. Autoclave at 121 C for 15 min.

After the tubes cool and with caps loose, pass them into an anaerobic

---

[‡]Resazurin solution—11 mg resazurin in 44 ml distilled H_2O.
[†]Salt solution:

$CaCl_2$...0.2 g
$MgSO_4$..0.2 g
K_2HPO_4 ....1.0 g
KH_2PO_4 ....1.0 g
$NaHCO_3$ ....10.0 g
NaCl ....2.0 g

Mix $CaCl_2$ and $MgSO_4$ in 300 ml distilled H_2O until dissolved. Add 500 ml H_2O, and swirl while adding the remaining salts. Continue swirling until all salts are dissolved. Add 200 ml H_2O, and store in refrigerator.

glove box (85% N_2, 10% H_2, 5% CO_2). Fasten caps securely and remove tubes from glove box. Store in a refrigerator at 4 C or at ambient temperature.

P.L.E.T. Selective Agar (14)

Heart infusion agar	40 g
Polymyxin B	30,000 units
Lysozyme	40 mg
Disodium ethylenediaminetetraacetate (EDTA)	300 mg
Thallous acetate	40 mg
Distilled water	1000 ml

Mix agar and water; autoclave at 121 C for 20 min. Cool to approximately 45 C and aseptically add appropriate amounts of stock solutions of remaining ingredients that have been sterilized by filtration. Mix thoroughly and dispense into sterile petri plates.

Determine the degree of selectivity by streaking the new batch of medium with cultures of both *B. anthracis* and *B. cereus* before the medium is used. *B. anthracis* should produce typical, macroscopic colonies within 48 hr at 37 C, but most strains of *B. cereus* should be inhibited markedly under the same conditions. Variations from these results should prompt checking on the potency of inhibitors before producing a new batch of this medium.

Employ a heavy inoculum and spread the entire surface of the medium. Incubate at 37 C for a least 48 hr. Examine colonies that grow on this selective medium after 24 and 48 hr, and subculture colonies with the morphology described for *B. anthracis* to 5% blood agar plates to determine the hemolytic reaction of the isolate. Note: Because this is an inhibitory medium, transfer only the growth from the uppermost portion of the colony to avoid secondary contamination of the subculture.

Serum-Glucose Agar (9), Modified

Basal medium:

Tryptose or Trypticase soy broth	5 g
Beef extract	3 g
Agar	15 g
Distilled water	1000 ml

Mix thoroughly and heat to dissolve agar. Autoclave at 121 C for 15 min. Cool to 50 C.

Serum glucose:

Horse or ox serum, free of brucella agglutinins	50 ml
Glucose	10 g

Dissolve glucose in serum which has been inactivated by heating at 56 C for 30 min. Filter sterilize. Store at 4 C.

Complete Medium:

Add 50 ml serum glucose to 1000 ml basal medium. Pour into petri plates.

Serum-Peptone Agar

Tryptose or Trypticase soy broth	5 g
Beef extract	3 g
Agar	15 g
Distilled water	1000 ml

Mix thoroughly and heat to dissolve agar. Autoclave at 121 C for 15 min. Cool to 50 C, and add 50 ml of inactivated agglutinin-free horse or ox serum. Pour into petri plates.

Snyder's Medium (20)

Peptone (Difco)	20 g
NaCl	10 g
Glucose	1 g
Distilled water	1000 ml

Mix thoroughly and dispense. Autoclave at 121 C for 15 min. This material can be used as solid medium by adding 2% agar.

Note: Peptones found satisfactory by the originators are Difco's peptone, proteose peptone #3, and tryptose. Tryptone and neopeptone were not satisfactory.

Starch Agar

Purple broth base (Difco)	16.0 g
Cornstarch	10.0 g
Agar	15.0 g
Distilled water	1000 ml

Mix thoroughly, and heat to boiling. Autoclave at 121 C for 15 min. Cool to 50 C, and pour 20–25 ml per plate.

Steadham Urea Broth

Peptone	1.0 g
Dextrose	1.0 g
NaCl	5.0 g
KH_2PO_4	0.4 g
Urea	20.0 g
Phenol red (sodium; 1% solution)	1.0 ml
Tween 80	0.1 ml
Distilled water	1000 ml

Final pH = 5.8

Sterilize by filtration through a membrane filter (0.22-μm pore size) and despense 1.5-ml quantities into 13 × 100 mm screw-capped tubes. Medium may be stored for up to 2 months without adversely affecting results of the test.

Stuart Leptospira Medium* (21)

25x Phosphate Buffer

Na_2HPO_4	16.6 g
KH_2PO_4	2.172 g

Dilute to 1 liter.

20x Salts Solution

```
NaCl..........................................................................................38.5 g
NH4Cl..........................................................................................5.35 g
MgCl2·6H2O..........................................................................................3.81 g
Asparagine..........................................................................................2.64 g
Thiamine hydrochloride..........................................................................................0.4 g
```

Dilute to 1 liter.

Medium

```
25× phosphate buffer..........................................................................................40 ml
20× salts solution..........................................................................................50 ml
Distilled water..........................................................................................910 ml
```

Mix thoroughly. Dispense in desired amounts in 20- × 125-mm screw-capped tubes, and autoclave at 121 C for 15 min. Allow to cool, and add 8% v/v sterile rabbit serum (0.8 ml serum to every 9.2 ml base).

Thayer-Martin Medium (16)

See *Chocolate Agar.*

Tinsdale Medium, Modified*

Base:

```
Proteose peptone #3..........................................................................................2.0 g
NaCl..........................................................................................0.5 g
Bacto-agar (Difco)..........................................................................................2.0 g
Distilled water..........................................................................................100 ml
```

Adjust to pH 7.4. Autoclave at 121 C for 15 min. Cool to 50 C.

Add enrichment:

```
Bovine serum..........................................................................................10 ml
1% (w/v) cysteine hydrochloride†..........................................................................................1.75 ml
1% (w/v) potassium tellurite†..........................................................................................3 ml
2.5% (w/v) sodium thiosulfate†..........................................................................................1.7 ml
```

Mix well, and pour 20 ml per plate. Allow surface of medium to dry before use. Store for no more than 7 days.

Transgrow (17)

See *Chocolate agar.*

Tryptose-Sulfite-Cycloserine Agar (TSC) (23)

```
Tryptose or Biosate..........................................................................................15.0 g
Phytone..........................................................................................5.0 g
```

---

†Prepare fresh solutions in sterile water; do not sterilize.

```
Yeast extract ...................................................................................................5.0 g
Sodium metabisulfite ...........................................................................1.0 g
Ferric ammonium citrate.......................................................................1.0 g
Agar....................................................................................................20.0 g
Distilled water.................................................................................1000 ml
```

Mix thoroughly to obtain uniform suspension, then adjust to pH 7.6. Dissolve and autoclave at 121 C for 10 min. Cool to 50 C. Add 40 ml of 1% filter-sterilized cycloserine. Pour into petri plates. Allow to dry for 24 hr before using.

Supplement: 80 ml of sterile 50% egg yolk emulsion can be added after the medium is autoclaved and cooled to 50 C.

Tetrathionate Broth

Basal medium:

```
Tetrathionate broth base...........................................................................4.6 g
Distilled water...................................................................................100 ml
```

Mix thoroughly, and heat to boiling. Continue to mix, and tube in 10 ml amounts. Cool to below 45 C.

Iodine solution:

```
Potassium iodide ....................................................................................5 g
Iodine ..................................................................................................6 g
Distilled water...................................................................................100 ml
```

Complete medium

Immediately before use, add 0.2 ml of iodine solution to 10 ml basal medium. Medium containing iodine must be used the day it is prepared.

Supplements

Brilliant green: Add 1 ml of 0.1% brilliant green per 100 ml cooled basal medium.

Urea Broth

```
Yeast extract (Difco)..........................................................................100 mg
Urea...................................................................................................20 g
Phenol red, 0.2%...................................................................................5 ml
Sorenson's phosphate buffer, M/15, pH 6.5 .............................................1000 ml
```

Mix and store at 4 C in a stoppered flask over approximately 1 ml of chloroform per 100 ml of medium. To use, aseptically dispense 1 ml into a sterile 13 × 100 mm tube.

Urea Semi-Solid Medium (4)

```
Thioglycollate without glucose or indicator (Difco 0432-01) .....................................9.6 g
Yeast extract (Difco) ............................................................................0.8 g
```

```
Distilled water...........................................................................................................400.0 ml
Urea broth (Difco) ......................................................................................15.5 g
Distilled water............................................................................................50.0 ml
```

Combine first three ingredients, dissolve by heating, autoclave at 121 C, and cool to about 60 C.

Mix the urea broth and water and sterilize by filtration. Combine both solutions aseptically and mix. This is the urea semi-solid medium. Dispense the medium aseptically in 7-ml quantities into 15- × 90-mm screwcapped tubes. Pass tubes with caps loose into an anaerobic glove box so that the atmosphere of approximately 85% N_2, 10% H_2, and 5% CO_2 replaces air in tubes. Tighten caps securely, and remove tubes from the glove box. Store the tubes of medium in a refrigerator at 4 C or at ambient temperature if necessary.

Vaginalis Agar (10)

```
Columbia Agar Base (BBL)..........................................................................42.5 g
Proteose peptone #3 (Difco) .....................................................................10.0 g
Distilled water............................................................................................1000 ml
```

Mix thoroughly, and heat to boiling. Autoclave at 121 C for 15 min. Cool to 50 C, and add 50 ml of sterile whole human blood preserved with citrate phosphate dextrose solution. Mix, and pour 20–25 ml per plate.

Xylose Lysine Desoxycholate Agar* (XLD) (22)

```
XL agar base................................................................................................45 g
Distilled water............................................................................................1000 ml
```

Mix thoroughly to dissolve ingredients completely. Autoclave at 121 C for 15 min. Cool to 50 C, and add 20 ml of a filter-sterilized solution containing 34% sodium thiosulphate, 4% ferric ammonium citrate, and 25 ml of a 10% filter-sterilized solution of sodium desoxycholate. Mix well, and adjust to pH 6.9. Pour into sterile petri plates.

Note: While this medium is commercially available as a complete medium with no need for supplementation, Taylor feels strongly that the heat-labile substances should be added to the sterilized, cooled base (personal communication).

General References

BLAZEVIC DJ and EDERER GM: Principles of Biochemical Tests in Diagnostic Microbiology. John Wiley and Sons, New York, 1975

FINEGOLD SM, MARTIN WJ, and SCOTT EG: Diagnostic Microbiology, 5th edition. The C.V. Mosby Co, St. Louis, 1978

HOLDEMAN LV, CATO EP, and MOORE WEC: Anaerobe Laboratory Manual 4th edition. VPI Anaerobe Laboratory, Blacksburg, Va, 1977

KONEMAN EW, ALLEN SD, DOWELL VR JR, and SOMMERS HM: Color Atlas and Textbook of Diagnostic Microbiology. J.B. Lippincott Co, Philadelphia, 1979

MacFADDIN JF: Biochemical Tests for Identification of Medical Bacteria. Williams and Wilkins Co, Baltimore, 1976

PARK G and SUGGS MT: Reagents, stains, and miscellaneous test procedures. *In* Manual of Clinical Microbiology, 2nd edition. Lennette EH, Spaulding EH, and Truant JP (eds.). American Society for Microbiology, Washington, DC, 1974

VERA HD and DUMOFF M: Culture media. *In* Manual of Clinical Microbiology, 2nd edition. Lennette EH, Spaulding EH, and Truant JP (eds.). American Society for Microbiology, Washington, DC, 1974

References

1. BLAZEVIC DJ and EDERER GM: Principles of Biochemical Tests in Diagnostic Microbiology. John Wiley and Sons, New York, 1975
2. BRETZ GB and FROBISHER M: Enrichment of Leoffler's Medium with Glycerol. CDC Bull. X, Number 5. Center for Disease Control, Atlanta, Ga, May 1951
3. CARY SG and BLAIR EB: New transport medium for shipment of clinical specimens. I. Fecal specimens. J Bacteriol 88:96–98, 1964
4. DOWELL VR JR, LOMBARD GL, THOMPSON FS, and ARMFIELD AY: Media for Isolation, Characterization, and Identification of Obligately Anaerobic Bacteria. Center for Disease Control, Atlanta, Ga, 1977
5. DUNKELBERG WD JR, SKAGGS R, and KELLOGG DS JR: Method for isolation and identification of *Corynebacterium vaginale (Haemophilus vaginalis)*. Appl Microbiol 19:47–52, 1970
6. ELLINGHAUSEN HC and MCCULLOUGH WG: Nutrition of *Leptospira pomona* and growth of 13 other serotypes: Fractionation of oleic albumin complex and a medium of bovine albumin and polysorbate 80. Am J Vet Res 26:45–51, 1965
7. ELLNER PD, STOESSEL CJ, DRAKEFORD E, and VASI F: A new culture medium for medical bacteriology. Am J Clin Pathol 45:502–504, 1966
8. FLETCHER W: Recent work on leptospirosis, tsutsugamushi disease, and tropical typhus in the Federated Malay States. Trans Roy Soc Trop Med Hyg 21:265–288, 1927-1928
9. FRANCIS E: Cultivation of *Bacterium tularense* on mediums new to this organism. Hyg Lab Bull #130:45–58, March 1922
10. GREENWOOD JR, PICKETT MJ, MARTIN WJ, and MACK EG: *Haemophilus vaginalis (Corynebacterium vaginale)*: Method for isolation and rapid biochemical identification. Health Lab Sci 14:102–106, 1977
11. HOLDEMAN LV and MOORE WEC (eds.): Anaerobe Laboratory Manual, 2nd edition. The Virginia Polytechnic Institute and State University Anaerobe Laboratory, Blacksburg, Virginia, 1972
12. JOHNSON RC and HARRIS VG: Differentiation of pathogenic and saprophytic leptospires. I. Growth at low temperatures. J Bacteriol 94:27–31, 1967
13. KELLY RT: Cultivation of *Borrelia hermsi*. Science 173:443–444, 1971
14. KNISELY RF: Selective medium for *Bacillus anthracis*. J Bacteriol 92:784–786, 1966
15. LENNETTE EH, SPAULDING EH, and TRUANT JP (eds.): Manual of Clinical Microbiology, 2nd edition. American Society for Microbiology, Washington DC, 1974
16. MARTIN JE JR, BILLINGS TE, HACKNEY JF, and THAYER JD: Primary isolation of *N. gonorrhoeae* with a new commercial medium. Public Health Reports 82:361–363, 1967
17. MARTIN JE JR and LESTER A: Transgrow, a medium for transport and growth of *Neisseria gonorrhoeae* and *Neisseria meningitidis*. HSMHA Health Reports 86:30, 1971
18. MCCLUNG LS and TOABE R: The egg yolk plate reaction for the presumptive diagnosis of *Clostridium sporogenes* and certain species of the gangrene and botulinum groups. J Bacteriol 53:139–147, 1947
19. NOGUCHI H and BATTISTINI TS: Etiology of oroya fever. I. Cultivation of *Bartonella baciliformis*. J Exp Med 43:851–864, 1926
20. SNYDER TL, PENFIELD RA, ENGLEY FBJR, and CREASY JC: Cultivation of *Bacterium tularense* in peptone media. Proc Soc Exp Biol Med 63:26–30, 1946

21. STUART RD: The preparation and use of a simple culture medium for leptospirae. J Pathol Bacteriol 58:343–349, 1946
22. TAYLOR WI: Isolation of shigellae. I. Xylose lysine agars; new media for isolation of enteric pathogens. Am J Clin Pathol 44:471–475, 1965
23. VERA HD and DUMOFF M: Culture media. *In* Manual of Clinical Microbiology, 2nd edition. Lennette EH, Spaulding EH, and Truant JP (eds.). American Society for Microbiology, Washington, DC, 1974

Part Four

INTRODUCTION

Libero Ajello, Ph.D.

More than ever the mycoses loom as disease agents of major public health concern. Over the years, in the absence of vaccines and other preventive measures, little has occurred to diminish the incidence and prevalence of actinomycotic and mycotic diseases in general (with the possible exception of dermatophyte infections in certain groups of the population). On the contrary, the increased longevity of the general population with a concomitant loss of resistance to infectious diseases, and the ever-broadening use of such compounds as antibiotics, steroids, and immunosuppressive drugs all have rendered patients susceptible to primary and secondary infections not only by the already well-known pathogenic fungi but by a whole series of moulds that had not been known to be pathogenic. Members of this latter group have come to be known as the opportunistic fungi.

An inkling of the magnitude of the burden exacted by the systemic actinomycetes and fungi is gained from the latest available data on mortality attributed to them. In 1976, 597 such deaths were recorded. These were caused by actinomycosis [11], aspergillosis [66], blastomycosis [2], candidiasis [244], coccidioidomycosis [66], cryptococcosis [123], histoplasmosis [49] and nocardiosis [36]. In addition 63 deaths were attributed to unspecified fungi (1).

An analysis of discharge records of 1875 hospitals participating in the Professional Activity Study of the Commission on Professional and Hospital Activities led to projected incidence rates of 23 cases of histoplasmosis per 1 million inhabitants to 0.2 per million for blastomycosis. Direct costs for hospitalization alone in 1976 stemming from actinomycosis, aspergillosis, blastomycosis, candidiasis, coccidioidomycosis, cryptococcosis, histoplasmosis, and sporotrichosis were estimated at $27,000,000 (2).

To reduce the suffering, mortality, and monetary losses caused by the actinomycetes and fungi, these infections need to be diagnosed promptly and correctly. The chapters in this section were prepared by recognized authorities in their fields to make these goals attainable by diagnostic laboratories. In them the authors present the most effective procedures for serological tests as well as those for isolating and identifying the etiologic agents.

1. CENTER FOR DISEASE CONTROL: Reported Morbidity and Mortality in the United States. Annual Summary, 1977. 26:1–80, 1978
2. FRASER DW, WARD JI, AJELLO L, and PLIKAYTIS BD: The growing problem of aspergillosis and other systemic mycoses. A national study. J Am Med Assoc (In press)

CHAPTER 47

COLLECTION AND ISOLATION OF HUMAN PATHOGENIC FUNGI

Ira F. Salkin

Introduction

Although fungi are ubiquitous in nature, fewer than 300 of the more than 100,000 species have been reported associated with infections in man. In this chapter are discussed the specialized procedures required in collecting and processing clinical specimens and in isolating and identifying zoopathogenic fungi (10, 19, 23, 31, 32, 47, 62, 80).

Collection of clinical specimens. Since fast-growing saprophytic fungi as well as zoopathogens are frequently found in clinical material, special precautions must be followed in collecting and handling such specimens to minimize contamination.

Direct observation of clinical specimens. Direct microscopic observation of clinical material, which is required in processing virtually all specimens, necessitates specific fungal stains and special techniques.

Primary isolation of fungal pathogens. Isolating and culturing the fungal agent generally require careful use of a number of simple and complex media, several containing particular antibiotics.

Identification procedures. Since taxonomic diagnosis of the zoopathogen is dependent on gross colony characteristics, microscopic morphology, and, to a limited degree, biochemical features, it also requires specific culturing procedures and/or diagnostic media.

Collection of Clinical Specimens

Aseptic techniques should be used in collecting clinical specimens from all patients with suspected mycotic infections. The area around the site of infection is usually contaminated with saprophytic fungi and bacteria, which frequently grow under the same cultural conditions as pathogenic fungi. Cultures inoculated with grossly contaminated specimens obtained with poor techniques will be overgrown by the contaminants, which will obscure the pathogen or suppress its development.

Whenever possible, sufficient material should be collected from the site for both direct microscopic observation and cultural studies. Swabs used to collect clinical specimens should be streaked over the surface of glass slides.

Superficial Mycoses and Dermatophytoses

In superficial mycoses and dermatophytoses, the surface of the affected area should first be scrubbed with cotton gauze moistened with 70% ethyl alcohol. If the skin lesions contain fissures or if the nails are cracked (so that alcohol may cause pain to the patient) surface contaminants can be largely removed by washing with sterile distilled water.

Since the lesions of pityriasis versicolor and hairs infected by certain species of *Microsporum* and *Trichophyton* fluoresce under a Wood's lamp (ultraviolet radiation at 3660 Å), this instrument can be extremely useful in selecting the sites from which specimens should be obtained. Specimens should not be collected from areas recently treated with topical antimycotic agents, where the fungi are no longer viable.

The periphery of the skin lesion is generally the site of active fungal development, whereas the center is the area of healing. The epidermal scales from these active borders should be collected with a sterile scalpel or the edge of a sterilized microscope slide. Alternatively, a small piece of plastic transparent tape can be pressed to the surface of the lesion to strip off the horny layer containing the fungus (41, 54). The tape can then be used for both direct microscopic examination and isolation procedures. The tops of newly formed vesicles can be clipped off and submitted to the laboratory.

Superficially infected hairs with nodules (white or black piedra) should be clipped off. Approximately 10–15 hairs will provide sufficient material for both microscopic and cultural studies. Hairs infected with dermatophytes should be plucked with forceps rather than clipped, since the basal area is most likely to contain the fungus. With such infections the hairs are generally loose in the follicles and can be easily removed without pain to the patient. Sterile combs or small sterile brushes (49) can be used instead of forceps to obtain hair from the scalp or from animal fur. If hairs are broken off close to the scalp, as in black dot lesions, clinical material can be recovered by scraping the area with a scalpel.

Scrapings from nails can be collected with a sterile scalpel. To avoid possible surface contamination, the initial scrapings should be discarded. If the patient has excessively thickened or split nails, and scraping might cause discomfort, the nails can be clipped and the clippings submitted to the laboratory.

Skin, hair, or nail specimens to be shipped to reference laboratories should be kept dry to inhibit the development of contaminating bacteria or saprophytic molds. Specimens can be submitted in clean paper envelopes; in clean, closed paper packets; in sterile, cotton-stoppered glass tubes; or sandwiched between surface-sterilized glass slides sealed at the edges with cellophane tape.

Specimens from subcutaneous lesions (sinus tracts, abscesses, ulcers, fistulas)

When possible, subcutaneous clinical material should be obtained by aspirating a closed lesion to minimize contamination. The specimen should be collected in a sterile, screw-capped tube. If only a small volume of material is obtained, a few drops of sterile broth can be used to keep it moist until it reaches the laboratory.

If the subcutaneous lesion is open, clinical material can be collected by curetting the sinus tract, abscess, ulcer, or fistula to obtain material from deep in the tract and tissue from the wall of the lesion. If cotton swabs are used, they should first be moistened with sterile water or saline; after use they should be sealed in a sterile screw-capped tube to prevent drying.

Sputum, bronchial, and gastric washings

Sputum should be collected after the patient's mouth is rinsed thoroughly and before or several hours after the patient has breakfasted to minimize the amount of food debris in the specimen. The specimen should contain sputum from the lungs, rather than salivary or nasopharyngeal secretions. Copious amounts of sputum should be collected in sterile, 1-oz (30-cc) or 4-oz (120-cc) widemouth screw-capped jars or 19- × 150-mm sterile screw-capped tubes. Since the specimen will probably be contaminated with bacteria and saprophytic fungi, repeated single fresh specimens conveyed immediately to the laboratory are preferable to 24-hr-old material.

Bronchial or gastric washings should also be sent immediately to the laboratory, either in the original vessels in which they were obtained or in sterile, screw-capped tubes or jars.

Blood and bone marrow specimens

For blood cultures, 10-ml samples of whole blood can be collected in sterile tubes containing anticoagulants. Alternatively, they can be inoculated directly at the patient's bedside onto a complex nutrient agar medium or into a nutrient broth (10 ml/50 ml of medium). For serologic studies, the same volume of blood is required, but no anticoagulants should be used.

As with blood specimens, a small quantity of bone marrow (approximately 0.3–0.5 ml) can either be cultured directly on an agar medium or transported immediately to the laboratory in a heparinized syringe.

Cerebrospinal, pleural, and pericardial fluid specimens

The largest practical volume (3–5 ml) of cerebrospinal fluid (CSF) should be collected in sterile, screw-capped tubes containing 0.01 g sodium citrate/5 ml of spinal fluid to prevent clotting. The same volume of CSF without anticoagulants should be submitted for serologic studies.

Pleural or pericardial fluid can be submitted in sterile, screw-capped tubes with or without sodium citrate.

Urine and fecal specimens

Urine can be collected either as a midstream clean catch or through a catheter, but the latter specimens should be carefully collected to avoid contamination from genitalia. The specimen can be submitted in sterile tubes or wide-mouthed, screw-capped jars. No preservatives should be used.

Normal or diarrheic fecal specimens should be collected in sterile screw-capped jars or wax-lined paper containers. Specimens obtained by an enema or those contaminated with urine are unsatisfactory for cultural studies.

Biopsy or autopsy tissue specimens

Tissue can be collected directly in a sterile, widemouthed, screw-capped jar or tube without formalin or other preservative. If the specimen cannot be sent to the laboratory immediately, it should be refrigerated, or a few drops of sterile saline or broth should be added to the tube to prevent desiccation. Alternatively, it can be collected between two pieces of sterile, moistened gauze and submitted in a petri dish or a sterile, widemouthed, screw-capped jar.

Specimens for mycotic keratitis (corneal ulcers)

Since the fungi associated with mycotic keratitis are usually found in the deep layers of the corneal structure, samples cannot be obtained simply by swabbing the affected region. They should be collected by scraping the bed and edges of the ulcer and should be shipped in two or three drops of sterile saline in sterile, screw-capped tubes.

Oral cavity specimens

Portions of plaque adhering to the oral mucosal lining (as in oral candidiasis or thrush) can be removed with a sterile swab or sterile tongue depressor. Since contamination by bacteria and saprophytes will be a serious problem, the specimen should be placed in a sterile tube and sent immediately to the laboratory. Because of these contamination problems, specimens from oral ulcers are best obtained in a surgical biopsy of the lesion.

Specimens from otomycosis (external ear)

For otomycoses, epithelial debris can be removed with sterile swabs, which are then inserted into sterile tubes for immediate transport to the laboratory.

Direct Observation of Clinical Specimens

The first step in processing virtually all clinical material should be direct microscopic examination of the specimen. Visible fungal structures may either indicate the etiologic agent or guide the laboratorian in selecting appropriate isolation media. If one can observe the location of the fungus in the specimen, portions most likely to yield the agent can then be inoculated onto media most likely to support the growth of the organism.

Skin, Nail, and Hair Specimens

A small portion of skin scrapings should be mounted in one or two drops of 10% KOH or NaOH on a glass slide and coverslip added. The preparation can be heated gently (not boiled) over a low flame and examined with reduced lighting under low and high powers of a compound microscope. The KOH or NaOH "clears" the material by breaking down host cells and proteinaceous debris and bleaching out pigments without seriously disrupting the morphologic features of the fungus. The fungus should be readily visible as a highly refractile body within the specimen. If initial observations are negative, the preparation should be reexamined 1 to 3 hr later when it is clearer.

Examination of skin specimens can be facilitated by staining the fungus with a mixture of 10% KOH and ink (Table 47.1). The fungus selectively takes up the ink stain, and the KOH clears the material. More intense staining is obtained by increasing the concentration of ink. Lactophenol cotton blue (LPCB; Table 47.1) can also be used.

The same procedures (mounting in KOH or KOH + ink and heating) can be used for direct observation of hairs or nail scrapings. However, these preparations generally require a day or more to clear. Chlorolactophenol (F. Blank, personal communication; Table 47.1) may be preferable to KOH as a mounting medium for hairs, as the former is less likely to disrupt the taxonomically critical arthrospore configuration. Fungi in nail scrapings, as in skin scrapings, are not localized, but dermatophytes in hairs are concentrated primarily in the basal areas.

With all specimens, hyphae must be differentiated from such artifacts as cotton or wool fibers and fat droplets. Although the "mosaic" or network of cholesterol crystals deposited around epidermal cells is very difficult to distinguish from hyphae, the former's lack of internal structure or of penetration through the epidermal cells and its crystalline composition differentiate it from hyphae.

Sputum, Pus, or Other Viscous Fluid Specimens

Sputum or pus can be processed like skin scrapings, i.e., mounted in one or two drops of 10% KOH (for a wet, unstained preparation) or 10% KOH + ink and examined under reduced light on a compound microscope. However, if the specimen is excessively viscous or the volume is quite large, mucolytic agents and concentration of the fungal cells may be required. Although KOH or NaOH are effective mucolytic additives, they so greatly reduce the viability of the fungi that the material cannot be used in direct isolation of the pathogen (4).

In contrast, Sandford et al. (71) reported that pancreatin effectively digests sputum and has no deleterious effect on fungi. Sputum or pus should be mixed with pancreatin, incubated at 37 C for 30 to 90 min or until liquefied, and centrifuged at 2500 rpm for 20 min. A portion of the sediment can be aseptically removed with a Pasteur pipette and examined microscopically.

Reep and Kaplan (60, 61) described a faster digestion and concentration procedure with N-acetyl-l-cysteine or dithiothreitol. The specimen is added to an equal volume of either mucolytic agent, mixed on a vortex mixer for 5 to 10 sec, and centrifuged at 950 rpm for 15 min. The supernatant is discarded, and a portion of sediment is aseptically removed for direct observation. Since neither agent seriously affects the viability of fungi, with the exception of *Paracoccidioides brasiliensis*, the same specimen can be used for isolation.

To facilitate visualization of the fungus within the specimen, a portion of the sediment can be mixed with LPCB or stained with the periodic acid-Schiff reagent (PAS, Table 47.1). However, the PAS technique is rather involved, requiring several different reagents and time-consuming steps. While it may be quite useful in demonstrating fungi in embedded tissue sections, it has only a limited value in direct microscopic observations of clinical specimens.

In testing for histoplasmosis, the best results are obtained by spreading a

TABLE 47.1—FUNGAL STAINS FOR DIRECT OBSERVATION

Acid-fast stain for Nocardia
   Heat fix slide.
   Flood slide for 3 min with Kinyoun carbolfuchsin (basic fuchsin, 4.0 g; liquefied phenol,
      8.0 ml; ethyl alcohol (95%), 20 ml; distilled water, 100 ml).
   Rinse with tap water.
   Decolorize for 2–5 sec with acid alcohol (3% concentrated hydrochloric acid in 95% ethyl
      alcohol).
   Wash in tap water.
   Counterstain for 1 min with methylene blue (0.1% methylene blue in 100 ml distilled water).
   Wash with tap water and blot dry.

Chlorolactophenol
   Chloral hydrate   2.0 g
   Lactic acid   1.0 g
   Phenol   1.0 g
   Distilled water   100.0 ml

Giemsa stain
   Fix slide in 100% methyl alcohol for 1–2 min.
   Air dry smear.
   Flood slide for 45 min with Giemsa stain (Fisher Scientific Co.).
   Wash with distilled water.
   Air dry smear.

Gram stain
   Heat-fix slide.
   Mix solutions of crystal violet (2 g in 20 ml of 95% ethyl alcohol) and ammonium oxalate
      (0.8 g in 80 ml distilled water), and flood slide for 1 min.
   Wash in tap water for 2 sec.
   Flood slide for 1 min with iodine solution (iodine, 1 g; potassium iodide, 2 g; distilled water,
      300 ml).
   Wash in tap water and blot dry.
   Decolorize for 30 sec with 95% ethyl alcohol.
   Blot dry.
   Counterstain for 10 sec with safranin solution (safranin O, 10 ml of a 2.5% solution in 95%
      ethyl alcohol; distilled water, 100 ml).
   Wash in tap water.
   Blot dry.

Lactophenol-cotton blue
   Phenol   20 g
   Lactic acid (85%)   20 g
   Glycerol   40 g
   Water   20 ml
   Cotton blue (C₄B Poirrier) 0.05 g

Potassium hydroxide + ink
   Potassium hydroxide (10%)   70 ml
   Glycerol   20 ml
   Parker Superquink permanent black ink 10 ml

Periodic acid-Schiff stain (80)
   Fix specimen on slide in absolute alcohol for 1 min.
   Flood slide for 5 min with 5% periodic acid.
   Wash in tap water for 2 min.
   Stain for 2 min in basic fuchsin (0.1% basic fuchsin in 95 ml distilled water + 5 ml of 95%
      ethyl alcohol).

TABLE 47.1—Continued

Wash in tap water.
Flood for 10 min in zinc hydrosulfite (1 g zinc hydrosulfite, 0.5 g tartaric acid, 100 ml distilled water).
Wash for 5 min in tap water.
Dehydrate, 2 min each, in 70%, 80%, 95%, and absolute ethyl alcohol.
Place in xylol for 2 min.
Mount.

portion of the concentrated specimen on a glass slide, fixing it with methyl alcohol for 10 min, and staining with the Giemsa procedure (Table 47.1) to observe the small, intracellular yeasts. For suspected actinomycete infections, the sediment can be air dried on a glass slide, heat fixed, and Gram stained (Table 47.1) to show the narrow, branching filaments of these bacteria. To detect *Nocardia* species, a portion can be acid-fast stained (Table 47.1) to reveal the characteristic partial acid-fast nature of these actinomycetes.

Sputum or pus may contain the typical "sulfur granules" of *Actinomyces* species. These can be collected by spreading a portion of the specimen on a glass slide and examining for the yellow-white, firm clumps up to 2.5 mm in diameter. A single granule can then be dissected away, placed in a drop of water, crushed under a cover-slip, and examined directly or Gram stained.

Cerebrospinal Fluid Specimens

Body fluids such as CSF usually contain low concentrations of fungal elements. Thus, as is true with sputum specimens, the first step in processing such material is to concentrate the fungal cells by gentle centrifugation at 2500 rpm for 20 min. A portion of the sediment can then be aseptically removed with a sterile Pasteur pipette for direct microscopic observation.

In testing for cryptococcosis, the sediment can be mixed with a drop of India ink or any colored colloidal medium to obtain contrast for the encapsulated cells of *Cryptococcus neoformans*. However, India ink frequently contains artifacts and even microorganisms which may interfere with the examination. In addition, lymphocytes or erythrocytes can be confused with *C. neoformans*, as they may appear to be surrounded by a slight "halo" or "capsule." One must examine the material carefully to observe the cell wall of the yeast within the capsule, which distinguishes it from human cells.

An India ink preparation of CSF can also be used in testing for other zoopathogenic agents associated with central nervous system infections. Alternatively, a portion of CSF sediment can be PAS stained. In cases of possible actinomycete infections the CSF should be air dried, heat fixed, and Gram stained. If actinomycetes are present, a portion should be acid-fast stained to differentiate *Nocardia* species.

Body Fluid Specimens

Specimens of body fluids can be examined directly as wet, unstained preparations or can be stained with LPCB. Alternatively, as with sputum or

CSF, specimens can be concentrated by centrifugation at 2500 rpm for 20 min and examined directly as unstained preparations or with LPCB, Gram, PAS, Giemsa, or other stains.

Fecal Specimens

A fecal specimen can be stained with LPCB or mixed with one or two drops of sterile water and examined on a glass slide as a wet, unstained preparation.

Blood and Bone Marrow Specimens

A few drops of bone or blood marrow specimen should be streaked on a glass slide, air dried, heat fixed, and Gram stained or fixed with methyl alcohol and stained according to the Giemsa procedure.

Tissue Specimens

Tissue from a subcutaneous lesion or biopsy specimen should be placed in a sterile petri dish and cut into small fragments with sterile scissors and forceps. One small piece is then pressed firmly on a glass slide to create an impression film, which is treated with LPCB, Gram, acid-fast, or PAS stain. As an alternative, tissue fragments can be placed in a homogenizer, and a portion of the resulting homogenate can be added to 10% KOH or 10% KOH + ink or stained (as described above) for microscopic observation. Since grinding with a mortar and pestle may create a potentially hazardous aerosol, tissue specimens should not be processed in this manner.

Specimens on Swabs

Swabs used to collect clinical specimens should be streaked on the surface of glass slides. If swabs are dry when received, they should be moistened with a few drops of sterile broth. The slides are then treated with LPCB, Gram, or other stains.

Primary Isolation of Fungal Pathogens

All clinical specimens should be cultured for fungi regardless of whether fungal elements are observed in them in direct examination. The material should be freshly collected and processed promptly to minimize contamination with fast-growing bacteria and saprobes and to ensure the viability of the zoopathogenic agent.

At Laboratories for Mycology and Mycobacteriology, New York State Department of Health, we use cotton-stoppered, 19- × 150-mm glass culture tubes containing 5–7 ml of nutrient agar. To expose the maximum surface area of the medium to the fungus in the specimen, the tubes are slanted so that the agar will solidify in a gentle slope. Cotton stoppers permit a greater exchange of gases and water vapor with the external environment than do screw-capped tubes. This limitation curbs the development in the culture tube of microaerophilic-anaerobic conditions or drastic alterations in the relative humidity, which can have pronounced effects upon the gross colony morphology and microscopic characteristics of fungi (13, 81). Cotton stoppers cause less aberration in these critical taxonomic features than do screw caps. If screw-capped tubes must be used, the caps should be loosely applied.

The probability of isolating the fungal agent is enhanced by streaking the specimen over a large area (as on a petri dish) to separate the pathogen from possible contaminants. Plastic petri dishes (10 cm) containing 15–20 ml of medium can be used with fluids, swabs, and tissue specimens.

However, these containers should be used cautiously, since they can create potentially hazardous conditions. For example, if *Coccidioides immitis* or *Histoplasma capsulatum* were present, the aerosol of spores created simply by opening the dish to identify the fungus or in handling the plates could present serious health hazards for laboratory personnel. In addition, the enormous quantities of spores formed by common saprophytic contaminants when grown as macrocolonies in petri dishes could lead to contamination of other clinical isolates and laboratory equipment.

Primary isolations can be made on a number of nutrient media (Table 47.2). Because no single medium supports the optimal growth of all zoopathogenic fungi, most clinical specimens should be inoculated onto two or more media to increase the probability of isolating the fungal agent.

Virtually all primary cultures should be incubated at 25–30 C. It is sometimes helpful to incubate additional cultures at 37 C, but this temperature is not optimal for many zoopathogens, and it may inhibit the growth of some—including almost all dermatophytes.

Because zoopathogenic fungi are exceptionally slow-growing organisms, primary cultures should be held at least 2 weeks and preferably 4 weeks or longer before being discarded as negative. A frequent error in many laboratories is discarding a culture once a common pathogen such as *Candida albicans* has been isolated. Cutures should be held the full 2 weeks or longer to permit the isolation of less frequently encountered or slower-growing agents.

Common Isolation Media

Sabouraud dextrose agar (SDA) medium

SDA was originally devised by Raimond Saboraud (62) to culture dermatophytes. Although it does not support optimal development or sporulation, it is the most frequently used medium, since the taxonomic descriptions of most pathogens are based upon their morphology in such cultures. Better growth and sporulation can be achieved by reducing the dextrose concentration in SDA and adjusting the pH to around neutrality (modified Sabouraud dextrose agar or MSDA) (23). Bacterial contamination can be controlled by adding penicillin, streptomycin, or other antibacterial agents to either SDA or MSDA (SDA+, MSDA+). On occasion Sabouraud dextrose broth (SD Br) can be used for primary isolation.

Cycloheximide-chloramphenicol medium

Although Whiffen (83, 84) reported considerable variation in the sensitivity of fungi to cycloheximide, zoopathogens consistently grew at higher con-

TABLE 47.2—NUTRIENT MEDIA FOR PRIMARY ISOLATION

*Blood agar**		
Heart infusion agar (Difco) or blood agar base (BBL)	40	g
Horse blood	52	ml
Distilled water	1000	ml
*Brain-heart-infusion agar**		
Brain-heart-infusion agar (Difco or BBL)	52	g
Distilled water	1000	ml
Cycloheximide-chloramphenicol agar		
Dextrose	20	g
Soytone (Mycobiotic Agar, Difco) or Phytone (Mycosel, BBL)	10	g
Agar	20	g
Chloramphenicol (Chloromycetin, Parke, Davis, and Co.)	40	mg
Cycloheximide (Actidione, Upjohn and Co.)	500	mg
Distilled water	1000	ml
*Cystine heart-hemoglobin agar**		
Cystine heart agar (Difco or BBL)	10.2	g
Hemoglobin (Difco or BBL)	2.0	g
Distilled water	200.0	ml
Dermatophyte test medium (Schering Corp.)		
Phytone (BBL)	10	g
Dextrose	10	g
Phenol red solution (0.5 g in 15 ml 0.1 N NaOH made up to 100 ml with distilled water)	40	ml
Cycloheximide (Actidione, Upjohn and Co.)	500	mg
Gentamicin sulfate (Schering Corp.)	100	mg
Chlortetracycline HCl (American Cyanamid)	100	mg
HCl (0.8 N)	6	ml
Agar	20	g
Distilled water	1000	ml
*Sabouraud's dextrose agar**		
Dextrose	40	g
Neopeptone (Difco) or polypeptone (BBL)	10	g
Agar	20	g
Distilled water	1000	ml
*Modified Sabouraud's dextrose agar (Difco) or SDA Emmons (BBL)**		
Dextrose	20	g
Neopeptone (Difco) or polypeptone (BBL)	10	g
Agar	20	g
Distilled water	1000	ml
Sabouraud's dextrose broth		
Dextrose	40	g
Neopeptone (Difco) or polypeptone (BBL)	10	g
Distilled water	1000	ml

* Can be prepared with 20 units of penicillin and 40 units of streptomycin per ml.

centrations of the drug than did phytopathogens or saprophytes. This response led to cycloheximide being incorporated into MSDA to suppress contamination by saprophytes (25, 26).

Rosenthal and Furnari (65) and McDonough (51) reported that this

MSDA + cycloheximide medium fortified with the antibacterial agent chloramphenicol is extremely useful for isolating dermatophytes and dimorphic pathogens. This formulation is produced commercially under the trade names Mycosel (BBL) and Mycobiotic agar (Difco).

However, it should be used carefully, as the response to cycloheximide is dependent upon the species and strain of microorganism, the duration of exposure, and the organism's ability to acquire resistance to the drug (67, 70). Several zoopathogens, in particular *Cryptococcus neoformans*, are sensitive to cycloheximide at the concentrations used in Mycosel and Mycobiotic agars. Obviously, neither should be used for primary isolation of these zoopathogens.

In contrast, the initial development of saprophytes such as *Cladosporium* sp. may be inhibited by cycloheximide, but they may develop after only a short incubation and interfere with the isolation of zoopathogens.

Dermatophyte test medium (DTM)

Dermatophyte test medium was developed by Taplin et al. (78) so that relatively untrained technicians could isolate and identify dermatophytes. It contains cycloheximide to suppress fungal contaminants, chlortetracycline and gentamicin to inhibit bacterial growth, and the pH indicator phenol red to differentiate dermatophytes. Taplin and co-workers acknowledged that the medium is not absolutely specific for dermatophytes, as it allows several saprophytic fungi to grow and induce a color change.

Our studies (66) and others (37) indicate that such nondermatophytic pathogens as *H. capsulatum* and *Blastomyces dermatitidis* also cause color conversion of DTM. Since these systemic pathogens may be associated with cutaneous lesions and have a gross appearance on DTM similar to that of dermatophytes, there is a very real possibility of misidentifying the organism(s). DTM should be used only with these limitations in mind.

Rich organic media

Cysteine heart agar + hemoglobin (CHHA), brain-heart infusion (BHI) agar or broth, blood agar (BA), and Sabhi (15, 29) provide extremely rich sources of nutrients for zoopathogens. These media, fortified with antibacterial agents, are useful for isolating pathogens such as *C. neoformans* and *H. capsulatum*, which can be difficult to isolate on standard media. These rich media without antibiotics are the principal means of isolating the pathogenic actinomycetes.

Primary Isolation Procedures

Once the specimen has been initially processed and examined microscopically, the material can be cultured as follows:

Skin, nail, and hair specimens

Skin, nail, and hair specimens are inoculated onto two or more tubes of either Mycobiotic or Mycosel agar and on one tube of SDA+ or MSDA+ (with the material slightly embedded in the agar) and incubated at 27 C. Since dermatophytic infections are generally associated with such specimens, Mycosel or Mycobiotic agar is used to suppress contaminating saprophytes. Two or more tubes are used because dermatophytes are sometimes difficult to isolate. Since other zoopathogens which may be sensitive to cycloheximide can be associated with cutaneous lesions, SDA + or MSDA+ is also used.

Malassezia furfur, the causative agent of pityriasis versicolor, is lipophilic (27, 28), and exogenous fatty acids must be supplied to culture it from skin scrapings. The scales are embedded in Mycosel or SDA+ slants; one or two drops of sterile olive oil are added with an asepto pipette, and the oil is spread over the agar surface with a transfer loop. The tubes are inclined at an angle to maintain the overlay of oil and incubated at 37 C.

Body fluid specimens

Sputum, pus, and other liquid specimens should be streaked over the surface of CHHA+ or BA+ plates and incubated at 27 C and 37 C. In addition, portions of material should be incubated on SDA and SDA+ tubes at 27 C. Finally, if an actinomycete infection is suspected or if branching bacterial filaments are observed on direct examination, the material can be streaked over BA or BHI plates and incubated aerobically and anaerobically (Gas-Pak, BBL) at 37 C.

Paraffin baiting has been described (43, 55, 56) as an alternative method for isolating *Nocardia*. A 2-ml portion of the specimen is mixed with 5 ml of a sterile carbon-free broth in a sterile culture tube. A paraffin-coated sterile glass rod is then added to each tube, and the system is incubated at 37 C. *Nocardia* grows in tufts on the paraffin bait.

Rippon (62) suggested that BA, although it permits bacterial and fungal contamination, is the medium of choice for isolating *H. capsulatum*. However, Smith and Goodman (74) found yeast extract-phosphate medium with concentrated ammonium hydroxide added to the surface (73) superior for selective isolation of *H. capsulatum* or *B. dermatitidis*.

The specimen is streaked over the surface of the yeast extract-phosphate medium in a plastic petri dish. One drop of concentrated ammonium hydroxide is immediately added to the surface and allowed to diffuse (not streaked) throughout the medium. The ammonium hydroxide inhibits most bacteria and yeasts and, to a lesser degree, saprophytic molds—facilitating the isolation of the resistant *H. capsulatum* and *B. dermatitidis*.

Petri dishes are advantageous with these fluid specimens because the material can be streaked over a large surface area to separate the pathogens from possible contaminants. Several different nutrient media are used to increase the probability of providing the optimal combination of nutrients for the pathogens. Since several pathogens found in fluids, e.g., *Aspergillus fumigatus* and *Actinomyces* spp., grow optimally at 37 C, and since this temperature restricts the growth of many contaminants, specimens are incubated at both 27 C and 37 C.

Cerebrospinal fluid specimens

The concentrated sediment of CSF is streaked onto CHHA+ or BA+ plates and incubated at 27 C and 37 C. Additional material is incubated on BHI agar tubes (or in BHI broth) and on SDA tubes at 37 C and on SDA+

and SD Br tubes at 27 C. As with sputum, pus, etc., the use of petri plates, several different media, and two different incubation temperatures raises the probability of isolating not only the fungal agent but also a wider range of zoopathogens associated with infections of the central nervous system.

Tissue specimens

Small pieces of tissue can be streaked with a forceps over the surface, slightly embedded into CHHA+ and BA+ in petri dishes, and incubated at 27 C and 37 C. Other portions should be incubated on SDA+ and SDA tubes at 27 C. Similar techniques can be used with tissue homogenates.

Swabs

Dry swabs received in the laboratory should be moistened by being immersed briefly in an SD Br tube. The moistened swabs are then streaked over the surface of a CHHA+ or BA+ plate and SDA+ tube and, together with the SD Br tube, incubated at 27 C.

Cultures

All yeast and mold cultures received in our reference laboratory for identification are routinely inoculated onto one tube of SDA+ or MSDA+ and one tube of Mycosel or Mycobiotic agar and incubated at 27 C. This set of media provides the best opportunity for any pathogens to grow and to display their characteristic gross and microscopic morphology.

Identification Procedures

The characteristics of and techniques used in taxonomic diagnosis of zoopathogenic fungi and actinomycetes are summarized below. Detailed methods of identification will be described in later chapters.

General Morphologic Characteristics

Identification of fungi is based primarily upon morphologic criteria, the first of which is the nature of the vegetative body, i.e., the structure formed as the organism grows. From the morphology of the body the fungi can be divided into three groups: (i) molds, i.e., fungi whose vegetative bodies are composed of interwoven filaments (hyphae) which form a mat (mycelium); (ii) yeasts or yeastlike forms, i.e., fungi whose vegetative bodies generally consist of a single, oval cell at 25 C; and (iii) dimorphics, i.e., fungi whose vegetative forms are environmentally mutable, being either mold or yeastlike under different specific environmental conditions.

A second critical characteristic is the spores formed through asexual reproduction. In this type of reproduction, as distinct from the union of two nuclei, propagating units are formed by mitotic nuclear division. Spores can be formed by the simple fragmentation of hyphae (arthrospores), by the splitting of one cell into two daughter cells (fission spores), and by the formation of an outgrowth from the parent cell (buds).

In addition, spores can develop by specialized mechanisms, either in a mass within a case on an aerial hypha (the sporangiospores within the sporangium on a sporangiophore), or singly or in relatively small numbers without a case at the tips or sides of specific hyphae (i.e., conidia on conidiophores).

The mechanism by which the spores are formed; their color, size, and shape; the presence or absence of septation, etc., are all important taxonomic characteristics. The asexual spores are often found in specialized protective structures, or "fruiting bodies," such as the pycnidium or hollow flask-shaped case formed by *Phoma*. In such instances the shape, color, size, etc., of the fruiting body are additional points of differentiation.

A third characteristic is the spores formed by sexual reproduction, i.e., by the union of two nuclei and the consequent formation of propagating units by meiotic nuclear division. In medically important fungi, these sexually formed spores may be simple, single, thick-walled structures situated on specialized hyphae (zygospores); housed in multiples of two, but usually eight, in a sac (ascospores within an ascus); or situated in groups of four on the surface of a club-shaped structure (the basidiospores on a basidium). Again, the size, shape, color, and septation of the spores, as well as of the fruiting structures which contain them, are useful in the taxonomic diagnosis of a few fungi.

General Characteristics for Identifying Yeasts

A combination of cultural and biochemical characteristics is used to identify yeasts. The ability of the yeast isolate to form hyphae or pseudohyphae, blastospores, and chlamydospores can be assessed by culture on Cornmeal + Tween 80, Cream of Rice (79), or Wolin-Bevis medium (87), as the technician prefers. This procedure is useful, for example, in differentiating *Torulopsis* and *Cryptococcus* from *Trichosporon* and *Candida*. The morphology of these structures is an important factor in distinguishing among the species of *Candida*.

A second cultural characteristic is germ-tube formation. Culturing isolates in normal human serum or glucose-beef-extract broth or on TOC and other solid media (9, 24, 30, 38, 88) is a quick, although not foolproof, means of differentiating *Candida albicans* and *C. stellatoidea* from other pathogenic yeasts.

Urease production by certain yeasts is a critical biochemical character, which can be assessed by the use of Christensen's agar (18) or urea broth (63).

A characteristic unique to *Cryptococcus neoformans* is the formation of a brown pigment on media containing *Guizotia abyssinica* seed extract or various diphenols. A number of media have been described (16, 17, 24, 33–35, 57, 58, 68, 72, 75, 77) to evaluate this character.

A biochemical procedure which has long been employed to provide definitive data for identification of yeasts is the carbohydrate assimilation test. The ability of a yeast to assimilate or utilize a particular carbohydrate as the sole carbon source in a chemically defined medium can be determined by either the auxanographic or broth technique. In the former, a dry carbohydrate in a paper disk is placed on a synthetic medium, with (44, 46, 59, 82) or without (52) a pH indicator, which has been heavily seeded with yeast suspension.

Growth of the yeast in the region adjacent to the disk (and color conversion of the pH indicator) indicates assimilation of the carbohydrate. A kit which provides the nutrient agar medium and carbohydrate-impregnated disks (Mini-tek) is available from BBL (Cockeysville, Md.).

In the broth procedure, the carbohydrate is incorporated into a defined nutrient broth, which is then inoculated with a yeast suspension (85, 86). Turbidity after 14–21 days indicates growth of the yeast and assimilation of the sugar. A modification of the Wickerham procedure in which the carbohydrate is incorporated into a nutrient agar base with a pH indicator can also be employed (1, 50, 59).

Disk or broth techniques can be used to determine the yeast's ability to assimilate KNO_3 as the sole nitrogen source within a defined medium. This same physiologic character can be assessed by the use of specially impregnated swabs (36).

The carbohydrate fermentation test provides additional biochemical data. Fermentation appears as acidification of the defined nutrient broth and formation of CO_2 bubbles within a Durham tube inserted in the broth medium (85).

Finally, several kits are commercially available (API 20 C from Analytab Products, Inc., Plainview, N.Y.; Micro-Drop from Clinical Sciences, Inc., Whippany, N.Y.; Randolph Mt-M or Mt-Y from Randolph Biologicals, Houston, Tex.; and Uni-Yeast-Tek from Flow Laboratories, Roslyn, N.Y.) for identification of unknown yeast isolates by a combination of morphologic and physiologic characters. Although the kits identify only a limited number of yeasts, recent reports (11, 12, 20, 45, 53, 64) indicate that they are useful for diagnosis of medically important species.

Identifying Molds

Gross colony and microscopic morphology are the primary characteristics which identify pathogenic molds. The most important factor is the asexual spores, whose arrangement is best observed in a slide culture. For this purpose a block of appropriate nutrient medium, approximately 1–2 cm on each side and 2- to 3-mm deep, is aseptically placed onto a sterile glass slide. The slide is placed on a bent glass rod in a sterile petri dish, and the upper edge of each side of the agar block is inoculated with the unknown mold. The block is then covered with a sterile cover slip, and sterile water is added to the petri dish to maintain moist conditions. The slide is removed at intervals and observed directly under the compound microscope.

Formation and/or evaluation of the salient features of asexual spores may require specific media. Czapek's medium is used for all *Aspergillus* spp., since the standard morphologic descriptions are based upon their appearance on this medium. Cornmeal and Czapek's agar are the best for dematiaceous molds. Malt agar and potato dextrose medium induce sporulation in a wide variety of molds. There are also several limited-function media which can be employed to identify a single genus or species or a small, select group of molds. For example, Aspergillus Differential Medium (69) is used to distinguish members of the *Aspergillus flavus* group from other *Aspergillus* species which may be associated with human infections, and Staib's (76) serum-albumin medium is used to identify and differentiate *Trichophyton rubrum*.

Spores formed through sexual reproduction are rarely used in identifying pathogenic fungi. The morphologic features of these structures and the methods used to observe them are considered in the chapters on specific mycoses.

As an alternative to the use of morphologic criteria or as an additional factor in the identification of several systemic fungal pathogens, one can employ immunologic methods (39). Exoantigens formed by the organism in culture can be tested with reference antisera in microimmunodiffusion tests.

Identifying Dimorphics

For identification of dimorphic pathogens, it is essential to obtain both the mold and yeast phases. While the former is relatively easy to obtain with standard methods and media at 25 C, the latter requires specialized media. Molds can generally be converted to yeasts on Kurung medium at 37 C (42). Campbell's (14), Kelley's (40), and CHHA media also provide an excellent nutrient base for inducing the "*in vivo*" yeast stage of these pathogens.

Identifying Actinomycetes

Although similar to fungi in that they form a branched filamentous network, actinomycetes are true bacteria. However, by historical precedent *Actinomyces* and *Nocardia* have been studied along with pathogenic fungi. They can be differentiated from fungi by their relatively small size (filaments are usually less than 1 μm in diameter). They grow best on rich organic nutrient sources without antibiotics, such as BHI, BA, or CHHA medium at 37 C. *Actinomyces* species are facultatively or obligately anaerobic and should be cultured under a high CO_2 environment in a Gas-Pak (BBL) jar.

These two genera can be differentiated from other bacteria and from each other by their appearance in Gram- and acid-fast-stained preparations, by colony morphology, and by responses in such biochemical tests as those for catalase production, carbohydrate fermentation, and casein-tyrosine-xanthine hydrolysis. However, the biochemical tests are numerous, and the morphologic features are variable and require experience for correct interpretation.

General Manuals for Identification

Several manuals or keys which are commonly used to identify pathogenic fungi are listed in the References (2, 3, 5–8, 21, 22, 48).

References

1. ADAMS ED JR and COOPER BH: Evaluation of a modified Wickerham medium for identifying medically important yeasts. Am J Med Technol 40:377–388, 1974
2. AINSWORTH GC, SPARROW FK, and SUSSMAN AS: The Fungi, an Advanced Treatise, Volume IVA. Academic Press, New York, 1973
3. AINSWORTH GC, SPARROW FK, and SUSSMAN AS: The Fungi, an Advanced Treatise, Volume IVB. Academic Press, New York, 1973
4. AJELLO L, GRANT VQ, and GUTSKE MA: The effect of tubercule bacillus concentration procedures on fungi causing pulmonary mycoses. J Lab Clin Med 38:486–491, 1951
5. ARX JA VON: The Genera of Fungi Sporulating in Pure Culture. J Cramer, Vanduz, Germany, 1974
6. BARNETT JA and BANKJURST RJ: A New Key to the Yeasts. North-Holland Publishing Co, Amsterdam, The Netherlands, 1974

7. BARNETT HL and HUNTER BB: Illustrated Genera of Imperfect Fungi, 3rd edition. Burgess Publishing Co, Minneapolis, 1972
8. BARRON GL: The Genera of Hyphomycetes from Soil. Williams and Wilkins Co, Baltimore, 1968
9. BEHESTI F, SMITH AG, and KRAUSE GW: Germ tube and chlamydospore formation by *Candida albicans* on a new medium. J Clin Microbiol 2:345–348, 1975
10. BODILY HL, UPDYKE EL, and MASON JO (eds.): Diagnostic Procedures for Bacterial, Mycotic, and Parasitic Infections, 5th edition. American Public Health Association, Inc, New York, 1970
11. BOWMAN P and AHEARN DG: The evaluation of commercial systems for the identification of clinical yeast isolates. J Clin Microbiol 4:49–53, 1976
12. BUESCHING WJ, KUREK K, and ROBERTS GD: Evaluation of the modified API 20C system for identification of clinically important yeasts. J Clin Microbiol 9:565–569, 1979
13. BURNETT JH: Fundamentals of Mycology. St Martin's Press, New York, 1968
14. CAMPBELL CC: Reverting *Histoplasma capsulatum* to the yeast phase. J Bacteriol 54:263–264, 1947
15. CAPLAN DM and MERZ WG: Evaluation of two commercially prepared biphasic media for recovery of fungi from blood. J Clin Microbiol 8:469–470, 1978
16. CHASKES S and TYNDALL RL: Pigment production by *Cryptococcus neoformans* from para- and ortho-diphenols: effect of the nitrogen source. J Clin Microbiol 1:509–514, 1975
17. CHASKES S and TYNDALL RL: Pigment production by *Cryptococcus neoformans* and other *Cryptococcus* species from aminophenols and diaminobenzenes. J Clin Microbiol 7:146–152, 1978
18. CHRISTENSEN WB: Urea decomposition as a means of differentiating *Proteus* and paracolon cultures from each other and from *Salmonella* and *Schigella* types. J Bacteriol 52:461, 1946
19. CONANT NF, SMITH DT, BAKER RD, and CALLAWAY JL: Manual of Clinical Mycology, 3rd edition. W.B. Saunders Co, Philadelphia, 1971
20. COOPER BH, JOHNSON JB, and THAXTON ES: Clinical evaluation of the Uni-Yeast-Tek system for rapid presumptive identification of medically important yeasts. J Clin Microbiol 7:349–355, 1978
21. ELLIS MB: Dematiaceous Hyphomycetes. Commonwealth Mycological Institute, Kew, England, 1968
22. ELLIS MB: More Dematiaceous Hyphomycetes. Commonwealth Mycological Institute, Kew, England, 1976
23. EMMONS CW, BINFORD CH, UTZ JP, and KWON-CHUNG KJ: Medical Mycology, 3rd edition. Lea and Febiger, Philadelphia, 1977
24. FLEMING WH III, HOPKINS JB, and LAND GA: New culture medium for the presumptive identification of *Candida albicans* and *Cryptococcus neoformans.* J Clin Microbiol 5:236–243, 1977
25. FUENTES CA, TRESPALACIOS F, BAQUERO GF, and ABOULAFIA R: Effect of actidione on mold contaminants and on human pathogens. Mycologia 54:170–175, 1952
26. GEORG LK, AJELLO L, and GORDON MA: A selective medium for the isolation of *Coccidioides immitis.* Science 114:387–389, 1951
27. GORDON MA: The lipophilic mycoflora of the skin. I. *In vitro* culture of *Pityrosporum orbiculare* n. sp. Mycologia 43:524–535, 1951
28. GORDON MA: Lipophilic yeastlike organisms associated with tinea versicolor. J Invest Dermatol 17:267–272, 1951
29. GORMAN JW: Sabhi, a new culture medium for pathogenic fungi. Am J Med Technol 33:151–157, 1967
30. GRIFFIN ER: The value of germ tube production test in rapid identification of *Candida albicans.* J Med Lab Technol 21:298–301, 1964
31. HALEY LD and CALLAWAY CS: Laboratory Methods in Medical Mycology, 4th edition. U.S. Government Printing Office, Washington, D.C., 1978
32. HAZEN EL, GORDON MA, and REED FC: Laboratory Identification of Pathogenic Fungi Simplified, 3rd edition. Charles C. Thomas Co, Springfield, Ill, 1970
33. HEALY ME, DILLAVOUS CL, and TAYLOR GE: Diagnostic medium containing inositol, urea, and caffeic acid for selective growth of *Cryptococcus neoformans.* J Clin Microbiol 6:387–391, 1977

34. HOPFER RL and BLANK F: Caffeic acid-containing medium for identification of *Cryptococcus neoformans*. J Clin Microbiol 2:115–120, 1975
35. HOPFER RL and GROSCHEL D: Six-hour pigmentation test for the identification of *Cryptococcus neoformans*. J Clin Microbiol 2:96–98, 1975
36. HOPKINS JM and LAND GA: Rapid method for determining nitrate utilization by yeasts. J Clin Microbiol 5:497–500, 1977
37. JACOBS PH and RUSSELL B: Dermatophyte test medium for systemic fungi. J Am Med Assoc 224:1649, 1973
38. JOSHI KR, GAVIN JB, and BREMMER DA: The formation of germ tubes by *Candida albicans* in various peptone media. Sabouraudia 11:259–262, 1973
39. KAUFMAN L and STANDARD P: Immuno-identification of cultures of fungi pathogenic to man. Curr Microbiol 1:135–140, 1978
40. KELLEY WH: A study of the cell and colony variations of *Blastomyces dermatitidis*. J Infect Dis 64:293–296, 1939
41. KNUDSEN EA: Fungal cultures from skin strippings. Sabouraudia 9:167–168, 1971
42. KURUNG JM and YEGIAN D: Medium for maintenance and conversion of *Histoplasma capsulatum* to yeastlike phase. Am J Clin Pathol 24:505–508, 1954
43. KURUP PV, RANDHAWA HS, and MISHRA SK: Use of paraffin bait technique in the isolation of *Nocardia asteroides* from sputum. Mycopathol Mycol Appl 51:363–367, 1970
44. LAND GA, DORN GL, FLEMING WG III, BEADLES TA, and FOXWORTH JH: Isolation and rapid identification of yeasts from compromised hosts. Mycopathology 65:123–131, 1978
45. LAND GA, HARRISON BA, HULME KL, COOPER BH, and BYRD JC: Evaluation of the new API 20C strip for yeast identification against a conventional method. J Clin Microbiol 10:357–364, 1979
46. LAND GAE, VINTON EC, ADCOCK GB, and HOPKINS JM: Improved auxanographic-methods of yeast assimilations: comparison with other approaches. J Clin Microbiol 2:206–217, 1975
47. LENNETTE EH, SPAULDING EH, and TRUANT JP (eds.): Manual of Clinical Microbiology, 2nd edition. American Society for Microbiology, Washington, DC, 1974
48. LODDER J: The Yeasts. A Taxonomic Study, 2nd edition. North-Holland Publishing Co, Amsterdam, The Netherlands, 1970
49. MACKENZIE DWR: "Hairbrush diagnosis" in detection and eradication of nonfluorescent scalp ringworm. Br Med J 2:363–365, 1963
50. MARTIN MV and SCHNEIDAU JD JR: A simple and reliable assimilation test for the identification of *Candida* species. Am J Clin Pathol 53:875–879, 1970
51. MCDONOUGH ES, GEORG LK, AJELLO L, and BRINKMAN S: Growth of dimorphic human pathogenic fungi on media containing cycloheximide and chloramphenicol. Mycopathol Mycol Appl 8:113–120, 1960
52. MICKELSEN PA, MCCARTHY LA, and PROPST MA: Further modifications of the auxonographic method for identification of yeasts. J Clin Microbiol 5:297–301, 1977
53. MILLER RE JR and LU L-P: Evaluation of the multitest microtechnique for yeast identification. Am J Med Technol 42:238–242, 1976
54. MILNE LJR and BARNESTSON RSTC: Diagnosis of dermatophytoses using vinyl adhesive tape. Sabouraudia 12:162–165, 1974
55. MISHRA SK and RANDHAWA HS: Application of paraffin bait technique to the isolation of *Nocardia asteroides* from clinical specimens. Appl Microbiol 18:686–687, 1969
56. MISHRA SK, RANDHAWA HS, and SANDHU RS: Observations on paraffin baiting as a laboratory diagnostic procedure in nocardiosis. Mycopathol Mycol Appl 51:147–157, 1973
57. PALIWAL DK and RANDHAWA HS: A rapid pigmentation test for identification of *Cryptococcus neoformans*. Antonie van Leeuwenhoek J Microbiol Serol 44:243–246, 1978
58. PALIWAL DK and RANDHAWA HS: Evaluation of a simplified *Guizotia abyssinica* seed medium for differentiation of *Cryptococcus neoformans*. J Clin Microbiol 7:346–348, 1978
59. RACHER JR: A comparison of two rapid methods for determining carbohydrate assimilation patterns of yeast-like fungi. Can J Med Tech 40:65–73, 1978
60. REEP BR and KAPLAN W: The effect of newer tubercule bacillus digestion and decontamination procedures on fungi causing pulmonary diseases. Mycopathol Mycol Appl 46:325–334, 1972
61. REEP BR and KAPLAN W: The use of N-acetyl-L-cysteine and dithiothreitol to process sputa for mycological and fluorescent antibody examinations. Health Lab Sci 9:118–124, 1972

62. RIPPON JW: Medical Mycology. W.B. Saunders Co, Philadelphia, 1974
63. ROBERTS GD, HORSTMEIER CD, LAND GA, and FOXWORTH JH: Rapid urea broth test for yeasts. J Clin Microbiol 7:584–588
64. ROBERTS GD, WANG HS, and HOLLICK GE: Evaluation of the API 20C microtube system for the identification of clinically important yeasts. J Clin Microbiol 3:302–305
65. ROSENTHAL SA and FURNARI D: The use of a cycloheximide-chloramphenicol medium in routine culture for fungi. J Invest Dermatol 28:367–371, 1957
66. SALKIN IF: Dermatophyte test medium: evaluation with nondermatophytic pathogens. Appl Microbiol 26:134–137, 1973
67. SALKIN IF: Adaptation to cycloheximide: *in vitro* studies with filamentous fungi. Can J Microbiol 26:1413–1419, 1975
68. SALKIN IF: Further simplification of *Guizotia abyssinica* seed medium for identification of *Crypotococcus neoformans* and *Cryptococcus bacillispora*. Can J Microbiol 25:1116–1118, 1979
69. SALKIN IF and GORDON MA: Evaluation of *Aspergillus* differential medium. J Clin Microbiol 2:74–75, 1975
70. SALKIN IF and HURD N: A quantitative evaluation of the antifungal properties of cycloheximide. Antimicrob Agents Chemother 1:177–184, 1972
71. SANDFORD LW, MASON KM, and HATHAWAY BM: The concentration of sputum for fungus culture. Am J Clin Pathol 44:172–176, 1965
72. SHAW CE and KAPICA L: Production of diagnostic pigment by phenoloxidase activity of *Cryptococcus neoformans*. Appl Microbiol 24:824–830, 1972
73. SMITH CD: Isolation and identification of *Histoplasma capsulatum* from soil. *In* Histoplasmosis. Balows A (ed.). Charles C. Thomas Co, Springfield, Ill, 1971, pp 277–283
74. SMITH CD and GOODMAN NL: Improved culture method for the isolation of *Histoplasma capsulatum* and *Blastomyces dermatitidis* from contaminated specimens. Am J Clin Pathol 63:276–280, 1975
75. STAIB F: *Cryptococcus neoformans* and *Guizotia abyssinica* (syn. *G. oleifer* D.C.) (Farbreaktion für *C. neoformans*). Z Hyg Infektionskr Med Mikrobiol Immunol Virol 148:466–475, 1962
76. STAIB F, QUANSAH-ENGELBERT B, and WEBER I: Serum-albumin agar used as an agar slant for the differentiation between *Trichophyton rubrum* and *Trichophyton metagrophytes:* specific red pigmentation of *T. rubrum*. Zentralbl Bakteriol Parasitenkd Infektionskr Hyg 240:525–528, 1978
77. STRACHAN AA, YU RJ, and BLANK F: Pigment production of *Cryptococcus neoformans* grown with extracts of *Guizotia abyssinica*. Appl Microbiol 22:478–479, 1973
78. TAPLIN D, ZAIAS N, REBELL G, and BLANK H: Isolation and recognition of dermatophytes on a new medium (DTM). Arch Dermatol 99:203–209, 1969
79. TASCHDJIAN CL, BURCHILL JJ, and KOZINN PJ: Rapid identification of *Candida albicans* by filamentation in serum and serum substitute. Am J Dis Child 99:212–215, 1960
80. VANBREUSEGHEM R, DE VROEY C, and TAKASHIO M: Practical Guide to Medical and Veterinary Mycology, 2nd edition. Masson Publ. USA, Inc, New York, 1978
81. WEBSTER J: Introduction to Fungi. The University Press, Cambridge, England, 1970
82. WEYMANN LH, STAGER CE, QADRI SGM, VILLARREAL A, and HUSSAIN QADRI SM: Evaluation of a modified dye pour-plate auxanographic method for the rapid identification of clinically significant yeasts. Med Microbiol Immunol 67:11–20, 1979
83. WHIFFEN AJ: The production, assay, and antibiotic activity of actidione, an antibiotic from *Streptomyces griseus*. J Bacteriol 56:283–291, 1948
84. WHIFFEN AJ: The activity *in vitro* of cycloheximide (Acti-dione) against fungi pathogenic to plants. Mycologia 42:253–258, 1950
85. WICKERHAM LJ: Taxonomy of Yeasts. U.S. Dept. of Agriculture Tech Bull 1029, 1951
86. WICKERHAM LJ and BURTON KA: Carbon assimilation tests for the classification of yeasts. J Bacteriol 56:363–371, 1948
87. WOLIN HK, BEVIS ML, and LAURORA N: An improved synthetic medium for the rapid production of chlamydospores by *Candida albicans*. Sabouraudia 2:96–99, 1962
88. YONG DCT, SMITKA C, PRYTULA A, and KANE J: The comparison of two agar media for germ tube and chlamydospore production by *Candida albicans*. Health Lab Sci 15:197–200, 1978

CHAPTER 48

CUTANEOUS MYCOSES (DERMATOMYCOSES)

Margarita Silva-Hutner, Irene Weitzman, and Stanley A. Rosenthal

INTRODUCTION

Dermatomycoses are fungal infections restricted to the skin of man and animals because the causative fungi are unable to invade deeper tissues or organs. Based on frequency of occurrence, and either clinical similarity of the lesions or degree of relatedness of the etiologic fungi, or both, the dermatomycoses can be further subdivided into: a) superficial, b) dermatophytic, and c) opportunistic.

Superficial mycoses are those in which the causative fungi colonize acellular layers of the skin and its appendages. These fungi have not been isolated with certainty from the external environment. The diseases they produce include macular lesions characterized by changes of the pigment of the skin (i.e., tinea versicolor and tinea nigra), and nodular infections along the hair shaft distal to the follicle (black piedra, white piedra).

Dermatophytic cutaneous mycoses are caused by the dermatophytes, a group of fungi of related phylogeny. They are *Ascomycetes* (family Gymnoascaceae), whose natural habitat is soil or human or animal skin and its appendages. Dermatophytes can invade the cellular layers of the epidermis and sometimes those of the dermis.

Opportunistic dermatomycoses are cutaneous infections produced by saprophytic fungi which are occasionally implanted traumatically into the skin. They must be diagnosed either by early biopsy or culture, or both, since the fungi are of low virulence and the lesions may heal spontaneously.

Section one of this chapter deals exclusively with the superficial dermatomycoses. The dermatophytic and the opportunistic dermatomycoses are discussed in sections two and three.

Section One: Superficial Mycoses

The superficial mycoses are cutaneous infections produced by fungi of such low pathogenicity that they are not only unable to attack the deeper tissues but do not even invade the living cellular layers of skin, hair, or nails. These diseases are nearly asymptomatic and cause the patient little physical discomfort. Psychological discomfort can be severe for esthetic reasons. The fungi in this group thus far recognized, and the diseases they cause, are listed in Table 48.1.

Lesions become evident for one of three reasons:

a. Development of pigmentary changes (hypopigmentation or hyperpigmentation) induced by the effect of the fungus on melanin deposition by cutaneous cells (16, 44) as in macular tinea versicolor, or by the dark color of the fungus itself as in tinea nigra.

b. Mild tissue irritation resulting in the formation of papules surrounding the follicular orifices as in papular and follicular tinea versicolor (48).

c. Production of nodular masses of fungal growth adherent to and often surrounding the hair shaft distal to the skin, as in the piedras (trichomycosis nodosa).

For clarity, each disease will be discussed in detail as a separate entity.

Tinea (Pityriasis) Versicolor

Causative organism

Malassezia (Pityrosporum) furfur, a lipophilic yeast, is characterized by spherical cells 2–8 μm in diameter. It reproduces by bud-fission, i.e., by extrusion of a bud through a polar opening in the cell wall of the flask-shaped mother cell (phialide) and subsequent formation of a septum between bud and mother cell. Recent studies by phase-contrast and electron micrography show a collarette or rim at the opening of the mother cell at the level of the septum (5, 47) and parallel indentations on the cell membrane which curve in a spiral swirl (10).

Many budding cells accumulate at the sporulating site to form spherical masses consisting of 10 to 12 elements; others extrude short septate wavy hyphae. These in turn can fragment into unicellular, budding elements.

The membranes of the yeast cells of *M. furfur* are thick, and characteristically corrugated with a series of "parallel" indentations which curve spirally to converge at one point. These indentations can be seen with ordinary light microscopy at higher magnification and can be better seen in stained cells or with

TABLE 48.1—FUNGI CAUSING SUPERFICIAL MYCOSES

ORGANISM	SYNONYMS	NAME OF DISEASE
1. *Malassezia furfur*	*Pityrosporum orbiculare*	tinea (pityriasis) versicolor
2. *Exophiala werneckii*	*Cladosporium werneckii*	tinea (keratomycosis) nigra
	Dematium werneckii	
	Pullularia werneckii	
3. *Piedraia hortae*		black piedra, tinea nodosa
4. *Piedraia quintanilhai*		black piedra in Central African mammals
5. *Trichosporon beigelii*	*T. cutaneum**	white piedra, chignon disease

* Systemic infections have been reported to be caused by *T. cutaneum*. Whether the agents belong in the same species or represent opportunistic invaders should be ascertained.

freeze-etching or scanning electron microscopy (4, 10). They are diagnostic for the genus; they are absent in species of *Brettanomyces, Candida, Cryptococcus,* and *Torulopsis* (54).

For many years the characteristics and growth requirements of this fungus in culture remained undefined because its strict lipid requirements did not permit growth on routine mycologic media. Lipid requirements on defined media were first demonstrated for a fungus by Benham in cultures of *M. furfur* that she had isolated from seborrheic skin (9). In 1951 Gordon cultured lipophilic yeast-like organisms from tinea versicolor, and in the same year he described *Pityrosporum orbiculare* as a new species (28, 29). This species was subsequently shown to be identical with *M. furfur* by Keddie et al. with electron microscopy and immunofluorescence (34, 37, 53). The name *M. furfur* has priority and is valid for the species. General acceptance of *M. furfur* as the cultural form of the etiologic agent of tinea versicolor was delayed by the rarity of filamentation *in vitro*. This deficiency may have been corrected by Dorn and Roehnert, who in 1977 formulated a defined culture medium that permits the *in vitro* formation of the mycelium of *M. furfur* (*P. orbiculare*) (25).

There has also been a delay in accepting *P. orbiculare* (*M. furfur*) and *P. ovale* as synonyms. The predominance of spherical budding cells (2–8 μm in diameter) in smears, scrapings, or primary cultures from certain lesions versus the predominance of oval or cylindrical budding cells (1 × 2 μm in diameter) in others has helped maintain the belief that *P. orbiculare* and *P. ovale* are two distinct species.

These two types of unicellular elements can also coexist in lesions and cultures and interconvert in cultures. This property is now attributed to the polymorphic nature of *M. furfur* (49, 50).

Clinical manifestations

Tinea versicolor is most commonly found on the upper trunk and arms (Fig 48.1). However, lesions may also occur on the face, scalp, neck, hands, lower trunk, and extremities, including the feet, toes, and even the toenails (57). Early lesions are discrete and range in size from approximately 2 mm to 2 cm. In older infections, lesions may become confluent and cover larger areas of skin. Occasionally in hot humid weather, a patient may show exacerbation in the form of rapidly spreading, confetti-like lesions concentric with hair follicles on the trunk. These are usually pinkish at first and appear irritated, but may later become hypopigmented, especially after exposure to light. This is now believed to be due to a decreased deposition of melanin on the melanosomes and a block in the transfer of melanosome granules to keratinocytes (16), and to the production of an inhibitor of tyrosinase by the fungus (44).

Untreated, active lesions of tinea versicolor may show a bronze-orange, yellow, or brownish fluorescence under the Wood's light (filtered ultraviolet light, peak wavelength 365 nm).

Although the lesions of tinea versicolor are scaly, they may appear smooth when undisturbed. Gentle scratching with a fingernail or a blunt instrument reveals a scaly surface. The scales are easily detached in strips resembling wood shavings or else as an entire impression of the lesion adhering to transparent vinyl tape (36). This property is used as a clinical diagnostic test to

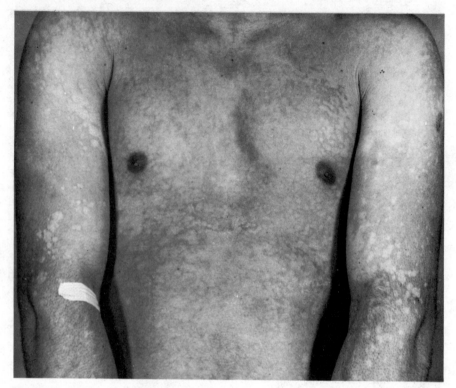

Figure 48.1—Tinea versicolor lesions on trunk and arms. Note hypo- and hyper-
        pigmented macules. Size reduced.

differentiate tinea versicolor from other macular lesions. The diagnosis is confirmed by direct microscopic examination of the scales and is based on demonstrating the characteristic yeast and mycelial forms of *M. furfur*. This yeast can
also be seen in reduced numbers and sometimes cultured from areas of se-
borrhea in the absence of lesions, indicating that it may be part of the normal
flora of the skin. Proliferation is favored either by the accumulation of essential lipids in certain areas or by the weakening of the host defenses associated
with Cushings' syndrome and other susceptibility factors (11, 31).

Epidemiology

   Age, sex, occupational, and racial distribution. Tinea versicolor is a rather
common disease seen predominantly in young adults, although it is also observed in other age groups. Some authors have reported a higher prevalence
among males, whereas others have reported a higher prevalence among females. The occurrence of tinea versicolor is also affected by personal hygiene
and the amount of perspiration. These factors could affect distribution of cases
by sex and perhaps also by occupation. No racial predilection has been reported.

Geographic distribution. Tinea versicolor has a world-wide distribution; it appears as frequently in temperate zones as in the tropics, but certain differences have been reported from the two climatic zones: (a) Patients in the tropics have lesions on the face, scalp, and hands more frequently than do those in temperate zones, where the disease is usually limited to areas covered by clothing. (b) Patients in temperate zones usually have lesions in a variety of colors depending on the age of the lesions and/or associated erythema. Thus the name tinea versicolor has been applied to the disease. In the tropics, lesions on a given patient will be all white, pink, yellow, or brown, giving rise to terms such as tinea alba, tinea rosea, tinea flava, and tinea fusca (7, 15). The term chromophytosis has been suggested to encompass these various manifestations.

Source of infection and contagion. As already noted, *M. furfur* may be part of the normal flora of the skin. Factors influencing the development of lesions are not well understood; the production of oily secretions, an impairment of host defenses, hormonal changes, and the bacterial flora may all play a role.

Collection and processing of specimens

A definitive microscopic examination of material taken from the lesion is all that is required at present for the laboratory diagnosis of tinea versicolor, because the parasitic morphology of *M. furfur* is diagnostic. Material can be obtained by one of three methods: (a) Scraping the surface of the lesion with a scalpel blade or the edge of a glass slide or tongue depressor; (b) applying transparent adhesive tape (35, 36) (certain adhesives and tape backings are more suitable than others—see below); (c) squeezing exudate from a pustular lesion (24).

If cultures are to be done, scales should be planted on suitable media at the moment of collection since *M. furfur* loses viability in skin scrapings *in vitro* (unlike dermatophytes).

Although antibodies have been demonstrated in human sera with immunofluorescence, serology is neither a necessary nor a practical diagnostic procedure.

Time of collection. The best time for collection is during a period of exacerbation of the lesions.

The number of specimens. One good specimen usually suffices to establish the diagnosis. If direct microscopic examination can be carried out in the office or clinic while the patient is waiting, the suitability of the specimen and/or collection site can be judged immediately. Active tinea versicolor lesions are positive throughout their surface and particularly so around hair follicles, i.e., near the external orifices of sebaceous ducts.

Diagnostic procedures

Microscopic examination. The KOH preparations described in Chapter 47 are suitable for examining clinical material for *M. furfur*. The fungus is made more visible by staining with Parker's "Super-Quink" ink (blue-black or black). This method was first described by Cohen, who detailed the formulation of the ink (18).

The use of adhesive cellophane tape was first studied by Keddie et al.

(35), who recommended tapes No. 681 and No. 473 of The Minnesota Mining and Manufacturing Company as superior in obtaining permanent mounts. The tape is pressed against the patient's lesion, adhesive side down, until enough scales adhere to it. This portion of the tape is then pressed directly (adhesive side down) on a clean microscope slide or onto a drop of mounting fluid and examined.

Primary isolation media. If cultures are desired, various media, some of which contain olive oil, have been recommended for isolation (28, 50). Not all olive oils are suitable, either because they may be deficient in essential fatty acids (myristic and palmitic) or because antifungal substances may be present.

Adding CP-grade myristic or palmitic acid (10 mg/100 ml) to isolation media may prove preferable (51). Incubate at 34 C–37 C, because this temperature range favors the growth of *M. furfur* and inhibits that of many other yeasts. Growth appears within 4 to 7 days as minute colonies resembling droplets of cream, which coalesce to form a wrinkled membrane. With aging the color darkens to a brownish tan.

Identification procedures. The criteria used to identify *M. furfur* include (a) cell morphology (Fig 48.2) and (b) nutritional growth requirements.

Budding yeast cells may be spherical (3–7 μm), or they may contain a

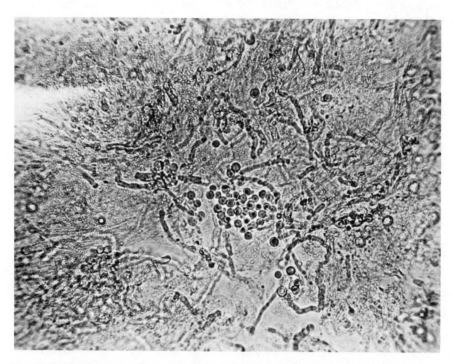

Figure 48.2—*Malassezia furfur* in scales from lesions of tinea versicolor (KOH preparation). Note short septate, blunt-ended hyphae and clusters of spherical cells, some with buds. ×430.

mixture of oval, bottle-shaped, or cylindrical cells (1–3 μm × 2–7 μm). The key morphological criteria are semi-endogenous successive monopolar budding and the presence of a collarette and a septum at the site of the bud scar. Physiologically, *M. furfur* requires that oil and taurocholate be added to routine mycological media; *M. pachydermatis* requires no additives (52). Both species grow well at 37 C.

Serologic procedures. Serologic procedures for obtaining routine diagnosis and prognosis of tinea versicolor are not necessary.

Specific quality control. Batches of olive oil should be checked for their ability to support the growth of a culture of *M. furfur.*

Tinea Nigra (Keratomycosis Nigricans Palmaris; Cladosporiosis)

Causative organism

Nomenclature. The causative organism of tinea nigra is a polymorphic dematiaceous fungus. Because of its polymorphism, this organism has been classified into various genera, among them, *Cladosporium* (14, 45), *Dematium* (23), and *Pullularia* (20), depending on the emphasis that each author has given to one or another of the various methods of conidial production which he has observed or accepted. At present, emphasis is being placed on the observation that this fungus produces annelloconidia, i.e., conidia produced by successive budding, leaving annellations (rings) on the annellophore (special type of conidiophore). On this basis von Arx proposed that *C. werneckii* be transferred to the genus *Exophiala* (59). This proposal has been accepted by several authors, after some of them clearly depicted annellophores in this fungus (19, 30, 43). The currently accepted name for the agent of tinea nigra is *Exophiala werneckii* (Parreiras-Horta) von Arx, 1970.

Characterization. *E. werneckii* is a dematiaceous fungus which produces hyphae and clusters of elongated budding cells in infected epidermal scales. When newly isolated, the fungus produces black, tar-like, glabrous colonies composed of unicellular and bicellular budding cells. As colonies age, grayish velvety sectors are produced which outgrow the glabrous areas. The colonies eventually become completely filamentous, sporulating by conidial formation (see below).

Clinical manifestations

Tinea nigra is characterized by the appearance of darkly pigmented macules or patches on the skin—most frequently on the palms (Fig 48.3) but sometimes on the soles or dorsa of the feet. They are either gray or brown—in shades that have been likened to that of a stain caused by silver nitrate. The color is not uniform, but tends to be darker toward the periphery of the lesion. The lesions are not scaly. Both palms may be affected simultaneously, but unilateral involvement is the general rule.

Epidemiology

The disease is probably acquired exogenously. Familial spread has not been reported. All races and age groups are apparently susceptible; males and

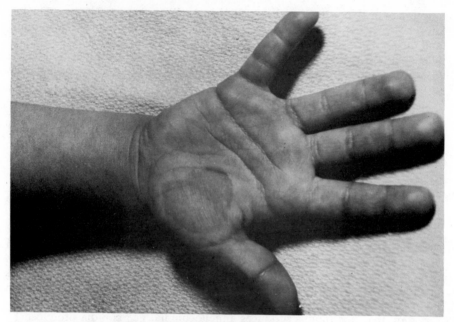

Figure 48.3—Lesion of tinea nigra on palmar surface of hand. Note dark pigmentation and absence of elevation of lesion. ×1.

females are equally infected. Tinea nigra is considered to be primarily a disease of the tropics but is sometimes found in temperate climates (2). Some cases seen in the temperate zone began while the patient was in the tropics.

Public health significance

The disease poses no threat to the health of the patient and is only of cosmetic importance if left untreated. Once medical help is sought, however, it is important that the physician distinguish tinea nigra from other pigmented lesions of the skin, especially from malignant melanoma, which it may closely resemble (61), since the incorrect diagnosis may subject the patient to mutilating surgery for the treatment of melanoma. Other dermatologic conditions which may clinically resemble tinea nigra are junction nevi and post-inflammatory pigmentary changes.

Collection and processing of specimens

Scales are collected by scraping the lesions. They should be examined and cultured promptly until more information is available of the viability of the fungus in scales.

Diagnostic procedures

Direct microscopic examination. Scales obtained from suspicious lesions are examined in potassium hydroxide (KOH) preparations (Fig 48.4 and 48.5).

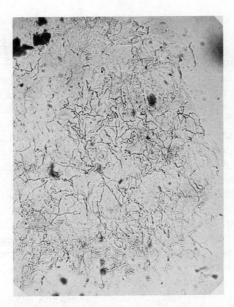

Figure 48.4—*Exophiala* (*Cladosporium*) *werneckii* in KOH preparation of skin scrapings from lesion of tinea nigra. Note abundance of long, branching, dematiaceous (dark-colored) hyphae and small clusters of ellipsoid spores, ×125.

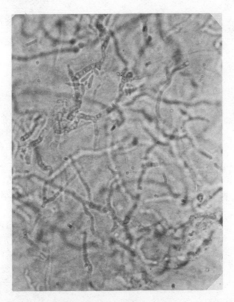

Figure 48.5—*E. werneckii* in KOH preparation of skin scrapings from lesion of tinea nigra. Higher magnification, ×560.

Fungal elements are usually present in large numbers and are seen as olive-colored, frequently branched, septate filaments, usually 1.5 × 5 μm in diameter. Hyphal fragments and budding cells are also seen. The pigmented filaments of this fungus in KOH preparations are readily differentiated from those of hyaline fungi. In fact, it is the pigmented nature of *E. werneckii*'s mycelium as it grows in the stratum corneum that makes the lesions dark.

Culture. Skin scrapings are cultured at 25 C on Sabouraud agar with and without antibiotics (Fig 48.6 and 48.7). *E. werneckii* grows slowly and appears in two distinct morphologic stages. At first it is seen as a black, shiny yeast colony, tar-like in appearance. After 2 or more weeks of additional incubation, velvety gray aerial mycelium appears on portions of the yeast growth and eventually predominates.

Microscopic morphology correlates well with the gross appearance of the colony. The initial yeast growth consists of olive-colored budding cells, both single and 2-celled. As the colony changes to the mycelial form, a corresponding change in microscopic morphology ensues, with the development of a preponderance of olivaceous, thick-walled hyphae that are septate at frequent intervals. It is on these hyphae that conidial sporulation occurs. It consists mainly of spherical clusters of one or 2-celled conidia (annelloconidia) that arise terminally or on short lateral conidiophores (annellophores) bearing successive annellations (rings) (19). Observation of this type of sporulation is the basis for reclassifying this fungus in the genus *Exophiala* (Barron's series Annellosporae) (6). In older cultures of the mycelial form, branching chains of conidia with terminal budding have also been seen and photographed (14).

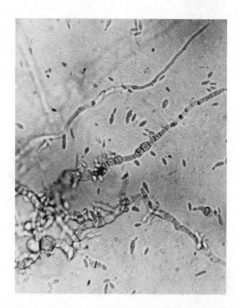

Figure 48.6—*E. werneckii* on Sabouraud agar. Note thin- and thick-walled hyphae and spores originating from short lateral conidiophores. ×560.

The presence of this type of sporulation has been the basis for recommending classification in the genus *Cladosporium* (Barron's series Blastosporae) (6). But *Cladosporium* is a monomorphic genus, and the agent of tinea nigra is indeed polymorphic in its sporulating ability. Branching conidial chains with terminal budding were depicted and described by Carmichael when he described the new genus *Exophiala* (12).

Black Piedra (Tinea Nodosa)

Causative organisms

The usual agent of black piedra is a dark-colored ascomycete, *Piedraia hortae*, characterized by its ability to form hard (stony) nodules along parasitized hairs. The nodule is composed of a fungal pseudotissue (pseudoparenchyma) that is actually an ascostroma (i.e., it harbors asci and ascospores). Asci are globose-to-oval and they are contained in special cavities or locules within the nodule. These characteristics place the genus *Piedraia* in the order Myrangiales of the Loculoascomycetes (family Saccardinulaceae) (41). A new species, *P. quintanilhai*, has been described recently in Central African mammals (58). *In vivo*, *P. hortae* forms oval asci containing two to eight aseptate, fusiform ascospores. These ascospores are hyaline to light brown, usually curved, sometimes S-shaped, and bear a filament at each end. Most ascospores range from 19–55 μm long by 4–8 μm wide (27, 42). *P. quintanilhai* was described by Van Uden (59) as a new species on the basis of the absence of polar filaments on the ascospore. Takashio and DeVroey (55) subsequently reported filamentless ascospores from nodules of black piedra from pelts of chimpanzees from Zaire.

P. hortae grows slowly on Sabouraud dextrose agar. Colonies are compact, heaped in the center, dark brown to black, and are either glabrous or covered with short aerial hyphae. Microscopically, thick-walled brownish hyphae and chlamydospores are observed. Ascospores do not usually form on

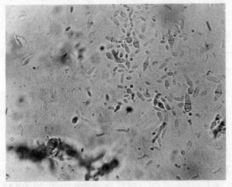

Figure 48.7—*E. werneckii* on Sabouraud agar. Note bicellular spores and bipolar budding. ×560.

routine culture media but can be induced with some strains by the transplantation technique of Takashio and Vanbreuseghem (56).

Clinical manifestations

Black piedra is characterized by the presence of discrete, hard and gritty,
dark-brown to black nodules which adhere firmly to the hairs of the scalp,
beard, and mustache. These nodules range in size from microscopic to 3 mm in
diameter. In humans, the fungus penetrates and disrupts the cuticle of the hair
shaft and grows around it, but deep penetration and complete disruption of
hair is not observed (17). In contrast, black piedra in animals can result in severe pilar damage, with the cortex and medulla being destroyed and the hair
being broken at the site of the nodule (32, 58).

Epidemiology

Black piedra occurs in humid tropical regions in South and Central
America, southeast Asia, and Africa. It has been reported in humans in the
South American counties of Surinam, Venezuela, Paraguay, Argentina, Uruguay, and Brazil and from the Southeast Asian countries of Indonesia, Malaysia, Thailand, and Indochina (27). Black piedra was observed in animals held
in captivity for prolonged periods (32, 58). The source of infection is believed
to be exogenous and of nonanimal origin—probably as a result of exposure to
an undetermined source in nature (32, 58). A combination of climatic conditions (abundant rainfall, high humidity, and a temperature of 26 C) and the
use of possibly contaminated plant oil in the hair probably result in the endemicity of this disease in Brazilian Indians in the Amazon area (27). It has been
suggested that infection may spread to neighboring hairs of an infected human
by the dissemination of free ascospores through the gaps in the nodule (17).
There are no reports of animal to animal transmission, but an epidemic reported on by Carrion in 1938 (13) and 1965 (15) which involved 45 boys in a
government orphanage in Puerto Rico leaves no doubt that person-to-person
transmission can occur. One of the authors of this chapter (MSH) recalls that
the boys involved in this epidemic used to share wet combs when "styling"
their own or each other's hair at the time this evidence of contagion was disclosed.

Public health significance

In areas of high humidity it is possible for piedra to become a public
health problem. Hygienic measures should be observed.

Collection and processing of specimens

Hairs containing nodules are required for laboratory studies.

Diagnostic procedures

Microscopic examination. Hair fragments containing the nodules are examined in a 10%-20% KOH preparation, after the slide is gently heated, for the
presence of compacted masses of septate brownish hyphae on the surface of
the hair and for the oval asci containing up to eight aseptate, curved, fusiform
ascospores (like a bunch of bananas) within the crushed nodule (Fig 48.8 and
48.9). The ascospores may bear a filament at each end.

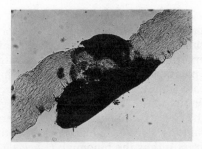

Figure 48.8—Black piedra nodule on hair from human scalp. Note fungal filaments along advancing border of nodule. KOH preparation. ×100.

Culture media. Sabouraud dextrose agar with chloramphenicol and cycloheximide has been used successfully to isolate *P. hortae* (17, 27), although the presence of cycloheximide has been reported to inhibit the growth of this fungus (3). Sabouraud agar with chloramphenicol is generally recommended to inhibit bacterial growth (3, 32).

White Piedra (Chignon Disease, Piedra Colombiana, Piedra Nostras)

Causative organism

Nomenclature. The agent of white piedra is the yeast *Trichosporon beigelii.* This microorganism was originally described as an alga, *Pleurococcus beigelii,*

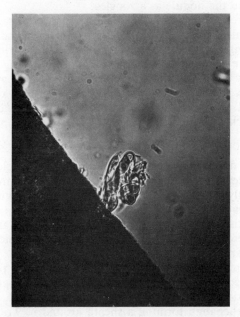

Figure 48.9—Ascospores within ascus of black piedra alongside nodule. KOH preparation. ×430.

in 1867 by Küchenmeister and Rabenhorst, who studied white nodules on chignons (detachable hair pieces worn on back of head or nape of neck) (39). Behrend described a culture from a nodular mustache infection in Germany (8). In comparing the morphology of the hair nodules with that of nodules on hairs from Colombian piedra and with the original drawings of Beigel of nodules from chignon disease (infestation), Behrend recognized the fungal nature of this agent and its identity in the three diseases and suggested the name *Trichosporon ovoides* for the causative fungus. In 1902 Vuillemin pointed out that this fungus was identical to *P. beigelii*, and he transferred this validly described species to *Trichosporon* (60); thus the binomial *T. beigelii* has priority. While Diddens and Lodder preferred *T. cutaneum* (a species described in 1926 from a cutaneous wound infection) (21), several authors have questioned this recommendation (22, 26). The variable patterns of carbohydrate assimilation and other characteristics listed for *T. cutaneum* in the second edition of *The Yeasts* are indicative of the probable heterogeneity of *T. cutaneum* (22). As Emmons points out (26), and in our experience, *T. beigelii* remains confined to the distal portion of the affected hairs without skin involvement.

Characteristics. T. beigelii has a distinct parasitic morphology, appearing as soft, white, ivory or beige, oval nodules, adhering to hairs in humans and to the fur of animals (1, 33). In the nodules, budding cells (blastoconidia) and fragmented hyphal elements (arthroconidia) intermingle in either mosaic arrangement or aligned perpendicular to the hair axis, forming a compact oval mass. The hyaline refringency of the fungal structures, absence of locules, asci, and ascospores, and softer consistency of these nodules clearly distinguish this agent from the agent of black piedra. As in the latter, associated micrococci sometimes surround the nodule as a zooglea.

T. beigelii grows on various routine media but is sensitive to cycloheximide. Colonies are fast growing (1-2 cm/week); they are creamy in consistency when young but soon become membranous and wrinkled, sometimes separating from the agar. Aerial hyphae may develop along the edges of the colony, particularly upon subculture. The fungus grows well at 37 C and forms pellicles on liquid media. Microscopically, the presence of arthroconidia, blastoconidia, and septate hyphae define the genus *Trichosporon*. Specific identification criteria will be described under identification procedures.

Clinical manifestations

The disease is manifested by the development of multiple white-to-beige-colored nodules occurring at intervals or coalescing along mustache or beard hairs, less frequently on scalp, axillary, or pubic hairs of humans (40, 46), or on fur. The nodules must be distinguished from those of black piedra, the nits of pediculosis capitis, keratin casts (38), trichorrexis nodosa, and trichomycosis axillaris. This differentiation, usually feasible by microscopic examination, is important for therapy and prognosis.

The microscopic appearance of the nodules of white piedra and black piedra has been described in earlier paragraphs. The nits of pediculosis capitis have a characteristic morphology and are usually eccentric, adhering to one side of the hair rather than forming a sheath around it. Trichorrexis nodosa appears as brush-like fibers teased out at intervals along the hair shaft. Peripilar keratin casts are freely movable cylinders of keratinized epidermal cells emerging from the follicle and moving distally on the hair as it grows. The concretions in trichomycosis axillaris can be red, yellow, or black, and they are usually longer and more cylindrical than those of the piedras; microscopically they are made up of corynebacteria rather than of fungal cells.

Epidemiology

Whereas *T. cutaneum* has been isolated from various parasitic and saprophytic habitats, the distribution of *T. beigelii* outside its parasitic niche has not been unequivocally demonstrated. *T. cutaneum* and *T. beigelii* must be further differentiated in order to understand the source of white piedra infections. White piedra is more prevalent than black piedra in temperate zones, and it is possibly more prevalent in males than in females because of its apparent predilection for the beard and mustache.

Public health significance

White piedra does not constitute a public health problem.

Collection and processing of specimens

Kind of specimens required. For laboratory diagnosis of white piedra, hairs with nodules are required.

Diagnostic procedures

Microscopic examination. The KOH preparations described in Methods are suitable for examining nodules of piedra. Hair should be cut into short pieces containing nodules. The characteristic morphology described above is diagnostic. Cultures will help identify the etiologic agent(s).

Primary culture media. Sabouraud glucose-peptone agar with 0.5% yeast extract is a suitable isolation medium. This medium should be used both with and without antibiotics.

Identification procedures. Teased mounts from the colony usually suffice for generic identification of the *Trichosporon sp.* The production of arthroconidia, blastoconidia, and septate hyphae is diagnostic. Enzymatic reactions are necessary for specific identification, and pure cultures are necessary for these studies. Although the presence of antibacterial agents in the medium may inhibit bacterial growth, it does not guarantee their absence. It is therefore important to streak a presumably pure culture on media such as brain heart infusion agar to encourage growth of any bacteria that may be still associated with the fungal culture. By picking an isolated yeast colony and restreaking it on another BHI plate, one can evaluate the purity of the culture.

Serologic procedures. No serologic procedures are used in the routine diagnosis of white piedra infections or in the identification of *T. beigelii.*

Section Two: Dermatophytoses

The principal etiological agents of the cutaneous mycoses are the dermatophytes. They, and the diseases they cause, the dermatophytoses, are the subject of this section. Unrelated filamentous fungi which are primarily soil saprophytes or plant pathogens may occasionally cause cutaneous mycoses, especially in the compromised host. These agents are discussed briefly in the next section under the heading "Opportunistic Dermatomycoses."

The dermatophytoses (ringworm) are fungal infections of the keratinous tissues (skin, hair, nails, feather, horns) of humans and animals caused by closely related fungi belonging to the imperfect genera: *Microsporum, Trichophyton,* and *Epidermophyton.* Both pathogenic and non-pathogenic species of these genera typically have an affinity for keratin and can use this insoluble scleroprotein. These fungi may exist as soil saprophytes or as zoopathogens, some of which are exclusively pathogenic for man.

Causative Organisms

The etiologic agents of the dermatophytoses belong to the genera *Microsporum, Trichophyton,* and *Epidermophyton.* Emmons' classification scheme is essentially based on the asexual spores of these three genera (25). This scheme, updated by Ajello (2, 4, 5), is the basis of the current classification of the imperfect state of the dermatophytes.

Many of the dermatophytes reproduce sexually. These species have perfect states belonging to the genera *Nannizzia* and *Arthroderma* of the family Gymnoascaceae of the Ascomycotina. The perfect states of the *Microsporum* species are found in the genus *Nannizzia* (Table 48.2) and of the *Trichophyton* species in the genus *Arthroderma* (Table 48.3). The perfect state for the *Epidermophyton* sp. has not been discovered. The majority of these fungi are heterothallic; sexual reproduction requires the pairing of compatible mating types (referred to as + and − or as A and a) on a suitable medium. The best results are obtained on soil and hair, but special nonkeratinous agar media are suitable substrates for most species (52, 73, 78).

Most of the *Microsporum* and *Trichophyton* species produce two kinds of conidia: large multiseptate spores called macroconidia, and small aseptate spores called microconidia. Some species, notably *T. terrestre,* produce conidia that are transitional between microconidia and macroconidia.

TABLE 48.2—ASCOMYCETOUS (PERFECT) STATE OF *MICROSPORUM* SPECIES

NANNIZZIA (PERFECT STATES)	*MICROSPORUM* (IMPERFECT STATES)
N. borellii	M. amazonicum
N. cajetanii	M. cookei
N. fulva	M. fulvum*
N. grubyia	M. vanbreuseghemii
N. gypsea	M. gypseum*
N. incurvata	M. gypseum*
N. obtusa	M. nanum
N. otae	M. canis
N. persicolor	M. persicolor
N. racemosa	M. racemosum

* Referred to as the *M. gypseum* complex.

TABLE 48.3—ASCOMYCETOUS (PERFECT) STATE OF *TRICHOPHYTON* SPECIES

ARTHRODERMA (PERFECT STATE)	*TRICHOPHYTON* (IMPERFECT STATE)	
A. benhamiae	T. mentagrophytes*	
A. ciferrii	T. georgiae	
A. flavescens	T. flavescens	
A. gertlerii	T. vanbreuseghemii	
A. gloriae	T. gloriae	
A. insingulare	T. terrestre ⎤	
A. lenticularum	T. terrestre ⎬	T. terrestre complex
A. quadrifidum	T. terrestre ⎦	
A. simii	T. simii	
A. uncinatum	T. ajelloi	
A. vanbreuseghemii	T. mentagrophytes*	

* *T. mentagrophytes* complex.

Differential features of *Microsporum, Trichophyton,* and *Epidermophyton* are discussed below and in Table 48.6 and 48.7.

Microsporum

The distinguishing feature of this genus is the roughened surface of the wall of the macroconidia, often described as verrucose, verruculose, or echinulate. The roughened wall may be very prominent, as in *M. canis,* or difficult to discern without an oil immersion lens, as in *M. persicolor.* Scanning electron microscopic studies have revealed that these are vesicles rather than spines, suggesting the term vesiculate rather than echinulate (53).

Microsporum species usually sporulate profusely and produce numerous macroconidia and smaller numbers of microconidia (*M. audouinii* and *M. ferrugineum* are notable exceptions since sporulation is usually rare or absent unless induced on special media). Macroconidia are typically borne singly on the conidiophores, are multiseptate (1–15 septa), spindle-shaped (fusiform), thin to thick-walled, and range from 6–160 μm long and from 6–25 μm wide. The *Microsporum* species are listed in Table 48.4.

TABLE 48.4—*MICROSPORUM* SPECIES

M. amazonicum	M. fulvum ⎤	M. gypseum complex
M. audouinii	M. gypseum ⎦	
M. boullardii	M. nanum	
M. canis	M. persicolor	
M. cookei	M. praecox	
M. distortum	M. racemosum	
M. ferrugineum	M. ripariae	
M. gallinae		
M. vanbreuseghemii		

Trichophyton

Macroconidia are smooth-walled and borne singly or in clusters on the conidiophores. These spores may be absent, rare, or abundant depending upon the species and culture media. They are usually multiseptate (1–12 septa), variable in shape (clavate, cylindrical, cylindrofusiform, and fusiform), thin to thick-walled, and range in size from 8–86 μm long by 4–14 μm wide (51). Microconidia are smooth-walled and may be globular, pear-shaped, club-shaped, or, on rare occasions, cylindrical. They may be borne singly along the sides of the hyphae (*en thyrse*) or in grapelike clusters (*en grappe*). Transitional forms between micro- and macroconidia are characteristic of some species or varieties. The *Trichophyton* species are listed in Table 48.5.

Perfect states of Microsporum and Trichophyton

Tables 48.2, 48.3, 48.4, and 48.5 list *M. gypseum, T. mentagrophytes* and *terrestre* as complexes rather than as single species. These complexes were revealed when mating studies among the so-called imperfect species led to the discovery of the perfect states and more than one perfect species. For example, *M. gypseum* (*M. fulvum* was formerly considered synonymous with *M. gypseum*) was found to be the imperfect state of three perfect species (71): *Nannizzia gypsea, N. incurvata,* and *N. fulva*. Thus, we refer to the imperfect state (including *M. fulvum*) as the *M. gypseum* complex. Similarly, a complex of species was recognized in the imperfect species *T. mentagrophytes* (perfect states *A. benhamiae* and *A. vanbreuseghemii*) and in *T. terrestre* (perfect states *A. quadrifidum, A. lenticularum,* and *A. insigulare*).

Epidermophyton

Macroconidia are smooth-walled, borne singly or in clusters, obovate to broadly clavate, have 0–4 septa, and range in size from 20–40 μm by 6–12 μm. They produce no microconidia. Until recently, this genus was monotypic; *E. floccosum* was the only species. However, a new species "*E. stockdaleae*" has been reported (54). (According to the rules on orthography, in the *International Rules of Botanical Nomenclature*, the correct spelling of this species should be *E. stockdali*.)

TABLE 48.5—*TRICHOPHYTON* SPECIES

T. ajelloi	
T. concentricum	T. rubrum
T. equinum	T. schoenleinii
T. flavescens	T. simii
	T. soudanense
T. georgiae	T. terrestre complex
T. gloriae	T. tonsurans
T. gourvilii	T. vanbreuseghemii
T. megninii	T. verrucosum
T. mentagrophytes complex	T. violaceum
T. phaseoliforme	T. yaoundei

Specific Identification

Identification of species of *Microsporum* and *Epidermophyton* is often based on colony characteristics and on the morphology of the macroconidia. These criteria alone are often insufficient for specific identification in the genus *Trichophyton*, since colonial and microscopic morphology vary and some isolates cannot sporulate when subcultured. Also, many dermatophytes, particularly on Sabouraud glucose agar, develop white fluffy tufts on the surface of the colony which may eventually overgrow the original culture. This condition is often called pleomorphism. Subcultures of these tufts show loss in pigmentation and sporulation. This phenomenon may result from mutation (76) or chromosomal aberration (24) and occurs most frequently in the *M. gypseum* complex, *M. canis, E. floccosum,* and the *T. mentagrophytes* complex.

Physiological tests are often required in conjunction with morphology to correctly identify species. Such tests include: perforation of hair *in vitro*; urease activity; special nutritional requirements; comparison of growth at room temperature and at 37 C; and pigment production on special media. Mating reactions may be helpful in identifying a species complex or an atypical isolate. However, this procedure is not usually practical or necessary in most diagnostic laboratories.

Mating reactions should be done at reference laboratories or by individuals engaged in research in this field, since specialized media, an extensive collection of cultures for each species, and isolates of each mating type are required.

The characteristic features of the pathogenic *Microsporum, Epidermophyton,* and *Trichophyton* species are listed in Tables 48.6 and 48.7. Key features of the rarely pathogenic *Microsporum* and *Trichophyton* species are described in Table 48.8.

Certain saprophytic or rarely pathogenic fungi (e.g., *T. terrestre*) superficially resemble some dermatophyte species. Many of these fungi also have one or more properties of the dermatophytes, such as: ability to turn Dermatophyte Test Medium (DTM) red; production of perforating organs *in vitro;* urease activity; and ability to grow on media containing cycloheximide. Table 48.9 lists some of these fungi, the dermatophytes for which they may be mistaken, and some differentiating characteristics.

Clinical Manifestations

Generalities

The clinical manifestations of dermatophytic infections (tineas, ringworm) may range from mild to severe depending on the virulence of the infecting agent, the anatomical location of the lesion(s), and host factors such as age, sex, and immune status. A single fungal species can infect many anatomical locations and produce various types of lesions. Conversely, different species can produce clinically identical lesions.

Traditionally, the diseases caused by dermatophytes have been named according to their anatomical location: tinea capitis (scalp), tinea barbae (beard),

TABLE 48.6—CHARACTERISTIC FEATURES OF PATHOGENIC *MICROSPORUM* AND *EPIDERMOPHYTON* SPECIES

SPECIES	COLONY ON SABOURAUD DEXTROSE AGAR	MICROSCOPIC MORPHOLOGY	DIFFERENTIAL FEATURES
Microsporum M. audouinii	Grayish-white to buff, flat, spreading, velvety; light salmon pink to light reddish brown on reverse	Usually no conidia, apiculate, terminal chlamydospores are the only characteristic feature; pectinate hyphae may be present	Poor growth and brownish discoloration on rice grains; sporulating strains have irregular fusiform and elongated macroconidia with few septa at irregular intervals
var. *rivalieri**	Grayish white; folded; pale apricot on reverse; more rapid growth than M. audouinii	Inflated, bulbous, pectinate hyphae	Pathogenic for guinea pigs; macroconidia produced on soil and hair by some isolates
var. *langeronii**	Rose to tan with radial grooves, more rapid growth than M. audouinii	May have more sporulation than M. audouinii	Pathogenic for guinea pigs
M. canis†	White to pale buff, fluffy or velvety with radial grooves; yellow orange to orange brown or colorless on reverse	Numerous fusiform macroconidia with thick walls, up to 15 septa; 18–125 μm × 5–25 μm, with asymmetric knobbed apex; few microconidia	Good growth and sporulation on rice grains
M. distortum	White to pale buff; usually with radial grooves; colorless to yellowish on reverse	Macroconidia are distorted and bizarre in shape, 20–60 μm × 7–27 μm; microconidia abundant	
M. ferrugineum	Yellowish to rust colored; heaped and folded; waxy; very slow grower	Usually no conidia; chlamydospores; irregular hyphae and long, straight coarse hyphae with prominent septa ("bamboo hyphae")	Some isolates produced spindle-shaped multi-cellular thick-walled macroconidia on freezing agar or on diluted SDA (75); light yellow colonies on Lowenstein-Jensen medium differentiates M. ferrugineum from dark reddish brown colonies of T. soudanense
M. gallinae	White, tinged with pink; slightly folded; downy; raspberry red diffusing pigment on reverse	Macroconidia fairly abundant, blunt tipped, 6–8 μm × 15–50 μm, 5–6 celled, cell wall usually smooth but slightly echinulate; pyriform microconidia	Conidia formation stimulated by growth on media containing yeast extract

TABLE 48.6—(Continued)

Species	Colony on Sabouraud Dextrose Agar	Microscopic Morphology	Differential Features
M. gypseum complex (M. gypseum and M. fulvum)	Pale buff to rosy buff, white border; flat; powdery, granular to floccose; rosy buff, cinnamon, or amber on reverse	Abundant macroconidia, 25–60 μm × 7.5–15 μm; ellipsoidal; fusiform to cylindrical, up to 6 septa, thin-walled; microconidia moderately abundant	
M. fulvum	Usually floccose	Macroconidia more cylindrical but with tapering ends	Perfect state: Nannizzia fulva
M. gypseum	Usually coarsely to finely granular	Macroconidia ellipsoidal to fusiform	Perfect states: N. incurvata, N. gypsea
M. nanum	White to buff; flat; powdery to downy; reddish brown on reverse	Abundant obovate to clavate macroconidia, 10.5–30 μm × 6.5–13 μm, usually 2-celled, microconidia rare	Grows more slowly than members of M. gypseum complex; also must differentiate from Trichothecium roseum
M. persicolor	Yellowish buff becoming peach to pink; flat; powdery to downy; reddish brown on reverse	Abundant microconidia, spherical to pyriform (few clavate), stalked, borne mostly in grapelike clusters, but also singly along the sides of hyphae; thin-walled macroconidia; often produces spirals	Differentiated from T. mentagrophytes by echinulations of macroconidia which are more evident when growing on cereal agar or soil and hair; pink to wine rose colonies on cereal agar or sugar-free peptone agar. Perfect state: N. persicolor
Epidermophyton E. floccosum	Yellowish olive to olive green; flat to radially folded; suedelike; brownish orange on reverse; white tufts common on surface of older cultures (pleomorphism)	Abundant broadly clavate, smooth-walled macroconidia, 20–40 μm × 6–8 μm, single or in clusters, 0–4 septa; no microconidia; chlamydospores common in older cultures	No microconidia

* Considered by some as a variety, by others as a distinct species.
† The description given here includes M. equinum, considered by some as a variety of M. canis, by others as a distinct species.

TABLE 48.7.—CHARACTERISTIC FEATURES OF PATHOGENIC *TRICHOPHYTON* SPECIES

	COLONY ON SABOURAUD DEXTROSE AGAR	MICROSCOPIC MORPHOLOGY	DIFFERENTIAL FEATURES
T. concentricum	Buff to beige; elevated and convoluted; glabrous to velvety; no undersurface color; slow growing	Microconidia and macroconidia usually absent; chlamydospores may be present	Fifty per cent of isolates are stimulated by thiamine, others are autotrophic
T. equinum	Cream colored; flat; fluffy; reverse yellow, becoming red or brown	Pyriform or spherical microconidia; macroconidia rare	Requires nicotinic acid; an autotrophic variety has been described (70)
T. gourvilii	Pink to red; heaped up; convoluted; glabrous; a brown pigment may diffuse into the medium	Macroconidia and microconidia usually found	
T. megninii	Pink to rose; radially folded; suede-like; wine red on reverse	Pyriform to clavate microconidia; macroconidia rare	Requires l-histidine
T. mentagrophytes	Cream, tan, or pink; flat; powdery to granular or fluffy; light tan, yellow, or red on reverse	Round to pyriform microconidia, often in clusters; macroconidia present in some isolates; coiled hyphae (spirals) usually seen	Urease positive; perforates hair *in vitro*; grows at 37°C
T. mentagrophytes var. *erinacei*	Cream colored; flat with central elevation; powdery becoming velvety; brilliant yellow on reverse; pigment diffuses into the medium	Microconidia numerous, elongated; macroconidia irregular in size, 2–6 celled; intermediate forms numerous	
T. rubrum	White; fluffy (seldom powdery); usually wine red on reverse, but sometimes yellow, orange, or melanoid; melanoid pigment diffuses into the medium	Pyriform microconidia usually along unbranched hyphae; macroconidia rare, thin, and elongate to clavate in granular cultures	Urease test usually negative; *in vitro* hair perforation test negative; cornmeal dextrose agar stimulates production of red pigment
T. schoenleinii	White to tan; elevated and convoluted; glabrous or waxy, becoming velvety on subculture; reverse lacks pigment; slow growing	Micro- and macroconidia rarely seen; chlamydospores often numerous; hyphal tips often show "nail head" morphology and branch to form antler-like structures (favic chandeliers)	Autotrophic for vitamins, differentiating it from *T. verrucosum*

TABLE 48.7—(Continued)

	COLONY ON SABOURAUD DEXTROSE AGAR	MICROSCOPIC MORPHOLOGY	DIFFERENTIAL FEATURES
T. simii	Pale to buff; flat or slightly convoluted; powdery; straw to salmon on reverse	Numerous macroconidia which may fragment or develop chlamydospores resembling chlamydospores; pyriform microconidia may be present; spirals may be found	
T. soudanense	Yellow orange (like dried apricots); flat with convolutions; suedelike texture; fringed (eyelash) periphery; yellow to orange yellow on reverse; slow growing	Pyriform microconidia are rare; macroconidia not reported; reflex branching characteristic	Reflex branching
T. tonsurans	Color varies with isolate (yellow, cream, white, pink, brown, gray, etc.); usually convoluted, sometimes flat; velvety to powdery; dark brown to mahogany red on reverse; slow growing	Clavate to elongate microconidia, some swollen into balloonlike forms and some 2-celled, attached to branched conidiophore by short sterigmata; macroconidia rare	Stimulated by thiamine
T. verrucosum	White to yellowish tan; heaped, flat, or convoluted; glabrous or downy; no reverse pigment; slow growing	Usually no micro- or macroconidia; chlamydospores usually numerous and form chains	All isolates require thiamine; most require inositol as well; growth stimulated at 37 C
var. *album*	White; heaped and folded; glabrous to downy		
var. *discoides*	Cream to tan; flat to discoid, velvety		
var. *ochraceum*	Yellow ochre; convoluted; glabrous		
T. violaceum	Violet or lavender; heaped and convoluted; glabrous or velvety; purple undersurface; slow growing	Microconidia and macroconidia usually lacking; chlamydospores may be found	Growth stimulated by thiamine
T. yaoundei	Initially buff, turning to chocolate brown; convoluted; glabrous; brown on reverse, diffusible; slow growing	Microconidia rare; macroconidia not found; chlamydospores seen	

TABLE 48.8—CHARACTERISTICS OF RARELY PATHOGENIC *MICROSPORUM* AND *TRICHOPHYTON* SPECIES

SPECIES	COLONY ON SABOURAUD AGAR	MICROSCOPIC
Microsporum		
M. cookei	Yellowish to reddish tan; flat; powdery, granular or downy; reverse dark purple-red	Macroconidia numerous and resembling *M. gypseum* but differentiated by presence of thick walls (1–5 μm); microconidia abundant
M. racemosum	White, cream or buff; flat; finely granular; reverse dark purple-red	Macroconidia abundant, fusiform to ellipsoidal, 41–77 μm × 9–16 μm, 3–8 septa, moderately thick walls, numerous microconidia, mostly stalked and produced in grapelike clusters
M. vanbreuseghemii	Pink to deep rose, light buff or yellowish; flat; coarsely granular to downy; reverse cream to pale yellow	Abundant cylindrofusiform macroconidia, 43.8–87.5 μm × 8–13.5 μm, thick-walled, up to 12 septa; numerous pyriform to obovate microconidia borne singly along sides of hyphae
Trichophyton		
T. ajelloi (*Keratinomyces*)	White, cream or orange-tan; flat; powdery; reverse typically blackish-purple or sometimes nonpigmented	Macroconidia numerous, cylindrofusiform, 42–54 μm × 8–10 μm, thick walled, multiseptate, (5–12 celled); microconidia rare
T. terrestre complex	White, pale yellow to pink; flat; granular to downy; reverse pale yellow, yellowish-brown, or pink to vinaceous red	Macroconidia clavate to cylindrical; thin-walled 2–6 celled; microconidia clavate to pyriform borne singly or in groups; intermediate forms transitional between micro- and macroconidia characteristic

tinea corporis (face and trunk), tinea axillaris (armpits), tinea cruris (groin), tinea pedis (feet), tinea manuum (hands), and tinea unguium (nails).

Terms describing the morphology of the lesions have also been coined: (a) tinea circinata, for infections showing discrete circular lesions with a raised border; (b) tinea imbricata, for lesions showing concentric layers of scales whose borders overlap like tiles on a roof (imbricate pattern); (c) kerion of Celsi, for raised, boggy, inflammatory lesions with a smooth, pink-to-red surface and pustules; (d) Majocchi's granuloma, for lesions involving deeper tissues around hair follicles; and (e) favus (or tinea favosa), for infections producing a honeycomb pattern of saucer-like depressions called scutula (tiny shields).

Specifics

Brief descriptions of the various clinical manifestations follow. Descriptions of hair infections are summarized in Table 48.10.

Tinea capitis. This infection is characterized by one or more areas of alopecia (bald spots) caused by the breaking-off of hairs invaded by the fungus. The disease occurs mostly in children, but certain fungi (i.e., *T. tonsurans* and *T. schoenleinii*) produce lesions that persist into adulthood. The clinical picture is influenced by the infecting fungus. The *Microsporum* species, *T. mentagrophytes* and *T. verrucosum,* produce arthrospores outside the hair so that infected hairs are covered with a grayish sheath (ectothrix infection). Hairs break off 2–5 mm above skin level. When seen under Wood's light (filtered ultraviolet light, peak wavelength 365 nm), *Microsporum*-infected hairs may emit a greenish fluorescence. The skin surface is also invaded by hyphae.

In *T. tonsurans* and *T. violaceum* infections, the arthrospores are produced inside the hair (i.e., endothrix infection). The hairs break off flush with the scalp, and the subsurface hairs coil into minute knots resembling dots under the scaly skin surface. These infections in patients with dark hair are called "black dot tinea." Certain patients respond to fungal infection of the scalp with an acute inflammatory reaction, resulting in raised, smooth-surfaced, pink-to-red, boggy, pustular lesions (kerions). Kerions are usually produced in response to zoophilic fungi such as *M. canis* and *T. mentagrophytes* variety *mentagrophytes* and *T. verruscosum* or to geophilic fungi such as *M. gypseum,* although other dermatophytes may elicit them on occasion.

TABLE 48.9—SOME SAPROPHYTIC FUNGI MISTAKEN FOR DERMATOPHYTES

SAPROPHYTE	DERMATOPHYTE	SAPROPHYTE DIFFERENTIATED FROM THE DERMATOPHYTE BY:
1. *Chrysosporium tropicum*	*T. mentagrophytes*	Larger microcondidia (3–4 μm × 6–7 μm) may be slightly roughened, pyriform to clavate, with a broadly truncate base
2. *C. keratinophilum*	*M. nanum*	Aseptate conidia, typically smooth (may be slightly roughened); colony granular
3. *Trichothecium roseum*	*M. nanum*	Smooth conidial walls; conidia produced in short chains at apex of simple conidiophore and remain as a group if undisturbed (slide culture recommended)
4. *Trichophyton terrestre*	*T. mentagrophytes*	Transitional forms of spores intermediate between microconidia and macroconidia; species studied show poor or no growth at 37 C (51). Perfect states: *A. quadrifidum, A. lenticularum, A. insingulare*
5. *Fusarium* species	*T. rubrum*	Crescent- or boat-shaped macroconidia; microspores characteristically in short chains or clusters
6. *Drechslera* sp. and *Helminthosporium* sp.	*Microsporum* or *Epidermophyton*	Dark colonies and spores

TABLE 48.10—GENERAL CHARACTERISTICS OF HAIR INFECTIONS BY DERMATOPHYTES IN HUMANS

DISEASE NAME AND VARIATIONS	SITE AND TYPE OF INFECTION	MOST PREVALENT IN:	USUALLY CAUSED BY:
A. Tinea capitis	Scalp	Children	
Gray patch ringworm	Bald, scaly spot with straight hair stumps	Children	*M. canis, M. audouinii*
Black dot tinea	Bald, scaly spot with coiled hair stumps (black dots)	Children and adults	*T. tonsurans, T. violaceum*
Kerion Celsi	Raised, inflammatory, and pustular bald area	Children	*M. canis, M. gypseum, T. mentagrophytes, T. tonsurans, T. verrucosum, T. violaceum*
B. Favus	Scalp and glabrous skin; honeycombed clusters of saucer-shaped depressions; mousy odor; permanent hair loss	Children and adults	*T. schoenleinii*
C. Tinea barbae	Bearded area	Adult men	
Dry	Scaly with straight hair stumps		*T. megninii, T. mentagrophytes*
Suppurating	Inflammatory; pustular	Dairy farmers	*T. verrucosum*

1. Observe colony for the development of surface and reverse pigments, characteristic topography, texture, and rate of growth. Consult identification charts (Tables 48.7–48.9) to arrive at a presumptive identification.
2. Prepare one or more teased mounts and search for identifying structures under various powers of the compound microscope (Figures 48.21–48.35; Tables 48.7–48.9). If this search is insufficient, then proceed to step 3.
3. Prepare, incubate, mount, and similarly examine slide cultures. If this step is still inconclusive, then proceed to step 4.
4. Perform the following physiological tests as necessary (see text for details of procedure).
   A. Hair perforation
   B. Urease production
   C. Nutritional requirements (if a *Trichophyton* is suspected)
   D. Growth on rice grains (if a *Microsporum* is suspected) (teased mounts from growth on media used on tests C and D often reveal identifying structures that had been absent on routine media)
   E. Effect on growth of incubation at 37 C
   F. Production of asci and ascospores (or at least mating reaction) when paired with known dermatophyte tester strains
5. Arrive at final identification.

Figure 48.10—Sequence of procedures for identification of dermatophytes in pure culture.

Tinea barbae. This infection occurs in two clinical forms: dry and suppurative. In dry lesions (sycosis barbae), the beard involvement resembles the gray patches of alopecia described for tinea capitis. The hairs break off a few millimeters above the skin surface, leaving a straight hair stump surrounded by a sheath of arthrospores. The most common agent of dry tinea barbae in the United States is *T. mentagrophytes*, although cases produced by *T. rubrum* have been reported (21). When the *T. mentagrophytes* infection is of animal origin, kerions are produced on the bearded area. In Europe, particularly Portugal, France, and Belgium (50, 68), dry tinea barbae is produced by *T. megninii.*

Suppurative tinea barbae is most often seen among dairy farmers who contract *T. verrucosum* infections from cattle. The kerions are raised, erythematous, pustular, and boggy. Infected hairs are broken off a few millimeters above the skin, but are also loosened by the inflammatory process and often fall out spontaneously. Since some of the remaining hairs may not be infected, it is essential to collect many to increase the chances that some of them will contain fungal elements. It is also important to culture a large number of hairs (10 or 12). As mentioned elsewhere, *T. verrucosum* grows fastest at 37 C. Primary cultures should be incubated at this temperature.

Tinea corporis. This term usually refers to dermatophyte infections of the glabrous skin, excluding nails or intertriginous areas. As in tinea capitis, the lesions of tinea corporis vary depending on the patient's age and on the causative fungus. In children, face lesions commonly accompany fungous infections of the scalp, particularly those produced by *M. canis* or *M. audouinii.* Acute lesions of this sort are circinate, i.e., circular, with a raised, active border. Similar lesions may also appear on the wrists, neck, and throat area, but rarely on

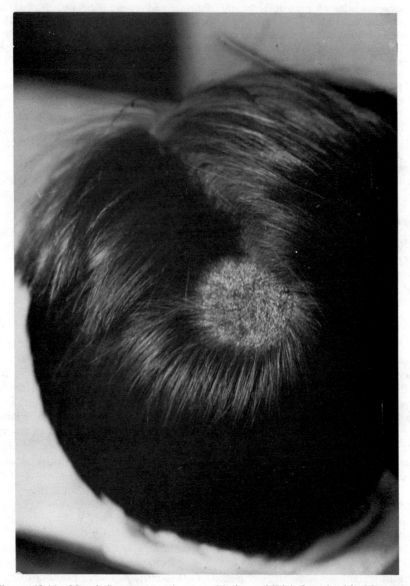

Figure 48.11—Non-inflammatory tinea capitis in a child infected with *Microsporum canis*. Note circular area of alopecia with scaly surface and remaining hair stumps, each showing a grayish sheath (ectothrix arthrospores). (See also Fig 48.12 and 48.13).

the face, of the mother or other young adults in contact with an infected child. These lesions are seldom seen in the elderly, who are more likely to suffer from chronic tinea corporis.

In contrast to acute tinea circinata, chronic dematophyte lesions of the

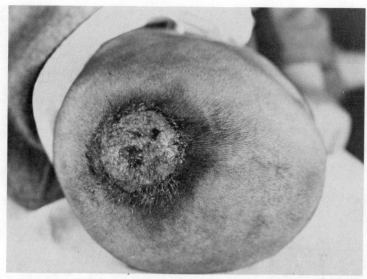

Figure 48.12—Inflammatory (kerion type) lesion also produced by *M. canis* in another child.

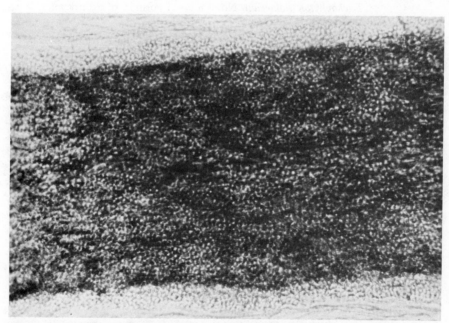

Figure 48.13—Photomicrograph of hair with ectothrix type of infection by *M. canis*. Note mosaic of spherical arthrospores surrounding hair and extending as a sheath beyond its perimeter. KOH preparation. ×1000.

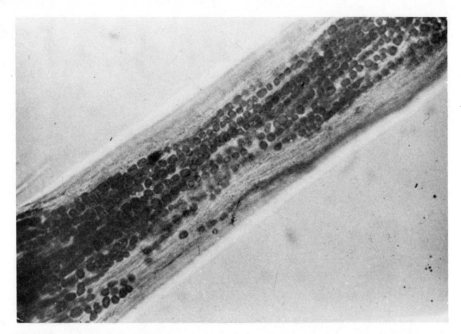

Figure 48.14—Photomicrograph of hair with endothrix type of infection produced by *Trichophyton violaceum.* Note internal position of arthrospores. Polychrome-blue stain. ×600.

glabrous skin are more often found throughout the trunk and extremities, occasionally invading the face, and they are frequently associated with tinea pedis and tinea manuum. On a world-wide basis, *T. rubrum* is the most common agent of this type of generalized, chronic infection. In localized geographic areas, other species, such as *T. tonsurans, T. schoenleinii,* and *T. concentricum,* may predominate. The clinical picture of *T. tonsurans* lesions is less generalized, showing local spreading areas of induration and a granulomatous reaction. Lesions caused by *T. schoenleinii* occur on the glabrous skin and the scalp of both children and adults. These lesions are characteristically funnel- or saucer-shaped depressions (scutula) centered around hair follicles. They may occur in clusters over extensive areas.

Tinea imbricata, caused by *T. concentricum,* is a distinct type of tinea corporis in which the lesions appear as concentric circles of imbricate (overhanging) scales, like tiles on a roof. The lesions cover the trunk, face, and extremities.

Tinea unguium. The toe- or fingernail undergoes one or more of the following changes as a result of the infection: is discolored (yellow or white), loses hardness and is easily crumbled, thickens, becomes grooved, separates from the nail bed, and/or accumulates subungual debris. The most frequent cause of tinea unguium is *T. rubrum.* Superficial chalk-white discolorations are pro-

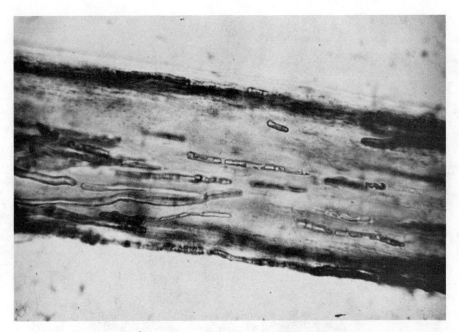

Figure 48.15—Photomicrograph of hair from case of favus (*T. schoenleinii* infection). Note internal septate hyphae and "air tunnels," i.e., digested portions of hair replaced by trapped air. KOH preparation. ×600.

duced most often by *T. mentagrophytes. E. floccosum* nail infections are less frequent.

In addition to dermatophytes, other fungi such as species of *Aspergillus, Candida, Fusarium,* and *Scopulariopsis* can infect nails causing a clinically similar condition called onychomycosis (see following section on opportunistic dermatomycosis).

Tinea cruris. Lesions in the groin area are characterized by sharply demarcated, raised edges on which scales and vesicles may appear. *T. rubrum* and *E. floccosum* are the most common agents. These lesions, which are red or tawny-brown, must be differentiated from clinically similar lesions caused by *Candida* and from erythrasma.

Tinea pedis. This disease varies widely in its clinical manifestations. The most common is the interdigital (intertriginous) type, with maceration, peeling, itching, and painful fissuring. The spaces between the fourth and fifth toes are most frequently attacked. The soles may have hyperkeratotic patches or blisters. The most common agents of tinea pedis are *T. mentagrophytes* and *T. rubrum.* The former frequently causes inflammatory, vesicular lesions, while *T. rubrum* more often causes hyperkeratotic, chronic lesions. *E. floccosum* is third in frequency.

Tinea manuum. This condition appears most frequently as a unilateral, diffuse hyperkeratosis of the palm and fingers. Other clinical manifestations

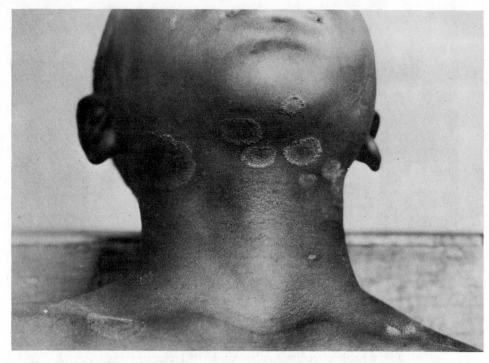

Figure 48.16—Tinea faciei and corporis in a child infected with *M. audouinii.* Note abrupt, raised, scaly, and vesicular border of the lesions. These are usually contracted from a sibling with tinea capitis.

are exfoliation, papules, and follicular patches. The most frequent agent is *T. rubrum,* less frequently *T. mentagrophytes.* Tinea manuum must be differentiated from "dermatophytid" reactions, which appear on the fingers in response to a dermatophyte infection on another part of the body. These lesions are sterile and allergic.

Epidemiology

Prevalence

Since ringworm and other superficial fungous infections are not reported to public health departments, the true number of such infections is not known. On the basis of sales of antidermatophyte medications, the prevalence of infection appears considerable (3). A recent clinical and laboratory survey (41) of over 20,000 persons in the United States has given some data on the approximate prevalence of fungal infections. These data show that fungal infections constitute the second largest group of skin conditions in the general population (81 per 1,000), second only to diseases of the sebaceous glands (85 per 1,000). This means about 15.7 million persons in the United States have at least one fungous infection.

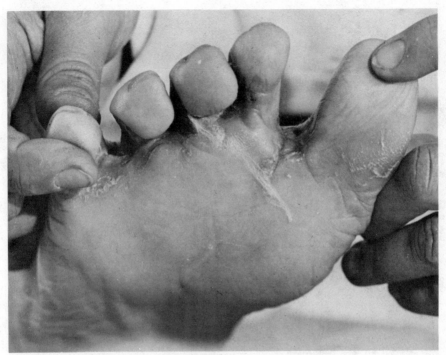

Figure 48.17—Tinea pedis. Non-inflammatory, scaly, desquamating lesions of inter-digital and sub-digital areas seen in chronic cases.

Table 48.11 lists the estimated prevalence of the most common superficial fungous diseases. In addition, the table shows that males were more frequently infected than females, with an overall ratio > 3:1. In the case of tinea cruris, the ratio was almost 14:1.

Contagion

Tinea capitis. This highly contagious disease spreads rapidly within a family or a school community. The great Eastern United States epidemic caused

TABLE 48.11—PREVALENCE OF SUPERFICIAL FUNGOUS INFECTIONS IN THE UNITED STATES*

	RATE PER 1,000 PERSONS	TOTAL NUMBER OF CASES (in millions)	MALE TO FEMALE RATIO
Tinea pedis	38.7	7.5	6:1
Tinea unguium	21.8	4.2	2:1
Tinea versicolor	8.4	1.6	2:1
Tinea cruris	6.7	1.3	14:1
Other tineas	5.5	1.1	
Totals	81.1	15.7	4:1

* Constructed from data of Johnson and Roberts (41).

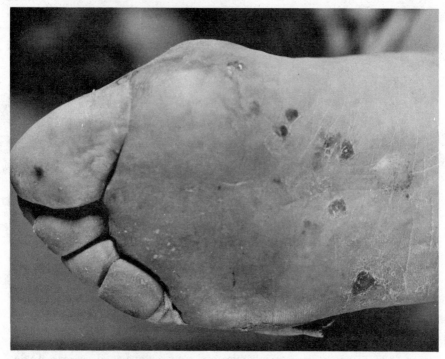

Figure 48.18—Blister formation in acute tinea pedis caused by *T. mentagrophytes.*

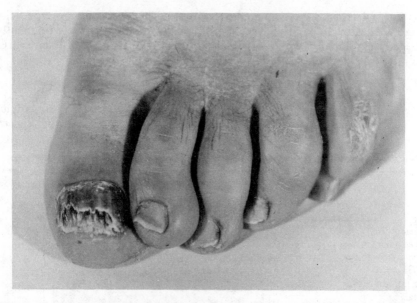

Figure 48.19—Onychomycosis of large toe nail. Note smooth surface of nail with thickened, darkened, subungual debris.

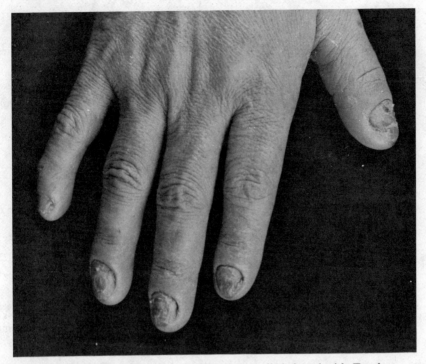

Figure 48.20—Onychomycosis of five fingernails infected with *T. rubrum.*

by *M. audouinii* during the 1940's (49) is an example of the extent of contagion and spread of tinea capitis. *M. audouinii* is an anthropophilic fungus. Thus, the person-to-person chain of transmission has to be broken to terminate an epidemic.

In recent years, *M. canis* and *T. tonsurans* have replaced *M. audouinii* as the principal causes of ringworm of the scalp in the same area, although they are less prevalent than was *M. audouinii* at the height of the epidemic mentioned.

The advent of griseofulvin as an effective antidermatophyte agent has apparently greatly changed the prevalence of tinea capitis. Many cases are treated without specific diagnosis of the etiologic agent. Furthermore, since the disease is not reported to public health authorities, its actual incidence and the prevalence of a particular etiologic fungus are difficult to ascertain. *M. canis* is frequently contracted from cats, and to a lesser degree from dogs, monkeys, and other furry pets. Public health officers should know that animals can now be effectively treated, rather than destroyed, in combating the source of *M. canis* infections.

Another recent change in the epidemiology of tinea capitis in North America is the increasing prevalence of *T. tonsurans* as an etiologic agent. This fungal species is believed to have been brought into the United States from Mexico, Central and South America, and the Caribbean area. There is also a

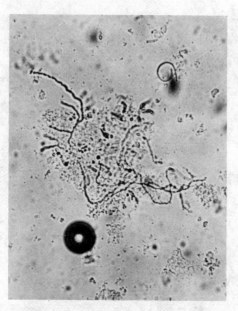

Figure 48.21—Photomicrograph of dermatophytic hyphae in KOH preparation of skin scrapings. Note branching, septate hyphae beginning to fragment into arthrospores. ×150. (See Fig 48.22).

long-standing focus of *T. tonsurans* infections in adults in the French areas of the province of Quebec in Canada (16).

Tinea pedis. The epidemiology of tinea pedis is still a controversial subject. Some believe that contact with dermatophytes incites clinical disease. Others feel that host factors, such as immunologic status, are the determinants of infection and that exogenous exposure to dermatophytes is relatively unimportant. There is evidence to support both points of view.

The following facts support the theory that exogenous exposure to dermatophytes is important in transmitting tinea pedis:

(a) *Viable dermatophytes are readily shed from the feet of persons with tinea pedis.* These fungi have been recovered from areas where people walk barefooted (i.e., the floors of shower rooms) and from towels, shoes, and socks (7, 31, 32, 37).

(b) *Epidemiologic data suggest person-to-person transmission.* The incidence of tinea pedis increased threefold when communal showers were installed in a coal mine for use by the workers (34). Within families of patients with *T. rubrum* infections, other infections of this same species tend to occur (47). However, when extreme precautions are taken to prevent contact between a person with tinea pedis and other members of his household, no cross-infection occurs (26).

(c) *Strains of dermatophytes isolated within families are similar.* The growth characteristics of the isolates of *T. rubrum* isolated from

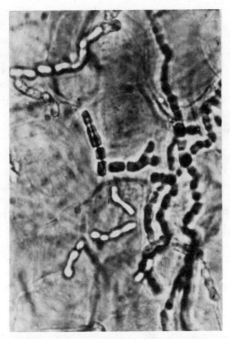

Figure 48.22—More advanced stage in arthrospore formation. KOH preparation. ×1000.

various persons within a family are often morphologically similar (26).

The following facts support the theory that exogenous exposure to dermatophytes is *not* important in transmitting tinea pedis:

(a) *Experimental infection has failed.* The fungus-free feet of volunteers were placed in foot baths containing high concentrations of viable dermatophytes, either from culture material or in scales directly from the feet of patients with tinea pedis. Clinical fungous infection of the feet was not induced in any of 68 subjects thus exposed (11). Only when the feet were deliberately damaged (blistered with cantharidin) before exposure could "takes" be induced (10).

(b) *Person-to-person transmission has rarely been demonstrated.* Contrary to the epidemiologic data cited above supporting the importance of direct contact in transmitting tinea pedis, other similar studies support the opposite view. A survey of 88 dermatologists in the United States (72) on the contagiousness of tinea pedis and tinea cruris among their patients revealed only four instances out of surely hundreds of thousands where family transmission was strongly suspected.

Hopkins et al. (39) examined groups of soldiers at an army base during World War II and found that the species of dermatophytes occurred in about the same ratio in all groups examined. If contagion were important in the spread of tinea pedis, one would expect a particular species to predominate within an individual group of soldiers. This has not been the case, except for one instance involving *T. mentagrophytes* infection (*A. benhamiae,* mating type '-') among American soldiers in the Mekong Delta in Vietnam (9, 17, 58). In this case, however, an exogenous source of infection was implicated, rather than human-to-human transmission. This was aggravated by factors such as poor hygiene, excess moisture, and occlusive clothing, particularly combat boots.

(c) *Dermatophytes are found on clinically normal feet.* Most surveys indicate that dermatophytes can be isolated from feet which do not have clinically apparent infection, with the incidence of isolation ranging from 1% to 40% (64).

Tinea cruris. Person-to-person transmission of tinea cruris apparently occurs rarely (72), although Beare, Gentles, and Mackenzie (14) think the disease can be transmitted by sharing towels and clothing.

Tinea corporis. There is little evidence that tinea corporis is transmissible, except for the fact that acute infections are frequently associated with episodes of tinea capitis in the immediate contacts of the patient with glabrous skin le-

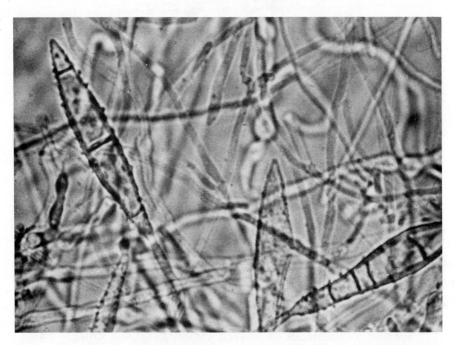

Figure 48.23—Macroconidia of *M. audouinii* on Sabouraud honey agar plus yeast extract. Note rough-walled, fusiform spores with septa at irregular intervals and with thickened outer walls. Lactophenol preparation. ×1000.

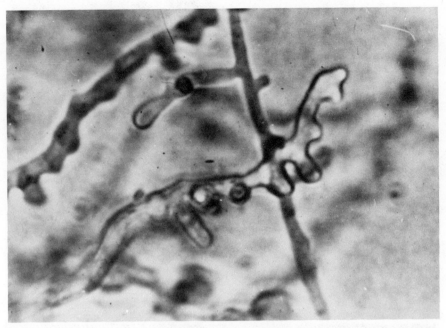

Figure 48.24—Pectinate organs (curved hyphae with many short side branches). These structures are abundantly produced on Sabouraud agar by cultures of *M. audouinii* and aid in its identification. Lactophenol preparation. ×1000.

sions. Chronic tinea corporis is not considered contagious, but evidence of the special susceptibility of a given patient.

Tinea unguium. There is little evidence of contagion in tinea unguium, particularly since some patients continue for many years with only two or three toenails or fingernails involved and without the infection spreading to any of the adjacent nails.

Ecology

The dermatophytes and related nonpathogenic species may be grouped into three categories based on host preference and natural habitat (Table 48.12). Certain species infect humans and rarely infect animals; these are the anthropophilic dermatophytes. Others, the zoophilic species, primarily infect animals. The geophilic dermatophytes are essentially soil organisms and usually have a world-wide distribution.

Anthropophilic dermatophytes. These fungi are found in the genera *Microsporum, Trichophyton,* and *Epidermophyton.* They infect humans almost exclusively. Some of the rare animal infections have been traced to sustained close human contact. There is no evidence of a saprophytic niche in nature. Infection in humans is attributed directly to close contact or indirectly to fomites (combs, brushes, chair backs, floors, bed linens, etc.) or aerosols, which may

TABLE 48.12—GROUPING OF THE DERMATOPHYTES AND RELATED KERATINOPHILIC FUNGI ON
THE BASIS OF NATURAL HABITAT AND HOST PREFERENCE

ANTHROPOPHILIC	ZOOPHILIC	GEOPHILIC
M. audouinii	M. canis	M. amazonicum
M. ferrugineum	M. distortum	M. boullardii
T. concentricum	M. gallinae	M. cookei
T. gourvilli	M. persicolor	M. fulvum
T. megninii	T. equinum	M. gypseum
T. mentagrophytes	T. mentagrophytes	M. nanum
var. interdigitale	(var. mentagrophytes,	M. racemosum
T. rubrum	var. quinckeanum,	M. ripariae
T. schoenleinii	and var. erinacei)	M. vanbreuseghemii
T. soudanense	T. verrucosum	T. ajelloi
T. tonsurans		T. georgiae
T. violaceum		T. gloriae
E. floccosum		T. phaseoliforme
		T. simii
		T. terrestre complex
		T. vanbreuseghemii
		E. stockdaleae

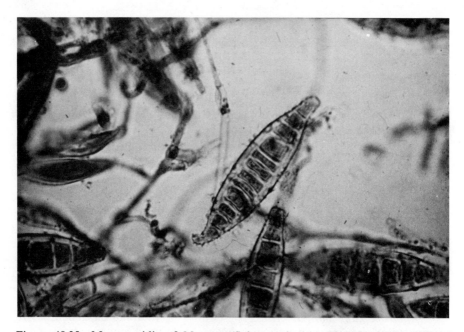

Figure 48.25—Macroconidia of *M. canis* (Sabouraud agar). Note knob-like ends of
fusiform spores with rough walls thickest at level of medial septa. These
occur at regular intervals unlike those of *M. audouinii* (Fig 48.23). Lactophenol-blue preparation accounts for darker staining of cytoplasm.
×1000. Compare with Figure 48.26.

carry the infected scales and hair to others. *M. audouinii, T. rubrum, T. tonsurans, T. mentagrophytes* var. *interdigitale,* and *E. floccosum* are examples.

Zoophilic dermatophytes. These fungi of the genera *Microsporum* and *Trichophyton* are primarily animal parasites. Human infections are acquired directly by contact with the animal or indirectly by contact with infected hair, feathers, or scales from the animal. Commonly recognized zoophilic fungi include *M. canis, T. mentagrophytes* var. *mentagrophytes,* and *T. verrucosum.*

Geophilic dermatophytes and closely related species. This category includes

TABLE 48.13—DERMATOPHYTES CAUSING NATURAL INFECTIONS IN DOMESTIC AND WILD ANIMALS*

ANIMAL	DERMATOPHYTE
1. Cat	
Frequent:	*M. canis,*[†] *M. distortum* (New Zealand), *M. gypseum* complex, *T. mentagrophytes*
Rare or unconfirmed:	*M. audouinii, M. gallinae, M. vanbreuseghemii, T. rubrum, T. schoenleinii, T. verrucosum, T. violaceum*
2. Dog	
Frequent:	*M. canis,*[†] *M. gypseum* complex, *T. mentagrophytes*
Rare or unconfirmed:	*M. audouinii, M. cookei, M. distortum, M. gallinae, M. nanum, M. persicolor, M. vanbreuseghemii, T. ajelloi, T. equinum, T. rubrum, T. simii, T. verrucosum, T. violaceum, E. floccosum*
3. Horse	
Frequent:	*M. gypseum, T. equinum,*[†] *T. mentagrophytes, T. verrucosum*
Occasional:	*M. canis* (includes *M. equinum*)
Rare or unconfirmed:	*M. distortum*
4. Cattle	
Frequent:	*T. verrucosum*[†]
Occasional:	*T. mentagrophytes*
Rare or unconfirmed:	*M. canis, M. gypseum* complex
5. Pig	
Frequent:	*M. nanum*[†]
Occasional:	*T. mentagrophytes*
Rare or unconfirmed:	*M. canis*
6. Nonhuman Primates	
Frequent:	*M. canis,*[†] *T. mentagrophytes, T. simii*[†] (India)
Occasional:	*M. gypseum*
Rare or unconfirmed:	*M. audouinii, M. cookei, M. distortum, M. gallinae, M. gypseum* complex, *T. rubrum*
7. Fowl	
Frequent:	*M. gallinae,*[†] *T. simii* (India)
Rare or unconfirmed:	*M. gypesum* complex, *T. verrucosum*
8. Rodents	
Frequent:	*M. gypseum* complex, *T. mentagrophytes*[†]
Occasional:	*M. canis, M. persicolor*
Rare or unconfirmed:	*M. gallinae, M. vanbreuseghemii*

* Modified from Rebell and Taplin (56), Rippon (59), and Ainsworth and Austwick (1).

[†] Most common etiologic agent.

members of the genera *Microsporum* and *Trichophyton* and may include a new species of *Epidermophyton, E. stockdalae* isolated from the soil (54). These fungi generally inhabit the soil and are often associated with keratinaceous material acting as an enrichment medium. Exposure to soil is the main source of infection for humans and animals, although direct and indirect contact with infected humans and animals is also a mode of transmission.

Members of the *M. gypseum* complex are representative geophilic dermatophytes. *M. nanum,* included in this category, has been reported as zoophilic since it primarily infects pigs (8) and is isolated from pig yards. However, the presence of typical macroconidia in pig yards suggests its saprophytic existence in soil, especially since macroconidia are not formed *in vivo* (8). Included among the geophilic species are those *Microsporum* and *Trichophyton* species isolated from the fur of small, wild mammals that do not have lesions (*M. amazonicum,* for example) or from the feathers and nests of birds (*M. ripariae*). Additional studies may indicate a soil origin for these fungi or a change in category.

Dermatophyte species that naturally infect domestic and wild animals are listed in Table 48.13 (1, 56, 59).

To date, the perfect state of the dermatophytes has been obtained in some of the geophilic and zoophilic species and in only one of the anthropophilic species.

Geographic distribution

Although certain species of dermatophytes are most prevalent in or near the geographic regions where they were first described (Table 48.14), their presence is not restricted to that area. The increasing frequency and speed of

TABLE 48.14—GEOGRAPHIC DISTRIBUTION OF THE DERMATOPHYTES*

SPECIES	AREA OF FREQUENT ISOLATION
Epidermophyton floccosum	Cosmopolitan
Microsporum audouinii	United States, Africa, Western Europe
M. canis	Scandinavia, England, United States
M. ferrugineum	Japan, China, Russia, Africa
M. gypseum complex	Cosmopolitan
Trichophyton concentricum	Southeast Asia, South Pacific Islands, Central and South America, and Mexico
T. gourvilii	Africa
T. megninii	Portugal, Sardinia
T. mentagrophytes	Cosmopolitan
T. rubrum	Cosmopolitan
T. simii	India
T. schoenleinii	Mediterranean area, Western Russia, Europe
T. soudanense	Africa
T. tonsurans	Cuba, Mexico, United States, South America
T. verrucosum	Cosmopolitan
T. yaoundei	Africa

* Modified from Rippon (59).

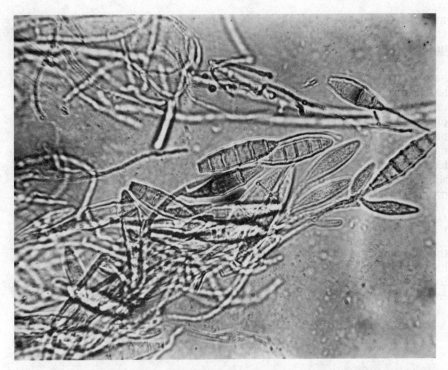

Figure 48.26—Macroconidia of *M. gypseum* on Sabouraud agar. Note shorter, blunter
shape of spores, fewer numbers of septa, and uniformity in thickness of
spore wall. Compared to *M. canis* (Figure 48.25). Lactophenol preparation. ×450.

travel and migration have helped distribute these exotic dermatophytes, so
that cases are encountered far from the original geographic niche for a given
species. Therefore, it is important for laboratories to maintain the ability to
identify exotic as well as domestic species, since the former will occasionally be
isolated.

Among the "foreign" species which have been reported in the United
States are *T. soudanense* (40, 62), and *T. simii* (61). In addition, three isolates of
T. yaoundei (identification of first isolate confirmed at Center for Disease Control, Atlanta, Georgia) have been recovered by M. Zuckrow in New York City
(personal communication) from tinea capitis in children born abroad: a
brother and sister from Zaire and a child from Zambia. *T. megninii* was reported in Canada (43).

Knowledge of the geographic origin or ethnic contacts of a patient can
provide clues leading to the identification of an unusual isolate.

Collection and Processing of Specimens

The proper collection of a specimen of hair, skin, or nails for mycologic
diagnosis of a cutaneous lesion requires the following steps: (a) clinical examination of the lesion to observe its characteristics and determine the type of

specimen to collect; (b) selection of the proper instruments for obtaining a suitable specimen; (c) obtaining enough material for both microscopic and cultural studies.

Dermatophytes can survive for long periods in dried specimens of skin, hair, and nails; therefore, it is neither urgent nor necessary to culture these materials at the time specimens are collected. It is inadvisable, however, to store the specimens in impermeable containers, such as tightly sealed glass vials or plastic wrapping. The high humidity thus generated encourages the growth of bacteria, yeast, and saprophytic fungi, making the cultural isolation of the dermatophyte more difficult. If the laboratory is distant, specimens can be collected and mailed between glass slides, or better still in paper envelopes; glass slides are often crushed by postal cancellation devices unless the slides are properly packaged for mailing.

Hair infections (tinea capitis, tinea barbae)

Clinical examination. Lesions usually appear as an area of baldness or thinning hair growth (scalp or beard). This is because the fungus invades the hair follicles and penetrates the hair near its base, weakening it until the hair fractures and leaves a straight stump or a "dot." The "dot" is formed by the coiled end of the fractured hair at the follicular opening.

Collection of specimens.

(a) Examine the lesion under Wood's light to see if infected hairs fluoresce. The fluorescence appears as a green, green-blue, or silver-

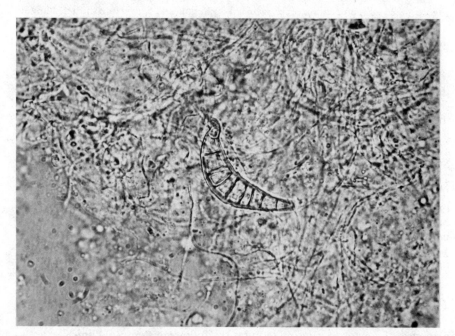

Figure 48.27—Macroconidium of *M. distortum* on Sabouraud agar. Note characteristic boomerang (bent) shape of spore. Lactophenol preparation. ×600.

green color. This can be a clue to the etiologic agent and helps select infected hairs for study. Once a lesion has been shown to fluoresce, the disappearance of fluorescence indicates healing. Not all infected hairs fluoresce, depending on the species of fungus causing the infection.

(b) Using fine forceps, such as eyebrow tweezers, pluck individual hair *stumps* (i.e., hairs that have broken off close to the skin as result of the infection). Fluorescent hairs, if present, are choice materials. The coiled hairs of "black dot tinea" can be lifted with eyebrow tweezers or shaved off with a scalpel. However, the use of a scalpel is discouraged since it creates a fungal aerosol (30).

(c) Collect 5–10 such stumps and place them between two glass slides or inside a petri dish. Half of the material can be used for direct examination, the other half for culture.

Glabrous skin infections

Clinical examination. The lesions should be examined for raised borders, scales, vesicles, and/or areas of maceration and fissures. These constitute the active sites of fungal invasion and are the best areas from which to collect material for mycologic study.

Collection of specimens. Scales should be collected on a slide or petri dish

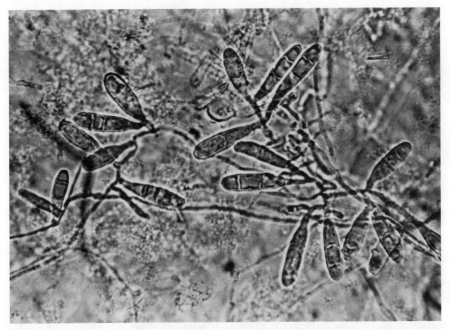

Figure 48.28—Macroconidia of *Epidermophyton floccosum* on Sabouraud agar. Note clusters of clavate (club-shaped) macroconidia with 1–3 septa, smooth walls and rounded distal ends. Lactophenol-blue preparation. ×450.

by scraping the site of infection with a dull, sterile scalpel or spatula. These instruments should be held perpendicular to the surface of the skin to tear off,
rather than cut, the material being collected. Firm strokes usually dislodge
enough scales or vesicle tops. If the vesicles are large (as on the soles of the
feet), the roof of one or more should be cut off with sterile scissors and used for
microscopic examination and culture.

Nail infections

Clinical examination. Inspection of the nails will reveal whether the infection is: (a) superficial (chalky), (b) paronychial (starting from the cuticle fold),
or (c) eponychial (occurring under the nail with accumulation of subungual
debris and/or separation of the nail from the nail bed).

Collection of specimens. The point or side of a scalpel is adequate for collecting material from the first two types of nail infections, since the fungal elements are readily accessible to direct scraping. If the nails are hard and thick,
however, one must bore a small hole or groove using the tip of a pointed scalpel; nail clippings are less suitable for mycologic examination. The surface material from the hole or groove should be discarded, since it does not contain
fungal elements or may contain contaminants or nonviable dermatophyte
hyphae. It is in the waxy, yellowish subungual debris that the viable fungal

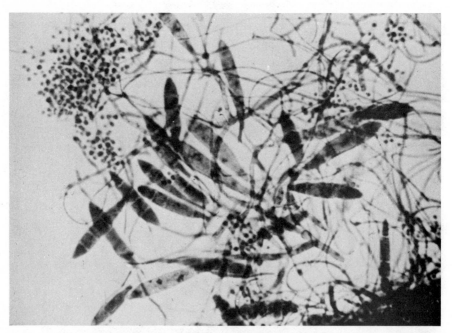

Figure 48.29—Micro- and macroconidia of *T. mentagrophytes* var. *mentagrophytes* on
Sabouraud agar. Note clusters of detached spherical microconidia, thin
walled fusiform macroconidia, and loosely spiraled hyphae (see also
Fig 48.30). Lactophenol-blue preparation. ×600.

elements of the pathogen are found. For this reason, do not use the debris under the nail near the tip.

Diagnostic Procedures

Direct microscopic examination (KOH)

Hair. (a) Pick 2–3 hair stumps and place them close together on a clean slide. (b) Add a drop of 80% alcohol to wet the hairs and facilitate penetration of the KOH (this step is optional). (c) A drop of 10% KOH should follow. Twenty percent or higher is too strong, since the hair quickly disintegrates, making it difficult to determine if the infection is ectothrix or endothrix. (d) Cover with a glass or plastic coverslip. (e) To accelerate clearing, warm but do not boil the preparation. (f) Gently press down on the coverslip through a double layer of paper toweling to attain a thin preparation for better visibility. The paper towel avoids wetting the upper surface of the coverslip and absorbs the KOH squeezed out by pressure; crystallized, dried KOH obscures vision. (g) Search for the following:

> (i) A mosaic of round arthrospores surrounding hair as a stocking or sheath indicates an ectothrix infection.
> (ii) Individual arthrospores 2–3 μm indicate *M. canis* or *M. audouinii.*
> (iii) Individual arthrospores 5–8 μm indicate megaspore ecotothrix (i.e., *T. verrucosum, T. megninii,* and *M. gypseum).*
> (iv) Small arthrospores 3–5 μm but retaining a linear arrangement indicate ectothrix microides (*T. mentagrophytes* complex).
> (v) Round arthrospores in a mosaic pattern contained within the hair shaft are endothrix (*T. tonsurans* and *T. violaceum*).
> (vi) Rectangular arthrospores in a linear arrangment or hyphae and "air tunnels" within the hair shaft indicate favus (*T. schoenleinii*).

Glabrous skin. The KOH preparations described for hair infections can also be used in examining epidermal scrapings. Place three to five bits of epidermis on a slide; add the alcohol and KOH. After putting a coverslip over this material, maceration is encouraged by gentle heating over a flame or hot plate. A thin preparation can be obtained by pressing the coverslip with a paper towel.

Search for areas of squamous epithelium (pavementlike, empty, hyaline cells). Flatten these areas down to a single layer to see the fungal elements better. In dermatophyte infections, these elements will appear as hyaline, septate, branching hyphae (2–4 μm) which may fragment into arthrospores. These arthrospores are cylindrical at first, but become spherical after disarticulation of the mother hypha. It is important to learn to differentiate between fungal hyphae and artifacts such as "mosaic fungus," cotton fibers, collagen fibers, etc. (45).

Nails. Twenty percent KOH preparations are preferred for clearing nail material for microscopic examination. Proceed as with other cutaneous specimens. Once a suitably thin preparation has been obtained, search for fungal hyphae and/or arthrospores. Chains of beadlike, spherical arthrospores are common in nail infections, but long, thin, hyaline hyphae are also found.

Selection and inoculation of primary culture media

The standard medium used in medical mycology is Sabouraud glucose (dextrose) agar. This medium, basically a glucose-peptone agar with a pH of 5.6, has been modified repeatedly since Sabouraud's original formulation in attempts to substitute reagents that are more chemically defined and more easily obtained from commercial sources (Sabouraud used crude maltose or honey as a source of glucose, and a special peptone, Chasaing's, no longer available). The various formulations in use at present are given in Table 47.2.

Another modification is the addition of 0.5% yeast extract for the isolation of more fastidious dermatophytes such as *T. verrucosum*.

Sabouraud agar, as described above, is generally unsatisfactory for isolating dermatophytes from heavily contaminated materials. To prevent bacterial or fungal overgrowth, antibiotics are added according to various formulations (see Table 47.2). A recent formulation is Dermatophyte Test Medium (DTM), which contains bacterial antibiotics, cycloheximide, and phenol-red indicator. Dermatophytes change the color of the medium from yellow to red. However, DTM has its limitations; it can cause changes in growth and color of some saprophytic fungi resembling dermatophytes (*Trichothecium roseum* and *Chrysosporium* species, for example) and of certain nondermatophytic pathogens (48, 69). Two media should be used for primary cultures—one with antibiotics,

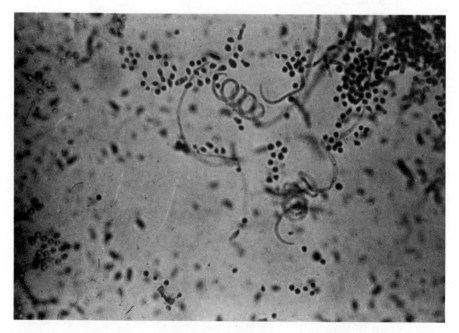

Figure 48.30—Tighter coils produced by hyphae of *T. mentagrophytes* are also seen by this variety on Sabouraud agar. Lactophenol-blue preparation. ×450.

the other without—since certain yeasts and filamentous fungi causing cutaneous infections may be inhibited by antibiotics.

Culture of hairs. Four to six hair stumps should be inoculated on suitable primary isolation media, with and without antibiotics. The bulb end of the hair should be inserted directly into the agar to ensure contact of the fungal elements with the growth medium.

Culture of skin. Four to six small fragments of epidermal scrapings should be deposited on the surface of the primary culture media. Allow adequate space (2–3 cm) between fragments to facilitate subculture of the dermatophyte and diminish the chances of overgrowth by contaminants.

Culture of nails. Four to six very small nail fragments should be distributed among at least two primary isolation media, one with and one without antibiotics. The nail fragments should be slightly embedded (2–3 cm apart) into the agar surface.

Cultures are usually incubated at 23–30 C, but if *T. verrucosum* is suspected (material from cattle or dairy farmers), cultures should also be incubated at 37 C.

Cultures should be examined for growth in 6–7 days. If growth is present, make subcultures from the periphery of the colony to minimize contamination. Routine cultures may be discarded in 2–3 weeks if no growth is visible and direct examination is negative. However, if *T. verrucosum* or the more exotic dermatophytic fungi are suspected, or if the direct examination was positive, the cultures may be held up to 4 weeks.

Identification procedures

Figure 48.10 is a flow sheet indicating the steps that may be necessary to arrive at the definitive identification of a dermatophyte isolate. The techniques for performing these tests are described below. Further aids to identification are found in Figures 48.11–48.35 and in Tables 48.15 and 48.16.

A presumptive identification of *E. floccosum*, most species of *Microsporum*, and some species of *Trichophyton* can frequently be made by gross examination of the colony.

TABLE 48.15—*In Vitro* Hair Perforations by Dermatophytes*

PERFORATIONS FORMED		PERFORATIONS NOT FORMED
M. canis	M. vanbreuseghemii	T. rubrum
M. audouinii (rarely)	T. ajelloi	T. schoenleinii
M. gypseum complex	T. terrestre	T. verrucosum
M. nanum	T. simii	T. violaceum
M. persicolor	T. mentagrophytes	
M. cookei	T. tonsurans (variable)	

* The hair perforation test is most useful in distinguishing between isolates of *T. rubrum* and *T. mentagrophytes*.

Colony characteristics of dermatophytes

(a) *Color of surface and reverse*. Colloquial names for colors (i.e., beige, buff, pink, brick-red) are often used to describe colonies, although interpretations may vary with the observer. Various attempts have been made to establish color standards to permit comparison and uniformity in color designation (55).

(b) *Topography*. This term refers to a colony's contours, margin, elevation, folding, etc.

(c) *Texture*. This term refers to whether the surface of the colony appears velvety, downy, feltlike, waxy, granular, or powdery.

(d) *Rate of growth*. This is usually determined by measuring colony diameter after a given interval of growth (1–3 weeks). Growth rate ranges from 1 mm/week (slow) to 10 mm/week (fast).

Tables 48.6–48.8 offer detailed information on colony characteristics.

Microscopic morphology

Further confirmatory (and sometimes definitive) identification can be made through microscopic examination of teased mounts, plastic tape mounts, and/or slide cultures.

(a) *Teased mounts*. Observation of the morphology and arrangement of the conidia produced by dermatophytes is essential for species identification. Sufficient information often may be obtained by preparing and examining a teased mount. This is accomplished by using two stiff needles to tease apart a small fragment from the aerial mycelium in a drop or two of mounting fluid on a slide. The mounting fluid is usually lactophenol-cotton blue or colorless lactophenol. The mount can then be examined microscopically after adding a coverslip.

(b) *Plastic tape mounts*. Adequate microscopic preparations may also be made from petri dish cultures of heavily sporulating fungi by using transparent pressure-sensitive tape, such as No. 800 acetate-backed tape, Minnesota

TABLE 48.16—UREASE PRODUCTION BY DERMATOPHYTES

UREASE POSITIVE*	UREASE NEGATIVE	UREASE VARIABLE
E. floccosum	T. rubrum	T. mentagrophytes
M. audouinii	T. soudanense	var. erinacei
M. canis	T. concentricum	T. verrucosum
M. gypseum	M. ferrugineum	
T. megninii	M. gallinae	
T. mentagrophytes		
T. schoenleinii		
T. tonsurans		
T. violaceum		

* Within 5–7 days.

Mining and Manufacturing Company. This method is described in Rebell and Taplin (67) as follows:

A flag of tape is fastened to a wooden applicator stick and the sticky surface touched to the surface of the thallus [colony] just proximal to the advancing periphery. The tape is then pressed sticky side down on a slide with a drop of lacto-phenol cotton blue stain and examined under the microscope directly. The tape selectively removes branches of hyphae bearing conidia [since these lie at the surface of the colony] and avoids the taxonomically valueless vegetative mycelium.

(c) *Slide cultures.* A slide-culture technique is often necessary when the aerial hyphae and spores must not be disturbed so that conidial ontogeny (manner of origin and development) and spore arrangement can be observed. Three of several slide-culture techniques will be described. Each of the techniques described requires a heat-sterilized culture chamber, consisting of a petri dish, filter paper, a piece of bent glass tubing, a slide, and a coverslip. Culture media recommended for slide cultures should be poor in nutrients to stimulate sporulation and inhibit vegetative mycelium. Cornmeal dextrose agar and potato dextrose agar are suitable.

(i) *Method One*: Lay the glass slide across a piece of bent glass tubing. Then dispense melted agar onto the slide by a pipette, enough agar to cover an area equivalent to a 22 mm × 40 mm coverslip. After the agar solidifies, inoculate the fungus in two parallel streaks on the surface of the agar. Sterile distilled water is added to the bottom of the petri dish, and

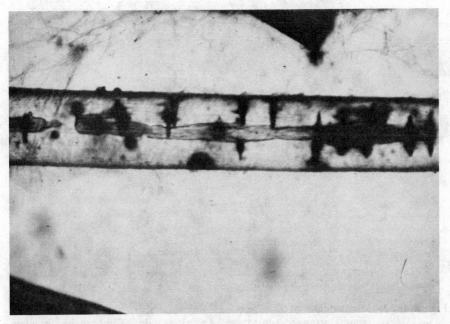

Figure 48.31—Wedge-shaped hair perforations produced by *T. mentagrophytes* during standard *in vitro* test (see text for details). ×600.

the preparation is incubated until the fungus reaches the proper state of development. When this is attained, dry the agar by leaving the petri dish cover slightly ajar. After the agar dries, a few drops of absolute alcohol is added to the area of growth to wet it down, followed by mounting fluid and a coverslip.

(ii) *Method Two*: This technique includes the same preparation of the slide as above. However, with this technique two preparations may be obtained. Cut out a 10-mm square of agar from a solidified agar plate, place it on the slide, and inoculate the four edges of the agar square. Alternatively, a round slab of agar may be cut out from the poured plate by using the rim of a test tube ("cookie-cutter" technique). Place a sterile coverslip over the inoculated agar slab. Add sterile water to the bottom of the petri dish to provide moisture.

When the culture is ready to be examined, remove and invert the coverslip, and wet down the growth with a few drops of alcohol. Place the culture growth side down on a slide containing a drop of the mounting fluid. Make a second preparation from the slide by removing the block of agar, wetting down the growth adherent to the slide, and adding the mounting fluid and a coverslip.

(iii) *Method Three* (44): Using tweezers, dip sterile slides into sterile, melted medium and allow them to drain briefly. A very thin layer of agar is obtained. Place the slides on a bent glass support within a sterile petri dish and inoculate them into the center of the agar surface. Add sterile water to the bottom of the petri dish. To observe growth without disturbing it, remove the dish lid during incubation and scan by low power.

When characteristic structures are seen, take the slide out. Completely remove the agar from both sides of the slide, leaving only a small edge of agar around the growth. The edge of a microscope slide is suitable for removing the agar. Place the slide on a glass support (growth side down, to protect it from dust) and allow it to dry for 24 hr at 37 C.

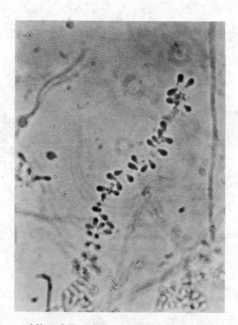

Figure 48.32—Microconidia of *T. rubrum* on Sabouraud agar. Note pyriform shaped conidia arranged "en thyrse," i.e., along sides of unbranched hyphae which characteristically shrivel and become inconspicuous as spores mature. Lactophenol-blue preparation. ×1000.

If the colony has a central elevation, remove it with a scalpel or needle. Then dip the slide in a solution of ethyl ether (two parts), absolute ethanol (two parts), and nonflexible collodion (one part). (Flexible collodion cannot be used since it contains castor oil and camphor which interfere with staining slides. A suitable nonflexible collodion is available from Fisher Scientific Co., Fairlawn, N.J., Cat. #C-407.) Drain off the excess collodion rapidly, and place the slide on a support at 37 C to dry. The collodion fixes the growth to the slide and keeps any spores in the position in which they are formed. After this procedure, the slides can be stored for long periods. To stain the slides, immerse them in 0.5% lactophenol-cotton blue for 10–15 min, wash then in 70% ethanol for about 2 min, and dehydrate them successively with acetone, acetonexylene (1:1), and xylene. Permanently mount the slides using the preferred natural resin or synthetic sealer (Canada balsam, Clarite, Histoclad, etc.).

Examination of one or more of the above slide preparations may disclose the characteristic microscopic morphology of the species. When such an examination does not provide sufficient information for species identification, more tests are necessary to determine certain physiological characteristics.

Physiological tests

(a) *Hair perforation* (6). Several fragments of human hair (preferably a child's) about 1 cm in length are sterilized by autoclaving at 120 C for 10 min in petri dishes. Using 100 mm diameter dishes, add about 25 ml of sterile distilled water and two to three drops of sterile 10% yeast extract. Inoculate with several fragments of the organism under study (from growth on Sabouraud agar) and incubate at 25 C (room temperature) for up to 4 weeks.

After 7 to 10 days of incubation, aseptically remove hairs which are cov-

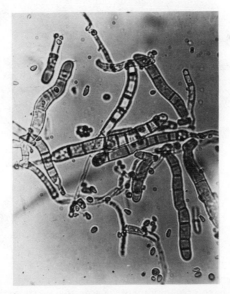

Figure 48.33—Pencil-shaped and curved macroconidia characteristic of *T. rubrum* (granular variety). ×1000.

ered with mycelia for microscopic examination. Mount hairs in lactophenol-cotton blue stain or other mounting medium, and examine them under low power. Perforations appear as wedge-shaped erosions occurring at irregular intervals along the hair shaft. The observation of wedge-shaped perforations constitutes a positive test. A negative test is seen when hyphae grow on the surface of the hair, but with no perforations.

If perforations are not seen after 10 days, the microscopic examination should be repeated at intervals or until 28 days have passed. Table 48.15 lists the *in vitro* hair perforation reactions of some *Microsporum* and *Trichophyton* species.

(b) *Urease formation* (65). Either urea agar (urea agar base [BBL or Difco] + 1.5%–2.0% agar, prepared according to manufacturer's directions) or urea broth (Christensen's) can be used. The latter is more reliable than the agar formulations for the demonstration of urease formation (42).

Inoculate the medium with the fungus under study and incubate it for 7 days at 25 C. Insure that screw-capped tubes are not tightly closed. The appearance of a purple-red color in the medium indicates a positive test result; no color change or slight changes to orange or pale pink are negative results.

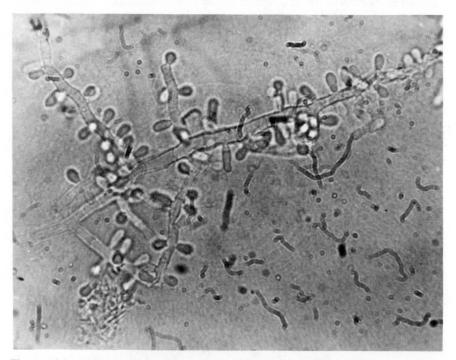

Figure 48.34—Microconidia of *T. tonsurans*. Note right-angled branching and "pine-tree" shape of conidiophore whose main axis is thickened, also note clavate shape and firm attachment of each conidium with septum at its base. ×1000.

Strains of *T. mentagrophytes* (positive) and *T. rubrum* (negative) whose reactions are known should be inoculated simultaneously as controls. Table 48.16 lists those dermatophytes whose urease activity has been thoroughly studied.

(c) *Special nutritional requirements.* Certain species of *Trichophyton* have either absolute or partial growth requirements for specific vitamins and amino acids (15, 35, 63) (Table 48.17). Based on this information, Georg and Camp (36) devised an identification scheme that helps differentiate these species from other dermatophytes that resemble them morphologically. The media used in this test are available commercially as "Trichophyton agars 1-7." Although details for the preparation of these media are described later, their general composition is summarized below:

Medium 1: Casein basal medium (vitamin-free)
Medium 2: Casein basal medium plus inositol
Medium 3: Casein basal medium plus thiamine and inositol
Medium 4: Casein basal medium plus thiamine
Medium 5: Casein basal medium plus nicotinic acid
Medium 6: NH_4NO_3 basal medium
Medium 7: NH_4NO_3 basal medium plus histidine

The results obtained when certain dermatophytes are cultured on these media are summarized on Table 48.17. It is important to use small inocula to avoid carrying over nutrients that would nullify this test.

(d) *Growth on rice grains.* The inability of *M. audouinii* to grow well on a substrate composed exclusively of boiled or autoclaved polished white rice grains is a useful clue to the identification of this poorly-sporulating species (23). The medium is easily prepared as a simple mixture of 1 part raw rice

TABLE 48.17—GROWTH RESPONSE OF CERTAIN DERMATOPHYTE SPECIES ON TRICHOPHYTON AGARS 1–7*

	TRICHOPHYTON AGARS No.[†]						
SPECIES	1	2	3	4	5	6	7
T. verrucosum, 84%	0	±	4+	0			
T. verrucosum, 16%	0	0	4+	4+			
T. schoenleinii	4+	4+	4+	4+			
T. concentricum, 50%	4+	4+	4+	4+			
T. concentricum, 50%	2+	2+	4+	4+			
T. violaceum	±			4+			
T. tonsurans	±			4+			
T. rubrum	4+			4+			
T. mentagrophytes	4+			4+			
T. equinum	0				4+		
T. megninii						0	4+
M. gallinae						4+	4+

* After Georg (35).

† (1) Casein basal medium (vitamin-free), (2) casein basal medium plus inositol, (3) casein basal medium plus thiamine and inositol, (4) casein basal medium plus thiamine, (5) casein basal medium plus nicotinic acid, (6) NH_4NO_3 basal medium, (7) NH_4NO_3 basal medium plus histidine.

grains to 3 parts water in a flask or tube. The rice is subsequently "cooked" by boiling or autoclaving. On the surface of the soft-cooked rice grains, most *Microsporum* species grow well and produce characteristic colonies closely resembling those grown on Sabouraud agar. The exception is *M. audouinii*, producing only negligible growth with a brownish discoloration.

(e) *Effect on growth of incubation at 37 C.* Place small inocula of about equal size on the surface of two slants of Sabouraud agar. One tube is incubated at 22 C–24 C (room temperature) and the other at 37 C. After they are incubated for 1 or 2 weeks, the tubes are compared for amount of growth (colony diameter and elevation).

(f) *Production of the perfect state* (sexual state resulting in gymnothecia [cleistothecia], asci, and ascospores). Certain dermatophytes may defy classification using routine procedures, because they are atypical or so similar they constitute an imperfect species complex (i.e., the *T. terrestre* complex, the *T. mentagrophytes* complex, and the *M. gypseum* complex). In the latter case, it is not usually necessary for diagnostic purposes to determine the perfect species; identification of the imperfect state is sufficient.

Occasionally, it may be difficult to differentiate the saprophytic, imperfect species (i.e., *T. terrestre*) from the pathogenic species, *T. mentagrophytes*. In such a case, definitive identification would be based on obtaining the perfect state. Since most of the perfect species are heterothallic, the formation of gym-

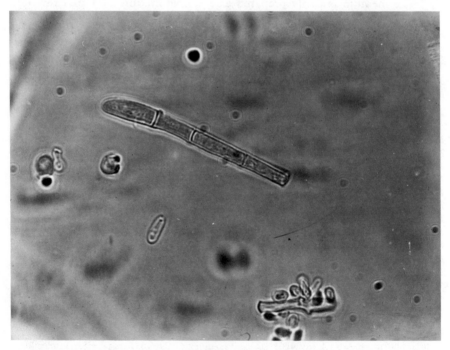

Figure 48.35—Clavate (club-shaped) macroconidium of *T. tonsurans.* ×1000.

nothecia with asci and ascospores requires pairing, mating, or crossing the unknown isolate with tester strains comprising the two mating types (+ and − or A and a) of a species on a suitable culture medium (52). This is done by cutting a cube from an agar culture of each of the two isolates to be crossed and pairing them side by side on the appropriate medium.

For example, to determine if an atypical isolate is a member of the *M. gypseum* complex, pair the unknown isolate with each of several strains representing the two mating types of *N. gypsea, N. incurvata,* and *N. fulva.* Also, pair the unknown with itself to determine if it is self-fertile or a mixture of compatible mating types. Cross the + and − tester strains of each perfect species with each other to determine if they are still fertile. Incubate the paired isolates at 22 C–25 C for 3 to 5 weeks and then examine for the presence of gymnothecia.

Gymnothecia appear to the naked eye as tiny white to yellowish bumps on the agar surface. The gymnothecia are mounted on a slide in lactophenol-blue, crushed, and examined microscopically for the presence of asci and ascospores. Identification of the unknown is usually based on the particular cross resulting in these structures. Exceptions, however, may occur (77). The search for sexually compatible tester strains may involve hundreds of pairings. Therefore, a specialized laboratory and investigator to perform this test are needed.

(g) *Epilogue.* While we have outlined a rather extensive series of identification procedures, many will be unnecessary to identify most isolates. The great majority of dermatophytes can be identified by the first two or three steps in the flow sheet (Fig. 48.10); the remaining dermatophytes may require physiological tests for definitive identification.

Section 3: Opportunistic Dermatomycoses

Causative Organisms

Nondermatophytic filamentous fungi reported as probable etiologic agents of cutaneous infection are listed in Table 48.18 (12, 13, 18–20, 22, 27, 28, 29, 33, 38, 46, 57, 60, 66, 74, 79–82). This list is not exhaustive since the literature is replete with reports of isolation of adventitious fungi, particularly from abnormal nails (19, 20, 33, 46, 57, 66, 81, 82).

Clinical Manifestations

Some of these fungi, notably *Alternaria sp.* (18), *Aphanoascus fulvescens* (60), *Hendersonula toruloidea* (19, 33), and *Scytalidium hyalinum* (20), have been reported to produce skin lesions clinically indistinguishable from a dermatophyte infection.

Several investigators have reported a dematiaceous (dark-colored) fungus, *Hendersonula toruloidea,* originally described as a plant pathogen of trees, as the etiologic agent of a disease clinically indistinguishable from ringworm, especially in patients from the tropics. Gentles and Evans (33) reported that this fungus was isolated from eight patients and diagnosed as tinea pedis or onychomycosis. In each case, the direct examination was positive for fungal hyphae and *H. toruloidea* was isolated repeatedly in media without cycloheximide. In each case, no dermatophyte was isolated. Since this first report, additional isolations of this species from skin and nails have been reported (19).

Most of the nondermatophytic filamentous fungi infecting the nail cause distal subungual onychomycosis (81). Fungi other than *T. mentagrophytes* producing leukonychia (white spots on the surface of the nail) are *Acremonium (Cephalosporium) roseogriseum, Aspergillus terreus,* and a member of the *Fusarium oxysporum* group (81, 82).

English (27) reported on the saprophytic invasion of the skin by filamentous nondermatophytic fungi. In each of three cases of macerated toe webs, characteristic spores were seen in the direct microscopic examination of the skin scrapings (*Aspergillus* conidial heads, conidia characteristic of *Petriellidium (Allescheria) boydii,* and *Fusarium sp.*). The cultures grew out the expected fungi, respectively, *A. niger, P. boydii,* and *F. solani.*

Relationship of disease to fungus

These opportunistic fungi are normally saprophytes or plant pathogens: hence, their isolation in culture is not, in itself, proof of pathogenicity. A fun-

TABLE 48.18—CUTANEOUS INFECTIONS BY ADVENTITIOUS FILAMENTOUS FUNGI

1. Nails	*Alternaria* sp.
	Aspergillus (A. candidus, A. flavus, A. fumigatus, A. glaucus, A. nidulans, A. niger, A. sydowii, A. terreus, A. terricola, A. ustus, A. versicolor)
	Botryodiplodia theobromae
	Acremonium (Cephalosporium) (A. acremonium, A. oxysporum, A. roseogriseum)
	Cladosporium (Hormodendrum) (C. cladosporioides, C. nigrescens)
	Hendersonula toruloidea
	Penicillium (P. chrysogenum)
	Paecilomyces lilacinus (Penicillium lilacinum)
	Scopulariopsis brevicaulis
2. Skin of hands and feet	*Petriellidium (Allescheria) boydii*
	Alternaria (A. alternata, A. tenuis)
	Aphanoascus fulvescens
	Aspergillus niger
	Drechslera spicifera
	Fusarium moniliforme
	Fusarium solani
	Fusarium oxysporum var. *redolens*
	Hendersonula toruloidea
	Scytalidium hyalinum
3. Face	*Alternaria* sp.
	Paecilomyces lilacinus
4. Hair	*Alternaria* sp.

gus that is repeatedly isolated, especially in large numbers, from a patient may be suspected of playing a potentially pathogenic role if one or more of the following additional criteria are met: (a) observation on direct microscopic examination of an adequate number of fungal elements whose morphology is compatible with the organism isolated; (b) observation of a histopathologic reaction in response to the fungal invasion; (c) repeated failure to isolate a dermatophyte on selective media; and (d) disappearance of the fungus and a clinical cure.

Epidemiology

At least one of these opportunistic cutaneous invaders, *H. toruloidea*, remains stable in dry skin scales for 6 months (19), suggesting an epidemiology similar to that of tinea pedis.

Diagnostic Procedures

The techniques used to collect, examine, and culture specimens for dermatophyte infections are all applicable to the diagnosis of opportunistic cutaneous mycoses. For the reasons outlined above, give close attention to the presence and morphology of the fungus in direct microscopy.

Since most of these fungi are sensitive to cycloheximide, include media lacking this agent for routine culture.

Identification Procedures

Most isolates of *H. toruloidea* grow rapidly. The color of the colony has been described as mouse-gray on the surface, with a brownish-gray to black reverse. In slide-culture preparations, coiled hyphae and chains of thick-walled two-celled arthrospores are characteristic features. Campbell (19) studied 25 isolates and found two cultural types differing in growth rate, abundance of aerial mycelium, and arthrospores. All isolates were nonpathogenic for guinea pigs, but Wildfeuer (79) succeeded in infecting rabbits.

References for Section One

1. AJELLO L: Survey of tree shrew pelts for mycotic infection. Mycologia 56:455–458, 1964
2. AJELLO L: The black yeasts as disease agents. *In* Proceedings of the Fourth International Conference on the Mycoses: The Black and White Yeasts. Scientific Publication No 536. Pan American Health Organization, Washington, DC, 1978, pp 9–16
3. AJELLO L and PADHYE AA: Dermatophytes and the agents of superficial mycoses. *In* Manual of Clinical Microbiology. Lennette EH, Spaulding EH, and Truant JP (eds.). American Society for Microbiology, Washington, DC, 1974, pp 469–481
4. BARFATANI M, MUNN RJ, and SCHJEIDE J: An ultrastructural study of *Pityrosporum orbiculare*. J Invest Dermatol 43:231–233, 1964
5. BARNES WG, SAUER GS, and ARNOLD JD: Scanning electron microscopy of tinea versicolor organisms (*Malassezia furfur-Pityrosporum orbiculare*). Arch Dermatol 107:392–394, 1973
6. BARRON GL: The Genera of Hyphomycetes. Williams & Wilkins Co, Baltimore, Md, 1968
7. BASSET M, GROSSHANS E, and PRADINAUD R: Le polymorphisme du pityriasis versicolor en Guyane Francaise. Bull Soc Fr Mycol Med 3:75–76, 1974

8. BEHREND G: II. Über Trichomycosis nodosa (piedra). Berl Klin Wochenschr 27:464–467, 1890

9. BENHAM RW: Cultural characteristics of *Pityrosporum ovale*—a lipophilic fungus. Nutrient and growth requirements. Proc Soc Exp Biol 46:176–178, 1941

10. BREATHNACK AS, GROSS M, and MARTIN B: Freeze-fracture replication of cultured *Pityrosporum orbiculare*. Sabouraudia 14:105–113, 1976

11. BURKE RC: Tinea versicolor: Susceptibility factors and experimental infection in human beings. J Invest Dermatol 36:389–402, 1961

12. CARMICHAEL JW: Cerebral mycetoma of trout due to a *Phialophora*-like fungus. Sabouraudia 5:120–123, 1967

13. CARRION AL: *In* Report of the Director of the School of Tropical Medicine. Bachman GW. Columbia Univ Press, New York, 1938, p 25

14. CARRION AL: Yeastlike dematiaceous fungi infecting the human skin. Arch Dermatol 61:996–1009, 1950

15. CARRION AL: Dermatomycoses in Puerto Rico. Arch Dermatol 91:431–438, 1965

16. CHARLES CR, SIRE DJ, JOHNSON BL, and BEIDLER JG: Hypopigmentation in tinea versicolor: A histochemical and electron-microscopic study. Int J Dermatol 12:49–57, 1973

17. CHONG KC, ADAM BA, and SOO-HOO TS: Morphology of *Piedraia hortai*. Sabouraudia 9:157–160, 1975

18. COHEN MN: A simple procedure for staining tinea versicolor (*M. furfur*) with fountain pen ink. J Invest Dermatol 22:9–10, 1954

19. COLE GT: Conidiogenesis in the black yeasts. *In* Proceedings of the Fourth International Conference on the Mycoses: The Black and White Yeasts. Scientific Publication No. 536. Pan American Health Organization, Washington, DC, 1978, pp 66–78

20. DEVRIES GA: Contribution to the Knowledge of the Genus *Cladosporium* Link ex Fr. Uitgeverig and Drukkerij Hollandia, Baarn, The Netherlands, 1952, pp 100–101

21. DIDDENS HA and LODDER J: Die Anaskosporogenen Hefen, II Halfte, Amsterdam, 1942

22. DO CARMO-SOUZA L: *In* The Yeasts, second edition. Lodder J. North-Holland, Amsterdam, 1970, pp 1309–1352

23. DODGE CW: *Dematium werneckii* (Parreiras-Horta) Dodge, n. comb. *In* Medical Mycology. Dodge CW. C.V. Mosby Co, St. Louis, 1935, pp 676–678

24. DOMPMARTIN D and DROUHET E: Folliculites a *Pityrosporum ovale*: Action de l'econazole. Bull Soc Fr Mycol Med 6:15–20, 1977

25. DORN M and ROEHNERT K: Dimorphism of *Pityrosporum orbiculare* in a defined culture medium. J Invest Dermatol 63:244–248, 1977

26. EMMONS CW, BINFORD CH, UTZ JP, and KWONG-CHUNG JK: Medical Mycology, third edition. Lea & Febiger, Philadelphia, 1977, pp 182–183

27. FISCHMAN O: Black piedra among Brazilian Indians. Rev Inst Med Trop 15:103–106, 1973

28. GORDON MA: The lipophilic mycoflora of the skin. I. *In vitro* culture of *Pityrosporum orbiculare* nov. sp. Mycologia 43:524–535, 1951

29. GORDON MA: The lipophilic yeast-like organisms associated with tinea versicolor. J Invest Dermatol 17:267–272, 1951

30. GUSTAFSON RA, HARDCASTLE RV, and SZANISZLO PJ: Budding in the dimorphic fungus *Cladosporium werneckii*. Mycologia 67:942–951, 1975

31. JUNG EG and TRUNIQER B: Tinea versicolor in Cushing's syndrome. Dermatologica 127:18–22, 1963

32. KAPLAN W: The occurrence of black piedra in primate pelts. Trop Geogr Med 11:115–126, 1959

33. KAPLAN W: Piedra in lower animals. J Am Vet Med Assoc 134:113–117, 1959

34. KEDDIE FM: Electron microscopy of *Malassezia furfur* in tinea versicolor. Sabouraudia 5:134–137, 1966

35. KEDDIE F, ORR A, and LIEBES D: Direct staining on vinyl plastic tape. Demonstration of the cutaneous flora of the epidermis by the strip method. Sabouraudia 1:108–112, 1961

36. KEDDIE F, SHADOMY J, SHADOMY S, and BARFATANI M: Intrafollicular tinea versicolor demonstrated on monomer plastic strips. J Invest Dermatol 41:103–106, 1963

37. KEDDIE FM AND SHADOMY S: Etiological significance of *Pityrosporum orbiculare* in tinea versicolor. Sabouraudia 3:21–25, 1963

38. KOHN SR: Hair casts or pseudonits. J Am Med Assoc 238:2058–2059, 1977

39. KUCHENMEISTER and RABENHORST: *In* Zwei Parasiten an den todten Haaren der Chignons. Rabenhorst L. Hedwigia 6(4):49, 1867

40. LONDERO AT, RAMOS CD, and FISCHMAN O: White piedra of unusual location. Sabouraudia 5:132–133, 1966

41. LUTTRELL ES: Loculoascomycetes. *In* The Fungi: An Advanced Treatise, Volume IVA. Ainsworth GC, Sparrow FK, and Sussman AS (eds.). Academic Press, New York and London, 1973, pp 135–219

42. MACKINNON JE and SCHOUTEN GB: Investigaciones sobres las enfermedades de los calbelos denominadas "piedra." Arch Soc Biol Montevideo 10:227–266, 1942

43. MCGINNIS MR: Human pathogenic species of *Exophiala, Phialophora* and *Wangiella. In* Proceedings of the Fourth International Conference on the Mycoses: The Black and White Yeasts. Scientific Publication No. 536. Pan American Health Organization, Washington, DC, 1978, pp 37–59

44. NAZZARO PORRO M and PASSI S: Identification of tyrosinase inhibitors in cultures of *Pityrosporum.* J Invest Dermatol 71:205–208, 1978

45. PARREIRAS HORTA P: Sobre um caso de tinha preta e um novo cogumelo (*Cladosporium werneckii*). Rev Med Cirurg Brasil 29:269–274, 1921

46. PATTERSON JC, LAINE SL, and TAYLOR WB: White piedra occurring on the pubic hair of a native caucasian North American. Arch Dermatol 85:534–536, 1962

47. PIERARD J and DOCKX P: The ultra-structure of tinea versicolor and *Malassezia furfur.* Int J Dermatol 11:116–124, 1972

48. POTTER BS, BURGOON CF, and JOHNSON WC: *Pityrosporum* folliculitis. Arch Dermatol 107:388–391, 1973

49. RANJANDICHE M: Polymorphisme de *Pityrosporum ovale* (Bizzozero) Castellani and Chalmers *in vivo* and *in vitro.* Bull Soc Fr Mycol Med 5:79–84, 1976

50. SALKIN IF and GORDON MA: Polymorphism of *Malassezia furfur.* Can J Microbiol 23:471–475, 1977

51. SHIFRINE M and MARR AG: The requirement of fatty acids by *Pityrosporum ovale.* J Gen Microbiol 32:263–270, 1963

52. SLOOFF WC: Genus *Pityrosporum* Sabouraud. *In* The Yeasts, A Taxonomic Study, second edition. Lodder J (ed.). North-Holland Publishing Co., Inc., New York, 1970, p 1174

53. STERNBERG TH and KEDDIE FM: Immunoflourescence studies in tinea versicolor. Arch Dermatol 84:999–1003, 1961

54. SWIFT JA and DUNBAR SF: Ultrastructure of *Pityrosporum ovale* and *Pityrosporum canis.* Nature 206:1174–1175, 1965

55. TAKASHIO M and DEVROEY C: Piedra noire chez des chimpanzes du Zaire. Sabouraudia 13:58–62, 1975

56. TAKASHIO M and VANBREUSEGHEM R: Production of ascospores by *Piedraia hortai* in vitro. Mycologia 63:612–618, 1971

57. TAPLIN D and REBELL G: Tinea versicolor (pityriasis versicolor). *In* Clinical Dermatology, Vol 3. Demis DJ, Dobson RL, and McGuire J (eds.). Harper & Row, New York, 1972, Unit 17-2, pp 1–9

58. VAN UDEN N, DEBARROS MACHADO A, and CASTELO BRANCO R: On black piedra in Central African mammals caused by the ascomycete *Piedraia quintanilhai* nov. spec. Revista Brasiliera e Porgugesa de Biologia em Geral 3:271–276, 1963

59. VON ARX JA: The Genera of Fungi Sporulating in Pure Culture. J.Cramer, 3301 Lehre, Germany, 1970, p 180

60. VUILLEMIN P: Trichosporum et trichospories. Arch Parasitol 5:38–66, 1902

61. YAFFEE AS: Tinea nigra palmaris resembling malignant melanoma. N Engl J Med 283:1112, 1970

Glossary for Section One

alba: white

Cladosporium: dematiaceous fungal genus in which the conidia are produced successively in branching chains (Greek *klado*, branch) in the direction of the apex, i.e., the youngest conidium is most distal; conidia separate from adjacent ones by means of disjunctors; basal conidia become shield-shaped and bicellular with age.

dandruff: a combination of dander (an old dialectal English word for scales of the scalp) and an old Norse word (*hrufa*) for crust, scab or scales.

dimorphic: having two forms.

flava: yellow (Latin *flavus*, yellow).

furfur: a classical Latin word originally meaning bran, then later scurf and scales on the scalp; in the name *Malessezia furfur*, the term relates to the scurfy appearance of the disease this fungus causes.

furfuraceous: like bran; finely scaly.

fusca: from New Latin meaning dark or tawny.

hyaline: non-pigmented, transparent; from Greek *hyalos*, glass.

locule: a cavity, especially one in a stroma, from Latin *loculus*, a cavity.

macule: from Latin meaning spot, stain or blemish, in dermatology, a perceptible change in skin color, not raised above or depressed below the surrounding skin.

melanin: colored complexes of protein, most commonly tan, brown or black, resulting from the polymerization of tyrosine and hydroxyphenylalanine by tyrosinase.

nigra: black.

orbiculare: resembling (*−are*) a small (*−cul−*) disc (*orbi−*), hence annular, circular or round. Appears in the name *Pityrosporum orbiculare*.

papule: from Latin *papula*, a small swelling; a solid small (*−ule*), skin lesion raised above the surface of the skin, ranging roughly up to pea-size.

phialide: conidiogenous cell in which spores are produced at the apex in basipetal succession (youngest at the base), usually semi-endogenously.

pilar: referring or related to hair (Latin *pilus*, hair).

piedra: Spanish word for stone, referring to stony concretions on hair.

pityriasis versicolor: a scaly condition (*pityriasis*) which changes color (*versicolor*).

pseudoparenchyma: a false (*pseudo−*) parenchyma, a soft tissue of higher plants (from Greek *enchyma*, an infusion); looking like true parenchyma, but formed from hyphae.

seborrheic blepharitis: inflammation of the eyelids (*blephar-*) associated with a flow(*-rrhea*) of sebum.

trichomycosis nodosa: a fungous (*-mycosis*) condition of the hair (*trich-*) that has the clinical appearance of many knots (*nodosa*).

Besides the general texts cited in the bibliography, the following sources were consulted in preparation of this glossary:

AINSWORTH GC and BISBY GR: Dictionary of the Fungi, 5th edition. Commonwealth Mycological Institute, Kew, Surrey, England, 1963

LEIDER M and ROSENBLUM M: A Dictionary of Dermatologic Words, Terms, and Phrases, revised edition. Dome Laboratories, Inc, West Haven, Conn, 1976

SNELL WH and DICK EA: A Glossary of Mycology. Harvard Univ Press, Cambridge, Mass, 1957

References for Sections Two and Three

1. AINSWORTH GC and AUSTWICK PKC: Fungal Diseases of Animals. Commonwealth Agricultural Bureaux, Farnham Royal, Slough, England, 1973

2. AJELLO L: A taxonomic review of the dermatophytes and related species. Sabouraudia 6:147–159, 1968

3. AJELLO L: The medical mycological iceberg. *In* Proc First Int Symp Mycoses. Sci Publ No 205. Pan Am Health Organ, Washington, DC, 1970, pp 3–12

4. AJELLO L: Milestones in the history of medical mycology: The dermatophytes. *In* Recent Advances in Medical and Veterinary Mycology. K. Iwata (ed.). Univ of Tokyo Press, Tokyo 1977, pp 3–11

5. AJELLO L: Taxonomy of the dermatophytes. A review of their perfect and imperfect states. *In* Recent Advances in Medical and Veterinary Mycology. K. Iwata (ed.). Univ of Tokyo Press, Tokyo, 1977, pp 289–297

6. AJELLO L and GEORG LK: *In vitro* hair cultures for distinguishing between atypical isolates of *Trichophyton mentagrophytes* and *Trichophyton rubrum*. Mycopathologia (Den Haag) 8:3–17, 1957

7. AJELLO L and GETZ ME: Recovery of dermatophytes from shoes and shower stalls. J Invest Dermatol 22:17–21, 1954
8. AJELLO L, VARSAVSKY E, GINTNER OJ, and BUBASH G: The natural history of *Microsporum nanum*. Mycologia 56:873–884, 1964
9. ALLEN AM and TAPLIN D: Epidemiology of dermatophytosis in Vietnam. *In* Compt Rend Commications Ve Congres. Drouhet E (ed.). ISHAM, Paris, 1971, pp 102–103
10. BAER RL and ROSENTHAL SA: The biology of fungous infections of the feet. J Am Med Assoc 197:1017–1020, 1966
11. BAER RL, ROSENTHAL SA, LITT JZ, and ROGACHEFSKY H: Experimental investigations on the mechanism for producing acute dermatophytosis of the feet. J Am Med Assoc 160:184–190, 1956
12. BAKERSPIGEL A: The isolation of *Phoma hibernica* from a lesion on a leg. Sabouraudia 7:261–264, 1970
13. BANG PEDERSEN N, MARDH PA, HALLBERG T, and JONASSON N: Cutaneous alternariosis. Br J Dermatol 94:201–209, 1976
14. BEARE JM, GENTLES JC, and MACKENZIE DWR: Mycology. *In* Textbook of Dermatology. Rook A, Wilkinson DS, and Ebling FJG (eds.). Blackwell Scientific Publications, Oxford, 1972, pp 694–805
15. BENHAM RW: Nutritional studies of the dermatophytes—effect on growth and morphology. Trans NY Acad Sci 15:102–106, 1953
16. BLANK F and STRACHAN AA: Infections due to *Trichophyton tonsurans* (and *T. sulfureum*) in rural eastern Quebec. Mycopathologia 18:207–212, 1962
17. BLANK H, TAPLIN D, and ZAIAS N: Cutaneous *Trichophyton mentagrophytes* infections in Vietnam. Arch Dermatol 99:135–144, 1969
18. BOTTICHER WW: *Alternaria* as a possible human pathogen. Sabouraudia 4:256–258, 1966
19. CAMPBELL CK: Studies on *Hendersonula toruloidea* isolated from human skin and nail. Sabouraudia 12:150–156, 1974
20. CAMPBELL CK and MULDER JL: Skin and nail infections by *Scytalidium hyalinum* sp. nov. Sabouraudia 15:161–166, 1977
21. CHAMPION RH and WHITTLE CH: Sycosis barbae due to *Trichophyton rubrum*. Trans St John's Hosp Dermatol Soc 44:114–119, 1960
22. COLLINS MS and RINALDI MG: Cutaneous infection in man caused by *Fusarium moniliforme*. Sabouraudia 15:151–160, 1977
23. CONANT NF: Studies on the genus *Microsporum*. I. Cultural studies. Arch Dermatol 33:665–683, 1936
24. EL-ANI AS: The cytogenetics of the conidium in *Microsporum gypseum* and of pleomorphism and the dual phenomenon in fungi. Mycologia 60:999–1015, 1968
25. EMMONS CW: Dermatophytes. Natural grouping based on the form of the spores and accessory organs. Arch Dermatol 30:337–362, 1934
26. ENGLISH MP: *Trichophyton rubrum* infections in families. Br. Med J 1:744–746, 1957
27. ENGLISH MP: Invasion of the skin by filamentous non-dermatophyte fungi. Br J Dermatol 80:282–286, 1968
28. ESTES SA, MERZ WG, and MAXWELL LG: Primary cutaneous phaeohyphomycosis. Arch Dermatol 113:813–815, 1977
29. FARMER SG and KOMOROWSKI RA: Cutaneous micro-abscess formation from *Alternaria alternata*. Am J Clin Pathol 66:565–569, 1976
30. FRIEDMAN L, DERBES VJ, HODGES EP, and SINSKI JT: The isolation of dermatophytes from the air. J Invest Dermatol 35:3–5, 1960
31. GENTLES JC: The isolation of dermatophytes from the floors of communal bathing places. J Clin Pathol 9:374–377, 1956
32. GENTLES JC: Athlete's foot fungi on the floors of communal bathing places. Br Med J 1:746–748, 1957
33. GENTLES JC and EVANS EGV: Infection of the feet and nails with *Hendersonula toruloidea*. Sabouraudia 8:72–75, 1970
34. GENTLES JC and HOLMES JG: Foot ringworm in coal miners. Br J Ind Med 14:22–29, 1957
35. GEORG LK: Dermatophytes, new methods in classification. U.S. Dept. Health, Education, and Welfare, Center for Disease Control, Atlanta, Ga, 1957

36. GEORG LK and CAMP LB: Routine nutritional tests for the identification of dermatophytes. J Bacteriol 74:113–121, 1957
37. GIP L: Estimation of incidence of dermatophytes on floor areas after barefoot walking with washed and unwashed feet. Acta Derm Venereol 47:89–93, 1967
38. HIGASHI N and ASADA Y: Cutaneous alternariosis with mixed infection of *Candida albicans*. Arch Dermatol 108:558–560, 1973
39. HOPKINS JG., HILLEGAS AB, CAMP E, LEDIN RB, and REBELL G: Dermatophytosis at an infantry post. J Invest Dermatol 8:291–316, 1947
40. JOHNSON JA and ROSENTHAL SA: Superficial cutaneous infection with *Trichophyton soudanense*. Arch Dermatol 97:428–431, 1968
41. JOHNSON MLT and ROBERTS J: Prevalence of dermatological disease among persons 1–74 years of age: United States. *In* USDHEW, Advance Data from Vital and Health Statistics, No. 4. Washington, DC, 1977, pp 1–3
42. KANE J and FISCHER JB: The differentiation of *Trichophyton rubrum* and *T. mentagrophytes* by use of Christensen's urea broth. Can J Microbiol 17:911–913, 1971
43. KANE J and FISCHER JB: Occurrence of *Trichophyton megninii* in Ontario. Identification with a simple cultural procedure. J Clin Microbiol 2:11–114, 1975
44. LANGERON M and VANBREUSEGHEM R: Precis de Mycologie, 2nd edition. Masson et Cie, Paris, 1952, pp 416–417
45. LEWIS GM and HOPPER ME: An Introduction to Medical Mycology. The Year Book Publications, Inc, Chicago, Ill, 1939, pp 208–211
46. LIAUTAUD B, GROSSHANS E, and BASSET M: Les onychomycoses a champignons saprophytes. La Presse Medicale 25:1163–1166, 1971
47. MANY H, DERBES VJ, and FRIEDMAN L: *Trichophyton rubrum:* Exposure and infection within household groups. Arch Dermatol 88:226–229, 1960
48. MERZ WG, BERGER CL, and SILVA-HUTNER M.: Media with pH indicators for the isolation of dermatophytes. Arch Dermatol 102:545–547, 1970
49. MITCHELL JH: A survey of tinea capitis. Arch Dermatol 60:495–496, 1949
50. MUIJS D: *Trichophyton rosaceum.* Ned Tijdschr Geneeskd 60:1985–1992, 1916
51. PADHYE AA and CARMICHAEL JW: The genus *Arthroderma* Berkeley. Can J Bot 49:1525–1540, 1971
52. PADHYE AA, SEKHON AS, and CARMICHAEL JW: Ascocarp production by *Arthroderma* and *Nannizzia* species on keratinous and non-keratinous media. Sabouraudia 11:109–114, 1973
53. PIER AC,, RHOADES KR, HARES TL, and GALLAGHER J: Scanning electron microscopy of selected dermatophytes of veterinary importance. Am J Vet Res 33:607–613, 1972
54. PROCHACKI H and ENGELHARDT-ZASADA C: *Epidermophyton stockdaleae sp. nov.* Mycopathologia 54:341–345, 1974
55. RAYNER RW: A Mycological Colour Chart. Commonwealth Mycological Institute, Kew, Surrey, England, 1970, p 5 (References)
56. REBELL G and TAPLIN D: Dermatophytes—Their Recognition and Identification. Univ of Miami Press, Coral Gables, Fla, 1970
57. RESTREPO A, ARANGO M, VELEZ H, and URIBE L: The isolation of *Botryodiplodia theobromae* from a nail lesion. Sabouraudia 14:1–4, 1976
58. RIPPON J: Biochemical-genetic determinants of virulence among dermatophytes. *In* Mycoses, Proc 3rd Int Conf on the Mycoses. Sci Publ No 304. Pan Am Health Organ, Washington, DC, 1975, pp 88–97
59. RIPPON JW: Medical Mycology. The Pathogenic Fungi and the Pathogenic Actinomycetes. WB Saunders Co, Philadelphia, Pa, 1974
60. RIPPON JW, LEE FC, and McMILLEN S: Dermatophyte infection caused by *Aphanoascus fulvescens.* Arch Dermatol 102:552–555, 1970
61. RIPPON JW and MALKINSON FD: *Trichophyton simii* infection in the United States. Arch Dermatol 98:615–619, 1968
62. RIPPON JW and MEDINICA M: Isolation of *Trichophyton soudanense* in the United States. Sabouraudia 3:301–304, 1964
63. ROBBINS WJ: Growth requirements of dermatophytes. Ann NY Acad Sci 50:1357–1361, 1950
64. ROSENTHAL SA: The epidemiology of tinea pedis. *In* The Diagnosis and Treatment of Fungal

Infections. Robinson HM Jr (ed). Charles C. Thomas, Springfield, Ill, 1974, pp 516–526

65. ROSENTHAL SA and SOKOLSKY H: Enzymatic studies with pathogenic fungi. Dermatologia Internationalis 4:72–79, 1965

66. ROSENTHAL SA, STRITZLER R, and VILLANFANE J: Onychomycosis caused by *Aspergillus fumigatus.* Arch Dermatol 97:685–687, 1968

67. ROTH F JR: Microscopic preparations from cultures to show aleuriospores. *In* Dermatophytes. Their Recognition and Identification, revised edition. Rebell G and Taplin D. University of Miami Press, Coral Gables, Fla, 1970, p 114

68. SABOURAUD R: Contribution a l' etude de la trichophytie humaine. Trichophyties pilaires de la barbe. Ann Dermatol Syphiligr 4:814–835, 1893

69. SALKIN IF: Dermatophyte test medium: evaluation with nondermatophytic pathogens. Appl Microbiol 26:134–137, 1973

70. SMITH JMB, JOLLY RD, GEORG LK, and CONNOLE MD: *Trichophyton equinum var. autotrophicum;* its characteristics and geographical distribution. Sabouraudia 6:296–304, 1968

71. STOCKDALE PM: The *Microsporum gypseum* complex (*Nannizzia incurvata* Stockd., *N. gypsea* (Nann.) *comb. nov., N. fulva sp. nov.*). Sabouraudia 3:114–126, 1963

72. SULZBERGER MB, BAER RL, and HECHT R: Common fungous infections of the feet and groin. Negligible role of exposure in causing attacks. Arch Dermatol 45:670–675, 1942

73. TAKASHIO M: Sexual reproduction of some *Arthroderma* and *Nannizzia* on diluted Sabouraud agar with or without salts. Mykosen 1:11–17, 1972

74. TAKAYASU S, AKAGI M, and SHIMIZU Y: Cutaneous mycosis caused by *Paecilomyces lilacinus.* Arch Dermatol 113:1687–1690, 1977

75. VANBREUSEGHEM R, DeVROEY C, and TAKASHIO M: Production of macroconidia by *Microsporum ferrugineum,* Ota, 1922. Sabouraudia 7:252–256, 1970

76. WEITZMAN I: Variation in *Microsporum gypseum.* I. A genetic study of pleomorphism. Sabouraudia 3:195–203, 1964

77. WEITZMAN I and PADHYE AA: Is *Arthroderma simii* the perfect state of *Trichophyton quinckeanum?* Sabouraudia 14:65–74, 1976

78. WEITZMAN I and SILVA-HUTNER M: Non-keratinous agar media as substrates for the ascigerous state in certain members of the Gymnoascaceae pathogenic for man and animals. Sabouraudia 5:335–340, 1969

79. WILDFEUER A: Die Wirkung von Pimaricin gegen *Hendersonula toruloidea.* Exp Untersuch Arzeneimittle Forschung 22:101–104, 1972

80. ZAIAS N: Superficial white onychomycosis. Sabouraudia 5:99–103, 1966

81. ZAIAS N: Onychomycosis. Arch Dermatol 105:263–274, 1972

82. ZAIAS N, OERTEL I, and ELLIOTT DF: Fungi in toe nails. J Invest Dermatol 53:140–142, 1969

Glossary for Sections Two and Three

alopecia: any loss of hair. From the Greek for fox *(alopex),* an animal that commonly suffers from a mange which causes a loss of hair.

anthropophilic: infecting humans, either exclusively or principally.

apiculate (of a spore): having a short projection at the apex.

Arthroderma: a genus of the Gymnoascaceae characterized by the appearance of the cells of the outer peridial hyphae which are spiny and swollen at each end, and smooth and constricted in the middle, appearing dumb-bell shaped. All known species have either *Trichophyton* or *Chrysosporium* as the asexual state.

arthrospore (arthroconidium): asexual spore, characteristically cylindrical but often becoming rounded; formed by spontaneous separation at the septa or by fracture across the wall of sterile intermediate cells.

ascospore: one of usually eight sexual spores formed within a round or elongated sac (the ascus) as the result of nuclear fusion and meiosis. Ascospores may be uni- or multicellular. From Greek *askos,* bag or wineskin + *spora,* seed.

ascus: a specialized sac-like structure containing ascospores characteristic of the *Ascomycetes,* and formed as the result of nuclear fusion and meiosis.

aseptate: having no cross-walls (septa).

autotrophic: literally, capable of growing without organic substances as sources of energy. In medical mycology common usage has modified this meaning to signify the ability to grow in a vitamin-free medium, which may contain organic compounds.

bulbous: bulb-like; enlarged at the base.

bulla (-ae): a blister; from Latin *bulla* meaning anything that becomes round by swelling, like a bubble.

chandelier: from French *chandelier,* candelabrum. Repeated terminal branching of filaments in *T. schoenleinii* resulting in structures resembling antlers or candelabra; often referred to as favic chandeliers.

chlamydospore: from Greek *chlamydo-,* cloak; thick-walled spore, intercalary or terminal, which is formed by modification of a preexisting hyphal cell.

clavate: club-shaped.

cleistotheium: a closed (cleisto-) fruiting body (ascocarp) of an ascomycete, within which asci and ascospores develop. The ascospores are released with the disintegration or splitting of the ascocarp.

condiophore: a specialized hypa which bears conidia.

condium: an asexual, exogenous, deciduous spore; from Greek *konidion,* dust.

cycloheximide: an antifungal antibiotic produced by species of *Streptomyces;* Actidione[R].

cylindrofusiform: essentially cylindrical but with a slight tapering at both ends.

dematiaceous: belonging to the family Dematiaceae, in which the condidia or conidiophores (or both) are pigmented, generally olivaceous, dark brown or black.

dermatophyte: a plant (-phyte) capable of infecting the skin (dermato-). Generally applied to the fungi that infect the skin and its appendages exclusively, but there is nothing in the word to so limit it.

dermatophytid: a pustular eruption, allergic in nature, induced by, and usually distant from a primary infection by a dermatophyte.

disarticulate: to separate at the septa.

discoid: like a disc, i.e., solid, round and flat (or only slightly raised).

echinulate; covered with small spines; prickly.

ectothrix: outside (ecto-) of the hair (-thrix). Refers to the location of arthrospores in infected hairs.

endothrix: inside (endo-) the hair (-thrix). Refers to the location of arthrospores in infected hairs.

en grappe: in a cluster, resembling bunches of grapes (referring to microcondidia).

en thyrse: arranged singly along a hypha (referring to microconidia).

eponychial: on top of (epi-) the nail (-onych-).

favic chandeliers: see chandelier.

favus: a disease caused by *T. schoenleinii.* The word itself is Latin for honeycomb. The lesions are covered with scutula which may be crowded together to resemble a honeycomb.

floccose: from Latin, meaning wooly (literally, full of flocks of wool). The word appears in the name, *E. floccosum.*

fluorescence: the property of emitting light when exposed to light, the wavelength of the emitted light being longer than that of the light absorbed.

fusiform: spindle-shaped; narrowing toward both ends.

geophilic: term applied to fungi whose natural habitat is principally in soil (Greek *Ge-,* earth, ground or soil).

glabrous: from Latin, *glaber,* meaning smooth, and by extension, without hair (skin) or without aerial hyphae (fungal colonies).

globose: spherical.

griseofulvin: an antibiotic obtained from *Penicillium griseofulvum* and other fungi with specific activity against dermatophytes and related fungi.

gymnothecium: a fruiting body (ascocarp) made up of a loose network of interwoven hyphae through which mature ascospores sift out (Greek *gymno,* naked).

heterothalic: Greek *heteras,* other, different + *thallos,* a shoot. In the restricted sense used in this chapter, it refers to species consisting of self-sterile individuals requiring the union of two compatible thalli for sexual reproduction.

kerion: direct transliteration of the Greek word for honeycomb, beeswax, and honey. Used by Hippocrates for tumors resembling honeycombs but it is now applied to inflammatory tumefactions developing on superficial fungous infections, especially on the scalp, where such lesions may show many sites of purulence, vaguely simulating a honeycomb.

macroconidium: the larger of two distinctively different-sized types of conidia in cultures of fungi. May be single-celled or have one or more septa.

megaspore: Sabouraud's term for the large-spore (5–8 μm) ectothrix morphology in hair, as, for example, with *T. verrucosum.*

melanoid: from the Greek, *melas,* meaning dark or black.

microconidium: smaller of two distinctively different-sized conidia in cultures of fungi. Usually single-celled, and spherical, ovoid, pyriform or clavate in shape.

microides: Sabouraud's term for small (2–3 μm), ectothrix spores in chains, as with infections of the scalp caused by *T. mentagrophytes.*

Nannizzia: a genus of the Gymnoascaceae characterized by the appearance of the outer cells of the peridial hyphae which are only slightly swollen at the ends, have one or more slight constrictions along its length and are uniformly roughened. All known species have *Microsporum* as the asexual state.

obovate (obovoid): inversely ovate, i.e. narrower at the base.

onychomycosis: a fungous infection *(-mycosis)* of a nail *(onycho-).*

ovate: ovoid, like a hen's egg; narrower at the top.

paronychial: near or next to *(par-)* a nail *(-onych-),* said of the skin and other tissue surrounding a nail.

pectinate hyphae: hyphae with unilateral tooth-like projections, like those of a comb.

perfect state: morphological and biological representation (as, for example, by cleistothecia) of sexual reproduction in a fungus. Asexual reproduction is called the imperfect state.

pleomorphic: literally, having two or more spore forms; polymorphic. In the more restricted sense as used in this chapter, it refers to a degenerative change in a fungus which converts the colony into a white, fluffy one, no matter what the original appearance, and that microscopically has lost, either completely or in part, the ability to form characteristic and diagnostic spores.

pyriform: pear-shaped. (Latin *pirum,* pear; medieval Latin, *pyrum).*

reflex branching: branching backwards, that is in a direction opposite to that of the elongating filament (e.g., forming a reflex angle). Characteristic of *T. soudanense.* (Latin *reflectere,* to bend backward).

ringworm: this term, which is used to designate superficial fungal infections, harks back to the 15th century. It derives from the ancient belief that these infections are caused by worm-like organisms which induced the elevated border and from the fact that the lesions were often circinate or circular. Since the term has erroneous implications, it should be discarded by physicians and microbiologists, but is probably too firmly established.

scutulum: Latin meaning little *(-ulum)* shield *(scut-).* Used to describe a concave crust, seen especially in favus, composed essentially of fungal filaments and arthrospores.

septate: having cross-walls (septa).

septum: cross-wall in a hypha or spore.

suppuration: process of forming or discharging pus.

sycosis barbae: a new Latin formation from Greek roots meaning a figgy *(syc-)* condition *(-osis)* of the beard *(barba,* Latin).

verrucose; Latin, wart; i.e., bearing wart-like bulges.

verruculose: delicately verrucose.

vesicle: from Latin (vesicula) or French (vésicule) meaning small blister. On skin it is limited to about 1 cm in diameter; if larger, is referred to as a bulla. In mycology it refers to the swollen apex of a conidiophore or to blister-like protuberances on another cell.

Wood's light: an ultraviolet lamp with a nickel-oxide containing filter that permits the passage of light with a maximum wavelength of about 365 nm; used in medical mycology to detect, by their fluorescence, hairs infected by certain fungi and also lesions of pityriasis versicolor. Named after Robert W. Wood, American physicist.

zoophilic; applied to fungi that have a predilection to infect lower animals, rather than man.

Besides the general texts cited in the bibliography, the following sources were consulted in preparation of this glossary:

AINSWORTH GC and BISBY GR: Dictionary of the Fungi, 5th edition. Commonwealth Mycological Institute, Kew, Surrey, England, 1963

LEIDER M and ROSENBLUM M: A Dictionary of Dermatologic Words, Terms, and Phrases, revised edition. Dome Laboratories, Inc, West Haven, Conn, 1976

SNELL WH and DICK EA: A Glossary of Mycology. Harvard Univ Press, Cambridge, Mass, 1957

CHAPTER 49

SUBCUTANEOUS MYCOSES

G. D. Roberts

Introduction

Traditionally, the term "subcutaneous mycoses" refers to infections which involve the skin and subcutaneous tissues. Usually the infections remain localized to these areas without further spread.

The primary mode of transmission is usually by traumatic implantation of the etiologic agent into the skin or subcutaneous tissues. The etiologic agents include both hyaline and dematiaceous fungi, which usually exist in nature as saprobes. The common subcutaneous infections included in this chapter are sporotrichosis and chromoblastomycosis.

Sporotrichosis

Etiologic Agent

The single etiologic agent of sporotrichosis is *Sporothrix schenckii*, a mould that has a yeast form in tissue or at 37 C on enriched media and a filamentous form in nature and on various media at room temperature.

In general, the filamentous culture appears within 3–5 days of incubation at 25–30 C. Young colonies are moist, wrinkled, white to tan, and glabrous in appearance. With age, some colonies darken to brown and eventually to black; marked irregular folding becomes prominent, and the texture of the colonial surface becomes leather-like (Fig 49.1). Some cultures remain glabrous and may be mistaken for yeasts unless a careful microscopic examination is made.

Microscopic examination reveals small (2 μm in diameter), delicate, branched hyphae with numerous single, simple conidiophores arising at right angles to the hyphae. Small ovate to pyriform, hyaline to slightly pigmented, conidia are clustered at the apices of the conidiophores (Fig 49.2). Very close examination shows that individual conidia are connected to the conidiophore by a small thread-like attachment. The clustering arrangement of conidia is referred to as a "flowerette" or "rosette" type of sporulation. As the culture matures and begins to show slight pigmentation, single conidia develop individually along the sides of hyphae and are connected by a small thread-like attachment (sterigmata) (Fig 49.3). Conidia may resemble those seen in the flowerette arrangement or they may be somewhat triangular in shape. Conidia

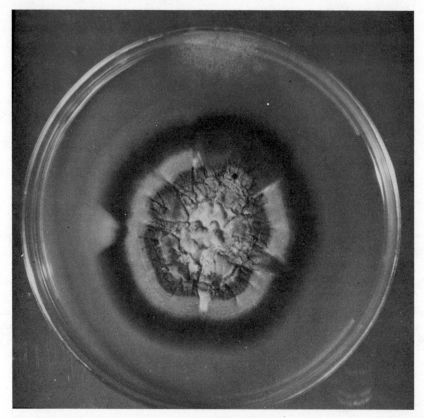

Figure 49.1—*Sporothrix schenckii.* Colony exhibiting dark pigmentation with folding and radial grooves. (Courtesy of American Society of Clinical Pathologists, *Atlas of Clinical Mycology,* Volume V.)

in this "sleeve" arrangement are usually darkly pigmented since their development parallels pigmentation of the colony. Cultures may exhibit one or both types of sporulation; however, either is characteristic of *S. schenckii.*

The final identification of this mould is based on the conversion of its filamentous form to a yeast form. Colonies of the yeast form of *S. schenckii* are moist and creamy in texture, shiny, and cream to tan or grayish-white in color. The colonies often resemble those of bacteria.

Microscopically, the yeast form is composed of a mixture of small, round to oval cells (5–10 μm in diameter) and elongated (1–3 $\times$ 3–10 μm) cells. Yeast cells may have single buds but more often exhibit multiple budding (Fig 49.4).

The definitive laboratory identification of *S. schenckii* is based on obtaining both the filamentous and yeast forms *in vitro.*

Clinical Manifestations

The clinical presentation of typical lymphocutaneous sporotrichosis seems to be characteristic of this disease. Commonly, the patient has a recent history of trauma to the upper or lower extremities. Frequently, the finger or dorsum of the hand is abraded or punctured by thorns or barbs of plant material or by splinters from wood, and the etiologic agent is introduced into the integument. Many times the patient fails to remember the traumatic injury but gives a history of handling plant material.

After an incubation period of 6–12 days, a small papule develops into a pustule which eventually ulcerates. Multiple subcutaneous nodules then develop along the lymphatics which drain the infected area. Many of the subcutaneous nodules become discolored and rupture spontaneously to form a chain of draining ulcers (Fig 49.5). Although the lesions are usually painless, they may become painful if secondarily infected by bacteria. This characteristic clinical picture persists with the chronic infection until therapy is instituted.

Many other sites of infection have been reported including the scalp, face, eyelids, nose, neck, and axilla. In some instances the lesion may remain localized without further spread by the lymphatic drainage.

Other forms of sporotrichosis including articular, pulmonary, osseous, nasal, sinusitis, and disseminated infections have been recognized; however, they occur much less frequently and the diagnosis is made entirely on the recovery of the etiologic agent or its demonstration in histopathologic section of infected tissue.

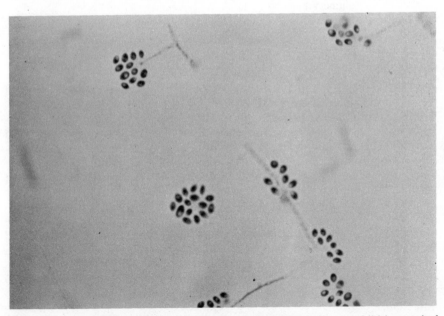

Figure 49.2—*Sporothrix schenckii,* filamentous form. Slide culture exhibiting typical "flowerette" clustering of conidia on single conidiophores. (Courtesy of American Society of Clinical Pathologists, *Atlas of Clinical Mycology,* Volume V.)

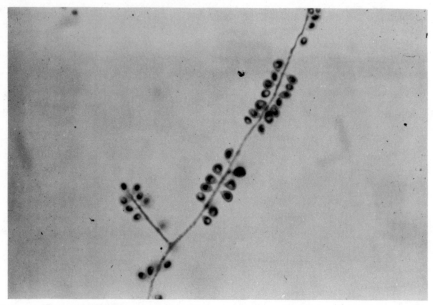

Figure 49.3—*Sporothrix schenckii,* filamentous form. Slide culture demonstrating "sleeve" arrangement of conidia along the sides of a hypha. (Courtesy of American Society of Clinical Pathologists, *Atlas of Clinical Mycology,* Volume V.)

Epidemiology

S. schenckii is found in nature as a saprobe in most of the world. The most common source in nature is the surface of plant material. It has been recovered from rose bushes, barberry bushes, straw, prairie hay, corn husks, sphagnum moss, cactus, tree bark, timber, and soil. The most frequently reported source has continually been the rose bush, and most clinical cases have resulted from traumatic contact with it. Bites by animals and insects have been implicated in the transmission of the infection; however, such cases have not been well-documented.

S. schenckii is a cosmopolitan fungus. Cases have been reported in Europe, Asia, the Americas, and Australia. It is more commonly found in the warm temperature zones of the world such as Mexico, Central America, and South America. However, many cases have been reported in Canada and in almost every part of the United States.

Sporotrichosis has been diagnosed in persons of all ages ranging from 10 days to 70 years of age; no single age group has shown marked susceptibility to infection.

The disease occurs more often in males than females at a ratio of approximately 7 to 3 (8). Most reported cases have occurred in males whose occupations required outdoor exposure or in females who engaged in horticultural activities. Hence, it appears well established that the infection is occupation-related.

Public Health Significance

Sporotrichosis is a definite occupational hazard to those persons who manually handle plant material that is contaminated with *S. schenckii*. Persons who are most likely to become infected include: florists, farmers, packers, gardeners, horticulturists, and others who might come in contact with contaminated material. Animals such as dogs, cats, rats, horses, and mules have been found infected also. Even though the infection is rarely debilitating, the risk of dissemination in the compromised patient is always present, and this type of infection is usually fatal.

Prevention is best accomplished by the use of gloves and protective clothing when handling materials that are likely to be contaminated with *S. schenckii* in addition to the avoidance of trauma. In addition, children should be cautioned not to play with hay that is likely to be contaminated, since it has been associated with several outbreaks. Treating lumber with fungicides is recommended in industries where the infection has occurred.

Since nasal sinus and pulmonary infections have occurred after the aerosolization of sphagnum moss, it is recommended that masks be worn during prolonged exposure to that material.

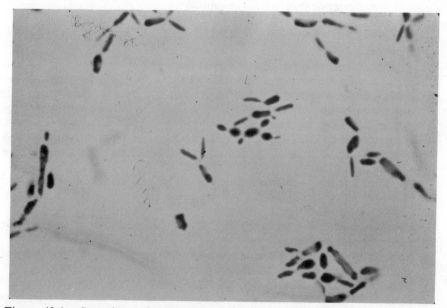

Figure 49.4.—*Sporothrix schenckii,* yeast form. Preparation showing elongated budding yeast cells. (Courtesy of American Society of Clinical Pathologists, *Atlas of Clinical Mycology,* Volume V.)

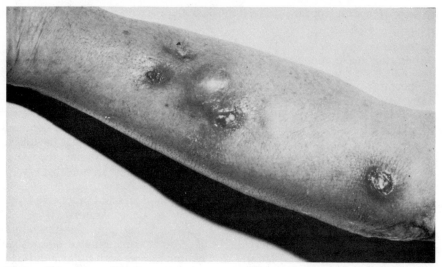

Figure 49.5—Sporotrichosis. Clinical manifestation of lymphocutaneous infection. Chain of nodules and ulcerating lesions are exhibited. (Courtesy of American Society of Clinical Pathologists, *Atlas of Clinical Mycology*, Volume V.)

Collection and Processing of Specimens

Types of specimens required

Cultural.

(1) Lymphocutaneous infection—Material from within subcutaneous nodules is best for the recovery of *S. schenckii*. A sterile needle and syringe should be used in aseptically aspirating an unopened nodule for subsequent culture. Exudate from draining ulcerated lesions may also be satisfactory for culture; however, such specimens are usually contaminated with bacteria. If curettage is desired, the ulcer bed is preferable; if a biopsy is necessary, a firm subcutaneous nodule or the active border of an ulcerative lesion is satisfactory.

(2) Articular infection—Synovial fluid should be aspirated from the infected joint with a sterile needle and syringe and then concentrated by centrifugation before culturing.

(3) Osseous infection—Curettage or biopsy of the infected bone will provide adequate material for culture.

(4) Pulmonary infection—Three subsequent first morning sputum or induced sputum specimens are satisfactory for culture.

(5) Disseminated infection—*S. schenckii* has been recovered from the blood of patients having disseminated infection; however, cultures are usually negative and are not recommended.

Serological. Although several serologic procedures are available for diagnosing sporotrichosis, there is little indication that they are widely used. Most cases of sporotrichosis are of the lymphocutaneous type and produce symptoms which are easily recognized by clinicians. In addition, cultures are highly reliable and provide information usually within 3–5 days.

More extracutaneous forms of the infection are being recognized but they are not easily diagnosed and serologic tests may provide useful information for this diagnosis.

If serologic testing is desired, serum is preferable to other body fluids.

Time of collection

Cultural. All specimens for culture should be taken from lesions which appear infected; otherwise, the time of collection is not important.

Serological. Serum for serologic testing should be collected as soon as clinical signs of infection are present. Specimens should be transported to the laboratory as soon as possible.

Number of specimens

Cultural. Enough specimens should be collected for culture to provide a representative picture of the infected sites.

Serological. Follow-up samples may be collected at 2–3 week intervals if desired.

Diagnostic Procedures

Microscopic examination

S. schenckii, in clinical specimens such as exudates, appear as spherical or ovate to elongate cells (1–3 × 3–10 μm) with single or multiple buds.

The direct microscopic examination of exudates from infected lesions has proven to be of little diagnostic value. The number of yeast form cells present in exudates is very small and this makes their microscopic detection difficult. The use of phase contrast microscopy or conventional staining methods has helped little. However, special fungal stains, including the methenamine silver or periodic acid Schiff-diastase stains, increase the chances of their detection in clinical specimens. It is interesting to note that although the yeast cells cannot be readily seen in a clinical specimen, they can easily be cultured from that same specimen.

The direct fluorescent antibody stain (6) has been highly useful for the detection of *S. schenckii* in clinical specimens but the availability of reagents is limited and the test therefore is not generally used in the routine microbiology laboratory.

Culture media

S. schenckii grows well and is easily recovered on most of the common mycologic media used in the diagnostic laboratory. Since specimens may be contaminated with bacteria or saprobic fungi, it is usually necessary to use a medium that contains antibacterial and the antifungal antibiotic, cycloheximide. Sabouraud's dextrose agar containing chloramphenicol and cycloheximide is an adequate culture medium.

Cultures should be incubated at 25–30 C and observed daily for the presence of typical colonies that develop after 3–5 days of incubation.

Identification procedures

The characteristic colonial morphology and the microscopic presence of delicate hyphae with conidia arranged in the flowerette or sleeve arrangement allows one to make a tentative identification of *S. schenckii*. However, since some saprobic fungi may resemble the filamentous form of this mould, it is necessary that both the saprobic (filamentous) and parasitic (yeast) forms be obtained in the laboratory. *In vitro* conversion to the yeast form may be accomplished by placing a large inoculum of the filamentous culture onto the surface of a fresh, moist slant of brain-heart infusion agar containing 5%–10% sheep blood. Slants may be moistened by adding 0.5–1 ml of sterile distilled water before inoculating the medium. Cultures are incubated at 37 C, and transfers to fresh media are made as soon as growth appears. The inoculum for the transfer should be taken from the portion of growth that appears most creamy in consistency. Several transfers may be necessary before complete conversion to the yeast form is accomplished, although conversion may occur in as short a time as overnight incubation.

Colonies of the yeast form appear tannish and are creamy in texture. Microscopically, the cells are round to oval to elongate and have one to several buds present. Demonstration of the yeast and filamentous forms of the isolate provides a definitive identification of *S. schenckii*.

An alternative to the *in vitro* conversion method is animal inoculation, which involves injecting intratesticularly a small amount of a suspension of the isolate in its filamentous form. Within a week or 10 days, the animal develops orchitis, and the yeast form should be readily visible on direct microscopic examination. The presence of yeast cells confirms the presence of *S. schenckii*.

Serologic procedures

The tube agglutination test developed by Norden (7) and the slide latex test developed by Blumer et al. (4) are highly reliable.

The fluorescent antibody staining procedure for the rapid diagnosis of sporotrichosis is highly recommended (6). It helps to quickly detect *S. schenckii* yeast cells in smears made from lesion exudates; however, its use is limited to a few large institutions.

Antimicrobial Susceptibility and Resistance

Virtually all cases of lymphocutaneous sporotrichosis respond to potassium iodine therapy. However, extracutaneous infections require treatment with amphotericin B. Fungal susceptibility tests using filamentous organisms are not reliable since numerous variables of the test have not been standardized. It is known that *S. schenckii* is resistant to 5-fluorocytosine and most isolates are resistant to amphotericin B at a minimum inhibitory concentration of 1.56 to 12.5 μg/ml (5). Antimicrobial susceptibility testing using *S. schenckii* is unnecessary and therefore not recommended.

Evaulation of Laboratory Findings

The cultural recovery of *S. schenckii* from synovial fluid or subcutaneous nodules and exudates from patients with a clinically compatible picture is diagnostic of sporotrichosis. The recovery of the fungus from respiratory secretions does not necessarily indicate active infection; however, a growing number of cases of pulmonary infection have been reported. The clinical significance of the isolate should certainly be determined by the clinician.

Tube agglutination titers of ≥80 are good presumptive evidence of active infection, whereas lower titers reflect probable nonspecific reactions and are disregarded. This test is highly specific, and elevated serum titers correlate well with culturally proven infection. The test is positive in 95%–100% of the extracutaneous infections and in 75% of the lymphocutaneous infections.

Latex agglutination titers of ≥4 are considered to be good presumptive evidence of active disease. The test detects more than 90% of the culturally proven cases of sporotrichosis, including lymphocutaneous infections.

Chromoblastomycosis (Chromomycosis)

Etiologic Agents

The etiologic agents of chromoblastomycosis are dematiaceous fungi thought to be closely related; however, the proper classification of these fungi was uncertain for many years. Currently most investigators place the etiologic agents in three genera, *Phialophora, Fonsecaea,* and *Cladosporium;* all are based on the type or types of conidiophores that they produce and are described below.

Phialophora type. Sporulation is characterized by the presence of specialized conidiophores that are vase shaped and terminate with a collarette. Conidia are formed at the end of the phialide, and as they are extruded, mulcilaginous material is deposited at the tip to give it a flared appearance. Conidia are characteristically arranged in clusters around the top of the phialide (Fig 49.6).

Acrotheca (Rhinocladiella) type. Sporulation is characterized by the production of oval conidia along the top and sides of a single, simple conidiophore (Fig 49.7).

Cladosporium type. Sporulation is characterized by the development of simple, slender conidiophores that bear conidia in branched chains (Fig 49.8). The length of the chain varies; however, conidia that have become detached show a scar (disjunctor) where they were previously attached to adjacent conidia.

The genus *Phialophora* contains fungi that possess only the *Phialophora* type of sporulation. *P. verrucosa* is the only member of this genus known to cause chromoblastomycosis.

The genus *Cladosporium* contains fungi that exhibit only the *Cladosporium* type of sporulation. *C. carrionii* is the one member of this genus known to cause chromoblastomycosis.

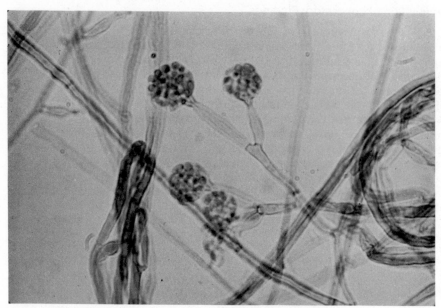

Figure 49.6—*Phialophora verrucosa.* Slide preparation exhibiting flask-shaped or tubu-
lar phialides with flared tips containing a cluster of conidia. (Courtesy of
American Society of Clinical Pathologists, *Atlas of Clinical Mycology,*
Volume V).

Some of the etiologic agents of chromoblastomycosis exhibit the acrotheca type of sporulation; moreover, some may have any combination of the
three types of sporulation. The genus *Fonsecaea* includes those fungi that have
the *Cladosporium* type of sporulation present with either or both the acrotheca
and phialophora types also present in the same culture. This genus includes *F.
pedrosoi* and *F. compactum*; the latter is the rarest etiologic agent of chromoblastomycosis.

(1) *P. verrucosa*

Colonies are slow growing, dark olive-gray to black in color, dome shaped when
young, and exhibit a flattened and velvety appearance with age.

Microscopic examination reveals the presence of vase-shaped or flask-shaped
phialides with flared cup-shaped tips; however, some may be elongated. Phialides usually occur singly but may appear branched on a single stalk. Conidia 1.5–3 μm × 2.5–4
μm are formed within the phialide and deposited at the tip where they are held together as a ball-like mass surrounded by an adhesive material (Fig 49.6).

(2) *C. carrionii*

Colonies are slow growing, flat to folded, velvety in appearance, and gray-green to
olive-black.

Microscopic examination reveals numerous elongate, dematiaceous conidiophores
that give rise to long flexuous chains of delicate conidia (Fig 49.8). Only the *Cladosporium* type of sporulation is seen. Conidia are regular in form (1.5–3.0 μm × 2.7–7.5
μm).

(3) *F. pedrosoi*

Colonies are slow growing, flat to folded, velvety to fluffy, and vary in color from
olive to dark brown to black.

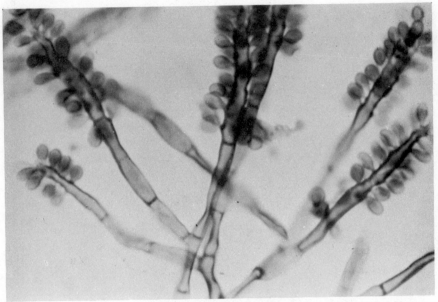

Figure 49.7—*Fonsecaea pedrosoi*. Slide exhibiting acrotheca type of sporulation with conidia surrounding a simple conidiophore. (Courtesy of American Society of Clinical Pathologists, *Atlas of Clinical Mycology*, Volume V.)

Microscopic examination reveals any of the three types of sporulation present. The abbreviated *Cladosporium* type with short chains of conidia usually predominates; however, many isolates show an accompanying acrotheca type of sporulation (Fig 49.7 and 49.9). The *Phialophora* type of sporulation, when present, resembles that of *P. verrucosa*.

(4) *F. compactum*

Colonies are very slow growing, heaped, brittle, and dark olive to black. After 3–4 weeks, tufts of brown to black aerial hyphae develop on the surface.

Microscopic examination may reveal the three types of sporulation previously mentioned. Branching conidial chains of the Cladosporium type are predominant. The conidia are usually wider and shorter than those of *F. pedrosoi* and appear more closely packed together in the spore heads (Fig 49.10).

Clinical Manifestations

Chromoblastomycosis is a chronic, usually well localized, mycotic infection that involves the skin and subcutaneous tissues. In most instances lesions develop on an exposed area of the body, e.g., hands, feet, legs, arms, shoulders, face, neck, and buttocks. Most lesions, however, are confined to the lower extremities.

The infection occurs as a result of trauma which introduces the etiologic agent into the integument. The primary lesion begins as a small erythematous papule that develops small satellite lesions around its periphery. These lesions aggregate, become red to violet in color, and eventually become ulcerated. The

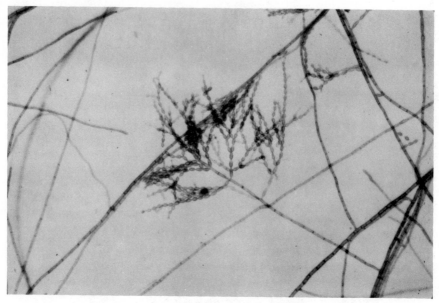

Figure 49.8—*Cladosporium carrionii.* Slide showing long chains of conidia attached to simple, slender conidiophores. (Courtesy of American Society of Clinical Pathologists, *Atlas of Clinical Mycology,* Volume V.)

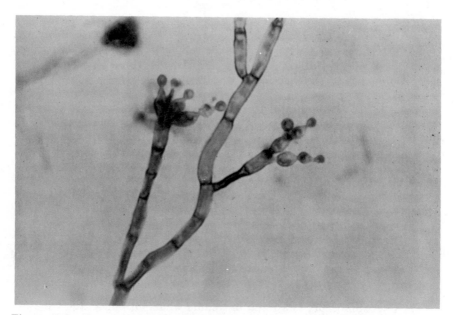

Figure 49.9—*Fonsecaea pedrosoi.* Microscopic examination exhibiting abbreviated cladosporium type of sporulation. (Courtesy of American Society of Clinical Pathologists, *Atlas of Clinical Mycology,* Volume V.)

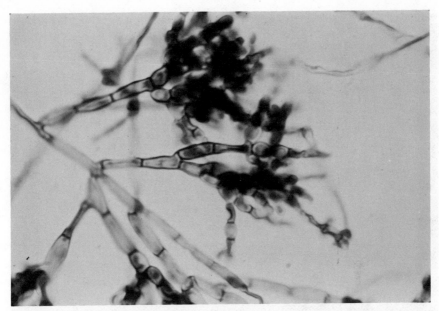

Figure 49.10—*Fonsecaea compactum.* Microscopic examination exhibiting closely packed spore heads having the cladosporium type of sporulation. (Courtesy of American Society of Clinical Pathologists, *Atlas of Clinical Mycology,* Volume V.)

ulcerated lesions later develop into crusted, dry, verrucous, darkly pigmented areas with well-defined indurated margins. Characteristically these lesions are described as "cauliflower-like" and nodular. The infection progresses very slowly and may be well-localized to a limb even after several years (Fig 49.11). Most lesions are painless unless complicated by bacterial superinfection. Chromoblastomycosis does not usually disseminate to other parts of the body.

Epidemiology

The etiologic agents of chromoblastomycosis are known to exist as saprobes in nature. They are most commonly found in soil and on wood and plant debris. They have been recovered from tree bark, rotting wood, forest soil containing decaying plant debris and decaying palm trees.

Chromoblastomycosis has a worldwide distribution, although some areas of the world are definitely more endemic than others. Most cases have been found within the tropical and subtropical regions of the world.

P. verrucosa, a common etiologic agent of chromoblastomycosis, has been found in Uruguay, Costa Rica, Venezuela, Ecuador, Brazil, Colombia, Paraguay, Japan, and the United States.

C. carrionii, a common cause of chromoblastomycosis in Australia, has also been found in Venezuela, Mexico, South Africa, Malagasy, and India.

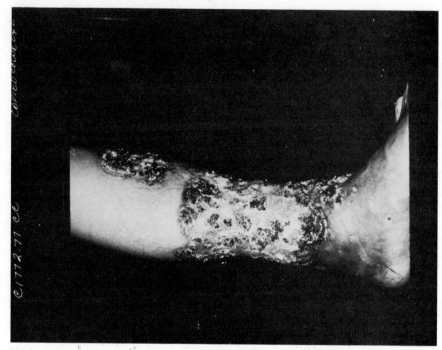

Figure 49.11—Chromoblastomycosis. Clinical case with "cauliflower" type of lesion with well defined indurated margins. (Courtesy of American Society of Clinical Pathologists, *Atlas of Clinical Mycology,* Volume V.)

F. pedrosoi, the most common etiologic agent of chromoblastomycosis, has been found in numerous countries including: Brazil, Venezuela, Argentina, Paraguay, Nicaragua, Colombia, Peru, Puerto Rico, the United States, Mexico, Guadelupe, Costa Rica, Honduras, Panama, and Cuba. It has also been found in Russia, Bulgaria, Poland, Finland, and Czechoslovakia, and in Japan, Ceylon, India, Singapore, Iraq, and China. African countries in which *F. pedrosoi* has been found include Madagascar, Algeria, Republic of Congo, Ivory Coast, Rwanda, and Cameroon.

F. compactum, the least common etiologic agent of chromoblastomycosis, has been found in Puerto Rico, Paraguay, Costa Rica, Panama, Venezuela, Brazil, Colombia, Bolivia, India, China, and Russia.

Chromoblastomycosis most often occurs among persons 30 to 50 years old; however, it has affected persons 3 to 82 years of age.

Most cases of chromoblastomycosis occur in males since their outdoor occupations provide exposure to soil and plant material.

Public Health Significance

Chromoblastomycosis is an important, but not a life-threatening, public health problem for persons whose occupations require that they work outdoors. The infection results from the contamination of traumatic wounds on exposed areas of the body, most often the extremities. The infection is rarely painful and may take as long as 40 years for an entire limb to become involved. The infection is debilitating only when it reaches an advanced stage. This usually is seen in patients who are members of the working group and consequently chromoblastomycosis usually poses a threat to their occupational livelihood.

Chromoblastomycosis can best be prevented by educating persons in endemic areas to wear shoes and cover the extremities and other exposed body parts. Early diagnosis and treatment can eliminate the infection before it spreads and involves large areas of the body.

Collection and Processing of Specimens

Cultural confirmation of the etiologic agent is preferable for the diagnosis of chromoblastomycosis; however, microscopic demonstration of the tissue form of the etiologic agents in tissue or exudates is adequate to make the diagnosis. Deep biopsy is preferable for culture since the subcutaneous tissue is less likely to be contaminated with bacteria or saprophytic fungi. Scrapings and exudate are often satisfactory for culture; however, they are most likely to be contaminated.

All specimens for culture should be taken from obvious lesions. If chromoblastomycosis is suspected, the lesion should be cultured and direct microscopic examination made as soon as possible.

Diagnostic Procedures

Microscopic examination

Direct examination of specimens. Scrapings or crusts from lesions or exudates should be examined by direct microscopic examination. Zaias et al. (9) recommend that diagnostic black dots from the surface of lesions are the preferred specimens for direct microscopic examination and culture.

Potassium hydroxide (10%) preparations of any of the above mentioned materials allow one to detect the presence of the round, thick walled, dark brown to chestnut, sclerotic bodies, that multiply by fission. Sclerotic bodies are usually 6–12 μm in diameter, occur singly or in groups and have fission planes in one or more planes. It is common to observe dark brown hyphae fragments in crusts or exudates taken from superficial areas of the lesion. No stain is necessary since the bodies are darkly pigmented and easily visible.

Examination of stained histologic sections. Special fungal stains are not usually necessary for the detection of sclerotic bodies in histologic sections. Most often they are found within the center of granulomas or abscesses. Hematoxylin-eosin does not stain the sclerotic cells and they retain their natural appearance (Fig 49.12).

Culture media

Most material from lesions of chromoblastomycosis is contaminated and it is necessary to use culture media containing antibiotics for the successful re-

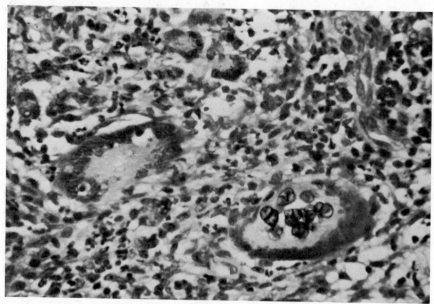

Figure 49.12—Chromoblastomycosis. Histopathologic section stained with hematoxy-
        lin-eosin showing typical sclerotic bodies. (Courtesy of American So-
        ciety of Clinical Pathologists, *Atlas of Clinical Mycology*, Volume V.)

covery of the etiologic agent. Sabouraud's dextrose agar containing chloramphenicol or other antibacterial antibiotics and cycloheximide is satisfactory for
the recovery of any of the etiologic agents of chromoblastomycosis.

Cultures should be incubated for at least six weeks at 25–30 C. Many cultures will show no evidence of growth until after three weeks of incubation;
however, they should be examined frequently to insure a prompt diagnosis.

Identification procedures

Definitive identification of the etiologic agents of chromoblastomycosis
may be difficult. Colonial morphology is of no value in determining the identification of the organisms. The microscopic appearance of the predominant
type of sporulation and the presence or absence of other types of sporulation
are necessary criteria for the definitive identification of the etiologic agents.

Temperature tolerance or biochemical tests are not helpful for the identification of members of the genera *Phialophora, Cladosporium* and *Fonsecaea.*
Gelatin liquefaction can be used to distinguish pathogenic *Cladosporium* species from the saprobic members of the same genus since only the latter liquefy
gelatin.

Serologic procedures

Serologic testing has no role in the diagnosis of chromoblastomycosis.
Precipitating antibodies have been detected in patients having chromoblas-

tomycosis, but antigens are difficult to prepare, are not standardized, and are not available for routine testing.

Antibiotic Susceptibility and Resistance

Most cases of chromoblastomycosis are resistant to chemotherapy. Amphotericin B appears to be ineffective; however, thiabendazole (2) and flucytosine (3) show some promise as therapeutic agents. Routine antimicrobial susceptibility testing for the etiologic agents of chromoblastomycosis is not recommended.

Evaluation of Laboratory Findings

The presence of sclerotic bodies in biopsy specimens seen on histopathologic examination provides a definitive diagnosis of chromoblastomycosis. The recovery of the etiologic agent in the presence of a compatible clinical and histological picture is diagnostic of chromoblastomycosis. However, these black moulds are commonly found in nature and their presence on normal skin may be expected and clinical correlation must be exhibited before their significance can be determined.

References

1. AL-DOORY YA (ed.): Chromomycosis. Mountain Press Publishing Co, Missoula, Mont, 1972
2. BAYLES MAH: Chromomycosis: Treatment with thiabendazole. Arch Dermatol 104:476–485, 1971
3. BAYLES MAH: 5-fluorocytosine treated chromomycosis. Br J Dermatol 91:715–, 1974
4. BLUMER SO, KAUFMAN L, KAPLAN W, MCLAUGHLIN DW, and KRAFT DE: Comparative evaluation of five serological methods for the diagnosis of sporotrichosis. Appl Microbiol 26:4–8, 1973
5. BRANESBERG JW and FRENCH ME: In vitro susceptibility of isolates of *Aspergillus fumigatus* and *Sporothrix schenckii* to Amphotericin B. Antimicrob Agents Chemother 2:402–404, 1972
6. KAPLAN W and IVENS MS: Fluorescent antibody staining of *Sporotrichum schenckii* in cultures and clinical materials. J Invest Dermatol 35:151–159, 1960
7. NORDEN A: Sporotrichosis: Clinical and laboratory features and a serologic study in experimental animals. Acta Pathol Microbiol Scand (Suppl) 89:1–119 1951
8. ROBERTS GD: The epidemiology of sporotrichosis. *In* The Epidemiology of Human Mycotic Diseases. Al-Doory Y (ed.). Charles C. Thomas, Springfield, Ill, 1975, p 232
9. ZAIAS N and REBELL G: A simple and accurate diagnostic method in chromoblastomycosis. Arch Dermatol 108:545–546, 1973

CHAPTER 50

SYSTEMIC MYCOSES

Lorraine Friedman and Judith K. Domer

Introduction

Systemic mycoses are caused by a wide variety of fungi, most of which are acquired by inhalation of organisms normally resident in soil or similar niches in man's environment. For histoplasmosis, coccidioidomycosis, paracoccidioidomycosis, and blastomycosis, there is (or there is presumed to be) an initial infection of the lower respiratory tract which usually is inconsequential or of such a benign nature as to go unrecognized. These stages of infection are often referred to as primary. When clinically manifest, as in primary histoplasmosis or coccidioidomycosis, they are indistinguishable from other common diseases such as influenza.

Occasionally, the organism may spread from an initial site of infection, following phagocytosis of either spore or yeast, and cause systemic disease. When the spread is from one organ to another or several, the disease is said to be disseminated. Any organ may become involved but different fungal species seem to have different predilections. The diseases are nevertheless clinically indistinguishable from one another as well as from other diseases such as tuberculosis, various granulomas, lymphomas, and other malignancies.

A major problem in the diagnosis of all systemic fungous diseases is the lack of any specific clinical feature, especially when there are no accompanying cutaneous lesions to trigger suspicion. With few exceptions, the onset is insidious and disease may be well advanced before severe symptoms appear, and the symptoms will depend entirely upon the area of localization of the organism.

Progression from the above described benign primary mycosis to serious potentially fatal systemic disease is a relatively uncommon event, for most healthy individuals have a remarkable capacity to handle their primary infections well; they usually heal spontaneously. In fact, infection is the rule and disease the exception.

This ratio is subverted, however, in the case of individuals whose natural defenses have been weakened by coexisting disease such as certain kinds of malignancies. Also, prolonged treatment with corticosteroids, antileukemics or other immunosuppressants that depress cell-mediated immunity, increases susceptibility to disease for the cell-mediated immune system seems to provide the major defense against systemically pathogenic fungi.

949

The humoral system is stimulated by fungal antigens but it is generally considered that the resultant antibodies are of little or no benefit to the host, although they are utilized diagnostically and prognostically.

Such sharply defined categories of disease have not been established for blastomycosis and paracoccidioidomycosis, although epidemiological data suggest primary benign forms of each. Neither do aspergillosis and zygomycosis fit the clinical spectrum previously described. A primary benign form is not known and there are few epidemiological data to suggest that one occurs. Exposure must be widespread, however, inasmuch as the etiologic agents are ubiquitous, probably more so than the agents of the above diseases. Clinical disease is usually systemic. There are clearly factors that predispose but the nature of host defense is not well understood.

The incidence and prevalence of any systemic mycosis are difficult to determine. None is contagious and reporting is not mandatory. In the case of histoplasmosis and coccidioidomycosis, skin-testing surveys have revealed vast numbers of infected individuals with no more than a residual sensitivity to antigens as a token of the experience. There can be no doubt, however, that systemic mycotic diseases (as opposed to infection) do constitute an important public health problem. Despite impressive advances in antibacterial antibiotic therapeutics, treatment of systemic mycoses remains seriously inadequate. Moreover, the prevalence of mycotic disease has increased concurrent with modern modes of therapy that prolong the lives of individuals suffering with cancer and other chronic diseases.

For the purpose of this chapter, only the above diseases and their agents will be discussed in detail, with limited comment on some that exceptionally have systemic manifestations. It should be emphasized, however, that many other fungi display a capacity to cause systemic disease. The list of isolated instances of such disease caused by fungi previously unknown as human or animal pathogens is extensive, and there is no taxonomic common denominator. Albeit not systemic, the diversity of fungi with pathogenic potential can be impressively exemplified by a case of mucocutaneous ulcer caused by a mushroom, *Schizophyllum commune* (109).

Cryptococcosis, which almost always is systemic, and candidiasis will be covered in the chapter on yeast infections.

Various texts and general references provide additional information regarding the systemic mycoses (24, 40, 52, 112, 129).

Coccidioidomycosis

The etiologic agent, *Coccidioides immitis,* is a dimorphic fungus in that it grows as a mould under ordinary saprobic conditions but is unicellar (nonfilamentous), although not a yeast, as a parasite. The precise taxonomic position is unknown. A sexual form, which would provide a definitive answer, has never been observed.

Based upon features of asexual growth, some have speculated (8) that *C. immitis* is a zygomycete, because asexual spores are formed within a sack (sporangium) during one phase of growth, a feature distinctive of zygomycetes. (In fact, it is on this basis that the term, sporangium, rather than mature spherule, is used by some to identify the large endosporulating forms by which the organism reproduces *in vivo;* this is the term applied to the asexual sporulation structures of the Zygomycetes.)

Other characteristics, however, suggest that this fungus is an ascomycete, viz., the hyphae are septate; there are electron-dense Woronin-like bodies adjacent to the septa; and there is occasional formation of spiral hyphae in culture, comparable to those produced by some dermatophytes (4).

There are various ways of categorizing the spectrum of coccidioidomycosis but in general they cover primary pulmonary infection, asymptomatic; primary pulmonary infection, symptomatic; progressive disease (extrapulmonary or disseminated coccidioidomycosis, progressive pulmonary, coccidioidal granuloma); or one of several chronic pulmonary residuals. These categories are not sharply delineated, however, and often merge, one into the other.

Cutaneous lesions are a common manifestation of disseminated coccidioidomycosis but primary cutaneous disease does not often occur. About 60 percent of primary pulmonary lesions cause no symptoms. In those that are symptomatic there is fever, slight dry cough, and chest pain. Night sweats may be present. Pleural effusion is common. Erythema nodosum and the Valley fever complex constitute those primary infections marked by intense allergic reactions.

In the majority of primary infections, recovery occurs in 2 or 3 weeks without sequelae, but approximately 5 percent may develop residual cavitary disease, sometimes nodules (coin lesions), or abscess.

In an even lesser percent, chronic progressive pulmonary disease may develop. Disseminated (extrapulmonary) progressive disease occurs in only a small number of individuals, although this number is increased considerably when infection occurs beyond the third trimester of pregnancy, and in black and Philippine males.

Progressive disease, if it is to occur, occurs usually as a gradual progression from a primary infection. A period of latency between infection and disease, such as in tuberculosis, apparently can occur but rarely. It is not uncommon, however, for the primary infection that precedes a progressive disease to have been inapparent. The course of untreated progressive coccidioidal disease may be chronic and of many years' duration, or fulminant and terminating fatally within a few months.

Signs and symptoms of disseminated coccidioidal disease depend upon the area of localization. Irrespective of localization, the histopathological response may be granulomatous, or suppurative or a mixture of the two. It is thought that the larger fungal cells (spherules) evoke a granulomatous response whereas the smaller ones (endospores) stimulate the polymorphonuclear reaction. For a review of the pathogenesis and clinical manifestations of this disease the reader is referred to one of several texts [e.g., (95, 97) for humans; and (63) for animals].

The mechanism by which this fungus brings about destruction of tissue is not clearly understood. By analogy with tuberculosis, delayed hypersensitivity engendered in the host may be contributory.

The geographic distribution of coccidioidomycosis is restricted rather sharply to the semi-arid regions of the Western hemisphere. These are parts of Mexico, Guatemala, Honduras, Venezuela, Paraguay, Colombia and Argentina; and in the United States, in several areas of southern California (e.g., San Joaquin Valley), southern Arizona, Nevada, New Mexico, parts of Utah, and southwest Texas. (The ecology, including distribution, of *C. immitis* was reviewed in reference 3.)

Maddy first pointed out the similarity of these endemic areas to the Lower Sonoran life zone, a biologic zone that is characterized by hot summers and few winter freezes, a low altitude, and an alkaline soil (85). Only a few animals and plants, including *C. immitis* survive. Outside of this environment, *C. immitis* appears unable to compete with other soil organisms and thus the endemic area does not enlarge even though without doubt the organism has been transplanted.

Within the conditions described, the fungus presumably multiplies when the soil is wet, forming arthrospores, which are disseminated by the wind when the soil dries, and may be inhaled. Since these weather conditions are seasonal, the disease likewise is seasonal to some extent, although arthrospores, once formed, are extremely hardy, are able to survive for long periods of time, and may be infectious at any time. Cases occurring outside the endemic area are thought to result from infection by spores carried on materials transported outside the area. The confines of the endemic areas have been determined by skin-testing of incoming noninfected populations (e.g., cattle), by actual isolation of organisms from soil, and by finding infected animals such as rodents.

The public health importance of this disease is unquestioned. In some highly endemic areas, such as the lower half of the San Joaquin Valley and in southern Arizona, 70 percent or more of inhabitants become infected. As previously stated, 40 percent of those can be expected to develop symptoms. The importance of symptomatic primary coccidioidomycosis can be amply documented by the statistics of Scogins (118). He reported 1063 man-days lost during one year at one Air Force base in Arizona, with 32 cases requiring hospitalization for an average of 12 days each. More man-days were lost because of coccidioidomycosis than because of upper respiratory infections such as the common cold. Other data support these observations; in the state of California during 1972, 1973, and 1974, there were 415, 415, and 526 new cases reported, respectively; Arizona reported 537, 542, and 571 for 1969, 1970, and 1971 (96). The importance of progressive coccidioidomycosis is further intensified by the long periods of hospitalization and continued significant mortality. Furthermore, in the state of California, several land-mark cases have firmly placed coccidioidomycosis among those conditions that may entitle an individual to workmen's compensation (80). The importance of coccidioidomycosis is such that vaccination undoubtedly would be widely used should an effective vaccine become available.

Knowledge of a relatively strong resistance to second infection as a consequence of recovery to a naturally acquired infection encourages continued search for an effective means of artificial immunization, not so much perhaps to entirely prevent coccidioidomycosis as to ameliorate the course of a naturally acquired infection and to reduce the incidence of the dread progressive form. To this point a vaccine of killed spherules has been tried on a limited scale, but with minimal success (96). Large doses are toxic and lesser doses do not consistently induce signs of immunologic stimulation. Whether or not resistance can be engendered with these kinds of materials, despite failure to detect antibody or delayed hypersensitivity, can be determined only by actual massive field trials, a criterion not easily met. Meanwhile, efforts are underway to isolate and concentrate the effective immunogen(s) that might permit inoculation with larger and perhaps less toxic doses (23).

Collection and Processing of Specimens

The specimen to be collected depends entirely upon the area of localization, and procurement is not different from that for any other systemic disease. An excellent monograph has been published by the American College of Chest Physicians that details diagnosis of the mycoses and should be referred to for collection of specimens (129).

It should be emphasized that for any systemic mycosis 24-hr sputum specimens should not be collected, that early morning specimens should be sent to the laboratory daily or at two- to three-day intervals, and that a minimum of six specimens should be submitted. Bronchial aspirates can be submitted when sputum is not produced or cannot be induced. When bronchial aspirates or sputa prove negative, nodes or direct lung biopsy can be obtained. Empyema fluid or cavitary aspirates may be collected. Pus from any draining sinus tract, if not copious, can be collected by means of a sterile gauze held in place for a period of time and the gauze can be cultured, or the wall of the tract can be scraped deep within the sinus. Skin or mucous lesions frequently accompany progressive coccidioidomycosis and these can be scraped or biopsied. When the meninges are the site of dissemination, it should be obvious that cerebrospinal fluid is the appropriate specimen to collect. Blood cultures usually are sterile.

Any specimen, irrespective of the site, should be cultured with a minimum of delay. If delay is unavoidable, the specimen should be stored in a refrigerator. The *in vivo* forms do not have the hardiness rightfully attributed to the saprophytic phase.

In the case of primary coccidioidomycosis with influenza-like symptoms, diagnosis usually rests with serology. Any cough is usually nonproductive and the benignancy of the condition does not warrant drastic measures such as lung biopsy. Even when other forms of coccidioidomycosis are suspected, sera should be collected. Detection of antibodies may assist in diagnosis, is indispensable for determining prognosis, and provides a means whereby effectiveness of chemotherapy can be monitored.

Diagnostic Procedures

In tissues or body fluids, *C. immitis* usually occurs in the form of spherical bodies called spherules ("sporangia"). These structures can range from 5 to 200 μm in diameter, but usually reach a diameter of only 30 to 60 μm. At maturity, the spherules have a thick wall (up to 2 μm thick) and are filled with globular or irregularly shaped spores called endospores that range from 2 to 5 μm in diameter. A mature spherule may contain anywhere from a few to several hundred endospores, sometimes dispersed peripherally and other times throughout the spherule. After sporulation is completed, the spherule's wall ruptures and the endospores are released; the liberated spores gradually enlarge and develop eventually into mature endosporulating spherules.

Direct mounts of clinical materials such as sputum, pus, pleural fluid and gastric washings can be examined microscopically as wet unstained preparations for the presence of spherules. If the sample is dense with host cells, a drop of 10% KOH may be added and the preparation gently heated to clear the specimen but the use of KOH creates artifacts.

Mature spherules are usually easily recognized by their thick refractile walls and the presence of endospores. Without KOH, however, granulocytes and mononuclear cells remain intact and can be confused with spherules, especially to the observer intent upon finding C. immitis. Large mononuclear cells filled with granules bear a striking resemblance to mature spherules filled with endospores. The granules, however, will not germinate whereas endospores will, and this can be determined by a few hours' incubation of the microscopic preparation (without KOH), kept moist to prevent dehydration during the incubation. If the cell is coccidioidal, hyphae will protrude in all directions.

Endospores recently released from a parent cell are virtually impossible to differentiate from host cell constituents, other debris, and small contaminating yeast in the case of specimens from a contaminated source.

Diagnosis of coccidioidomycosis by direct microscopic examination is contingent upon finding the fungus in its reproductive stage, viz. mature endosporulating spherules. It is possible, however, by observation of immature spherules (that stage of growth intermediate in size between endospore and a mature, endospore-filled spherule) to make a reasonably reliable presumptive diagnosis of a systemic mycosis, albeit unidentified as to species. Absence of budding would point to coccidioidomycosis as opposed to blastomycosis and absence of a capsule as well as no budding would tend to rule out cryptococcosis. Hyphae, rather than spherules, or a mixture of the two, may be seen in sputum from old cavitary lesions.

Regardless of the direct findings, cultures and/or animal inoculations should always be made. Specimens from a contaminated source should be inoculated onto a nutrient all-purpose medium such as Sabouraud's dextrose agar or brain heart infusion agar containing cycloheximide and antibacterial antibiotics. (See discussion of histoplasmosis and chapter on collection and isolation.) Specimens from a noncontaminated source can be inoculated onto these media without the added antimicrobials although the presence of an antibacterial antibiotic is useful in preventing growth of bacterial contaminants that occasionally are present in clinic and hospital-collected specimens.

The container for the agar medium is a point of considerable debate. Because of the highly infectious nature of the arthrospores, which would be the morphologic form obtained in culture, it is usually recommended that only test tubes with slanted agar surfaces be used. Usually it is recommended that such tubes be at least 25 × 150 mm in order to provide a broad agar surface. Use of Petri plates is definitely *not* recommended by most authorities. This is probably wise with specimens from noncontaminated sources, if coccidioidomycosis is suspected, or if the diagnostic facility can afford the luxury of tubed agar as well as plates routinely. In most hospital laboratories, Petri plates are replacing test tubes for use in isolation of fungi, in part perhaps because of availability of safety facilities. Furthermore, previously recommended procedures such as flooding a slant by inoculation of saline through a cotton plug is neither safe nor convenient. Cotton plugs have all but disappeared from the current laboratory, and this method of preparing a saline suspension for microscopic examination was never without some hazard. Spores of this mould are difficult to wet and in fluid media tend to form dry clumps that can easily release airborne spores during handling. Many isolates of *C. immitis* sporulate prolifically in culture. The spores are easily aerosolized and are highly infectious. Even the ideal of performing all mycologic maneuvers within a safety cabinet cannot be attained easily because of the desirability of performing microscopic examination of suspicious colonies. One rule to follow is that of transfer or examination while growth is still young; sporulation and, therefore, hazard is far less than with older cultures.

Cultures of *C. immitis* usually are incubated at ambient room temperature rather than at 37 C, although many laboratories have incubators set at 28 to 30 C. Irrespective of temperature, however, this fungus grows as a mould on ordinary laboratory media, albeit nonfilamentous *in vivo*.

Colonies of *C. immitis* usually appear by the 3rd to 5th day. Early growth may be moist, slightly convex, grayish in color, and may have a slightly granular surface. *C. immitis* characteristically forms abundant aerial mycelium, rapidly growing and white.

There is considerable variation among isolates. Some isolates remain glabrous, producing little aerial mycelium, especially in the central portion. Microscopic examination (which, as previously stated, should be done while cultures are young) of aerial growth typically reveals the formation of rectangular or barrel-shaped arthrospores (2–10 μm in diameter) that characteristically alternate with smaller empty cells. The empty cells rupture easily to free the arthrospores, often leaving remnants of the empty cells on the ends of the arthrospores.

There is variation also in microscopic appearance, however, as has been amply documented in the studies cited. Arthrospores may be thin-walled, elongated and lacking the alternate empty cells, and they may be round rather than rectangular. Furthermore, contaminating saprophytic fungi can be isolated that bear a marked similarity to typical *C. immitis* (e.g., *Oidiodendron* sp., *Auxathron* sp., *Malbranchea* sp.) (39, 120).

To identify *C. immitis,* conversion of hyphal forms to endosporulating spherules is necessary. This usually is accomplished by the inoculation of suspicious colonies into animals. A suspension of young growth can be prepared by flooding the surface of an agar culture with physiological saline containing a wetting agent such as Tween 80 (0.2% to 0.5%). Growth should be gently rubbed and suspended with a stiff inoculating wire. (These procedures are hazardous and should be performed within a safety unit.) The suspension can be transferred to a rubber stoppered "vaccine" bottle for easy withdrawal with a needle and syringe. Mice of either sex or male guinea pigs can be used. A guinea pig should be inoculated intratesticularly with about 0.1 ml of suspension. If the fungus is *C. immitis*, a marked orchitis usually will develop within 2 weeks, at which time fluid may be withdrawn from the testes with a sterile syringe for microscopic examination. If orchitis does not develop, the animal should be held for 2 more weeks then sacrificed and the testes examined.

If mice are used, several should be inoculated intraperitoneally with no more than 1 ml of the suspension. One can be sacrificed at the end of a week, and any exudate or lesion (usually omental) examined microscopically. If the first mouse is negative, the same procedure can be repeated with other of the mice at two and four weeks. Depending upon the virulence of the isolate, the infectious process will have remained confined to the peritoneal cavity or will have spread to the viscera, especially lungs. The finding of mature spherules containing endospores verifies the cultural identification of *C. immitis*. Although it is customary to culture any lesions, the mere recovery of the organism in culture is not sufficient for identification. Some saprophytic simulants can survive *in vivo* for days to weeks and can be cultured from organs at autopsy.

A major diagnostic problem is that most laboratories do not have experimental animals readily available. A system that offers promise is that of *in vitro* conversion to spherules. It has long been known that some isolates can be induced to form endosporulating spherules as well as hyphae and arthrospores *in vitro* by careful control of conditions of growth. Recently Sun, Huppert, and Vukovich developed this procedure for routine utilization in a clinical laboratory, but the procedure has not yet been widely tested (127).

The question is frequently asked whether failure of an isolate to grow at human body temperature is sufficient to rule out identification as *C. immitis*. Certainly such a behavior would suggest the isolate not to be *C. immitis* because *C. immitis* characteristically grows well at 37 C as a mould, but two recognized authorities (D. Pappagianis and M. Huppert, personal communication) have indicated they would not accept such a criterion, because of the repeated aberrant behavior of *C. immitis* in unanticipated ways.

An "exoantigen" test has been developed by Standard and Kaufman that offers promise for serologic identification of cultures, especially for those laboratories that lack animal facilities. Briefly, the method consists of extracting cultures about 1 week old and then testing the extract by immunodiffusion against known positive serum (71, 72, 123). In a total of perhaps a hundred cultures reported by several investigators (e.g., 32), the system seems to be highly sensitive and specific, justifying a presumptive identification of *C. immitis*.

Serology in the diagnosis or prognosis of coccidioidomycosis was the subject of a statement by the American Thoracic Society and has been reviewed by Kaufman (19, 66). It is covered in another chapter in this text (Chapter 54).

Antimicrobic Susceptibility and Resistance

The primary treatment for coccidioidomycosis has been with the polyene, amphotericin B. Although this substance is highly toxic, inevitably causing renal damage with prolonged use, resistance has not been a problem. Accordingly, susceptibility testing is not routinely performed.

Because of some therapeutic failures, despite *in vitro* susceptibility, and because of toxicity, other modes of therapy have been avidly sought. Among the agents recently introduced are a synthetic imidazole, miconazole (Janssen, New Brunswick) and a methyl ester of amphotericin B (124). (Another recently introduced antifungal compound, 5-fluorocytosine, is not being used with coccidioidomycosis.)

When susceptibility testing is requested, there are several systems that can be used. A broth-agar dilution method is described in the Center for Disease Control's methods manual (52). More recently, Holt has published detailed methods for susceptibility testing, including a disk method as well as one that is a tube dilution (59). The basal medium is synthetic and this appears to be important inasmuch as complex media may obscure results (58). At best, antifungal testing lacks the superb degree of standardization that has been accomplished with antibacterial agents.

Serum assays can be performed, at least for amphotericin B (10, 55), but are not without problems such as instability (9), and are not within the capabilities of most laboratories.

Evaluation of Laboratory Findings

To our knowledge, *C. immitis* has never been isolated from a patient in the absence of disease. This fungus does not colonize the respiratory tract, as may *Cryptococcus neoformans,* and does not occur as an airborne contaminant. At least the latter always exists as a possibility, especially in areas of high endemicity, but current information would suggest the possibility to be remote. Isolation from a clinical specimen, therefore, should be assumed *prima facie* as evidence for coccidioidomycosis.

As stated previously, diagnosis of primary coccidioidomycosis usually must be made by serology because of the inability of most patients to produce sputum. Fortunately, the antibody produced in this stage of disease (precipitin) is highly specific, does not persist for any significant period of time beyond recovery and is not detected in healthy individuals. Therefore, a positive test is acceptable evidence of coccidioidomycosis.

Histoplasmosis

The causative organism, *Histoplasma capsulatum,* is an intracellular parasitic yeast of the reticuloendothelial system of man and other warm-blooded animals. It is one of the dimorphic fungi, in that in tissue or on artificial media at 37 C it grows as a budding yeast; and in soil or on artificial media incubated at room temperature, it grows as a mould. Until recently, *H. capsulatum* was classified as an imperfect fungus, but the perfect state has now been described and this fungus is known to be an Ascomycete (76). The name given to the perfect state was *Emmonsiella capsulata.*

H. capsulatum var. *duboisii* is the causative agent of "large form" African histoplasmosis. The term, large-form, derives from the fact that the yeast cells of this variety are characteristically much larger in tissue than those of *H. capsulatum* var. *capsulatum*. It is considered a variety rather than a separate species, however, since the perfect state is identical to *Emmonsiella capsulata* and isolates of *H. capsulatum* var. *duboisii* can be mated with isolates of *H. capsulatum* var. *capsulatum* (77).

Histoplasmosis can assume any one of several clinical forms. Since the usual portal of entry is the lung, infection is initiated there. The fungus appears to be ingested almost immediately, however, by alveolar macrophages and quickly spreads hematogenously to other organs such as the spleen, liver, and bone marrow. Even though systemic spread occurs regularly, most infected individuals can deal with the fungus adequately and never show signs or symptoms of disease, or if clinical symptoms do occur, they are characteristic of only an influenza-type syndrome and the infection resolves without specific treatment.

The preponderance of subclinical or mild but acute disease is known as a result of skin-testing and autopsy surveys (33, 94, 125). In the autopsy surveys, calcifications were found in lungs and spleen that were unrelated to the cause of death and that obviously had been there for some time.

The clinical manifestations of disease can be broadly categorized into three syndromes: 1) primary histoplasmosis which can be either acute or minimally symptomatic, 2) progressive disease which can involve virtually any organ in the host, but only rarely involves skin or brain, and 3) chronic forms of the disease which are usually limited to the lung and in which cavitation often occurs. There is lymph node involvement in virtually all cases, including primary disease. Progressive disseminated disease is indistinguishable from miliary tuberculosis, and chronic cavitary disease is frequently mistaken for carcinoma of the lung. The acute form of histoplasmosis usually goes undiagnosed because of the unremarkable and mild nature of the disease and because it is often difficult to obtain appropriate specimens for culture. Lesions in tissue are granulomatous with epitheleoid cells, occasional giant cells, and macrophages containing ingested yeasts. Such lesions can resolve with or without calcification. The disease is not contagious.

The mechanism of tissue destruction in histoplasmosis is not clearly understood but by analogy with tuberculosis the delayed hypersensitivity engendered in the host may be contributory. Certainly, the tissue reaction in histoplasmosis is more akin to that of tuberculosis, and cavitation is more frequent than that of the other mycoses. This kind of hypersensitivity is a prominent feature of this mycosis.

African or large form histoplasmosis is characterized by cutaneous lesions that may extend into subcutaneous tissue and eventually bone. Pulmonary manifestations with or without calcification are relatively rare, but lesions have been described in lung, spleen, liver, and lymph nodes (21). The reason for the difference in pathogenesis from classical histoplasmosis is not known.

The natural reservoir for *H. capsulatum* var. *capsulatum* is the soil, particularly soil enriched with bat or bird feces (38). Birds themselves do not seem to become infected, but bats have been shown to have ulcers in their gastrointestinal tracts resulting from *H. capsulatum* var. *capsulatum* infection. Dilution of the excrement with soil and conversion to humus is important; *H. capsulatum* var. *capsulatum* will not grow on fresh feces. It is believed that the high nitrogen content of the droppings provides the soil with necessary nutrients for the fungus. Roosting places for chickens, blackbirds, and starlings have been implicated most often as the point sources of infection in individual cases, as well as in epidemics.

When infested soil is disturbed, aerosols containing the spores of *H. capsulatum* var. *capsulatum* are generated, and inhalation of spores of the appropriate size results in infection. In a rural environment, most point-source infections and epidemics have occurred from infected soil enriched with chicken manure, while in an urban environment, infections are usually associated with starling or blackbird roosts (44, 116).

Outbreaks have been reported as resulting from a variety of outdoor activities, e.g., excavations and environmental clean-up campaigns (27, 41, 47, 98, 101). Ironically, one of the latter epidemics occurred because school students were participating in Earth Day activities by cleaning their school's courtyard and driveways.

Portions of the United States and other countries have areas of high endemicity. In general, endemic areas are located geographically in tropical or subtropical climates and include most of the great river valleys of the world with the possible exception of the Nile River valley. An important endemic area outside of the tropics is the Ohio and Mississippi River valley in central United States. A part of the endemic area for histoplasmosis in the United States coincides with that for blastomycosis. The ecology and distribution of the *H. capsulatum* have been reviewed by Ajello (3).

It is difficult to assess the public health importance of histoplasmosis. Infection with *H. capsulatum* var. *capsulatum* is widespread, and it has been estimated that 40 million people in the United States have been infected (45). It has been estimated, also, that there are 500,000 new infections per year with 800 deaths. Eighty or ninety percent of the adults in highly endemic areas are skin-test positive. It is impossible to determine the extent of disease from these infections because the preponderance are mild and go undiagnosed.

There are presently no generally accepted preventive measures available, although attempts have been made to eradicate *H. capsulatum* from soil foci implicated in outbreaks (134). The most successful of the agents tested was 3% formalin.

Collection and Processing of Specimens

The specimen depends upon the site of localization, but those most frequently processed are sputum, peripheral blood, bone marrow, and node biopsy.

Any clinical specimen suspected of containing *H. capsulatum* must be handled promptly, more so probably than with any of the other systemically pathogenic fungi, and should never be allowed to stand at room temperature or held for long periods of time in a refrigerator.

Sputum should be collected after the first morning coughing spell and following a thorough cleansing of the mouth. Twenty-four hour specimens are of no value. If the patient is producing little or no sputum, attempts can be made to induce it by standard aerosol inhalation techniques. Multiple sputum specimens, six collections on consecutive days or at 2 to 3 day intervals, should be obtained. If sputum is negative or difficult to obtain, bronchial aspirates should be obtained by the attending physician. Empyema fluid or cavitary aspirates can be obtained under appropriate circumstances as well.

Hematogenous spread occurs with virtually every respiratory infection caused by *H. capsulatum* var. *capsulatum,* so that the culturing of venous blood specimens can be a useful aid in diagnosis. Yeast cells sometimes appear in the peripheral circulation in large numbers in terminal histoplasmosis, but they are released also into the circulation in primary histoplasmosis, albeit in smaller numbers and perhaps more intermittently; and daily blood cultures may serve as a means of diagnosing even the primary type pulmonary disease. (A patient usually will tolerate frequent withdrawals of venous blood whereas repeated marrow taps, or even one, is not lightly undertaken.)

Microscopic examination of peripheral blood in primary disease, however, is not a worthwhile effort, although organisms rarely have been seen and all technicians should be aware of such a possibility. Organisms frequently can be seen in peripheral blood of patients with progressive disseminated diseases, especially in the terminal stage of disease.

There is nearly always lymph node involvement in histoplasmosis, even in primary pulmonary disease. Therefore, when sputum and blood cultures are negative, biopsy specimens of mediastinal (preferably) or scalene lymph nodes may be obtained.

Bone marrow is an excellent specimen for the diagnosis of histoplasmosis. Usually a sternal tap is performed.

If the disease is widely disseminated in, for example, immunosuppressed individuals, there may be mucocutaneous lesions or lesions in the kidney, in which cases biopsy and urine, respectively, should be obtained for culture.

Specimens should always be collected for serological testing (prior to any skin-testing), to provide assistance in diagnosis, prognosis, and patient management.

Diagnostic Procedures

Unstained preparations such as with KOH are of virtually no value in the diagnosis of histoplasmosis. Blood smears prepared from the buffy coat or bone marrow in acute or disseminated disease, urine sedimented from individuals with progressive disease, impression smears of biopsies (e.g., lymph nodes or mucosal lesions), or scrapings of mucosal lesions, should be stained with a polychrome methylene-blue eosin stain, such as the Wright or Giemsa, prior to microscopic examination.

One looks for intracellular yeast cells in monocytes, macrophages, and rarely polymorphonuclear leukocytes. The yeast cells are small, 2–4 μm in diameter, and characteristically appear as round bodies consisting of a central stained area with a surrounding halo-like area. This capsular appearance gave rise to the name of the organism, but the yeast is not, in fact, encapsulated and the "halo" is actually an artifact created by shrinkage of the cytoplasm from the cell wall, which does not stain.

Another intracellular parasite which must be ruled out in a differential diagnosis is *Leishmania donovani*. When stained preparations are examined under an oil immersion lens, *L. donovani* cells will be found to contain a kinetoplast, an accessory body located to one side of the nucleus and consisting of two portions united by a fibril. The *H. capsulatum* var. *capsulatum* yeast cells contain no such body.

Direct examination of sputum, stained or unstained, is usually of little value in the diagnosis of histoplasmosis. One exception is examination with an FA conjugate specific for *H. capsulatum*.

Biopsies and other tissue specimens should be prepared for histologic examination and stained with hematoxylin and eosin, PAS, or GMS. The latter two emphasize the cell wall, and, in fact, this emphasis sometimes creates the illusion of an increase in the total size of the cell. Since it is sometimes difficult to obtain material containing sufficient viable cells for recovery in culture, diagnosis may rest upon histologic examination. This is especially true when observation of fungi is an unanticipated event, a portion of the tissue was not cultured, and there is reluctance to subject the patient to an additional surgical procedure in order to obtain another specimen. Attempts should be made to culture all specimens.

In tissue *H. capsulatum* var. *duboisii* is a large yeast, 8–15 μm in diameter and often found within macrophages and giant cells. It has similar staining properties to those of *H. capsulatum* var. *capsulatum*. The main differential, however, is with another fungus, *Blastomyces dermatitidis*, that also causes disease in Africa. The main difference, which is not readily apparent, is that budding of the *H. capsulatum* var. *duboisii*, when seen, is by a narrow attachment to the parent cell as opposed to the broad base of *B. dermatitidis*.

The culture media onto which the specimens are plated depend to some degree on the source of the specimens. Specimens obtained under sterile conditions can be plated on blood, brain-heart infusion or similarly enriched agar media that do not contain inhibitory substances, whereas for contaminated specimens, inoculations must include media containing substances inhibitory to bacteria (e.g., chloramphenicol) and to saprophytic fungi (cycloheximide). It should be noted that tissue forms of most of the dimorphic fungi are inhibited by cycloheximide in selective media when incubated at 37 C.

For primary isolation from a contaminated specimen, we inoculate Petri plates of a cycloheximide-chloramphenicol agar, brain-heart infusion agar (BHI) with chloramphenicol, Littman agar (chloramphenicol and oxgall), and Sabouraud's agar with and without chloramphenicol. If the fungus in the specimen is *H. capsulatum*, it will grow poorly, if at all, on Littman's agar.

There are other commercially available media which work equally well for the primary isolation of fungi and this list is not meant to be exhaustive. The important point is to use a battery of general and selective media that will provide adequate coverage for all of the systemically pathogenic fungi (refer to the chapter on isolation and identification for other media). This battery of cultures should be incubated at room temperature.

It is possible to treat contaminated specimens first with antibacterial antibiotics and then plate onto media without antibiotics; or antibiotics can even be added directly to the medium, under circumstances when antibiotic-containing media are not readily available. Specimens obtained from normally sterile environments can be plated onto an enriched medium without inhibitory substances and incubated at 37 C. All cultures should be closed in some way to prevent drying, e.g., placed in plastic bags or taped, especially those to be incubated at 37 C or any to be held longer than 2 weeks.

One to two weeks usually are required for colonies to appear on any of the media, but all cultures should be kept for 4 to 6 weeks before being considered negative.

If *H. capsulatum* is the causative agent, it will grow as a mould on the media incubated at room temperature, and as a yeast on media incubated at 37 C. The mould begins as a small white cottony growth, which, as it grows concentrically, may remain white and cottony, sometimes with the mycelial mat appearing to crack with age, or may become powdery with a buff to tan coloration.

The mycelial mat consists of septate hyphae with one or both of two types of conidia, viz. macroconidia (sometimes erroneously referred to as chlamydospores) and microconidia. The microconidia are usually 2–6 µm in size, have smooth walls and may vary in shape from round to pyriform. Their attachment and arrangement on the hyphae may vary as well. For example, they may be in clusters or single; and may be attached to the lateral sides of hyphae by short "stalks" (conidiophores) or occur terminally. Microconidia are generally regarded as the infectious particle, as they are small enough to penetrate into the alveolar spaces where they can be ingested by alveolar macrophages, convert from their conidial to a yeast form, and establish an infection.

The macroconidia are the most distinctive morphologic feature of the mould form, in that they are typically tuberculate, and the tubercle-like appendages can be visualized even at low magnification on the surface of the macroconidium. The size of macroconidia ranges from 8–25 µm. Smooth-walled macroconidia may occur as well, and a single culture may contain one or both types of macroconidia.

To make an unequivocal identification of *H. capsulatum,* the mould form must be converted to the yeast form. This is done by transplanting some of the mycelium to the agar surface of a slant of enriched medium (e.g., BHI or glucose-cysteine-blood agar), and incubating at 37 C. For best results, we have added approximately 0.5 ml of BHI broth to the tube prior to inoculation. The inoculum is placed in the agar above the fluid level. After 4 to 7 days, peripheral areas of the mycelial mat should begin to look pasty. Such areas should then be transferred to fresh medium. Most mycelial cultures will convert to the yeast form after about 4 weeks of weekly transfers. Rarely, however, will the conversion be complete; usually there will be a mixture of small (2 to 4 µm), thin-walled yeasts, some of which will be budding (singly), and of hyphal forms. There is nothing distinctive to differentiate the yeast form of *H. capsulatum* from those of other yeast species except that they are not encapsulated. They are easily differentiated, however, from the thick-walled yeast form cells of *B. dermatitidis.* The yeast form will convert to the mycelial form simply by changing the temperature of incubation to about 25 C.

Animal inoculation can be used as an aid in the identification of an isolate suspected of being *H. capsulatum* but which has resisted conversion to the yeast form. In such cases, mycelial growth is homogenized in saline in a safety hood and injected intraperitoneally into mice. Mice should be autopsied after a few weeks (usually 2 and 4 weeks). Smears of the cut surface of the spleen or of any gross lesions should be stained with Wright or Giemsa stains. Histologic sections and cultures may also be made.

For those laboratories lacking animal facilities or in an instance of resistance to *in vitro* conversion, a culture can be presumptively identified as *Histoplasma* by an "exoantigen" test which is currently being evaluated (see section on *Coccidioides*).

Contaminated clinical specimens, such as sputum, can be inoculated directly into mice. A specimen should be mixed first with antibacterial antibiotics such as penicillin and streptomycin, or chloramphenicol. High concentrations of chloramphenicol inhibit *H. capsulatum,* however. Otherwise, the quantity of antibiotic is not critical but 20 units of penicillin and 40 units of streptomycin or 0.5 mg of chloramphenicol per ml of specimen are customarily used. One ml of the specimen-antibiotic mixture should be injected intraperitoneally and animals monitored as above. If animals appear ill the first few days following inoculation, they are probably ill with a bacterial infection and should be treated with antibacterial antibiotics.

Arthroderma tuberculata and *Sepedonium* species, other fungi which produce tuberculate conidia that mimic those of *H. capsulatum* (73), can be distinguished from *H. capsulatum* because they cannot be converted to a yeast phase. Mycelial cultures of *H. capsulatum* that do not form tuberculated spores are indistinguishable from *B. dermatitidis* but their yeast phases are different— the latter being larger, thicker walled, and buds, when seen, having a broader base of attachment. The mycelial form of *H. capsulatum* var. *duboisii* is indistinguishable from that of *H. capsulatum* var. *capsulatum.* In the yeast form of the former, a few large yeasts are frequently mixed with small yeasts but the smaller forms are indistinguishable from those of *H. capsulatum* var. *capsulatum.*

Prior to the introduction of the "exoantigen" test, attempts were made to adapt fluorescent antibody techniques to the identification of isolated organisms, as well as to the demonstration of the organism in tissue (51, 69). Kaplan (64) presented an excellent review of the development of such techniques. This method is complicated by the presence of many cross-reacting antibodies in antisera, and adsorptions of the antisera must be carefully performed. Moreover, the staining properties of cells with antisera seems to be dependent upon the age of the cell, with young cells staining well and older cells staining poorly.

As with *H. capsulatum*, there are no standard serologic procedures available for routine use in the identification of *H. capsulatum* var. *duboisii.* Both *H. capsulatum* var. *capsulatum* and *H. capsulatum* var. *duboisii* share antigens in common and there are conflicting data regarding the production of specific reagents capable of distinguishing the two (60, 102).

As of writing there are three commercially available antigens for detection of antibody to *H. capsulatum*—yeast and mycelial forms for use in complement fixation (Microbiological Associates) and a latex particle for agglutination (Inolex; Hyland). Especially the latter, because of its relative simplicity, is widely used.

As mentioned previously, there are serotypes and mating types of *H. cap-*

sulatum but they have not been shown to be useful for epidemiologic investigations. There are several techniques available for the isolation of *H. capsulatum* from soil that may prove useful in identifying point sources of an outbreak. These have been reviewed by Smith (121).

Perhaps the easiest method is to prepare a 1:10 dilution of soil with sterile water and shake vigorously for 5 min in a stoppered container. Allow the specimen to sit undisturbed for 5 min and then draw off most of the supernatant fluid with the tip of a pipette located near the interface of the large soil particles and supernatant fluid. Chloramphenicol, 0.2 mg per 10 ml of suspension, should be added and 1.0 ml of the resultant mixture injected intraperitoneally into each of four white outbred laboratory mice. Since large inocula of *H. capsulatum* are required to kill mice, and since small inocula may be disposed of eventually by the normal host defenses of the mouse, the mice should be sacrificed at about 2 and 4 weeks, and bits of liver and spleen spread onto Sabouraud's agar plates, some of which should be incubated at 37 C and others between 25 C and 30 C. With heavily contaminated specimens, it may be necessary to continue antibiotic treatment of the mice, either intraperitoneally or incorporated into the drinking water to prevent overwhelming bacterial infection.

Antimicrobic Susceptibility and Resistance

Currently the only effective and available agent for the treatment of histoplasmosis is amphotericin B, although others are under investigation. Insofar as is known, there are no isolates of *H. capsulatum* resistant to amphotericin B. Since the drug is so toxic, and many individuals with acute pulmonary forms of histoplasmosis will recover spontaneously with only bed rest and symptomatic treatment, therapy with amphotericin B is not automatically instituted upon diagnosis of histoplasmosis, but is reserved primarily for individuals with obvious progressive disease, 80–90 percent of whom will die without therapy, and for those with chronic cavitary disease. Procedures for sensitivity and bioassay are not performed routinely but methods are cited under coccidioidomycosis.

Evaluation of Laboratory Findings

A definitive diagnosis of histoplasmosis depends upon isolation and identification of the causative organism in culture, or the demonstration of *typical* intracellular yeast forms in histologic sections. A presumptive diagnosis often can be made on the basis of serologic tests, but the use of serology for the purpose of diagnosis is somewhat more complex than with coccidioidomycosis.

H. capsulatum antigens as a group tend to be less specific but cross-reactivity is a problem that can be resolved by parallel testing with other fungous antigens. Less easily overcome is the problem of low titers in many individuals without active disease.

Low titers are common in previously infected but normal healthy individuals and titers can be boosted by skin-testing (a procedure that is gradually being discontinued as an aid to diagnosis of histoplasmosis). Residual and boosted titers are minimal, however, and titers higher than can be accounted for by a previous infection point to a diagnosis of histoplasmosis.

In fact, serology is frequently the only way of diagnosing acute primary disease, but for any form of this disease serology should be used as a screen, notwithstanding that failure to detect antibody does not rule out histoplasmosis. At the least, a positive serology will stimulate a concerted effort to obtain a positive culture. Serology also serves, however, as a basis for patient management—for prognosis and to monitor any chemotherapy. A more detailed discussion of the use of serology can be found in Chapter 54.

North American Blastomycosis

The etiologic agent, *Blastomyces dermatitidis,* is one of the dimorphic fungi capable of causing disease in man and lower animals. It is described as dimorphic because in tissue sections or exudates, as well as on artificial media at 37 C, it appears as a large, budding yeast form, but grows as a typical mould on artificial media at room temperature, i.e., 25–30 C. The perfect stage, *Ajellomyces dermatitidis,* has been described by McDonough and Lewis (88). It is an ascomycete with characteristics typical of the members of the family Gymnoascaceae.

Blastomycosis is usually a chronic granulomatous and suppurative disease initiated in the lung, but more often diagnosed on the basis of extrapulmonary lesions. The extrapulmonary lesions are usually the result of hematogenous dissemination from the lung. Clinical forms of the disease have been divided arbitrarily into systemic (including pulmonary and disseminated) and cutaneous.

Chronic pulmonary blastomycosis is difficult to differentiate from carcinoma or tuberculosis. Cavitations may occur but are uncommon (24). Lesions are characterized by suppuration and epithelioid cell granulomatous reactions with giant cells. An acute pulmonary form that is benign and self-limited has been described, but the incidence of such a mild form or of subclinical infections is unknown (115).

Dissemination of the *B. dermatitidis* may result in its hematogenous spread to one or more organ systems, usually bone, skin, viscera, the genitourinary tract, or the central nervous system (CNS), or there may be widespread generalized disease. Dissemination may occur concurrent with progressive disease of the lung, or there may have been spontaneous resolution of infection within the lung, often with no sign of earlier involvement of the pulmonary site. The gastrointestinal tract is almost never involved. CNS involvement is uncommon. The prostate may be involved in up to 15% of the cases. The histopathological responses are essentially the same as previously described.

Cutaneous lesions are the most common clinical observation in blastomycosis, but they are only rarely the result of direct inoculation into the skin. Rather, as previously stated, they are considered by most to result from hematogenous spread from a primary infection in the lungs. The cutaneous lesions may take months or even years to develop, and begin as small pustules which break down in the middle and spread peripherally. An irregularly shaped ulcer results with raised erythematous margins containing microabscesses. Such lesions occur most frequently on the face, hands, feet, and ankles.

The geographic distribution is predominantly within North America, but confirmed cases have been reported during the past two decades in Africa as well. The African and American isolates are closely related, since they are antigenically similar, but they may not be the same species since attempts to pair them have resulted in the production of sterile cleistothecia only (87, 126).

The endemic area in the United States seems to overlap with that of histoplasmosis but delineation has been difficult because of the lack of a sensitive and specific skin-testing reagent, and the failure to find its natural habitat. There have been only two published reports of isolation from soil, and one from pigeon manure (30, 31, 117). In fact, sparse knowledge of case distribution and circumstances of infection have probably impeded efforts to isolate *B. dermatitidis* from sources in nature.

Furcolow et al. studied the distribution of human and canine cases in the United States between 1885 and 1968, however, and suggested that the endemic area for blastomycosis may be even broader than that for histoplasmosis, extending farther eastward and more northerly (46).

There have been four documented outbreaks in the United States, two in North Carolina, one in Illinois, and one in Minnesota, but *B. dermatitidis* was not cultured from the environment in any, although attempts were made to do so (18, 74, 122, 128). (See 3 for a review of its ecology.)

The public health significance of blastomycosis has lessened in the past two decades. Illness and mortality have been considerably reduced through early diagnosis and the advent of chemotherapy. The disease remains, however, among the systemic mycoses of serious consequence. There are no known preventive measures.

Collection and Processing of Specimens

The predominant clinical specimens in which one is likely to find *B. dermatitidis* are various biopsied tissue, sputum, pus, prostatic fluid, urine, and joint fluids, although this depends, of course, upon the localization. Blood and lymph node biopsies are unlikely to yield positive material. The potential of prostatic secretions takes on added significance when considering that 90% of blastomycosis patients are male. As with all suspected fungal infections, sputum should be freshly collected. The handling and processing of these specimens do not differ significantly from those described for histoplasmosis, with the exception that *B. dermatitidis* is not as difficult to recover from sputum as is *H. capsulatum*.

Diagnostic Procedures

Direct examination of unstained materials such as sputum or pus is valuable as an aid in the diagnosis of blastomycosis. A presumptive diagnosis can be made on the basis of finding the typical yeast form cells of *B. dermatitidis* in the specimen. They lack a capsule, are large, 8–15 μm, and have a thick refractile wall sometimes referred to as "double-contoured." Single buds are attached to the mother cell by a broad base, 4–5 μm, and often remain attached until they have reached a size equal to that of the mother cell.

There have been two reports of the detection of hyphal forms in clinical material but such forms appear to be rare (22, 53). In tissue specimens, the yeast form cells can be revealed by staining with the PAS or GMS procedures following standard histologic processing.

The isolation media and cultural conditions are identical to those described for *H. capsulatum.* Samples plated onto media containing cycloheximide should not be incubated at 37 C as this antimicrobial inhibits the yeast form. All room temperature cultures should be held for 4–6 weeks before being considered negative.

Positive identification depends upon the demonstration of both the yeast and mycelial (mould) forms of the fungus. If cultures are incubated at 25–30 C the mycelial form will usually develop in 1 to 3 weeks. Colony characteristics vary and one isolate may have white cottony aerial mycelium while another may be tan. The aerial growth may be abundant or may be moist and closely adherent to the agar surface, even forming coremia which appear as protruding spicules. These characteristics are not specific and mimic many other fungi, including saprophytes but especially *H. capsulatum.* Globose, smooth-walled conidia (asexual spores) 2–10 μm, are produced at the ends of regularly septate hyphae or attached to the sides by slender conidiophores ("stalked"). Conidia may be abundant or only sparse.

To convert the mycelial form to the yeast form, the culture should be inoculated onto a slant of enriched medium, e.g., brain-heart infusion agar, and incubated at 37 C. After a few days, the colony, or portions thereof, will begin to appear glabrous or waxy. Such portions should then be transferred to fresh medium and incubated again at 37 C. Several such transfers may be required to obtain complete conversion. Moreover, moisture seems to be important in the conversion, and it is helpful to pipette about 0.5 ml of liquid medium onto each slant prior to inoculating the agar surface (see discussion of histoplasmosis).

An occasional isolate of *B. dermatitidis* is difficult to recover from clinical material, does not produce typical colonies *in vitro,* or does not readily convert to the yeast phase *in vitro.* In such instances, mice can be inoculated intraperitoneally with clinical material, as described under histoplasmosis, or with a suspension of the isolate. The animals should be sacrificed 1 to 4 weeks (at intervals) following inoculation and the peritoneal cavities examined for localized abscesses. Yeast typical of *B. dermatitidis* usually can be seen in the pus, and culture at 37 C will yield yeast phase growth.

A procedure for immunologic identification of cultures ("exoantigen" test, see section on *Coccidioides immitis*) is said to be valuable for presumptive identification of cultures (72), but its sensitivity and specificity for *Blastomyces* has not yet been confirmed.

Serologic procedures can be performed in any laboratory set up to perform complement fixation; antigens are commercially available (Microbiological Associates). Furthermore, these tests are available through most Public Health laboratories. The fungal reagents developed to date have been cross-reactive with other of the systemically pathogenic fungi, mainly *H. capsulatum* but this poses no serious problem inasmuch as it is customary to perform a battery of tests using both antigens. The main problem is that many patients, even with culturally proven blastomycosis, may not have detectable levels of antibody. This is especially true when the disease process is not extensive. When antibodies are present, however, a valid assumption is that the patient has blastomycosis and the laboratory should be able to isolate the organism. Apart from usefulness as a diagnostic aid, serological data provide invaluable assistance in judging the extent of invasion, prognosis, and a means of monitoring chemotherapy.

Among the newer serologic procedures is an immunodiffusion test that reportedly detects 80% of proven cases of blastomycosis but it is not in routine use (70).

A fluorescent-antibody test has been developed for the identification of the yeast form of *B. dermatitidis* in tissue or culture, but it is used only in special laboratories, and the serum is not commercially available (65).

Antimicrobic Susceptibility and Resistance

There are two drugs that can be used against *B. dermatitidis,* amphotericin B and 2-hydroxy-stilbamidine (Hydroxy-stilbamidine isothionate). Both drugs are administered intravenously. The latter drug is less toxic than amphotericin B and is particularly useful in patients with skin lesions and noncavitary pulmonary involvement. There are no known resistant strains to either antifungal, although therapeutic failure may result if treatment is withheld because of an improper diagnosis; the disease may have progressed to the point where therapy is not effective. Susceptibility testing is not routinely performed, but there are methods for testing (described under coccidioidomycosis).

Evaluation of Laboratory Findings

The finding of typical yeast forms in unstained wet mounts of clinical material is sufficient evidence to begin antifungal therapy. This presumptive diagnosis, however, should be confirmed by positive culture, which usually can be obtained without difficulty.

The usefulness of serology in diagnosis and prognosis is not widely acclaimed by clinicians, largely, as stated above, because blastomycosis patients so often have negative serology. Even with this mycosis, however, serology does provide assistance, although perhaps not to the same extent as with histoplasmosis and coccidioidomycosis. The presence of antibodies is, nevertheless, presumptive evidence of blastomycosis that should spur efforts to obtain cultural isolation. Even a negative serology is of assistance in proper patient evaluation inasmuch as absence of antibody indicates minimal invasion. Serology is discussed in greater detail in Chapter 54.

Since there is no commercially available skin-test reagent, the skin-test cannot be used as a diagnostic aid.

Paracoccidioidomycosis (South American Blastomycosis)

Paracoccidioides brasiliensis, a dimorphic fungus occurring in tissue or on artificial media at 37 C as a yeast and at 25–30 C as a mould, is the causative agent of paracoccidioidomycosis. This fungus is characterized as "imperfect" since a sexual stage has not been described.

The disease is chronic and progressive, suppurative, and granulomatous, with a wide variety of clinical manifestations. Since one of the most prominent features of the disease in a high percentage of the cases is lesions of the oral and nasal mucosa, it was believed for many years that the primary portal of entry was mucocutaneous via traumatic introduction of the fungus (82, 83). It has become increasingly clear in recent years, however, as the result of animal experimentation and studies of autopsy and case histories that the primary portal of entry is the lung, and that all other manifestations result from hematogenous spread.

The main difficulty in defining the evolution of the disease is that there appears to be a long interval (months or years) between initial contact with the etiologic agent and the appearance of clinically recognizable disease. Giraldo et al. have presented a study of 46 patients seen in Colombia between 1971 and 1974, and have developed a model of pathogenesis in which they propose that primary exposure to the pathogen via the respiratory route initiates infection, that the infection stage is asymptomatic and may never proceed beyond that, but that infection may proceed to disease in a certain percentage of individuals (50).

These investigators further hypothesized that if the infected individuals are young, disease usually takes the form of an acute syndrome, the severity of which depends on the degree of organ involvement; but if the individuals are older, disease usually takes the form of a chronic syndrome and can either be localized to the lung or may involve other tissues, notably mucocutaneous tissue, the lymphatics and viscera.

The most common sites of paracoccidioidomycosis are pulmonary, gastrointestinal, and mucocutaneous. Gastrointestinal involvement and prominent cervical lymphadenopathy are features that distinguish this disease from blastomycosis. The cutaneous and mucocutaneous lesions are typically ulcers or crusted granulomas and must be distinguished from lesions resulting from cutaneous tuberculosis, yaws and cutaneous leishmaniasis. Microscopic examination of exudates of such lesions, however, results in the observation of the typical yeast form cells of *P. brasiliensis.*

This mycosis is confined primarily to the subtropical forest areas of South America. A few cases have been reported from Central America and Mexico. Ten cases have been reported in the United States but all originated in Latin America (16, 92). Initially, the disease was called the Brazilian disease because of its prevalence in that country.

The ecologic niche of *P. brasiliensis* is unknown, but based upon circumstantial evidence, it is believed to reside in soil, and, in fact, has been isolated from soil on at least one occasion (28). The disease predominates in males, many of whom are agricultural workers. Paracoccidioidomycosis is not communicable. Skin-test antigens, which would aid in a definition of specific endemic areas, are currently in a developmental stage and are not generally available for epidemiologic studies.

The public health importance of paracoccidioidomycosis cannot be doubted. Mackinnon dramatically emphasized this in his literature survey of nearly 5000 cases, most of which came from Brazil (84). The importance is further emphasized by the marked chronicity, frequent disability and requirement for lengthy treatment. Cases usually do not come to the attention of a physician until the appearance of secondary manifestations resulting from systemic spread. There is no way of knowing how many individuals have been infected. There are no preventive measures.

Collection and Processing of Specimens

Sputum, scrapings or pus from mucocutaneous or cutaneous ulcers, and biopsy material are the commonest specimens processed. *P. brasiliensis* usually is not recoverable from blood. Processing of these specimens does not differ from that described for the other systemic mycoses (see discussion of histoplasmosis and Chapter 47).

Diagnostic Procedures

Microscopic examination of unstained clinical material is especially valuable as an aid in the diagnosis of paracoccidioidomycosis. The demonstration of typical, large yeast forms (30 μm is not uncommon) with multiple buds attached circumferentially by narrow "stalks," is virtually pathognomonic. The mother cells and attached small buds may give the appearance of a "pilot's wheel." The budding cells are usually slightly ovate and have a thinner wall than the mother cell. Older cells have thicker walls but they seldom attain the thickness characteristic of *B. dermatitidis.*

Biopsy specimens can be fixed and stained by standard histologic techniques. Typical budding forms can be seen in sections stained with hematoxylin and eosin, but are visualized better with special stains, such as PAS and GMS.

P. brasiliensis will grow on the mycologic media routinely used in diagnostic laboratories, e.g., Sabouraud's or modified Sabouraud's agar. It has been demonstrated recently, however, that yeast extract agar is superior for recovery of this fungus from sputum, primarily because growth of *Candida* sp. is limited (108). Specimens acquired under aseptic conditions from normally sterile sources can be plated directly onto blood agar or other enriched media, and incubated at 37 C, but all other cultures should be incubated initially at 25–30 C.

P. brasiliensis, like the other dimorphic pathogenic fungi, is identified on the basis of its morphology and colony characteristics when incubated at both room temperature and 37 C.

At room temperature (usually 25–30 C) the fungus slowly grows as a white mould with dense but short aerial hyphae. With age, the colony may turn brown. Sporulating cultures are the exception rather than the rule but when conidia are present, they are indistinguishable from those produced by *B. dermatitidis.*

Restrepo found that more isolates sporulated on the yeast extract medium than on Sabouraud's agar, producing arthrospores as well as conidia; and that primary isolates and recent stock cultures sporulated better than old cultures (107).

To confirm the identification of *P. brasiliensis* the mycelial form must be converted to the yeast form, or vice versa. The procedures are as described for *H. capsulatum* and *B. dermatitidis.* In the yeast form, the typical large forms with multiple buds must be seen. The mycelial form of *P. brasiliensis* is the slowest growing of the fungi that cause systemic disease and, in fact, because of this very slow growth rate, laboratories sometimes have difficulty in isolating the fungus in its mycelial form. For this fungus, therefore, perhaps more than any other of the dimorphics, considerable reliance is placed upon isolation at 37 C rather than room temperature, but only if the specimen is not contaminated with other moulds.

A procedure for immunologic identification of cultures ("exoantigen" test, see section on *Coccidioides immitis*) is said to be valuable for presumptive identification of cultures (72), but its sensitivity and specificity for *Paracoccidioides* have not been confirmed.

Laboratory animals are relatively resistant to infection with *P. brasiliensis,* *in vitro* conversion is relatively easy, and its yeast form is so characteristic, that animal inoculation is seldom used.

Serologic procedures are covered elsewhere. Suffice it to say that they are valuable adjuncts to the diagnosis of paracoccidioidomycosis, but that commercial preparations are not available and the tests are performed mainly in special laboratories.

There are no commercially available skin-test antigens for detecting sensitivity to *P. brasiliensis.* There are several preparations, including culture filtrates and polysaccharide fractions, that have been and are being used experimentally, however.

Antimicrobic Susceptibility and Resistance

The major chemotherapeutic agents employed in paracoccidioidomycosis are the sulfonamides and amphotericin B. Therapy with sulfadiazine or sulfisoxazole is relatively inexpensive and easy to administer, and so is used primarily for the less advanced forms of the disease (42). Sulfonamide treatment, however, appears to be more suppressive than curative and relapses are frequent when used on advanced cases. Treatment with amphotericin B usually results in more rapid healing of dermal lesions and more effective regression of visceral lesions. Miconazole has been reported to be effective in at least one case (132).

Susceptibility testing is not usually performed but methods are cited under coccidioidomycosis.

Evaluation of Laboratory Findings

A definitive diagnosis rests on the isolation and identification of *P. brasiliensis* in culture, but evidence of infection sometimes rests upon the demonstration of *typical* yeast form cells in clinical specimens or on the demonstration of precipitin reaction with the patient's serum.

Aspergillosis

Unlike previously discussed agents of systemic fungus disease, the pathogenic aspergilli are not dimorphic. They grow as moulds both *in vitro* and *in vivo*. Their hyphae are septate and branched. Cleistothecia (structures bearing sexually formed spores) are formed by some species, placing them among the Ascomycetes. Those species having a sexual stage are placed in different genera (Eurotium, Sartoya, Emericella). For most species, however, sexual reproduction has not been observed and identification is contingent upon colony characteristics such as pigment and morphology.

There are nearly 150 recognized species and varieties, all of which are normally saprophytic in the environment or plant pathogens. Of this large number, relatively few, perhaps a half dozen, cause most of the cases of aspergillosis in man and lower animals.

Sites of infection include nail (uncommon), external auditory canal, and the respiratory tract, including the paranasal sinuses. In 1963, Wahner and associates presented an excellent review of cases depicting pulmonary aspergillosis (133). Since that time there have been many additional reports that attest to the spectrum of pulmonary aspergillosis, e.g., Young et al., Prystowsky et al., Varkey and Rose, and Pennington (99, 103, 130, 136).

Common manifestations of pulmonary infection are bronchopneumonia, bronchitis, abscess, and granuloma; or infection may be localized, with only saprophytic growth of the fungus, usually within a pre-existing cavity (aspergilloma, "fungus ball"). Occasionally there is dissemination, with involvement of many organs, including the meninges; in exception, aspergillomas seem to remain localized and rarely become invasive. In most individuals, aspergillosis is secondary to another disease but may, nevertheless, be the primary cause of death. A lesion usually is characterized by tissue and vascular invasion, especially the latter, with thrombosis, infarction, and hemorrhage. The mechanism of this invasive property is not known. Aspergilli do form toxins (e.g., aflatoxin) that are known to be lethal or highly carcinogenic to some species (e.g., trout, turkeys), but there is no direct evidence that such metabolites are toxic to man, or that they are produced *in vivo*. Neither is there evidence that an *Aspergillus* "endotoxin," described many years ago by Henrici and later confirmed (20), contributes to the pathogenicity of the aspergilli.

Pulmonary aspergillosis may be manifest also as an allergic condition—in atopic subjects, as asthma and pulmonary infiltrates with eosinophilia (100). In nonatopic individuals, allergy to aspergilli can result in a clinical picture (allergic alveolitis) analogous to farmer's lung disease. In the latter and with pulmonary infiltration, antibody of the Arthus type is thought to be operative.

The public health significance of aspergillosis is limited. There is no threat to the normal individual. As with many other mycoses, patients with leukemia and lymphoma appear to be more susceptible. Clinical and experimental evidence suggests anti-neoplastic as well as corticosteroid therapy also contribute to increased susceptibility. Attempts to prevent disease by immunization are not feasible. It would seem desirable, however, to protect highly susceptible patient populations from excessive exposure by attempting to reduce high concentrations of *Aspergillus* sp. spores in hospital environments. In at least one instance, an increase in aspergillosis was associated with highly contaminated fireproofing materials used in the construction of a new hospital (2).

Collection and Processing of Specimens

Specimens are usually tissue, either biopsy or autopsy, or sputum, and the processing does not differ from that of any other systemic mycosis (see discussion of histoplasmosis and Chapter 47.)

Sera can be tested for antibodies with a variety of serological procedures (see Chapter 54.)

Diagnostic Procedures

Tissue should be sectioned and stained by hematoxylin and eosin and PAS, Gridley, or GMS. We prefer the latter one.

The *Aspergillus* sp. will be seen in the form of hyphae but a major problem is differentiating their hyphae from those of a Zygomycete. The traditional distinction is that *in vivo* hyphae in the latter are relatively broad, irregularly branched and non-septate, whereas those in aspergillosis are relatively narrow, dichotomously branched and septate. Frequently, however, such sharp distinctions are not apparent. (Refer to section on zygomycosis for details on differences.)

Furthermore, Ascomycetes other than *Aspergillus* but having the same *in vivo* morphology as the *Aspergillus* sp. may be encountered as agents of disease, especially in the present era of longterm life-support for patients with chronic diseases.

Any specimen, but especially one from a contaminated source, should be examined microscopically as a "wet" preparation. Aspergilli, as well as other moulds, usually appear as hyphae that must be distinguished from the pseudohyphae of a yeast. Cells of the latter will be separated by constrictions (pseudohyphae are, in fact, a series of elongated buds) whereas hyphae of the type formed by the aspergilli will consist of cells separated by cross-walls (septations). It should be noted, however, that some yeasts, including *Candida*, can form true (septate) hyphae. The hyphae of aspergilli cannot be differentiated from those of other moulds—other than zygomycetes (phycomycetes), which are nonseptate and the septate mycelium of dematiaceous fungi.

Conidiophores with spores sometimes form *in vivo* and can be seen in section, especially if the tissue derives from an area exposed to air such as a pulmonary cavity.

Media to be inoculated should include one that contains antibacterial substances but not cycloheximide because most species grow poorly and some not at all in the presence of this antifungal agent. Sabouraud dextrose agar containing chloramphenicol is commonly used. Littman oxgall agar with chloramphenicol has the added advantage of restricting colony size of contaminating moulds as well as aspergilli, which may facilitate isolation. (See section on histoplasmosis and Chapter 47).

Petri dishes can be used. However, most cultures in plates sporulate readily and prolifically and provide an annoying source of contamination in the laboratory.

Media should be heavily inoculated but at least one area, preferably a separate slant or plate, should be streaked for isolated colonies.

Aspergilli grow relatively rapidly at either ambient room or 37 C temperature. Colonies will be grossly visible and usually sporulating within 2 or 3 days.

All species of *Aspergillus* reproduce asexually in essentially the same way. The spore-bearing unit consists of an unbranched hypha (conidiophore) that is swollen at the tip forming a "vesicle." Flask-shaped structures (sterigmata, phialides) protrude from the surface of the vesicle (over the entire area or only the apical portion, depending upon the species), giving the impression of a head covered with pins and having a long neck. Depending upon the species, there may be secondary sterigmata, formed from the first and giving the appearance in cross view of a second row of sterigmata. Spore-bearing structures having secondary sterigmata are referred to as biseriate, whereas the term uniseriate is used to identify those having only the single row. Conidia (spores) are formed on the tips of the sterigmata, each sterigma giving rise to an unbranched chain of spores. The entire reproductive structure (sometimes referred to as the conidial head) of aspergilli superficially resembles that of the penicillia but the latter lack a vesicle.

Inexperienced workers sometimes confuse an *Aspergillus* sp. with a zygomycete species in that an immature sporangium and sporangiophore of the latter may resemble a conidiophore with a vesicle, and inadvertent attachment of freed sporangiospores to the surface of an immature sporangium results in a further artifactual resemblance to an aspergillus. Such confusion is unwarranted, however, inasmuch as hyphae of all aspergilli are septate whereas those of the Zygomycetes are not.

Specific identification is much more difficult. Of the nearly 150 species, however, only a few have been reported as etiologic agents of invasive disease. These include *A. amstelodami, A. oryzae, A. restrictus, A. sydowi, A. terreus,* and *A. fischeri* (48, 137). Those most frequently causing disease, primarily pulmonary, are *A. fumigatus* and *A. flavus.*

Speciation is based upon the morphology of the conidial head (whether the chains of spores form long compact "columns," whether they are loose and "shaggy," etc.); type of seriation of the sterigmata; and other morphologic and certain physiologic characteristics. Cleistothecia, when present, aid also in identification. Perhaps one of the most useful characteristics, at least for the less experienced, is pigmentation of the conidial heads. This is especially definitive when the isolate is grown on Czapek's agar. Colors vary from some shade of green or brown, to white or black.

For a definitive taxonomical treatment of the aspergilli, the reader is referred to the monograph of Raper and Fennell, who have divided the species of aspergilli into 18 taxonomic groups (104). Three of the most important pathogenic species will be described here.

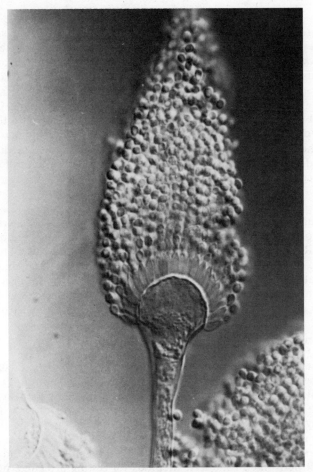

Figure 50.1—A photomicrograph of an *Aspergillus* conidial head that is columnar and
uniseriate (89).

A. fumigatus

Conidial heads are typically columnar and usually compact, usually blue-
green or very dark green (an albino variant was reported by McGinnis et al. in
1971); no sterigmata on the lower half of the vesicle; sterigmata nonseptate
and uniseriate (89). It is stated by Emmons et al. (1977) that *A. fumigatus* is
one of the few aspergilli capable of growth at 50 C (40). A number of species
resemble *A. fumigatus* to the extent that Raper and Fennell have included
them, as well as *A. fumigatus*, in an *A. fumigatus* group. Also, certain members
of the *A. versicolor* group are indistinguishable, especially by color, from *A.
fumigatus* except that the sterigmata are strictly biseriate.

A. flavus

Conidial heads are globose to radiate or columnar, usually to such an extent that the gross appearance of the colony is rougher and less velvety than that of *A. fumigatus*. Individual heads are almost visible to the naked eye and they are usually bright yellow green. This gross appearance is characteristic. Vesicles are covered with sterigmata over virtually the entire surface. Sterigmata are both uniseriate and biseriate. Conidial walls are rough. Closely related to and in the same group with *A. flavus* are several species that can be differentiated by having only uniseriate sterigmata or by changing to a brownish green when grown on Czapek's agar. A recently described medium is said to assist in differentiating the *A. flavus* group and other species of interest in medical mycology (114).

A. niger

Conidial heads are strikingly black, even when young, and sterigmata are biseriate. Probably any *Aspergillus* having these characteristics will be reported as *A. niger*. Raper and Fennell, however, described several closely related species that are differentiated by length of conidiophore, size and shape of conidia, and rate of growth on Czapek's agar (104). Only *A. niger* has conidiophores not exceeding 4 mm in length, conidia 5 μm or less and flattened horizontally at maturity; and grows relatively slowly on Czapek's agar.

Antimicrobial Susceptibility and Resistance

Treatment of invasive aspergillosis has been especially difficult and has proved successful mainly when the invasion is not advanced. The drug of choice remains the polyene, amphotericin B, but there has been some success claimed also with 5-fluorocytosine. Recently, Arroyo, Medoff, and Kobayashi reported a synergistic effect by using a combination of the two in the therapy of experimental aspergillosis (7).

In vitro susceptibility of isolates does not vary significantly and sensitivity testing is not performed routinely. Methods for testing are cited, however, in the discussion of coccidioidomycosis.

Evaluation of Laboratory Findings

Aspergillosis is an uncommon mycotic infection in man. Aspergilli, even *A. fumigatus* and *A. flavus*, are widely distributed in nature and are common contaminants in the laboratory. Isolation from a specimen derived from a contaminated source such as sputum is not, therefore, *per se* evidence of etiology. In the absence of histologic evidence, caution is required in making a diagnosis of aspergillosis. Repeated isolation is suggestive but not conclusive because these fungi are known to colonize persons suffering from a variety of chronic disorders. In a patient population predisposed to fungus infection, however, even a single isolation should alert the physician to the possibility of aspergillosis. Diagnosis is further complicated in that isolation often is difficult in patients known to have aspergillosis. Multiple positive cultures, for example, are uncommon (136).

At present, the best evidence of aspergillosis rests upon observing septate hyphae in histopathologic section, or in uncontaminated body fluids from which colonies of aspergilli can be cultured. That *in vivo* morphology alone cannot be relied upon is exemplified by the case reported by McGinnis et al. in which the initial diagnosis by tissue was erroneously zygomycosis (89). In short, unequivocal diagnosis of aspergillosis is difficult and frequently is not made antemortem. Appropriate serological tests are described in Chapter 54.

Zygomycosis (Mucormycosis)

Fungus diseases caused by moulds, the mycelium of which consists of hyphae that are coenocytic (nonseptate except in the older hyphae), have been variously designated medically as mucormycosis, phycomycosis and, more recently, as zygomycosis. The reason for these shifts in terminology is based upon an effort to keep medical terms current with changes in fungal taxonomy.

The term, phycomycosis, was introduced to cover all diseases caused by organisms of the now defunct class Phycomycetes. This class had lumped together a large group of quite dissimilar fungi, including nonfilamentous unicellular forms as well as moulds; and only related to each other by *not* having a distinct dikaryotic growth cycle.

Species pathogenic for man were found only among the Zygomycetes [also referred to as Aplanatae (6)], previously a subgrouping of the Phycomycetes but now generally accorded class status and consisting of two large orders, Entomophthorales and Mucorales. Both orders contain fungi pathogenic to man. For the most part, disease that is systemic has been caused by fungi in the order Mucorales and the term mucormycosis is valid to connote diseases caused by such agents. Fungi within the order Entomophthorales have been isolated almost exclusively from disease processes restricted to subcutaneous tissues and seen primarily in the tropics ("subcutaneous tropical phycomycosis"). The relatively new medical term zygomycosis must, perforce, cover diseases in both these distinctive categories. The separation becomes less distinct, however, with the recent report of *Conidiobolus incongruous,* a fungus of the order Entomophthorales, isolated from systemic disease (75).

For a discussion of varying views on appropriate medical terminology to designate these diseases, the reader is referred to the review by Ajello, Dean, and Irwin and the text by Emmons et al. (5, 40).

Systemic disease occurs mainly in three forms: cerebral, pulmonary, and intestinal. The first, which is most frequent and seems to be more often associated with diabetes, usually begins in the nose or nasopharynx (rhinomucormycosis), extends into the sinuses or orbits, or directly to the meninges and brain by way of septic thromboses, although there is at least one recorded instance of cranial zygomycosis acquired by trauma (29). The pulmonary form may resemble pneumonia, abscess or infarct; tends to occur concurrent with a leukemia or lymphoma; and not infrequently is an incidental observation at autopsy. Lesions involving the gastrointestinal tract are uncommon and presumably arise by ingestion of the organism (1). Involvement of other organs may occur, even skin, usually as a result of dissemination from a lung lesion, although primary cutaneous infection has been reported (131).

A succinct review of the common clinical forms is that of Meyer, Rosen, and Armstrong (90). For a disease so rare, however, publications have been numerous. In an excellent editorial on pulmonary zygomycosis, Murray makes the point that with early recognition and treatment, which is now possible, survivors, which have been rare in the past, may soon no longer warrant a publication (91).

An understanding of the basic mechanism of pathogenicity of these organisms has lagged behind that of diagnosis and treatment. These fungi, like many other opportunistic pathogens, are abundant in the environment. Many individuals are exposed and the organisms are transient residents of the human integument, yet infection leading to disease rarely occurs. Invasive disease is seen predominantly in patients with severe underlying illness, especially leukemia, lymphoma and diabetic ketoacidosis. Increased susceptibility in experimentally induced diabetes has been shown repeatedly and in one investigation, induced leukopenia also proved to be a factor but only during the early phase of disease (12, 105).

Once predisposing conditions permit initiation of infection, this group of fungi has a remarkable capacity to invade blood vessels, seemingly without restriction. Irrespective of the organ of involvement, a characteristic feature is the abundant growth into arteries, penetrating the thick walls and causing thromboses and infarcts. Small arteries can be seen filled with hyphae, penetrating into adjacent tissue, and cutting off blood supply to the organ. The mechanism of this striking vascular damage is as yet without satisfactory explanation.

That a specific immunity can be engendered in normal individuals, conferring a substantial resistance, has been shown experimentally but the nature of this resistance has not been clearly defined (25).

The incidence of systemic zygomycosis is not known but, as stated previously, clearly the disease is uncommon. It is not contagious yet occurrence of even a single case is frightening, because of the usually rapid course and high mortality. It is generally agreed, however, that incidence has increased, as have other diseases caused by opportunistically pathogenic organisms, but there are some indications that this trend may have reversed by virtue of improved ventilation systems that protect the predisposed hospital population (113). Also, there is little doubt that cures are occurring with greater frequency as physicians have learned when to suspect, how to diagnose, and what to do (54, 91).

Collection and Processing of Specimens

Specimens will consist of those usually obtained for diagnosis of pulmonary disease; mucosal scrapings if there is concurrent nasal, sinus, or orbital involvement; and sometimes brain tissue. Occasionally a lesion will be located such that brain biopsy will be possible.

Diagnostic Procedures

Histological sections can be stained with the special stains used for fungi although it has been our experience that the PAS stain is not as satisfactory for fungal hyphae as is the GMS stain, especially the hyphae of the zygomycetes. Mycelium is often difficult to find and when only fragments and cross-sections are seen, only the cell wall may be prominent, remindful of a nematode in section. The usual problem, however, is that of differentiating the zygomycete mycelium from that of the aspergilli.

All zygomycete hyphae appear in tissue as broad and nonseptate, usually in pieces shorter than those of the aspergilli. Apparently growth *in vivo* is tortuous and the straight plane of sectioning results in a slivering of the hyphae. Zygomycete hyphae are also relatively more distorted, wrinkled and even folded, than those of the aspergilli. In fact, one common mistake is to confuse the artifact created by a hyphal fold, for a septum. Branching, when it is seen, tends to occur at right angles as compared to the dichotomous branching of the aspergilli. Sporulation usually does not occur *in vivo,* although sporangia have been seen in nasal cavity tissue (79).

Hyphae can be observed *in vivo* also by direct microscopic examination of "wet" preparations, treated with KOH if necessary for visualization. In such preparations, entire lengths of hyphae can be seen but still having a bizarre appearance, viz. bulging irregular walls, and exceptional broadening or clubbing terminally. The cytoplasm may appear granular.

Zygomycetes will grow on routinely used media but some, including a few pathogenic isolates, require transfer to special agars for sporulation (e.g., malt, Czapek's solution, hay infusion) or bits of agar medium afloat on water (5, 78). Sabouraud's agar is satisfactory for primary isolation but cycloheximide should not be added because most isolates are sensitive to this antifungal agent. Our preference for the isolation of Zygomycetes from specimens from a contaminated source is Littman's oxgall agar with chloramphenicol. One area of agar surface should be heavily inoculated (numbers of organisms are often sparse) and another (preferably a separate plate or tube) should be streaked for isolated colonies. Incubation is usually at room temperature although all Zygomycetes of pathogenic potential seem to be thermophilic.

Growth is rapid, and cultures should be observed daily, else there will be confluent growth over the entire surface. If the isolate is of the order Mucorales, growth is usually apparent within 1 to 3 days and aerial mycelium is abundant, often filling the container and usually grey or light tan depending upon the species. Microscopic examination will reveal that the hyphae are nonseptate and, if mounted in water or saline, streaming of the protoplasm usually can be seen. If the isolate is of the order Entomophthorales, asexual production will be by means of spores discharged forcibly into the air (ballistospores); fungi of the order Mucorales lack this characteristic. In the Mucorales, one or more asexual spores are borne within a sack (sporangium).

Species known to cause systemic disease occur chiefly in three genera, *Absidia, Rhizopus* and *Mucor. Cunninghamnella elegans, C. bertholetiae,* and *Saksenaea vasiformis* have been implicated only rarely (29, 78, 135). *Mortierella wolfii* is a common cause of systemic disease in animals but has not been reported as a cause of such disease in human beings.

All zygomycetes reproduce sexually but this is of little value in the identification of agents of systemic disease; many are heterothallic and zygospores are not produced. Identification rests with recognition of asexually produced spores.

Species of *Absidia, Mucor,* and *Rhizopus* have large numbers of spores within the sporangia. In all three genera a sporangium is located at the end of a supporting hypha (sporangiophore) but separated from the supporting hypha by a septum which forms a protrusion (columnella) into the sporangium. In some species a columnella may be flat and the sporangiophore and columnella will appear as an open umbrella after disruption of the sporangium. Rhizoids (root-like structures) are formed by species of both *Absidia* and *Rhizopus* but not *Mucor,* and are located at intervals (nodes) along a hypha (stolon, "runner"). In the case of *Rhizopus* sp., the rhizoids are located at nodes from which the sporangiophores arise; the rhizoids are opposite the sporangiophores and do, indeed, appear as roots. The sporangiophores usually arise in a cluster from a node but do not branch. The species of *Absidia* are distinguishable from the *Rhizopus* sp. only in that the sporangiophores are not located opposite rhizoids; they are internodal.

Species of *Mucor* never form either rhizoids or stolons; sporangiophores arise directly from the mycelium, usually singly rather than in clusters, but there may be branching (see Figure 50.2).

The genus *Saksenaea* is strikingly characterized by sporangia that are flask or sausage-shaped (36). *Cunninghamella* is one of the genera of Mucorales that form single-spored sporangia in which the walls of the spore and sporangium become indistinguishably fused and the entire structure is referred to as a conidium (but identification as a zygomycete is unequivocal by observation of nonseptate hyphae). The conidia are found crowded onto the surface of the swollen tip (vesicle) of a sporangiophore. The taxonomy of this group has recently been reported upon by Weitzman and Crist (135).

The number of pathogenic species within these genera fortunately is limited. Ajello recognizes the following Mucorales as agents of human disease: *Absidia corymbifera (A. ramosa), Mucor pusillus, M. ramosissimus, Rhizopus arrhizus, R. microsporus, R. oryzae, R. rhizopodiformis* and *Saksanaea vasiformis* (5). *Cunninghamnella elegans* and *C. bertholetiae* must be added to this list and still others are listed in the texts by Rippon (112) and by Emmons et al. (40). Some, however, have not been incriminated as agents of human disease that is systemic. In any case, the most common agents of systemic human disease are *R. oryzae* and *R. arrhizus,* with *A. corymbifera* perhaps next in rank.

Most laboratories will have difficulty in identifying even the latter three species. Descriptions of pathogenic species can be found in any standard text of medical mycology and keys can be consulted, e.g., Ellis and Hesseltine on *Absidia;* and Inui, Takeda, and Iizuka for the genus *Rhizopus* (35, 62). Gilman's text of soil fungi (49) also is useful as are the many publications of C. W. Hesseltine (e.g., 56). Even with these resources, however, speciation is difficult, and identification of any presumed pathogen ought to be confirmed by an authority. The comments below are intended only as a guide.

A. corymbifera has the characteristics described for the genus but is distinguished from other *Absidia* species by having uniquely branched sporangiophores: a single, long sporangiophore arises from a stolon; towards the apex but before the sporangium, a cluster of 5 or 6 sporangiophores are formed by repeated branching, each of different length but each producing a sporangium at about the same height. This formation (a corymb) is best seen in an undis-

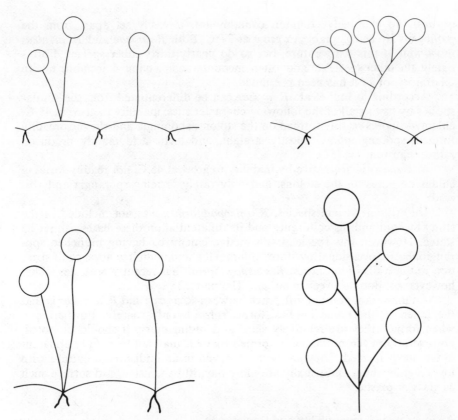

Figure 50.2—Sporulation patterns of some Mucoraceae. (a) All species of *Absidia:* sporangiophores arising from a stolon ("runner") at points between (internodally) rhizoids (root-like structures). (b) *A. corymbifera*, branching of sporangiophores but with sporangia located at approximately the same plane, forming a corymb. (c) All species of *Rhizopus:* sporangiophores arising from stolon opposite location of rhizoids. (d) All species of *Mucor:* absence of stolons and rhizoids. Sporangiophores branching and formed from aerial hyphae.

turbed culture using a low magnification. Colonies are gray in color. Growth and sporulation are excellent at 37 C–45 C, although it is not clear that this level of thermotolerance is unique to this species.

There are numerous species of *Rhizopus* and all grow rapidly and vigorously, forming a relatively coarse, sturdy, gray, aerial mycelium. Sporangial heads of most, including the pathogens, are such a dark brown as often to be visible to the naked eye. All species are said to lack the ability to utilize either sodium or potassium nitrate as a sole source of nitrogen, a characteristic which, in fact, sets this genus apart from all others of the order Mucorales (62).

Distinction between species, however, is not easy. *R. stolonifera (R. ni-*

gricans), an extremely common contaminant, is easily set apart from the pathogens by being unable to grow at 37 C. Both *R. oryzae* and *R. arrhizus* grow well at this temperature, but so do nearly thirty other species. Fortunately, the other species are not often encountered in a clinical or public health laboratory, or so it has been presumed.

According to Inui et al., *R. oryzae* can be differentiated from the similar species by having all of the following characteristics: inability to grow at 45 C, chlamydospores readily formed on the stolons, sporangia and rhizoids readily formed, sporangiophores mostly straight, and lactic acid mainly produced rather than fumaric (62).

R. arrhizus is distinctive by inability to grow at 45 C, not readily forming chlamydospores on the stolons, and only rarely forming sporangia and rhizoids.

Unfortunately, one species, *R. rhizopodiformis,* was not included in the study by Inui and his colleagues and its differential on these bases cannot be stated. However, this species is distinctive chiefly by having branched sporangiophores, occasional pyriform columnella, and complete absence of striation in the walls of its spores. *R. rhizopodiformis* has recently been described, however, by Bottone, Weitzman, and Hanna (15).

An important point of difference between *R. oryzae* and *R. arrhizus* is that the latter, as the name implies, forms rhizoids only sparely. Furthermore, when formed they are relatively short and rudimentary. It should be noted, however, that even prominently formed rhizoids may not be readily apparent to the inexperienced. They are best visualized in an undisturbed culture with low magnification, and usually are more plentiful against a hard surface such as glass or plastic.

Antimicrobial Susceptibility and Resistance

Amphotericin B is the drug of choice. Despite reported variations in *in vitro* susceptibility, sensitivity testing is not performed routinely; responses *in vivo* have been good provided disease is caught sufficiently early, otherwise treatment is of little avail (11). Methods for such testing are cited under the discussion of coccidioidomycosis.

Evaluation of Laboratory Findings

The best diagnostic evidence of zygomycosis is observation of typical invasive forms in histopathological section and confirmation by isolation in culture.

Diagnosis cannot be made by culture alone, especially if the specimen is from a contaminated source. But even if the specimen is of an ordinarily sterile body fluid or tissue, there is always the possibility that the fungus is a contaminant. Observation *in vivo*, as well as culture, is mandatory. Unfortunately, cultures may be negative even when aseptate mycelium is seen in tissue. Apparently, the zygomycetes do not very well tolerate the trauma of homogenization as may be necessary with tissue. Diagnosis often rests, then, upon observation of typical Zygomycete hyphae seen in section but, as stated elsewhere, the typical morphology may not be evident and then usually the query is aspergillosis versus zygomycosis. In such a case, signs and symptoms may provide circumstantial evidence.

Some Uncommon Systemic Mycoses

Sporotrichosis is seen usually as a subcutaneous disease, acquired by traumatic inoculation through the skin. Occasionally, however, pulmonary infection occurs as a consequence of inhaling the organism. When this occurs, the resulting disease usually resembles tuberculosis or one of the other progressive pulmonary mycoses, although a more acute form has been reported (111).

Diagnosis is aided by the patient's having antibodies and a positive skin-test with sporotrichin, but isolation of the organism in culture is required. Sputa should be inoculated onto a battery of media as described under histoplasmosis. Culture of blood is usually not a fruitful procedure and, in fact, is not necessary; isolation from sputum is relatively easy. The agent, *Sporothrix (Sporotrichum) schenkii,* and sporotrichosis are further discussed in another chapter.

Another seldom encountered systemic manifestation of a disease that usually is subcutaneous is that caused by the fungus variously designated as *Monosporium apiospermum, Allescheria boydii,* or, more recently, *Petriellidium boydii*—all one and the same fungus. The reason for these variations in terminology is related to changes in knowledge of taxonomy.

The first designation, *M. apiospermum,* was, and still is, proper for the imperfect form of the fungus, i.e., when sexual reproduction does not occur. For many years the relationship of *M. apiospermum* to *A. boydii* was not realized, and the disease was called monosporiosis, after the genus of the imperfect form. Several decades ago, however, *M. apiospermum* was discovered to be the imperfect form of *A. boydii,* an ascomycete (37). Eventually the latter designation gained acceptance as did the term allescheriosis for the disease. Now another change is imminent.

Based upon the careful taxonomic studies of Malloch (86), *Petriellidium* gradually is gaining acceptance as the correct generic nomenclature. This action predictably will be followed by a push to designate the disease as petriellidiosis. Whatever the outcome, the point to be made is that this fungus is a soil saprophyte of limited pathogenic potential that may be expressed especially when accidentally implanted or under conditions of immunosuppression.

The most common form of disease has been that of a mycetoma (see chapter on mycetomas). Eye injuries also have been followed by infections with this organism (34). With increasing frequency but still rare, have been reports of systemic disease, often without preceding trauma. In a recently reported case (Bousley, 1977), hyphae were seen in two different samples of pleural fluid from which the fungus was cultured; the organism was never isolated from sputum and apparently was not present in the lungs.

In yet another case (81), sputum cultures had been positive (even though evidence of pulmonary involvement was not obtained) a month before the patient developed signs of neurologic abnormality and died. At autopsy, hyphae were seen in brain abscesses from which this fungus was cultured, but there were no fungi in the lung. This latter case seems to be an undeniable instance of a deep mycosis with portal of entry through the lung, without damage to the portal organ.

That systemic disease may be the consequence of accidental implantation is perhaps best exemplified by the report of Benham and Georg (13) in which the organism probably was introduced during administration of a spinal anesthetic.

Specimens to be collected depend upon the site of involvement. Diagnosis is relatively simple but, as with any saprophyte, is contingent upon observation of the fungus in situ as well as its isolation in culture, even if the specimen is an ordinarily sterile body fluid or tissue. Cultural isolation is mandatory because the septate hyphae of this fungus cannot be differentiated from those of any other ascomycete, and observation in the specimen by direct microscopic examination lends credibility that the fungus isolated was, in fact, the etiologic agent and not an airborne contaminant. It should be noted also that growth as a mycelial "ball" in viscera is not a characteristic feature of the organism, as it is in subcutaneous infection.

Immunological procedures would be an especially welcome diagnostic adjunct but trials have been limited (119).

Chemotherapeutic trials also have been limited, perforce the rarity of the disease. According to the data of Lutwick et al. (81), this fungus appears to have a degree of resistance to all currently available antifungal agents.

A third systemic mycosis of rarity is that of cerebral chromomycosis, caused usually by *Cladosporium bantianum* and discussed in the chapter on phaeohyphomycosis.

References

1. AHLUWALIA HS, LIE KJ, and ARULAMBALAM TR: Gastric phycomycosis: report of a case in Malaysia. J Trop Med Hyg 77:116–118, 1974
2. AISNER J, SCHIMPFF SC, BENNETT JE, YOUNG VM, and WIERNIK PH: Aspergillus infections in cancer patients. Association with fireproofing materials in a new hospital. J Am Med Assoc 235:411–412, 1976
3. AJELLO L: Comparative ecology of respiratory mycotic agents of disease. Bacteriol Rev 31:6–24, 1967
4. AJELLO L: Sexual reproduction among fungi pathogenic to man. A historical review. Mykosen 14:343–352, 1971
5. AJELLO L, DEAN DF, and IRWIN RS: The zygomycete *Saksenaea vasiformis* as a pathogen of humans with critical review of the etiology of zygomycosis. Mycologia 68:52–62, 1976
6. ALEXOPOULOS CJ: Introductory Mycology, 2nd edition. John Wiley & Sons, New York, 1962
7. ARROYO J, MEDOFF G, and KOBAYASHI GS: Therapy of murine aspergillosis with amphotericin B in combination with rifampin and 5-fluorocytosine. Antimicrob Agents Chemother 11:21–25, 1977
8. BAKER EE, MRAK EM, and SMITH CE: The morphology, taxonomy, and distribution of *Coccidioides immitis* Rixford and Gilchrist,. 1896. Farlowia 1:199–244, 1943
9. BANNATYNE RM and CHEUNG R: Discrepant results of amphotericin B assays on fresh versus frozen samples. Antimicrob Agents Chemother 12:550, 1977
10. BANNATYNE RM, CHEUNG R, and DEVLIN HR: Microassays for amphotericin B. Antimicrob Agents Chemother 11:44–46, 1977
11. BATTOCK DJ, GRAUZ H, BOBROWSKY M, and LITTMAN ML: Alternate days amphotericin

B therapy in treatment of rhinocerebral phycomycosis (mucormycosis). Ann Intern Med 68:122–137, 1968

12. BAUER H and SHELDON WH: Leukopenia with granulocytopenia in experimental mucormycosis (*Rhizopus oryzae* infection). J Exp Med 106:501–508, 1957

13. BENHAM RW and GEORG LK: *Allescheria boydii*, causative agent in a case of meningitis. J Invest Dermatol 10:99–110, 1948

14. BINFORD CH, THOMPSON RK, GORHAN ME, and EMMONS CW: Mycotic brain abscess due to *Cladosporium trichoides*, a new species. Am J Clin Pathol 22:535–542, 1952

15. BOTTONE EJ, WEITZMAN I, and HANNA BA: *Rhizopus rhizopodiformis*: emerging etiological agent of mucormycosis. J Clin Microbiol 9:530–550, 1979

16. BOUZA E, WINSTON DJ, RHODES J, and HEWITT WL: Paracoccidioidomycosis (South American blastomycosis) in the United States. Chest 72:100–102, 1977

17. BROWN JW III, NADELL J, SANDERS CV, and SARDENZA L: Brain abscess caused by *Cladosporium trichoides (bantianum)*: a case with paranasal involvement. J South Med Assoc 69:1519–1521, 1976

18. CENTER FOR DISEASE CONTROL: Blastomycosis in North Carolina. Morbid Mortal Weekly Rep 25:205, 1976

19. CHICK EW, BAUM GL, FURCOLOW ML, HUPPERT M, KAUFMAN L, and PAPAGIANIS D: The use of skin tests and serologic tests in histoplasmosis, coccidioidomycosis, and blastomycosis. A statement by the scientific assembly on microbiology and immunology, American Thoracic Society. Am Rev Respir Dis 108:3–6, 1973

20. CLAYTON YM, cited by CAMPBELL MJ and CLAYTON YM: Bronchopulmonary aspergillosis. Am Rev Respir Dis 89:186–196, 1964

21. COCKSHOTT WP and LUCAS AO: Histoplasmosis duboisii. Q J Med 33:223–238, 1964

22. COLLINS DN and EDWARDS MR: Filamentous forms of *Blastomyces dermatitidis* in mouse lung. Light and electron microscopy. Sabouraudia 7:237–240, 1970

23. COLLINS MS, PAPPAGIANIS D, and YEE J: Enzymatic solubilization of precipitin and complement fixing antigen from endospores, spherules and spherule fraction of *Coccidioides immitis*. *In* Coccidioidomycosis, Current Clinical and Diagnostic Status. Ajello L (ed.). Symposia Specialists, Miami, 1977

24. CONANT NF, SMITH DT, BAKER RD, CALLOWAY JL, and MARTIN DS: Manual of Clinical Mycology, 3rd edition. WB Saunders Co, Philadelphia, 1971

25. CORBEL MJ and EADES SM: Experimental phycomycosis in mice; examination of the role of acquired immunity in resistance to *Absidia ramosa*. J Hyg Camb 77:221–233, 1976

26. COREMANS N DE J: Un test biochimique de differencation de *Histoplasma duboisii* Vanbreuseghem 1952 d'avec *Histoplasma capsulatum* Darling 1906. C R Seances Soc Biol 157:1130–1132, 1963

27. D'ALESSIO DJ, HEEREN RH, HENDRICKS SL, OGILVIE P, and FURCOLOW ML: A starling roost as the source of an urban epidemic histoplasmosis in an area of low incidence. Am Rev Respir Dis 92:725–731, 1965

28. DE ALBORNOZ MD: Isolation of *Paracoccidioides brasiliensis* from rural soil in Venezuela. Sabouraudia 9:248–253, 1971

29. DEAN DF, AJELLO L, IRWIN RS, WOELK WK, and SKARULIS GJ: Cranial zygomycosis caused by *Saksenae vasiformis*. J Neurosurg 46:97–103, 1977

30. DENTON JF and DiSALVO AF: Isolation of *Blastomyces dermatitidis* from natural sites at Augusta, Georgia. Am J Trop Med Hyg 13:716–722, 1964

31. DENTON JF, McDONOUGH ES, AJELLO L, and AUSHERMAN RJ: Isolation of *Blastomyces dermatitidis* from soil. Science 133:1126–1127, 1961

32. DiSALVO AF, SEKHON AS, LAND GA, and FLEMING WH: An evaluation of the exoantigen test for the identification of *Histoplasma* species and *Coccidioides immitis* cultures. J Clin Microbiol, in press, 1980

33. EDWARDS PQ and PALMER CE: Nationwide histoplasmin sensitivity and histoplasmal infections. Public Health Rep 78:241–249, 1963

34. ELLIOT ID, HALDE C, and SHAPIRO J: Keratitis and endophthalmitis caused by *Petriellidium boydii*. Am J Ophthalmol 83:16–18, 1977

35. ELLIS JJ and HESSELTINE CW: Species of *Absidia* with ovoid sporangiospores II. Sabouraudia 5:59–77, 1966

36. ELLIS JJ and HESSELTINE CW: Two new families of Mucorales. Mycologia 66:87–95, 1974

37. EMMONS CW: *Allescheria boydii* and *Monosporium apiospermum*. Mycologia 36:188–193, 1944
38. EMMONS CW: Isolation of *Histoplasma capsulatum* from soil. Public Health Rep 64:892–896, 1949
39. EMMONS CW: Fungi which resemble *Coccidioides immitis*. *In* Coccidioidomycosis. Ajello L (ed.). Univ of Arizona Press, Tucson, 1967, pp 333–337
40. EMMONS CW, BINFORD CH, UTZ JP, and KWON-CHUNG KJ: Medical Mycology, 3rd edition. Lea & Febiger, Philadelphia, 1977
41. FAIGEL HC: Caution: ecology can be hazardous to your health. Clin Pediatr 10:245, 1971
42. FAVA NETO C: The immunology of South American blastomycosis. Mycopathol Mycol Appl 26:349–359, 1965
43. FELGER CE and FRIEDMAN L: Experimental cerebral chromoblastomycosis. J Infect Dis 3:1–7, 1962
44. FURCOLOW ML: Epidemiology of histoplasmosis. *In* Histoplasmosis. Sweany HC (ed.). Charles C Thomas, Springfield, Ill, pp 113–148, 1960
45. FURCOLOW ML: Environmental aspects of histoplasmosis. Arch Environ Health 10:4–10, 1965
46. FURCOLOW ML, CHICK EW, BUSEY JF, and MENGES RW: Prevalence and incidence studies of human and canine blastomycosis. Am Rev Respir Dis 102:60–67, 1970
47. FURCOLOW ML, TOSH FE, LARSH HW, LYNCH HJ, and SHAW G: The emerging pattern of urban histoplasmosis. N Engl J Med 264:1226–1230, 1961
48. GERBER J, CHOMICKI J, BRANDSBERG JW, JONES R, and HAMMERMAN KJ: Pulmonary aspergillosis caused by *Aspergillus fischeri* var. *spinosus*. Report of a case and value of serologic studies. Am J Clin Pathol 60:861–866, 1973
49. GILMAN JC: A manual of soil fungi. Iowa State College Press, Ames, 1945
50. GIRALDO R, RESTREPO A, GUITIERREZ F, ROBLEDO M, LONDONO F, HERNANDEZ H, SIERRA F, and CALLE S: Pathogenesis of paracoccidioidomycosis: a model based on the study of 46 patients. Mycopathol Mycol Appl 58:63–70, 1976
51. GORDON MA: Fluorescent staining of *Histoplasma capsulatum*. J Bacteriol 77:678–681, 1959
52. HALEY LD and STANDARD PG: Laboratory Methods in Medical Mycology. U. S. Dept. Health, Education, and Welfare, Center for Disease Control, Atlanta, Ga, 1973
53. HARDIN HF and SCOTT DI: Blastomycosis. Occurrence of filamentous forms *in vivo*. Am J Clin Pathol 62:104–106, 1974
54. HAUCH TW: Pulmonary mucormycosis. Another cure. Chest 72:92–94, 1977
55. HERD PA and MARTIN HF: A semiquantitative spectrophotometric assay for amphotericin B in blood. Clin Biochem 7:359–365, 1974
56. HESSELTINE CW: Genera of Mucorales with notes on their synonomy. Mycologia 47:344–363, 1955
57. HESSELTINE CW and ELLIS JJ: The genus *Absidia*: Gongronella and cylindrical-spored species of *Absidia*. Mycologia 56:568–601, 1964
58. HOEPRICH PD and HUSTON AC: Effect of culture media on the antifungal activity of miconazole and amphotericin B methyl ester. J Infect Dis 134:336–341, 1976
59. HOLT RJ: Laboratory tests of antifungal drugs. J Clin Pathol 28:767–774, 1975
60. HOTCHI M, SCHWARZ J, and KAPLAN W: Limitations of fluorescent antibody staining of *Histoplasma capsulatum* in tissue sections. Sabouraudia 10:157–163, 1972
61. HUPPERT M, SUN SH, and BAILEY JW: Natural variability in *Coccidioides immitis*. *In* Coccidioidomycosis. Ajello L (ed.). Univ of Arizona Press, Tucson, 1967
62. INUI T, TAKEDA Y, and IIZUKA H: Taxonomic studies on the genus *Rhizopus*. J Gen Appl Microbiol 11(Suppl):1–121, 1965
63. JUNGERMAN PF and SCHWARTZMAN RM: Veterinary Medical Mycology. Lea & Febiger, Philadelphia, 1972
64. KAPLAN W: Application of the fluorescent antibody technique to the diagnosis and study of histoplasmosis. *In* 2nd National Conference on Histoplasmosis. Balows A (ed.). Charles C Thomas, Springfield, Ill, 1971, pp 327–340
65. KAPLAN W and KAUFMAN L: Specific fluorescent antiglobulins for the detection and identification of *Blastomyces dermatitidis* yeast-phase cells. Mycopathol Mycol Appl 19:173–180, 1963
66. KAUFMAN L: Serodiagnosis of fungal diseases. *In* Manual of Clinical Immunology. Rose

NR and Friedman H (eds.). American Society for Microbiology, Washington, DC 1976, pp 363–381

67. KAUFMAN L and BLUMER S: Occurrence of serotypes among *Histoplasma capsulatum* strains. J Bacteriol 82:729–735, 1966

68. KAUFMAN L and CLARK MJ: Value of the concomitant use of complement fixation and immunodiffusion tests in the diagnosis of coccidioidomycosis. Appl Microbiol 28:641–643, 1974

69. KAUFMAN L and KAPLAN W: Preparation of a fluorescent antibody specific for the yeast phase of *Histoplasma capsulatum*. J Bacteriol 82:729–735, 1961

70. KAUFMAN L, MCLAUGHLIN DW, CLARK MJ, and BLUMER S: Specific immunodiffusion test for blastomycosis. Appl Microbiol 36:244–247, 1973

71. KAUFMAN L and STANDARD P: Improved version of the exoantigen test for identification of *Coccidioides immitis* and *Histoplasma capsulatum* cultures. J Clin Microbiol 8:42–45, 1978

72. KAUFMAN L and STANDARD P: Immuno-identification of cultures pathogenic to man. Current Microbiol 1:105–140, 1978

73. KEDDIE F, SHADOMY J, and BARFANTI M: Brief report on the isolation of *Arthroderma tuberculatum* from a human source. Mycopathol Mycol Appl 20:1–2, 1963

74. KITCHEN MS, REIBER CD, and EASTIN GB: An urban epidemic of North American blastomycosis. Am Rev Respir Dis 115:1062–1066, 1977

75. KONG DS and JONG SC: Identity of the etiological agent of the first deep entomophthoraceous infection of man in the United States. Mycologia 68:181–183, 1976

76. KWON-CHUNG KJ: Sexual state of *Histoplasma capsulatum*. Science 175:326, 1972

77. KWON-CHUNG KJ: Perfect state (*Emmonsiella capsulata*) of the fungus causing large-form African histoplasmosis. Mycologia 67:980–990, 1975

78. KWON-CHUNG KJ, YOUNG RC, and ORLANDO M: Pulmonary mucormycosis caused by *Cunninghamnella elegans* in a patient with chronic mylogenous leukemia. Am J Clin Pathol 64:544–548, 1975

79. LA TOUCHE CJ, SUTHERLAND TW, and TELLING M: Histopathological and mycological features of a case of rhinocerebral mucormycosis (phycomycosis) in Britain. Sabouraudia 3:148–150, 1964

80. LEVAN NE: Workman's compensation legislation and coccidioidomycosis; legal and sociocultural considerations. *In* Coccidioidomycosis, Current Clinical and Diagnostic Status. Ajello L (ed.). Symposia Specialist, Miami, Fla, 1977

81. LUTWICK LI, GALGIANI JN, JOHNSON RH, and STEVENS DA: Visceral fungal infections due to *Petriellidium boydii (Allescheria boydii)*. In vitro drug sensitivities. Am J Med 61:632–640, 1976

82. MACHADO FILHO J and LISBOA MIRANDA J: Consideracoes relativas a blastomicose sulamericana: localizacoes, sintomas inciais vias de penetrocal e disseminacae em 313 casos consecutivos. O Hospital 58:99–131, 1960

83. MACHADO FILHO J and LISBOA MIRANDA J: Consideracoes relativas a blastomicose sulamericana. Da participascas pulmonar entre 338 casos consecutivos. O Hospital 58:431–439, 1960

84. MACKINNON JE: On the importance of South American blastomycosis. Mycopathol Mycol Appl 41:187–193, 1970

85. MADDY KT: The geographic distribution of *Coccidioides immitis* and possible ecologic implications. Arizona Medicine 15:178–188, 1958

86. MALLOCH D: New concepts in the *Microascaceae* illustrated by two new species. Mycologia 62:727–740, 1970

87. MCDONOUGH ES: Blastomycosis - epidemiology and biology of its etiologic agent *Ajellomyces dermatitidis*. Mycopathol Mycol Appl 41:195–201, 1970

88. MCDONOUGH ES and LEWIS AL: *Blastomyces dermatitidis*: production of the sexual stage. Science 156:528–529, 1967

89. MCGINNIS MR, BUCK DL, and KUTZ B: Paranasal aspergilloma caused by an albino variant of *Aspergillus fumigatus*. J South Med Assoc 70:886–888, 1971

90. MEYER RD, ROSEN P, and ARMSTRONG D: Phycomycosis complicating leukemia and lymphoma. Ann Intern Med 77:871–879, 1972

91. MURRAY HW: Pulmonary mucormycosis, one hundred years later (editorial). Chest 72:1–2, 1977
92. MURRAY HW, LITTMAN ML, and ROBERTS RB: Disseminated paracoccidioidomycosis (South American blastomycosis) in the United States. Am J Med 56:209–220, 1974
93. NEGRONI P: El *Paraccidioides brasiliensis*. Vive saprofiticamente en el suelo Argentina. Pren Med Argent 53:2831–2932, 1966
94. OKUDAIRA M, STRAUB M, and SCHWARZ J: The etiology of discrete splenic and hepatic calcifications in an endemic area of histoplasmosis. Am J Pathol 39:599–611, 1961
95. PAPPAGIANIS D: Coccidioidomycosis. *In* Immunological Diseases, 2nd edition. Samter M (ed.). Little, Brown and Co, Boston, 1971
96. PAPPAGIANIS D and LEVINE HB: The present status of vaccination against coccidioidomycosis in man. Am J Epidemiol 102:30–41, 1975
97. PAPPAGIANIS D and SMITH CE: Coccidioidomycosis. *In* Communicable and Infectious Diseases, 7th edition. Top FJ Sr and Wehrle PF (eds.). CV Mosby, St. Louis, 1972
98. PARROTT T Jr, TAYLOR G, POSTON MS, and SMITH DT: An epidemic of histoplasmosis in Warrenton, North Carolina. South Med J 48:1147–1150, 1955
99. PENNINGTON JE: Aspergillus pneumonia in hematologic malignancy. Arch Intern Med 137:769–771, 1977
100. PEPYS J: Pulmonary aspergillosis, farmer's lung, and related diseases. *In* Immunological Diseases. Samter M (ed.). Little, Brown, and Co, Boston, 1971
101. PERKINS RL, SASLAW S, and OCKNER SA: Migration histoplasmosis. Ann Intern Med 57:363–372, 1962
102. PINE L, KAUFMAN L, and BOONE CJ: Comparative fluorescent antibody staining of *Histoplasma capsulatum* and *Histoplasma duboisii* with a specific anti-yeast phase *H. capsulatum* conjugate. Mycophathol Mycol Appl 24:315–326, 1964
103. PRYSTOWSKY SD, VOGELSTEIN B, ETTINGER DS, MERZ WG, KAIZER H, SULICA VI, and ZINKHAM WH: Invasive aspergilloma. N Engl J Med 295:655–658, 1976
104. RAPER KB and FENNELL DI: The Genus *Aspergillus*. Williams and Wilkins, Baltimore, 1965
105. REINHARDT DJ, KAPLAN W, and AJELLO L: Experimental cerebral zygomycosis in alloxan diabetic rabbits. I. Relationship of temperature tolerance of selected Zygomycetes to pathogenicity. Infect Immun 2:223–230, 1970
106. RESTREPO-M A: La prueba de immunodiffusion en gel de agar en el diagnostico de la paracoccidioidomicosis. Sabouraudia 4:223–230, 1966
107. RESTREPO-M A: A reappraisal of the microscopical appearance of the mycelial phase of *Paracoccidioides brasiliensis*. Sabouraudia 8:141–144, 1970
108. RESTREPO-M A and CORREA-R I: Comparison of two culture media for primary isolation of *Paracoccidioides brasiliensis* from sputum. Sabouraudia 10:260–265, 1972
109. RESTREPO-M A, GREER DL, ROBLEDO M, OSORIO O, and MONDRAGON H: Ulceration of the palate caused by a basidiomycete *Schizophylum commune*. Sabouraudia 11:201–204, 1971
110. RESTREPO-M A and MONCADA LH: Characterization of the precipitin bands detected in the immunodiffusion tests for paracoccidioidomycosis. Appl Microbiol 28:138–144, 1974
111. RIDGEWAY NA, WHITCOMB FC, ERICKSON EE, and LAW SW: Primary pulmonary sporotrichosis. Report of two cases. Am J Med 32:153–160, 1962
112. RIPPON JW: Medical Mycology: the Pathogenic Fungi and the Pathogenic Actinomycetes. WB Saunders Co., Philadelphia, 1974
113. ROSEN PP and STERNBERG SS: Decreased frequency of aspergillosis and mucormycosis. N Engl J Med 295:1319–1320, 1976
114. SALKIN IF and GORDON MA: Evaluation of aspergillus differential medium. J Clin Microbiol 2:74–75, 1975
115. SAROSI GA, HAMMERMAN KJ, TOSH FE, and KRONENBERG RS: Clinical features of acute pulmonary blastomycosis. N Engl J Med 290:540–543, 1974
116. SAROSI GA, PARKER JD, and TOSH FE: Histoplasmosis outbreaks: their patterns. *In* Histoplasmosis. Proceedings of the 2nd National Conference on Histoplasmosis. Balows A (ed.). Charles C Thomas, Springfield, Ill, 1971, pp 123–128
117. SAROSI GA and SERSTOCK DS: Isolation of *Blastomyces dermatitidis* from pigeon manure. Am Rev Respir Dis 114:1179–1183, 1976
118. SCOGINS JT: Comparative study of time loss in coccidioidomycosis and other respiratory

diseases. Proceedings of the Symposium on Coccidioidomycosis. U. S. Dept. Health, Education, and Welfare, PHS publication No 575, 1957

119. SEELIGER HPR: Recent applications of immunologic techniques in the diagnosis of the deep mycoses. *In* Systemic Mycoses, a CIBA Foundation Symposium. Wolstenholme GEW and Porter P (eds.). Little, Brown, and Co, Boston, 1967

120. SIGLER L and CARMICHAEL JW: Taxonomy of Malbranchea and some other hyphomycetes with arthroconidia. Mycotaxon 4:349–488, 1976

121. SMITH CD: Isolation and identification of *Histoplasma capsulatum* from soil. *In* Histoplasmosis. Proceedings of the 2nd National Conference on Histoplasmosis. Balows A (ed.). Charles C Thomas, Springfield, Ill, 1971, pp 277–283

122. SMITH JG JR, HARRIS JS, CONANT NF, and SMITH DT: An epidemic of North American blastomycosis. J Am Med Assoc 158:641–646, 1955

123. STANDARD PG and KAUFMAN L: Immunological procedure for the rapid and specific identification of *Coccidioides immitis* cultures. J Clin Microbiol 5:149–153, 1977

124. STEVENS DA, LEVINE HB, and DERENSKI SC: Miconazole in coccidioidomycosis. II. Therapeutic and pharmacologic studies in man. Am J Med 60:191–202, 1976

125. STRAUB M and SCHWARZ J: The healed primary complex in histoplasmosis. Am J Clin Pathol 25:727–741, 1955

126. SUDMAN MS and KAPLAN W: Antigenic relationship between American and African isolates of *Blastomyces dermatitidis* as determined by immunofluorescence. Appl Microbiol 27:496–499, 1974

127. SUN HS, HUPPERT M, and VUKOVICH KR: Rapid in vitro conversion and identification of *Coccidioides immitis*. J Clin Microbiol 3:186–190, 1976

128. TOSH FE, HAMMERMAN KJ, WEEKS RJ, and SAROSI GA: A common source epidemic of North American blastomycosis. Am Rev Respir Dis 109:525–529, 1974

129. UTZ JP, BECKER A, BUECHNER HA, CAMPBELL GD, EINSTEIN HE, and SEABURY JH: The Pulmonary Mycoses: Diagnostic and Therapeutic Guidelines. Committee on Fungus Diseases of the American College of Chest Physicians. ER Squibb & Sons, Inc, 1976

130. VARKEY B and ROSE HD: Pulmonary aspergilloma. A rational approach to treatment. Am J Med 61:626–631, 1976

131. VELIATH AJ, RAO R, PRABHU MR, and AURORA AL: Cutaneous phycomycosis (mucormycosis) with fatal pulmonary dissemination. Arch Dermatol 112:509–512, 1976

132. VINCKIER F: *Blastomyces brasiliensis* (paracoccidioidomycosis). Acta Stomatol Belg 70:399–409, 1973

133. WAHNER HW, HEPPER NGG, ANDERSEN HA, and WEED LA: Pulmonary aspergillosis. Ann Intern Med 58:472–485, 1963

134. WEEKS RJ and TOSH FE: Control of epidemic foci of *Histoplasma capsulatum*. *In* Histoplasmosis. Proceedings of the 2nd National Conference on Histoplasmosis. Balows A (ed.). Charles C Thomas, Springfield, Ill, 1971, pp 184–189

135. WEITZMAN I and CRIST MY: Studies with clinical isolates of Cunninghamnella. I. Mating behavior. Mycologia 71:1024–1033, 1979

136. YOUNG RC, BENNETT JE, VOGEL CL, CARBONE PP, and DE VITA VT: Aspergillosis. The spectrum of the disease in 98 patients. Medicine 49:147–173, 1970

137. YOUNG RC, JENNINGS A, and BENNETT JE: Species identification of invasive aspergillosis in man. Am J Clin Pathol 58:555–557, 1972

General References

BUECHNER HA, SEABURY JH, CAMPBELL CC, GEORG LK, KAUFMAN L, and KAPLAN W: The current status of serologic, immunologic, and skin tests in the diagnosis of pulmonary mycoses. Chest 63:259–270, 1973

LENNETTE EH, SPAULDING EH, and TRUANT JP (eds.) Manual of Clinical Microbiology, 2nd edition. American Society for Microbiology, Washington, D.C., 1974

CHAPTER 51

YEAST INFECTIONS

Donald G. Ahearn and Ronald L. Schlitzer

Causative Organisms

We use the term "yeast" to denote any unicellular, white or pastel-pigmented fungus that typically reproduces by budding, although budding fungi that produce profuse aerial mycelia or intense melanoid pigments are arbitrarily excluded.

The traditional classification of yeasts is based on morphologic and physiologic properties. The presence and type of ascospores or basidiomycetous structures are of prime importance. Secondary characteristics include cellular morphology and fermentation and assimilation reactions (28).

Over 500 species of yeasts are currently recognized (43). About 25 species, mostly of the families Cryptococcaceae of the Deuteromycota, commonly are associated with man. Of these, *Candida albicans* and *Cryptococcus neoformans* are responsible for most reported yeast infections. In the last 20 years, other yeasts (mainly *C. tropicalis, C. parapsilosis,* and *Candida [Torulopsis] glabrata*) have emerged as opportunistic pathogens.

Most yeast infections are caused by *Candida* spp. This ill-defined form-genus includes oxidative and fermentative species that lack arthrospores and have pseudo-mycelium to true mycelium absent, rudimentary or well-developed. True hyphae are filaments in which septation occurs after terminal extension. Pseudohyphae are filaments composed of catenulate budding cells. At maturity, pseudohyphae may be indistinguishable in gross appearance from true hyphae. The pseudohyphae of yeasts may vary in appearance with growth conditions and among isolates; however, one type of pseudohypha may be common for a particular species. The genus *Candida* includes fungi of ascomycetous and basidiomycetous phylogeny.

Some common types of pseudohyphae are:

mycotorula—blastospores occurring in grape-like clusters at septal nodes of pseudohyphae;

mycotoruloides—blastospores at septal nodes of pseudohyphae in short irregular branched chains;

candida—sparsely branched chains of blastospores mostly at ends of pseudohyphal chains;

mycocandida—strongly branched pseudohyphae often with single budding blastospores symmetrically arranged at septal nodes (Fig 51.1).

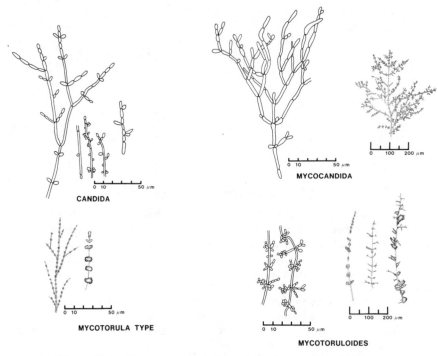

Figure 51.1—Common types of pseudohyphae produced by yeasts.

C. albicans is the most common etiologic agent of yeast infections. Typically, initial growth of *C. albicans* on most media is by unicellular budding—with cells globose to oval and 3.5–12 μm in diameter at their widest point. Smaller variants (averaging 3–4 μm in diameter at their widest point) are sometimes found in initial cultures of clinical specimens. Such isolates may not readily form hyphae.

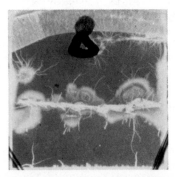

Figure 51.2—Macroscopic appearance of *C. albicans* on cornmeal agar at 96 hr. Spike-like strands of cells develop from proliferation of blastospores along mycotorula-type pseudohyphae.

Colonies are hyaline at first and have an entire border, but on media such as cornmeal agar, macroscopic spike-like strands of cells often project from the periphery of the colony (Fig 51.2). These form from single mycotorula elements encased by their blastospores. Microscopically the filaments are generally of the mycotorula-type pseudohyphae, but mycotoruloides or candida-type structures may be present.

Most isolates produce characteristic germ tubes and chlamydospores. Germ tubes, which in routine screening tests are formed along with pseudohyphal cells, are not constricted at their point of origin (Fig 51.3). Chlamydospores vary by strain in size and number produced but are generally thick-walled and at least 2–3 times the size of the yeast cell (Fig 51.4). They are most often produced in terminal clusters on branches of candida-type pseudohyphae.

Various sexual stages or life cycles have been described for several isolates of *C. albicans*, but these reports have not been generally accepted. The cell wall of *C. albicans* appears to be two-layered rather than lamellar, its mode of budding is of the ascomycetous type, and the guanine plus cytosine content of its deoxyribonucleic acid (DNA) is about 35%. These properties suggest an ascomycetous relationship.

C. tropicalis appears to be the second most common cause of systemic candidiasis, but no definitive records are available. Typical isolates of *C. tropicalis* rapidly produce hyphae of the mycotoruloides type and generally ferment earlier and more vigorously than *C. albicans*. The range of variation for *C. albicans* and *C. tropicalis* species is broad enough that they sometimes cannot be differentiated in routine tests. For example, sucrose-negative forms are present in both species, and a few strains of *C. tropicalis* may produce chlamydospore-like cells. Results of DNA reassociation studies of the two species show that they are distinct (3).

C. parapsilosis is generally more restricted than *C. albicans* or *C. tropicalis* in its pseudohyphal development and fermentation. In laboratory studies with mice or rabbits, *C. parapsilosis* is also less invasive than the others. On cornmeal agar, short candida to mycocandida psuedohyphae are present by 96 hr.

Candida glabrata (syn. *Torulopsis glabrata*) can often be differentiated from the above *Candida* spp. by size alone. Typical cells are globose and 2–5 μm in diameter; no hyphae are formed. Occasionally short chains of budding cells are observed. Ascospores have been found in the type species of *Torulopsis*, making the nomenclatural status of the genus uncertain (42). *Torulopsis* had been separated arbitrarily from *Candida* by lack of hyphae, a variable characteristic for many isolates of both genera (28). Therefore, Yarrow and Meyer (45) amended the classification of *Candida* to include the former species of *Torulopsis*. Like *C. tropicalis* and *C. parapsilosis*, *C. glabrata* has the characteristics of an ascomycetous yeast.

Cr. neoformans (Sanfelice) Vuillemin is the type species of the form genus *Cryptococcus*. This genus appears to be composed entirely of heterobasidiomycetous yeasts. *Cr. neoformans* has globose to spheroidal cells ranging from 5 to 12 μm in diameter on most media. Generally, the cells are encapsulated with a starch-like polysaccharide, but some isolates have a negligible capsule. Colonies are typically mucoid, hyaline to cream-colored, and have an

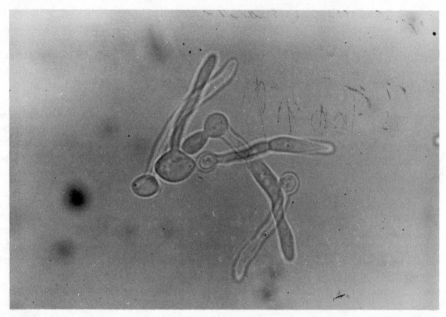

Figure 51.3—Germ tubes of *C. albicans* produced in bovine serum after 2 hr at 37 C, ×1400.

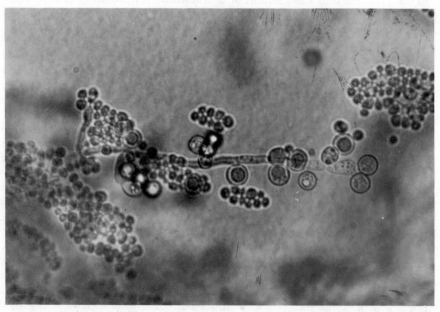

Figure 51.4—Chlamydospores of *C. albicans* on cornmeal agar with Tween 80, ×600.

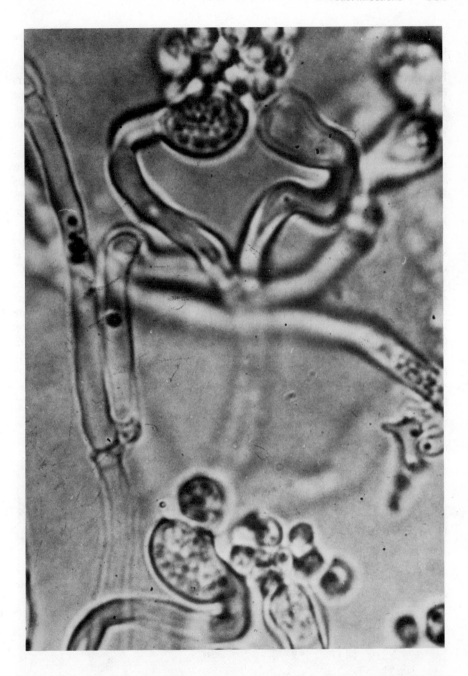

Figure 51.5—Basidia and basidiospores of *Filobasidiella neoformans* on malt extract agar after 3 weeks, ×1400.

entire border. Hyphae are rarely formed, and are usually seen deep within the colony or subsurface in the agar.

Kwon-Chung (23) first demonstrated that isolates of *Cr. neoformans* had a basidiomycetous life cycle. When the Coward strain (serotype D) of Shadomy (37) was crossed with an isolate of *Cr. neoformans* from Denmark (serotype D), profuse aerial hyphae, clamp connections, basidia, and globose basidiospores in chains were produced (Fig 51.5). A new taxon—*Filobasidiella neoformans* Kwon-Chung—was established.

Later Kwon-Chung (24) found a second sexual stage, *F. bacillispora* (distinguished by rod-shaped basidiospores), by mating isolates of *Cr. neoformans* serotypes B and C. In old cultures hyphal isolates may produce ustilaginous basidia (17). Kwon-Chung (26) demonstrated that a low percentage of self-fertile isolates are produced during the sexual cycle of the heterothallic *Cr. neoformans.*

Cr. uniguttulatus (Wolfram and Zach) Phaff and Fell, a nonpathogenic species, has phenotypic properties similar to those of *Cr. neoformans* and is distinguished by its inability to use dulcitol (galactitol) and to grow at 37 C. Kwon-Chung (25) found the perfect stage of this species and described it as *Filobasidium uniguttulatum.* Basidiospores of the *Filobasidium* spp. are in a terminal whorl rather than being catenulate as in *Filobasidiella* (Fig 51.6). The imperfect stages of both *F. uniguttulatum* Kwon-Chung and *F. capsuligenum* (van der Walt et van Kerken) de Miranda may be confused with *Cr. neoformans. Filobasidium capsuligenum* is variable for fermentation (particularly primary isolates), assimilates dulcitol, and may grow weakly at 37 C. The currently known species of *Filobasidium* do not show phenol oxidase activity.

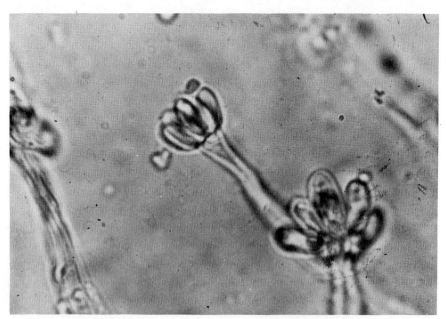

Figure 51.6—Basidia and basidiospores of *Filobasidium capsuligenum,* ×1400.

Rare and Questionable Pathogens

Yeast species such as *C. krusei* (endocarditis), *C. pseudotropicalis* (disseminated candidiasis), *C. guilliermondii* (endocarditis, candida arthritis), *C. viswanathii* (meningitis), *Rhodotorula rubra* (fungemia), *Trichosporon cutaneum* (fungemia), and even *Saccharomyces cerevisiae* (brewer's lung) have been implicated as opportunistic pathogens. The taxonomy of some of the form species at the time of the reports and the lack of histopathologic documentation raise some questions concerning the validity of associating the species with the disease. All isolates of a species may not be pathogenic, particularly since form species often include phenotypically similar fungi of diverse phylogeny.

Host debilitation is a prime factor in yeast infections, and current medical practice probably enables the incidence of opportunistic yeast infections with "rare" etiological agents to continue to rise. The common and prolonged use of catheterization combined with extensive chemotherapy has resulted in numerous cases of transient fungemia and secondary tissue invasion by some of the above species (2).

Clinical Manifestations

Candidiasis caused by *C. albicans* presents a diversified clinical picture which includes superficial infections of the skin, oral thrush, systemic and disseminated infections involving almost all internal organs, and mucocutaneous candidiasis. The high incidence of vaginitis caused by *C. albicans* reflects the fact that it is probably the most common type of yeast infection. The syndromes produced by this species overlap those produced by all other yeasts. Candidiasis caused by other species (perhaps with the exception of vulvovaginitis) is usually systemic, particularly endocarditis, peritonitis, funguria, and fungemia. Hematogenous chorioretinitis commonly accompanies systemic candidiasis, and it may be useful to check patients for characteristic eye lesions with direct ophthalmoscopy in order to detect early candidiasis (15, 31). Precipitating antibodies (as detected by immunodiffusion) may be found in the sera of patients with systemic candidiasis.

Primary infection with *Cr. neoformans* is pulmonary and is often mild or subclinical. Symptoms of more serious infections mimic those of tuberculosis or pneumonia. Disseminated cryptococcosis with involvement of the abdominal viscera, bones, and skin may occur. The yeast has a predilection for the central nervous system, and cerebral meningitis is the most commonly diagnosed form of infection.

Epidemiology

C. albicans, the most prevalent agent of candidiasis, is almost always associated with an animal host. It may appear in large numbers as a saprophyte throughout the oral-gastrointestinal tract of numerous warm-blooded vertebrates. It is isolated rarely from normal skin. Person-to-person transmission of candidiasis can occur, e.g., between sexual partners or from mother to child at birth. In general, however, candidiasis caused by *C. albicans* is endogenous in origin and develops with stress or debilitation of the host.

Other agents of candidiasis are also part of the normal flora, but *C. tropicalis* and *C. parapsilosis* commonly appear as normal flora of the skin and in nature. The rising incidence of *Candida* endocarditis and fungemia caused by *C. parapsilosis* has been associated in part with the use of contaminated materials (especially by drug addicts). *C. parapsilosis* is a common inhabitant of the nail region but is rarely an agent of onychomycosis.

Elevated incidence and susceptibility to yeast infections have long been known to accompany malnutrition, diabetes, and pregnancy. In the past 10 years, systemic candidiasis has been recognized as a hospital-acquired infection associated with many diseases, particularly cancer (4). Extensive chemotherapy with antibiotics or immunosuppressives, hyperalimentation, and indwelling catheterization are predisposing conditions for candidiasis. The prognosis for untreated systemic candidiasis is poor, and the disease itself may be pathognomonic of a grave underlying affliction.

In contrast to the agents of candidiasis, *Cr. neoformans* is rarely isolated from asymptomatic patients and is found in high concentrations in pigeon excreta in the environment (mainly serotypes A and D). *Cr. neoformans* apparently does not cause disease among pigeons, nor has bird-to-man transmission been documented. Although the species is handled frequently in clinical laboratories, no laboratory-acquired infections have been reported.

It has been speculated that the large cell size of *Cr. neoformans* grown in culture prevents its reaching the alveoli where primary infection can occur. Maintaining *Cr. neoformans* in soil or in pigeon droppings yields viable cells small enough (1–2 μm) to reach these sites. The basidiospores of *F. neoformans* are also of a size to be infectious. The presence of the sexual stages of the *Filobasidella* species in the environment has not been documented.

The ecology and natural habitat of the serotypes of *Cr. neoformans* are not fully understood. Bennett et al. (9) reported that serotype A was the most prevalent form of *Cr. neoformans* in the United States, constituting 203 of 272 isolates associated with infections and 85 of 89 isolates from the environment. Serotypes B and C, which include the mating types of *F. bacillispora*, were not isolated from the environment. The absence of these types from 67 soil and pigeon-droppings samples from Southern California was striking because 25 of 49 isolates associated with infections in that area were serotypes B or C. In a study of 47 isolates from pigeon excreta in Georgia, 51% were the alpha mating type (serotype A) of *F. neoformans* (12). No mating types of *F. bacillispora* and none of the *a* of *F. neoformans* were isolated from the pigeon droppings or found among 80 clinical isolates. Approximately 50% of the clinical isolates also could be induced to form the perfect state.

Cryptococcosis occurs worldwide, but its incidence is not yet known. Ajello (5) conservatively estimated that 330 cases of cryptococcal meningitis occur annually in the United States. The high fatality rate associated with meningitis infections makes cryptococcosis a significant public health problem.

Antimicrobial Sensitivity and Resistance

The polyene antibiotics nystatin and amphotericin B are prescribed most often for yeast infections. Both alter the permeability of the yeast cell membrane, are poorly absorbed in the intestinal tract, and are toxic. Nystatin is used topically, in vaginal suppositories, and in oral tablets. The minimal inhibitory concentration for most *Candida* spp. in M-20 medium (Difco) is between 1 and 3 μg/ml. Amphotericin B may be effective with intravenous injection for systemic infections, but it must be carefully administered because of its renal toxicity. The minimal inhibitory concentration for most yeasts in M-20 (Difco) is less than 1.0 μg/ml. Combining the polyenes with rifampin or 5-fluorocytosine gives significant synergistic inhibition (7, 8).

Fluorocytosine, a systemic antifungal drug, is readily absorbed, relatively non-toxic, and may be effective against *Candida* and *Cryptococcus* species at concentrations of <5 μg/ml. *Candida* spp. and *Cr. neoformans* readily develop resistance to fluorocytosine (33).

Imidazole compounds such as chlormidazole, clotrimazole, miconazole, and enconazole have been used with relative success against topical yeast infections. The mode of action appears to be against the cell membrane. Clotrimazole and miconazole have been examined for systemic use. Clotrimazole may produce adverse side effects (gastric intolerance, psychic disturbances), but such problems have not been reported for miconazole. The pharmacology of the imidazoles was reviewed by Holt (19).

Collection and Processing of Specimens

The protean nature of yeast infections means that numerous types of specimens are submitted for isolation of yeasts. Such material should be collected, transported, and, in most instances, processed with the same procedures and care used in detecting other mycotic agents. Since most of the pathogenic yeasts may be part of the normal flora, specimens such as sputa, bronchial aspirates, and urine usually must be analyzed as a series of specimens obtained at different times in order to obtain multiple yeast isolates and establish probable significance. In particular, body fluids of immobilized patients undergoing hyperalimentation should be monitored for any conversion from negligible to significant concentrations of yeasts.

Blood specimens should be collected in hypertonic broth media containing sodium polyanethol sulfonate or in biphasic broth-agar slant bottles at a 1:10 ratio of blood to broth. Heart infusion, brain heart infusion broth, and their respective agars are satisfactory. Bottles should be incubated at room temperature, vented, and examined daily for 4–6 weeks before being discarded as negative for yeast. Biphasic bottles should be agitated periodically to give the yeasts direct access to the agar surface. The blood cultures should be subcultured within 24 hr and after 5 days of incubation regardless of the macroscopic appearance of the culture medium. The mean recovery time of yeasts from positive blood cultures is 2–6 days, but in unvented bottles *Candida* spp. may take 3–4 weeks before growth is visible.

Cerebrospinal fluids (more than 3.0 ml) should be centrifuged at 1500–2000 rpm for 15 min. Without decanting, a portion of the sediment should be removed with a Pasteur pipette and a nigrosin or India ink preparation made. Portions of the sediment can be plated onto medium or the specimen resuspended and aliquots plated to media and broth. Alternately, the resuspended specimen can be filtered (0.45 μm) and the filter placed (organism side up) on an agar surface. Also, the filter can then be washed with 0.5–1.0 ml of sterile saline, and the fluid can be plated. Any remaining specimen should be saved and refrigerated for additional tests if warranted (cryptococcal antigen or antibody determination).

Other fluid specimens (such as synovial or those obtained through thoracentesis or ventricular or paracentesis) can be processed and cultured as described for spinal fluids or sputum specimens. Gastric lavage specimens should be adjusted to pH 4.5–5.5 with NaOH.

Sputum cultures may not show a true picture of the microbiota of the lower respiratory tract, because sputa can be contaminated by oropharyngeal secretions. Transtracheal aspirates or fiberbronchoscopic aspirates may more reliably reflect the flora of the lower respiratory tract.

If such specimens are not available, collected or induced sputum specimens should be carefully obtained. For example, having the subject brush teeth, rinse the mouth, and gargle with an antiseptic mouth wash will help minimize contamination by oral flora.

Respiratory tract specimens should be collected early in the morning and processed immediately before saprophytic *Candida* spp. develop hyphal forms in the specimen. The nature and volume of the sputum should be recorded. Viscous, purulent, blood-tinged material is most desirable. Portions of such material (0.5 ml) should be cultured directly and examined microscopically in wet mounts.

Specimens too viscid for direct plating can be diluted with sterile phosphate-buffered saline, homogenized, and placed on a mechanical shaker to accelerate liquification. Antibiotics can be added to the specimen. It may be necessary to digest sputum with N-acetyl-L-cysteine (0.5%) or dithiothreitol, but the procedure should be done carefully to avoid lowering the concentration of yeasts present. The type, concentration, temperature, and length of exposure to the digestant dictate the total number of viable yeasts recovered. The sputum specimen must be digested rapidly and concentrated and neutralized immediately for optimal recovery. Treating sputum with NaOH or using the procedure for recovering mycobacteria is not recommended for recovering yeasts.

Urine specimens (bladder aspirated, catheterized, or clean catch) are mixed in the container. A calibrated loop is used to streak the specimen on mycologic media for quantitating yeasts. The urine specimen is then centrifuged at 2000 rpm for 15 min. The supernatant is discarded, and the sediment is streaked on media with and without antibiotics. The pellet from centrifuged specimens should be examined with light or phase microscopy. At the same time, smears for PAS or Gram stains should be prepared. The report on urine cultures should include the number of different colony types and indicate the relative percentage of yeast and hyphal fragments per high-power microscopic field. Direct examination of nigrosin preparations may reveal yeast cells of *Cr. neoformans* from patients with disseminated cryptococcosis.

Diagnostic Procedures

Microscopic Examination

Budding yeasts and hyphal cells may be found in materials such as skin and mucous membrane scrapings after PAS or Gram staining. Yeasts are usually strongly gram-positive, but gram-negative variants are sometimes found in clinical specimens. Smears for KOH preparations and PAS stains should be prepared from purulent and caseous material. Spinal, joint, and pericardial fluids should be centrifuged at 1500-2000 rpm and the sediment examined. Smears of the sediment should be mixed with formalized nigrosin or India ink and examined for encapsulated yeasts. The direct fluorescent antibody technique is a valuable tool for the rapid detection of most isolates of *Cr. neoformans* in almost all types of specimens (21).

Isolation

Commercially prepared Sabouraud's dextrose agar or yeast extract-malt extract agar (malt extract 3 g, yeast extract 3 g, peptone 5 g, dextrose 10 g, and agar 20 g/liter) is adequate for the isolation of most yeasts. Chloramphenicol (0.05–0.2 g/liter), gentamicin (0.02 g/liter), or some other suitable antibiotic should be added to inhibit bacteria. Commercial mycologic media containing cycloheximide allow most isolates of *C. albicans* to grow, but cycloheximide inhibits numerous other yeasts, particularly cryptococci.

The pH of the isolation media can be adjusted to between 4.5 and 5.5 instead of adding antibiotics. At lower pH's, the agar concentration should be raised to 2.3%–2.5% to assure solidification.

Most yeasts can be isolated on blood agar. Brain heart infusion agar is unreliable for recovery of cryptococci. Several slants of the isolation medium should be inoculated and incubated at 25 and 35 C. Visible yeast colonies of most species are present by 48–72 hr, but the slants should be held for several weeks before being discarded as negative. Most pathogenic yeasts grow well at 37 C by 96 hr.

The selective medium of Shields and Ajello (38), which contains an aqueous extract of the seeds of *Guizotia abyssinica*, or preferably the DOPA medium of Chaskes and Tyndall (13) allows the rapid detection of most *Cr. neoformans* spp. Alpha mating types of serotypes A and D generally have active phenol oxidases and produce black colonies on these media.

Some isolates of the *a* mating type of serotypes A and D and the less common serotypes B and C show only negligible to latent phenol oxidase activity after a week. Rare isolates of *Cr. albidus* and *Cr. laurentii* on the *Guizotia* seed medium may show slight phenol oxidase activity comparable to that of the less active *Cr. neoformans*.

Primary isolates should be streaked on the isolation agar and on blood agar to assure purity prior to further studies. All discrete colonies should be examined since infection by multiple species is possible.

Serology

Whole cell agglutination tests for *Candida* species and fluorescent antibody (FA) reagents for the more common serotypes of *Cr. neoformans* have proven valuable for rapid identifications (21, 40). Unfortunately these reagents are not commonly available. Serologic tests for detecting systemic candidiasis have also been developed but are performed at only a few research centers.

These tests including agar gel diffusion, whole cell agglutination, latex agglutination, and counterimmunoelectrophoresis methods are promising, but techniques and reagents must be standardized before they can be fully evaluated (29).

Animal Inoculation

Pathogenicity for mice can be used in identifying *Cr. neoformans.* Swiss white mice 3–4 weeks old are inoculated intracerebrally with 0.05 ml or intraperitoneally with 0.2 ml of a phosphate-buffered saline suspension containing 10^6–10^7 viable cells. The cerebral hemispheres of animals that die after 72 hr are scraped lightly with an inoculating needle, and the adhering tissue is mixed on a slide with the formalin-nigrosin mixture for microscopic examination for encapsulated cells (Fig 51.7). Isolates of *Cr. neoformans* vary in their virulence. Mice may survive experimental infections for several months or longer without signs of disease, although brain smears may reveal budding yeasts.

Of the agents of candidiasis, only *C. albicans* and *C. tropicalis* normally are lethal for mice, through primary invasion of the kidneys. *C. albicans* is usually more virulent, with intravenous inoculation of 10^6 viable cells being sufficient to cause death of the mouse (18–23 g) within 10 days. Inocula of virulent isolates of *C. tropicalis* must usually contain 5×10^6–10^7 viable cells in order to cause fatal infections within 2 weeks. The signs of disease and histo-

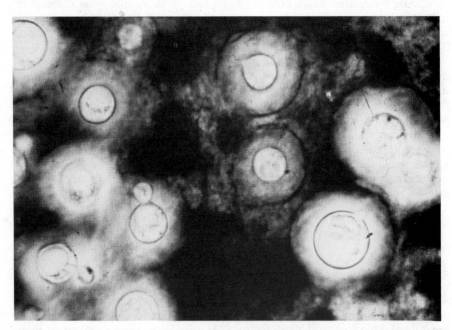

Figure 51.7—Encapsulated cells of *Cr. neoformans* in nigrosin-stained smear of mouse brain, ×1400.

pathologic findings are similar for both yeasts. Avirulent isolates of both species are sometimes found.

Germ Tubes

Most isolates of *C. albicans* (syn. *C. stellatoidea*) readily produce germ tubes in sera or serum substitutes within 3 hr at 37 C. An economical screening test can be performed as follows: colonies from a 24- to 72-hr culture on isolation agar are picked directly with the tip of a Pasteur pipette. The pipette is placed in a test tube containing 0.3–0.5 ml of serum, and the material is incubated at 37 C for 3 hr. The cells are transferred with the pipette to a slide for microscopic examination.

Agar media can be used also for germ tube production (18). Cells of some isolates from media containing cycloheximide may have reduced germ tube capacity. *C. albicans* may produce both germ tubes and pseudohyphal cells in these tests, but only the germ tubes have diagnostic significance. Some isolates of *C. tropicalis* produce elongated pseudohyphal cells similar to germ tubes, but they can be differentiated with careful microscopic examination (10). Germ tube-positive isolates of *C. tropicalis* have been described (41), but the cultures are not available for examination.

The percentage of germ tubes produced by a given isolate is highly variable and is affected by the physiological state of the inoculum and the type of induction medium (14, 32). Several fields should be scanned before negative results are recorded. Atypical isolates of *C. albicans* (poor fermentation, latent development of pseudohyphae, and negligible chlamydospores) are being seen more and more often in clinical specimens. These isolates may not produce germ tubes in routine screening tests (32).

Pseudomycelium and Chlamydospore Production

Either cornmeal agar with Tween 80 or the yeast morphology agar of Wickerham (44) can be used to induce production of hyphae. The plates are inoculated with a cut into the agar that is covered with a sterile cover slip. Most isolates of *C. albicans* produce pseudohyphae and chlamydospores within 48 hr, but some produce sparse and latent filaments or are negative for chlamydospores. Similarly, a few *Candida* isolates may not produce characteristic pseudohyphae. Oxgall agar (Difco) or other commercial media can be used to induce chlamydospore production. Rarely, small chlamydospores are formed by some isolates of *C. tropicalis.*

Induction of Perfect Stages

Yeast extract-malt extract isolation agar will induce ascosporulation in numerous ascomycetous yeasts and will support development of the basidial stage of some heterobasidiomycetous yeasts. Malt extract or Diamalt (Standard Brands, 50 g with 30 g agar/liter) agar also supports the development of sexual stages. No one medium is adequate to induce the production of ascospores by all species. Various methods for inducing ascospore production are described in Lodder (28).

Assimilation and Fermentation Tests

Various procedures are available for determining the assimilation of carbohydrates or KNO_3 by yeasts (1, 27, 28, 36, 44). Commercially prepared systems for presumptive identification can also be used with reasonable degrees of accuracy (11). The widely used defined basal media of Wickerham (44) are available commercially. The analyst must be thoroughly familiar with the procedure and and must include known cultures as controls if any system is to be effective.

Fermentation of carbohydrates is a less stable criterion than carbohydrate assimilation for identification. A few fungi (e.g., *Malessezia pachydermatis*, *Brettanomyces* spp.) may grow on the isolation agars and in the fermentation broth but not in the assimilation media. A dye can be added to the fermentation broth to make it easier to see acid and gas. Only gas is considered to be an indication of fermentation. Material for the traditional fermentation and assimilation tests is incubated at room temperature; however, the incubation time and temperature vary with the method. Fermentation results obtained at 37 C may differ from those obtained at room temperature (e.g., *C. albicans* and *C. parapsilosis* may produce gas in sucrose at 37 C). Fermentation tests may take as long as 2 weeks, but with sufficient inocula most medically important isolates produce typical patterns within 5 days.

Auxanographic assimilation tests are usually more rapid than broth tests, but some latent reactions may not be obvious. Latent reactions are best observed in broth cultures incubated with agitation.

It is not uncommon for primary isolates to vary from the typical pattern of carbohydrate utilization by lacking an enzymatic function (especially alpha- or beta-glucosidase activity). Often after specimens are maintained in culture, these enzymatic functions are readily expressed. A schematic for tentative identification of clinical yeasts is presented in Figure 51.8. The salient diagnostic characteristics of the animal-associated yeasts are presented in Table 51.1.

Interpretation of Laboratory Findings

Recent studies involving ultrastructure comparison, DNA reassociation, and comparative zone electrophoresis of enzymes indicate that the standard criteria for classifying certain yeasts are not totally reliable (3, 6, 30, 34). These new procedures probably will allow researchers to determine which of the traditional characteristics that can be determined practically in the clinical laboratory are most reliable. Until that time, most clinical yeast isolates can be identified with the standard tests, but variations (such as failure to express a property) should be expected.

A key for the presumptive identification of some of the more common animal-associated yeasts is presented below.

TABLE 51.1—CHARACTERISTICS OF COMMON ANIMAL-ASSOCIATED YEASTS*

SPECIES	DEXTROSE A	DEXTROSE F	CELLOBIOSE A	CELLOBIOSE F	DULCITOL A	GALACTOSE A	GALACTOSE F	INOSITOL A	LACTOSE A	LACTOSE F	MALTOSE A	MALTOSE F	MELIBIOSE A	RAFFINOSE A	RAFFINOSE F	SUCROSE A	SUCROSE F	TREHALOSE A	TREHALOSE F	XYLOSE A	KNO₃ A	UREASE TEST	37 C	CYCLO-HEXIMIDE
C. albicans	+	+	−	−	−	+	V	−	−	−	+	+	−	−	−	+†	−†	+	V	+†	−	−	+	+
C. glabrata	+	+	−	−	−	−	−	−	−	−	−	−	−	−	−	−	−	+	+	−	−	−	+	−
C. guilliermondii	+	+	+	+	+	+	V	−	−	−	+	−	+	+	+	+	+	+	+†	+	−	−	+	V
C. krusei	+	+	−	−	−	−	−	−	−	−	−	−	−	−	−	−	−	−	−	−	−	+†	+	−
C. parapsilosis	+	V	−	−	−	+	V	−	−	−	+	+	−	−	+	+	−†	+	V	V	−	−	+	V
C. pseudotropicalis	+	+	+†	+†	−	+	−	−	+	+	−	−	−	+	−	+†	+	−	−	+	−	−	+	V
C. tropicalis	+	+	V	−	−	V	+	−	−	−	+	+	−	−	+	+	+†	+	+	+	−	−	+	V
Cr. albidus	+	−	+	−	V	+	−	+	V	−	+	−	V	+	−	+	−	+	−	+	+	+	−†	V
Cr. laurentii	+	−	+	−	+	+	−	+	+	−	+	−	V	V	−	−	−	+	−	+	−	+	−†	−
C. neoformans	+	−	+	−	+	V	−	+	−	−	V	−	−	V	−	+	−	+†	−	+	−	+	+†	−
Cr. terreus	+	−	V	−	V	+	−	+	−	−	+	−	−	−	−	+	−	+	−	+	+	+	−	−
Cr. uniguttulatus	+	−	+	−	−	V	−	+†	−	−	+	−	−	V	−	+	−	V	−	+	−	+	−	−
F. capsuligenum	+	V	V	−	+	+	−	+†	−	−	+	V	−	−	−	+	−	+†	−	−	+	+	+†	−
R. rubra	+	−	−	−	−	+	−	−	−	−	+	−	−	+	−	+	−	+	−	+	+	+	V	V
S. cerevisiae	+	+	V	V	−	V	+†	−	−	−	+	+	V	V	V	−	+	V	V	−	−	−	+	V
Tr. cutaneum	+	−	−	−	V	V	−	V	+	−	+	−	+†	V	−	+	−	V	−	V	−	V	V	V
Tr. pullulans	+	−	+	+	−	+	−	+	V	−	+	−	−	+†	−	+	−	+	−	V	+	+	V	V

* Reactions determined by Wickerham procedure with agitation used for assimilations: (F) fermentation, (A) assimilation, (V) common strain variation, (+) growth, (−) negative

† Rare strain variation

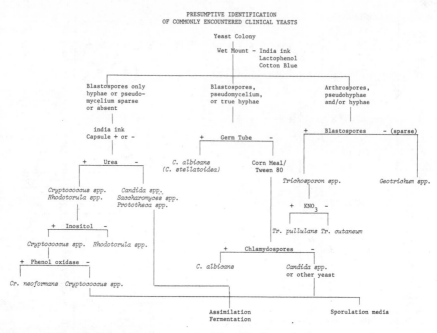

Figure 51.8—Schemata for presumptive identification of yeasts commonly found in clinical specimens.

KEY TO COMMON ANIMAL-ASSOCIATED YEASTS*

1. Germ tube test positive — *C. albicans*
   Germ tube test negative — 2
2. Pseudohyphae absent or sparse — 3
   Pseudohyphae well developed — 8
3. Inositol positive (*Cryptococcus*)[†] — 4
   Inositol negative (*Rhodotorula*, *Saccharomyces* or *Candida* spp.) — 16
4. Potassium nitrate positive — 5
   Potassium nitrate negative — 6
5. Maltose and sucrose positive — *Cr. albidus*
   Maltose variable, sucrose negative — *Cr. terreus*
6a. Maltose, sucrose, and dulcitol positive; lactose and melibiose negative — 7
   b. Maltose, sucrose and lactose positive; melibiose and dulcitol variable — *Cr. laurentii*
   c. Maltose and sucrose positive; lactose, melibiose, and dulcitol negative — *Cr. uniguttulatus*

---

*Unless specified reactions are assimilations, the key is based on absence of ascospores. C = *Candida;* Cr = *Cryptococcus;* R = *Rhodotorula;* Tr = *Trichosporon;* TTC = 2,3,5 triphenyl-tetrazolium chloride.

7. Fermentation absent, DOPA reaction   *Cr. neoformans*
   usually positive
   Fermentation weak to latent, DOPA   *Filobasidium capsuligenum*
   reaction negative
8. Arthrospores produced (*Trichosporon*)   9
   Arthrospores not produced, inositol   10
   negative, rarely positive (*Candida*)
9. Potassium nitrate negative, lactose   *Tr. cutaneum*
   and melibiose positive
   Potassium nitrate positive, lactose   *Tr. pullulans*
   variable, melibiose positive
10. Potassium nitrate positive   *Candida* spp.
    Potassium nitrate negative   11
11. Lactose fermented   *C. pseudotropicalis*
    Lactose negative   12
12. Raffinose and melibiose positive   *C. guilliermondii*
    Raffinose negative   13
13. Trehalose positive   14
    Trehalose negative (glucose positive;   *C. krusei*
    galactose, sucrose, and maltose negative)
14. Cellobiose positive, maltose fermented   *C. tropicalis*[†]
    Cellobiose negative   15
15. Maltose and sucrose fermentation   *C. tropicalis*
    usually positive, TTC reduced
    Maltose fermentation negative, sucrose   *C. parapsilosis*
    fermentation variable (generally
    negative)
    Maltose fermented, sucrose not fermented, *C. albicans*
    TTC not reduced (repeat germ tube test)
16. Carotenoid pigments present   *Rhodotorula*-like complex[‡]
    Carotenoid pigments not present   17
17. Only dextrose and trehalose fermented   *C. glabrata*
    Dextrose, galactose, maltose, and   Possible imperfect state
    sucrose fermented   of *Saccharomyces* spp.

[†]See Addendum.
[‡]Carotenoids are visually prominent in *Sporobolomyces, Sporidiobolus, Rhodosporidium, Phaffia,* and some strains of *Cryptococcus.*

Miscellaneous Yeastlike Microorganisms

Prototheca

Prototheca spp. produce hyaline yeast-like colonies on most mycological media at 37 C. They vary in their sensitivity to cycloheximide. Cells are round to oval and range from about 2–16 μm in diameter. Reproduction is by intracellular cleavage (Fig 51.9). The microscopic appearance in culture is charac-

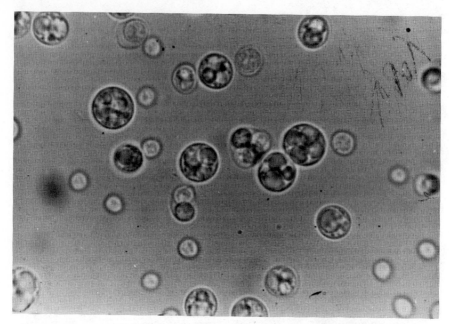

Figure 51.9—Vegetative cells of *Prototheca wickerhamii,* ×1400.

teristic and similar to that in tissue sections. The microorganisms possess properties similar to those of algae and fungi, but their phylogeny is not established. The species may be readily distinguished with fluorescent antibody reagents (39) or with assimilation tests (Table 51.2).

TABLE 51.2—PHYSIOLOGICAL CHARACTERISTICS OF SPECIES OF *GEOTRICHUM* AND *PROTOTHECA*

	DEXTROSE		GALACTOSE		SUCROSE		TREHALOSE		XYLOSE	CELLOBIOSE	PROPANOL	UREASE TEST	KNO$_3$
	A	F	A	F	A	F	A	F	A	A	A		
Geotrichum													
G. candidum	+	V	+	−	−	−	−	−	+	−	/*	−	−
G. capitatum	+	−	+	−	−	−	−	−	−	−	/	−	−
G. fermentans	+	V	+	V	−	−	−	−	+	+	/	−	−
G. penicillatum	+	V	+	V	−	−	−	−	+	−	/	−	−
Prototheca													
P. wickerhamii	+	−	+	−	−	−	+	−	−	−	−	−	−
P. zopfii	+	−	+	−	−	−	−	−	−	−	+	−	−
P. stagnora	+	−	+	−	+	−	−	−	−	−	−	−	−

* Not determined

Kaplan (22) reported in a comprehensive review that of 18 known cases of human cutaneous to subcutaneous protothecosis, 12 were caused by *P. wickerhamii,* one by *P. zopfii,* and five by unidentified species. The disease was most common in cattle and is sometimes disseminated and usually caused by *P. zopfii.*

Geotrichum

The genus *Geotrichum* usually is characterized by scanty aerial mycelium and reproduction by arthrosporulation (Fig 51.10). The genus includes asexual forms of the ascomycetes *Endomyces* and *Dipodascus. G. candidum* may be present in sputa and feces and is commonly found in dairy and fruit wastes. It has been associated with conjunctivitis, cutaneous lesions, septicemia, and acute bronchitis as a rare secondary invader (20). Infections are rarely documented, and the status of the disease is often questionable (16).

Von Arx et al. (43) reclassified *Tr. capitatum, Tr. fermentans,* and *Tr. penicillatum* in *Geotrichum.* These fungi all possess hyphal septa with plasmodesmata (multipored septa) and ascomycetous-type cell walls.

Malassezia (Pityrosporum)

Isolates of *Pityrosporum orbiculare* and *P. ovale* are recognized as yeast stages of *Malassezia furfur* (35). The fungus grows as a yeast in media enriched with olive oil. The cells are generally small, globose to elongate, about 1.5–5.5

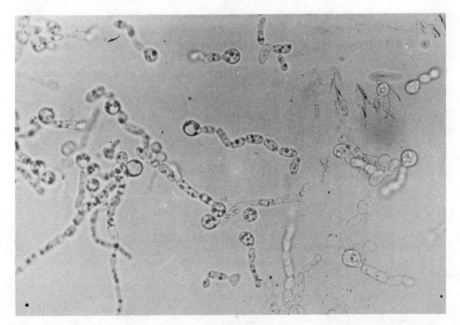

Figure 51.10—Arthrospores of *G. penicillatum* on cornmeal agar after 24 hr, ×1100.

μm in diameter at their widest point. Generally, repeated budding occurs at one pole at the same location, and the released buds leave successive scars which form a collarette.

A second species, *M. pachydermatis,* grows well on complex media with no oil added but does not grow in defined assimilation media. This species is usually isolated from canines, but cultures are obtained occasionally from humans. In old cultures the various forms may produce a few hyphae.

Addendum

Since this manuscript was prepared, several pertinent reports have been published. The genus *Cryptococcus* was found to include two species that produced thick-walled ascospores. These species, *Cr. lactativorus* and *Cr. cereanus,* have been placed in the genus *Sporopachydermia* (34a). A third species, *Cr. melibiosum,* also has ascomycetous characters, but a sexual stage is yet to be found. The legitimacy of the genus *Cryptococcus* has been questioned. Species with xylose in their cell walls have been transferred to *Apiotrichum,* whereas those containing fucose have been placed in *Rhodotorula* (43a). The distinction of genera is based also on the type of budding. The practical assignment of species to the appropriate genera on the basis of chemical analyses will be difficult, but cell wall differences appear to correlate well with other biochemical distinctions between basidiomycetous and ascomycetous yeasts.

Candida lusitaniae, an occasional isolate from clinical specimens, has been implicated as an adventitious pathogen (19a). Strains of this species show variable fermentation of maltose and superficially may resemble *C. parapsilosis* or *C. tropicalis. C. lusitaniae* is distinguished from both of these species by several physiologic properties, most notably its ability to ferment cellobiose and to assimilate rhamnose. Isolates of *C. lusitaniae* and *C. obtusa* are heterothallic and mate to produce one to four clavate ascospores per ascus. The perfect stage has been described as *Clavispora lusitaniae* (34b).

References

1. AHEARN DG. Identification and ecology of yeasts. *In* Opportunistic Pathogens. Prier JE and Friedman H (eds.). Univ Park Press, Baltimore, 1974, pp 129–146
2. AHEARN DG and HOLZSCHU DL: The white yeasts as disease agents: historical perspective. *In* Proceedings of the 4th International Congress on Mycoses. Pan American Health Organization, Washington, DC, Sci Publ No. 356, 1978, pp 119–123
3. AHEARN DG, MEYER SA, MITCHELL G, NICHOLSON MA, and IBRAHIM AI: Sucrose-negative variants of *Candida tropicalis.* J Clin Microbiol 5:494–496, 1977
4. AISNER J, SCHMPFF SC, SUTHERLAND JC, YOUNG VM, and WIERNIK PH: *Torulopsis glabrata* infections in patients with cancer, increasing incidence and relationship to colonization. Am J Med 61:23–28, 1976
5. AJELLO L: The medical mycological iceberg. *In* The Epidemiology of Human Mycotic Diseases. Al-Doory Y (ed.). Charles C Thomas, Springfield, Ill, 1975, pp 290–306
6. BAPTIST JN and KURTZMAN CP: Comparative enzyme patterns in *Cryptococcus laurentii* and its taxonomic varieties. Mycologia 68:1195–1203, 1976
7. BEGGS WH, SAROSI GA, and WALKER MI: Synergistic action of amphotericin B and Rifampin against *Candida* species. J Infect Dis 133:206–209, 1976
8. BENNETT JE: Flucytosine. Ann Intern Med 86:319–322, 1977

9. BENNETT JE, KWON-CHUNG KJ, and HOWARD DM: Epidemiologic differences among serotypes of *Cryptococcus neoformans*. Am J Epidemiol 105:582–586, 1977

10. BOWMAN PI and AHEARN DG: Evaluation of the Uni-Yeast-Tek kit for the identification of medically important yeasts. J Clin Microbiol 2:354–358, 1975

11. BOWMAN PI and AHEARN DG: Evaluation of commercial systems for the identification of clinical yeast isolates. J Clin Microbiol 4:49–53, 1976

12. BOWMAN PI and AHEARN DG: Ecology of *Cryptococcus neoformans* in Georgia. *In* Proceedings of the 4th International Congress on Mycoses. Pan American Health Organization, Washington, DC, Sci Publ No. 356, 1978, pp 258–268

13. CHASKES S and TYNDALL RL: Pigment production by *Cryptococcus neoformans* from para- and ortho-diphenols: effects of the nitrogen source. J Clin Microbiol 1:509–514, 1975

14. DABROWA N, TAXER SS, and HOWARD D: Germination of *Candida albicans* induced by proline. Infect Immun 13:733–734, 1976

15. EDWARDS JE JR, MONTGOMERIE JZ, FOOS RY, SHAW VK, and GUZE LB: Experimental hematogenous endophthalmitis caused by *Candida albicans*. J Infect Dis 131:649–657, 1975

16. EMMONS CW, CHAPMAN BH, UTZ JP, and KWON-CHUNG KJ: Medical Mycology, 3rd edition. Lea and Febiger, Philadelphia, Pa, 1977

17. ERKE KH: Light microscopy of basidia, basidiospores and nuclei in spores and hyphae of *Filobasidiella neoformans (Cryptococcus neoformans)*. J Bacteriol 28:445–455, 1976

18. FLEMING WH III, HOPKINS JM, and LAND GA: New culture medium for the presumptive identification of *Candida albicans* and *Cryptococcus neoformans*. J Clin Microbiol 5:236–243, 1977

19. HOLT RJ: Topical pharmacology of imidazole antifungals. J Cut Pathol 3:45–59, 1976

19a. HOLZSCHU DL, PRESLEY HL, MIRANDA M, and PHAFF HJ: Identification of *Candida lusitaniae* as an opportunistic yeast in humans. J Clin Microbiol 10:202–205, 1979

20. KAHANPAA A: *Geotrichum candidum* and pulmonary diseases. Reprint. Karstenia 15:5–12, 1976

21. KAPLAN WM: Practical application of fluorescent antibody procedures in medical mycology. Mycoses. Pan Am Health Organ Publ No. 304, pp 178–186, 1975

22. KAPLAN W: Protothecosis and infections caused by morphologically similar green algae. *In* Proceedings of the 4th International Congress on Mycoses. Pan American Health Organization, Washington, DC, Sci Publ No. 356, 1978, pp 218–232

23. KWON-CHUNG KJ: A new genus, *Filobasidiella*, the perfect state of *Cryptococcus neoformans*. Mycologia 67:1197–1200, 1975

24. KWON-CHUNG KJ: A new species of *Filobasidiella*, the sexual state of *Cryptococcus neoformans* B and C serotypes. Mycologia 68:942–946, 1976

25. KWON-CHUNG KJ: Perfect state of *Cryptococcus uniguttulatus*. Int J Syst Bacteriol 27:293–299, 1977

26. KWON-CHUNG KJ: Heterothallism vs. self-fertile isolates of *Filobasidiella neoformans (Cryptococcus neoformans)*. *In* Proceedings of the 4th International Congress on Mycoses. Pan American Health Organization, Washington, DC, Sci Publ No. 356, 1978, pp 204–213

27. LAND GA, VINTON EC, ADCOCK GB, and HOPKINS JM: Improved auxanographic method for yeast assimilations: a comparison with other approaches. J Clin Microbiol 2:206–217, 1975

28. LODDER J (ed.): The Yeasts. North-Holland Publishing Co, Amsterdam, 1970

29. MERZ WB, EVANS GL, SHADOMY S, ANDERSON S, KAUFMAN L, KOZINN PJ, MACKENSIE DW, PROTZMAN WP, and REMINGTON JS: Laboratory evaluation of serological tests for systemic candidiasis: a cooperative study. J Clin Microbiol 5:596–603, 1977

30. MEYER SA, ANDERSON K, BROWN RE, SMITH MT, YARROW D, MITCHELL G, and AHEARN DG: Physiological and DNA characterization of *Candida maltosa* a hydrocarbon-utilizing yeast. Arch Microbiol 104:225–231, 1975

31. MONTGOMERIE JZ and EDWARDS JE JR: Association of infection due to *Candida albicans* with intravenous hyperalimentation. J Infect Dis 137:197–201, 1978

32. OGLETREE FF, ABDELAL AT, and AHEARN DG: Germ tube formation by atypical *Candida albicans*. Antonie van Leeuwenhoek J Microbiol Serol 44:15–24, 1978

33. POLAK A and SCHOLER HJ: Mode of action of 5-fluorocytosine and mechanisms of resistance. Chemotherapy 21:113–130, 1975

34. PRICE CW, FUSON GB, and PHAFF HJ: Genome comparison in yeast systematics: delimitation of species within the genera *Schwanniomyces, Saccharomyces, Debaryomyces,* and *Pichia.* Microbiol Rev 42:161–193, 1978

34a. RODRIGUES DE MIRANDA L: A new genus: *Sporopachydermia.* Antonie van Leeuwenhoek J Microbiol Serol 44:439–450, 1978

34b. RODRIGUES DE MIRANDA L: *Clavispora,* a new yeast genus of the Saccharomycetales. Antonie van Leeuwenhoek J Microbiol Serol 45:479–483, 1979

35. SALKIN IF and GORDON MA: Polymorphism of *Malassezia furfur.* Can J Microbiol 23:471–475, 1977

36. SEGAL E and AJELLO L: Evaluation of a new system for the rapid identification of clinically important yeasts. J Clin Microbiol 4:157–159, 1976

37. SHADOMY HJ: Clamp connections in two strains of *Cryptococcus neoformans. In* Recent Trends in Yeast Research. Ahearn DG (ed.). Georgia State Univ, Atlanta, Ga, 1970, pp 67–72

38. SHIELDS AB and AJELLO L: Medium for selective isolation of *Cryptococcus neoformans.* Appl Microbiol 24:824–830, 1966

39. SUDMAN MS and KAPLAN W: Identification of the *Prototheca* species by immunofluorescence. Appl Microbiol 25:981–990, 1973

40. SWEET CE and KAUFMAN L: Application of agglutinins for the rapid and accurate identification of medically important *Candida* species. Appl Microbiol 19:830–836, 1970

41. TIERNO PM JR and MILSTOC M: Germ tube-positive *Candida tropicalis.* Am J Clin Pathol 68:294–295, 1977

42. VAN DER WALT JP and JOHANNSEN E: Ascospores in the type species of the genus *Torulopsis.* Antonie van Leeuwenhoek J Microbiol Serol 40:281–283, 1974

43. VON ARX JA, RODRIGUES DE MIRANDA L, SMITH MT, and YARROW D: The genera of yeasts and the yeast-like fungi. Studies in Mycology. No. 14, 42 pp.

43a. VON ARX JA and WEIJMAN ACM: Conidiation and carbohydrate composition in some *Candida* and *Torulopsis* species. Antonie van Leeuwenhoek J Microbiol Serol 45:547–555, 1979

44. WICKERHAM LJ: Taxonomy of Yeasts. U.S. Dept. Agriculture Tech Bull No. 1029. U.S. Dept. Agriculture, Washington, DC, 1971

45. YARROW D and MEYER SA: 1978 A proposal for the amendment of the diagnosis of the genus *Candida* Berkhout nom. cons. Int J Syst Bacteriol 28:611–615.

CHAPTER 52

PHAEOHYPHOMYCOSIS

Michael R. McGinnis

Introduction

Phaeohyphomycosis is the name given to a group of mycotic infections of humans and lower animals caused by dematiaceous fungi that develop in host tissue as dark-walled (dematiaceous), septate hyphae (2, 3). The term phaeohyphomycosis is derived from three Greek roots: phaio (dark), hyphe (web), and mykes (fungus), which were combined into a word that signifies a disease (osis) caused by any fungus whose tissue form is basically in the nature of septate, darkly pigmented hyphae. The term phaeohyphomycosis is not meant to be used solely for mycotic infections caused by members of the class Hyphomycetes. The invasion hyphae may appear as regularly shaped, short to elongate hyphal elements; as distorted and swollen mycelial filaments; or a mixture of both (Fig 52.1).

Phaeohyphomycosis is a distinct disease entity and should not be confused with chromoblastomycosis. The classical and diagnostically important tissue form of the agents of chromoblastomycosis is the thick-walled, darkly pigmented, muriform cell that is commonly referred to as a "sclerotic body." Some medical mycologists use the term "chromomycosis" (12, 34) for infections caused by the agents of chromoblastomycosis and phaeohyphomycosis. These two diseases are strikingly different with respect to their clinical expression and tissue form, and should not be merged under a common name. Chromoblastomycosis and phaeohyphomycosis involving nails, skin, and eyes will be discussed elsewhere within this manual.

Description of the Disease and Etiology

Infections caused by the agents of phaeohyphomycosis range from cutaneous and subcutaneous diseases to those that involve the vital organs of the body (3, 5, 13–18, 20–23, 25–27, 29–33, 36, 39, 40). Their clinical expressions are so varied that a definitive diagnosis rests solely upon the detection and demonstration of dematiaceous hyphal elements in the clinical material. Table 52.1 lists the currently known fungi that have caused confirmed cases of phaeohyphomycosis. These 22 species representing 10 genera, which are inhabitants of soil, wood, and decaying vegetative matter throughout the world, will be described later in this chapter.

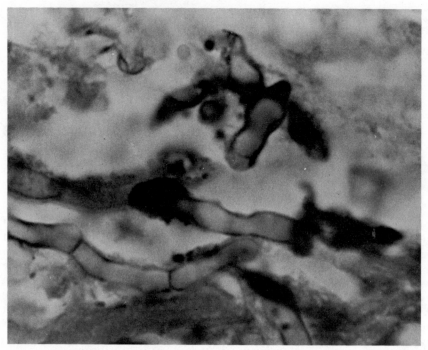

Figure 52.1.—Hyphae of a sterile mould in human brain tissue, GMS, 2400×.

Collection and Processing of Specimens

The agents of phaeohyphomycosis are ubiquitous fungi in nature and are sometimes encountered in the diagnostic laboratory as contaminants. The care exercised in the collection and handling of the clinical material is of utmost importance (8, 24, 35, 37, 41) in order to insure that the fungi isolated are not "contaminants." All clinical specimens for mycological study should be collected aseptically and transported promptly to the laboratory in a properly labelled sterile specimen container for immediate processing.

Mycological Procedures

Direct Examination

Once received by the diagnostic laboratory, the clinical specimen should be macroscopically examined for the presence of granules, necrotic tissue, blood, pus and caseous material. Suspicious portions of the clinical material are mounted in 10% KOH and examined microscopically for the presence of fungi. If granules are seen in the specimen, they should be mounted in sterile

TABLE 52.1—CURRENTLY KNOWN AGENTS OF HUMAN PHAEOHYPHOMYCOSIS

A. Phylum Deuteromycotina
  1. Class Hyphomycetes

Alternaria alternata	*Mycocentrospora acerina*
Alternaria sp. (sexual state *Pleospora*)	*Phialophora hoffmannii*
Cladosporium bantianum	*P. parasitica*
C. cladosporioides	*P. repens*
Curvularia geniculata	*P. richardsiae*
C. pallescens	*Wangiella dermatitidis*
Drechslera hawaiiensis	2. Class Coelomycetes
D. rostrata	*Phoma hibernica*
D. spicifera	*Phoma* sp.
Exophiala jeanselmei	B. Phylum Ascomycotina
E. moniliae	1. Class Pyrenomycetes
E. spinifera	*Chaetomium funicolum*
Mycelia Sterilia	

saline and not KOH, since the granule(s) may also have to be cultured in order to recover the pathogen. Tissue specimens must be homogenized prior to being examined microscopically for the presence of fungal elements. The presence of fungi in the clinical specimen is made known in a preliminary report to the physician in order to insure that appropriate therapy is initiated promptly.

To establish a diagnosis of phaeohyphomycosis, dematiaceous septate hyphae must be seen in the clinical material. Mounting media such as lactophenol cotton blue, which is used by some microbiologists to examine clinical materials, may mask the true color of the hyphae. Likewise, the observation of hyphae by phase-contrast microscopy in clinical specimens should be reviewed by bright field microscopy to determine if the cell walls are pigmented. A careful search of the specimen may be required before the dematiaceous nature of the hyphae becomes obvious. When reviewing tissue sections, it is important to look at both unstained and stained sections. This is best accomplished with unstained slides by placing a drop of immersion oil on a paraffin mounted section and then examining it with the microscope. Dematiaceous hyphae are generally readily visible utilizing this technique.

Cultural Procedures

Many of the agents of phaeohyphomycosis are sensitive to cycloheximide. When media containing this antimycotic agent are used, additional media, such as plain Sabouraud dextrose agar (2% dextrose) must also be used. Two 25- × 150-mm test tubes, one containing Sabouraud dextrose agar and the other Sabouraud dextrose agar plus cycloheximide and chloramphenicol make an ideal set of media for the primary recovery of these fungi. The culture tubes should be incubated at either 25 or 30 C, but not 37 C, since at higher temperatures many opportunistic pathogens may not grow. The culture tubes should not be discarded as negative until after four weeks. In phaeohyphomycosis, as well as in other mycoses, the repeated recovery of a fungus from clinical specimens collected over several days aids in assessing the role of the fungus in the disease process.

Public health laboratories serve a unique role in the diagnosis of phaeohyphomycosis. These laboratories represent the primary referral centers for the identification of the etiologic agents. Thus, public health laboratories must keep abreast of the agents of phaeohyphomycosis and be aware of specialists who can be called upon to assist in the identification of difficult isolates. In many instances, potentially significant fungi are discarded as mere contaminants simply because they were unfamiliar and could not be identified by the laboratory technologist. This is an unacceptable practice. These fungi should be sent to recognized specialists for identification.

There are many different species of fungi that are potential pathogens of man. Owing to the great variety and unpredictability of opportunistic pathogens, serologic procedures have not been developed for phaeohyphomycosis. The diagnosis of phaeohyphomycosis must rely upon the demonstration of dematiaceous hyphae within the host's tissue and the concurrent recovery of a compatible dematiaceous fungus.

Antimycotic Susceptibility

The agents of phaeohyphomycosis are extremely varied in their response to antimycotic drugs (19, 38). Susceptibility testing is a necessity, especially if the patient is not responding to therapy. Amphotericin B and 5-fluorocytosine are the drugs of choice, but in some instances, miconazole may be of value. Unfortunately, drug resistance is usually the rule and not the exception in this group of fungi.

Diagnostic Generic Characteristics

The identification of the various agents of phaeohyphomycosis is often extremely frustrating. During the past few years, a new direction for the identification of the Deuteromycotina (Fungi Imperfecti) has evolved (27). The genera and species of Hyphomycetes and similar fungi are now being classified primarily on the basis of how they produce their conidia. Traditional characteristics such as shape, septation and arrangement of conidia, and the general nature of the conidiophore are considered to be of secondary importance. The various methods of conidial development can be readily seen in mounts prepared from slide cultures, thus permitting an accurate identification of these fungi (1, 4, 6, 7, 10, 11).

Alternaria

Alternaria is a genus of dematiaceous Hyphomycetes that produces branched chains of muriform conidia that arise from a distinct conidiophore. Each new conidium develops through a pore in the apex of the preceding conidium. Thus, the youngest conidia are at the tip of the chain, while the most mature conidia are closest to the conidiophore.

1) *A. alternata* (Fr., 1832) Keissler, 1912. Synonymy: *A. tenuis* Nees, 1816–1817; *Torula alternata* Fr., 1832.
2) *Alternaria* sp. Sexual state: *Pleospora infectoria* Fuckel, 1870.

Chaetomium

Chaetomium is an Ascomycete genus whose species produce darkly pigmented perithecia that are covered with radiating hairs of various sizes and shapes. The perithecia are usually round to oval and have a single ostiole (opening) at the upper end of the fruiting body. The asci are usually not seen as they readily deliquesce, releasing their 8 one-celled, pigmented ascospores. Freshly mounted perithecia typically have masses of ascopores around their ostioles.

1) *C. funicolum* Cooke, 1873.

Cladosporium

Branched chains of dematiaceous blastoconidia with dark hilums (basal scars) that arise directly from a distinct conidiophore characterize the genus *Cladosporium*. Each blastoconidium is formed by being "blown-out" from the apex of the preceding conidium. The conidium closest to the conidiophore usually produces two conidia, one at each of its upper corners. These cells have the general appearance of shields and are commonly referred to as "shield-cells."

1) *C. bantianum* (Saccardo, 1912) Borelli, 1960. Synonymy: *Torula bantiana* Saccardo, 1912; *C. trichoides* Emmons, 1952.
2) *C. cladosporioides* (Fres., 1863) de Vries, 1952.

Curvularia

Curvularia is a genus of dematiaceous Hyphomycetes that form conidia with true septa. Each new conidium develops through a pore in the cell wall of the conidiophore. Such conidia are called poroconidia. The poroconidia are slightly curved with each of the end cells being lighter in color than the center cell(s).

1) *C. geniculata* (Tracy et Earle, 1896) Boedijn, 1933. Synonymy: *Helminthosporium geniculatum* Tracy et Earle, 1896. Sexual state: *Cochliobolus geniculatus* Nelson, 1964.
2) *C. pallescens* Boedijn, 1933.

Drechslera

The genera *Drechslera* and *Curvularia* are very similar in that they both produce poroconidia from sympodial conidiophores. Unlike *Curvularia,* the poroconidia of *Drechslera* have pseudosepta and are neither curved nor are the ends of the conidia lighter in color than the rest of the conidium.

1) *D. hawaiiensis* (Bugnicourt, 1955) Subram. et Jain ex M.B. Ellis, 1971. Synonymy: *Helminthosporium hawaiiense* Bugnicourt, 1955. Sexual state: *Cochliobolus hawaiiensis* Alcorn, 1978.
2) *D. rostrata* (Drechsler, 1923) Richardson et Fraser, 1968. Synonymy: *Helminthosporium rostratum* Drechsler, 1923.
3) *D. spicifera* (Bainier, 1908) v. Arx, 1970. Synonymy: *Curvularia spicifera* (Bainier, 1908) Boedijn, 1933; *Helminthosporium spiciferum* (Bainier, 1908) Nicot, 1953. Sexual state: *Cochliobolus spicifer* Nelson, 1964.

Exophiala

Until recently, a number of fungi now classified in the genus *Exophiala* were considered to be species of *Phialophora,* primarily because their flask-shaped conidiogenous cells (conidia producing cells) were believed to be phial-ides. *Exophiala* produces a flask-shaped to lageniform conidiogenous cell that tapers at its apex. As each conidium breaks free from the conidiogenous cell, a small amount of cell wall material is left behind, forming a ring around the tip. This repeated process results in a conidiogenous cell, that is, an annellide, that tapers towards its tip with a series of apical annellations (rings) (Fig 52.2).

1) *E. jeanselmei* (Lang., 1928) McGinnis et Padhye, 1977. Syn-onymy: *Torula jeanselmei* Langeron, 1928; *Phialophora jeanselmei* (Lang., 1928) Emmons, 1945; *Torula bergeri* Langeron, 1949; *P. gougerotii* (Matruchot, 1910) Borelli, 1955 in the sense of Borelli; *Rhinocladiella mansonii* (Castellani, 1905) Schol-Schwarz, 1968 in part, in the sense of Schol-Schwarz.

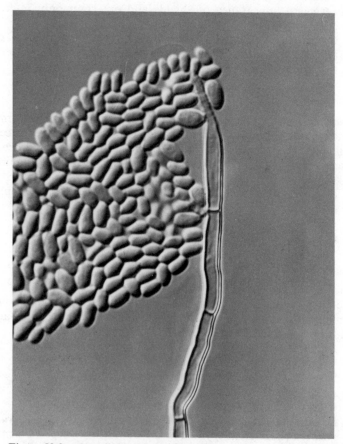

Figure 52.2.—Annellide and annelloconidia of *Exophiala spinifera,* 2400×.

2) *E. moniliae* de Hoog, 1977.
3) *E. spinifera* (Nielsen et Conant, 1968) McGinnis, 1977. Synonymy: *Phialophora spinifera* Nielsen et Conant, 1968; *Rhinocladiella spinifera* (Nielsen et Conant, 1968) de Hoog, 1977.

Mycocentrospora

Members of the genus *Mycocentrospora* develop distinctive conidia that are narrow and very long. The conidia are light brown, smooth walled and septate. Each new conidium develops at the tip of the conidiophore. As the conidium matures, a new growing point forms just below and to one side of the developing conidium. The conidiophore then increases in length, following which, the process is repeated. As a result of this type of growth, the conidiophore become geniculate. Such sympodial development of the conidiophore is one of the key characteristics of the genus *Mycocentrospora*, in addition to its unique conidia. *M. acerina* was originally misidentified as *Cercospora apii* (9) by Emmons et al. (13).
1) *M. acerina* (Hartig) Deighton, 1972.

Phialophora

The genus *Phialophora* is characterized by the production of flask-shaped phialides with a terminal collarette. In contrast to the annellides of *Exophiala*, this type of conidiogenous cell neither increases in length as each new conidium develops nor are annellations formed at its apex (Fig 52.3).

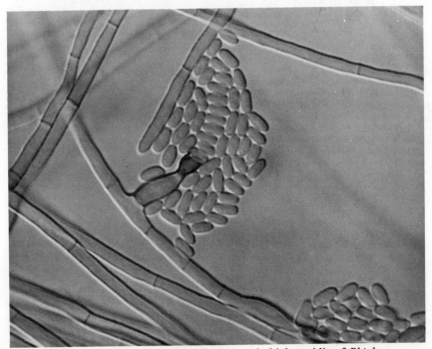

Figure 52.3.—Phialide with collarette and phialoconidia of *Phialophora verrucosa*, 2400×.

1) *P. hoffmannii* (Beyma, 1939) Schol-Schwarz, 1970. Synonymy: *Phialophora aurantiaca* Beyma, 1940; *P. luteo-viridis* (Beyma, 1939) Schol-Schwarz, 1970; *P. mutabilis* (Beyma, 1944–1945) Schol-Schwarz, 1970.
2) *P. parasitica* Ajello, Georg, Steigbigel et Wang, 1974.
3) *P. repens* (Davidson, 1935) Conant, 1937.
4) *P. richardsiae* (Nannf., 1934) Conant, 1937. Synonymy: *P. brunnescens* (Davidson, 1935) Conant, 1937; *P. calciformis* Smith, 1962.

Phoma

Members of the genus *Phoma* produce large, round to slightly lens-shaped, dematiaceous, asexual fruiting bodies called pycnidia. Inside the pycnidia, small, one-celled, cylindrical, hyaline conidia are formed. These conidia ooze out through an ostiole at the apex of the fruiting bodies.

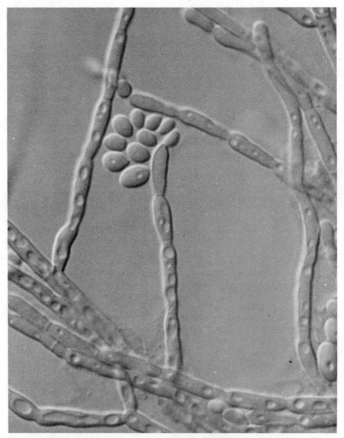

Figure 52.4.—Phialide without collarette and phialoconidia of *Wangiella dermatitidis*, 2400×.

1) *P. hibernica* Grimes, O'Connor et Cummins, 1935.
2) *Phoma* sp.

Wangiella

Wangiella is a newly described genus that is characterized by the development of phialides without collarettes. This fungus forms large amounts of toruloid (series of swollen cells) hyphae, true hyphae, and yeast-like cells with blastoconidia. The flask-shaped to cylindrical phialides develop from both the toruloid and true hyphae. The conidia are one-celled and tend to accumulate in loose globular aggregates at the tip of the phialides (Fig 52.4).

1) *W. dermatitidis* (Kano, 1934) McGinnis, 1977. Synonymy: *Hormiscium dermatitidis* Kano, 1934; *Fonsecaea dermatitidis* (Kano, 1934) Carrión, 1950; *Phialophora dermatitidis* (Kano, 1934) Emmons, 1963; *Exophiala dermatitidis* (Kano, 1934) de Hoog, 1977.

Diagnostic Cultural Characteristics

Diagnostic cultural characteristics are presented in Table 52.2 following the references.

References

1. AINSWORTH GC, SPARROW FK, and SUSSMAN AS (eds.): The Fungi: An Advanced Treatise. Vol. 4A and 4B, Academic Press, New York, 1973
2. AJELLOL L: Phaeohyphomycosis: Definition and etiology. *In* Mycoses. Proceedings of the Third International Conference on the Mycoses. Pan American Health Organization, Scientific Publication No. 304, Washington, DC, 1975, pp 126–130
3. AJELLO L, GEORG LK, STEIGBIGEL RT, and WANG CJK: A case of phaeohyphomycosis caused by a new species of *Phialophora*. Mycologia 66:490–498, 1974
4. ARX JA VON: The genera of fungi sporulating in pure culture, 2nd edition. J. Cramer, Leutershausen, 1974
5. BAKERSPIGEL A: The isolation of *Phoma hibernica* from a lesion on a leg. Sabouraudia 7:261–264, 1970
6. BARNETT HL and HUNTER BB: Illustrated genera of imperfect fungi, 3rd edition. Burgess Publishing Co, Minneapolis, 1972
7. BARRON GL: The genera of Hyphomycetes from soil. Williams & Wilkins Co, Baltimore, 1968
8. BREWER NS and WEED LA: Diagnostic tissue microbiology methods. Hum Pathol 7:141–149, 1976
9. DEIGHTON FC and MULDER JL: *Mycocentrospora acerina* as a human pathogen. Trans Br Mycol Soc 69:326–327, 1977
10. ELLIS MB: Dematiaceous Hyphomycetes. Commonwealth Mycological Institute, Kew, 1971
11. ELLIS MB: More Dematiaceous Hyphomycetes. Commonwealth Mycological Institute, Kew, 1976
12. EMMONS CW, BINFORD CH, UTZ JP, and KWON-CHUNG KJ: Medical Mycology, 3rd edition. Lea and Febiger, Philadelphia, 1977
13. EMMONS CW, LIE-KIAN-JOE, NJO-INJO TJOEI ENG, POHAN A, KERTOPATI S, and VAN DER MEULEN A: *Basidiobolus* and *Cercospora* from human infections. Mycologia 49:1–10, 1957
14. ESTES SA, MERZ WG, and MAXWELL LG: Primary cutaneous phaeohyphomycosis caused by *Drechslera spicifera*. Arch Dermatol 113:813–815, 1977
15. FARMER SG and KOMOROWSKI RA: Cutaneous microabscess formation from *Alternaria alternata*. Am J Clin Pathol 66:565–569, 1976

16. FUSTE FJ, AJELLO L, THRELKELD R, and HENRY JE: *Drechslera hawaiiensis*: Causative agent of a fatal fungal meningo-encephalitis. Sabouraudia 11:59–63, 1973

17. GARAU J, DIAMOND RD, LAGROTTERIA LB, and KABINS SA: *Alternaria* osteomyelitis. Ann Intern Med 86:747–748, 1977

18. KAUFMAN SM: *Curvularia* endocarditis following cardiac surgery. Am J Clin Pathol 56:466–470, 1971

19. KOBAYASHI GS and MEDOFF G: Antifungal agents: Recent developments. Annu Rev Microbiol 31:291–308, 1977

20. KOCH HA and HANEKE H: *Chaetomium funicolum* Cooke als möglicher Erreger einer tiefen Mykose. Mykosen 9:23–28, 1966

21. KWON-CHUNG KJ, SCHWARTZ IS, and RYBAK BJ: A pulmonary fungus ball produced by *Cladosporium cladosporioides*. Am J Clin Pathol 64:564–568, 1975

22. LAMPERT RP, HUTTO JH, DONNELLY WH, and SHULMAN ST: Pulmonary and cerebral mycetoma caused by *Curvularia pallescens*. J Pediatr 91:603–605, 1977

23. LIE-KIAN-JOE, NJO-INJO TJOEI ENG, KERTOPATI S, and EMMONS CW: A new verrucous mycosis caused by *Cerocospora apii*. Arch Dermatol 75:864–870, 1957

24. MATSEN JM and EDERER GM: Specimen collection and transport. Hum Pathol 7:297–307, 1976

25. MCGINNIS MR: *Exophiala spinifera*, a new combination for *Phialophora spinifera*. Mycotaxon 5:337–340, 1977

26. MCGINNIS MR: *Wangiella*, a new genus to accommodate *Hormiscium dermatitidis*. Mycotaxon 5:353–363, 1977

27. MCGINNIS MR: Human pathogenic species of *Exophiala*, *Phialophora*, and *Wangiella*. *In* Mycoses. Proceedings of the Fourth International Conference on the Mycoses. Pan American Health Organization, Scientific Publication No. 356, Washington, DC, 1978, pp 37–59

28. MCGINNIS MR:· Taxonomy of *Exophiala jeanselmei* (Langeron) McGinnis and Padhye. Mycopathologia 65:79–87, 1979

29. MCGINNIS MR and PADHYE AA: *Exophiala jeanselmei*, a new combination for *Phialophora jeanselmei*. Mycotaxon 5:341–352, 1977

30. MEYERS WM, DOOLEY JR, and KWON-CHUNG KJ: Mycotic granuloma caused by *Phialophora repens*. Am J Clin Pathol 64:549–555, 1975

31. NIELSEN HS and CONANT NF: A new human pathogenic *Phialophora*. Sabouraudia 6:228–231, 1968

32. PEDERSEN N, MARDH PA, HALLBERG T, and JONSSON N: Cutaneous alternariosis. Br J Dermatol 94:201–209, 1976

33. PIERACH C, GÜLMEN G, DHAR GJ, and KISER JC: *Phialophora mutabilis* endocarditis. Ann Intern Med 79:900–901, 1973

34. RIPPON JW: Medical Mycology. The Pathogenic Fungi and the Pathogenic Actinomycetes. W. B. Saunders Co, Philadelphia, 1974

35. ROBERTS GD: Laboratory diagnosis of fungal infections. Hum Pathol 7:161–168, 1976

36. SCHWARTZ IS and EMMONS CW: Subcutaneous cystic granuloma caused by a fungus of wood pulp *(Phialophora richardsiae)*. Am J Clin Pathol 49:500–505, 1968

37. SEABURY JH, BUECHNER HA, BUSEY JF, GEORG LK, and CAMPBELL CC: The diagnosis of pulmonary mycoses. Report of the committee on fungus diseases and subcommittee on criteria for clinical diagnosis. American College of Chest Physicians. Chest 60:82–86, 1971

38. SHADOMY S and ESPINEL-INGROFF A: Susceptibility testing of antifungal agents. *In* Manual of Clinical Microbiology, 2nd edition. Lennette EH, Spaulding EH, and Truant JP (eds.). American Society for Microbiology, Washington, DC, 1974, pp 569–574

39. SLIFKIN M and BOWERS HM: *Phialophora mutabilis* endocarditis. Am J Clin Pathol 63:120–130, 1975

40. YOUNG NA, KWON-CHUNG KJ, and FREEMAN J: Subcutaneous abscess caused by *Phoma* sp. resembling *Pyrenochaeta romeroi*. Am J Clin Pathol 59:810–816, 1973

41. WASHINGTON JA (ed.): Laboratory Procedures in Clinical Microbiology. Little, Brown and Co, Boston, 1974

TABLE 52.2—CULTURAL CHARACTERISTICS OF THE CURRENTLY KNOWN AGENTS OF PHAEOHYPHOMYCOSIS

ETIOLOGIC AGENTS	COLONY CHARACTERISTICS	MICROSCOPIC CHARACTERISTICS
A. Phylum Deuteromycotina 1. Class Hyphomycetes		
a) *Alternaria alternata*	Colonies rapid-growing, cottony, black to grey in color.	Condiophores dematiaceous, single or in small groups, branched or unbranched, 3–6 × 50 µm. Poroconidia dematiaceous; forming branching chains, obclavate to oval, smooth or rough, muriform, 9–18 × 20–60 µm, with a short cylindrical beak at the apex.
b) *Alternaria* sp. (sexual state *Pleospora infectoria*)	Colonies rapid-growing, cottony, black to grey in color.	Conidiophores dematiaceous, single or in small groups, branched or unbranched, 3–6 × 80 µm. Poroconidia dematiaceous, forming branching chains, obclavate to oval, distinctly rough, muriform, 9–18 × 20–70 µm, with a long gradually tapering beak making up approximately 1/2 of the conidium.
c) *Cladosporium bantianum*	Colonies rapid-growing, velvety, olive grey to olive brown in color.	Conidiophores dematiaceous and variable in length. Blastoconidia dematiaceous, forming branching chains, oval to elliptical, 1-celled, 2–2.5 × 4–7 µm.
d) *C. cladosporioides*	Colonies rapid-growing, velvety, olive green to olivaceous brown in color.	Conidiophores dematiaceous, smooth or rough, 2–6 × up to 350 µm. Blastoconidia dematiaceous, forming long branching chains, elliptical, 1-celled, 2–5 × 3–11 µm.
e) *Curvularia geniculata*	Colonies rapid-growing, velvety to cottony, grey to black or brown in color.	Conidiophores dematiaceous, single or in groups, branched or unbranched, septate, geniculate (occasionally), 3–6 µm thick. Poroconidia dematiaceous, except for the end cells, usually curved, typically 5-celled, smooth, 8–14 × 18–37 µm.

Etiologic Agents	Colony Characteristics	Microscopic Characteristics
f) *C. pallescens*	Colonies rapid-growing, cottony, brown to greyish brown in color.	Conidiophores dematiaceous, single or in groups, branched or unbranched, septate, geniculate (occasionally), 3–6 × up to 500 µm. Poroconidia pale, straight or slightly curved, 2-celled, 7–12 × 17–32 µm.
g) *Drechslera hawaiiensis*	Colonies rapid-growing, velvety to cottony, grey to blackish in color.	Conidiophores dematiaceous, single, geniculate, septate, 2–7 × up to 120 µm. Poroconidia pseudoseptate, dematiaceous, oblong to cylindrical, rounded at the ends, 3- to 8- (typically 6)-celled, 5–11 × 12–37 µm.
h) *D. rostrata*	Colonies rapid-growing, velvety, greyish brown in color.	Conidiophores dematiaceous, single or in groups, septate, geniculate, 6–8 × up to 200 µm. Poroconidia dematiaceous, obclavate, rostrate, 7- to 17-celled, 14–22 × 40–180 µm.
i) *D. spicifera*	Colonies rapid-growing, velvety, blackish brown in color.	Conidiophores dematiaceous, geniculate, septate, 4–9 × up to 300 µm. Poroconidia dematiaceous, oblong to cylindrical, rounded at the ends, 4-celled, 9–14 × 20–40 µm.
j) *Exophiala jeanselmei*	Colonies slow-growing, at first moist, becoming velvety, grey to blackish in color.	Conidiogenous cells dematiaceous, annellides, lageniform to cylindrical, tapering to a narrow apex with distinct annellations, 1.9–9.8 µm. Annelloconidia hyaline, 1-celled, subglobose to cylindrical, 1.5 × 2.8 µm, accumulating in a mass at the tip of the annellide. Yeast-like cells and toruloid hyphae typically present. Annelloconidia may be produced from reduced intercalary annellides.
k) *E. moniliae*	Colonies slow-growing, at first smooth, becoming velvety, greyish olivaceous in color.	Conidiogenous cells dematiaceous, annellides, strongly inflated to elliptical, tapering towards a narrow apex with distinct annellations, 3.8 × 10–20 µm. Annelloconidia hyaline, 1-celled, ellipsoidal, 1.9 × 3.1 µm, accumulating in a mass at the tip of the annellide. Yeast-like cells and toruloid hyphae typically present. Annelloconidia may be produced from reduced intercalary annellides.

ETIOLOGIC AGENTS	COLONY CHARACTERISTICS	MICROSCOPIC CHARACTERISTICS
l) *E. spinifera*	Colonies slow-growing, at first moist, becoming velvety, grey to blackish in color.	Conidiogenous cells dematiaceous, annellides, developing at the apex of dematiaceous spine-like conidiophores, lageniform to cylindrical, tapering to a narrow apex with distinct annellations, 2.2 × 7.8 µm. Annelloconidia hyaline, 1-celled, subglobose to cylindrical, 1.7 × 2.5 µm, accumulating in a mass at the tip of the annellide. Yeast-like cells and toruloid hyphae typically present. Annelloconidia may be produced from reduced intercalary annellides.
n) Mycelia Sterilia	Colonies slow-growing, cottony, olivaceous grey in color.	This agent of phaeohyphomycosis produces sterile hyphae and chlamydoconidia-like cells. The fungus was recovered and demonstrated in several clinical specimens from a patient with cerebral phaeohyphomycosis. It has not produced conidia, even following exposure to ultra-violet radiation, various temperatures, and numerous media designed to enhance the development of conidia.
o) *Mycocentrospora acerina*	Colonies slow-growing, raised with furrows, velvety, olivaceous black in color.	Conidiophores dematiaceous, unbranched, 0–3 septa, 5–7 µm up to 50 µm long, geniculate with broad flat scars. Conidia light brown, straight or curved, 4–24 septa (usually 8–11), 5–7 × 50–300 µm, without a basal appendage.
p) *Phialophora hoffmannii*	Colonies slow-growing, at first moist, becoming woolly to cottony, grey in color.	Conidiogenous cells hyaline to dematiaceous, phialides, cylindrical with reduced collarette, 1.1 × 3.3 µm. Phialoconidia hyaline, 1-celled, oblong to cylindrical, 1.3 × 4.2 µm, accumulating in a mass at the tip of the phialide. Yeast-like cells and chlamydoconidia typically present. Phialoconidia also produced from reduced intercalary phialides.

ETIOLOGIC AGENTS	COLONY CHARACTERISTICS	MICROSCOPIC CHARACTERISTICS
q) *P. parasitica*	Colonies slow-growing, at first moist, becoming cottony, olivaceous grey in color.	Conidiogenous cells hyaline to dematiaceous, phialides, cylindrical to obclavate, with collarette, 1-celled, 2.6×11.5 μm. Phialoconidia hyaline, 1-celled, cylindrical to allantoid, 1.3×3.4 μm, accumulating in a mass at the tip of the phialide. Yeast-like cells typically present. Phialoconidia also produced from reduced intercalary phialides.
r) *P. repens*	Colonies rapid-growing, cottony, olivaceous in color.	Conidiogenous cells hyaline to lightly dematiaceous, phialides, cylindrical, with collarette, 1.5×20 μm. Phialoconidia hyaline, 1-celled, ellipsoidal to cylindrical, 1.5×3.3 μm, accumulating in a mass at the tip of the phialide. Yeast-like cells usually present.
s) *P. richardsiae*	Colonies slow-growing, woolly, olivaceous grey in color.	Conidiogenous cells hyaline to dematiaceous, phialides, cylindrical, with flattened collarette, 2.4×10.5 μm. Phialoconidia hyaline, 1-celled, subglobose, 1.2×2.4 μm, accumulating in a mass at the tip of the phialide.
2. Class Coelomycetes		
a) *Phoma hibernica*	Colonies rapid-growing, woolly, dark brown in color.	Pycnidia have 1 to 3 ostioles, round to flask-shaped, dematiaceous, 70×76 μm. Conidia hyaline (pink in mass), 1-celled, oblong, 4.0×6.0 μm.
B. Phylum Ascomycotina		
1. Class Pyrenomycetes		
a) *Chaetomium funicolum*	Colonies slow-growing, woolly to velvety, grey in color.	Perithecia have 1 ostiole, round to oval, dematiaceous, 145×145 μm. Dichotomously branched, terminal hairs, 6 μm in diameter, forming a dense, compact mass. Lateral hairs comparatively numerous. Asci club-shaped, 8 spored, 8×34 μm. Ascospores hyaline when young, becoming dematiaceous when mature, egg-shaped to lemon-shaped, slightly pointed at both ends, 4.3×6.0 μm.

CHAPTER 53

MYCETOMAS

Libero Ajello and Glenn D. Roberts

Introduction

Mycetomas are tumors caused by a wide variety of exogenous, geophilic actinomycetes and fungi that develop in tissues in the form of mycelium organized into structures known as granules. The infections that these microorganisms cause, once they enter the body through some traumatic incident, are progressive and persistent. Not only do these etiologic agents invade cutaneous and subcutaneous tissues, they may also eventually attack and destroy bone. As the disease progresses the affected portion of the body enlarges, giving the appearance of a tumor.

Mycetomas are of two basic types: actinomycotic and eumycotic. The granules of the actinomycotic mycetomas are composed of mycelial filaments that are approximately 1 μm or less in diameter. In comparison, the granules produced by true fungi are made up of mycelium that is 2–3 or more μm in diameter. This mycelium may be quite irregular in size and form. Portions may also be differentiated into chlamydospores. In both actinomycotic and eumycotic granules, the mycelium of some of the etiologic agents may be embedded in a cement-like material. Such characteristics as color, size, presence or absence of cement, and tinctorial reaction are species dependent. Thus the granules, on the basis of their gross and microscopic features, provide an insight into the type of mycetoma under observation and the identity of the etiologic agent.

Actinomycotic mycetomas are caused by six species of aerobic actinomycetes of the genera *Actinomadura, Nocardia,* and *Streptomyces.* The species involved are cited in Table 53.1. The principal agents of the eumycotic mycetomas are presented in Table 53.2.

Description of Disease and Etiology

Mycetomas are invariably acquired through some traumatic incident that introduces the infectious elements of a potentially pathogenic actinomycete or fungus into the wound. These microorganisms inhabit soil where they live and grow as saprophytes (1, 2, 3, 5, 8, 9). Once the infection begins, the interaction between the host and the pathogen leads to the development of a generally

TABLE 53.1—ACTINOMYCOTIC AGENTS OF MYCETOMAS

(Phylum: Actinomycota,*	Class: Proactinomycetes)
Order: Actinomycetales	Family: Actinomycetaceae
Actinomadura madurae	*N. brasiliensis*
A. pelletieri	*N. caviae*
Nocardia asteroides	*Streptomyces somaliensis*

* Classification according to Margulis L: The classification and evolution of Prokaryotes and Eukaryotes. *In* Handbook of Genetics. Vol. 1. King RC (ed.). Plenum Publishing Corp, New York, 1974

painless, hard, subcutaneous tumor. The infection develops slowly and so insidiously that the victim frequently ignores it. As a result, very few patients seek medical attention when their mycetomas are in an early stage. In time, the tumor enlarges and the affected area becomes swollen and deformed. Internally, suppurative and fibrotic reactions occur in varying degrees. Abscesses and ramifying fistulous tracts develop in the subcutaneous tissues. These tend to follow the tendons. They also extend to the bones and eventually result in osteal destruction. The fistulous tracts characteristically erupt to the surface and discharge serosanguinous fluid that contains the granules that the pathogen has produced.

If the patient is not treated, the mycetomas continue to develop, involving more tissues with consequent tumefaction and bone and tissue destruction. New sinuses develop as the old ones close up and stop discharging fluid and granules. Mycetomas are basically localized infections. Generalized reactions to the diseases are rare. When such reactions are noted, they are almost invariably due to secondary bacterial infections. Mycetomas spread to contiguous tissue through dissemination of granules or granule fragments by way

TABLE 53.2 —PRINCIPAL ETIOLOGIC AGENTS OF EUMYCOTIC MYCETOMAS

Phylum:	Deuteromycota	Phylum:	Ascomycota
Class:	Hyphomycetes	Class:	Loculoascomycetes
Acremonium falciforme		*Leptosphaeria senegalensis*	
A. kiliense		*L. tomkinsii*	
A. recifei		*Neotestudina rosatii*	
Exophiala jeanselmei			
		Class:	Plectomycetes
Madurella grisea			
		*Emericella nidulans**	
M. mycetomatis			
		Class:	Pyrenomycetes
Class:	Coelomycetes		
		*Petriellidium boydii***	
Pyrenochaeta romeroi			

* Imperfect state: *Aspergillus nidulans*

** *Allescheria boydii* is one of its synonyms. Its imperfect state is generally referred to as *Monosporium apiospermum*, but more properly as *Scedosporium apiospermum*.

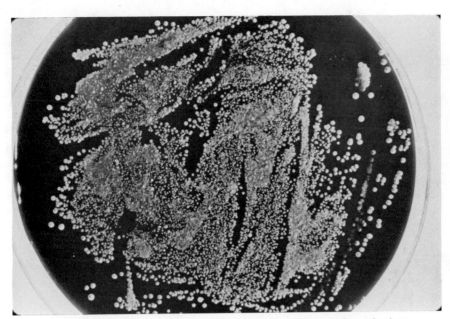

Figure 53.1—*Nocardia asteroides*. Small, round, heaped, dry colonies.
(All figures courtesy of American Society of Clinical Pathologists, *Atlas of Clinical Mycology*, Volume V.)

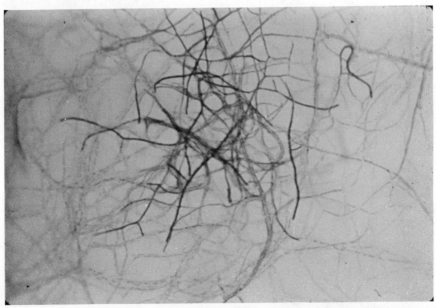

Figure 53.2—*Nocardia asteroides*. Slide preparation with long branched filaments and coccobacilli, some of which retain the acid-fast stain.

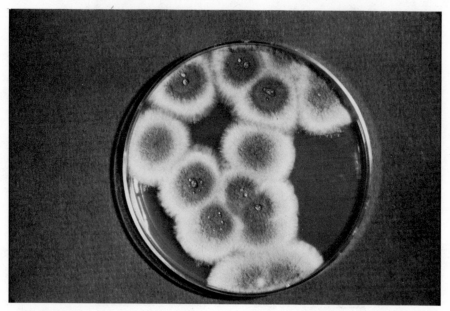

Figure 53.3—*Petriellidium boydii*. Group of floccose tan to gray-white colonies.

of the fistulous tracts. The number of granules that develop in a mycetoma may be enormous. Lymphatic spread of infection to regional lymph nodes has been shown in infections by *Madurella mycetomatis*, a *Nocardia* sp., *Petriellidium boydii*, and *Streptomyces somaliensis* (4, 7).

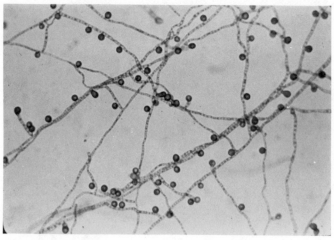

Figure 53.4—*Petriellidium boydii*. Slide preparation showing simple conidiophores with single pyriform conidia at their tips.

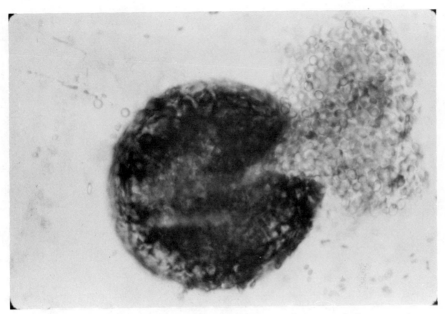

Figure 53.5—*Petriellidium boydii.* Mature ascocarp with extruded ascospores.

Collection and Processing of Specimens

In most mycetoma cases the serosanguinous fluid discharged by a drain-ing sinus is the material of choice for direct microscopic study and culture. This should be collected in a sterile petri dish and spread thinly over the sur-face of the bottom plate. If granules are present, they will be generally visible to the naked eye. These should be picked up with a sterile needle and washed repeatedly in several changes of sterile physiological saline. Such washing helps to reduce the number of possible adhering contaminating bacterial and mould cells. Thus the chances for successfully isolating the etiologic agent are enhanced.

The gauze wrappings or pads over a draining sinus tract should be exam-ined for trapped granules. If present, they can be picked up with a sterile needle and prepared as just described.

Mycological Procedures

Direct examination

The single granules or their aggregates measure, depending upon the spe-cies involved, from 20 μm to 3 mm or more in diameter. They may be white, yellow, red, or black. After their color and size have been noted, they should be placed in a drop of water or 10% KOH on a slide, pressed out under a cover slip (if soft) or between two slides (if hard) and examined microscopically.

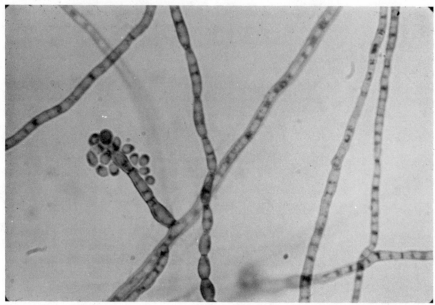

Figure 53.6—*Madurella mycetomatis.* Photomicrograph of a phialide with a cluster of conidia at the tip and moniliform hyphae.

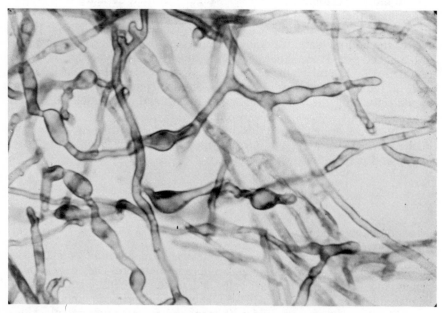

Figure 53.7—*Madurella grisea.* Slide preparation of sterile, large swollen hyphae.

Actinomycotic granules will be composed of mycelial elements 1 μm or less in diameter. Eumycotic granules will contain mycelium that averages 2–4 μm or more in diameter and chlamydospores.

Isolation

Eumycotic granules aspirated from unopened lesions or washed ones picked from exudates should be inoculated in several tubes of Sabouraud dextrose agar containing 0.05 mg/ml of chloramphenicol. Actinomycotic granules or material from mycetomas suspected of being caused by actinomycetes, however, should be cultured in antibiotic-free media, since these agents are susceptible to the inhibitory action of antibacterial antibiotics.

The use of cycloheximide to suppress the growth of saprophytic moulds is not advocated. Unfortunately, this antibiotic inhibits the growth of some of the eumycotic agents of mycetomas.

The inoculated tubes should be incubated at room temperature (25 C) and at 37 C. The cultures should be examined periodically for several weeks for signs of growth.

Identification of Etiologic Agents

Actinomycotic species

Actinomadura madurae

This species was formerly classified in the genera *Actinomyces, Discomyces, Nocardia, Streptomyces,* and *Streptothrix.* But new classification systems for the actinomycetes based on cell-wall constituents have led to the genus *Actinomadura* being created to accommodate this and related species (6). Colonies grow slowly and are white, becoming folded and rose with age as well as waxy in texture. Delicate, branched mycelium, < 1 μm in diameter. Chains of spores rarely produced. Best identified on the basis of its physiological properties (Table 53.3).

A. pelletieri

Slow-growing colonies, moist and at first pale pink, but becoming coral red with age. Surface irregularly folded. Mycelium delicate, 1 μm in diameter, nonacid-fast, branched, chains of arthroconidia occasionally formed. Optimal growth temperature, 37 C.

Nocardia asteroides

Colonies highly variable in their cultural and physiological expression. Because some isolates grow better at 25 C than at 37 C and vice versa, both temperatures should be used for isolation and identification studies. Surface color varies from white to pink to orange and to various shades of brown. Texture may be waxy or chalky or soft and moist. Narrow mycelium 1 μm in diameter; acid-fast. Chains of arthroconidia occasionally produced on aerial mycelium. Mycelium tends to fragment into rod- and coccus-shaped elements. Mycelial fragments are not all acid-fast.

TABLE 53.3.—DIAGNOSTIC PROPERTIES OF THE ACTINOMYCOTIC MYCETOMA AGENTS

SPECIES	ACID-FASTNESS	CASEIN DIGESTION	XANTHINE DIGESTION	HYPOXAN-THINE DIGESTION	ACID PRODUCTION ARABINOSE	ACID PRODUCTION XYLOSE
A. madurae	–	+	–	+	+	+
A. pelletieri	–	+	–	+	–	–
N. asteroides	+	–	–	–	–	–
N. brasiliensis	+	+	–	+	–	–
N. caviae	+	–	+	+	–	–
S. somaliensis	–	+	–	–	–	–

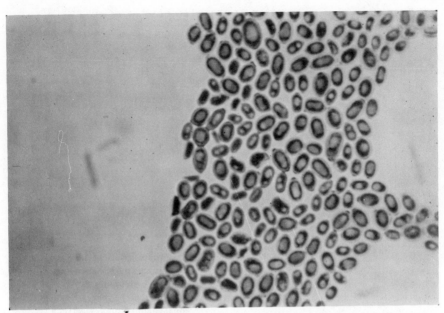

Figure 53.8—*Exophiala jeanselmei*, yeast form. Slide preparation showing dematiaceous budding yeast cells.

N. brasiliensis and N. caviae

Because of their great cultural variation, these two species are morphologically indistinguishable from *N. asteroides*. They are separated from each other on the basis of their physiological characteristics (see Table 53.3).

Streptomyces somaliensis

Slow-growing colonies, soft, folded surface, yellowing brown to dark grey. Mycelium 1 μm in diameter; nonacid fast; forms chains of spores on aerial mycelium.

All of the above species are best identified on the basis of their physiological properties and their acid-fast staining reactions (Table 53.3). The media required to carry out the physiological tests are described in the appendix to Chapter 56. The diagnostic characteristics of the actinomycete granules are presented in Table 53.4. The staining reactions of *A. madurae, A. pelletieri,* and *S. somaliensis* granules are based on the conventional hematoxylin-eosin stain. When fresh, all of the granules are soft; when desiccated they become hard.

Eumycotic Species

Acremonium falciforme (synonym: Cephalosporium falciforme)

Downy white colony with a diffusible violet pigment on reverse side. Mycelium 2–4 μm in diameter, septate. Conidiophores simple, septate, and variable in length; may be over 50 μm long. Conidia produced in dry or mucoid

TABLE 53.4—CHARACTERISTICS OF GRANULES FROM EUMYCOTIC MYCETOMAS

SPECIES	COLOR	SIZE	HISTOLOGICAL PROPERTIES (HEMATOXYLIN AND EOSIN STAIN)
Acremonium			
A. falciforme	White	200–300 μm D	No cement; border stained red; periphery pink.
A. kiliense	White	200–300 μm D	No cement; border stained red; periphery pink.
A. recifei	White	200–300 μm D	No cement; border stained red; periphery pink.
Emericella			
E. nidulans	White	65–160 μm D	No cement; mycelium stained pink
Exophiala			
E. jeanselmei	Black	200–300 μm D	No cement; vacuolate granule; periphery thick, made up of dark mycelium and chlamydospores.
Leptosphaeria			
L. senegalensis	Black	400–600 μm D	Cement present; periphery of polygonal chlamydospores; center a network of mycelium.
L. tompkinsii		500–1000 μm D	Cement present; periphery of polygonal chlamydospores; center a network of mycelium.
Madurella			
M. grisea	Black	350–500 μm D	No cement; periphery of polygonal chlamydospores; center a network of mycelium.
M. mycetomatis	Black	200–900 μm D	Two types of granules: 1. Compact type filled with cement; stains uniformly a rust brown. 2. Vesicular type: Cement in periphery, stains deep brown, filled with vesicles 6–14 μm in diameter, central zone light colored, composed of hyaline mycelium.
Neotestudina			
N. rosatii	White	300–600 μm D	Cement present on periphery; central area hematoxylin positive.
Petriellidium			
P. boydii	White	200–300 μm D	No cement; border stained red; periphery pink.
Pyrenochaeta			
P. romeroi	Black	300–600 μm D	No cement; periphery of polygonal chamydospores; center a network of mycelium.

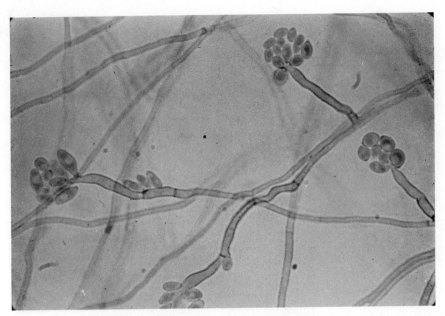

Figure 53.9—*Exophiala jeanselmei,* filamentous form. Photomicrograph of annellides and annelloconidia characteristic of this species.

clusters at tip of conidiophore. Conidia curved, with rounded upper ends, and a wide, straight base, 7–10 × 3–3.5 μm; some conidia may be uniseptate, hyaline, and smooth.

A. kiliense (synonyms: Cephalosporium kiliense, c. madurae)

Ochre, downy to floccose colony, frequently furrowed. Reverse, brownish. Mycelium variable in width, some 0.5–1.0 μm in diameter, majority 2–3 μm in diameter. Conidiophores simple, up to 70 μm long. Conidia held in mucoid clusters at tips of conidiophores, hyaline, smooth, ellipsoid to cylindrical, ends rounded, 3–6 μm × 1–1.5 μm. Chlamydospores, especially produced on corn meal agar, 4–8 μm in diameter.

Acremonium recifei (synonym: Cephalosporium recifei)

Colonies downy, white to greenish yellow to pale pink. Reverse, brownish. Mycelium 2–4 μm in diameter. Conidiophores simple, up to 60 μm long. Conidia in clusters, curved, base pointed, hyaline, smooth, 4–6 μm × 1–2 μm.

Exophiala jeanselmei (synonym: Phialophora jeanselmei)

Colonies slow growing, at first mucoid and yeast-like, greenish-black, with greyish black aerial mycelium eventually developing and producing a dome-shaped velvety colony. Early mucoid colonies are composed of unicellular blastospores, 2–4 μm in diameter. Mycelium of developed colonies, dematiaceous, simple, elongated, and tapered. Conidia, unicellular, spherical

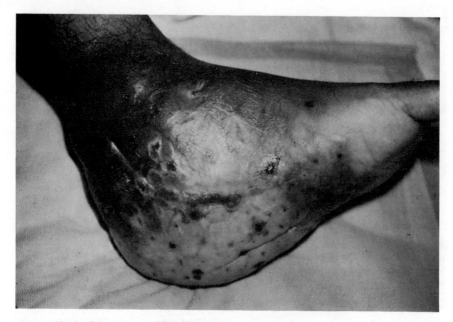

Figure 53.10—Mycetoma of foot with tumor-like lesion enlargement and numerous draining sinus tracts caused by *Nocardia brasiliensis*.

to subglobose 1.5–3.0 μm in diameter, generally accumulated in clusters at the top of the conidiophore. Conidiophore tip bears a series of superimposed rings or annellides. The rings are produced when the annelloconidia are cut off from the apex.

Emericella nidulans (imperfect state: Aspergillus nidulans)

Colonies downy, green because of prolific sporulation. When cleistothecia are produced, colony surface is cream to yellowish. Conidiophores up to 250 μm long, smooth, may be dematiaceous. Conidial heads short and columnar, deep yellow green to bluish green. Phialides in two series. Conidia globose, rough walled, 2.5–4 μm in diameter.

Cleistothecia globose, 300–400 μm in diameter. Generally enveloped by a broken layer of hülle cells that are globose to citriform. Ascospores orange red, lenticular of bivalve construction, 4.5–5.0 × 3.5 × 4.0 μm. Homothallic.

Madurella grisea

Dark, leathery, folded colony covered with a greyish surface down that becomes brownish with age. Dematiaceous mycelium 3–5 μm in diameter. Colonies sterile. Production of conidia is not known. Formation of pycnidia with pycnidiospores reported by several investigators. A possible relationship with *Pyrenochaeta romeroi* suspected, but not confirmed. Dextrose, galactose, maltose, and sucrose used as carbon sources. Lactose not used.

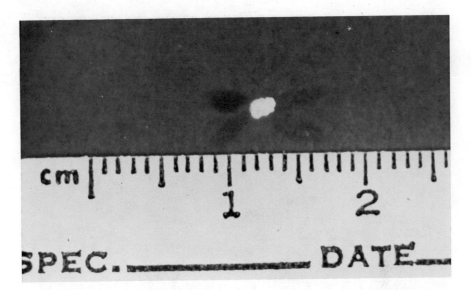

Figure 53.11—Granule of *Nocardia asteroides* removed from a draining sinus tract.

M. mycetomatis

Slow growing; optimum growth temperature, 37 C. Colonies velvety or powdery, smooth or folded surface, cream to ochre. Diffusable brown pigment produced. On Sabouraud's dextrose agar, colonies are generally sterile. Septate mycelium dematiaceous. On cornmeal agar, sporulation can generally be induced. Conidia, spherical, 3 μm in diameter, borne in clusters from tips of short phialides. Other conidia pyriform and with a truncate base, borne at the tops of a simple, branched conidiophore. Dextrose, galactose, lactose, and maltose used as carbon sources. Sucrose not used.

Pyrenochaeta romeroi

Colony woolly, greyish black with dark reverse. Optimal growth temperature 30 C. Septate, dematiaceous mycelium, no free asexual spores. Pycnidia produced singly or in groups on a variety of media, 50–126 × 40–100 μm, black with ostioles. Surface covered with rigid or flexible septate setae. Pycnidiospores hyaline, elliptical, unicellular, 1.5–2 × 0.75–1.0 μm, yellowish, borne in chains from the tips of short, simple conidiophores.

Leptosphaeria senegalensis

Rapid-growing colony, brownish downy colony. Reverse, black; some isolates develop a pink tint. Mycelium dematiaceous, no asexual spores. Dark perithecia produced 100–300 μm in diameter in old cultures. Hyaline, clavate asci in mature perithecia, 80–100 × 17–20 μm. Eight ascospores typically present in each ascus, multiseptate with three to five septa, oval 20–30 × 8–10 μm. Homothallic.

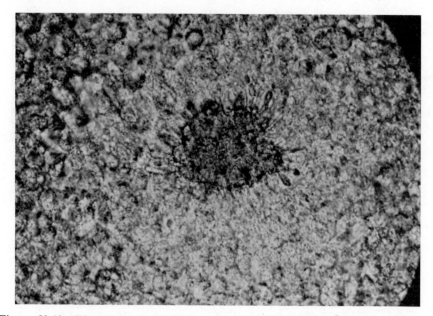

Figure 53.12—Direct microscopic mount of granule of *Nocardia brasiliensis* exhibiting small interwined filaments with clubbing at the periphery.

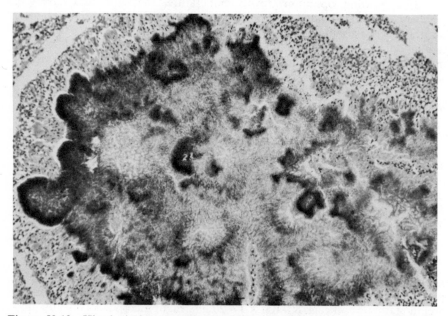

Figure 53.13—Histological section of actinomycotic granule stained with hematoxylin-eosin exhibiting numerous filaments present.

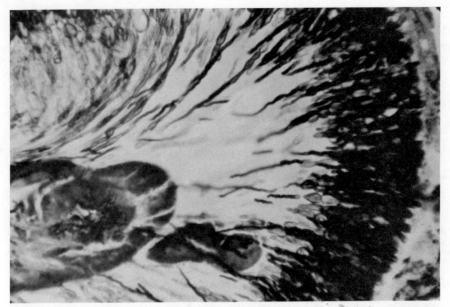

Figure 53.14—Histological section of eumycotic granule stained with methenamine silver exhibiting septate hyphae with swollen cell present. Mycetoma caused by *Petriellidium boydii.*

L. tompkinsii

Similar to *L. senegalensis.* But perithecia larger, 214–535 μm in diameter. Asci a bit larger, 80–115 × 20–25 μm. Ascospores 32–45 × 8–11 μm, fusoid, tapered at ends, six to seven septa. Homothallic.

Petriellidium boydii (synonym: Allescheria boydii)

Imperfect state generally referred to as *Monosporium (Scedosporium) apiospermum.* Fast-growing floccose colony that rapidly covers the slope of an agar slant. Grayish white. Septate mycelium hyaline. Asexual spores numerous, large (6.2–10.4 × 3.5–9 μm), unicellular; ovate with a truncated base borne singly or in small groups at the tips or sides of a simple, variable-length conidiophore. Bundles of spore-bearing conidiophores known as coremia produced on occasion.

Some isolates produce perithecia, especially when grown on cornmeal agar. Perithecia are black, spherical, and 100–200 μm in diameter. Asci are evanescent and seldom observed. Ascospores, elliptical, 4–5 × 7–8 μm, with attenuated ends. Homothallic.

Neotestudina rosatii (synonym: Zopfia rosatii)

Slow growing, with heaped periphery, flat, with radial folds. Glabrous, tan with deep brown reverse. Optimum growth temperature, 30 C. Mycelium, hyaline and septate. Black, spherical to kidney-shaped perithecia produced,

200–350 μm in diameter after 3 or more weeks' growth on cornmeal agar at 30 C. Asci spherical, 11–15 μm in diameter, filled with eight two-celled, brown ascospores that are smooth and slightly curved, 11.0 × 4.5 μm.

References

1. AJELLO G, BROWN J, MAHGOUB ES, and AJELLO L: A note on the isolation of pathogenic aerobic actinomycetes from Sudanese soils. Current Microbiology 2:25–26, 1979
2. AJELLO L: The isolation of *Allescheria boydii Shear*, an etiologic agent of mycetomas, from soil. Am J Trop Med Hyg 1:227–238, 1952
3. BORELLI D: *Madurella mycetomi* y *Madurella grisea*. Arch Venez Med Trop Parasit Med 4:195–211, 1962
4. EL HASSAN AM and MAHGOUB ES: Lymph node involvement in mycetoma. Trans R Soc Trop Med Hyg 66:165–169, 1972
5. GAMS W: Cephalosporium—Artige Schimmelpilze (Hyphomycetes). Gustav Fischer Verlag, Stuttgart, 1971
6. LECHEVALIER HA, LECHEVELIER MP, and GERBER NN: Chemical composition as a criterion in the classification of actinomycetes. Adv Appl Microbiol 14:47–72, 1971
7. OYSTON JK: Madura foot. A study of twenty cases. J Bone Joint Surg 43B:259–267, 1961
8. SEGRETAIN G and MARIAT F: Recherches sur la presence d' agents de mycetomes dans le sol et sur les epineux du Senegal et de la Mauritanie. Bull Soc Path Exot 62:194–202, 1968
9. THIRUMALACHAR MJ and PADHYE AA: Isolation of *Madurella mycetomi* from soil in India. Hindustan Antibiotics Bull 10:314–318, 1968

CHAPTER 54

MYCOSERODIAGNOSIS

Morris A. Gordon

Introduction

Using Mycoserology to Diagnose the Mycoses

In most instances, the diagnosis of a fungal infection is confirmed by demonstrating an appropriate etiologic agent, either by microscopically examining host material or by identifying the organism in cultures. However, in an appreciable proportion of cases of deep-seated mycoses, the incitant may not be found, its identification may be either delayed or in question, or the significance of its presence may not be clear. Under these circumstances, immunologic methods can often be used to obtain presumptive or even definitive evidence of a specific fungal disease.

In this chapter, my objective is to present for the benefit of laboratory workers who are acquainted with general serologic techniques the currently established, practical, and reproducible serologic methods generally accepted to be substantial aids in the laboratory diagnosis—and often prognosis—of deep-seated mycoses. In addition to descriptions of reagents and procedures, the chapter contains comments on clinical or epidemiologic indications for given tests, an assessment of specificity and sensitivity of each of the techniques, and interpretation of results as they relate to the available clinical information. Recommended tests for each of the mycoses are displayed in Table 54.1.

Benefits of serologic tests in cases of suspected mycoses include the following:

Diagnosis

1) A high titer or a significant rise in titer would help to establish the diagnosis when a fungus has not been demonstrated or when it has been demonstrated but not clearly identified. In some instances, the serologic findings may present the first clue to the existence of mycotic infection. 2) Serologic results may establish the significance of isolating a fungus, as with suspected candidiasis or aspergillosis. 3) In borderline cases serologic results, although not diagnostic, will generate further efforts to isolate the organism or to establish a rising titer.

Prognosis

Monitoring the titer may help in following the course of the disease (including effects of chemotherapy) for infections such as coccidioidomycosis and

TABLE 54.1—RECOMMENDED SERODIAGNOSTIC TESTS FOR DEEP MYCOSES

MYCOSIS	CF	ID	CIE	TP	TA	LA	CPA	IHA	IFA
Aspergillosis	u	S	sc						u
Blastomycosis	S	S							
Candidiasis		S	sc		S	u		u	u
Coccidioidomycosis	S	sc		S		sc			
Cryptococcosis					S	S	S		u
Histoplasmosis	S	S	u			S			
Mucormycosis		u							
Paracoccidioidomycosis	S	S	u						
Sporotrichosis	S	S			S	S			

CF = complement fixation
ID = immunodiffusion
CIE = counterimmunoelectrophoresis
TP = tube precipitin
TA = tube agglutination
LA = latex agglutination

CPA = charcoal particle agglutination
IHA = indirect hemagglutination
IFA = indirect fluorescent antibody
S = standard test
u = useful but not (yet) considered standard
sc = "screening" procedure

cryptococcosis. Of course, one must remember that with fungal and other infections the lack of a serologic reaction may result from primary or secondary immunologic unresponsiveness on the part of the subject, which in turn may result from the administration of immunosuppressants or the effects of the infection itself.

Serologic Methods Used in Mycology

No single serologic technique can be used for all of the mycoses. This discussion emphasizes the test or combination of tests most helpful in diagnosing each disease considered. Complement fixation (CF) and immunodiffusion (ID) are the most widely used procedures, and manuals of standard methods for applying these techniques to the systemic mycoses have been published (25, 26).

One of the procedures which we adopted in the ID test is using a pattern of large central wells for serum and large and small peripheral wells for antigen (38). This modification is particularly valuable for eliciting precipitin bands with weak sera which might otherwise give a negative result, since the smaller well in effect provides a 10-fold dilution of antigen.

In a further modification of this method, we test the serum both undiluted and approximately 10-fold concentrated, especially for *Candida* and *Aspergillus* antibody. Serum can readily be concentrated 10-fold by adding 1 ml to a small amount of Sephadex G-25 in an 11 × 75 mm tube (just enough to cover the curve at the bottom of the tube). After the mixture stands for 1 hr at room temperature, the supernatant is pipetted off.

Counterimmunoelectrophoresis (CIE) is useful in diagnosing several of the mycoses (13), but details of method differ with its various applications and will be referred to later. The same is true for latex particle agglutination (LPA). Other procedures which can be used for individual mycoses include tube precipitation (TP), tube agglutination (TA), charcoal particle agglutination (CPA), indirect fluorescent antibody (IFA), and indirect hemagglutination (IHA).

Reagents

One of the most serious handicaps of mycotic serology is a lack of standardized reagents. There is likewise little interlaboratory uniformity in performing procedures. It must therefore be emphasized that laboratories which do these tests should use adequate positive and negative control sera and, initially at least, should establish a program of exchanging homemade antigens with other competent and experienced laboratories for comparison. Such a practice is particularly useful for a technique like ID, because the similarity of two lots of a given antigen may be determined by lines of identity produced when they are plated against a standard antiserum.

Commercially available reagents for the procedures discussed are listed in the Appendix.

Skin Tests

Commercially available, diagnostically useful skin test materials for the mycoses are limited to coccidioidin and spherulin for coccidioidomycosis and histoplasmin for histoplasmosis. Each of these is injected and read according to the Mantoux technique, with 0.1 ml of an appropriate dilution (as specified by the manufacturer) being given intradermally. The coccidioidin and spherulin tests should be read at 24–36 hr, and the histoplasmin test should be read at 48–72 hr.

Spherulin has been reported to detect significantly more reactors than does coccidioidin (44), which would seem to call for differences in interpreting the reactions caused by each. A positive reaction with either is indicative of past or present infection with *Coccidioides immitis*, although cross-reactions with the agents of histoplasmosis and blastomycosis have been reported. A negative reaction does not rule out the disease, because the test is not usually positive until about 3 weeks after initial infection and is frequently negative in the presence of widely disseminated disease (anergy), in specimens from patients with residual pulmonary cavities, and in those from patients with impaired cellular immunity.

Coccidioidin does not induce humoral antibodies in man, nor does it cause the development of skin sensitivity in nonsensitive persons, but it can boost the level of skin sensitivity to coccidioidin in those who are already sensitive. A positive reaction may cause a transitory rise in titer of complement-fixing antibody to histoplasmin but not to coccidioidin. For a healthy person, a positive coccidioidin skin test implies resistance to infection. The test is also useful in defining endemic areas and in identifying and delineating a common-source epidemic.

A positive reaction to histoplasmin (induration of 5 mm or larger) also indicates past or present infection. There may be cross-reactivity with the agents of blastomycosis or coccidioidomycosis. The test is usually positive 1 to 3 weeks following exposure and may be negative in anergic individuals. False-negative reactions have been reported for a small percentage of patients with active pulmonary histoplasmosis (6). A positive skin-test reaction to histoplasmin may raise complement fixation titers to the mycelial antigen but not to the yeast form antigen. It may also elicit an *m* band in the ID test (see below). It is not known whether a positive histoplasmin skin test indicates heightened resistance to histoplasmosis. Epidemiologic considerations noted for coccidioidin also apply to histoplasmin.

Skin test antigens of *Blastomyces dermatitidis* have not proven useful in diagnosing blastomycosis, and blastomycin is no longer available commercially. Those for paracoccidioidomycosis, cryptococcosis, and sporotrichosis have not yet been shown to be clinically useful.

An immediate skin test reaction to aspergillin (concentrated culture filtrate of *Aspergillus fumigatus* or other *Aspergillus* species) is used as one of the diagnostic criteria for allergic bronchopulmonary aspergillosis. This test is also positive for some people with aspergilloma. The usefulness of the intradermal technique for epidemiological studies and for demonstrating a delayed reaction indicative of aspergillosis has not been determined.

Skin-test reactions to antigens of *Candida albicans* are used in determining the immune competence of human adults but are not useful in diagnosing candidiasis, because *C. albicans* is a component of the normal flora and as such appears to invoke an immune response in almost all healthy people.

Collection and Processing of Serologic Specimens

In general, 5 ml of serum must be drawn, processed, and shipped aseptically for serologic tests. Specimens can be preserved in 1:10,000 Merthiolate.

Spinal fluid specimens, drawn and handled aseptically, can be submitted for mycoserodiagnosis if there is suspected central nervous system involvement with either coccidioidomycosis or cryptococcosis. Merthiolate can be added if the specimen is not to be cultured. Generally, preserved specimens shipped by first class or special delivery mail need not be refrigerated en route. Non-preserved specimens may need to be refrigerated if delayed in transit. Specimen tube closures of whatever type should be liquid-tight *before* tape is applied to seal them.

Diagnostic Procedures

Aspergillosis

Pathogenic infestation or infection with *Aspergillus fumigatus* (or, occasionally, with one of four or five other species of this genus) may appear as asthma, allergic bronchopulmonary aspergillosis (ABA), aspergilloma ("fungus ball" in a preformed pulmonary cavity), or invasive aspergillosis—the last always in a compromised host. The most widely used serodiagnostic test for aspergillosis is immunodiffusion (ID), in which is used an extract of ruptured mycelium or a concentrate of acetone-precipitated broth culture filtrate of *Aspergillus fumigatus* as an antigen (aspergillin). If this antigen and similarly prepared antigens of *A. flavus* and *A. niger* are used in ID, infection with almost all known pathogens of this genus can be detected.

The ID test for aspergillosis is highly specific, particularly when reference serum is used to demonstrate lines of identity (7). The question yet to be answered is which type of aspergillosis is indicated. The test is positive in practically 100% of sera from patients with aspergilloma cases and in 50%–70% of the sera of those with ABA, but far less frequently for patients with invasive aspergillosis. The presence of three or four precipitin bands is highly indicative of either aspergilloma or the invasive type, whereas one or two bands may appear with either of these as well as with purely allergic manifestations of aspergillosis.

A word of caution: Some strains of *A. fumigatus* produce C-substance, which may form a precipitate with C-reactive protein in a patient's serum. Of course, such a precipitin band will not make a line of identity with control serum and will disappear after being soaked with 5% sodium citrate for 45 min.

Counterimmunoelectrophoresis (CIE) with aspergillin is a more sensitive test for aspergillosis than is ID, but may be less specific (9, 13, 49). It is useful for screening.

Complement fixation is sensitive but less specific than ID (36, 48). We have found, in particular, that there is cross-reaction with histoplasma antigen in cases of aspergillosis. More or less arbitrarily, a CF titer of 8 or higher is considered "significant."

Another promising quantitative test is the indirect fluorescent antibody (IFA) procedure (16), which is highly sensitive particularly in detecting ABA and aspergilloma. A titer of 32 to 64 or higher is considered significant.

Blastomycosis (North American)

The test most widely used in serodiagnosing blastomycosis is macro or micro complement fixation, but the procedure lacks sensitivity (i.e., is nonreactive for at least half of the known infections with *Blastomyces dermatitidis*). Immunodiffusion appears to be more sensitive (70%), especially with a concentrated, acetone-precipitated filtrate of yeast form *B. dermatitidis* cells (27). The ID procedure also has a potential of 100% specificity when reference reagents are used to detect lines of identity, whereas in complement fixation there is cross-reaction with antigens of *Histoplasma capsulatum* and *Coccidioides immitis*.

The CF antigen may be a suspension of ground (26) or whole yeast form cells of *B. dermatitidis*. In either case, box titration of antigen against patient's serum is helpful. A dilution of 1 : 160 (v/v) of whole cells appears to be optimal, at least for preliminary screening. A titer of 8 or higher is generally considered to be presumptive evidence of infection. Of course, a high or rising titer is more definitive. Since there is a significant amount of cross-reactivity between sera from patients with histoplasmosis and those from patients with blastomycosis, the CF test should be done with both antigens when there is a request for either.

The ID test for blastomycosis can be performed with a concentrated (acetone-precipitated) culture filtrate of either the mycelial form (blastomycin) or the yeast form. A positive reaction (one or two bands forming a line of identity with reference serum) denotes recent or current infection.

Candidiasis

C. albicans is an opportunistic pathogen, with infection usually arising from an endogenous source in a compromised host. *C. albicans* antibody can be detected with a tube agglutination test (with whole yeast cells as antigen) in normal humans from early adolescence onward. Thus, a positive TA result cannot be taken as evidence of active infection, although a very high titer (e.g., 160) or a rising titer may constitute presumptive evidence of infection.

The most commonly used serodiagnostic tests for systemic candidiasis are based on the so-called "somatic" antigen, a crude extract of disrupted yeast form cells of *C. albicans* type A. The ID procedure, which is the most widely used and, according to a recent comparison (31), the most reproducible, has a specificity of about 85%–90% and a sensitivity of about 95%. A positive result with this test should be considered strongly suggestive of systemic candidiasis, especially when it is accompanied by a fourfold or greater rise in tube agglutination titer. Counterimmunoelectrophoresis (CIE) is more sensitive but tends to be less specific in some laboratories (34). A slide latex agglutination test (45) appears to be at least as sensitive as the ID but is less specific. The former has the advantage of being quantitatable, as is the IFA test with specific anti-IgG conjugate and whole yeast cell antigen (29). The number and intensity of ID and CIE bands may also give a clue to the severity of infection.

An indirect hemagglutination (IHA) test has been used in detecting antigen (50) and antibody (32). In the latter report, IHA was found to detect mainly IgM antibodies, whereas IFA detected mainly IgG antibodies.

In recent studies, determining clumping factor was found to be inadequate for diagnosing visceral candidiasis (12), but the germ tube dispersion test was superior to agglutination and precipitin tests for correlating with infection among burn patients (33). It has also been pointed out (20) that the ID test often is positive in the absence of systemic candidiasis for patients with candidal vaginitis, those with subacute bacterial endocarditis, or those who have had open heart surgery.

C. albicans antigens have been found in some instances to cross-react with antisera to *Torulopsis glabrata*.

Coccidioidomycosis

The basis for suspecting that a patient has this disease should include a history of residence or travel in an endemic area and/or a positive skin test to coccidioidin or spherulin.

Quantitative macro or micro complement fixation is the definitive serologic procedure for diagnosing infection with *Coccidioides immitis* except in cases of early (1–3 weeks) primary infection or reactivation of infection, when CF antibodies (to IgG) are not yet detectable, but IgM (i.e., early antibody response) can be measured with a tube precipitin (TP) test. TP declines and becomes negative generally within 2 to 6 months. The CF titer generally varies directly with the severity of infection, and serial studies are important in prognosis.

Complement fixation is also used in detecting antibodies in the cerebrospinal fluid from patients with coccidioidal meningitis, but the titer in such situations is not prognostic, and results are negative for about a quarter of these patients. Pleural and joint fluids can also be used in this test.

The CF antigen is a pool of mycelial culture filtrates—"coccidioidin" (43). Recently spherulin, an extract of the parasitic phase grown *in vitro* (42), has been found to be more sensitive than coccidioidin, but it is has also been reported to be less specific (21). A slide latex agglutination (SLA) test with heated coccidioidin (60 C, 30 min) to sensitize the particles has been developed as a screening test for TP (IgM) antibodies, and an ID test with toluene extract of mycelium (35) has been developed as a screening test for CF (IgG) antibodies. A combination of CF and TP has been reported to be reactive for 85% of patients with active coccidioidomycosis, whereas a combination of ID and LA was reactive for 93% of such patients (22). Positive results with SLA or ID should be confirmed and quantitated, respectively, with results of TP and CF.

Few false positives are obtained with these tests. SLA is more sensitive but slightly less specific than TP. A CF titer of ≥ 2 may be diagnostic, but low titers may also indicate histoplasmosis or blastomycosis. A CF titer of ≥ 16 usually indicates disseminated disease. However, the CF test is negative for about 25% of patients with central nervous system disease, 30% of those with pulmonary cavity disease, and 70% of those with solitary pulmonary nodules.

Cryptococcosis

Cryptococcosis of the central nervous system (CNS) should be suspected for any patient with meningitis of unknown etiology, cerebral abscess, papilledema, or possible brain tumor, especially when symptoms include low-grade fever and chronic headache, disorientation, or personality changes.

For suspected CNS infections, tests should be performed for capsular polysaccharide antigen of *Cryptococcus neoformans* with the cerebrospinal fluid (CSF) and for both antigen and antibody with serum. Antigen is detectable in sera from patients in all but the earliest stages of CNS infection and also in sera from those with other forms of disseminated disease including severe pulmonary involvement. It is found in CSF only when the CNS is involved.

On the other hand, antibody is detectable in sera from patients in the early stages of meningitis, from those with mild or localized pulmonary disease, and from those whose involvement is limited to a solitary cutaneous nodule. Detectable antigen and antibody rarely coexist in the serum, and the antigen titer in serum or spinal fluid is prognostic—varying directly with degree of infection. Antibody titer also falls with remission of disease.

The most sensitive and an extremely specific test for cryptococcal antigen in CSF, serum, urine, and other body fluids is SLA, with particles sensitized with rabbit anticryptococcal globulin (4, 17). A CF test yielding parallel results (3) can also be used.

Serum specimens to be tested should first be inactivated at 56 C for 30 min. CSF and urine should be placed in boiling water for 10 min. The SLA test (which detects as little as 0.025 μg of polysaccharide per ml) and CF are more sensitive than the conventional India ink examination for detecting the presence of *C. neoformans* in CSF, and a well-controlled positive SLA is completely specific for active cryptococcosis. High-titered rheumatoid factor in serum can cause nonspecific agglutination of latex particles, but this factor is readily controlled (15).

The TA test (17) is a sensitive and probably the most specific known method for detecting antibody which denotes active infection with *C. neoformans*. Although the test usually gives negative results with patients' sera containing large amounts of cryptococcal antigen (which is true for most patients with cryptococcal meningitis by the time the identity of the infection is suspected), only rarely is neither antibody nor antigen detected. A charcoal particle test (14) is more sensitive for detecting cryptococcal antibody, but titers of 4 or lower may or may not be associated with active infection. An IFA test (47) produces many more positive results than does the TA, but it is much less specific for active cryptococcosis.

Histoplasmosis

Histoplasmosis in the United States is not limited to the Mississippi Valley; there are other endemic foci, and the infection is commonly associated with exposure to organic dust—particularly from old chicken houses, silos, bat caves, and blackbird roosts.

The uses and significance of CF tests for histoplasmosis are similar to those for coccidioidomycosis, although the system for interpreting titers and titer changes is less well-defined for the former than for the latter. In particular, the CF titer for histoplasmosis may decline slowly as the chronic pulmonary disease resolves. However, since *H. capsulatum* is often difficult to culture from sputum of patients with some forms of pulmonary histoplasmosis, serologic tests are often relied upon heavily in diagnosing this disease. The yeast form CF titer tends to be much lower in cavitary than in noncavitary cases. CF is also of particular value in diagnosing histoplasma endocarditis. A combination of a CF test with yeast form antigen and the ID test for specific (h, m, and y) antibodies can be used to detect essentially all cases of histoplasmosis (1).

Macro and micro CF tests are equally effective (24). The CF test with the yeast form antigen is more sensitive and more specific than that with mycelial antigen, and the latter is not necessary—especially when the ID test with histoplasmin is also used.

The yeast form antigen of *H. capsulatum*, as well as that of *B. dermatitidis*, consists of a saline suspension of washed whole cells, which are heat-killed and preserved in Merthiolate. The histoplasmin used in the ID test, which should contain *m*, *h*, and *c* antigens (19), is a concentrated acetone precipitate of mycelial phase broth culture supernate (30). The y antigen is a phenol extract of yeast form cells (46). The presence in patients' sera of *h* or *y* antibody denotes active histoplasmosis. An *m* band indicates present or past infection and can be recalled with a positive skin test. It appears consistently in association with early, acute infections, together with a *c* band in more severely affected patients (18).

The CF results may be negative for primary acute infection, or there may be cross-reaction with the agent of blastomycosis. A yeast form CF titer of 8 or higher is presumptive evidence of active histoplasmosis (although this diagnosis is not precluded by lower titers). A CF titer of 16 or higher is usually specific for histoplasmosis, and 32 is considered by some workers to be diagnostic for active disease. However, titers in this range are sometimes found in sera from aspergillosis cases.

A latex particle agglutination (LA) test is very sensitive for acute infections—with a titer of 16 or 32 considered very significant. However, negative results are often obtained for patients with chronic histoplasmosis (2). A recent report (11) cites apparent false-positive LA reactions in patients with tuberculosis. We have noted that sera from some patients with aspergillosis may fix complement with antigen of *H. capsulatum.*

A CIE test with the same antigen used in the ID gives more rapid results which correlate well with those of the ID (28).

Mucormycosis

The immunodiffusion test with soluble antigens extracted from sonicated mycelium of *Rhizopus*, *Mucor*, and *Absidia* species is useful in diagnosing rhinocerebral mucormycosis. These three genera cross-react so that, for example, for one infection caused by *R. oryzae*, an early serum specimen from the patient reacted only with *Mucor* antigen, whereas later specimens were also positive to *Rhizopus*. We found no precipitins in specimens from patients whose infections were diagnosed very early, and who were treated successfully with antifungal antibiotics, and whose underlying diabetes was controlled. A recent report (23) tends to confirm the specificity of this test and indicates that the three genera may be differentiated antigenically. Antibody was detected in 8 of 11 sera from suspected or proven cases of mucormycosis.

Paracoccidioidomycosis

Sources of this disease appear to be limited to Central and South America. Although the respiratory tract is probably the primary portal of entry, and chronic pulmonary involvement is not uncommon, a large percentage of these infections are manifested as ulcerative lesions of the skin and mucosae. Lymphadenopathy is often present. Clinical manifestations of this disease are discussed by Restrepo et al. (41).

A combination of CF and ID, both with yeast form filtrate antigens, detects more than 95% of cases of paracoccidioidomycosis (39). The two tests are equally sensitive, although CF is less specific—cross-reacting with some histoplasmosis infections, usually at a titer of 8 or less. Some sera from patients with paracoccidioidomycosis have been found to produce an *m* band with histoplasmin (40).

Yarzabal (51) used CIE in serodiagnosing this disease and discovered a specific cathodic antigenic fraction (i.e., it migrates in a direction opposite to that of most antigens), labeled "E," which is apparently found in specimens from nearly all patients with paracoccidioidomycosis (8).

CF titers are in direct proportion to the severity of the disease, and titers of 8 or higher are considered presumptive evidence of active infection.

Sporotrichosis

Diagnostic serology of sporotrichosis is more helpful for pulmonary or disseminated forms of the disease than for the more common cutaneous lymphatic form (which can readily be diagnosed by culture and whose antibody is not regularly detectable). The techniques commonly used for detecting antibody to *Sporothrix schenckii* are CF and ID, although a recent report (5) indicates that a slide latex agglutination (SLA) and a tube agglutination (TA) test have higher sensitivity. Both newer tests detected about 94% of proven cases of sporotrichosis, and an SLA titer of 4 or higher was considered presumptive evidence of this disease. The TA test showed some cross-reactivity with sera from patients with leishmaniasis.

Appendix: Commercial Sources of Reagents

Berkeley Biologicals, Berkeley, CA 94710: spherulin (skin test, CF).
Cutter Laboratories, Berkeley, CA 94710: coccidioidin (skin test).
Greer Laboratories, Lenoir, NC 28645: aspergillin (skin test, ID, CIE); aspergillus ID kit.
Hollister-Stier Laboratories, Yeadon, PA 19050: aspergillin (skin test, ID, CIE); aspergillus ID kit; candida ID antigen (supplied in 1:10 dilution; used at final dilution of 1:40).
Hyland Laboratories, Costa Mesa, CA 92626: coccidioides SLA and ID kits; histoplasma SLA kit.
Inolex Corporation, Glenwood, IL 60425: histoplasmin tube LA antigen and control serum.
Meridian Diagnostics, Inc., Cincinnati, OH 45244: ID, CIE, and CF antigens and control sera for histoplasmosis, blastomycosis, coccidioidomycosis, and aspergillosis; ID and CIE for Candida; cryptococcosis SLA kit.
Microbiological Associates, Bethesda, MD 20014: CF kit and individual reagents for histoplasmosis (both antigens), blastomycosis, coccidioidomycosis, and aspergillosis; ID kit and individual reagents for histoplasmosis, blastomycosis, coccidioidomycosis, and aspergillosis; cryptococcosis SLA kit.
Microbiological Consulting Service, Long Beach, CA 90815: coccidioides CF antigen.
Parke-Davis, Detroit, MI 48208: histoplasmin (skin test).
Wampole Corporation, Cranbury, NJ 08512: cryptococcosis SLA kit.

References

1. BAUMAN DS and SMITH CD: Comparison of immunodiffusion and complement fixation tests in the diagnosis of histoplasmosis. J Clin Microbiol 2:77–80, 1975
2. BENNETT DE: The histoplasmin latex agglutination test. Clinical evaluation and a review of the literature. Am J Med Sci 251:175–183, 1966
3. BENNETT JE, HASENCLEVER HF, and TYNES BS: Detection of cryptococcal polysaccharide in serum and spinal fluid: value in diagnosis and prognosis. Trans Assoc Am Physicians 77:145–150, 1964
4. BLOOMFIELD N, GORDON MA, and ELMENDORF DF JR: Detection of *Cryptococcus neoformans* antigen in body fluids by latex particle agglutination. Proc Soc Exp Biol Med 114:64–67, 1963

5. BLUMER SO, KAUFMAN L, KAPLAN W, McLAUGHLIN DW, and KRAFT DE: Comparative evalution of five serological methods for the diagnosis of sporotrichosis. Appl Microbiol 26:4–8, 1973

6. BUECHNER HA, SEABURY JH, CAMPBELL CC, GEORG LK, KAUFMAN L, and KAPLAN W: The current status of serologic, immunologic, and skin tests in the diagnosis of pulmonary mycoses. Chest 63:259–270, 1973

7. COLEMAN RM and KAUFMAN L: Use of the immunodiffusion test in the serodiagnosis of aspergillosis. Appl Microbiol 23:301–309, 1972

8. CONTI-DÍAZ IA, SOMMA-MOREIRA RE, GEZUELE E, DE GIMÉNEZ AC, PENA MI, and MACKINNON JE: Immunoelectroosmophoresis-immunodiffusion in paracoccidioidomycosis. Sabouraudia 11:39–41, 1973

9. DEE TH: Detection of *Aspergillus fumigatus* serum precipitins by counterimmunoelectrophoresis. J Clin Microbiol 2:482–485, 1975

10. DEE TH and RYTEL MW: Detection of candida serum precipitins by counterimmunoelectrophoresis: an adjunct in determining significant candidiasis. J Clin Microbiol 5:453–457, 1977

11. DISALVO AF and CORBETT DS: Apparent false positive histoplasmin latex agglutination tests in patients with tuberculosis. J Clin Microbiol 3:306–308, 1976

12. EVERETT ED, LAFORCE FM, and EICKHOFF TC: Serologic studies in suspected visceral candidiasis. Arch Intern Med 135:1075–1078, 1975

13. GORDON MA, ALMY RE, GREENE CH, and FENTON JW II: Diagnostic mycoserology by immunoelectroosmophoresis: a general, rapid, and sensitive microtechnic. Am J Clin Pathol 56:471–474, 1971

14. GORDON MA and LAPA E: Charcoal particle agglutination test for detection of antibody to *Cryptococcus neoformans*. Am J Clin Pathol 56:354–359, 1971

15. GORDON MA and LAPA E: Elimination of rheumatoid factor in the latex test for cryptococcosis. Am J Clin Pathol 61:488–494, 1974

16. GORDON MA, LAPA EW, and KANE J: Modified indirect fluorescent-antibody test for aspergillosis. J Clin Microbiol 6:161–165, 1977

17. GORDON MA and VEDDER DK: Serologic tests in diagnosis and prognosis of cryptococcosis. J Am Med Assoc 197:961–967, 1966

18. GORDON MA and ZIMENT I: Epidemic of acute histoplasmosis in western New York State. NY State J Med 67:235–243, 1967

19. HEINER DC: Diagnosis of histoplasmosis using precipitin reactions in agar gel. Pediatrics 22:616–627, 1958

20. HOLDER IA, KOZINN PJ, and LAW EJ: Evaluation of candida precipitin and agglutination tests for the diagnosis of systemic candidiasis in burn patients. J Clin Microbiol 6:219–223, 1977

21. HUPPERT M, KRASNOW I, VUKOVICH KR, SUN SH, RICE EH, and KUTNER LJ: Comparison of coccidioidin and spherulin in complement fixation tests for coccidioidomycosis. J Clin Microbiol 6:33–41, 1977

22. HUPPERT M, PETERSON ET, SUN SH, CHITJIAN PA, and DERREVERE WJ: Evaluation of a latex particle agglutination test for coccidioidomycosis. Am J Clin Pathol 49:96–102, 1968

23. JONES KW and KAUFMAN L: Development and evaluation of an immunodiffusion test for diagnosis of systemic zygomycosis (mucormycosis): preliminary report. J Clin Microbiol 7:97–103, 1978

24. KAUFMAN L, HALL EC, CLARK MJ, and McLAUGHLIN D: Comparison of macrocomplement and microcomplement fixation techniques used in fungus serology. Appl Microbiol 20:579–582, 1970

25. KAUFMAN L, HUPPERT M, FAVA NETTO C, POLLAK L, and RESTREPO A: Manual of Standardized Serodiagnostic Procedures for Systemic Mycoses. Part I: Agar Immunodiffusion Tests. Pan American Health Organization, Washington, DC, 1972

26. KAUFMAN L, HUPPERT M, FAVA NETTO C, POLLAK L, and RESTREPO A: Manual of Standardized Serodiagnostic Procedures for Systemic Mycoses. Part II: Complement Fixation Tests. Pan American Health Organization, Washington, DC, 1974

27. KAUFMAN L, McLAUGHLIN DW, CLARK MJ, and BLUMER S: Specific immunodiffusion test for blastomycosis. Appl Microbiol 26:244–247, 1973

28. KLEGER B and KAUFMAN L: Detection and identification of diagnostic *Histoplasma capsulatum* precipitates by counterelectrophoresis. Appl Microbiol 26:231–238, 1973

29. LEHNER T, BUCKLEY HR, and MURRAY IG: The relationship between fluorescent, agglutinating, and precipitating antibodies to *Candida albicans* and their immunoglobulin classes. J Clin Pathol 25:344–348, 1972

30. MCMILLEN S and DEVROE S: Specific precipitin bands in the serology of histoplasmosis. Am Rev Respir Dis 87:438–440, 1963

31. MERZ WG, EVANS GL, SHADOMY S, ANDERSON S, KAUFMAN L, KOZINN PJ, MACKENZIE DW, PROTZMAN WP, and REMINGTON JS: Laboratory evaluation of serological tests for systemic candidiasis: a cooperative study. J Clin Microbiol 5:596–603, 1977

32. MÜLLER HL and HOLTMANNSPÖTTER H: Vergleichende Titerbestimmungen mit dem *Candida*-hämagglutinationstest und dem *Candida*-immunfluoreszenztest. Mykosen 18:91–96, 1975

33. OBLACK D, SCHWARZ J, and HOLDER IA: Comparative evaluation of the *Candida* agglutination test, precipitin test, and germ tube dispersion test in the diagnosis of candidiasis. J Clin Microbiol 3:175–179, 1976

34. ODDS FC, EVANS EGV, and HOLLAND KT: Detection of *Candida* precipitins, a comparison of double diffusion and counterimmunoelectrophoresis. J Immunol Meth 7:211–218, 1975

35. PAPPAGIANIS D, SMITH CE, KOBAYASHI GS, and SAITO MT: Studies of antigens from young mycelia of *Coccidioides immitis*. J Infect Dis 108:35–44, 1961

36. PARKER JD, SAROSI GA, DOTO IL, and TOSH FE: Pulmonary aspergillosis in the south central United States. Am Rev Respir Dis 101:551–557, 1970

37. PICARDI JL, KAUFFMAN CA, SCHWARZ J, and PHAIR JP: Detection of precipitating antibodies to *Histoplasma capsulatum* by counterimmunoelectrophoresis. Am Rev Respir Dis 114:171–176, 1976

38. PROCTOR AG: Serologic methods in mycology. *In* Progress in Microbiological Techniques. Collins CH (ed.). Plenum Press, New York, 1967, pp 213–226

39. RESTREPO A and MONCADA LH: Serologic procedures in the diagnosis of paracoccidioidomycosis. Proceedings of the International Symposium on Mycoses. Sci Publ Pan Am Health Organ 205:101–110, 1970

40. RESTREPO A and MONCADA LH: Characterization of the precipitin bands detected in the immunodiffusion test for paracoccidioidomycosis. Appl Microbiol 28:138–144, 1974

41. RESTREPO A, ROBLEDO M, GIRALDO R, HERNANDEZ H, SIERRA F, GUTIERREZ F, LONDOÑO F, LÓPEZ R, and CALLE G: The gamut of paracoccidioidomycosis. Am J Med 61:33–42, 1976

42. SCALARONE GM, LEVINE HB, PAPPAGIANIS D, and CHAPARAS SD: Spherulin as a complement-fixing antigen in human coccidioidomycosis. Am Rev Respir Dis 110:324–328, 1974

43. SMITH CE, SAITO MT, BEARD RR, KEPP RM, CLARK RW, and EDDIE BU: Serological tests in the diagnosis and prognosis of coccidioidomycosis. Am J Hyg 52:1–21, 1950

44. STEVENS DA, LEVINE HB, DERESINSKI SC, and BLAINE LJ: Spherulin in clinical coccidioidomycosis. Comparison with coccidioidin. Chest 68:695–702, 1975

45. STICKLE D, KAUFMAN L, BLUMER SO, and MCLAUGHLIN DW: Comparison of a newly developed latex agglutination test and an immunodiffusion test in the diagnosis of systemic candidiasis. Appl Microbiol 23:490–499, 1972

46. TOMPKINS VN: Soluble antigenic constituents of yeast phase *Histoplasma capsulatum*. Am Rev Respir Dis 92:126–133, 1965

47. VOGEL RA, SELLERS TF, and WOODWARD P: Fluorescent antibody techniques applied to the study of human cryptococcosis. J Am Med Assoc 178:921–923, 1961

48. WALTER JE and JONES RD: Serologic tests in diagnosis of aspergillosis. Dis Chest 53:729–735, 1968

49. WARNOCK DW: Detection of *Aspergillus fumigatus* precipitins: a comparison of counterimmunoelectrophoresis and double diffusion. J Clin Pathol 30:388–389, 1977

50. WEINER MH and YOUNT WJ: Mannan antigenemia in invasive candida infections in man. J Clin Invest 58:1045–1053, 1976

51. YARZABAL LA: Anticuerpos precipitantes especificos de la Blastomicosis sudamericana revelados por immunoelectroforesis. Rev Inst Med Trop São Paulo 13:320–327, 1971

General References

GORDON MA: Practical serology of the systemic mycoses. Int J Dermatol 9:209–214, 1970

GORDON MA: Current status of serology for diagnosis and prognostic evaluation of opportunistic fungus infections. *In* Proceedings of the 3rd International Conference on Mycoses. Pan American Health Organization, Scientific Publication 304, Washington, DC, 1975, pp 144–153

GORDON MA: Immunological responses to fungal infection. *In* Chemical Rubber Company Handbook Series in Clinical Laboratory Science: Immunology. Baumgarten A and Richards FF (eds.), 1979, pp 159–164

KAUFMAN L: Current status of immunology for diagnosis and prognostic evaluation of blastomycosis, coccidioidomycosis, and paracoccidioidomycosis. *In* Proceedings of the 3rd International Conference on Mycoses. Pan American Health Organization, Scientific Publication 304, Washington, DC, 1975, pp 137–143

KAUFMAN L: Serodiagnosis of fungal diseases. *In* Manual of Clinical Immunology. Rose NR and Friedman H (eds.). American Society for Microbiology, Washington, DC, 1976, pp 363–381

CHAPTER 55

SUSCEPTIBILITY TESTS AND BLOOD LEVEL DETERMINATIONS OF ANTIMYCOTIC AGENTS

Arvind A. Padhye

Introduction

The methods of susceptibility testing with antifungal agents are aimed at defining the minimal amounts of a drug that will either inhibit the growth of a fungal pathogen or kill it *in vitro*. The experimental design used in evaluating the antifungal agents is similar to that used for antibacterial agents, even though there are certain differences that make testing with antimycotics somewhat different. The basic properties of an antifungal agent to be tested and the growth characteristics of the fungal pathogen involved should be taken into account in the design of the experimental method.

The antifungal drugs that are most widely used in the United States for treating systemic mycotic diseases are amphotericin B and 5-fluorocytosine. Nystatin is widely used for topical or oral therapy for mucocutaneous infections caused by yeasts. Griseofulvin, administered orally, is the drug of choice for treating the dermatophytoses or ringworm infections.

Amphotericin B is a heptaene antibiotic which belongs to the polyene group and is characterized by an aliphatic acid containing multiple conjugated double bonds. It is primarily used against such systemic mycotic diseases as blastomycosis, candidiasis, coccidioidomycosis, cryptococcosis, histoplasmosis, and a variety of opportunistic fungal diseases (40). It is most commonly administered by intravenous infusion, and, in certain instances, by the intrathecal route or by bladder infusion.

Nystatin, a tetraene polyene, is limited in its use to topical application or oral administration because of its toxicity. When the drug is administered orally, as in the treatment for intestinal candidiasis, it does not produce significant serum levels because it is poorly absorbed from the gastrointestinal tract.

5-Fluorocytosine (5-FC) is a fluoropyrimidine and is a stable, water soluble, antifungal compound administered orally for treating systemic infections incited by pathogenic yeasts (2, 30).

Griseofulvin, produced by several species of *Penicillium*—especially *P. griseofulvum*—is a white, bitter, thermostable compound of neutral pH. When administered orally, the antibiotic is quickly absorbed from the gastrointestinal tract and is deposited in the keratinous layers of the skin, hair, and nails.

Imidazole derivatives such as clotrimazole (a chlorinated imidazole) and

1057

miconazole (a phenyl-imidazole derivative) have a wide spectrum of activity against pathogenic fungi. Both drugs are available in the United States as investigational drugs. In Europe both are available commercially as oral and topical preparations. Miconazole is also available in an intravenous formulation.

Clotrimazole is insoluble in water but soluble in organic solvents such as ethyl alcohol. Oral administration is generally associated with severe gastrointestinal distress (nausea, vomiting). When the drug is given orally, it is absorbed into the blood stream erratically and usually is found in low concentrations in serum. These serious drawbacks have limited its use primarily to that of a topical agent. Clotrimazole powder can be dissolved in 95% ethanol, sterilized by filtration, and stored at −30 C without an appreciable loss of potency. Further dilutions in sterile distilled water cause clotrimazole to precipitate and produce turbidity, which may hinder reading the results of its *in vitro* activity.

Miconazole, unlike clotrimazole, is available for investigational purposes as a colloidal dispersion for intravenous injection. Clinical studies have shown that it is effective against dermatophytes (23) and to a limited extent against some of the pathogens that cause systemic infections (13). Recently, treatment of patients with aspergillosis, cryptococcosis, or sporotrichosis with miconazole intravenously was shown to be ineffective (12). *In vitro* sensitivity testing with miconazole nitrate is done by dissolving the powder in ethanol, with further dilutions being made with sterile distilled water.

The discussion that follows with respect to susceptibility testing procedures is devoted in great detail to three antifungal antibiotics (viz. amphotericin B, nystatin, and 5-fluorocytosine). Diffusion disks commonly used with the antibacterial agents are not available commercially in this country for *in vitro* testing with these antimycotics, although Boyer (8) showed that the procedure is reliable and quick and easy to perform. He showed that tests with diffusion disks, in the case of 5-FC, are as reliable as any of the other methods currently in use.

The broth dilution method for yeasts and yeast-like fungi and semisolid test media for the filamentous pathogens is widely used for the *in vitro* determination of minimum inhibitory concentrations (MICs) and minimum fungicidal concentrations (MFCs) (31). The important factors that must be carefully considered in susceptibility testing are: 1) solubilization of the antifungal agent, 2) the type of medium used, 3) the initial inoculum, and 4) the temperature and duration of incubation.

Antibiotic Solubilization

The two polyenes —amphotericin B and nystatin—are light sensitive and subject to thermal decay upon incubation. Both are insoluble in water and unstable in the presence of acid. Accordingly, certain rules must be followed in preparing test solutions of these antibiotics.

Amphotericin B and nystatin are solubilized in dimethylsulfoxide (DMSO) or dimethylformamide. The solutions must be protected from light to avoid decay and should be allowed to stand and self-sterilize for at least 30 min before use. The 5000 μg/ml stock solution of these two antibiotics may be stored in the dark at 4 C for up to a week without appreciable loss of potency. It should also be remembered that with each batch of these antibiotics, the potency varies slightly, and 1 mg of these antibiotics does not always correspond to 1000 μg. Accordingly, appropriate amounts should be weighed to obtain a 5000 μg/ml stock solution.

In contrast, 10,000 μg/ml stock solutions of 5-FC powder are prepared in distilled water (1 mg = 1000 μg/ml), and sterilized by filtration. The solutions can be stored at −30 C indefinitely if not contaminated with bacteria. The stock solution is not sensitive to light as are the two polyenes.

Media

The selection of the medium depends upon the drug to be tested. The MIC of a given antifungal agent against a yeast pathogen can best be determined by use of the broth dilution method. The method can also be adapted for testing with filamentous fungal pathogens. *In vitro* tests with amphotericin B and nystatin are performed in antibiotic medium 20 (M-20, Difco) or antibiotic medium 3 (M-3, Difco) (36). The acidic pH that develops as a result of fermentation or assimilation of glucose when testing yeasts adversely affects the polyenes. For this reason, broth media such as Sabouraud dextrose broth (which has an acidic pH) cannot be used in tests involving the polyenes.

Initially, *in vitro* studies with 5-FC were hampered by the fact that the free cytosine present in nonsynthetic culture media competed with the drug and totally inhibited its antifungal activity. Yeast nitrogen base (YNB, Difco) supplemented with glucose and asparagine is the medium of choice for susceptibility tests with 5-FC. This medium is most conveniently prepared as a 10× concentrate, sterilized by filtration, and stored at 4 C. A 1× strength solution of the 10× stock medium is prepared by making a 1:10 dilution in sterile distilled water.

Preparation of Inocula

Inocula for yeast cultures are prepared from 24- to 48-hr-old growth on Sabouraud dextrose agar. Suspensions are prepared in sterile saline and adjusted to a transmission of 95% measured at 530 nm (Bausch and Lomb 20 Colorimeter). This results in a concentration of approximately 10^5 cells/ml.

An alternative method is to prepare inocula by the "Wickerham card" technique, in which the yeast suspension to be adjusted is diluted in a tube of sterile saline that is then held in front of a white card bearing several sharply ruled lines. The desired end point is achieved when there is obvious turbidity but the lines on the card are sharply defined when viewed through the suspension. A similar suspension is also prepared with the control organism.

For testing yeasts, a specific control culture of *Saccharomyces cerevisiae*, ATCC 9763 or ATCC 2601, is used in many laboratories.

Temperature and Duration of Incubation

Since polyenes are unstable at high temperatures and also decay when held for long periods, the yeast susceptibility tests are read after 48 hr of incubation at 30 C. For filamentous fungi, the results are read usually after 96 hr of incubation at 30 C or when growth in the control tubes is visible.

Drug Dilutions and Performance of the Test

The procedure described below is that of Shadomy and Espinel-Ingroff (31). It uses sufficient drug material for one test fungus (in duplicate) and the control test fungus.

Using 1 × YNB for 5-FC or M-3 for amphotericin B, 10 ml of the 100 μg/ml solution are prepared. A 1:50 dilution from the 5000 μg/ml stock solution of amphotericin B in M-3 broth medium or a 1:100 dilution of 10,000 μg/ml solution of 5-FC yields 10 ml of the 100 μg/ml dilution.

Place 12 sterile disposable tubes (16 ×125 mm) in a rack, and add 5.0 ml of the appropriate broth medium to tubes 2 through 12. The first tube contains 10 ml of the 100 μg/ml concentration of the drug. Five milliliters of broth from tube 1 are aseptically withdrawn and mixed with 5 ml of broth in tube 2. The procedure is repeated through tube 12. For each transfer, fresh pipettes must be used to avoid carryover of the test drug. From tube 12, 5 ml are withdrawn and discarded. This procedure gives twofold serial dilutions in concentrations ranging from 100 μg/ml to 0.05 μg/ml. One ml is transferred from each dilution tube to each of four 12- × 75-mm sterile, disposable tubes. The remaining 1 ml volumes in the large tubes are retained as contamination controls for each of the serial dilutions. One milliliter of drug-free broth is added to each of four additional sterile 12- × 75-mm tubes to be used as growth controls.

Two tubes of each concentration of drug are inoculated with 0.05 ml of a standardized suspension of the test fungus. The remaining two tubes of each concentration are inoculated with 0.05 ml of the standardized suspension of *S. cerevisiae*. In addition, two tubes of drug-free medium are inoculated to serve as growth controls for the test fungus. The remaining two tubes are inoculated with *S. cerevisiae*.

Tubes are incubated at 30 C for 48 hr or until growth is visible in the growth control tubes. Tests with 5-FC should not be read in less than 48 hr. As shown by Block et al. (7) and Shadomy et al. (32), the MIC is profoundly influenced (especially in the case of 5-FC) by incubation temperature, inoculum size, and the duration of incubation. The duration of incubation is therefore critical in susceptibility testing with 5-FC.

Tests with nystatin and amphotericin B are performed in a similar manner with the M-3 broth medium.

After 48 hr of incubation at 30 C, the tubes are examined for growth of the fungi in the drug-free broth medium. The MIC is the lowest concentration of drug that inhibits visible growth. The MFC is determined by subculturing approximately 0.01 ml from each negative dilution tube and from the growth control tubes onto plates of Sabouraud dextrose agar with further incubation of the plates at 30 C for an additional 48 hr. The MFC is the lowest concentration of drug from which subcultures show no growth or which yield fewer than three colonies per plate.

Amphotericin B inhibits growth and exerts a cidal effect for most of the common yeasts at a concentration of 0.39 μg/ml or less. An MIC of 1.56 μg/ml for amphotericin B suggests probable clinical resistance, as a concentration of 1.56 μg/ml of amphotericin B in a patient's serum or cerebrospinal fluid cannot be routinely obtained.

Nystatin is inhibitory and fungicidal for most isolates of *Candida* spp. at concentrations of 3.13 μg/ml or less. Prolonged incubation or incubation at high temperature (such as 37 C) affects the MIC values in the case of the polyenes and gives erroneous results (29). As amphotericin B ages, its fungistatic and cidal activity falls.

Most isolates of susceptible yeasts are inhibited by 5-FC at concentrations below 12.5 μg/ml and reveal a fungicidal effect at 25.0 μg/ml. Many isolates of *C. neoformans* and *C. albicans* show intermediate susceptibilities (MICs between 25–50 μg/ml). The isolates of these two species develop resistance to 5-FC *in vitro* and *in vivo*. The rapidity with which this profound drug resistance develops both *in vitro* (6, 7, 32) and *in vivo* (37) and the failure to isolate cryptococci with intermediate degrees of 5-FC susceptibility suggest that the drug resistance occurs via a single mutational step similar to that seen with streptomycin (9) and isoniazid (34). This pattern is in contrast to that described for amphotericin B (1).

In the case of amphotericin B, resistance among *C. neoformans* and other pathogenic yeasts against amphotericin B is both rare and modest. It probably involves multiple mutational steps as is seen with penicillin resistance among the staphylococci (9). The mechanisms of 5-FC resistance in the case of yeasts can be summarized as follows. 5-FC enters yeast cells via a permease enzyme, is deaminated to form 5-fluorouracil intracellularly, and then enters the pathway for the synthesis of ribonucleic acid. This pattern can be antagonized by the natural pyrimidine analogue at both the uptake and deamination steps (38).

Susceptibility Tests Against Filamentous Fungi

The semisolid agar dilution method is applicable primarily for testing the susceptibility of filamentous fungi to amphotericin B. It is of value in testing isolates of the pathogenic *Aspergillus* spp. and *Cladosporium bantianum (trichoides)* for susceptibility to 5-FC.

Nystatin is active primarily against yeasts and inhibits the growth of filamentous fungi only at higher concentrations; thus it is less likely to be the drug of choice for treating mycotic infections caused by filamentous fungi. Since nystatin is not absorbed from the gastrointestinal tract when given orally, it is of very little value for treating systemic mycoses caused by filamentous fungal pathogens. The following discussion of drug susceptibility tests for filamentous or dimorphic pathogens is therefore restricted to only two antifungal agents—amphotericin B and 5-FC.

Media

The two media required for amphotericin B tests are an enriched brain-heart infusion broth (BHIB, Difco) and modified Sabouraud-brain heart infusion (SABHI). Tests with 5-FC are done with yeast nitrogen broth supplemented with glucose, asparagine, and sterile 0.5% agar.

Drug Dilutions

The stock solutions of amphotericin B and 5-FC are prepared as described earlier for the broth dilutions.

Preparation of Inocula

The sporulating culture of the test fungus (usually 10–12 days old) is harvested in sterile saline containing 0.05% Tween 80. The colony is gently scraped with a sterile needle to suspend the spores and pieces of hyphae in the saline. The suspension is adjusted to a transmission of 85% to 90% as measured at 530 nm on a Bausch and Lomb Spectronic Colorimeter. Approximately 3–4 ml of the adjusted inoculum suspension is required for each test.

Susceptibility Testing with Amphotericin B

One milliliter of the 10,000 μg/ml amphotericin B stock solution is diluted with 1 ml of dimethylsulfoxide to yield a 2-ml solution of 5000 μg/ml. One milliliter is pipetted from this solution to 24 ml of modified BHIB to give a concentration of 200 μg/ml.

Twelve (16 × 125 mm) disposable tubes are placed in a rack, and 5 ml of modified BHIB are added to each of tubes 2 through 12. Five milliliters of the 200 μg/ml solution of amphotericin B are added to the BHIB broth in tubes 1 and 2. The contents of tube 2 are thoroughly mixed, and the drug is serially diluted by pipetting 5-ml amounts from tubes 2 through 12. A fresh pipette is used for each transfer. Five milliliters of solution are discarded from tube 12. This gives serial dilutions that range from 200 μg/ml (tube 1) to 0.10 μg/ml (tube 12).

In sequence, starting from tube 1, add 5 ml of melted modified SABHI agar to each of the drug dilutions, mix, and immediately dispense 2-ml amounts to small test tubes. Do not hold any drug dilution at 50 C longer than required, for the drug quickly decays at high temperature. The small medium tubes are allowed to solidify in a vertical position. The control tubes are prepared similarly without any drug.

After the medium has hardened, the tubes are inoculated with 0.05 ml of the adjusted spore inoculum. Two tubes for each concentration are inoculated with the test fungus and are incubated at 30 C for 48 hr or until the control tubes show positive growth. Reading the end points is critical because of variations in growth. Isolates of *B. dermatitidis* and *H. capsulatum* are inhibited between 0.05 and 0.2 μg/ml. The MIC is the lowest concentration that completely inhibits growth. The MFC is determined in a procedure similar to the one described for the broth dilution.

Susceptibility Testing of Filamentous Fungal Pathogens with 5-FC

A solution of 1000 μg/ml of 5-FC is prepared in 10× YNB. To the 12 disposable tubes arranged in a rack, 0.5 ml of 10× YNB is added to tubes 1 and 2. The contents of tube 2 are mixed, and 0.5 ml is withdrawn and added to the broth in tube 3. The procedure is repeated through tube 12. Finally, 0.5 ml is discarded from tube 12.

To each dilution tube (1 through 12), 4.5 ml of melted 0.5% agar are added. The contents in 1.5-ml volumes are dispensed into small tubes. This process dilutes the drug 1 : 10 to yield a final concentration range from 100 μg/ml to 0.05 μg/ml.

The small agar tubes, when hardened, are inoculated with the adjusted spore suspension of the fungal pathogen to be tested, and the test is read when growth is evident in the control tubes.

Isolates of *Aspergillus fumigatus* show a wide range of inhibitory end points, but most isolates are inhibited at 50 μg/ml or less. *C. bantianum* isolates show MICs between 2.0 to 10 μg/ml and MFCs between 100 to 150 μg/ml. Some of the etiologic agents of chromoblastomycosis (viz. *Fonsecaea pedrosoi*) are inhibited from 2 μg/ml to 130 μg/ml (5, 27, 28, 39).

A new method for testing the susceptibility of filamentous fungi with antifungal agents was recently described (39). It is a modification of Erricsson's and Sherris's agar dilution technique that provides for the determination of both the MIC and MFC of antifungal agents for the various filamentous fungi. The method involves use of membrane millipore filters on which a suspension of the test fungus is inoculated. Eight test cultures can be tested simultaneously to determine MICs and MFCs, and the procedure can be performed relatively quickly.

The susceptibility methods used by Kitahara et al. (18, 19) with 5-FC and other antifungal agents against *Aspergillus* spp. involved Salvin's medium. They compared Salvin's medium with other synthetic and semisynthetic media such as Czapek-Dox and yeast nitrogen base (YNB) and found that the MIC for amphotericin B in the case of the *Aspergillus* spp. was much lower in Salvin's medium or Czapek-Dox medium than in YNB.

The MICs for 5-FC were also markedly different with the various media. When the incubation temperature was 25 C, the MICs for all the drugs (amphotericin B, 5-FC, and rifampin) were lower than those obtained at 37 C. The initial inocula also influenced the MICs. Much lower MICs were seen with an initial inoculum of 10^3 organisms/ml than with 10^5 organisms/ml.

Susceptibility Tests with the Combination of Amphotericin B and 5-FC

Recent studies on the synergistic action of amphotericin B *in vitro* with either tetracycline, rifampin, 5-FC, or polymyxin have created the hope of treating systemic mycotic infections without the serious side effects associated with amphotericin B alone. Amphotericin B is a polyene macrolide that binds to sterols in eukaryotic cell membranes. The relative specificity of amphotericin B for fungi apparently results from its greater avidity for ergosterol, the principal sterol in fungal cell membranes, than for cholesterol, the principal sterol in animal cell membranes.

Antibiotics that interfere with RNA or protein synthesis in fungal cell extracts often do not affect fungi, probably because the intact cells do not take them up. Medoff and coworkers (20, 21, 22, 24, 25, 26) used small doses of amphotericin B to facilitate the entry of some of those agents into fungi. They showed that in combination with concentrations of amphotericin B well below its minimum inhibitory concentration for each test organism, the antifungal effects of 5-FC, tetracyclines, and rifampin are increased against *B. dermatitidis, C. albicans, C. neoformans,* and *H. capsulatum.*

The increased activity of the drug combinations is secondary to a potentiation of the effects of the second effects by amphotericin B. For example, when rifampin is used in combination with low concentrations of amphotericin B, RNA synthesis is inhibited. On the other hand, when tetracycline is used with amphotericin B, protein synthesis is inhibited. Medoff et al. called the effect of the drug combinations synergistic when it amounts to more than the additive effects of the two agents alone (25).

Although it is difficult to prove synergism *in vivo*, Block and Bennett (4) showed that amphotericin B in combination with 5-FC has at least an additive, and perhaps a synergistic, effect against *C. neoformans* infections in mice. Titsworth and Gruneberg (35) obtained similar results in mice infected with *C. albicans.* Huppert et al. (15) reported that the combination of amphotericin B and tetracycline was somewhat synergistic against *Coccidioides immitis* infections in mice, even though the results were not spectacular.

These new developments make it necessary to develop a method of *in vitro* susceptibility testing for the new drug combinations; such a procedure for the combination of amphotericin B and 5-FC (33) is described below.

Medium

Yeast nitrogen base supplemented with asparagine (1.5 g/liter) and glucose (10.0 g/liter) is used as the test medium. The medium is sterilized by filtration. To avoid inactivation of the amphotericin B, 5 ml of a nonchelating buffer containing 15.89 g of 2(N-morpholino) propane sulfonic acid and 10.8 g of 2-amino-2 (hydroxymethyl)-1,3-propanediol, combined in a final volume of 100 ml of distilled water and sterilized by autoclaving, is added to 100 ml of yeast nitrogen base.

Amphotericin B is solubilized in DMSO to yield a stock solution of 100 μg/ml. 5-FC is dissolved in saline to give a stock solution of 10,000 μg/ml and sterilized by filtration.

Procedure

In most tests of synergy, 5-FC is titrated from 100 to 0.05 μg/ml in twofold increments both in the absence of and presence of graded amounts of amphotericin B by a classical checkerboard (box) titration scheme—with both 5-FC and amphotericin B being serially diluted in twofold increments and all concentrations being combined. The concentrations range from 100 to 0.05 μg/ml of 5-FC and from 5.0 to 0.005 μg/ml of amphotericin B. Tests are performed in duplicate. MIC and MFC are determined in a manner similar to the one described earlier for the broth dilution method.

A reduction of the MIC for 5-FC by at least a fourfold factor in the presence of an otherwise subinhibitory concentration of amphotericin B is regarded as synergistic potentiation of the former drug by the latter. A twofold reduction of the 5-FC MIC is regarded as possible potentiation. A twofold or greater increase in the MIC of 5-FC is regarded as antagonism. Similar criteria are used in evaluating MFC end points.

The 48 isolates that were tested by Shadomy et al. (33) were 32 *C. neoformans*, seven *C. albicans*, seven *C. tropicalis*, and seven *C. parapsilosis* isolates. Evidence of synergy, as indicated by a fourfold or greater reduction of the MIC of 5-FC in the presence of subinhibitory concentrations of amphotericin B, was seen with 11 of the 46 isolates (24%) at the fungistatic level and with three isolates (7%) at the fungicidal level. Indifferent results were obtained for 44 isolates at the fungistatic level and for 35 isolates at the fungicidal level. Antagonism was observed with three isolates.

Therefore, the synergistic phenomenon, although observed with the combination of 5-FC and amphotericin B, is not evident for every isolate of a yeast species. Thus, before treatment with the above combination of drugs is initiated, the involved pathogen must be tested in the laboratory to determine the synergistic effect of the combination.

Recently, Dougherty et al. (10) reported a microdilution transfer plate technique to determine the *in vitro* synergy of such antimicrobial agents as rifampin and amphotericin B against *C. albicans*. Their results correlated well with those of the conventional methods. The technique was found to be reproducible and enabled one to produce a checkerboard gradient in a fast, convenient, and responsible way.

Many methods have been described for determining MICs and MFCs more quickly. Hopfer and Groschel (14) used a Bactec 225 to study the effect of amphotericin B on CO_2 production by yeasts. A radiometric procedure for yeast susceptibility testing that required 3 hr of incubation was developed. The drug concentration causing at least a 44% decrease in CO_2 production correlated to the broth dilution minimum inhibitory concentration in 85% of the 44 isolates.

Acid production by certain yeast species through the fermentation of glucose was used as the basis of an *in vitro* test for measuring susceptibility of those yeasts to 5-FC by Fisher and Armstrong (11). Serial dilutions of 5-FC in yeast nitrogen base broth (with bromothymol blue indicator dye) were made on microtiter plates. Eighteen hours after inoculation, the lowest concentration of 5-FC that completely inhibited the production of acid was recorded as the MIC. The procedure was found to be a rapid, inexpensive alternative method to a turbidimetric assay which required 48 to 72 hr of incubation.

Determining Antifungal Agents in Body Fluids

Several methods have been described for the bioassay of amphotericin B and 5-FC in biological fluids. These methods, modifications of either turbidimetric or radial diffusion plate procedures, have involved various indicator fungi including *C. albicans, C. tropicalis, Curvularia lunata, Paecilomyces variotii,* and *Saccharomyces cerevisiae.*

The lower limits of sensitivity are usually in the range of 0.05 to 0.1 μg/ml for amphotericin B and 0.4 to 0.1 μg/ml for 5-FC. The bioassay methods for amphotericin B and 5-FC described below are those of Shadomy and Espinel-Ingroff (31).

Bioassay for Amphotericin B

Medium

The medium for the radial diffusion bioassay for amphotericin B and 5-FC is yeast morphology agar (M-12, Difco). It is prepared as a 100-ml quantity per 250 ml flask, autoclaved at 15 lb for 15 min, and cooled to about 55 C. The pH before sterilization is adjusted to 6.5.

Assay plates

The disposable NUNC Bioassay transparent polystyrene plates measuring 23 × 23 cm are suitable for bioassay.

Stock solution

A stock solution of 10,000 μg/ml of amphotericin B is prepared in alkaline 50% isopropyl alcohol. The solution is allowed to stand for at least 30 min in the dark for autosterilization.

Drug dilution

From the amphotericin B stock solution, serial dilutions ranging from 5 μg/ml to 0.031 μg/ml are prepared in pooled human sera.

Assay indicator organism

A 7-day-old sporulating culture of *P. variotii* on Sabouraud dextrose agar is scraped and suspended in sterile distilled water, and the suspension is adjusted to 65% to 70% at 530 nm transmission. One milliliter of this adjusted suspension is added to the 100 ml of the cooled medium, and the assay plate is poured and allowed to solidify.

Sterile, stainless steel antibiotic assay cylinders are placed at equal distances on the plate. A micropipette is used to add 0.1 ml of each dilution to the cylinders. The last two cylinders are controls loaded with 0.1 ml of normal drug-free serum. The patient's serum or other body fluid specimens are treated similarly. The plate is incubated at 30 C for 48 hr.

After incubation, the zones of growth inhibition are measured, and the average values of the zones of inhibition of each dilution are plotted on semilogarithmic graph paper, with the concentration of the drug in micrograms per milliliter as the ordinate (Y axis) and the zones of inhibition in millimeters as the abscissa (X axis). The slope of the curve is determined, and the antibiotic level in the patient's serum is read from the graph.

Bioassay for 5-FC

The procedure for 5-FC bioassay is similar to that for amphotericin B except for the following differences:

The test fungus for 5-FC bioassay is *Saccharomyces cerevisiae* (the same species that is used for the susceptibility test). However, sensitive strains of *C. albicans, C. tropicalis,* or *C. pseudotropicalis* can be substituted for *S. cerevisiae.*

A stock solution of 10,000 μg/ml is prepared in sterile normal saline. The serial dilutions for 5-FC range from 80 to 2.5 μg/ml instead of the 5 to 0.031 μg/ml for amphotericin B.

Estimating Amphotericin B in Sera of Patients Treated with 5-FC and Amphotericin B

The medium used is the yeast morphology agar (M-12, Difco). To 100 ml of M-12 medium, autoclaved and cooled, 0.1 ml of cytosine (cytosine H_2O, Nutritional Biochemical Corporation) of 10,000 μg/ml strength is added to give a final concentration of 10 μg/ml of cytosine. Each flask is seeded with 1 ml of the suspension of *Chrysosporium pruinosum* that was adjusted to 65%–70% transmission at 530 nm.

Stock Solution

A 1000 μg/ml solution of amphotericin B in alkaline isopropyl alcohol is prepared and diluted with alkaline isopropyl alcohol to give 5 ml of 50 μg/ml solution. A 1:10 dilution is made in serum from 50 μg/ml to yield 5 μg/ml solution in serum. Further serum dilutions range from 1 μg/ml to 0.31 μg/ml (1, 0.5, 0.25, 0.125, 0.0625, and 0.031 μg/ml). The rest of the procedure is similar to that described earlier for the amphotericin B bioassay.

The antifungal activity of 5-FC in patient's serum treated with a combination of amphotericin B and 5-FC is nullified by the inclusion of cytosine in the assay medium. The zones of inhibition which develop result from the presence of amphotericin B in the patient's serum. Since the test organism is quite sensitive to amphotericin B, measurable zones of inhibition are produced even at low concentrations of amphotericin B.

Estimating 5-FC in Sera of Patients Treated with 5-FC and Amphotericin B Combined

The concurrent use of amphotericin B and 5-FC complicates the measurement of 5-FC in the serum. Since the fungi used in the above bioassay systems are uniformly susceptible to amphotericin B, one cannot differentiate the effect of 5-FC from that of amphotericin B when the two are combined.

Attempts to circumvent this problem have included using dialysis to separate the two drugs (3). Kasper and Drutz (16) used yeast nitrogen base (YNB) agar supplemented with 5% dextrose as the medium of choice, because they found that 5-FC diffuses readily through the YNB agar from the filter paper disks, whereas amphotericin B apparently does not. They used a sensitive isolate of *C. albicans* (ATCC 24433) as the test organism to seed the medium and incubated test material for 6 rather than 48 hr. The standard solutions of drugs were prepared in pooled human AB sera.

Concentrations of 5-FC of 20 µg/ml or less were most useful in preparing standards, since higher concentrations produced such large zones that they overlapped the zones of other antibiotic concentrations. For the same reason, they preferred a 1:10 dilution of serum in sterile saline to insure readable zone sizes. After evaluating the disk diffusion, cut-well, and Kirby-Bauer methods, the authors preferred the disk diffusion method.

Inactivation of amphotericin B in sera of patients treated with both the drugs can also be achieved by heating the serum to 100 C and holding for 45 min (17). 5-FC is unaffected by this treatment, and its serum levels can subsequently be assayed with either tube dilution or disk diffusion methods. 5-FC is resistant to heating for as long as 60 min and is unaffected by temperature as high as 121 C.

Amphotericin B is inactivated by heating for 45 min at 100 C, and thus its antifungal activity can be easily abolished in serum containing both drugs. Since serum must be used if this heat inactivation is to occur, the mechanism of inactivation is related to the denaturation of proteins to which amphotericin B is strongly bound. Although protein denaturation results in turbidity, it does not interfere with performing the test or interpreting the results.

References

1. BENNETT JE: Susceptibility of *Cryptococcus neoformans* to amphotericin B. Antimicrob Agents Chemother, pp 405–410, 1967
2. BENNETT JE: Chemotherapy of systemic mycoses. N Engl J Med 290:320–323, 1974
3. BLOCK ER and BENNETT JE: Pharmacological studies with 5-fluorocytosine. Antimicrob Agents Chemother 1:476–482, 1972
4. BLOCK ER and BENNETT JE: The combined effect of 5-fluorocytosine and amphotericin B in the therapy of murine cryptococcosis. Proc Soc Exp Biol Med 142:476–480, 1973
5. BLOCK ER, JENNINGS AE, and BENNETT JE: Experimental therapy of cladosporiosis and sporotrichosis with 5-fluorocytosine. Antimicrob Agents Chemother 3:95–98, 1973
6. BLOCK ER, JENNINGS AE, and BENNETT JE: 5-Fluorocytosine resistance in *Cryptococcus neoformans*. Antimicrob Agents Chemother 3:649–656, 1973
7. BLOCK ER, JENNINGS AE, and BENNETT JE: Variables influencing susceptibility testing of *Cryptococcus neoformans* to 5-fluorocytosine. Antimicrob Agents Chemother 4:392–395, 1973
8. BOYER JM: Impregnated disc method for antifungal antibiotic testing. Antimicrob Agents Chemother 9:1070–1071, 1976
9. DEMEREC M: Origin of bacterial resistance to antibiotic. J Bacteriol 56:63–74, 1948
10. DOUGHERTY PF, YOTTER DW, and MATTHEWS TR: Microdilution transfer plate technique for determining in vitro synergy of antimicrobial agents. Antimicrob Agents Chemother 11:225–228, 1977
11. FISHER BD and ARMSTRONG D: Rapid microdilution colorimetric assay for yeast susceptibility to fluorocytosine. Antimicrob Agents Chemother 12:614–617, 1977
12. FISHER JF, DUMA RF, MARKOWITZ SM, SHADOMY S, ESPINEL-INGROFF A, and CHEW

WH: Therapeutic failures with miconazole. Antimicrob Agents Chemother 13:965–968, 1978

13. HOEPRICH PD and GOLDSTEIN E: Miconazole therapy for coccidioidomycosis. J Am Med Assoc 230:1153–1157, 1974

14. HOPFER RL and GROSCHEL D: Amphotericin B susceptibility testing of yeasts with a bactecradiometric system. Antimicrob Agents Chemother 11:277–280, 1977

15. HUPPERT M, SUN SH, and VUKOVICH KR: Combined amphotericin B-tetracycline therapy for experimental coccidioidomycosis. Antimicrob Agents Chemother 5:473–478, 1974

16. KASPER RL and DRUTZ DJ: Rapid, simple bioassay for 5-fluorocytosine in the presence of amphotericin B. Antimicrob Agents Chemother 7:462–465, 1975

17. KAUFFMAN CA, CARLETON JA, and FRAME PT: Simple assay for 5-fluorocytosine in the presence of amphotericin B. Antimicrob Agents Chemother 9:381–383, 1976

18. KITAHARA M, SETH VK, MEDOFF G, and KOBAYASHI GS: Antimicrobial susceptibility testing of six clinical isolates of Aspergillus. Antimicrob Agents Chemother 9:908–914, 1976

19. KITAHARA M, SETH VK, MEDOFF G, and KOBAYASHI GS: Activity of amphotericin B, 5-fluorocytosine and rifampin against six clinical isolates of Aspergillus. Antimicrob Agents Chemother 9:915–919, 1976

20. KOBAYASHI GS, CHEUNG SC, SCHLESSINGER D, and MEDOFF G: Effects of rifampin derivatives, alone and in combination with amphotericin B, against Histoplasma capsulatum. Antimicrob Agents Chemother 5:16–18, 1974

21. KOBAYASHI GS, MEDOFF G, SCHLESSINGER D, KWAN CN, and MUSSER WE: Amphotericin B potentiation of rifampin as an antifungal agent against the yeast phase of Histoplasma capsulatum. Science 177:709–710, 1972

22. KWAN CN, MEDOFF G, KOBAYASHI GS, SCHLESSINGER D, and RASKAS HJ: Potentiation of the antifungal effects of antibiotics by amphotericin B. Antimicrob Agents Chemother 2:61–65, 1972

23. MANOHAR V, RAMANANDA RAO G, SIRSI M, and KRISHNAMURTI N: Miconazole in the treatment of superficial mycoses. Mycopathologia 59:57–60, 1976

24. MEDOFF G, COMFORT M, and KOBAYASHI GS: Synergistic action of amphotericin B and 5-fluorocytosine against yeastlike organisms. Proc Soc Exp Biol Med 138:571–574, 1971

25. MEDOFF G and KOBAYASHI GS: Amphotericin B: old drug, new therapy. J Am Med Assoc 232:619–620, 1975

26. MEDOFF G, KOBAYASHI GS, KWAN CN, SCHLESSINGER D, and VENKOV P: Potentiation of rifampin and 5-fluorocytosine as antifungal antibiotics by amphotericin B. Proc Natl Acad Sci USA 69:196–199, 1972

27. MORRISON WL, CONNER B, and CLAYTON Y: Successful treatment of chromoblastomycosis with 5-fluorocytosine. Br J Dermatol 90:445–449, 1974

28. NSANZUMUHIRE H, VOLLUM D, and POLTERA AA: Chromomycosis due to Cladosporium trichoides treated with 5-fluorocytosine. Am J Clin Pathol 61:257–263, 1974

29. RHOADES ER, FELTON FG, WILKUS J, and MUCHMORE HG: Susceptibility of human and environmental isolates of Cryptococcus norformans to amphotericin B. Antimicrob Agents Chemother 1967, pp 736–738, 1968

30. SHADOMY S: What's new in antifungal chemotherapy. Clin Med 79:14–18, 1972

31. SHADOMY S and ESPINEL-INGROFF A: Susceptibility testing of antifungal agents. In Manual of Clinical Microbiology, 2nd edition. Lennette EH, Spaulding EH, and Truant JP (eds.). American Society for Microbiology, Washington, DC, 1974, pp 569–574

32. SHADOMY S, KIRCHOFF CB, and INGROFF AE: In vitro activity of 5-fluorocytosine against Candida and Torulopsis species. Antimicrob Agents Chemother 3:9–14, 1973

33. SHADOMY S, WAGNER G, INGROFF AE, and DAVIS BA: In vitro studies with combinations of 5-fluorocytosine and amphotericin B. Antimicrob Agents Chemother 8:117–121, 1975

34. SZYBALSKI W and BRYSON V: Bacterial resistance studies with derivatives of isonicotinic acid. Am Rev Tuberc 65:768–770, 1952

35. TITSWORTH E, and GRUNEBERG E: Chemotherapeutic activity of 5-fluorocytosine and amphotericin B against Candida albicans in mice. Antimicrob Agents Chemother 4:306–308, 1973

36. UTZ CJ, WHITE S, and SHADOMY S: New medium for in vitro susceptibility studies with amphotericin B. Antimicrob Agents Chemother 10:776–777, 1976

37. UTZ JP, TYNES BS, SHADOMY HJ, DUMA RJ, KANNAN MM, and MASON KN: 5-Fluorocytosine in human cryptococcosis. Antimicrob Agents Chemother 1968, pp 344–346, 1969

38. WAGNER G and SHADOMY S: Effects of purines and pyrimidines on the fungistatic activity of 5-fluorocytosine in *Aspergillus* species. Antimicrob Agents Chemother 11:229–233, 1977
39. WAGNER G, SHADOMY S, PAXTON LD, and INGROFF AE: New method for susceptibility testing with antifungal agents. Antimicrob Agents Chemother 8:107–109, 1975
40. WEINSTEIN L: Antibiotics IV. Miscellaneous antimicrobial, antifungal, and antiviral agents. *In* The Pharmacological Basis of Therapeutics, 4th edition. Goodman LS and Gilman A (eds.). The MacMillan Co, New York, 1970, pp 1299–1302

CHAPTER 56

OPPORTUNISTIC MYCOSES

Norman L. Goodman

Introduction

A wide variety of fungi cause infection and disease in the compromised host—who can be defined as a patient with a primary, underlying disease or one who receives therapy which impairs, to varying degrees, his natural resistance to infection or disease. This compromised state renders the host vulnerable to infection by many fungi which normally exist in a saprobic or commensal state in the environment. Since these fungi usually do not cause pathologic changes in the uncompromised host, they are referred to as opportunistic fungi.

It is difficult for the microbiologist-clinician team to determine whether and when a fungus is causing disease when it is found in clinical specimens. Thus, it is imperative that proper specimens be collected and that communications between laboratory personnel and physicans be well-established.

It is becoming more apparent that any fungus in the environment of a compromised patient can cause infection through inhalation, injection, or implantation. However, most opportunistic infections and diseases are caused by a relatively small group of fungi including yeasts (e.g., *Candida* spp., *Cryptococcus* spp., *Torulopsis glabrata*) and moulds (e.g., *Aspergillus* spp. and *Zygomycetes*).

Yeast Infections

The most common fungal infections for the compromised host are caused by yeasts. *Candida albicans* and other *Candida* spp. are most frequently reported to cause infection and disease, followed by *Cryptococcus* spp., *Torulopsis glabrata,* and *Trichosporon* spp. Morphologic features that differentiate frequently isolated yeasts are summarized in Table 56.1.

Candidiasis

Candidiasis is the collective name used for a wide variety of diseases caused by members of the genus *Candida*. Species of this genus are aerobic, grow well on most enriched bacteriological and mycological media when incubated at 25–30 C, with colonies reaching 1–3 mm in 2–3 days. Mature colo-

TABLE 56.1—MAJOR MORPHOLOGICAL DIFFERENTIAL FEATURES OF YEAST FREQUENTLY
ISOLATED FROM CLINICAL SPECIMENS

	ON CORN MEAL AGAR				
	PSEUDO-HYPHAE	TRUE HYPHAE	CHLAMYDO-SPORES	GERM TUBES	CAPSULE
Candida albicans	+	−	+	+	−
C. stellatoidea	+	−	+	V	−
C. parapsilosis	+	−	−	−	−
C. pseudotropicalis	+	−	−	−	−
C. krusei	+	−	−	−	−
C. guillermondii	+	−	−	−	−
Cryptococcus species	−	−*	−	−	+
Torulopsis glabrata	−	−	−	−	−
Rhodotorula species	−	−*	−	−	+
Trichosporon species	−	+	−	−	−

V = variable
* = rare

nies are usually white but may be cream-colored or tan. Colonies are usually creamy in consistency, but may be glabrous or membranous. Some may be rough and have rhizoid-like fringes with submerged pseudohyphae.

Microscopically, they appear as budding cells which may be oval, round, or oblong, which measure 2–3 × 15 μm, and which occur singly, in clusters, or in chains (pseudohyphae). Abundant pseudohyphae are usually produced on nutritionally deficient solid media. Pseudohyphal production is characteristic of the genus when isolates are cultured on morphologic media (43).

The clinical manifestations of candidiasis vary. This infection may involve the skin (intertrigo, paronychia, eczema, generalized cutaneous candidiasis) (12, 20, 57), mucous membranes (thrush, vaginitis) (5, 37), and the internal organs (e.g., lung, heart, urinary tract, meninges, brain) (23, 49, 51, 61). Infection commonly occurs as a result of inoculation via the intestinal tract, contaminated inhalation therapy equipment, deeply installed intravenous tubes, or indwelling urinary tract catheters (53, 69). The incidence of *Candida* infections among severely burned patients has increased markedly (39). Candidiasis is often associated with the use of broad-spectrum antibiotics. *Candida albicans* is the principal species which causes infection, although at least six other species have been incriminated as disease agents. *Candida tropicalis, C. parapsilosis,* and *C. guillermondii* have frequently been associated with fungemia, endocarditis, and urinary tract infections (49, 53, 61).

Candidiasis may occur as a nosocomial infection with considerable significance in terms of patient care and medical costs. Because knowledge about this disease is limited, it appears that preventing these infections requires proper aseptic maintenance of instruments used on the compromised or severely ill patient, controlled use of antibiotics and immunosuppressants, as well as close monitoring of the fungal flora of the debilitated patient.

Collection and processing of specimens

Collection of specimens for the laboratory diagnosis of candidiasis is critical. The critical question to be answered in a suspected case of candidiasis is whether the fungus is only colonizing or is causing disease. Since these organisms commonly inhabit the patient and the environment, the specimen *must* be collected from the site of infection and processed immediately.

Specimens collected for diagnosing candidiasis are usually scrapings from the skin or mucous membranes, sputum, tissue, urine, and blood. Where possible, specimens should be collected aseptically, placed into sterile containers, and taken directly to the laboratory. Tissue should be placed in a minimal amount of sterile water or saline for transport. Tissue specimens should never be frozen. Urine should be collected by the suprapubic route when feasible. Catheterized specimens are suitable only when catheterization is performed aseptically. Clean-catch specimens are rarely suitable for evaluating the presence of *Candida* spp. in the urine. Multiple specimens of sputum and urine are usually necessary to establish *Candida* infection.

Diagnostic procedures

The clinical specimen should be examined immediately or as soon as possible after collection for presence of yeast and yeast-like fungi and then cultured on appropriate media.

Direct examination of clinical specimen. The identification of yeasts in a clinical specimen begins with the direct microscopic examination of samples of the specimen. Direct examination of the specimen allows categorization rather than identification of the organism(s) present. More importantly, the relative number of organisms present can be determined. The presence of pseudohyphae in a freshly collected specimen is presumptive evidence of infection by *Candida* spp. Appropriate procedures for the direct examination of specimens depend on the type of specimen.

1. Sputum, other mucous secretions, or exudate. Select the mucoid or purulent parts of the specimen for examination. Add a drop of the material to a clean microscope slide, and cover with a clean cover glass. If the specimen is opaque or excessively bloody, a drop of 10% KOH can be added. Warm the slide gently for 10–15 sec and allow 5–10 min for the KOH to clear the specimen.

2. Scrapings. Place a small number of tissue fragments on a clean microscope slide, and add a drop of 10% KOH. Cover with a clean cover slide. Warm gently for 10–15 sec, and allow 15–30 min for the KOH to clear the specimen.

3. Urine and other body fluids. Centrifuge specimens to concentrate the sediment. After centrifugation, decant the supernatant, place a drop of the concentrated sediment on a clean glass slide, and cover the specimen with a clean cover slide.

4. Tissue. Large pieces of tissue should be checked for lesions containing fungi. Direct microscopic examination of tissue is difficult without special stains such as the periodic acid-Schiff or Gomori methenamine silver method.

However, material from lesions can be examined in the same manner described for sputum.

Microscopic examination of specimens should be done with the low power (10×) and high power (40×) objectives. The light intensity should be reduced by decreasing the aperture of the iris diaphragm. The phase microscope is very helpful in differentiating artifacts from fungi.

Candida spp. in specimens such as those listed above will appear as budding yeast or pseudohyphae. *Candida albicans* will usually form pseudohyphae when it invades tissue, which makes the presence of these structures clinically significant.

Culture procedures. Even though *Candida* species commonly found in clinical specimens grow well on most enriched laboratory media, the routine isolation medium is Sabouraud agar. It can be used in slants or plates, depending on whether the specimen is likely to contain several types of organisms. If so, plated media should be inoculated to assure obtaining isolated colonies. Specimens with mixed flora should also be planted on Sabouraud agar containing antibiotics (e.g., penicillin, streptomycin, and cycloheximide) to inhibit bacterial and mould growth. Some species of *Candida* are inhibited by cycloheximide. Cultures should be incubated at 25–30 C. Colonies of *Candida* spp. usually appear in 2–3 days; however, all cultures should be incubated for 4 weeks before they are reported to be negative.

Identification. Identification of *Candida* spp. requires the use of morphologic characteristics and results of biochemical tests. The initial step in identifying Candida species is obtaining a pure culture. Microscopic examination of wet preparations of organisms from an isolated colony in water or lactophenol cotton blue will provide evidence of a pure culture. When pure cultures are obtained, the following procedures can be used to determine the species of *Candida* in the specimen.

1. Morphology. The initial step in identifying yeasts should be determining their morphology. This determination usually prevents unnecessary biochemical testing and reduces the time for identification. Species of *Candida* commonly found in clinical specimens produce pseudohyphae when grown on special morphology medium.

The most commonly used medium is cornmeal agar. Streak the inoculum on the surface of the medium. Cover part of the streak with a clean, sterile cover glass and incubate at 25 C–30 C. After 24–48 hr of incubation, observe microscopically for the presence of pseudohyphae. Also, observe for chlamydospores, since *Candida albicans* often produces such structures in this length of time. Those versed in the morphology of *Candida* can often determine the species on the basis of its microscopic morphology; however, additional tests are usually required for speciation.

2. Germ tube test. The most reliable, rapid, presumptive test for the identification of *Candida albicans* is the germ tube test. To perform this test, prepare a dilute suspension of yeast from a pure culture in 0.5–1.0 ml of serum. This may be done by touching the tip of a sterile pasteur pipette to a colony and thoroughly emulsifying the cells in the serum. Incubate the inoculated serum at 37 C for 2 hr, remove 1 drop of suspension, place onto a clean microscope slide, cover the drop with a clean cover slide, and observe for germ

tubes. Germ tubes must be distinguished from pseudohyphal elements which may have been carried over in the inoculum. Always use a positive control made from a known culture of *Candida albicans*. *Note:* this test should be read at 2 hr, because species other than *Candida albicans* produce germ tubes after longer incubation.

3. Biochemical tests. Definite identification of *Candida* spp. is dependent upon results of biochemical testing. A pure culture of the organism is required for proper performance of these tests. This can be assured by restreaking primary isolates on blood agar.

Carbon Assimilation. The assimilation test is to determine the ability of a yeast to utilize a carbohydrate as the sole source of carbon. This requires a chemically defined medium containing essential salts and a nitrogen source. This test is essential for the definitive speciation of *Candida* isolates and should be used with all isolates considered to be of clinical significance. Assimilation patterns for the *Candida* species commonly isolated from clinical specimens are given in Table 56.2.

There are numerous methods for determining carbon assimilation. A standard plate method is shown in the Appendix to this chapter. There are many commercial systems available for determining the biochemical reactions of *Candida* spp. and other yeasts. While these systems are perfectly acceptable, each should be standardized to a given laboratory, and the tables provided for reading the test for that specific system *must* be used.

Fermentation. The ability of yeasts to ferment carbohydrate is a useful tool in speciating them. A positive fermentation test is indicated by the production of CO_2 gas. Therefore, any system used for determining fermentation must have some method of trapping gas.

The standard method for determining fermentation is the use of tubed media containing the Durham tube insert to collect gas. This method is described in the Appendix to this chapter. Again, a pure culture is needed. Also, best results can be obtained by using an inoculum from a nonenriched medium such as cornmeal agar.

Candida species vary considerably in their ability to ferment carbohydrate. Fermentation patterns for the candida species frequently isolated from clinical specimens are shown in Table 56.2.

Evaluation of laboratory findings

Isolation of *Candida albicans* or other *Candida* spp. from clinical specimens does not confirm the existence of disease. Demonstrating the presence of the organism in tissue is the only way to prove invasion. The presence of the organism at the site of infection (as demonstrated by multiple culture or direct microscopic examination) supports a tentative diagnosis of candidiasis. Multiple positive blood cultures are usually considered proof of candidiasis; however, it has been well-documented that patients with candidiasis often have negative blood cultures.

Cryptococcosis

Four species of cryptococci are considered to be of medical importance. They are: *Cryptococcus neoformans, C. laurentii, C. terreus,* and *C. albidus. Cryptococcus neoformans* is the most common cause of disease; however, the other species occur frequently in the environment and make a differential identification necessary (15, 19).

The cryptococci are aerobic and grow well on most bacteriological and mycological media when incubated at 25 C–30 C. Growth is rapid, with colonies usually being visible in 24–48 hr, although organisms from patients on in-

TABLE 56.2—MAJOR BIOCHEMICAL DIFFERENTIAL REACTIONS OF *CANDIDA* SPECIES FREQUENTLY ISOLATED FROM CLINICAL SPECIMENS

ORGANISM	CARBON ASSIMILATION												FERMENTATION						UREASE
	Gl	Ma	Su	La	Ga	Me	Ce	In	Xy	Ra	Tr	Du	Gl	Ma	Su	La	Ga	Te	
Candida albicans	+	+	+	–	+	–	–	–	+	–	+	–	+	+	–	–	+	V	–
C. stellatoidea	+	+	–	–	+	–	–	–	+	–	+	–	+	+	–	–	–	–	–
C. tropicalis	+	+	+	–	+	–	V	–	+	–	+	–	+	+	+	–	+	+	–
C. parapsilosis	+	+	+	–	+	–	–	–	+	–	+	–	+	–	–	–	V	–	–
C. pseudotropicalis	+	–	+	+	+	–	+	–	+	+	–	–	+	–	+	+	+	–	–
C. krusei	+	–	–	–	–	–	–	–	–	–	–	–	+	–	–	–	–	–	V
C. guillermondii	+	+	+	–	+	+	+	–	+	+	+	+	+	–	+	–	+	+	–

Note: All above *Candida* species do not assimilate nitrate.

Gl = Glucose   La = Lactose   Ce = Cellobiose   Ra = Raffinose
Ma = Maltose   Ga = Galactose   In = Inositol   Tr = Trehalose
Su = Sucrose   Me = Melibiose   Xy = Xylose   Du = Dulcitol
+ under assimilation indicates growth
+ under fermentation indicates gas production
V indicates variable (may be + or –)

tensive anticarcinogenic therapy may grow more slowly. Colony color may vary from white to pale pink, and consistency may vary from mucoid to butyrous.

Microscopically, cryptococcus cells are unicellular, budding yeast 5–20 μm in diameter. Characteristically, the yeast are surrounded by a polysaccharide capsule. The capsule width varies, depending on the medium in which the organism is grown. In enriched media and in tissue, capsule width is 5–30 μm. Nonencapsulated *C. neoformans* may be found in patients undergoing intensive treatment with potent chemotherapeutic agents such as 5-fluorouracil.

Cryptococcus neoformans is the most common cause of cryptococcosis, although other species have rarely been shown to be the etiologic agent (38). *Cryptococcus neoformans* can cause primary disease, but its role as the etiologic agent of secondary infection is well-documented and appears to be more prevalent as there are more compromised patients.

Cryptococcosis is an acute, subacute, chronic pulmonary, systemic, or meningeal infection. The pulmonary form is generally mild and often not recognized. Acute or chronic meningeal cryptococcosis is the most commonly recognized form of the disease. Skeletal and cutaneous manifestations have been associated with disseminated cryptococcosis. Cryptococcosis is considered to be of pulmonary origin. Pulmonary cryptococcosis is characterized by cough and production of mucoid sputum. The patient may develop low-grade fever and suffer weight loss. However, these symptoms may be masked in patients with other primary disease. Hematogenous spread of the organism is frequent, with subsequent involvement of other internal organs, the bones, skin, and brain (41, 42, 50). Cerebral cryptococcosis is manifested by the development of severe headaches, which may have an insidious or acute onset, vertigo, and vomiting. The patient may become disoriented, apathetic, overtalkative, or comatose. The course of the meningeal form of the disease is usually rapid and fatal if not treated.

The cryptococci exist as saprophytes in nature. They have been isolated from soil, water, fruit, and milk (17, 19). *Cryptococcus neoformans* has been repeatedly isolated from soil contaminated with pigeon manure and from the nests of pigeons (18). Cryptococcosis is distributed worldwide. There appears to be no significant difference in the case distribution related to age or race. More males than females are affected (20). One must be cautious in interpreting epidemiologic information of cryptococcosis, since there are as yet no reliable tools for identifying subclinical infections.

In the last decade, cryptococcosis has been recognized as a major opportunistic disease. Secondary infection by *C. neoformans* has been reported in a wide variety of compromised hosts ranging from immunosuppressed renal transplant patients to those with sarcoidosis (41, 60, 69, 70). Thus, this organism apparently does not have a predilection for any particular group of compromising diseases.

Because reporting of fungal diseases is inadequate, data on the public health significance of cryptococcosis are lacking. Hammerman et al. (33) estimated that 349 hospitalizations per year with 6,782 hospital days and 70 deaths are directly linked with cryptococcosis. There are indications that more compromised patients are having cryptococcosis, making this one of the foremost opportunistic fungal diseases.

Since little is known of the epidemiology of cryptococcosis, appropriate preventive measures have not been established. Avoiding contact between compromised patients and areas known to harbor these fungi should provide some protection.

Collection and processing of specimens

Specimens most commonly collected for cryptococcosis are spinal fluid, sputum, bronchial washes, urine, tissue, and blood. All specimens should be collected aseptically and transported immediately to the laboratory. Clear spinal fluid and urine should be concentrated by centrifugation or filtration.

Serological tests for cryptococcosis have proved to be of diagnostic value. The presence of cryptococcal polysaccharide antigen in spinal fluid and serum is strongly associated with disease. Anticryptococcal antibody may be present. Serum and spinal fluid should be collected and tested for the presence of the antigen and antibody. Multiple specimens collected during the course of treatment may show a rising or falling titer, which may indicate the course of the disease.

Diagnostic procedures

Direct examination of clinical specimen. In most cases, *C. neoformans* and other *Cryptococcus* spp. from clinical specimens will have a capsule. This capsule can be visualized with a background stain such as India ink or Nigrosin. Place a filled loop or small drop of fluid specimen or concentrated sediment on a clean microscope slide. Add a small drop of India ink or Nigrosin. Cover with a clean cover slide and observe with the low or high power objective. If the preparation is too dark or too dense, dilute with a small drop of water.

Cryptococcal cells should appear as small, round, budding yeasts inside a capsule. The capsule may vary in size from very large to practically nonexistent. The cryptococci do not generally develop a mycelium on Sabouraud agar or on cornmeal agar. Germ tubes are not formed when incubated in serum (see Table 56.1).

Culture procedure. Enriched media such as brain heart infusion agar with 5% sheep blood and Sabouraud agar are the media of choice for isolating cryptococci from clinical specimens. Antibiotics may be incorporated in the media to inhibit bacterial growth; however, cycloheximide should *not* be used, because the cryptococci will not grow in its presence.

Nigerseed or birdseed agar (see Appendix) is recommended for isolating *C. neoformans* from contaminated specimens. *Cryptococcus neoformans* will form a dark brown colony on this medium, whereas other *Cryptococcus* spp. form light-brown colonies, and other yeast colonies have no brown pigment.

Biochemical tests. Definitive speciation of cryptococci is based on results of biochemical testing. All species of the genus *Cryptococcus* possess the enzyme urease. The standard method of determining urease production is to streak Christenson's urea medium and incubate at 25 C–30 C. If the area turns deep red, the test for urease is positive. However, because other yeasts also produce urease, a positive urease test is not adequate to identify the organism as a cryptococcus.

Characteristically, the cryptococci are nonfermenting yeasts. Their ability to assimilate inositol is one of the primary characteristics that differentiate them from species of *Rhodotorula*. Testing for nitrate reduction is also useful in speciating cryptococci. Characteristics of the cryptococci frequently found in clinical specimens are shown in Table 56.3. Results shown in this table are obtained by the standard method of determining assimilation and fermentation (as described in the Appendix to this chapter).

Serologic procedures. Reliable serologic procedures have been developed for detecting and quantitating capsular antigen and antibody to *C. neoformans* (9, 27, 36, 66).

The cryptococcus latex agglutination test is an indirect agglutination procedure involving latex particles sensitized with anticryptococcal rabbit globulin. When cryptococcal polysaccharide antigen in serum or spinal fluid comes into contact with the anticryptococcal globulin-sensitized latex, the globulin-polysaccharide complex reacts and causes the latex to agglutinate. Because rheumatoid factor in the patient's serum may interfere with the latex test (8), appropriate controls must be used to rule out this interference in a positive test. A commercial kit for testing for cryptococcal antigen is available from several sources.

Antibodies to *C. neoformans* can be detected with the complement fixation test or with agglutination, using whole yeast cells of *C. neoformans* (9, 27, 36, 66).

Evaluation of laboratory findings

The isolation and identification of *Cryptococcus neoformans* from a clinical specimen is usually considered to be diagnostic of disease. This interpretation may be questionable when the isolate is from sputum or specimens from external areas of the body where the fungus may be present as a commensal or transient colonizer.

Demonstration of encapsulated yeasts in spinal fluid, sputum, exudate, or other clinical specimens from a compromised patient is highly presumptive evidence of cryptococcosis. However, since all cryptococci may be encapsulated, an encapsulated yeast is not necessarily *C. neoformans.*

Serologic results may be helpful in diagnosing cryptococcosis. A high cryptococcal antigen or antibody titer may indicate severe infection. Often a patient with cryptococcosis will have a high antigen titer, and a low or absent antibody titer. For this reason, it is useful to test for cryptococcal antigen and antibody when cryptococcosis is suspected. However, because the compromised host may not be capable of producing antibody, the value of this test for diagnostic purposes must be assessed accordingly.

Torulopsosis

Torulopsosis is one of the less common opportunistic yeast infections and is most commonly caused by *Torulopsis glabrata.*

Torulopsis glabrata grows well on most enriched media when incubated at 25–30 C. Growth is rapid, with colonies becoming evident in 24-48 hr. On Sabouraud agar, the colonies are usually cream-colored, soft, smooth, and glistening.

TABLE 56.3—DIFFERENTIAL CHARACTERISTICS OF *CRYPTOCOCCUS* SPECIES FREQUENTLY ISOLATED FROM CLINICAL SPECIMENS

	CARBON ASSIMILATIONS												NO₃⁻ ASSIM.	UREASE
	GL	MA	SU	LA	GA	ME	CE	IN	XY	RA	TR	DU		
Cryptococcus														
neoformans	+	+	+	–	+	–	+	+	+	+	+	+	–	+
albidus var. albidus	+	+	+	+	V	–	+	+	+	+	+	V	+	+
albidus var. diffluens	+	+	+	–	V	–	+	+	+	+	+	V	+	+
gastricus	+	+	V	V	+	–	+	+	+	–	+	–	–	+
laurentii	+	+	+	+	+	+	+	+	+	+	+	+	–	+
luteolus	+	V	–	–	V	–	+	+	+	+	+	+	–	+
terreus	+	+	+	+	V	–	+	+	+	–	V	V	+	+
unigutulatus	+	+	+	–	V	–	V	+	+	V	V	–	–	+

Gl = Glucose   Ce = Cellobiose   La = Lactose   Ra = Raffinose
Ma = Maltose   In = Inositol   Ga = Galactose   Tr = Trehalose
Su = Sucrose   Xy = Xylose   Me = Melibiose   Du = Dulcitol
V = variable

Note: *Cryptococcus* species do *not* ferment the above sugars.

Microscopically, the cells are oval to spherical and are 2–4 × 4–6 μm in size. No capsules, hyphae, or pseudohyphae are formed.

Torulopsis glabrata is often part of the normal flora of the soil and of the oral cavity, gastrointestinal tract, and urogenital tract of humans and animals (2, 13, 29, 63).

This organism has been reported more and more often among severely compromised patients who are immunosuppressed, have indwelling IV or urinary tract catheters, and/or are on long-term, broad-spectrum antibiotic therapy. Infections with this organism have been reported as esophagitis (44), endometritis (29), cystitis (35, 44), pyelonephritis (44), fungemia (3, 29, 35, 40, 44, 58), and pneumonia (3, 10).

Clinically, patients with torulopsosis initially have fever and chills, and symptoms similar to septic shock caused by gram-negative bacteremia have been reported. This reaction is usually associated with the entry of large numbers of the fungus into the blood system through indwelling catheters.

The rising incidence of this disease for severely compromised patients indicates a need for better means to prevent the entry of *T. glabrata* into the internal organs. In part, this goal can be reached by close monitoring of IV and urinary tract catheters and more judicious use of broad-spectrum antibiotics.

Collection and processing of specimens

Procedures for specimen collection and processing are the same as those described in the section on candidiasis.

Diagnostic procedures

Direct examination of clinical specimens. Clinical specimens should be examined microscopically for the presence of budding yeast immediately after they are collected. Opaque specimens should be cleared with 10% KOH. Tissue should be stained with special fungal stains (as discussed in the section on candidiasis).

Torulopsis glabrata will appear as single budding yeast, 2–4 × 4–6 μm in size. However, because other yeasts also have this morphology, direct observation of such a yeast in the specimen does not confirm the presence of *T. glabrata.*

Culture methods. Torulopsis glabrata grows well on most enriched laboratory media. The routine isolation medium is Sabouraud agar. Uncontaminated specimens such as tissue and spinal fluid can be planted on slants; however, plated medium should be used if multiple organisms are present when the wet preparation is checked. Specimens with mixed flora should be planted on Sabouraud agar containing antibiotics to inhibit bacterial growth. When incubated at 25–30 C, colonies of *T. glabrata* appear in 2–3 days.

Identification of *T. glabrata* is based on results of morphologic and biochemical tests. The small, single-budding yeast does not have a capsule or pseudohyphae (Table 56.1). Biochemical characteristics are shown in Table 56.4.

No serologic tests have been developed for torulopsosis.

TABLE 56.4—DIFFERENTIAL CHARACTERISTICS OF SELECTED YEASTS FREQUENTLY ISOLATED FROM CLINICAL SPECIMENS

	CARBON ASSIMILATION												NO₃⁻ ASSIM.	FERMENTATION						UREASE
	Gl	Ma	Su	La	Ga	Me	Ce	In	Xy	Ra	Tr	Du		Gl	Ma	Su	La	Ga	Tr	
Torulopsis glabrata	+	–	–	–	–	–	–	–	–	–	+	–	–	+	–	–	–	–	+	–
Rhodotorula rubra	+	+	+	–	V	–	V	–	+	+	+	–								+
Trichosporon																				
cutaneum (beigelii)	+	+*	+*	+	+	V	+	+*	+	V	V	V	–	–	–	–	–	–	–	+*
capitatum	+	–	–	+	+	–	–	–	–	–	–	–	–	–	–	–	–	–	–	–
penicillatum	+	–	–	–	+	–	–	–	+	–	–	–	–	+	–	–	–	+	–	–

Gl = Glucose
Ma = Maltose
Su = Sucrose
V = Variable
* = Rarely negative

La = Lactose
Ga = Galactose
Me = Melibiose

Ce = Cellobiose
In = Inositol
Xy = Xylose

Ra = Raffinose
Tr = Trehalose
Du = Dulcitol

Evaluation of laboratory findings

Single isolations of *T. glabrata* from open lesions, sputum, or other specimens from areas that may harbor this fungus as a commensal have little clinical significance. However, multiple isolations from and observation of numerous organisms in clinical specimens at least indicate colonization and potential infection. Multiple isolations from blood cultures, tissue, and other specimens collected aseptically indicate infection. The presence of the organism in tissue at the site of infection confirms invasion and disease.

Mould Infections

Aspergillosis

Aspergillosis is a complex group of diseases caused by several species of Aspergillus.

Aspergillus fumigatus is the most common etiologic agent of aspergillosis, with *A. flavus, A. niger, A. clavatus,* and *A. terreus* also causing infection.

Aspergillus species grow well on most laboratory media when incubated at 25-30 C. The fungi grow rapidly, with colony diameters reaching 5-6 cm within 4-5 days. Colonial morphology varies greatly depending on the species and the medium on which it is grown. Microscopically, the hyphae are septate and branching. Conidiophores arising from the hyphae have ends which enlarge into vesicles covered with sterigmata, bearing chains of conidia. Some species produce asci and ascospores (55).

Aspergillosis may be associated with numerous clinical symptoms. Basically, however, three categories of disease are currently recognized. There are (1) allergic aspergillosis, which may give rise to asthma-like symptoms or bronchitis with plugging of bronchi with mucus, (2) aspergilloma or "fungus ball," caused by the growth of the fungus in preexisting cavities, and (3) invasive aspergillosis, in which the fungus actively invades tissue. In the compromised host, all three of the above forms may progress to dissemination of the fungus to any part of the body, including the skin (6, 57).

Clinical symptoms of aspergillosis usually include fever and cough, and are usually accompanied by blood-tinged sputum in aspergilloma.

The aspergilli are ubiquitous fungi which have all at some time been isolated from the soil, air, plant, and animal substrates (14, 20). There is no apparent differential association of aspergillosis with age, sex, or race. The disease is noncommunicable and is distributed worldwide. Persons are infected by inhaling spores of the fungus in the environment or by being inoculated with material contaminated by the fungi. When healthy individuals inhale spores, there are no apparent adverse effects; however, in individuals with defective immune responses or other impaired defense mechanisms, the organisms may become invasive and cause disease ranging from mild allergy to dissemination and death.

Aspergillosis is a relatively common cause of secondary disease in the compromised host. Some estimate that 5% of leukemia patients have aspergillosis (10, 48). This disease has been reported as a complication for a high percentage of transplant patients (24, 31), as well as for those with many forms of cancer (47, 69). Although there are no accurate data on the incidence of this disease among compromised patients, individual reports indicate that it is a major cause of prolonged hospitalization.

Preventing aspergillosis hinges on protecting the compromised host from exposure to the *Aspergillus* spores, either by keeping him/her away from sources of the organism—such as compost piles, hay, etc.—or by assuring that the patient's environment is free of the fungus (e.g., filtering air and scrupulously monitoring inhalation equipment and injection fluids).

Collection and processing of specimens

Collection of proper specimens from patients with suspected aspergillosis depends on the type and site of the lesion(s). As is the case with all opportunistic organisms, contamination with *Aspergillus* spores that are transient or present as saprophytes must be avoided. When possible, tissue from the infected site should be excised under aseptic conditions and maintained under sterile, moist conditions for mycologic and histopathologic evaluation. Specimens such as sputum and exudate, which usually contain contaminating organisms, should be collected as aseptically as possible and processed immediately.

When attempting to obtain a diagnosis from sputum specimens, multiple specimens should be collected, preferably on consecutive days. As indicated above for yeasts, the subject's mouth should be thoroughly cleansed before the specimen is collected.

Because of the hyphal growth in tissue, aspergilli are usually not recovered from blood, spinal fluid or urine. If the specimen must be stored before processing, it should be kept refrigerated at 4–5 C, but storage time should be minimal, since many *Aspergillus* species can grow at this temperature. Specimens should *not* be frozen.

Diagnostic procedures

Direct examination of clinical specimens. Small portions of the specimen should be observed directly for the presence of hyphae or hyphal elements. Opaque specimens should be clarified with 10% KOH (see section on candidiasis). Tissue should be stained by the PAS and methenamine silver method. Sputum and other transparent exudates may be observed directly or stained by the lactophenol cotton blue method.

Aspergilli grow *in vivo* in the hyphal form only; therefore, if the fungus is growing in the specimen, it will appear as branching, septate hyphae, 5–6 μm in diameter. The hyphae may appear pleomorphic and have enlarged, rounded segments. Often, the hyphal growth will fragment and be distributed throughout the specimen.

Culture methods. The aspergilli grow well on all enriched laboratory media. The medium of choice for isolation and preliminary identification of these fungi from clinical specimens is Sabouraud agar. Plated media should be used when culturing specimens that are likely to contain mixed flora. *Aspergillus* species grow relatively rapidly on Sabouraud agar, with colonies appearing in 3–4 days when incubated at 25–30 C. As indicated above, colonial morphology and pigmentation vary greatly depending on the species. All aspergilli produce septate hyphae and conidiophores enlarged at the tips to form vesicles; the latter are covered with sterigmata, which in turn bear chains of conidia.

The criteria for identifying an isolate include: colony texture; color; rate of growth; conidiophore morphology, including the number of rows of sterigmata; conidial characters, relative to size, shape, and arrangement on heads; and characteristics, of any cleistothecia and ascopores. These characteristics, as exhibited on Czapek-Dox agar, are essential for speciation.

The monograph by Raper and Fennel on *The Genus Aspergillus* (55) should be consulted for a detailed description of all the groups and species. Other references containing less detailed keys may also be useful (12, 20, 57).

Serologic procedures. Patients with allergic aspergillosis and aspergillomas usually have serum precipitins (11). The numbers of precipitin bands vary from one to four or more. Few or no precipitin bands are found in patients with invasive aspergillosis; however, these patients are usually anergic. Results of complement fixation tests usually agree with those of the immunodiffusion test and may be obtainable earlier in the course of the disease (11, 52, 67).

Evaluation of laboratory findings

Since aspergilli can readily be isolated from the environment, and infection by these fungi is usually in a compromised host, the presence of these fungi in clinical specimens must be interpreted cautiously. Unless the aspergilli are observed growing in tissue, there is always some doubt as to the etiologic status of the fungus.

When an infection is suspected and the organism is isolated from sputum or other specimens that may contain transient aspergilli, results of serologic tests may be helpful. Demonstration of precipitins or complement-fixing antibodies to aspergilli indicates active disease and gives added weight to the importance of isolating the fungus from clinical specimens. Multiple isolations of aspergilli, even without positive serology, should warrant a call to the patient's physician to determine the former's clinical and immunological status.

Zygomycosis

Zygomycosis is the preferred name for a group of diseases caused by several species of fungi assigned to the class Zygomycetes.

Under an obsolete system of classification, the Zygomycetes were included in the class Phycomycetes. The latter class included a wide variety of fungi with fundamental differences. Recognizing these differences, modern mycologists reclassified the members of the class Phycomycetes into six new classes (4). The class Zygomycetes was created to accommodate most fungi that have an aseptate mycelium and form zygospores. A disease caused by Zygomycetes should thus properly be referred to as zygomycosis.

Zygomycetes cause several different types of infection in man: rhinocerebral, pulmonary, and subcutaneous zygomycosis, and rhinozygomycosis entomophthorae. Each of these diseases is caused by its own characteristic etiologic agent.

Rhinocerebral zygomycosis is a fungal infection of the paranasal sinuses, the meninges and the brain. It is one of the most fulminating of mycotic diseases. Death may occur within 2 to 10 days following infection. Most cases have occurred among people with diabetic ketoacidosis; however, these fungi can also cause disease among other types of patients (1, 46). Symptoms include unilateral headaches, diplopia, proptosis of the eyes, and lethargy. Lesions frequently develop in the palate, pharynx, and nasal mucosa. Through local extension and intravascular invasion, the disease spreads to the meninges and the brain.

To date only two species of fungi have been proven responsible for this acute mycotic disease: *Rhizopus arrhizus* Fischer 1892 and *Rhizopus oryzae* Went and Geerlings 1895. These two zygomycetes exist as free-living saprophytes in nature. When most people inhale their spores, the fungi do not develop and are eliminated from the body. However, in some diabetics, favorable conditions for the germination and phenomenal growth of these fungi are present, and they quickly invade the nasopharyngeal area and attack the meninges and the brain (7).

Primary pulmonary zygomycosis is rare. It is usually diagnosed at autopsy by the presence of wide mycelium in the tissues.

Subcutaneous zygomycosis is a tropical disease of Africa, Asia, and Latin America caused by *Basidiobolus meristosporus* Dreschsler 1955. This fungus invades subcutaneous tissues and the fascia of muscles. The most frequently involved areas of the body are the arms, buttocks, chest, and neck. The infected areas become indurated and swollen. Although some cases heal spontaneously, others may persist for several years.

B. meristosporus is commonly found in decaying vegetation and in chameleon and turtle feces. Infection is apparently contracted when the skin comes in contact with soil contaminated by the spores or mycelium of this fungus.

Rhinozygomycosis entomophthorae is a modification of the name given by Martinson and Clark (45) to subcutaneous infections caused by *Entomophthora coronata* (Constantin 1897) Kevorkian 1937. This benign disease is characterized by nasal obstruction. The infection apparently starts in the inferior turbinate, then spreads to the submucosa and paranasal sinuses, palate, cheek, pharynx, nasal dorsum, and upper lip. The lesions of the face are smooth or lobulated tumors.

E. coronata infections are apparently contracted from inhaling spores. This fungus is widely distributed in nature and has been isolated from garden and forest soils. Human infections have been reported from Africa and the Caribbean area. Equine infections known to occur in the United States are characterized by the development of chronic granulomatous lesions of the nose and lips.

Collection and processing of specimens

Biopsy specimens are the most satisfactory type for detecting and culturing the etiologic agents. Exudates from the nasal sinuses and oral lesions can be obtained from patients with rhinocerebral zygomycosis.

Direct examination of clinical specimens. Direct examinaiton of smears or histological sections will reveal the presence of broad (6–15 μm in diameter), aseptate mycelial fragments of varying length. The mycelium is best observed with the hematoxylin and eosin stain. The Gridley and other fungus stains are not as satisfactory, although of value.

Culture procedures. The zygomycetes involved in these diseases can usually be readily isolated. Adding chloramphenicol to isolation media is recommended to prevent growth of contaminating bacteria. Cycloheximide cannot be used, as it inhibits the growth of zygomycetes.

R. arrhizus and *R. oryzae* grow rapidly, quickly filling the tube with aerial mycelium. Early growth is grayish white, but as the colony begins to sporulate, the surface becomes yellowish brown.

Microscopic examination will reveal a nonseptate, hyaline mycelium 15–20 μm in diameter. Spores are borne in sporangia at the tips of long sporangiophores.

R. arrhizus bears single or clustered sporangiophores that range from 25–1000 μm in length. The terminal sporangia are 70–250 μm in diameter. They have a columella that varies in form from oval to hemispheric, measuring 30–96 $\times$ 26–112 μm. The sporangiospores are irregularly spherical or oval, are striated, and measure 5.5–6 $\times$ 4.5 μm.

R. oryzae produces clusters of dark sporangiophores (325–700 μm long and 12–16 μm wide) subtended by yellowish-brown rhizoids. These rhizoids bear large spherical sporangia 100–160 μm in diameter. The easily ruptured sporangia release numerous brown spores of striated and irregular form which measure 6–8.5 μm in length and 5–6 μm in width. Within each sporangium is found a flat-domed hyaline columella (45–120 μm in diameter). Good growth is obtained at both 25 C and 37 C.

B. meristosporus is a fast-growing organism which forms a thin glabrous layer of radially folded mycelium on the agar surface. Colony color is gray to pale yellow. The aseptate filaments are 8–20 μm in diameter. As asexual and sexual reproduction progresses, the colony surface is gradually covered with a white growth which is made up of conidiophores, chlamydospores, and zygospores.

Primary globose conidia 20–45 μm in diameter are borne on the inflated tip of a simple, elongated conidiophore 60–200 μm long. The inflated distal end of the conidiophore is 30–60 μm long and 15–30 μm wide. Conidia are forcibly shot off the conidiophore. The primary conidia often function as sporangia. Five to 90 sporangiospores are produced through progressive cleavage of the conidial cytoplasm.

Zygospores result from the union of two contiguous cells in mycelium or conidia. They are globose to elongate, measure 23–35 μm long and 20–32 μm wide, and are surrounded by a smooth slightly yellowish wall 2–3 μm thick. Two beak-shaped remnants of the copulation tubes ornament the zygospores.

B. meristosporus grows at 37 C, in contrast to other members of this genus.

Studies by Greer and Friedman (28) have shown that early workers erred in identifying the etiologic agent of subcutaneous zygomycosis as *B. ranarum.*

E. coronata grows well at room temperature or at 25 C on Sabouraud dextrose agar free of cycloheximide. It does not develop at 37 C. Young colonies on Sabouraud dextrose agar are pale yellow, glabrous, and radially furrowed. The colony surface soon becomes white and powdery.

The mycelium of *E. coronata* (6–15 μm wide) is essentially aseptate; septa rarely form. Simple elongate conidiophores (60–90 μm long and 8–12 μm wide) are produced, on the tips of which are formed single globose conidia (10–20 μm in diameter). These are forcibly discharged and are found stuck to the top of petri dish covers or on the sides of test tube cultures.

The conidia are capable of reproducing secondary conidia either singly or multiply. These secondary conidia are also forcibly discharged from the mother cell. Some conidia rather than replicating themselves develop numerous hair-like appendages.

Zygospore-like spores have been reported, but their true nature has yet to be established (21).

Evaluation of laboratory findings

The presence of broad aseptate mycelium in clinical materials from the nasopharyngeal area should be quickly reported, because it may indicate that the patient has rhinocerebral zygomycosis—the most fulminating and usually fatal mycotic disease known. Prompt diagnosis permits specific therapy which may save the patient's life.

Opportunistic Fungi Infrequently Causing Disease

It is becoming more evident that given the right environment any fungus can cause disease in the severely compromised host. Therefore, it is incumbent on the physician and laboratorian to critically evaluate the isolation of any fungus from clinical specimens from such a patient.

The most frequently isolated fungi have been discussed in detail; however, there are others that, although less frequently isolated, have caused disease in compromised patients.

Trichosporon capitatum and *T. cutaneum* have been documented to cause secondary pulmonary disease and brain abscesses in humans (25, 64, 68). See Tables 56.1 and 56.4 for morphologic and biochemical characteristics.

Geotrichum candidum is frequently isolated from clinical specimens and has been reported as the etiologic agent of secondary infections in humans (57, 62).

Petriellidium (Allescheria) boydii, a fungus commonly found in soil and a frequent cause of mycetoma, has been shown to colonize and invade tissue in patients with residual cavities from tuberculosis and fungal diseases and to cause invasive disease in other compromised hosts (32, 56, 57).

Other fungi reported occasionally to cause secondary infections in the compromised are *Rhodotorula* spp. (48, 54) and *Penicillium* spp. (16).

The methods for isolating and identifying these fungi from clinical specimens are as specified above. As indicated, the presence of these organisms as transient or commensal flora must be ruled out. Multiple observations and isolations of these fungi from carefully collected specimens lend strong support to a diagnosis; however, in most cases, the presence of the organism in tissue must be documented for a definite diagnosis.

Appendix: Media for Identifying Yeasts

a. Cornmeal agar. (for yeast morphology).
   Use commercially available cornmeal agar without dextrose.

b. Serum medium for rapid identification of *Candida albicans*.
   Dispense 0.5 ml of bovine serum, fetal calf serum, or pooled human serum in 10- × 75-mm tubes. Stopper and freeze. Thaw before use. Inoculate with small loopful of culture from a pure colony grown on an unenriched medium. Incubate at 37 C for 2 hr. Withdraw a small portion, and examine microscopically for germ tubes.

c. Christensen's urea medium for urease production by yeast-like fungi.
   1. Dissolve 29 g of urea agar base (Difco) in 100 ml of distilled water. Sterilize by filtration.
   2. Dissolve 15 g of agar in 900 ml of boiling water. Sterilize by autoclaving. Cool to 50 C–55 C, and add 100 ml of urea agar base.
   3. Mix, distribute in tubes, and slant.

d. Carbohydrate assimilation medium (Wickerham).
   Basal medium (10×)

Yeast nitrogen base	6.7 g
Distilled water	100 ml

   Sterilize by filtration, and store in refrigerator.
   1. Prepare 2% sterile agar, and dispense 13.5 ml into tubes. Store in refrigerator.
   2. Prepare assimilation medium by adding 1.5 ml of 10× basal medium to 13.5 ml cooled (50 C) agar. Mix and pour in petri dish.
   3. Immediately add 0.3 ml of suspension of organism to liquid medium in plate.
   4. Mix organism in medium by gently swirling plate.
   5. Allow medium to solidify.
   6. Add carbohydrate disks to surface of medium (maximum of six evenly spaced disks per 100-mm plate).

e. Sugar fermentation media for yeast.
   Basal fermentation broth (Wickerham)

Yeast extract	5.5 g
Peptone	7.5 g
Distilled water	1000 ml

   Add 1 ml of 1.6% aqueous solution of brom-cresol purple.
   1. Place 6-ml quantities into each of 12- × 100-mm screw-capped tubes containing 6- × 50-mm inserts (Durham tubes).
   2. Autoclave.
   3. Add 1 ml of a 6% carbohydrate solution that has been filter sterilized to the base medium. (Use 14% raffinose).

f. Birdseed agar (Staib's medium).

Guizottia abyssinica seeds	70.00 g
(Niger or thistle seed)	
Creatinine	0.78 g
Dextrose	10.00 g
Chloramphenicol	0.05 g
Agar	20.00 g
Distilled water	1.00 liter
Diphenyl	100.0 mg

   1. Grind seed to powder in blender. Add 300 ml of water, mix thoroughly, and autoclave at 115 C for 10 min.
   2. Filter through gauze, and bring volume of filtrate to 1 liter.
   3. Add all ingredients except diphenyl, and autoclave for 15 min.
   4. Cool to 50 C.
   5. Add diphenyl to 10 ml of 95% ethyl alcohol, and aseptically add to medium.
   6. Mix and dispense.

References

1. ABRAMSON E, WILSON D, and ARKY RA: Rhinocerebral phycomycosis in association with diabetic ketoacidosis. Ann Intern Med 66:735–742, 1967
2. AHERN DG, JANNACH JR, et al.: Speciation and densities of yeasts in human urine specimens. Sabouraudia 5:110–119, 1966
3. AISNER J, SCHIMPFF SC, SUTHERLAND JC, YOUNG VM, and WIERNIK PH: *Torulopsis glabrata* infection in patients with cancer: increasing incidence and relationship to colonization. Am J Med 61:23–28, 1976
4. ALEXOPOULOS CJ: Introductory Mycology, 2nd edition. John Wiley & Sons, New York, 1962
5. ARONSON K and SOLTANI K: Chronic mucocutaneous candidiasis: a review. Mycopathologia 60:17–25, 1976
6. Aspergilloma and residual tuberculosis cavities—the results of a resurvey. British Thoracic and Tuberculosis Association Report, 1970
7. BAUER H, AJELLO L, ADAMS E, and USEDA HERNANDEZ D: Cerebral mucormycosis: pathogenesis of the disease. Am J Med 18:822–831, 1955
8. BENNETT JE and BAILEY JW: Control for rheumatoid factor in the latex test for cryptococcosis. Am J Clin Pathol 56:360–365, 1971
9. BINDSCHADLER DD and BENNETT JE: Serology of human cryptococcosis. Ann Intern Med 69:45–52, 1968
10. BODEY GP: Fungal infections complicating acute leukemia. J Chronic Dis 19:667–687, 1966
11. COLEMAN RM and KAUFMAN L: Use of immunodiffusion test in the serodiagnosis of aspergillosis. Appl Microbiol 23:301–308, 1972
12. CONANT NF, SMITH DT, BAKER RD, and CALLAWAY JL: Manual of Clinical Mycology, 3rd edition. WB Saunders Co, Philadelphia, 1971
13. COOKE WB: Some effects of spray disposal of spent sulfite liquor on soil mold populations. Proceedings of Industrial Waste Conference, Purdue Univ, 45:35–48, 1961
14. COOKE WB: Our Mouldy Earth. U.S. Dept. Interior, Federal Water Pollution Control Admin, Cincinnati, Ohio, 1971
15. DENTON JF and DiSALVO AF: The prevalence of cryptococcus in various natural habitats. Sabouraudia 6:213–217, 1968
16. DiSALVO AF, FICKLING AM, and AJELLO L: Infection caused by *Penicillium marneffi*. Am J Clin Pathol 60:259–263, 1973
17. EMMONS CW: Isolation of *Cryptococcus neoformans* from soil. J Bacteriol 62:685–690, 1951
18. EMMONS CW: Saprophytic sources of *Cryptococcus neoformans* associated with the pigeon (Columba livia). Am J Hyg 62:227–232, 1955
19. EMMONS CW: Natural occurrence of opportunistic fungi. Lab Investigations 11 (Part 2):1026–1032, 1962
20. EMMONS CW, BINFORD CH, UTZ JP, and KWON-CHUNG KJ: Medical Mycology, 3rd edition. Lea and Febiger Pub, Philadelphia, 1977
21. EMMONS CW and BRIDGES CH: *Entomophthora coronata*, the etiologic agent of phycomycosis in horses. Mycologia 53:307–312, 1961
22. FINDLEY GH and ROUX HF: Skin manifestations in disseminated aspergillosis. Br J Dermatol 85:94–97, 1971
23. FRANKLIN WG, SIMON AB, and SODEMAN TM: Candida myocarditis without valvulitis. Am J Cardiol 38:924–928, 1976
24. GALLIS HA, BERMAN RA, CATE TR, HAMILTON JD, GUNNELLS JC, and STICKELS DL: Fungal infection following renal transplantation. Arch Intern Med 135:1163–1172, 1975
25. GEMEINHARDT H: The pathogenicity of *Trichosporon capitatum* in lungs of man. Zentralbl Bakteriol Parasitenkd Infektionskr 196:121–133, 1965
26. GOLBERT TM and PATTERSON R: Pulmonary allergic aspergillosis. Ann Intern Med 72:395–403, 1970
27. GORDON MA and VEDDER DK: Serologic tests in diagnosis and prognosis of cryptococcosis. J Am Med Assoc 197:961–967, 1968
28. GREER DL and FRIEDMAN L: Studies on the genus *Basidiobolus* with classification of the species pathogenic for man. Sabouraudia 4:231–241, 1966
29. GRIMLEY PM, WRIGHT LD JR, and JENNINGS AE: *Torulopsis glabrata* infection in man. Am J Clin Pathol 43:216–223, 1955
30. GROSSMAN M: Aspergillosis of bone. Br J Radiol 48:57–59, 1975

31. GURWITH MH, STINSON EB, and REMINGTON JS: Aspergillus infection complicating cardiac transplantation: report of five cases. Arch Intern Med 128:541–545, 1971
32. HAINER JW, OSTROW JH, and MACKENZIE DWR: Pulmonary monosporiosis: report of a case with precipitating antibody. Chest 66:601–603, 1974
33. HAMMERMAN KJ, POWELL KE, and TOSH FE: The incidence of hospitalized cases of systemic mycotic infections. Sabouraudia 12:33–45, 1974
34. IRANI FA, DOLOVICH J, and NEWHOUSE MT: Bronchopulmonary and pleural aspergillosis. Am Rev Respir Dis 103:552–553, 1971
35. KAUFFMAN CA and TAN JS: Torulopsis glabrata renal infections. Am J Med 57:217–224, 1974
36. KAUFMAN L and BLUMER S: Value and interpretation of serological tests for the diagnosis of cryptococcosis. Appl Microbiol 16:1907–1912, 1968
37. KIRKPATRICK CH and SMITH TK: Chronic mucocutaneous candidiasis: immunologic and antibiotic therapy. Ann Intern Med 80:310–320, 1974
38. KRUMHOLZ RA: Pulmonary cryptococcosis: a case due to Cryptococcus albidus. Am Rev Respir Dis 105:421–424, 1972
39. LAW EJ, KIM OJ, STIERITZ DD, and MACMILLAN BG: Experience with systemic candidiasis in the burned patient. J Trauma 12:543–552, 1972
40. LEES AW, RAO SS, GARRETT JA, and BOOT PA: Endocarditis due to Torulopsis glabrata. Lancet 1:943–944, 1971
41. LEWIS JL and RABINOVICH S: The wide spectrum of cryptococcal infections. Am J Med 53:315–322, 1972
42. LITTMAN ML and WALTER JE: Cryptococcosis: current status. Am J Med 45:922–932, 1968
43. LODDER J: The Yeasts. N Holland Pub, Amsterdam, 1970
44. MARKS MT, LANGSTON C, and EICKHOFF TC: Torulopsis glabrata, an opportunistic pathogen in man. N Engl J Med 283:1131–1135, 1970
45. MARTINSON FD and CLARK BM: Rhinophycomycosis entomophthorae in Nigeria. Am J Trop Med Hyg 16:40–47, 1967
46. MEYER R, ROSEN P, and ARMSTRONG D: Phycomycosis complicating leukemia and lymphoma. Ann Intern Med 77:871–879, 1972
47. MEYER RD, YOUNG LS, ARMSTRONG D, and YU B: Aspergillosis complicating neoplastic disease. Am J Med 54:6–15, 1973
48. MIRSKY HS and CUTTNER J: Fungal infections in acute leukemia. Cancer 30:1348–1352, 1972
49. MYEROWITZ RL, PAZIN GJ, and ALLEN CM: Disseminated candidiasis: changes in incidence, underlying diseases and pathology. Am J Clin Pathol 68:29–38, 1977
50. NOTTEBART HC, MCGEHEE RF, and UTZ JP: Cryptococcus neoformans osteomyelitis: case report of two patients. Sabouraudia 12:127–132, 1974
51. PARKER JC, MCCLOSKEY JJ, SOLANKI KV, and GOODMAN NL: Candidosis: the most common post-mortem cerebral mycosis in an endemic fungal area. Surg Neurol 6:123–128, 1976
52. PEPYS J, RIDDELL RW, CITRON KM, CLAYTON YM, and SHORT EI: Clinical and immunologic significance of Aspergillus fumigatus in the sputum. Am Rev Respir Dis 80:167–180, 1959
53. PLOUFFE JF, BROWN DG, SILVA J JR, ECK T, STRICOF RL, and FEKETY FR: Nosocomial outbreak of Candida parapsilosis fungemia related to intravenous infusions. Arch Intern Med 137:1686–1689, 1977
54. PORE RS and CHEN J: Meningitis caused by Rhodatorula. Sabouraudia 14:331–335, 1976
55. RAPER KB and FENNEL DI: The Genus Aspergillus. Williams & Wilkins Co, Baltimore, Md, 1965
56. REDDY PC, CHRISTIANSON CS, GORELICK DF, and LARSH HW: Pulmonary monosporosis: an uncommon pulmonary mycotic infection. Thorax 24:722–726, 1969
57. RIPPON JW: Medical Mycology, The Pathogenic Fungi and The Pathogenic Actinomycetes. WB Saunders Co, Philadelphia, 1974
58. RODRIQUES RJ, SHINYA H, WOLF WL, and PUTTLITZ D: Torulopsis glabrata fungemia during prolonged intravenous alimentation therapy. N Engl J Med 284:540–543, 1971
59. ROSE HD and STUART JL: Mycotic aneurysm of the thoracic aorta caused by Aspergillus fumigatus. Chest 70:81–84, 1976

60. SCHROTER GPJ, TEMPLE DR, HUSBERG BS, WEIL R, and STARZL TE: Cryptococcosis after renal transplantation: report of ten cases. Surgery 79:268–277, 1976
61. SEELIG MS, SPOTH CP, KOZINN PJ, TONI EF, and TASCHDJIAN CL: Candida endocarditis after cardiac surgery, clues to early detection. J Thorac Cardiovasc Surg 65:583–601, 1973
62. SHEEHY TW, HONEYCUTT BK, and SPENCER T: Geotrichum septicemia. J Am Med Assoc 235:1035–1037, 1976
63. STENDERUP A and PEDERSON GT: Yeasts of human origin. Acta Pathol Microbiol Scand 54:462–472, 1962
64. TASCHDJIAN C, KOZIN PJ, and TONI EF: Opportunistic yeast infections, with special reference to candidiasis. Ann NY Acad Sci 174:606–622, 1970
65. VALDIVIESO M, LUNA M, BODEY GP, RODRIGUEZ V, and GROSCHEL D: Fungemia due to *Torulopsis glabrata* in the compromised host. Cancer 38:1750–1756, 1976
66. WALTER JE and JONES RD: Serodiagnosis of clinical cryptococcosis. Am Rev Respir Dis 97:275–282, 1968
67. WALTER JE and JONES RD: Serologic tests in diagnosis of aspergillosis. Dis Chest 53:729–735, 1968
68. WATSON KC and KALLICHURUM K: Brain abscess due to *Trichosporon cutaneum*. J Med Microbiol 3:191–193, 1970
69. WILLIAMS DM, KRICK JA, and REMINGTON JS: Pulmonary infection in the compromised host. Am Rev Respir Dis 114:359–394, 1976
70. YOUNG RC, BENNETT JE, GEELHOED GW, and LEVINE AS: Fungemia with compromised host resistance: a study of 70 cases. Ann Intern Med 80:605–612, 1974
71. YOUNG RC, BENNETT JE, VOGEL CL, CARBONE PP, and DEVITA VT: Aspergillosis: the spectrum of the disease in 98 patients. Medicine 49:147–173, 1970

Part Five

CHAPTER 57

PARASITOLOGY: INTRODUCTION AND METHODS

James W. Smith, Kenneth W. Walls, Marilyn S. Bartlett,
and Dorothy Mae Melvin

Introduction

Parasitic diseases continue to be a significant problem in the world, particularly in underdeveloped and emerging countries in tropical and subtropical areas (26). In addition, diseases such as malaria (which had been under fairly good control in some areas) are once again increasing in prevalence because control efforts have relaxed and insect vectors have become resistant to insecticides. As worldwide travel by United States citizens has increased and as more foreign nationals visit the United States each year, the opportunities to be exposed to parasites have multiplied.

There are no good figures on the prevalence of parasites in the United States because many parasitic diseases are not reportable. A recent survey of the types of parasites seen in fecal specimens submitted to state public health laboratories (8) gives some index of the relative frequency of different parasites. (Table 57.1). It should be emphasized that these figures are based on those for specimens submitted for parasitic examination because of some clinical suspicion of parasitic diseases; they are not prevalence figures. Data are not available on whether these were infections acquired in the United States or in foreign countries. In addition, laboratories differ in their proficiency in performing parasitology tests, so these figures vary somewhat from state to state. A recent summary of malaria cases in the United States (9) shows that there has been a gradual and continuing increase in the number of malaria cases seen each year.

Review of data from the proficiency testing programs of the Centers for Disease Control and the College of American Pathologists (27) suggests that laboratories have difficulty identifying fecal parasites—particularly the protozoa—although proficiency testing grades have improved in recent years. In addition to problems with laboratory proficiency, physicians are receiving less education in parasitic diseases—with the average time being 7 hr of lecture and 4 hr of laboratory to cover the entire spectrum of parasitic diseases. Ten percent of the students receive no lectures in parasitology. Thus, some physicians may have little knowledge of when to suspect parasitic diseases, which parasitic diseases to suspect, and how to diagnose suspected parasitic diseases. In addition, they may not know the proper types of specimens to obtain and how they are best submitted.

TABLE 57.1—INCIDENCE OF INTESTINAL PARASITES IN 388,745 FECAL SPECIMENS EXAMINED BY STATE HEALTH DEPARTMENT LABORATORIES,* 1976

	NUMBER	% OF SPECIMENS[†]	% OF ALL IDENTIFICATIONS
Protozoa	48,353		61.1
Giardia lamblia	14,773	3.8	18.7
Entamoeba histolytica	2,486	0.6	3.1
Dientamoeba fragilis	1,588	0.4	2.0
Balantidium coli	21		
Isospora belli	3		
Nonpathogenic	29,482	7.6	37.3
Nematodes	29,107		36.8
Ascaris lumbricoides	9,207	2.4	11.6
Trichuris trichiura	8,796	2.3	11.1
Enterobius vermicularis	7,088	1.8	9.0
Hookworm	3,216	0.8	4.1
Strongyloides stercoralis	757	0.2	1.0
Trichostrogylus sp.	22		
Heterodera sp.	21		
Trematodes	396		0.5
Clonorchis/Opisthorchis	210	0.05	0.3
Schistosoma mansoni	143	0.04	0.2
Fasciolopsis buski	5		
Heterophyes heterophyes	3		
Fasciola hepatica	1		
Metagonimus yokogawai	1		
Paragonimus westermani	1		
Cestodes	1,205		1.5
Hymenolepis nana	946	0.2	1.2
Taenia sp.	209	0.5	0.3
T. solium	6		
T. saginata	45		
Taenia sp. unknown	158	0.04	0.2
Hymenolepis diminuta	23		
Diphylloboththrium latum	25		
Dipylidium caninum	2		

* Adapted from Center for Disease Control: Intestinal Parasite Surveillance Annual Summary 1976, Issued August 1977. Does not include laboratories in Guam, Puerto Rico, or Virgin Islands.

† Percentages are not calculated for parasites identified less than 100 times.

In most instances, the diagnosis of a parasitic infection must be confirmed in the laboratory, usually by demonstrating a stage of the parasite in a specimen from the patient and identifying the parasite based on morphologic characteristics. In some instances, serologic tests or culture procedures may be helpful. Serologic procedures are particularly helpful for parasitic diseases in which tissue is invaded.

In this chapter, we outline the laboratory procedures commonly used for diagnosing parasitic infections and refer to other more specialized procedures which may be used in specific clinical situations. We do not attempt to give a detailed history of each parasite and disease, because such a discussion is beyond the scope of this chapter, and the material is available in many other excellent text books of parasitology or tropical medicine (3, 5, 12, 14, 16, 17, 18, 20, 37). Pathology has also been covered thoroughly in other publications (4, 11, 19, 32). The brief outline of parasites and the diseases they cause emphasizes the types of specimens to examine, the ways to examine the specimens, and the criteria for identifying the parasites.

Serology of Parasitic Infections

Serologic tests are particularly useful in diagnosing parasitic infections which are not readily diagnosed by morphologic examination of blood or feces. A wide variety of serologic tests have been described which vary in sensitivity and specificity depending on the type of test and the antigen used. Different tests may vary in the duration of infection before positive results can be detected and in the rate at which antibody disappears. Laboratories performing serologic tests for parasitic diseases should use accepted procedures with appropriate controls and should thoroughly test procedures before performing them on clinical specimens. Interpretive criteria will depend on the exact test used.

Criteria for interpreting various commercial tests should be based on the manufacturer's information and on literature specific for that test. Values mentioned in this book are shown in Table 57.2 and are for the tests performed at the Centers for Disease Control (CDC); they are not necessarily the same as those for various commercial tests. As with other serologic tests, it is ideal to be able to demonstrate a fourfold rise in titer in paired specimens, but many parasitic infections may be chronic and such a rise cannot be demonstrated. In these instances, a single titer measurement must be used as a diagnostic criterion. The tests most widely used in this country by diagnostic laboratories are those for toxoplasmosis, amebiasis, and trichinosis; commercial reagents are available for these and some additional tests. Most other serologic tests are available from the CDC. Serum specimens sent to the CDC must be submitted through the state health department laboratories; in urgent situations, the CDC can be requested to report results by telephone.

Newer methods of serodiagnosis are rapidly being developed and may make it easier to perform serologic tests for parasitic disease as well as to interpret the results obtained with them. Specific details for performing serologic tests are not included here, but the reader is referred to original articles or reference texts.

Numerous serologic procedures have been suggested for serodiagnosis of parasitic infections. Of these, complement fixation (CF), indirect hemagglutination (IHA), and indirect immunofluorescence (IIF) are widely used because they can be adapted to test nearly every infection for which an antigen is available. An enzyme-linked immunosorbent assay (ELISA) is being increasingly used, and counterelectrophoresis (CEP) or double diffusion is useful for some infections.

Complement fixation, once the most popular method, is rapidly being replaced because of major drawbacks associated with it. Both the complement and the red blood cells used in the test are labile and easily affected by adverse conditions. Also, many substances are anticomplementary and interfere with the test. However, CF remains a useful procedure for some parasitic diseases, apparently measuring different antibodies than those detected with IHA or IIF. CF may be useful for diagnosing acute disease such as Chagas' disease or toxoplasmosis. In general, CF titers rise slightly later than those measured with other tests and revert to negative or minimal levels sooner. The results of CF in conjunction with those of another test may indicate that the infection is acute.

The microcomplement fixation test as described by Casey et al. (6) is perhaps the most commonly used procedure in the United States. CF requires more training and experience than other serologic tests, and some general considerations must be taken into account when CF is used to test for any infectious agent. The patient's serum must be clear and not hemolyzed. Icteric or lipidic sera will frequently be anticomplementary. Antigens are frequently difficult to prepare. The amount of antigen necessary is relatively large; consequently, extraneous materials such as growth media or tissue components frequently contaminate the specific antigen and may cause anticomplementary activity or contribute to cross-reactions and nonspecific reactions. In laboratories which

TABLE 57.2—THE TEST OF CHOICE AND SIGNIFICANT TITERS FOR SELECTED PARASITIC INFECTIONS AS PERFORMED AT THE CENTER FOR DISEASE CONTROL

	IHA	BFT	IIF	CF	DAT	OTHERS
Amebiasis	1:128					
Ascariasis						1:32—ELISA
Chagas disease				1:32		
Cysticercosis	1:128					
Echinococcosis	1:128					
Filariasis	1:128*	1:5*				
Leishmaniasis					1:64	
Malaria			1:64			
Paragonomiasis				1:16		
Pneumocystosis			1:16			
Schistosomiasis			Pos			
Strongyloidiasis	1:64					
Toxocariasis						1:32—ELISA
Toxoplasmosis			1:256			
Trichinosis		1:5				

* Both must be positive.
IHA—indirect hemagglutination
BFT—bentonite flocculation
IIF—indirect immunofluorescence
CF—complement fixation
DAT—direct agglutination
ELISA—enzyme linked immunosorbent assay

are too warm (as in tropical areas without air conditioning), there may be false hemolysis of erythrocytes or inactivation of complement. Finally, accurate determination of end point is usually by the subjective interpretation of the degree of hemolysis. Fortunately, if the test is properly performed, most of these problems may be overcome. In addition to being the test of choice for Chagas' disease and paragonomiasis, CF is still regularly used to test for schistosomiasis, amebiasis, and toxoplasmosis.

In the IIF test, antigen on microscope slides is used to bind antibody. The slide is reacted with fluorescein-conjugated antihuman globulin which binds to attached antibody and is detected microscopically by the fluorescence. Although somewhat simpler to perform than CF, IIF has two major disadvantages. For relatively large numbers of specimens, the latter is more time-consuming to perform because serum dilutions must be prepared and transferred to spots on microscope slides, and each dilution must be read visually under an ultraviolet microscope. In addition, the determination of the end point is subjective.

Procedural problems are not as numerous with IIF as with CF. The condition of the patient's serum is not critical; neither minor hemolysis nor bacterial growth interferes with the reaction. As a result, specimens collected under adverse conditions in the field or blood specimens collected on filter paper are adequate.

The antigens used for IIF can be less refined than those needed for CF and may consist of whole organisms or microtome sections of adult worms. The type of fluorescence or the portion of the antigen which fluoresces may indicate the stage of infection or may signal a nonspecific reaction or cross-reaction which could not be identified with other procedures. The disadvantage of IIF antigens is that they must be visualized, which means that extracts or fractionated antigens cannot be used. Two new methods, the defined antigen substrate spheres (DASS) (10) and a dip-stick fluorescent immunoassay (FIAX) (36), allow soluble antigens to be attached to a fixed substrate which can then be visualized or fluorometrically measured when reacted in a modified IIF test. These tests may make possible the use of purified, fractionated antigens in the immunofluorescence procedure. Fluorescein conjugated antihuman globulins need only react specifically with human globulin, be reasonably potent, and not react with the antigen being used in the test. Virtually all commercial products meet these criteria. In some situations, it is desirable to measure antibody of a single class—IgG, IgM, or IgA. The conjugates needed are more difficult to prepare, and the available products should be carefully screened to assure specificity and potency. Results of IIF testing generally are sensitive, specific, and reproducible.

Passive agglutination tests with particles such as bentonite, erythrocytes, or latex spheres which have been coated with antigen are widely used. Perhaps the simplest and most adaptable procedure in parasitic serology is the IHA test in which erythrocytes are coated with antigen and agglutinate in the presence of antibody. Few reagents are required, and the variables are few and easily identified. The condition of the patient's serum is not critical, and hemolysis and minor bacterial contamination have little effect on the reaction. The presence of complement or occasionally therapeutic agents may cause the serum to hemolyze or agglutinate the carrier erythrocytes. Heat inactivation of the serum should solve the former problem, but usually the problems resulting from therapy can only be overcome by testing a second specimen.

Various erythrocytes have been used. Sheep erythrocytes have most commonly been used but have the disadvantage that many infectious diseases and other conditions cause the development of "heterophile" antibodies which cause nonspecific agglutination of the sheep erythrocytes. Human O, Rh+ erythrocytes are frequently used to overcome this nonspecific agglutination. Turkey erythrocytes, because of their size and distinct settling patterns, have also been used.

The reactivity of the erythrocytes and the settling patterns are largely dependent upon the presensitization procedure used. With most techniques, the erythrocytes are treated with tannic acid to change the surface characteristics of the erythrocytes and permit better adsorption of antigens. Too much tannic acid causes the "tanned cells" to autoagglutinate, while too little does not permit proper adsorption of antigens.

One of the major advantages of IHA is that a wide variety of antigens can be used including excretions, secretions, extracts, metabolic products, and fractions of organisms. Since soluble components are adsorbed to the erythrocytes, the antigens can be more highly purified than for IIF and can be smaller molecular units than utilized in CF. Unfortunately, not all antigens will adequately adsorb to the erythrocytes, and some may cause autoagglutination.

Other procedures such as bentonite flocculation, cholesterol-lecithin agglutination, and direct agglutination have been used for specific diseases but have not been as universally accepted as CF, IIF, and IHA.

Methods for Parasite Detection

General Considerations

Many types of specimens can be submitted for parasitic examination. The most common are fecal specimens for helminths and protozoa, perianal preparations for *Enterobius* (pinworm) eggs, and blood films for malaria, trypanosomes, and microfilariae. Proper type(s) of specimens must be appropriately collected at the proper time to allow identification of the suspected parasite. Other specimens which can be used for examination include sputum, urine, vaginal or urethral swabs, aspirates, cerebrospinal fluid, sigmoidoscopic material, and tissue. Methods for collecting them will not be described in this chapter; instead, the reader is referred to manuals (15, 22, 35) and parasitology texts (3, 5, 12, 14, 16–18, 20, 37).

Fecal Specimens for Intestinal Parasites

Collection of fecal specimens

Feces should be collected in clean dry containers with close-fitting lids (e.g., cardboard ice cream cartons). Specimens should not be contaminated with water, urine, or soil. Such contamination can cause diagnostic forms to degenerate or introduce free-living organisms which may confuse diagnosis.

Specimens containing bismuth, barium, or mineral oil are unsatisfactory, as are specimens obtained after the subject has taken antidiarrheal or antacid compounds. Specimens should not be collected for at least 1 week after such medications are used. Antibiotic therapy may lower the numbers of detectable protozoa, especially amebae. Specimen containers should be labeled with patient identification and time of passage.

Multiple specimens should be collected because some parasites are passed intermittently. Usually three specimens collected at 2- to 3-day intervals are adequate.

Collection of purged specimens

If possible, normally passed stools should be collected and examined before using purgatives; however, purged specimens may be useful for recovering protozoa. Saline cathartics such as sodium sulfate or buffered phosphosoda should be used for purgation. All samples obtained with the aid of a purgative should be collected and submitted for examination immediately. The laboratory should be notified before the subject is given the purgative.

Handling fecal specimens

Specimens should be delivered to the laboratory and examined as soon after collection as possible—preferably within 2 hr. The time interval between passage and examination is most critical for soft or liquid specimens, because they are most likely to contain trophozoite stages which degenerate quickly. If greater delay is unavoidable, specimens should be preserved in a fixative such as polyvinyl alcohol (PVA) fixative. Formed feces can be held at room temperature or refrigerated prior to examination. Fecal specimens should never be placed in an incubator because the heat speeds the rate at which the parasites degenerate.

A two-vial preservation technique (one vial of 10% Formalin and one of PVA-fixative) is valuable not only for specimens that must be mailed to the laboratory but for those collected in hospitals and clinics in which there may be delays in transporting specimens to the laboratory and examining them. One part of feces is thoroughly mixed with 3 parts of 10% buffered Formalin and another portion is thoroughly mixed with 3 parts PVA-fixative. The PVA-fixative contains Schaudinn's fixative and polyvinyl alcohol (a synthetic resin) as an adherent.

Representative portions and portions of the specimen which contain mucus or blood should be mixed well with the fixatives in order to preserve any organisms which might be present. Specimens should be examined macroscopically for adult forms such as proglottids and for mucus or blood. The consistency of the specimen should be noted (liquid, soft, formed).

Preparation of wet mounts

With fresh specimens—especially soft or liquid ones—prepare direct wet mounts to look for motile trophozoites. Wet mounts can also be prepared from Formalin-fixed specimens and from concentrates obtained by various concentration techniques. In the latter instances protozoan cysts and helminth eggs and larvae can be detected, but these methods are not satisfactory for detecting protozoan trophozoites.

To prepare a wet mount, a bit of specimen should be removed with an applicator stick and mixed in a drop of physiological saline on a 2- × 3-inch glass slide. A second portion can be mixed with a drop of iodine (e.g., that of Dobell and O'Connor or Lugol's diluted 1:5). Cover each with a #1 thickness, 22 mm² coverslip. Mounts can be sealed with a petroleum jelly-paraffin mixture (Vaspar) to retard drying and allow oil immersion to be used if needed. The density should be such that newspaper print can just be read through the mount.

Saline and iodine mounts are also prepared from the concentrate as described above.

Examination of wet mounts

Wet mounts should be systematically scanned with a 10× or 20× objective covering the entire preparation. Higher magnifications (40× or 100× objectives) may be necessary in order to identify protozoan cysts.

Saline wet mounts of fresh feces are particularly useful for detecting motile organisms such as larvae or protozoan trophozoites. The type of motility of flagellate trophozoites is often sufficient to determine species. Motility of amebic trophozoites can also be evaluated in this type of mount, but permanent stains are usually necessary for detailed morphologic study and species identification. Protozoan cysts can often be more readily detected in unstained saline mounts because of their refractility; however, stained preparations (either temporary iodine stains or permanent stains) are needed to see morphologic details. On the other hand, helminth eggs can best be identified from unstained mounts; stains tend to obscure characteristics of eggs.

Unstained wet mounts of Formalin-fixed feces are also useful in detecting and identifying helminth eggs and larvae and in detecting protozoan cysts. Chromatoid bodies, fibrils, and sometimes nuclei can be seen in Formalin-fixed cysts, but iodine stains are usually needed for observing nuclear structure. Iodine stains the nuclei and fibrils of cysts but does not stain chromatoid bodies. Glycogen stains brown or red-brown. Cysts are less refractile in iodine mounts than in saline or unstained mounts and may be more readily overlooked.

Protozoan trophozoites can sometimes be recognized in Formalin-fixed material and, in the case of flagellates, can be identified on the basis of visible morphology. However, amebic trophozoites cannot be reliably identified in this type of mount and permanent stains are necessary.

Fecal Concentration Procedures

Various fecal concentration procedures have been described. They allow easier detection of parasite forms by decreasing the amount of background material and by concentrating the parasites on the basis of differences in specific gravity of the parasite forms and the fecal material. The two general methods involve sedimentation (in which parasites are concentrated in the sediment by gravity or centrifugation) and flotation (in which parasites float on a solution of high specific gravity).

A disadvantage of flotation methods is that the high specific gravity of the solution causes opercula to pop and may cause distortion of protozoan cysts and larvae; however, this can be prevented by first fixing the specimen in formalin as described for the zinc sulfate procedure.

The two methods described here are the Formalin-ether method of Ritchie (24) and a modification of the zinc sulfate flotation method (13) which uses Formalin-fixed feces (1). The Formalin-ether method generally allows good recovery of parasite forms, although *Giardia lamblia* cysts and *Hymenolepis nana* eggs may not concentrate well. The primary disadvantage of this method is that it requires the use of ether, which may present storage and usage hazards. The Formalin-zinc sulfate method allows most parasites to be recovered but is not satisfactory for recovering schistosome eggs and those of certain other species because they do not float; it is also less than ideal for recovering hookworm eggs. However, it has the advantage of providing a clearer background without the grit often found in sedimented specimens. Either method should be satisfactory for routine diagnostic fecal parasitology.

Formalin-ether for fresh specimens

1) Mix a sample of stool about the size of a marble in saline so that the resulting suspension will yield approximately 1 ml of sediment from 10 ml of suspension.
2) Strain 10 ml of suspension through wet cheesecloth into a 15-ml conical centrifuge tube. (Conical paper cups with the tips cut off are convenient funnels).
3) Centrifuge at 2500 rpm (650 $\times$ *g*) for 1–2 min. Decant supernate. Sediment should be approximately 1 ml. If there is not enough sediment, add more suspension from original specimen. If there is too much sediment, resuspend and pour off a portion, add additional saline, and centrifuge again.
4) Resuspend the sediment in fresh saline, centrifuge, and decant.
5) Add about 9 ml of 10% Formalin to the sediment. Mix thoroughly, and allow to stand at least 5 min.
6) Add 3 ml ether, stopper tube, and shake in an inverted position for at least 30 sec. Remove stopper carefully.
7) Centrifuge at 2000 rpm (450–500 $\times$ *g*) for 1–2 min. After centrifugation, there will be four layers (from top to bottom: ether, debris, Formalin, sediment).
8) Ring the debris plug with an applicator stick, and pour off the top three layers. Debris which clings to the sides of the tube can be removed with a cotton-tipped applicator stick.
9) Mix the sediment with the few drops of fluid remaining in the tube, and transfer drops to a slide to make unstained and iodine wet mounts for microscopic examination. Mounts can be sealed with Vaspar if desired.

Formalin-ether for preserved specimens

1) Mix formalinized specimen.
2) Depending upon the amount of specimen, strain a quantity through *wet* gauze into a conical 15-ml tube to give about 0.5 to 0.75 ml of sediment.
3) Add water to make 10 ml of suspension, mix, and centrifuge at 2000 to 2500 rpm (500–650 $\times$ *g*) for 1 to 2 min.
4) Decant supernatant. If desired, wash again. If sediment amount is incorrect, adjust by adding more specimen or pouring off specimen and adding water.
5) Add 9 ml of 10% Formalin, and mix thoroughly.
6) Add 4 ml of ether, stopper tube, and shake in an inverted position for at least 30 sec. Remove stopper with care.
7) Centrifuge at 2000 rpm (450–500 $\times$ *g*) for 1 to 2 min.

8) After centrifugation, there will be four layers (ether, debris, Formalin, sediment). Ring the debris plug with an applicator stick, and pour off the top three layers. Remove debris from sides of tube with a cotton swab.
9) Mix sediment in small amount of fluid remaining in tube. Prepare unstained and iodine wet mounts from sediment for microscopic examination. Mounts can be sealed with Vaspar if desired.

Zinc sulfate flotation

The original zinc sulfate flotation procedure was developed by Faust et al. (13) in 1938 for recovering helminth eggs and larvae and protozoan cysts. Since that time, various modifications have been described. The modified procedure described below is performed with feces-Formalin suspensions which have stood at room temperature at least 30 min.

The specific gravity of the zinc sulfate solution is critical to the efficiency of this technique. It *should* be 1.200 but *must not be* lower than 1.195 nor higher than 1.200.

Place fecal Formalin suspensions in round-bottomed tubes.

1) Centrifuge Formalin-feces suspensions at approximately 1800 rpm (400–450 × g) for 3.5 min. Allow the centrifuge to come to a full stop.
2) Decant the supernatant from each tube, and drain the last drop against a clean section of paper towel.
3) Place the tubes of sediment in a rack which holds them upright and steady.
4) Add zinc sulfate to each tube to within 1 inch of the rim.
5) Using two applicator sticks, mix the packed sediment thoroughly so that no coarse particles remain.
6) Immediately centrifuge at 1500 rpm (400 × g) for 1 min.
7) As soon as the centrifuge stops, carefully transfer the tubes to the rack. Avoid disturbing the surface films, which now contain the floating parasites.
8) Allow the tubes to stand for 1 min.
9) Place a drop of saline and a drop of iodine on a 2- × 3-inch glass slide.
10) With a wire loop which has a horizontal bend, transfer a loop of the surface film to the slide. Deposit next to the drop of saline. Deposit a second loop of the surface film next to the drop of iodine. In making the transfer, carefully touch the surface film, but do not penetrate the surface.
11) Using the heel of the loop, mix first the fecal drop and the saline, then the drop and the iodine.
12) Flame the loop before proceeding to the next tube.
13) Superimpose a clean 22- × 22-mm, No. 1 coverslip on each drop. Avoid trapping air bubbles.
14) Place each prepared slide in a petri dish containing moist paper towel to retard evaporation, or seal with Vaspar.
15) Examine the mounts within an hour. A longer holding period may cause distortion and make identifying some stages more difficult.

Permanent Stains

Either fresh or PVA-fixed feces can be used to prepare fecal smears for staining. If smears are prepared from fresh feces, they must not be allowed to dry before placing in Schaudinn's fixative. Prepare smears by spreading a portion of feces in an even film on a 1- × 3-inch clean glass slide. If the material is too watery to adhere to the slide, a drop of Mayer's albumin or normal (parasite-free) feces can be mixed with the specimen.

Films of PVA-fixed feces are prepared by thoroughly mixing the material before removing the samples. The smear should be spread in an even square so that it extends to the top and bottom edges of the slide to keep the film from peeling. Slides of PVA-fixed material should dry at least 4 hr at 35 C (preferably overnight) before staining.

Staining

The Wheatley modification of the trichrome stain is most widely used in the United States, although hematoxylin stains are used in many laboratories. Trichrome stain has the advantage of using stable reagents and requiring a relatively short time; it is the only stain discussed further here.

Trichrome stain for PVA-preserved feces:
1. Transfer drop of well-mixed sample to center of glass slide.
2. Using an applicator stick, spread uniformly into a rectangle so that smear extends to the sides of the slide.
3. Dry thoroughly, preferably overnight.

Stain Schedule

Reagent	Time	Purpose
1. 70% alcohol plus iodine	10–20 min	Remove mercuric chloride (hydration)
2. 70% alcohol	3–5 min	Remove iodine (hydration)
3. 70% alcohol	3–5 min	Wash (hydration)
4. Trichrome stain	6–8 min	Stain
5. 90% alcohol acidified	5–10 sec	Destain
6. 95% alcohol	Rinse	Stop destaining
7. 95% alcohol	5 min	Dehydration
8. Carbol-xylene	10 min	Clearing and dehydration
9. Xylene	10 min	Clearing

Trichrome stain for fresh unpreserved fecal smears:
1. Prepare thin uniform smears; mix a portion of firm feces in saline before smearing; apply an adhesive such as serum, egg albumin, or uncontaminated feces before smearing watery specimens.
2. Place fresh smears immediately into Schaudinn's fixative. Do not allow to dry. Smears should fix for at least 1 hr at room temperature or for 5 min at 50 C; however, they can be left in fixative for several days.
3. Stain as described for PVA-fixed fecal smears except use times as noted below.

1) Schaudinn's fixative	5 min at 50 C or 1 hr at room temp
2) 70% alcohol plus iodine	1 min
3) 70% alcohol	1 min
4) 70% alcohol	1 min
5) Trichrome stain	2–8 min
6) 90% alcohol acidified	Brief dip
7) 95% alcohol	Rinse
8) 95% alcohol	Rinse
9) Carbol-xylene	1 min
10) Xylene	1–3 min

Trichrome stains should be examined with an oil immersion objective. Specimens can be screened with a 50x oil immersion objective, but identification should be made with the 100x objective.

Trichrome Stain Reaction The appearance of trichrome-stained fecal films varies with the specimen, thickness of the smear, and age of the stain used. Nuclear structures and cytoplasm should be readily differentiated. Usually chromatin stains red to red-purple, and cytoplasm stains green to blue. Inclusions in cytoplasm may stain green to red. Background material usually stains green to blue-green.

Egg Counts

Egg counts have been used to estimate the intensity of infection with helminths which have a relatively constant output of eggs. Although developed primarily for estimating hookworm burden, egg counts have been used for other nematodes including *Ascaris* and *Trichuris*. Counts are an estimate at best because the daily output of eggs can vary, and the number of eggs recovered will be affected by the consistency of the specimen and the diet and immune system of the host. Egg counts can be helpful in determining the role of helminth infection in the disease (e.g., anemia) and the desirability of treatment or in assessing the success of treatment. Stoll's egg-counting technique (33) is a dilution technique. Both the standard smear of Beaver (2) and the Kato thick smear (21) depend upon a smear containing a measured amount of feces. If standard smears (2) contain about 2 mg of feces per coverslip, the number of eggs per gram can be estimated by multiplying the number of eggs per coverslip by 500. If no eggs are detected in a 2-mg preparation, the estimate should be reported as < 500 eggs/g. Detailed methods for performing counts are outlined in the Centers for Disease Control manual (22).

Perianal Preparations

Collection of perianal preparations

Perianal preparations are most useful in detecting *Enterobius* (pinworm) infection, although they can also be helpful in diagnosing *Taenia* infections. Either cellulose tape (Fig 57.1) or Vaseline-paraffin swabs can be used. Specimens should be collected between 9 p.m. and midnight or in the early morning before the patient has bathed or defecated. Several specimens should be collected over a number of days to rule out infection, because the female worms may not migrate each day. With one cellulose-tape preparation, only 55% of pinworm infections will be detected (25), although 90% can be diagnosed with three specimens. Persons with more severe infections will have a higher proportion of positive specimens.

Examination of cellulose-tape preparations

Cellulose-tape preparations should be examined with the 10× objective and reduced light. Any finding should be confirmed with the high dry objective. The entire tape (including the edges) should be screened. For easier examination, tape can be cleared with toluene (i.e., pull the tape back, add a drop of toluene, and smooth the tape into position with applicator sticks or a piece of gauze or cotton). *Enterobius* eggs remain viable and infective for weeks, so all specimens must be handled carefully.

Culture Methods for Protozoa

Culture methods for various intestinal, blood, and tissue protozoa have been described (34), although they are not widely used by diagnostic parasitology laboratories in the United States. Many amebae, including *Entamoeba histolytica*, can be grown in various diphasic media which have a slant overlaid with a broth. When inoculated with feces, bacteria are supplied by the inoculum, but when culturing bacteria-free material such as amebic liver abscess drainage, the medium must also be inoculated with bacteria such as *Clostridium perfringens*. Cultural procedures for intestinal protozoa are reviewed in the Centers for Disease Control manual (22). Cultural methods for malaria are research rather than diagnostic procedures, but cultures can aid in diagnosing leishmanial and trypanosomal infections.

Blood Specimens

Collection of blood for thick and thin smears.

Films without an anticoagulant such as those prepared from a finger stick are preferred because staining will be better. Blood containing an anticogulant can be used; however, films should be prepared within 1 hr. Malarial stages in peripheral blood vary in number and type according to the part of the cycle and some specimens contain so few parasites that they may be overlooked; at other times ring forms may predominate and make species identification difficult. The best time to obtain blood for smears is about midway between paroxysms of chills and fever. With suspected *P. falciparum* malaria (especially in the early acute stage), the parasites may be more numerous at the height of fever. Some microfilariae (e.g., *Wuchereria bancrofti)* may be found only at certain times of the day.

Preparation of blood films

Prepare both thick and thin blood films. Use only clean unscratched slides. A thick film should cover an area about the size of a dime and should not be so thick that it will flake off during the staining process. Newspaper print should be readable through a properly made thick film. To prepare a thick film, place two or three small drops of blood on a clean glass slide, and with the corner of another slide swirl or "puddle" the drops into a thick film. Allow the film to dry at room temperature in a horizontal position. Thick films must not be heated because heat will fix the erythrocytes. Thick films can be stained after they dry overnight or at least for several hours.

Thin films should have a large portion which is one cell layer thick, with the erythrocytes slightly separated. Prepare a thin film by placing 1 drop of blood toward the end of a clean glass slide. A second slide held at an acute angle is used to spread the film. Back the spreading slide into the drop of blood, and allow the blood to spread along the width of the slide. With a smooth, even motion, push the spreader slide toward the other end leaving a thin film.

Thin films must be fixed before they are stained. They should be immersed in methyl alcohol for a few seconds and allowed to air dry. Thick films

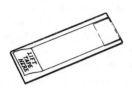

a. Cellulose – tape slide preparation

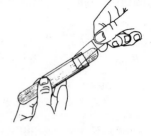

b. Hold slide against tongue depressor one inch from end and lift long portion of tape from slide

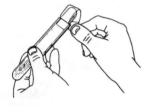

c. Loop tape over end of depressor to expose gummed surface

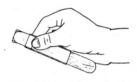

d. Hold tape and slide against tongue depressor

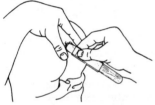

e. Press gummed surfaces against several areas of perianal region

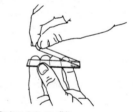

f. Replace tape on slide

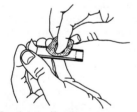

g. Smooth tape with cotton or gauze

Note: Specimens are best obtained a few hours after the person has retired, perhaps at 10 or 11 P.M., or the first thing in the morning before a bowel movement or bath.

Figure 57.1—Use of cellulose-tape slide preparation for diagnosis of pinworm infections (adapted from Brooke, Donaldson, and Mitchell, 1949).

should not be fixed so that the aqueous stain will lyse the unfixed red cells. It is easiest to make thick and thin films on separate slides, although the thick film may be on one end and the thin film on the other. In such combined films, care must be taken not to expose the thick films to alcohol vapors (which might fix them).

Staining of blood films

Giemsa is the preferred stain for blood films because it stains malaria parasites better than does Wright's stain. In addition, Wright's stain (which contains alcohol) cannot be used to stain thick films, whereas the aqueous Giemsa stain allows dehemoglobinization of thick films during the staining process.

For best staining of malarial parasites, blood films should be stained within 2 or 3 days after they are prepared. Erythrocytes in thick films become fixed if staining is delayed too long and will not lyse.

Fresh buffered Giemsa stain should be prepared from stock Giemsa each day. Stock solution is troublesome to make and is best purchased already prepared. Giemsa is prepared with 1 part stock Giemsa and 50 parts phosphate buffered water, pH 7.0–7.2 (add 100 ml of M/15 phosphate buffer, pH 7.0–7.2, to 900 ml of distilled water). Stain 45 min. Rinse thin films briefly in buffered water and air dry. Thick films should be washed for a longer time.

The powers used for examination depend on parasites being looked for. Films should be screened with low power (10×) to detect microfilariae and with 50× oil immersion and 100× oil immersion to detect blood protozoa. Thick films should be examined for no less than 5 min and thin films for no less than 30 min before they are reported to be negative.

Giemsa Stain Reaction.

Giemsa stains leukocyte nuclei purplish-blue and cytoplasm and cytoplasmic granules various colors, depending on the type of leukocyte. Malarial parasites have blue cytoplasm and red to red-violet chromatin. Pigment varies from golden brown to brown to black. Schüffner's stippling appears as fine red or pink granules if the pH of the stain is correct.

Miscellaneous Procedures

Specimens other than those discussed must be treated individually depending on the type of specimen and organisms which may be present (Table 57.3). In most cases, direct preparations should be examined. Fluids should be centrifuged and the sediment examined. Sputum can be examined directly for the presence of *Paragonimus* eggs and can be mixed with PVA-fixative on a slide for later staining to detect the presence of *E. histolytica.* Urine sediment can be examined directly for the presence of *Trichomonas vaginalis* or *Schistosoma haematobium* eggs. Cerebrospinal fluid should be examined in direct wet mounts for the presence of free-living amebae and trypanosomes. Giemsa-stained films can be prepared from various fluids with or without prior centrifugation. Vaginal and urethral swabs, duodenal drainage and aspirates, and sigmoidoscopic material should be examined in direct mounts. Permanent stains can be made from smears of these materials fixed in Schaudinn's fixative, or portions can be preserved in PVA-fixative for later staining. Tissue should be examined with both direct mounts of crushed fragments of the tissue in saline and in stains of impression smears. Histologic sectioning and staining methods can be used for biopsied tissue obtained for diagnosing trichinosis or other tissue parasite infections.

Calibration and Use of an Ocular Micrometer

An ocular micrometer is a disk on which is etched a scale in units from "0" to "50" or "100." In order to determine the micrometer value of each unit in a particular eyepiece and at a specific magnification, the unit must be calibrated with a stage micrometer. A stage micrometer has a scale 2 mm long ruled in fine intervals of 0.01 mm (10 μm).

To calibrate the ocular micrometer

1) Insert the micrometer in the eyepiece so that it rests on the diaphragm with the etched scale facing away from the eye. In many new microscopes, it can be dropped in and secured with a ring retainer. (It is helpful to have an extra ocular in which the micrometer may be left.)
2) Place the stage micrometer on the microscope stage.
3) Focus on the etched scale. Since the micrometer must be calibrated for each objective, begin with the lowest magnification (e.g., 10×).
4) Align the two scales so that the "0" points are superimposed (Fig 57.2)
5) Find a point far down the scales at which a line of the stage micrometer coincides with a line of the ocular micrometer. Count the number of ocular units and the number of stage units from zero to these coinciding lines.
6) Multiply stage micrometer units by 1000 to convert millimeters to micrometers.
7) Divide stage micrometer units by ocular units to determine the value of an ocular unit.

Repeat the calibration for each objective. Keep a record of the unit value for each objective for each microscope used.

To use the micrometer

Insert the eyepiece containing the calibrated ocular micrometer in the microscope. Count the number of ocular units which equal the structure to be measured. Multiply by the micrometer value of the ocular unit for the objective being used. If an ocular micrometer is properly used, parasites which are similar in appearance but different in size can be readily differentiated (Fig 57.3).

Quality Control

The quality control for procedures in the parasitology laboratory is similar to that in other laboratory areas. New reagents should be checked for proper reactivity—preferably in parallel—before being used. Specific gravity of zinc sulfate solutions should be checked and appropriately readjusted at least once a week. Permanent stains of fecal smears should be controlled with a control smear of known staining qualities each time a batch of slides is

TABLE 57.3—NONFECAL SPECIMENS FOR DIAGNOSIS

SPECIMEN	INFECTIOUS AGENT	STAGE
Sputum	*Paragonimus westermani*	Eggs
	Ascaris lumbricoides, hookworm, or *Strongyloides stercoralis* (rare)	Larvae
	Entamoeba histolytica	Trophozoites
Anal swab or cellulose tape preparation	*Enterobius vermicularis*	Eggs
	Taenia spp.	Eggs
Duodenal aspirate	*Strongyloides stercoralis*	Larvae
	Giardia lamblia	Trophozoites
Muscle biopsy	*Trichinella spiralis*	Larvae
Cyst fluid	*Echinococcus granulosus*	Hydatid sand
	Entamoeba histolytica	Trophozoites
Rectal biopsy	*Schistosoma japonicum* or *Schistosoma mansoni*	Eggs
Urine or urinary bladder biopsy	*Trichomonas vaginalis*	Trophozoites
	Schistosoma haematobium	Eggs
Liver biopsy	*Schistosoma* spp.	Eggs
	Nonhuman ascarids (visceral larval migrans)	Larvae
	Entamoeba histolytica	Trophozoites
	Echinococcus granulosus	Hydatid cyst
	Capillaria hepatica	Eggs
	Trypanosoma cruzi	Amastigotes
	Leishmania donovani	Amastigotes
Other tissue biopsy	*Taenia solium*	Cysticercus
	Multiceps multiceps	Coenurus
	Echinococcus granulosus	Hydatid cyst
	Onchocerca volvulus	Adult or microfilaria
	Other filariae	Adult
	Trypanosoma cruzi	Amastigotes
	Entamoeba histolytica	Trophozoites
	Pneumocystis carinii	Cysts and Trophozoites
	Toxoplasma gondii	Cysts and Tachyzoites
	Leishmania	Amastigotes
Cerebrospinal fluid	*Trypanosoma* spp.	Trypomastigotes
	Free-living amebae	Trophozoites
	Toxoplasma gondii	Tachyzoites
Blood	*Plasmodium* spp.	Trophozoites, Schizonts, Gametocytes
	Babesia spp.	Trophozoites
	Toxoplasma gondii (rare)	Tachyzoites
	Leishmania donovani (rare)	Amastigotes
	Filaria species	Microfilariae
	Trypanosoma spp.	Trypomastigotes

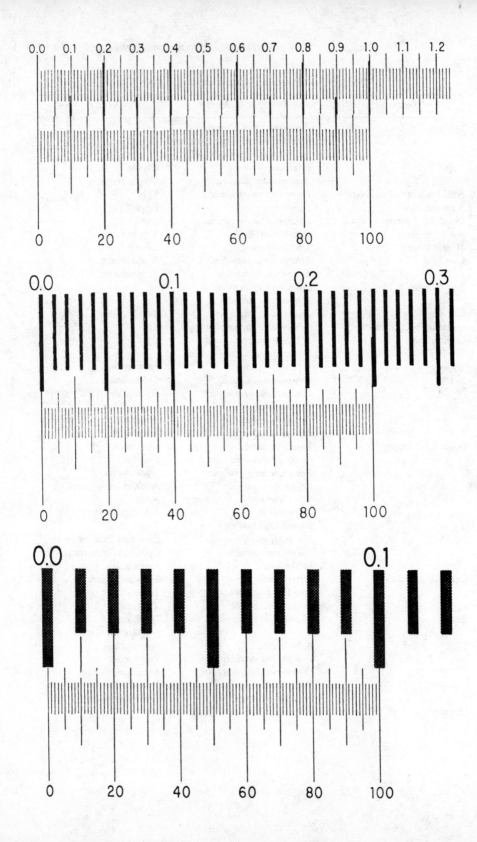

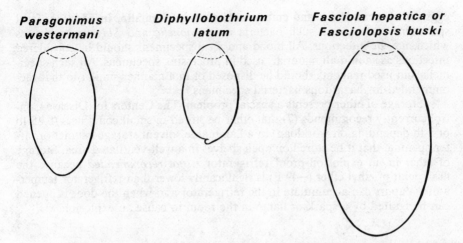

| Paragonimus westermani | Diphyllobothrium latum | Fasciola hepatica or Fasciolopsis buski |

Figure 57.3—Size comparison of *Paragonimus westermani, Diphyllobothrium latum,* and *Fasciola hepatica/Fasciolopsis buski* eggs. Note that these eggs have similar shapes but differ markedly in size. Measuring them with a properly calibrated ocular micrometer would assure accurate identification.

stained. Positive material is recommended, but feces that does not contain parasites can be used. Host cells such as epithelial cells and inflammatory cells in the negative specimen can be used to check the stain quality.

The laboratory should have a set of reference materials which can be reviewed periodically. Positive slides and Formalin-fixed materials are particularly useful but color atlases (23, 31), and collections of color photomicrographs (28, 29, 30) are also helpful. Participation in a proficiency testing program allows an external control of the quality of work performed.

Safety

Many specimens submitted for parasitic examination are potentially infectious. Blood or tissue specimens containing malaria parasites, trypanosomes, *Leishmania* species, or *Toxoplasma* organisms may cause infections if there is a break in the skin. Fresh fecal specimens containing protozoan cysts; trophozoites of *Dientamoeba fragilis;* eggs of *Enterobius vermicularis, Hymenolepis nana,* or *Taenia solium;* or specimens containing filariform larvae of *Strongyloides stercoralis* can be infectious. Older fecal specimens may contain filariform larvae of hookworm, *Strongyloides stercoralis,* or *Trichostrongylus* spp., or embryonated eggs of *Ascaris lumbricoides* or *Trichuris trichiura. Ascaris*

←——————————————————————————————————

Figure 57.2—Calibration of an ocular micrometer. This illustrates the appearance of the ocular micrometer (lower scale) and stage micrometer (upper scale) under low power (top), high dry (middle), and oil immersion (bottom). In these examples, one ocular unit has the following values: low power, 10 μm; high power, 2.5 μm; oil immersion, 1 μm.

eggs sometimes survive and embryonate even in Formalin. In addition, fecal specimens can contain such bacteria as *Salmonella* and *Shigella* or viruses which may be infectious. All blood and fecal specimens should be considered infectious as should all materials used in processing specimens. All such specimens and used reagents should be disposed of in a manner similar to that recommended for hazardous bacterial specimens.

Storage of ether presents a special problem. The Centers for Disease Control currently recommends (7) that ether be stored in small containers (0.25 lb or 1 lb depending on workload) in a flammable solvent storage cabinet or, after opening, that it be stored on open shelves in a well-ventilated area. Storage of ether in an explosion-proof refrigerator *is not recommended* because the flash point of ethyl ether (−49 F) is significantly lower than refrigerator temperature. Vapors can accumulate in the refrigerator and when the door is opened can be ignited by a spark or flame in the room to cause an explosion.

References

1. BARTLETT MS, HARPER K, SMITH N, VERBANAC P, and SMITH JW: Comparative evaluation of a modified zinc sulfate flotation technique. J Clin Microbiol 7:524–528, 1978
2. BEAVER PC: The standardization of fecal smears for estimating egg production and worm burden. J Parasitol 36:451–455, 1950
3. BELDING DL: Textbook of Parasitology, 3rd Edition. Appleton-Century-Crofts, New York, 1965
4. BINFORD CH and CONNER DH (eds.): Pathology of Tropical and Extraordinary Diseases, Vol. I. Armed Forces Institute of Pathology, Washington, DC, 339 pp, 1976
5. BROWN HW: Basic Clinical Parasitology, 4th Edition. Appleton-Century Crofts, New York, 1975
6. CASEY HL: Standardized Diagnostic Complement Fixation Method and Adaptation to Micro Test. Public Health Memo #74. U.S. Govt. Printing Office, 1965
7. CENTER FOR DISEASE CONTROL: Laboratory Safety at the Center for Disease Control. U.S. Dept. of H.E.W., CDC, Atlanta, Ga. D.H.E.W. Publ. no. CEC 76-8118 PI 57-157, 1974
8. CENTER FOR DISEASE CONTROL: Intestinal Parasite Surveillance Annual Summary, 1976. Atlanta, Ga, 1977
9. CENTER FOR DISEASE CONTROL: Malaria Surveillance Annual Summary, 1978. Atlanta, Ga, 1979
10. DEELDER AM and PLOEM JS: An immunofluorescence reaction for *Schistosoma mansoni* using the defined antigen substrate spheres (DASS) system. J Immunol Methods 4:239–251, 1974
11. EDINGTON GM and GILLES HM: Pathology in the Tropics. Edward Arnold Pub, London, 1969
12. FAUST EC, BEAVER PC, and JUNG RC: Animal Agents and Vectors of Human Diseases, 4th Edition. Lea and Febiger, Philadelphia, 1975
13. FAUST EC, D'ANTONI JS, ODOM V, MILLER MJ, PERES C, SAWITZ W, THOMEN LF, TOBIE JE, and WALKER JH: A critical study of clinical laboratory techniques for the diagnosis of protozoan cysts and helminth eggs in feces. Am J Trop Med Hyg 18:169–183, 1938
14. FAUST EC, RUSSELL PF, and JUNG RC: Craig and Faust's Clinical Parasitology, 8th Edition. Lea and Febiger, Philadelphia, 1970
15. GARCIA LS and ASH LR: Diagnostic Parasitology: Clinical Laboratory Manual. 2nd Edition. C.V. Mosby Co, St. Louis, 1979
16. HUNTER GW III, FRYE WW, and SWARTZWELDER JC: Tropical Medicine. 5th Edition. W.B. Saunders Co., Philadelphia, 1976
17. MAEGRAITH B: Adams and Maegraith's Clinical Tropical Diseases, 6th Edition. Blackwell, London, 1976

18. MANSON-BAHR PH: Manson' Tropical Disease 16th Edition. The Williams & Wilkins Co, Baltimore, 1966
19. MARCIAL-ROJAS RA: Pathology of Protozoal and Helminthic Diseases. The Williams & Wilkins Co, Baltimore, 1971
20. MARKELL EK and VOGE M: Medical Parasitology, 4th Edition. W.B. Saunders Co, Philadelphia, 1976
21. MARTIN LK and BEAVER PC: Evaluation of Kato thick-smear technique for quantitative diagnosis of helminth infections. Am J Trop Med Hyg 17:382–391, 1968
22. MELVIN DM and BROOKE MM: Laboratory Procedures for the Diagnosis of Intestinal, Parasites. Center for Disease Control. U.S. Dept. of H.E.W. PB 297958 Natl. Tech. Inform. Serv. Springfield, VA 22161, 1975
23. PETERS W and GILLES HM: A Colour Atlas of Tropical Medicine and Parasitology. Wolfe Medical Publications Ltd, London, 1977
24. RITCHIE LS: An ether sedimentation technique for routine stool examinations. Bull US Army Med Dept 8:326, 1948
25. SADUN EH and MELVIN DM: The probability of detecting infections with *Enterobius vermicularis* by successive examination. J Pediatr 48:438–441, 1956
26. SCHULTZ MG: Current concepts in parasitology. Parasitic diseases. N Engl J Med 297:1259–1261, 1977
27. SMITH JW: Identification of fecal parasites in the special parasitology survey of the College of American Pathologists. Am J Clin Pathol 72:371-373, 1979
28. SMITH JW, ASH LR, THOMPSON JH, MCQUAY RM, MELVIN DM, and ORIHEL TC: Diagnostic Parasitology—Intestinal Helminths. American Society of Clinical Pathologists, Chicago, 1976
29. SMITH JW, MCQUAY RM, ASH LR, MELVIN DM, ORIHEL TC, and THOMPSON JH: Diagnostic Parasitology—Intestinal Protozoa. American Society of Clinical Pathologists, Chicago, 1976
30. SMITH JW, MELVIN DM, ORIHEL TC, ASH LR, MCQUAY RM, and THOMPSON JH: Diagnostic Parasitology—Blood and Tissue Parasites. American Society of Clinical Pathologists, Chicago, 1976
31. SPENCER FM and MONROE LS: The Color Atlas of Intestinal Parasites. Charles C. Thomas Co, Springfield, Ill, 1961
32. SPENCER H, DAYAN AD, GIBSON JB, HUNTSMAN RG, HUTT MSR, JENKINS GC, KOBERLE F, MAEGRAITH BG, and SALFELDER K: Tropical Pathology. Springer-Verlag, New York, 1973
33. STOLL NR: Investigations on the control of hookworm disease. XV. An effective method of counting hookworm eggs in feces. Am J Hyg 3:59–70, 1923
34. TRAGER W: Cultivation of parasites in vitro. Am J Trop Med Hyg 27:216–222, 1978
35. U.S. NAVAL MEDICAL SCHOOL: Medical Protozoology and Helminthology. National Naval Medical Center, Bethesda, Md, 1965
36. WALLS KW and BARNHART ER: Titration of human serum antibodies to *Toxoplasma gondii* with a simple fluorometric assay. J Clin Microbiol 7:234–235, 1978
37. WARREN KS and MAHMOUND AAF (eds.): Geographic Medicine for the Practitioner: Algorithms in the Diagnosis and Management of Exotic Diseases. Univ. of Chicago Press, Chicago, 150 pp, 1978

CHAPTER 58

BLOOD AND TISSUE PARASITES

Dorothy Mae Melvin, Kenneth W. Walls, and James W. Smith

Introduction

The blood and tissue parasites are a diverse group including malaria, he-moflagellates, *Toxoplasma, Pneumocystis, Babesia,* filaria, and *Trichinella.* In addition, the tissues of man may be accidentally parasitized by larval stages of helminths such as *Echinococcus* and *Toxocara* that normally infect lower animals. In the past two decades, free-living amebae have also been found to cause serious tissue damage in humans.

Laboratory procedures for diagnosis of these parasites vary to some degree with the specific body location, the phase or stage of infection, and the growth pattern of the organism.

Protozoa

Malaria

Four species of malaria parasitize man: *Plasmodium vivax, P. falciparum, P. malariae,* and *P. ovale.* In the United States, autochthonous cases of malaria are rare, but over 1900 cases were reported in 1980 among foreign students, immigrants, and Americans who had lived or visited in endemic areas (16), and the number appears to rise each year (Fig 58.1). Occasionally persons transfused with infected blood and drug addicts who have shared needles with infected persons also are infected. The most severe infections are caused by *P. falciparum* and are often fatal if untreated. *P. vivax* infection is most common, followed by *P. falciparum, P. malariae,* and *P. ovale* infection, in that order. Recently, some travelers who were not given prophylactic medicines or failed to take those prescribed have been infected (15).

The life cycles of the four *Plasmodium* species are similar and involve sexual development (sporogony) in the vector and asexual development (schizogony) in humans. The vector for human malaria is a female *Anopheles* mosquito; over 60 species have been incriminated in different parts of the world.

Figure 58.2 shows the basic stages in the life cycle of malaria. Sporozoites, which are the end product of sporogony in the mosquito, are introduced into the human host as the mosquito bites. These forms enter the blood stream and are transported to the liver where they penetrate the parenchymal cells and undergo extensive development and multiplication. This is the exoerythrocytic phase of the cycle and causes no damage or symptoms.

After one complete growth phase, which requires 1 to 2 or more weeks depending on species, the merozoites (end products of asexual growth) are released from the liver cells into the circulating blood and initiate the erythrocytic phase of the malaria life cycle. Although the exoerythrocytic phase in the liver is not cyclic (that is, the merozoites produced do not enter other liver cells) (18), residual organisms (hypnozites) are present in the livers of persons infected with *P. vivax* and *P. ovale.* These residual exoerythrocytic stages are responsible for relapses which may occur with infections with these two species (17). With *P. malariae* and *P. falciparum* infections, residual liver stages are not present, nor do these species cause relapsing illness. However, symptoms may recur, but they stem from subpatent blood infections and are called recrudescences. Recrudescences associated with *P. malariae* infections are

MILITARY AND CIVILIAN CASES OF MALARIA, UNITED STATES, 1959-1976

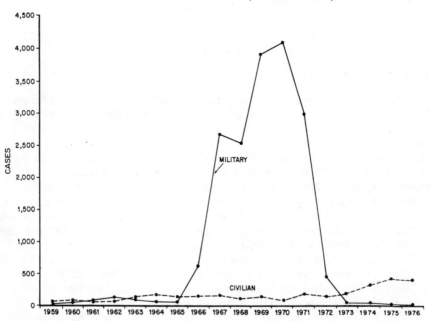

Figure 58.1—Reported malaria cases in the United States (Malaria Surveillance Annual Summary, 1976, Center for Disease Control, September 1977).

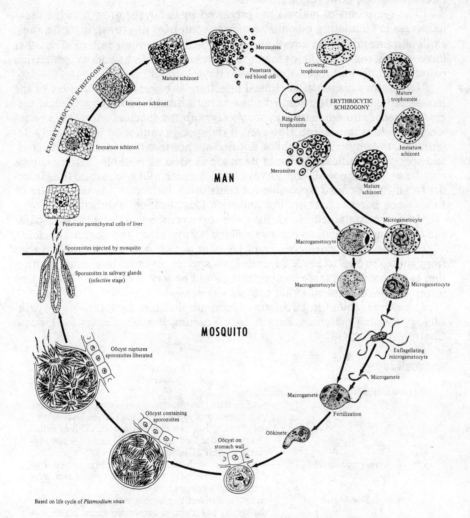

Figure 58.2—Life cycle of malaria. Courtesy of Parasitology Training Materials, Parasitology Training Branch, Centers for Disease Control, Atlanta, Ga.

common and may occur years after the initial clinical episode. With blood-induced infections, such as those acquired through transfusion or contaminated hypodermic needles, there is no liver phase and thus relapses do not occur. Recrudescences, however, are possible.

The symptoms of malaria are produced by the cyclic growth of the asexual stages in circulating blood. *P. malariae* completes its growth in 72 hr; thus, chills and fever occur on days 1 and 4, the so-called quartan pattern. The other three species complete their growth in approximately 48 hr and have a tertian pattern of chills and fever occurring on days 1 and 3.

Laboratory diagnosis of clinical infections is based on morphology of the parasitic stages found in stained films of peripheral blood. Since clinical disease, therapy, and epidemiology may vary with the species concerned, species identification is important. However, if the species cannot be immediately determined, the physician should be notified at once that the patient has malaria, and specific identification should be made as soon as possible. Serologic tests may be useful for population surveys and for epidemiologic studies (i.e., in order to find the donor responsible for transfusion-induced malaria) and are of value when parasitemias are low and slide identification is difficult.

In properly stained blood films, the three components of a malaria parasite are demonstrated: cytoplasm, which stains blue; chromatin (nucleus), which stains red or purple-red; and pigment, which does not stain but varies from golden brown to black depending on species. In order to identify a structure as a parasite, all three components should be seen (except with young ring forms, in which pigment is not usually visible).

The stages found in circulating blood are listed as the following in parasitology training materials, Parasitology Training Branch, Center for Disease Control, Atlanta, Ga:

Asexual stages

1. Trophozoites—growing, undivided parasite
   a. *Ring* —youngest trophozoite stage consisting of a vacuole surrounded by cytoplasm with a chromatin mass.
   —occasionally has two chromatin dots. (This is called "fragmentation" of the chromatin and does not represent nuclear division.)
   b. *Growing Trophozoite* —older form with distinctive cytoplasm and one chromatin mass. May be ameboid or compact. Pigment granules present.
   c. *Mature Trophozoite* —largest and oldest trophozoite stage and usually fills the rbc. It has a single chromatin mass. Pigment is present.
2. Schizonts—dividing form
   a. *Immature Schizont* —stage with two or more chromatin masses. Cytoplasm is undivided. Pigment beginning to clump.
   b. *Mature Schizont* —division of nucleus and cytoplasm is complete and stage is composed of a cluster of individual parasites called merozoites. Pigment is clumped.
   C. *Merozoite* —individual parasite produced as a result of asexual division (schizogony). Consists of a mass of cytoplasm and a single chromatin mass. This is the stage which is released when the rbc ruptures and the one which

penetrates other rbc. It is rarely seen outside the red cell in blood films.

Sexual stage or gametocyte

Develops in rbc and circulates until it dies. This is the infective stage for the mosquito and in the mosquito, develops into a gamete.
1. *Macrogametocyte*   —female sex cell.
2. *Microgametocyte*   —male sex cell.

Speciation is based on the appearance of asexual and sexual forms in stained blood films and recognition of the growth stages is important for reliable diagnoses (Table 58.1).

In stained thin films, the features used in identifying malaria species are as follows:
1. Appearance of the red cell
   a) Size—enlarged or normal
   b) Presence or absence of Schüffner's stippling
2. Appearance of the parasite
   a) Cytoplasm of growing trophozoites
      (1) ameboid or compact outline
      (2) staining intensity (light or dark blue)
   b) Number of merozoites produced in the mature schizont
   c) Amount and color of pigment
   d) Shape of gametocytes.

Detailed morphologic criteria for identifying malaria species in thin films are shown in Table 58.1. Features such as double chromatin dots and multiply infected red cells can be seen with any species, although they are more common with *P. falciparum* infections; thus, the examiner should not place undue weight on these characteristics in identification. Morphology of parasites in thin films is shown for *P. vivax* (Plate I), *P. ovale* (Plate II), *P. malariae* (Plate III), and *P. falciparum* (Plate IV).

In addition to the appearance of the parasite and the red cell, the stages present may also aid in species identification. For example, with *P. falciparum* infections, only ring-form trophozoites and gametocytes are found in peripheral blood films except with overwhelming infections in which growing trophozoites and schizonts may be present. All of the asexual stages as well as gametocytes are associated with infections of the other three species, and with those caused by *P. vivax* a wide range of growth stages is common.

The most difficult species to identify is *P. ovale*, since it has characteristics that resemble those of both *P. vivax* and *P. malariae*. Both the parasitized red cell and the parasite must be considered; therefore, *P. ovale* cannot be reliably diagnosed from thick films. Thin films, often several, are essential to establish an accurate identification of *P. ovale*. The trophozoites resemble those of *P. malariae* in that they tend to be dense and compact and to contain dark brown pigment. The number of merozoites produced is also about the same as that for *P. malariae*. On the other hand, the parasitized cells are enlarged and contain Schüffner's stippling, resembling those found in *P. vivax* infections. However, with *P. ovale* infections, 20% or more of the parasitized red cells may be oval and/or fimbriated (having irregular projections of the cell border). With *P. vivax* infections, 6% or less may be oval; thus, an occasional oval parasitized

TABLE 58.1—COMPARISON OF *PLASMODIUM* SPECIES AFFECTING MAN

	APPEARANCE OF ERYTHROCYTE			APPEARANCE OF PARASITE			
SPECIES	SIZE	SCHÜFFNER'S STIPPLING	CYTOPLASM	PIGMENT	NUMBER OF MEROZOITES	STAGES FOUND IN CIRCULATING BLOOD	
Plasmodium vivax	Enlarged. Maximum size (attained with mature trophozoites and schizonts) may be 1½–2 times normal erythrocyte diameter.	+ With all stages except early ring forms.	Irregular, ameboid in trophozoites. Has "spread-out" appearance.	Golden-brown, inconspicuous.	12–24 Average is 16.	All stages. Wide range of stages may be seen on given film.	
Plasmodium malariae	Normal.	– (Ziemann's dots rarely seen.)	Rounded, compact trophozoites with dense cytoplasm, Band-form trophozoites occasionally seen.	Dark-brown, coarse, conspicuous.	6–12 Average is 8. "Rosette" schizonts occasionally seen.	All stages. Wide variety of stages usually not seen. Relatively few rings or gametocytes generally present.	
Plasmodium ovale	Enlarged. Maximum size may be 1¼–1½ times normal red blood cell diameter. Approximately 20% or more of infected red blood cells are oval and/or fimbriated (border has irregular projections).	+ With all stages except early ring forms.	Rounded, compact trophozoites, Occasionally slightly ameboid. Growing trophozoites have large chromatin mass.	Dark-brown, conspicuous.	6–14 Average is 8.	All stages.	
Plasmodium falciparum	Normal. Multiply infected red blood cells are common.	– (Maurer's dots occally seen.)	Young rings are small, delicate, often with double chromatin dots. Gametocytes are crescent or elongate.	Black, Coarse and conspicuous in gametocytes.	6–32 Average is 20–24.	Rings and/or gametocytes. Other stages develop in blood vessels of internal organs but are not seen in peripheral blood except in severe infections.	

Smith JW, Melvin DM, Orihel TC, Ash LR, McQuay RM, and Thompson JH: Diagnostic Parasitology—Blood and Tissue Parasites. American So-

cell is of no diagnostic significance. Although both species cause enlargement of the red cell, the enlargement is less marked with *P. ovale* than with *P. vivax*. With *P. vivax,* cell enlargement may be 1.5 to 2 times normal size and in *P. ovale* it is usually 1.25 to 1.5 times. This variation can sometimes be helpful in speciation. Because maximal erythrocyte enlargement usually accompanies the mature trophozoite and schizont stages, measurements should be made on erythrocytes containing these stages. Twenty-five to 50 parasitized cells should be measured for a reliable size determination. With *P. vivax,* erythrocytes will probably measure 12 to 15 μm in diameter, and with *P. ovale,* from 10 to 12 μm. When diagnosis of *P. ovale* infection is in doubt, additional blood films should be made at 6-hr or 12-hr intervals in an effort to obtain diagnostic forms. *P. ovale* infections are often confused with those caused by *P. vivax* unless sufficiently distinctive characteristics are present. However, since these two infections are treated and handled in much the same way, this is not a serious clinical error.

Mixed infections with two (or, rarely, three) species of *Plasmodium* occur occasionally. However, they must be diagnosed cautiously since artifacts and atypical appearances may be confusing. Characteristic forms of both species suspected must be seen in order to diagnose mixed infections.

Morphology in thick films differs from that in thin films. In thick films, red cells are lysed, and identification is primarily dependent on morphology of the parasites. Rings are often incomplete and appear as punctuation marks (", !, ?). Trophozoites are more compact, which makes it difficult to differentiate those of *P. vivax*. Gametocytes of *P. falciparum* are stubbier. Although red cells are generally lysed, there may be some which are partially fixed near the periphery of the thick film. Enlargement of parasitized red cells and Schüffner's stippling may be evident in the partially fixed red cells. In areas in which red cells are lysed, Schüffner's stippling may sometimes be evident as a pink halo around the trophozoites but does not show the distinct granularity seen in thin films. Morphology in thick films is shown for *P. vivax* (Plate V), *P. malariae* (Plate VI), and *P. falciparum* (Plate VII).

Occasionally, only a few rings and no older forms may be seen in a blood smear. Since the appearance of the ring forms is essentially the same for all four species, "Malaria, species undetermined" should be reported in such instances. Additional films should be made at 12 and 24 hr in an effort to identify species. With *P. vivax, P. malariae,* and *P. ovale* infections, older stages will probably be found in the later films. Species identification should not be made unless species-specific characteristics are seen. Infections with numerous rings and no other forms can be diagnosed as *P. falciparum.* Young rings of *P. falciparum* are smaller than those of other species—as small as 1/6 the diameter of the erythrocyte—whereas those of other species are rarely less than 1/3 the diameter of an erythrocyte.

Malaria serology

Both the indirect immunofluorescence (IIF) and indirect hemagglutination (IHA) tests are useful for the diagnosis and seroepidemiology of malaria. The IIF is more sensitive in the early stages of infection and is preferred for the diagnosis of individual cases. Using a thick smear antigen (54), Wilson et al. (59) showed that the sensitivity and specificity of IIF are slightly superior to those of IHA. In addition, if the serum is obtained early in the course of a *primary* infection, IIF can be used to identify the infecting species. This is, however, an unusual circumstance, and serology should not be relied upon for this purpose. A titer of 1:128 is considered indicative of having had malaria at some time (Table 57.2).

In areas where malaria is endemic and the numbers of patients are larger, IHA may be the test of choice. First described by Stein and Desowitz (22) and later by Rogers et al. (44), IHA is slightly less sensitive than IIF but has the advantage of being simple to perform. However, the decreased sensitivity limits its effectiveness, and false-negative results are common. Perhaps the greatest usefulness of IHA is as a measure of the prevalence of malaria in a particular area to determine the need for or to follow the results of malaria control. Serologic testing for malaria has not been widely used because of the lack of available antigens. Parasitized monkey (or human) blood has been the source of antigen until recently, when organisms have been cultivated *in vitro* (51, 53, 55). If these methods are further refined and can be adapted to commercial levels of production, serologic tests for malaria will become available on a worldwide basis.

Artifacts

Malaria is sometimes erroneously diagnosed when artifacts or host cells are confused with parasites. Platelets probably are the most troublesome. Single platelets adhering to red cells in thin films can be confused with rings or young growing trophozoites. Clumps of platelets may be mistaken for mature schizonts or, if they are elongated, the gametocytes of *P. falciparum.* In thick films, fragments of white cells and platelets may be mistakenly identified as parasites.

Artifacts which present problems include precipitated stain, dust, dirt, bacteria, yeasts, molds, and occasionally fibers from cotton or gauze pads used to clean the patient's finger.

These problems can be eliminated or reduced if the films are correctly prepared and stained and if the examiner identifies as parasites only structures which have blue cytoplasm and red or purple-red chromatin. In all stages except rings, brown or black pigment should always be present.

Babesia

Babesia species are intraerythrocytic parasites of various animals including horses, dogs, and rodents. In the past decade, cases of babesiosis in humans have been reported, and the incidence is apparently rising (45).

The morphology of *Babesia* organisms varies slightly with the species involved, but in general they resemble malaria parasites. In fact babesiosis is often misdiagnosed as malaria in stained films. The species most commonly reported from man is *B. microti,* a rodent parasite. The ring-form parasites are sometimes slightly ameboid or oval, but are morphologically similar to those of *P. falciparum* (Fig 58.3). It is difficult to differentiate the rings of these two, but those of *Babesia* tend to be smaller and more delicate. There are no pigment and no gametocytes with *Babesia;* however, forms with four tiny trophozoites—tetrads—may be found and are helpful in identifying the organisms as *Babesia.*

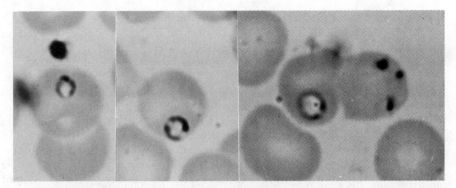

Figure 58.3—*Babesia microti*, Giemsa stain, oil immersion. Ring forms of *B. microti* are present in 1, 2, and 3. The parasitized erythrocyte on the right of 3 contains three small *B. microti* organisms.

To date, the serodiagnosis of babesiosis with IIF is in the developmental stage. Antigen from *B. microti* obtained from the blood of infected hamsters has been used successfully to measure antibody in proven cases (46). The IIF test appears to be an acceptable procedure. The limited number of cases restricts the evaluation of sensitivity, but tests of large numbers of other diseases indicate that the specificity is excellent. Serologic procedures are available in reference laboratories such as those of the Centers for Disease Control (CDC), to which sera should be submitted for diagnosis.

Toxoplasmosis:

A sporozoan of the coccidian group, *Toxoplasma gondii* often affects humans. Three particularly important types of infection may occur in humans: congenital, ocular, and acquired (42). Pregnant patients who acquire acute infections (often asymptomatic) transmit the infection across the placenta to the fetus. Disease manifestations depend on the stage of fetal development at the time of infection. Although the fetus is less likely to be infected early in pregnancy, the effects on those infected are more severe. Damage produced in the first and second trimester is worst—often leading to abortion or stillbirth or to severe congenital abnormalities. The central nervous system is often affected with development of calcifications and necrosis which may lead to hydrocephalus. Ocular infection may progress to chorioretinitis and to blindness. Infants may be asymptomatic at birth and develop disease, particularly chorioretinitis, during childhood or adolescence. The acquired disease is usually mild and not diagnosed, although a clinically acute infection with lymphadenopathy or pneumonia may occur which somewhat resembles infectious mononucleosis. Patients who develop acute toxoplasmosis as children or adults may develop chorioretinitis years later. In addition, the infection may remain latent and become active when the patient is immunocompromised, leading to neurologic and pulmonary disease.

The life cycle of *T. gondii* has been clarified in the past decade. *Toxoplasma* is an obligate intracellular parasite which has an intestinal cycle in cats and other felines and an extraintestinal cycle in various mammalian and avian hosts including man. Gametogony, oocyst production and sporogony occur in the feline intestinal mucosal epithelium and oocysts, the infective stage, are passed in the feces; thus, this stage of the disease resembles isosporiasis. In extraintestinal disease, the *Toxoplasma* organisms divide by a process of endodyogeny in which two daughter cells are formed in the mother cell; then the mother cell disintegrates. The organisms are able to invade and proliferate in almost any cells. With the development of immunity, cysts containing numerous organisms may be found in tissues, especially skeletal and cardiac muscle and the central nervous system (Fig 58.4). These cysts may persist as a latent infection for many years.

Infection may be acquired by ingesting cysts in inadequately cooked meat or by ingestion of oocysts from feces from infected cats. A recent outbreak at an indoor riding stable suggests that oocysts may also be inhaled in dust contaminated with cat feces (14).

Diagnosis is usually established serologically, though occasionally organisms may be found in material from biopsies or by inoculating laboratory animals with infected tissue (Fig 58.4).

Since the Sabin-Feldman dye test was introduced (49), serology has been a valuable adjunct to the clinical diagnosis of toxoplasmosis. Although it was too complex to be widely used, the dye test was rapidly accepted as a useful diagnostic aid. The significance of titers was firmly established, and this test served as the standard against which newer tests were compared.

Because the dye test is difficult to perform, the IHA test was introduced (28) as a simpler, more rapid, less expensive substitute for which reagents are commercially available; thus, it can be performed in any laboratory. There is a close—but not absolute—relationship between IHA and dye test titers (the tests apparently measure different antibodies). Some acute-phase sera do not react with IHA but give significant titers with the dye test; thus, diagnosis based on IHA results should be made cautiously. On the other hand, IHA efficiently measures older, established antibodies and is a good test for determining the immune status of pregnant patients.

More recently, the IIF test (31, 52) has become the test of choice. Its sensitivity and specificity are comparable to those of the dye test. The availability of commercial reagents and the ease with which the test can be performed make it feasible for most clinical laboratories. In addition, IIF can measure IgM antibody and thus can be used to indicate early infection in an adult or congenital toxoplasmosis in a neonate. The IIF test is particularly useful for individual clinical cases, but because it must be read microscopically, it is not as convenient for screening large numbers of prenatal patients.

The sensitivity, specificity, and reproducibility of the accepted procedures, particularly IIF and dye test, are such that a single titer may give useful clinical information, although a fourfold rise in titer is more helpful. In general, a titer of 1:256 is considered significant and 1:1024 in a compatible clinical situation is considered diagnostic. Patients with clinically inapparent disease or those with chronic ocular toxoplasmosis may have low titers. In addition, any toxoplasma IgM antibody titer in an infant is considered significant while an IgM titer of 1:64 or greater is required in an adult. Thorough familiarity with the ramifications of toxoplasmosis serology is advised before making clinical decisions based on serologic data.

Although most commercial reagents for IHA and IIF are of high quality, the quality can vary markedly. Each kit or reagent should be checked against controls. Any laboratory which begins to use a procedure should become thoroughly familiar with the technique before offering it as a diagnostic service.

Two new procedures have been introduced recently—enzyme-linked immunospecific assay (ELISA) and a dip-stick indirect immunofluorescent assay (FIAX). Both give results highly comparable to those obtained with IIF. Commercial kits may be available soon, although they must be evaluated further before they replace the accepted tests.

Pneumocystis carinii

Pneumocystis carinii (27) is an organism of uncertain taxonomy, but it is probably a sporozoan. It may cause pulmonary infections among malnourished and premature infants. However, in the United States, most infections are among immunocompromised persons such as transplant recipients and those being treated for leukemia, lymphoma, and other malignancies. The incidence of infection has risen as chemotherapy for malignancies and immunosuppression of transplant recipients have improved with some outbreaks following changes in therapy protocols.

Because the organism has only recently been grown in culture (34, 37), and serologic tests are not well-developed, the epidemiology of these infections has not been clearly defined. Most overt infections probably arise from latent infections which are activated when the patient becomes immunocompromised. Spread of infection by the respiratory route has been demonstrated in experimental animals (58), and there are probably asymptomatic carriers who serve as sources of infection.

The organisms develop in two forms—cysts and trophozoites. The growing trophozoites are extracellular but are attached to cells and are capable of dividing by binary fission (Fig 58.5). The cysts are formed from trophozoites which become rounded and produce a cyst wall. Division also occurs within the cyst, and the mature cyst contains eight organisms.

The infection usually produces an interstitial pneumonia, with alveoli filled with a foamy exudate containing organisms. The amount and character of the cellular response vary with the underlying condition of the patient and the severity and length of the infection. For immunocompromised patients, *Pneumocystis* pneumonia must be differentiated from other opportunistic pulmonary infections such as cytomegalovirus pneumonia, tuberculosis, histoplasmosis, nocardiosis, aspergillosis, cryptococcosis, and Legionnaires' disease, as well as from noninfectious conditions such as tumor infiltration and reaction to chemotherapeutic agents.

Diagnosis is usually established by demonstrating organisms in material from the lungs. The best specimen is lung tissue taken from the affected area by an open lung biopsy. Such material not only allows pneumocystosis and other infections to be diagnosed but is also satisfactory for diagnosing non-

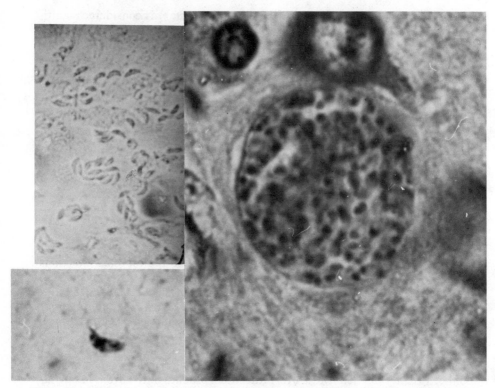

Figure 58.4—Toxoplasmosis. 1, tachyzoites in peritoneal exudate of a mouse, unstained, (oil immersion × 1000). 2, Tachyzoite, Giemsa stain (oil immersion × 1600). 3, Cyst in brain of infected mouse, (oil immersion × 1250).

infectious diseases. In some instances, material obtained by transthoracic needle biopsies or needle aspirations, transbronchial biopsies, brush biopsies, or bronchial washings have allowed some infections to be diagnosed but have not been as effective as material from open biopsies. Expectorated sputum is not usually satisfactory material for analysis. The urgency with which a diagnosis is needed depends on the condition of the patient and the rapidity with which the disease is progressing. Biopsy specimens can be examined as impression smears and/or sections depending on the size of the specimen and the capabilities of the laboratory. Impression smears stained with Giemsa allow the internal structures of cysts and free trophozoites to be seen. Smears should be prepared from secretions. Impression smears are prepared after blotting excess fluid from the tissue on sterile paper or gauze and touching the tissue to the slide repeatedly and firmly. If tissue is too wet when impression smears are made, organisms may remain in the alveoli and do not adhere to the slide. If the amount of tissue available is limited, a small circle of impressions should be made in the center of multiple slides and circled with a diamond-tipped marker.

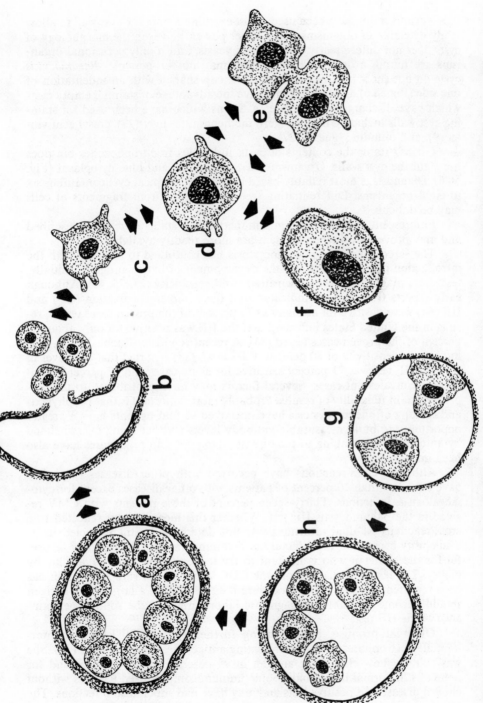

Figure 58.5—Life cycle of *Pneumocystis carinii:* a, mature cyst. b, ruptured cyst. c and d, growing trophozoites. e, dividing trophozoite. f, g, and h, immature cysts.

Various stains have been used. Most examiners stain the cyst wall to allow ready detection of organisms under lower power; however, the morphology of cysts does not differ greatly from that of yeasts, and if only occasional organisms are found, a definite identification may not be possible. *Pneumocystis* cysts do not show budding and are often cup-shaped with an indentation of one side (Fig 58.6). Cyst wall stains have the advantage of staining empty cysts which have discharged their contents. Stains which have been used for staining cyst walls include Gram-Weigert, methenamine silver (27), cresyl echt violet (9), and toluidine blue O (27).

Giemsa stains the contents of cysts and stains free trophozoites but does not stain the cyst walls. Organisms have red nuclei and blue cytoplasm (Fig. 58.6). Diagnosis is most reliably based on finding a typical cyst containing six to eight organisms. Differentiating free trophozoites from fragments of cells may be difficult.

Fluorescent antibody and immunoperoxidase stains have been described and may prove useful when antisera are more readily available.

The serodiagnosis of pneumocystosis has continued to improve with the introduction of the IIF test and the development of better antigens. Initially, tests were plagued by lack of sensitivity and specificity (23, 25, 43). Although early reports from Europe indicated that the complement fixation (CF) and IIF tests were positive for as many as 75 percent of the proven cases tested, results in the United States indicated that the IIF was positive for only about 32 percent of the proven cases tested (36). A recent report by Ruebush et al. (47) indicated a sensitivity of 80 percent. Pifer et al. (38) reported that at a level of 1:16 the IIF test was 71 percent sensitive for acute cases and 97 percent sensitive for convalescent cases. Several factors may have contributed to this improvement in reliability of results. Probably most important is that prophylaxis and therapy of pneumocystosis have improved so that patients have a greater opportunity to build measurable antibody levels without being overwhelmed by antigen or succumbing to the disease. Reagents and procedures have also been improved.

Although cross-reactions have occurred with other diseases (36), they have been less than 10 percent of patients with other diseases except for cytomegalovirus infections. Thirty-seven percent of these patients with CMV reacted in the pneumocystis IIF test. Whether this measurement reflected true cross-reactivity or dual infections was not determined. Still restricted in its availability because of the difficulty in obtaining antigen, the test may be useful for the clinician who is hesitant to try to demonstrate the organisms by biopsy. The test is available from the CDC. Recently, *in vitro* cultivation has been reported (34, 37). If the procedure is successful on a large scale, antigen should become available to diagnostic laboratories for the routine performance of the IIF test.

Of great promise, but requiring further evaluation, is the counterimmunoelectrophoresis test for circulating antigen described by Pifer (38). She was able to show circulating antigen in 95 percent of proven cases and for none of 120 normal individuals. Some immunocompromised patients without clinical disease had positive tests and may have had subclinical infections. The test may prove useful for diagnosis and prognosis.

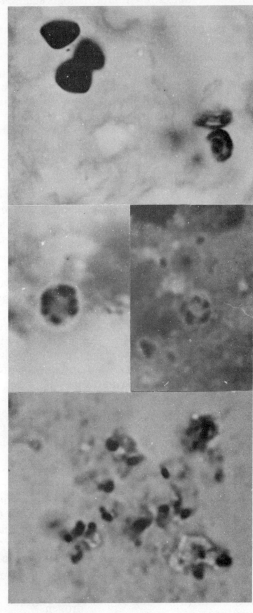

Figure 58.6—*Pneumocystis carinii*, oil immersion. 1, Free trophozoites stained with Giemsa. Dark nuclei and adjacent lighter cytoplasm are evident. 2 and 3, Cysts of *P. carinii*, Giemsa stain. Note the halo due to the unstained cyst wall. 4, Cysts of *P. carinii*, methenamine silver stain. The cyst at the lower left shows the rounded darker staining area often seen in cysts. The cyst at the upper right is cup shaped.

Hemoflagellates

Hemoflagellates include trypanosomes and *Leishmania* species. Hemoflagellates may be present in any of four different morphologic stages, with the stages produced varying among species (Fig 58.7, Table 58.2). Terminology has recently been revised, and the forms are named according to their flagellation. The amastigote (leishmania) does not have a flagellum and is an obligate intracellular parasite. The promastigote (leptomonas) has a free flagellum but no undulating membrane. The epimastigote (crithidia) has an undulating membrane which arises anterior to the nucleus and has a free flagellum. The trypomastigote (trypanosome) has a free flagellum and an undulating membrane which extends the length of the organism.

Four species of trypanosomes infect man. Two are found in Africa and two in the Western Hemisphere.

African trypanosomes

Trypanosoma gambiense, (West Africa) and *Trypanosoma rhodesiense* (East Africa) are etiologic agents of African sleeping sickness. According to Hoare (26), the correct species names should be *Trypanosoma brucei gambiense* and *Trypanosome brucei rhodesiense,* but for simplicity, the *brucei* has been omitted here.

T. rhodesiense appears to be more virulent than *T. gambiense* and often causes death before the classical sleeping stage of encephalitis is reached. *T. rhodesiense* parasitizes large game animals and cattle in Africa and is probably a zoonosis of humans.

The two African trypanosomes have similar life cycles. They are transmitted by blood-sucking flies of the genus *Glossina* (tsetse flies), and humans acquire infections by receiving the trypomastigote stage during a fly bite. Only the trypomastigote has been found in the human host, and it may be present in blood, lymph nodes, spleen, and spinal fluid. The parasites do not actually invade cells but are injurious to many areas of the body.

Diagnosis of African trypanosomiasis is based on finding the trypomastigotes in wet mounts or stained films of peripheral blood or lymphatic material during the early phases of infection. In later chronic phases of *T. gambiense* infections, organisms may be present in the spinal fluid. Patients with *T. rhodesiense* infections rarely survive long enough for organisms to reach the central nervous system.

Although organisms can be detected in wet mounts, specific characteristics are visible only in stained preparations, and (as with malaria) Giemsa stain is preferred. Thick blood films are usually recommended for diagnosis, but the organisms may be somewhat distorted. More distinctive morphology can be seen in thin films (Fig 58.8). Since the organisms are intercellular, the thicker portions of the thin film should be examined. Repeated daily blood films may be necessary to establish a diagnosis.

In stained films, stumpy forms (averaging 20 μm in length) and slender forms (approximately 30 μm long) may be seen. In general, the parasites are elongated, with the nucleus located in the center or slightly posterior. A small, discrete kinetoplast is located subterminally. Although variations occur, the

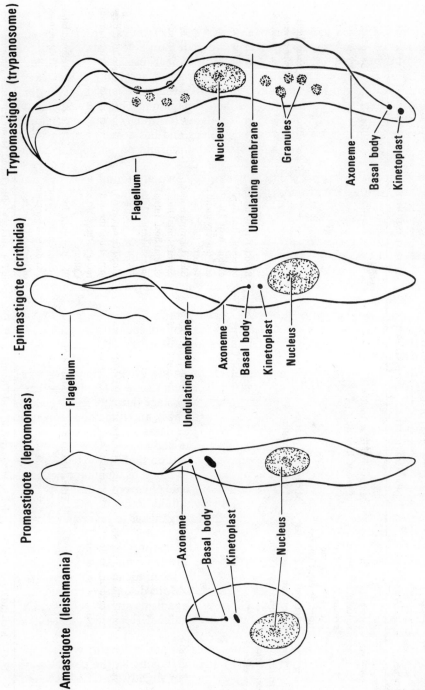

Figure 58.7—Hemoflagellate forms. With permission from Smith JW, Melvin DM, Orihel TC, Ash LR, McQuay RM, and Thompson JH: Diagnostic Parasitology—Blood and Tissue Parasites. American Society of Clinical Pathologists, Chicago, 1976.

TABLE 58.2—BLOOD AND TISSUE FLAGELLATES FOUND IN MAN

SPECIES	DEVELOPMENTAL STAGES				TRANS-MISSION	VECTORS
	AMASTIGOTE	PROMASTIGOTE	EPIMASTIGOTE	TRYPOMASTIGOTE		
Leishmania						
L. donovani	Intracellular, in reticuloendothelial system, lymph nodes, liver, spleen, bone marrow, etc. Culture.	Midgut and pharynx of vector. Culture	—	—	Bite	Sand flies (*Phlebotomus, Lutzomyia*)
L. tropica and *braziliensis*	Intra- and extracellular in skin and mucous membranes of man.	Midgut and pharynx of vector. Culture.	—	—	Bite	Sand flies (*Phlebotomus, Lutzomyia*)
Trypanosoma						
T. gambiense	—	—	Salivary glands of vector. Culture.	Blood, lymph nodes, cerebrospinal fluid of final host. Intestine and salivary gland of vector.	Bite	Tsetse fly (*Glossina*)
T. rhodesiense	—	—	Salivary glands of vector. Culture.	Blood, lymph nodes, cerebrospinal fluid of final host. Intestine and salivary glands of vector.	Bite	Tsetse fly (*Glossina*)
T. cruzi	Intracellular in viscera, myocardium, brain of man. Tissue culture.	Intracellular in man but transitional.	Midgut of vector. Culture.	Blood (temporary) of man. Intestine and rectum, feces of vector. Culture.	Feces of vector into wound.	Reduvid bugs (Triatominae)
T. rangeli	—	Transitional only.	Midgut of vector. Culture.	Blood of man. In hemolymph, salivary glands, and proboscis of vector. Culture.	Bite	Reduvid bugs (Triatominae)

Smith JW, Melvin DM, Orihel TC, Ash LR, McQuay RM, and Thompson JH: Diagnostic Parasitology—Blood and Tissue Parasites. American Society of Clinical Pathologists, Chicago, 1976.

posterior end is often blunt or bluntly tapered. Occasionally, an organism without a free flagellum is found. *T. gambiense* and *T. rhodesiense* are morphologically identical. When few organisms are present, the blood may be concentrated by fractional centrifugation and wet mounts or stained slides prepared from the sediment.

Cultivation on special blood agar and animal inoculation have been used in some cases but are generally less successful than direct blood or lymph examinations.

The recently developed IIF test has been used by some for serodiagnosis of African trypanosomiasis; however, the difficulty in preparing antigens and the relative unavailability of reagents and equipment in endemic areas has prevented its widespread application for diagnosing these infections. With the introduction of new, simpler techniques such as ELISA (57), it may be possible to develop a procedure which can be used in endemic areas.

American trypanosomes

Two species of trypanosomes affect humans in the Western Hemisphere— *Trypanosoma cruzi* (Central and South America, from Mexico to Argentina) and *Trypanosoma rangeli* (Central America and Northern South America). *T. rangeli* is apparently a nonpathogenic parasite of man, but *T. cruzi* causes a serious human infection, i.e., Chagas' disease.

T. cruzi infection occurs among humans and wild mammals. In the southern United States, a number of animals including opossums, raccoons, armadillos, etc., have been found infected, but only a few human cases have been reported. However, other human infections may have gone undetected.

T. cruzi is transmitted by species of Triatomid bugs. The infective forms (the young trypomastigote stage) are located in the hind gut of the bug and are passed in the feces. As the bug feeds, it defecates, and organisms are rubbed into the bite wound when the area is scratched. In the human host, *T. cruzi* occurs in the blood in the trypomastigote stage and in tissue (reticuloendothelial cells, the central nervous system, or myocardium) as the amastigote stage. Division takes place only in the amastigote stage. The trypomastigotes can be detected in wet mounts of blood (occasionally in lymphatic material) during the initial acute phase of the disease, which may be for 2 to 4 weeks, and during later febrile periods. However, the probability of detecting organisms during these febrile periods is rather low, because parasitemias are usually scanty.

The trypomastigotes have a large kinetoplast and typically have "C" and "S" shapes rather than the more delicate curves of typical African trypanosomes (Fig 58.7). The organisms distort rather badly in thick films, so thin films made somewhat thicker than usual are more useful. Since the parasites are intercellular, overlapping and piling of the red cells will not interfere with diagnosis, and the thicker areas of the film should be examined.

Since direct examination of blood often fails to reveal organisms, other methods of diagnosis which are more reliable include cultivation of blood (usually the centrifuged sediments), lymphatic material, or biopsied tissue; animal inoculations with the same materials; or serologic procedures. Cultivation procedures or animal inoculations are not done in most clinical laboratories, and specimens from patients suspected of having Chagas' disease are usually

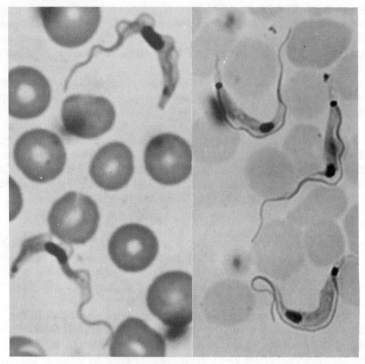

Figure 58.8—Trypanosomes, Giemsa stain, oil immersion. The photomicrograph on the left shows trypomastigotes of the type seen in *Trypanosoma gambiense* or *T. rhodesiense.* On the right are trypomastigotes of *T. cruzi.*

sent to reference laboratories for analysis. Serologic procedures are more widely used but currently are performed only in reference laboratories such as those at the CDC.

The serodiagnosis of Chagas' disease has been extensively studied. Both the IHA and CF tests have been successfully used. Although more easily performed and requiring fewer reagents, the IHA test is less specific than the CF test (19), and as a consequence IHA has been most extensively used as an epidemiologic tool.

Complement fixation with a delipidized antigen from cultured organisms has been recommended by the Pan American Health Organization as the test of choice. It is highly sensitive and specific and is of particular value for analysis of specimens from patients with acute Chagas' disease. Rising CF titers are highly indicative of current infection. Due to the chronicity of Chagas' disease, stable low to moderate titers by CF or IHA are difficult to interpret.

Other tests such as IIF (24) and direct agglutination (1, 56) have been reported to be of value; neither, however, offers sufficient advantages over CF and IHA to be recommended as a substitute.

Xenodiagnosis, or use of uninfected Triatomid bugs, is considered an ef-

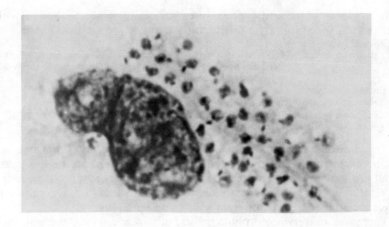

Figure 58.9—*Leishmania donovani*, Giemsa stain, oil immersion. This macrophage contains numerous amastigotes of *L. donovani*. Note the rod-shaped structures in the amastigotes.

fective and reliable procedure but is not practical or feasible for the average laboratory. Amastigote forms may be recovered in bone marrow or other biopsied tissue; however, these must be distinguished from similar stages of *Leishmania* which inhabit the same tissues. Tissue examinations are not usually relied upon in diagnosing Chagas' disease.

T. rangeli is also transmitted by Triatomid bugs, but the organisms are in the foregut of the bug and are injected as the bug bites. The young trypomastigote is the infective stage for vertebrate hosts, including monkeys, dogs, cats, and other animals, as well as humans. The process of development of the infection in humans is not completely known, but so far only the trypomastigote stage in blood has been described and presumably is the only stage present in the mammalian host. Parasitemias tend to be scanty, and the organisms are difficult to detect in blood films. In Giemsa-stained smears, the parasite resembles the African trypanosomes. It is undulated, about 30 μm long, and has a long, free flagellum. The nucleus is usually anterior to the center of the body; the subterminal kinetoplast is smaller than that of *T. cruzi* but is a distinct, readily seen structure. The posterior of the trypomastigote tapers to a more or less pointed end. It can usually be differentiated from *T. cruzi* without much difficulty. Cultivation techniques and animal inoculations can also be used for diagnosis.

Leishmania

The classification and nomenclature of *Leishmania* species affecting man are not clearly defined (33). Regardless of the differences in nomenclature and species, the organisms fall into two broad categories: the visceral forms and the cutaneous forms. Diagnostic procedures generally relate to body location rather than to species. For simplicity, only four species are listed here.

1. Visceral form
    Leishmania donovani—India, Mediterranean area, and other parts of the Eastern Hemisphere, and South and Central America. (The species in the Western Hemisphere may not be *L. donovani.*)
2. Cutaneous forms
    Leishmania tropica—Eastern Hemisphere
    Leishmania braziliensis—Western Hemisphere (Central and South America)
    Leishmania mexicana—Mexico, Central America

The clinical manifestations of the cutaneous forms vary somewhat, and a number of specific names have been given to these variations. It is possible that all are variants or subspecies of the same primary species; for more details, refer to the parasitology textbooks and specific literature. Diagnostic procedures are similar despite different species designations.

There are only two morphologic stages of *Leishmania*: the amastigote, which is the stage found in humans, and the promastigote stage, which is found in the vector.

The life cycles of the *Leishmania* are basically the same regardless of species. In visceral infection, the organisms are present in reticuloendothelial cells of the viscera and (less commonly) in monocytes and leucocytes in the blood or in monocytes or macrophages of the skin. In cutaneous infection, they are found primarily in monocytes and macrophages of the skin. The amastigotes are taken up by the vector, i.e., species of *Phlebotomus* or *Lutzomyia* (sandflies) (10), where they transform to promastigotes and multiply. In approximately 1 week, infective promastigotes are present in the proboscis of the fly and are injected when it bites again. After gaining access to the human host, they develop in either cutaneous or visceral tissue.

Although serologic methods are available for visceral leishmaniasis, the most conclusive diagnosis is by demonstrating organisms in biopsied tissue: spleen, liver, bone marrow, or lymph nodes. Probably the most common tissue obtained is bone marrow. Impression smears can be prepared and stained with Giemsa. Amastigotes may be visible intracellularly or, if the cells have ruptured, extracellularly. The presence of the rod-shaped kinetoplast allows differentiation from *Toxoplasma* and *Histoplasma* (Fig 58.9). The biopsied tissue can be sectioned in the usual histiological fashion. Cutaneous forms may be found in stained preparations of material scraped or aspirated from the edges of the lesions. Both the visceral and cutaneous forms may be cultured on blood agar. Cultures are grown at room temperature and should be examined for promastigote stages after 10 days. Cultures should be examined at weekly intervals up to 60 days before they are discarded as negative. Hamster inoculation has been used as a diagnostic procedure but takes 4 to 6 weeks before organisms can be demonstrated. Both cutaneous and visceral forms cause visceral infections in the hamster. For examination, the hamster must be sacrificed and impression smears or sections made of the spleen and liver. Amastigotes of all the species are identical, and species cannot be determined on the basis of morphology.

An intradermal skin test, the Montenegro test, may be useful in diagnosing cutaneous and mucocutaneous leishmaniasis but is unsatisfactory for visceral infections.

The sharing of common antigens by the three major *Leishmania* species make species differentiation by serologic means difficult. Usually, the homologous reaction is stronger than the heterologous, but this criterion cannot be used as the basis for speciation. IHA and IIF have been successfully used but have decreased in popularity since the direct agglutination (DA) test was developed (2).

If a trypsinized suspension of cultured promastigotes of the three species is used, the DA is more sensitive than IHA or IIF (2). Tests for different species vary slightly in reactivity; titers of 1:32, 1:128, and 1:64 are considered diagnostic for *L. donovani, L. tropica,* and *L. braziliensis,* respectively. Cross-reactions occur with sera from patients with Chagas' disease, but they have much lower titers and cause little confusion in diagnosis. Serologic tests are available from the CDC.

Free-Living Amebae

At least two groups of free-living amebae, *Naegleria* and *Acanthamoeba* are capable of causing disease in humans.

Organisms of the genus *Naegleria* most often cause infection. They are ameboflagellates—that is, they exist either as amebae or as flagellates but can divide only in the ameboid form. They divide by promitosis (during division, the nuclear membrane persists). *Naegleria* species cause acute meningoencephalitis, which usually has a rapidly fatal course. Butt (11) used the term "primary amebic meningoencephalitis" (PAM) to describe this disease, thus differentiating it from the central nervous system disease caused by *Entamoeba histolytica* which is secondary to infection of the colon, liver, or lung. About 100 cases have been reported throughout the world. Most of the patients acquired the amebic infection from swimming in warm water, but face washing with contaminated water has also caused infection. The amebae penetrate the olfactory bulbs and progress to the subarachnoid space. To date, few individuals with PAM have survived. A 14-year-old Australian boy survived after treatment with amphotericin B (13), a 6-year-old boy from England recovered after being treated with amphotericin B and sulfadiazine (5), and a 9-year-old girl from California recovered after being treated with amphotericin B and miconazole. Amebae were detected in the cerebrospinal fluid of two of these patients early in the disease, and treatment was begun immediately. Treatment was initiated for the third before symptoms appeared. This suggests that early treatment is essential for recovery. The pathogenic *Naegleria* are 10 to 15 μm in size and have prominent nucleoli, contractile vacuoles, and lobose pseudopodia.

Amebae of the genus *Acanthamoeba* have been implicated in at least five cases of encephalitis or meningoencephalitis and in chronic skin ulcers. The route of infection has not been definitely established, but in one instance a cutaneous lesion may have been the primary focus of infection, with subsequent hematogenous spread to the central nervous system. The disease is more slowly progressive than that caused by *Naegleria,* but the outcome is fatal. The *Acanthamoeba* are 15 to 35 μm in diameter, have large central nucleoli, and exhibit classic mitosis. Often the pseudopods are sharp and spiny—hence the name *Acanthamoeba.* There is no flagellate form.

If a patient has signs of meningeal irritation, headache, vomiting, stiff neck, a history of swimming in warm water, and cerebrospinal fluid that has elevated proteins and low glucose levels but in which no bacteria are found, free-living amebae should be considered.

The two genera have different drug susceptibilities. *Naegleria* are susceptible to amphotericin B but resistant to sulfa, whereas sulfadiazine is quite active against some strains of *Acanthamoeba in vitro.* In order to establish appropriate therapy, it is important to document infection by detecting amebae microscopically and in subsequent culture and to differentiate the amebae on the basis of nutritional requirements, type of mitosis, and presence or absence of a flagellate stage. Amebae are best demonstrated by direct microscopy of cerebrospinal fluid with a phase contrast microscope, and they must be differentiated from macrophages.

Culture methods are useful for isolating and identifying the organisms. *Naegleria* require a medium containing a low concentration of NaCl (0.40% rather than 0.85%) and living cells such as bacteria or tissue culture cells or other enrichment such as serum. *Acanthamoeba* amebae can be cultured in tryptic digest soy broth (20). All cultures must be aerobic and incubated at 37 C.

Helminths

The blood and tissue helminths include filariae, *Trichinella*, the larval stages of *Taenia solium,* and the larval stages of organisms that parasitize lower animals (e.g., *Echinococcus* spp. and *Toxocara canis*).

Filariae

Filariae are helminths belonging to the class Nematoda. Adult males and females inhabit the tissues or serous cavities of humans. Seven species are considered to be human parasites: *Wuchereria bancrofti, Brugia malayi, Loa loa, Mansonella ozzardi, Dipetalonema perstans, Dipetalonema streptocerca,* and *Onchocerca volvulus.* The two latter species have microfilariae in tissue only and are diagnosed by examining skin snips or biopsies. The other five release the diagnostic stage into the peripheral blood and so are considered with the blood parasites (Table 58.3).

The filariae have similar life cycles and are transmitted by blood-sucking insects—mosquitoes for *W. bancrofti* and *B. malayi* or flies for the other species. The stage picked up by the vector is a prelarval form called a microfilaria, which develops to the infective larval stage in the thoracic muscles of the vector, and in 1 to 2 weeks is present in the sheath of the proboscis (mouth parts). When the fly or mosquito bites again, the infective larvae actively migrate from the arthropod into the bite wound. In about a year, the parasites are mature, and the female begins to discharge microfilariae. Unlike infections caused by other blood parasites, filarial infections are not transferred by transfusion with infective blood or through contaminated needles. The microfilariae are not infective for humans, and filariasis can be acquired only from the vector. Geographical distribution of each species is well-known (Table

58.3), so the areas of residence and travel can be used to determine the type of infection to which the patient may have been exposed (50).

The diagnostic stage is a microfilaria, which is a worm-like organism whose body consists of a column of nuclei interspersed with anatomical features such as nerve ring, excretory pore, excretory cell, innerbody, anal pore, anal cell, and a series of four R-cells which are precursors of the lower digestive system (Fig 58.10). In addition, three of the species are enveloped in a sheath.

Laboratory diagnosis of the species other than *O. volvulus* or *D. streptocerca* depends on finding microfilariae in blood in either wet mounts or stained films. With three of the five species, the presence of microfilariae in peripheral blood is periodic, and blood for diagnosis must be taken at the time of peak parasitemia. Microfilariae of *Loa loa* tend to be more numerous during the day (diurnal periodicity), and blood should be taken between 10 a.m. and 2 p.m. Both *W. bancrofti* and *B. malayi* have a nocturnal periodicity, and blood should be collected at night. *W. bancrofti* specimens should be obtained around midnight (between 10 p.m. and 2 a.m.).

Blood can be collected by finger prick or venipuncture for examination. Small amounts of anticoagulants, such as EDTA, do not seem to adversely affect the microfilariae, so blood anticoagulated with EDTA can be used for wet mounts and for stained films without any problems. Occasionally, however, if the blood stands for a few hours, the sheath of the microfilaria may be shed.

Wet mounts are used in initial screening procedures to detect organisms. The blood can be examined directly undiluted or diluted with saline. Since the organisms are intercellular, they can be readily seen moving among the cells. If microfilariae are not found in direct mounts, concentrations such as those by the Knott's technique or the saponin technique can be used. Knott's technique with 2% Formalin is probably more widely used. It is an effective procedure but the microfilariae are dead and could be confused with artifacts such as fibers. In the saponin procedure, the microfilariae remain viable.

Species identifications cannot be made from wet mounts, and stained films to demonstrate the anatomical features are essential to establish a specific diagnosis. Only thick films are prepared; thin films are of little or no value. Not all of the anatomical characteristics can be seen in a single type of stain, but rarely would all of these features be needed to establish a species diagnosis. Differential diagnosis is generally based on presence or absence of a sheath, and presence or absence of nuclei in the tip of the tail and the configuration of the tip of the tail. Occasionally, the length of the cephalic space and/or the stain reaction can be used. The characteristics for each species are presented in the accompanying key (Table 58.3, Fig 58.10).

The visibility of these characteristics varies with the stain used, and a variety of stain techniques have been developed for microfilariae including Giemsa, hematoxylin, azure, methyl green, and pyronin stains. The most commonly used stain is Giemsa, but in doubtful cases, other stains may be needed for detailed staining of particular structures. The Giemsa procedure is the same as used for thick films for diagnosis of other blood parasites. With Giemsa-stained films, if a sheath is not visible, the presence of this structure

TABLE 58.3—FILARIAE THAT PARASITIZE MAN

	WUCHERERIA BANCROFTI	*BRUGIA MALAYI*	*LOA LOA*	*MANSONELLA OZZARDI*	*DIPETALONEMA PERSTANS*	*DIPETALONEMA STREPTOCERCA*	*ONCHOCERCA VOLVULUS*
Geographic distribution	Cosmopolitan; tropics and sub-tropics	Asia	West and Central Africa	South and Central America	Africa, South and Central America	West Africa	Africa, Central and South America
Adult habitat	Lymphatic system	Lymphatic system	Subcutaneous tissues	Mesenteries, body cavities	Mesenteries, perirenal, retroperitoneal tissues	Subcutaneous tissues	Subcutaneous tissues
Vector	Mosquitoes	Mosquitoes	*Chrysops* (deer fly)	*Culicoides* *Simulium*	*Culicoides* (midge)	*Culicoides* (midge)	*Simulium* (black fly)
Location of microfilariae	Blood	Blood	Blood	Blood	Blood	Skin	Skin
Periodicity	Nocturnal*	Nocturnal†	Diurnal	None	None	None	None
Morphology of microfilariae							
Sheath	Present	Present	Present	Absent	Absent	Absent	Absent
Length (µm)	230–300	175–260	250–300	175–240	190–200	180–240	Two sizes 285–370 150–290
Width (µm)	7.5–10	5–6	6–8.5	4–5	4–5	5–6	5–9
Tail and tail nuclei	Tapered to point; no nuclei in end of tail.	Tapered; terminal and subterminal nuclei.	Tapered; nuclei irregularly spaced to end of tail.	Long, slender tail; no nuclei in end of tail.	Tapered, bluntly rounded; nuclei to end of tail.	Tapered, bluntly rounded; nuclei to end of tail. Tail bent in hook shape.	Tapered to point; no nuclei in end of tail.

* Superiodic in Pacific Islands.
† Subperiodic form as well.
Smith JR, Melvin DM, Orihel TC, Ash LR, McQuay RM, Thompson JH: Diagnostic Parisitology—Blood and Tissue Parasites. American Society of Clinical Pathologists, Chicago, 1976.

cells are often indistinct. Giemsa will stain the sheath of *B. malayi* but will not stain the sheath of *Loa loa.* The sheath of *W. bancrofti* may or may not stain with Giemsa but does not stain as intensely as that of *Brugia.* Thus, in Giemsa-stained films, if a sheath is not visible, the presence of this structure cannot be ruled out. Sheaths are better demonstrated in hematoxylin stains, so if their presence is questioned, preparations should be stained with one of the hematoxylin stains.

Although the tip of the tail is very flexible and sometimes is bent or twisted so it cannot be seen, its appearance can be used for differentiating microfilariae. If the tail of *W. bancrofti* is bent, the nuclear column may appear to extend to the tip of the tail. For reliable identifications, several organisms should be examined. The preparation should be scanned under low power; then high-dry power and oil immersion should be used for more detailed study.

Lymph obtained from swollen lymph nodes can occasionally be used to diagnose *W. bancrofti* and *B. malayi* infections. With *Loa loa* infections, microfilariae have been reported in fluid from Calabar swellings (non-specific swellings which can occur on any part of the body in loaiasis).

Patients with chronic cases of filariasis, may not have microfilariae visible in blood (or lymph) smears. Serologic tests can be used but may not be conclusive.

Onchocerca volvulus adults are coiled in the subcutaneous tissues (Fig 58.11), and microfilariae migrate through the skin. They may migrate to the eye and are a significant cause of blindness in some parts of the world. Diagnosis is established by detecting microfilariae in skin by shaving off a piece of the skin and teasing it in saline. Infection caused by *Dipetalonema streptocerca* is diagnosed in a similar fashion. Microfilariae of these two species do not occur in the blood.

Several serologic tests including double diffusion and IIF have been used but the IHA is the most popular. The serology of filariasis is plagued by lack of sensitivity and specificity. The problem is the inability to obtain purified specific homologous antigens. An extract of adult *Dirofilaria immitis,* the dog filarial worm, is used. This antigen reacts with all genera of filarial worms. With this antigen, Kagan and Norman (30) report only 73 percent sensitivity using IHA. Ambroise-Thomas and Kien-Truong (4) reported 99 percent sensitivity using *Dipetalonema vitae* frozen sections in IIF. It is not unusual to find a low or negative serology in the presence of a measurable parasitemia. The apparent explanation of this is the adsorption or blocking of antibody by the excess of antigen in the blood. To overcome some of these problems, the bentonite flocculation (BFT) test (which is much less sensitive but more specific) is usually included. When both IHA and BFT tests are positive, there is an increased assurance of their significance. In spite of the problems, the IHA and BFT tests can assist the clinician faced with a patient with compatible travel history and symptomatology but with no microfilaremia. A titer of 1:128 IHA and 1:5 BFT in combination would be considered significant (Table 57.2). In most instances, active clinical disease is accompanied by much higher titers with both tests.

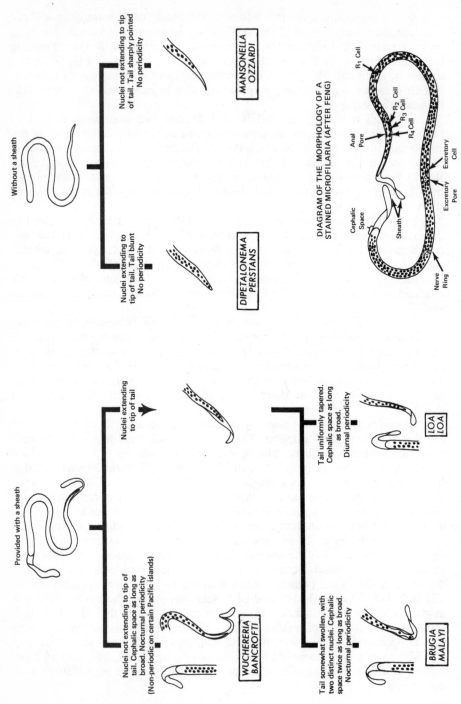

Figure 58.10—Key to microfilariae found in peripheral blood of man. From Parasitology Training Branch, Centers for Disease Con-

MALARIA IN MAN

Nine Color Plates with Explanatory Captions
Illustrating Various Forms and Phases of
Plasmodium Species Significant to Man

ACKNOWLEDGMENT.—The American Public Health Association and its Subcommittee on Diagnostic Procedures for Bacterial, Mycotic and Parasitic Infections are indebted, for permission to present these illustrations, to the U. S. Public Health Service (DHEW), in whose Publication No. 796 (*Manual for the Microscopical Diagnosis of Malaria in Man*, 1960 Edition) they last appeared.

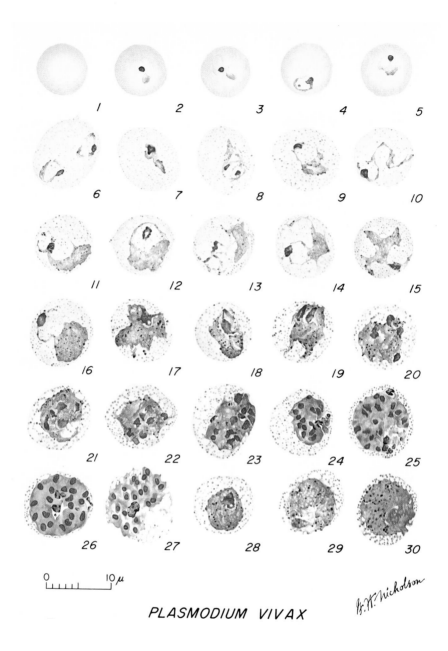

1   *2*   *3*   *4*   *5*

6   *7*   *8*   *9*   *10*

11   *12*   *13*   *14*   *15*

16   *17*   *18*   *19*   *20*

21   *22*   *23*   *24*   *25*

26   *27*   *28*   *29*   *30*

0   10 μ

PLASMODIUM VIVAX

G. W. Nicholson

PLATE I.—*Plasmodium vivax.*

Fig. 1.   Normal red cell.
Figs. 2–5.   Young trophozoites.
Figs. 6–16.   Growing trophozoites.
Figs. 17, 18.   Mature trophozoites.
Figs. 19–21.   Early schizonts.

Figs. 22, 23.   Developing schizonts.
Fig. 24–27.   Nearly mature and mature schizonts
Figs. 28, 29.   Nearly mature and mature
           macrogametocytes.
Fig. 30.   Mature microgametocyte.

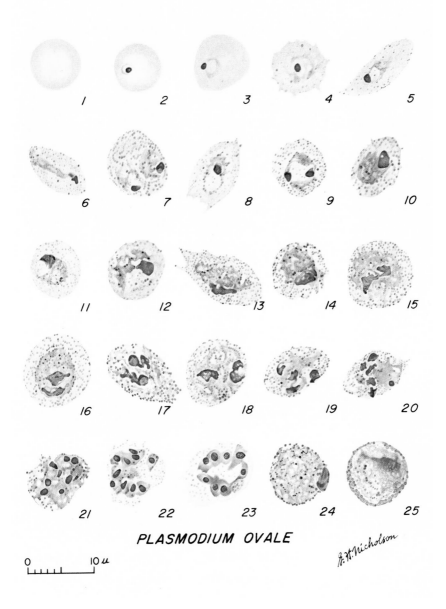

PLASMODIUM OVALE

0 |__|__|__|__|__| 10 μ

$\mathcal{H.H.Nicholson}$

PLATE II.—*Plasmodium ovale.*

Fig. 1. Normal red cell.	Figs. 16, 22. Developing schizonts.
Figs. 2–5. Young trophozoites.	Fig. 23. Mature schizont.
Figs. 6–12. Growing trophozoites.	Fig. 24. Adult macrogametocyte.
Figs. 13, 15. Mature trophozoites.	Fig. 25. Adult microgametocyte.

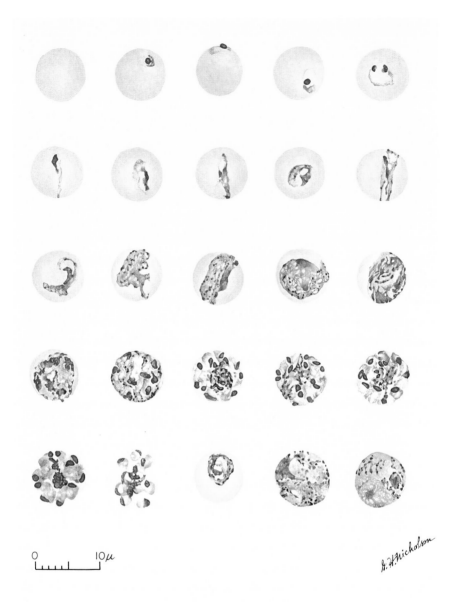

0 ⌊⌊⌊⌊⌊ 10μ

PLASMODIUM MALARIAE

PLATE III.—*Plasmodium malariae.*

Fig. 1. Normal red cell.
Figs. 2–5. Young trophozoites.
Figs. 6–11. Growing trophozoites.
Figs. 12, 13. Nearly mature and mature trophozoites.
Figs. 14–20. Developing schizonts.

Figs. 21, 22. Mature schizonts.
Fig. 23. Developing gametocyte.
Fig. 24. Mature macrogametocyte.
Fig. 25. Mature microgametocyte.

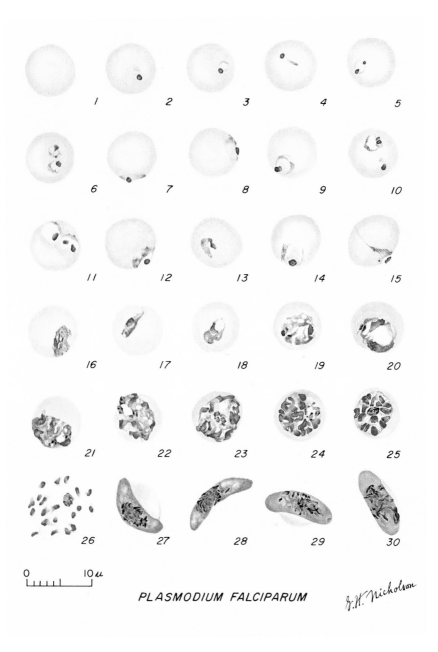

PLASMODIUM FALCIPARUM

0 ⌊⌊⌊⌊⌊ 10μ

PLATE IV.—*Plasmodium falciparum.*

Fig. 1.   Normal red cell.
Figs. 2–11.   Young trophozoites.
Figs. 12–15.   Growing trophozoites.
Figs. 16–18.   Mature trophozoites.

Figs. 19–22.   Developing schizonts.
Figs. 23–26.   Nearly mature and mature schizonts.
Figs. 27, 18.   Mature macrogametocytes.
Figs. 29, 30.   Mature microgametocytes.

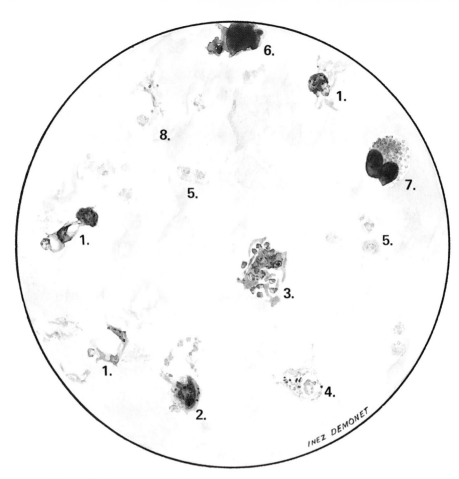

PLATE V—*P. vivax*, thick film
  1—Ameboid trophozoites.
  2—Schizont, two divisions of chromatin.
  3—Mature schizont.
  4—Microgametocyte.
  5—Blood platelets.
  6—Nucleus of neutrophil.
  7—Eosinophil.
  8—Blood platelet associated with cellular remains of young erythrocytes.

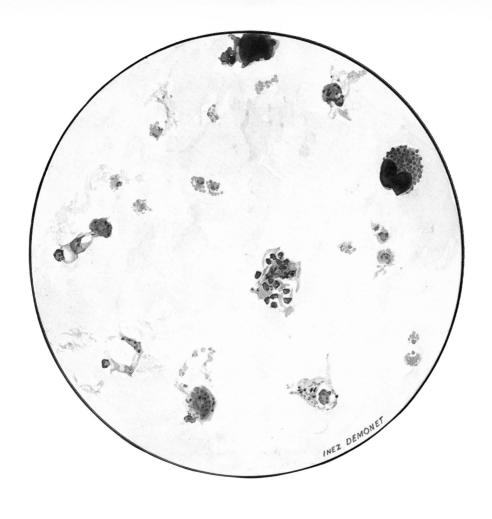

INEZ DEMONET

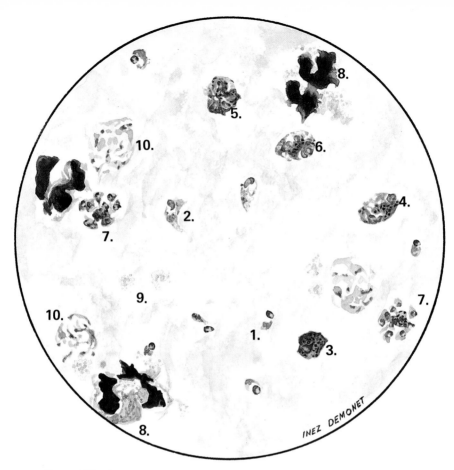

PLATE VI—*P. malariae,* thick film
 1—Small trophozoites.
 2—Growing trophozoites.
 3—Mature trophozoites.
 4
 5 } Immature schizonts with varying numbers of divisions of the chromatin.
 6
 7—Mature schizonts.
 8—Nucleus of leucocyte.
 9—Blood platelets.
10—Cellular remains of young erythrocytes.

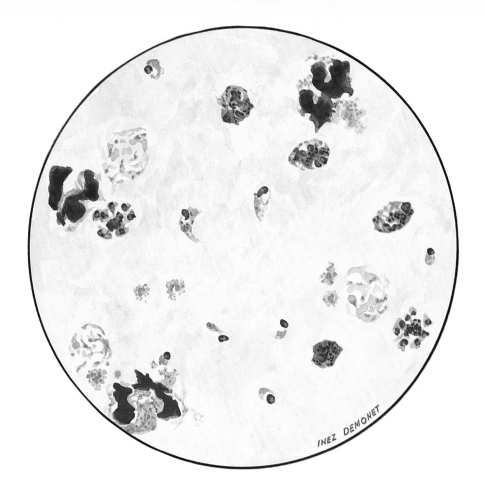

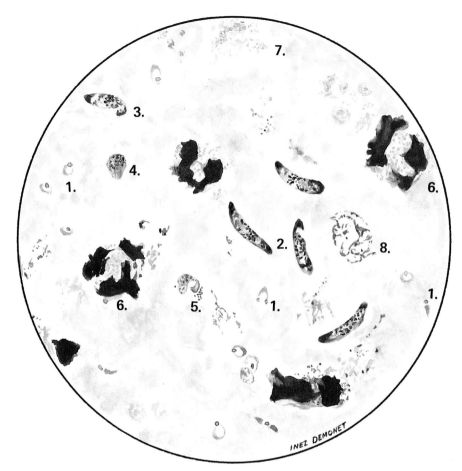

PLATE VII—*P. falciparum,* thick film
  1—Small trophozoites.
  2—Gametocytes, normal.
  3—Slightly distorted gametocyte.
  4—"Rounded-up" gametocyte.
  5—Disintegrated gametocyte.
  6—Nucleus of leucocyte.
  7—Blood platelets.
  8—Cellular remains of young erythrocyte.

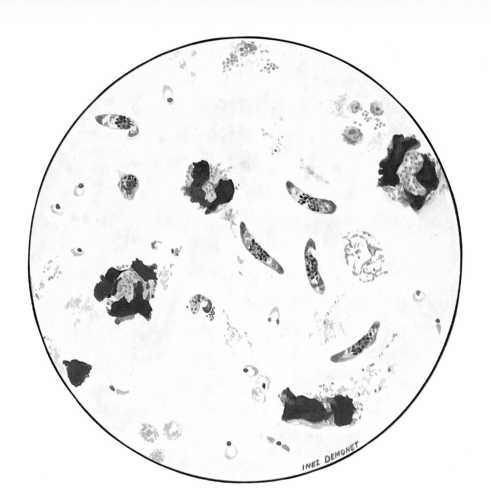

Trichinella

Trichinosis is not uncommon in the United States and is usually acquired by eating raw or improperly cooked pork containing infective larvae. Bear meat and hamburger contaminated with pork have been sources of infection in some cases.

Trichinella spiralis has both an intestinal phase (which is very short) and a tissue phase (which is much longer). The same host serves as both the definitive and intermediate host.

Man becomes infected by ingesting viable larvae in pork or other meat. In the mucosa of the small intestine, the parasites mature in about 2 to 4 days, and the females begin to deposit larvae. These gain access to the blood and are carried to all parts of the body. Those reaching skeletal or striated muscle continue developing, and in about 3 weeks become encysted in the muscle fibers. In humans, this is a blind alley, but in other animals such as hogs, rats, and bears, these encysted larvae may transmit the infection if the infected tissue is eaten by a susceptible host.

Trichinosis can be diagnosed by direct examination of biopsied tissue or more commonly by serologic methods. Biopsied tissue can be examined by teasing the tissue apart with needles, compressing it between slides and examining it for larvae, digesting it and examining the sediment for larvae, or sectioning and staining it in the usual fashion for histology. Larvae are large and can be readily recognized with low power.

Of all the parasitic serologic tests those for trichinosis are perhaps the best. Virtually every serologic technique has been used including BFT, IIF, and IHA (32, 35, 39). BFT uses an extract of trichina larvae from infected rat tissue and is simple to perform, highly sensitive, and nearly 100 percent specific. The test has been shown to become positive 3 weeks after infection, reach a maximum titer in about 2 months, and remain positive for several years. For this reason weakly positive titers should be interpreted with care to assure the presence of newly acquired antibody in contrast to old residual antibody. A fourfold or greater rise in titer allows diagnosis. There are two major disadvantages to the BFT test. Although simple to perform, strict quality control must be maintained because the bentonite suspension is unstable and can vary in sensitivity from resisting agglutination to autoagglutination. Also the BFT test does not react well with infected pig serum; thus, cannot be used to measure antibody in swine. IIF and IHA have both been suggested for this purpose; however, ELISA (48) appears to have the greatest promise. Rapid, simple, and sensitive, ELISA becomes positive in less than 1 week and titers directly correlate with the degree of infection.

Clinical trichinosis is usually accompanied by BFT titers of greater than 1:160, but because of the vagaries of the disease, a titer of 1:5 or greater should be considered important (Table 57.2).

Larva migrans

Larva migrans infections (6) may be caused by the larval stages of many species which ordinarily infect lower animals. Visceral larva migrans is usually

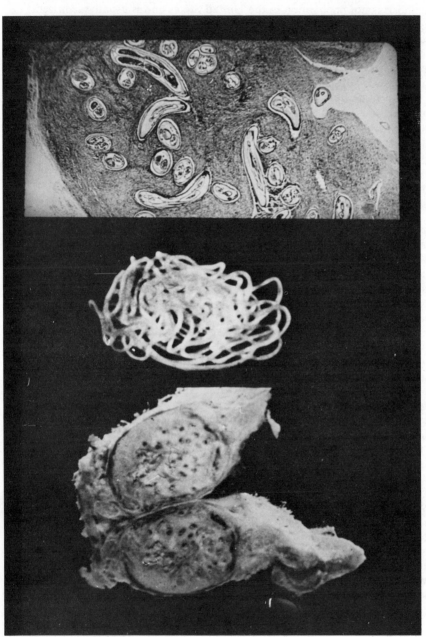

Figure 58.11—Onchocerciasis The photo on the left is a gross photograph of a subcutaneous nodule of onchocerciosis which has been bisected. In the center is an adult worm which has been digested from a similar nodule. On the right is a photomicrograph of a similar nodule showing sections of the worm encased in fibrous tissue. From Smith JW, Melvin DM, Orihel TC, Ash LR, McQuay RM, and Thompson JH: Parasitology—Blood and Tissue Parasites, American Society of Clinical Pathologists, Chicago, 1976.

caused by ingestion of embryonated eggs of *Toxocara canis*, the common roundworm infecting dogs. It occurs more often in children than in adults and may present some diagnostic problems. Patients usually have eosinophilia (7). Disease varies in severity from asymptomatic to serious disease with skin rash, pneumonitis, and central nervous system symptoms. Serologic methods may be used but must be evaluated in the light of clinical findings. Direct examination of tissue is not practical.

Until recently the serologic tests for visceral larval migrans (VLM) due to toxocariasis have been of questionable value. Cross-reactions with *Ascaris lumbricoides* were virtually 100 percent and differentiating the two depended upon the homologous reaction being stronger and the ability to adsorb the heterologous antibody. The differentiation of VLM and ascariasis may be important clinically. The most common procedure was a combination of IHA and BFT tests using a perienteric fluid antigen from *Ascaris* and an adult extract of *Toxocara* for both tests. Adsorption with the *Ascaris* antigen removes the *Ascaris* antibody. The tests are insensitive, reacting in only about 66 percent of patients (30) and showing considerable cross-reactions.

Recently, with cases of ocular VLM among children, Cypress (21) described an ELISA test using extracts of embryonated eggs as the antigens and showed remarkable specificity with some increase in sensitivity. Further evaluations in other laboratories have supported these data. As with earlier tests, there is cross-reactivity between *Toxocara* and *Ascaris*, but the difference between homologous and heterologous reaction is greater and the adsorption of the heterologous antibody is more complete. In ocular toxocariasis, a titer of 1:32 is considered significant (Table 57.2) and at least an 8-fold reduction in the *Ascaris* titer is necessary to indicate specificity. Although ELISA still lacks sensitivity, modification of the procedure may overcome this problem. ELISA has been of great value in differentiating ocular VLM from retinoblastoma. ELISA is now the preferred test for VLM as antigens become readily available.

Other larvae also cause human infections including animal hookworm species which cause "creeping eruption." Skin inflammation with serpiginous tracks develops in the area of larval penetration and migration. Since there are no good laboratory methods, either direct or serologic, most of these are diagnosed clinically.

Cysticercus

Cysticercosis is caused by the larval stage of *Taenia solium* which in the adult form parasitizes the human intestinal tract. The usual intermediate host for *T. solium* is the pig, and larval stages, or cysticerci, are found in various tissues. Man, however, can also be an intermediate host with cysticerci developing in various tissues including the eye, brain, and subcutaneous tissues. Cysticerci are fluid filled cysts approximately 1 cm in diameter which contain an invaginated scolex (Fig 58.12). Humans may acquire the infection by ingesting infective eggs passed in human feces. Relatively few cysticercosis cases are seen in the United States and the majority of these are imported from Mexico and Central America where the disease is most common. Cysticercosis

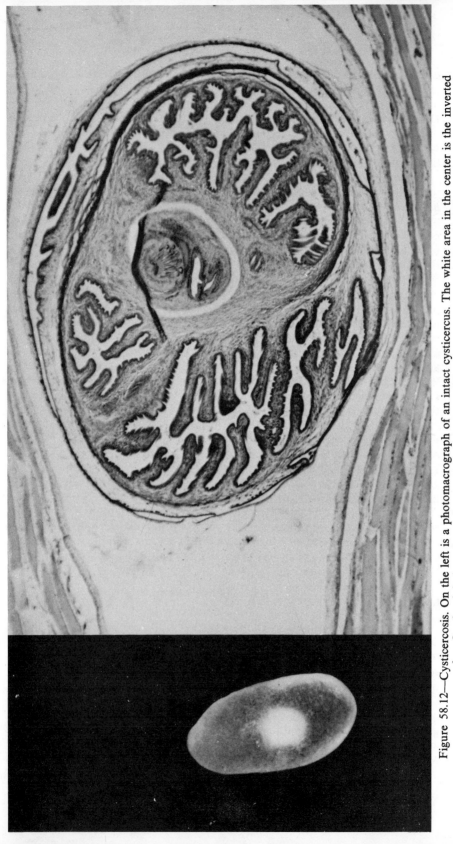

Figure 58.12—Cysticercosis. On the left is a photomacrograph of an intact cysticercus. The white area in the center is the inverted scolex. On the right is a photomicrograph of a section of a cysticercus in tissue. Hooklets may be seen in the inverted scolex. The clear areas to the sides of the inverted scolex are the fluid filled cyst.

is most frequently diagnosed by serologic means although it may occasionally be diagnosed by biopsy. Serologic techniques are not well developed at this time. Proctor et al. (40) in South Africa and Biagi et al. (8) in Mexico have reported excellent results using IHA in both animals and man. Significant cross-reactions occur between cysticercosis and echinococcosis sera and antigens. This close relationship between cestode infections has defied resolution although tests such as double diffusion and counterelectrophoresis have been investigated.

If the clinician is aware of the cross-reactions between cysticercosis and echinococcosis, the IHA test may provide a reliable diagnostic aid with titers of 1:128 or greater considered clinically important (Table 57.2). Serologic tests are available from the CDC.

Echinococcus

The definitive hosts for *Echinococcus* species are dogs, foxes, coyotes, and related animals. The usual intermediate hosts are sheep, cattle, or rodents, depending upon the specific species. Man becomes infected (hydatid disease) by ingesting eggs from feces of the definitive host and thus functions as an intermediate host. It generally takes years for the cysts to develop to a size where they become symptomatic. Larval stages (hydatid cysts) develop in the liver, lungs, and other areas of the body.

Diagnosis can be made either by finding scoleces in fluid from the cyst or by serologic testing. Immunodiagnostic procedures are the common means of diagnosis.

The serology of hydatid disease has been thoroughly evaluated and reported by Kagan (29). The IHA test is a sensitive and reactive procedure. There is a cross reactivity with about 50 percent of cysticercosis sera but very little problem with other diseases. Other tests, such as IIF (3, 12) and immunoelectrophoresis, have been used to increase specificity but each has its drawbacks.

The IHA reactivity may remain at low levels for long periods (years), while IIF tends to become negative within 1 year (3). Antigen for IIF is the scoleces from viable cysts and is somewhat more difficult to obtain than the hydatid fluid antigen used for IHA. In addition, the IHA test is a more rapid, simple procedure.

Counterelectrophoresis (CEP) has been used to demonstrate an antigen-antibody precipitin line known as "band 5" which is specific for echinococcosis (12). Although difficult to perform and requiring relatively large amounts of serum and antigen, CEP can be used to differentiate hydatidosis from cysticercosis. Unfortunately, the test requires a very reactive serum, frequently necessitating concentration to produce a band. The test is positive in only about 40 percent of proven cases.

A Casoni skin test for echinococcosis is available but is of little diagnostic value because it is undersensitive and once a patient reacts to the antigen the test will remain positive for life. Negatives must be questioned due to low sensitivity and positives give no temporal information; thus, skin test data are difficult to interpret.

With the IHA test, a titer of 1:128 should be considered significant and titers of 1:16,000 are not unusual (Table 57.2). Patients in whom the hydatid cyst is limited to the lung, or in whom the cyst is old and calcified, may have negative or low serologic titers. Complete surgical removal usually leads to a rapid decline of antibody in 2 to 3 months, and failure to observe the decline usually indicates incomplete cyst removal. Rupture of a cyst, either naturally or at surgery, may cause an allergic response with very high titers.

Sparganosis

Sparganosis is caused by the spargana (or plerocercoid) stages of diphyllobothrid species of lower animals, probably *Spirometra* species. The spargana of these species develop in various animals including frogs and snakes. The habit of using raw frog or snake tissue to treat "black eyes" may lead to ocular infections if the parasite migrates from the animal tissue into the eye. Man may also become infected by swallowing infected water crustacea *(Cyclops* spp.). Infections usually occur in the cutaneous tissue or in the eye and are generally diagnosed by examining surgically removed organisms.

Coenurosis

Coenurosis is the disease produced by larvae of the genus *Multiceps*—cestode parasites of dogs, wolves, and foxes. The larval stage, a coenurus, is a cystic form similar to the hydatid cyst of *Echinococcus* species. As in the hydatid cyst, multiple scoleces are produced, but there is only one cyst cavity and no daughter cysts. The usual intermediate hosts are herbivores (such as sheep) or rodents, depending on the specific species. The location of the coenurus also varies with the species and may be located in the brain, subcutaneous tissue, or somatic musculature. Humans are infected by ingesting eggs from dog feces. Infections of the eye and brain have been reported. Diagnosis is based on examination of surgically removed specimens.

References

1. ALLAIN DS and KAGAN IG: An evaluation of the direct agglutination test for Chagas' disease. J Parasitol 60:179–184, 1974
2. ALLAIN DS and KAGAN AG: A direct agglutination test for leishmaniasis. Am J Trop Med Hyg 24:232–236, 1975
3. AMBROISE-THOMAS P and KIEN-TRUONG T: L-immnonfluorescence dans le diagnostic serologique et le controle post-operataive de l'hydatidose humaine. I. Materiel et methods. Cah Med Lyon 46:2955–2962, 1970
4. AMBROISE-THOMAS P and KIEN-TRUONG T: Application of the Indirect Fluorescent Antibody Test on Sections of Adult Filariae to the Serodiagnosis, Epidemiology and Post Therapeutic Surveillance of Human Filariasis. WHO/FIL/72-101, World Health Organization, Geneva, 1972
5. APLEY J, CLARKE SKR, ROOME APCH, SANDRY SA, SAYGI G, SILK B, and WARHURST DC: Primary amoebic meningoencephalitis in Britain. Br Med J 1:596–599, 1970
6. BEAVER PC: The nature of visceral larva migrans. J Parasitol 55:3–12, 1969
7. BEAVER PC, SNYDER CH, CARRERA GM, DENT JH, and LAFFERTY J: Chronic eosinophilia due to visceral larva migrans. Report of three cases. Pediatrics 9:7–19, 1952

8. BIAGI F, NAVARRETE F, PINA A, SANTIAGO AM, and TAPIA L: Estudio de tres reacciones serologicas en el diagnostico de la cisticercosis. Rev Med Hosp Gen (Mex) 24:501–508, 1961

9. BOWLING MC, SMITH I, and WESCOTT SL: A rapid staining procedure for *Pneumocystis carinii*. Am J Med Technol 39:267–268, 1973

10. BRAY RS: Leishmaniasis. Annu Rev Microbiol 28:189–217, 1974

11. BUTT C: Primary amebic meningoencephalitis. N Engl J Med 274:1473, 1966

12. CAPRON A, YARZABAL LA, VERNES A, and FRUIT J: Le diagnostic immunologique de l'echinococcose humaine. Pathol-Biol 18:357–365, 1970

13. CARTER RF: Primary amebic meningoencephalitis, an appraisal of present knowledge. Trans R Soc Trop Med Hyg 66:193–213, 1972

14. CENTER FOR DISEASE CONTROL: Toxoplasmosis—Georgia. Morbidity and Mortality Weekly Report 26:409, 1977

15. CENTER FOR DISEASE CONTROL: Chemoprophylaxis of Malaria. Morbidity and Mortality Weekly Report (Supplement) 27:81, March, 1978

16. CENTER FOR DISEASE CONTROL: Morbidity and Mortality Weekly Report 29:613, January 9, 1981

17. COATNEY GR, COLLINS WE, WARREN McW, and CONTACOS PG: The Primate Malarias. U.S. Govt. Printing Office, Washington, DC, 1971

18. CONTACOS PG and COLLINS WE: Malaria relapse mechanism. Trans R Soc Trop Med Hyg 67:617–618, 1973

19. CUADRADO RR and KAGAN IG; The prevalence of antibodies to parasitic diseases with sera of young army recruits from the United States and Brazil. Am J Epidemiol 86:330–340, 1967

20. CULBERTSON CG: Soil amoeba infection. *In* Manual of Clinical Microbiology, 2nd Edition. Lennette EH, Spaulding EH, and Truant JP (eds.). American Society for Microbiology, Washington, DC, 1974, pp. 602–604

21. CYPESS RH, KAROL MH, ZIDIAN JL, GLICKMAN LT, and GITLIN D: Larva-specific antibodies in patients with visceral larva migrans. J Infect Dis 135:633–640, 1977

22. DESOWITZ RG, SAAVE JJ, and STEIN B: Application of the indirect hemaglutination test in recent studies on the immunoepidemiology of human malaria and the immune response in experimental malaria. Mil Med (Suppl) 131:1157–1166, 1966

23. EASTERLY JA: *Pneumocystis carinii* in lungs of adults at autopsy. Am Rev Respir Dis 97:935–937, 1968

24. FIFE EH JR and MUSCHEL LH: Fluorescent antibody technique for serodiagnosis of *Trypanosoma cruzi* infection. Proc Soc Exp Biol Med 101:540–543, 1959

25. GENTRY LO, RUSKIN J, and REMINGTON JS: *Pneumocystis carinii* pneumonia. Problems in diagnosis and therapy in 24 cases. Calif Med 116:6–10, 1972

26. HOARE CA: The Trypanosomes of Mammals; A Zoological Monograph. Blackwell Scientific Publications, Oxford, England, 1972

27. HUGHES WT: Current status of laboratory diagnosis of *Pneumocystis carinii* pneumonitis. *In* CRC Critical Reviews in Clinical Laboratory Sciences, 1975, pp. 145–170

28. JACOBS L and LUNDE MN: A hemagglutination test for toxoplasmosis. J Parasitol 43:308–314, 1957

29. KAGAN IG: A review of serologic tests for the diagnosis of hydatid disease. Bull WHO 39:25–37, 1968

30. KAGAN IG and NORMAN L: Serodiagnosis of parasitic diseases. *In* Manual of Clinical Immunology. Rose NR and Friedman HF (eds.). American Society for Microbiology, Washington, DC, 1976, pp. 382–409

31. KELEN AE, AYLLON-LEINDL L, LABZOFFSKY NA: Indirect fluorescent antibody method in serodiagnosis of toxoplasmosis. Can J Microbiol 8:545–554, 1962

32. LABZOFFSKY NA, BARATAWIDJAJA RK, KUITUNEN E, LEWIS FN, KAVELMAN DA, and MORRISSEY LP: Immunofluorescence as an aid in the early diagnosis of trichinosis. Can Med Assoc J 90:920–921, 1964

33. LAINSON R and SHAW JJ: Leishmaniasis of the New World: Taxonomic problems. Br Med Bull 28:44–48, 1972

34. LATORRE CR, SULZER AJ, and NORMAN LG: Serial propagation of *Pneumocystis carinii* in cell line cultures. Appl Environ Microbiol 33:1204, 1977

35. NORMAN L, and KAGAN IG: Bentonite, latex and cholesterol flocculation tests for the diagnosis of trichinosis. Public Health Rep 78:227–232, 1963
36. NORMAN L and KAGAN IG: Some observations in the serology of *Pneumocystis carinii* infections in the United States. Infect Immun 8:317–321, 1973
37. PIFER LL, HUGHES WT, and MURPHY MJ: Propagation of *Pneumocystis carinii* in vitro. Pediatr Res 11:305–316, 1977
38. PIFER LL, HUGHES WT, STAGNO S, and WOODS D: *Pneumocystis carinii* infection: Evidence of high prevalence in normal and immunosuppressed children. Pediatrics 61:35–41, 1978
39. PLONKA WS, GANCARZ Z, and ZAWADZKA-JEDRZEJEWSKA B: A rapid screening haemagglutination test in the diagnosis of human trichinosis. J Immunol Methods 1:309–312, 1972
40. PROCTOR EM and ELSDON-DEW R: Serological tests in porcine cysticercosis. S Afr J Sci 62:264–267, 1966
41. PROCTOR EM, POWELL SJ, and ELSDON-DEW R: The serological diagnosis of cysticerosis. Am Trop Med Parasitol 60:146–151, 1966
42. REMINGTON JS and DESMONTS G: Toxoplasmosis. *In* Remington JS and Klein JO: Infectious Diseases of the Fetus and Newborn Infant. W.B. Saunders Co, Philadelphia, 1976, pp. 191–332
43. RIFKIND D, FARIS TD, and HILL RB JR: *Pneumocystis carinii* pneumonia. Ann Intern Med 65:943–956, 1966
44. ROGERS WA JR, FRIED JA, and KAGAN IG: A modified indirect microhemagglutination test for malaria. Am J Trop Med Hyg 17:804–809, 1968
45. RUEBUSH TK II, CASSADAY PB, MARSH HJ, LISKER SA, VOORHEES DB, MAHONEY EB, and HEALY GR: Human babesiosis on Nantucket Island. Ann Intern Med 86:6–9, 1977
46. RUEBUSH TK II, JURANEK DD, CHISHOLM ES, SNOW PC, HEALY GR, and SULZER AJ: Human babesiosis on Nantucket Island. Evidence for self-limited and subclinical infections. N Engl J Med 297:825–827, 1977
47. RUEBUSH TK II, WEINSTEIN RA, BAEHNER RL, WOLFF D, BARTLETT M, GONZALES-CRUSSI F, SULZER AJ, and SCHULTZ MJ: An outbreak of *Pneumocystis* pneumonia in children with acute lymphocytic leukemia. Am J Dis Child 132:143–148, 1978
48. RUITENBERG EJ, STEERENBERG PA, and BROSI BJM: Microsystem for the application of ELISA to the serodiagnosis of *Trichinella spiralis* infections. Medikon Nederland 4:30–31, 1975
49. SABIN AB and FELDMAN HA: Dyes as microchemical indicators of a new immunity phenomenon affecting a protozoon parasite (*Toxoplasma*). Science 108:660–663, 1948
50. SASA M: Human Filariasis: A Global Survey of Epidemiology and Control. University Park Press, Baltimore, Md, 1976
51. SIDDIQUI WA, SCHNELL JV, and GEIMAN QM: *In vitro* cultivation of *Plasmodium falciparum*. Am J Trop Med Hyg 19:586–591, 1970
52. SULZER AJ, and HALL EC: Indirect fluorescent antibody tests for parasitic diseases. IV. Statistical study of variation in the indirect fluorescent antibody (IFA) test for toxoplasmosis. Am J Epidemiol 86:401–407, 1967
53. SULZER AJ, and LATORRE CR: A simplified method for *in vitro* production of schizonts of primate malarias useful as antigen in serologic tests. Trans R Soc Trop Med Hyg 71:553, 1977
54. SULZER AJ, WILSON M, and HALL EC: Indirect fluorescent antibody tests for parasitic diseases. V. An evaluation of a thick-smear antigen in the IFA test for malaria antibodies. Am J Trop Med Hyg 18:199–205, 1969
55. TRAGER W: A new method for intraerythrocytic cultivation of malaria parasites (*Plasmodium coatneyi* and *P. falciparum*). J Protozool 18:239–242, 1971
56. VATTUONE NH and YANOVSKY JF: *Trypanosoma cruzi*: Agglutination activity of enzyme-treated epimastigotes. Exp Parasitol 30:349–355, 1971
57. VOLLER A, BIDWELL DE, BARTLETT A, and EDWARDS R: A comparison of isotopic and enzyme-immunoassays for tropical parasitic diseases. Trans R Soc Trop Med Hyg 71:431–437, 1977
58. WALZER PD, SCHNELLE V, ARMSTRONG D, and ROSEN PO: The nude mouse: A new experimental model for *Pneumocystis carinii* infection. Science 197:177–179, 1977
59. WILSON M, FIFE EH JR, MATHEWS HM, and SULZER AJ: Comparison of the complement fixation, indirect immunofluorescence, and indirect hemagglutination tests for malaria. Am J Trop Med Hyg 24:755–759, 1975

CHAPTER 59

INTESTINAL AND ATRIAL PROTOZOA

James W. Smith and Marilyn S. Bartlett

Introduction

Several protozoa may inhabit the intestine and the atrial areas of man. Disease can be caused by *Entamoeba histolytica, Dientamoeba fragilis, Giardia lamblia, Trichomonas vaginalis, Balantidium coli,* or *Isospora belli.* Diagnosis is usually based on morphologic demonstration of protozoan cysts or trophozoites in appropriate specimens. In addition to these disease-causing protozoa, there are non-pathogenic protozoa, and it is important that they be recognized as commensals and differentiated from the potential pathogens mentioned above.

A recent review of results of the special parasitology proficiency testing program of the College of American Pathologists (27) shows that many laboratories have difficulty detecting and correctly identifying protozoa in fecal specimens.

The only atrial or intestinal protozoan for which serologic tests have been developed to a practical stage is *Entamoeba histolytica.* However, tests for giardiasis and trichomoniasis are being developed.

Amebae

Disease

The amebae belong to the class Rhizopoda and move by means of pseudopodia. *Entamoeba histolytica* is the most significant pathogen in this group, and ambebiasis is still the leading fatal intestinal parasitic infection in the United States (7). *Dientamoeba fragilis* can cause a less severe disease. In most instances, *E. histolytica* is a commensal in the intestinal lumen and does not cause disease. It can cause amebic colitis, which is characterized by alternating periods of constipation and diarrhea and asymptomatic intervals; occasionally it causes amebic dysentery, in which there is extensive ulceration of the colon with severe bloody diarrhea and toxicity. Amebic dysentery can be fatal if accompanied by such complications as perforation and peritonitis (1, 18). In instances of invasive amebiasis, such as with colitis and dysentery, the organisms may reach the blood stream and may cause metastatic abscesses in other organs (usually the liver). Liver abscesses develop in approximately 5 percent of people with untreated symptomatic intestinal disease (2). Amebiasis is acquired by ingesting cysts in contaminated food or water.

Dientamebiasis is a milder disease (31) not accompanied by liver abscesses. It is increasingly recognized as a cause of diarrhea, especially in California (8). There is no cyst stage, and it has been suggested the infection may sometimes be acquired by ingesting infected *Enterobius vermicularis* eggs (6). Recent taxonomic studies suggest that *D. fragilis* is a flagellate, but it will be included with the amebae in this discussion. Diagnosis is based on demonstrating the organism.

The other intestinal amebae (*E. coli, E. hartmanni, Endolimax nana,* and *Iodamoeba bütschlii*) are important in that they must be differentiated from the potentially pathogenic amebae (*E. histolytica* and *D. fragilis*). Size and morphologic characteristics of cysts and trophozoites allow identification of species. Size ranges of intestinal protozoa are shown in Figure 59.1.

Morphology

Morphologic characteristics of intestinal amebae are illustrated in Figures 59.2, 59.3, and 59.4 and are outlined in Tables 59.1 and 59.2. A self-study course is available (9).

Members of the genus *Entamoeba* have chromatin granules deposited on

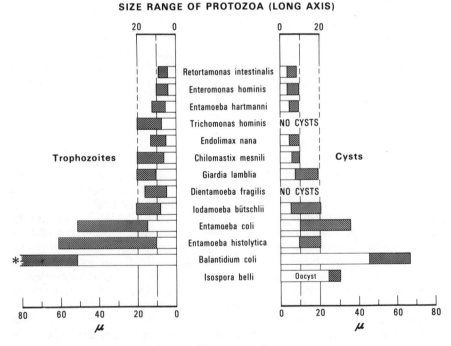

Figure 59.1—Size range of protozoa.

Figure 2
PROTOZOA FOUND IN STOOL SPECIMENS OF MAN

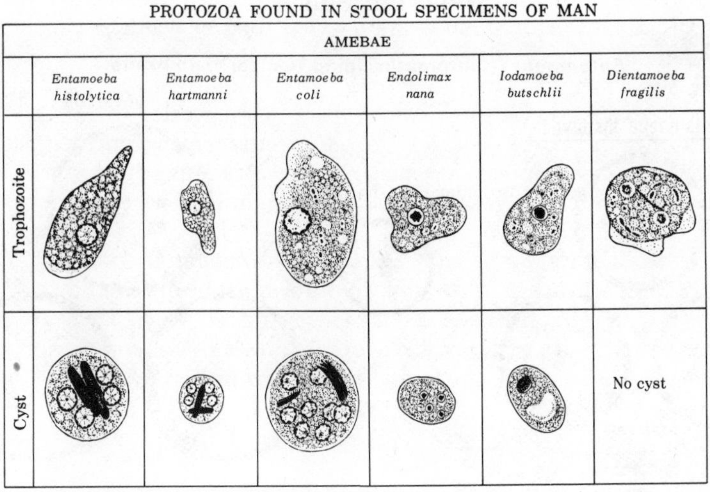

Figure 59.2—Protozoa found in stool specimens of man. Adapted with permission from Brooke MM and Melvin DM: Morphology of Diagnostic Stages of Intestinal Parasites of Man, U.S. Department of Health, Education, and Welfare Publ. No. (HSM) 72-8116.

the nuclear membrane (peripheral nuclear chromatin) and are the only amebae that infect humans which have this characteristic. *E. hartmanni* and *E. histolytica* are very similar and must be differentiated primarily on the basis of size. Trophozoites of *E. hartmanni* are smaller than 12 μm at the widest point, and cysts are smaller than 10 μm. Conversely, trophozoites of *E. histolytica* are generally larger than 12 μm, and cysts are larger than 10μm. Because of random variability in size, it is possible for a patient whose specimen contains numerous organisms of more than one species to have occasional organisms which slightly overlap the size range of the other species. A second species identification should not be made unless there is a distinct population of organisms of the second size. Trophozoites of *E. histolytica* vary from 12 to 60 μm at the widest point, with the largest organisms generally associated with invasive disease. Patients with amebic dysentery often harbor *E. histolytica* trophozites which have phagocytized erythrocytes in their cytoplasm. In general, the cytoplasm of *E. histolytica* does not contain ingested bacteria or yeasts, although commensal forms may contain some.

In saline wet mounts of fresh material, trophozoites of *E. histolytica* show directional movement, with elongated pseudopods of ectoplasm sharply demarcated from the more granular endoplasm; the organisms are often elongated. The nuclei are not visible. Trophozoites of *E. hartmanni*, although smaller, move similarly but more sluggishly. In contrast, trophozoites of *E. coli* are more rounded and do not show directional movement. In addition, there may be multiple blunt pseudopodia, and the ectoplasm is less sharply demar-

NUCLEI of AMEBAE

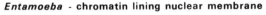

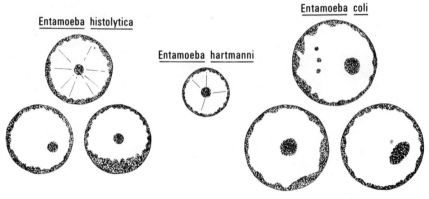

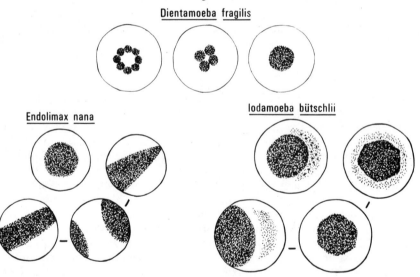

Figure 59.3—Nuclei of amebae.

cated from the endoplasm. Nuclei of *E. coli* may be visible in unstained saline wet mounts.

In stained preparations, the nuclei of *E. histolytica* typically have evenly distributed peripheral chromatin with a rounded central karyosome, and those of *E. hartmanni* are similar in appearance (Fig 59.2, 59.3, 59.4). In contrast, the nuclei of *E. coli* trophozoites have more irregularly distributed chromatin on the nuclear membrane and have larger, more irregular karyosomes, sometimes with fragments of chromatin material in the karyolymph

TABLE 59.1.— MORPHOLOGY OF TROPHOZOITES OF INTESTINAL AMEBAE

SPECIES	SIZE (DIAMETER OR LENGTH)	MOTILITY	NUCLEUS				CYTOPLASM	
			NUMBER	PERIPHERAL CHROMATIN	KARYOSOMAL CHROMATIN		APPEARANCE	INCLUSIONS
Entamoeba histolytica	12-60 μm Usual range, 15-20 μ-m* Over 20 μm†	Progressive, with hyaline, fingerlike pseudopods.	1 Not visible in unstained preparations.	Fine granules. Usually evenly distributed and uniform in size.	Small, discrete. Usually centrally located, but occasionally is eccentric.		Finely granular.	Erythocytes occasionally. Noninvasive organisms may contain bacteria.
Entamoeba hartmanni	5-12 μm Usual range, 8-10 μm	Usually nonprogressive, but may be progressive occasionally	1 Not visible in unstained preparations.	Similar to _E. histolytica._	Small, discrete, often eccentrically located.		Finely granular.	Bacteria.
Entamoeba coli	15-50 μm Usual range, 20-25 μm	Sluggish, nonprogressive, with blunt pseudopods.	1 Often visible in unstained preparations.	Coarse granules, irregular in size and distribution.	Large, discrete, usually eccentrically located.		Coarse, often vacuolated.	Bacteria, yeasts, other materials.
Endolimax nana	6-12 μm Usual range, 8-10 μm	Sluggish, usually nonprogressive, with blunt pseudopods.	1 Visible occasionally in unstained preparations.	None.	Large, irregularly shaped, blotlike		Granular, vacuolated.	Bacteria.
Iodamoeba bütschlii	8-20 μm Usual range, 12-15 μm	Sluggish, usually nonprogressive.	1 Not usually visible in unstained preparations.	None.	Large, usually centrally located. Surrounded by refractile, achromatic granules. These granules are often not distinct even in stained slides.		Coarsely granular, vacuolated.	Bacteria, yeasts, or other material
Dientamoeba fragilis	5-15 μm Usual range, 9-12 μm	Pseudopodia are angular, serrated, or broad lobed and hyaline, almost transparent.	2 (In approximately 20% of organisms only 1 nucleus is present.) Nuceli invisible in unstained preparations.	None.	Large cluster of 4-8 granules.		Finely granular, vacuolated.	Bacteria.

* For the commensal form. Usually found in asymptomatic or chronic cases; may contain bacteria.
† For the invasive form. Usually found in acute cases; often contain red blood cells.

Adapted with permission from Brooke MM and Melvin DM: Morphology of Diagnostic Stages of Intestinal Parasites of Man, U.S. Department of Health, Education, and Welfare Publ. No. (HSM) 72-8116, 1969.

TABLE 59.2—MORPHOLOGY OF CYSTS OF INTESTINAL AMEBAE

SPECIES	SIZE	SHAPE	NUCLEUS			CYTOPLASM	
			NUMBER	PERIPHERAL CHROMATIN	KARYOSOMAL CHROMATIN	CHROMATOID BODIES	GLYCOGEN
Entamoeba histolytica	10-20 μm. Usual range, 12-15 μm.	Usually spherical.	4 in mature cyst. Immature cysts with 1 or 2 occasionally seen.	Peripheral chromatin present. Fine, uniform granules, evenly distributed.	Small, discrete, usually centrally located. May be eccentric.	Present. Elongated bars with bluntly rounded ends or irregular bodies.	Usually diffuse. Concentrated mass often present in young cysts. Stains reddish brown with iodine.
Entamoeba hartmanni	5-10 μm. Usual range, 6-8 μm.	Usually spherical.	4 in mature cyst. Immature cysts with 1 or 2 often seen.	Similar to *E. histolytica*.	Similar to *E. histolytica*.	Present. Elongated bars with bluntly rounded end or irregular bodies often abundant.	Similar to *E. histolytica*.
Entamoeba coli	10-35 μm. Usual range, 15-25 μm.	Usually spherical. Occasionally oval, triangular, or of another shape.	8 in mature cyst. Occasionally, supernucleate cysts with 16 or more are seen. Immature cysts with 2 or more occasionally seen.	Peripheral chromatin present. Coarse granules irregular in size and distribution, but often appear more uniform than in trophozoites.	Large, discrete, usually eccentrically, but occasionally centrally located	Present, but less frequently seen than in *E. histolytica*. Usually splinterlike with pointed ends.	Usually diffuse, but occasionally well-defined mass in immature cysts. Stains reddish brown with iodine.
Endolimax nana	5-10 μm. Usual range, 6-8 μm.	Spherical, ovoid, or ellipsoidal.	4 in mature cysts. Immature cysts with less than 4 occasionally seen.	None.	Large (blotite), usually centrally located.	Occasionally, granules or small oval masses seen, but bodies as seen in *Entamoeba* species are not present.	Usually diffuse. Concentrated mass seen occasionally in young cysts. Stains reddish brown with iodine.
Iodamoeba bütschlii	5-20 μm. Usual range, 10-12 μm.	Ovoid, ellipsoidal, triangular, or of another shape.	1 in mature cyst.	None.	Large, usually eccentrically located. Refractile, achromatic granules on one side of karyosome. Indistinct in iodine preparations.	Granules occasionally present, but chromatoid bodies as seen in *Entamoeba* species are not present.	Compact, well-defined mass. Stains dark brown with iodine.

Adapted with permission from Brooke MM and Melvin, DM: Morphology of Diagnostic Stages of Intestinal Parasites of Man, U.S. Department of Health, Education, and Welfare Publ. No. (HSM) 72-8116, 1969.

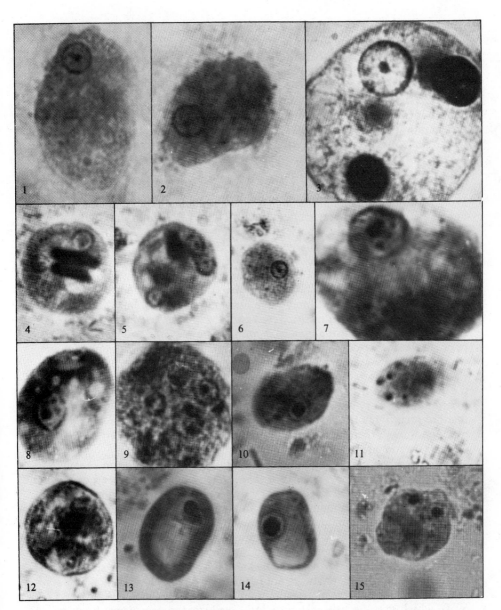

Figure 59.4—Intestinal amebae. All these trichrome-stained amebae are photographed at the same magnification. (1, 2) *Entamoeba histolytica* trophozoites. (3) *E. histolytica* trophozoite containing phagocytized erythrocytes. (4, 5) *E. histolytica* cysts with chromatoid bodies and glycogen vacuoles. Only some of the nuclei are visible at this focal plane. (6) *E. hartmanni* trophozoite. (7, 8) *E. coli* trophozoites. (9) *E. coli* cyst with four nuclei clearly evident at this focal plane. There are no chromatoid bodies. (10) *Endolimax nana* trophozoite. (11) *E. nana* cyst. (12) *Iodamoeba bütschlii* trophozoite with achromatic granules above and to the right of the karyosome. (13) *I. bütschlii* trophozoite with achromatic granules below the karyosome. (14) *I. bütschlii* cyst without evident achromatic granules. (15) *Dientamoeba fragilis* trophozoite with two nuclei.

space (Fig 59.2, 59.3, 59.4). However, nuclei do vary in appearance. *E. histolytica* or *E. hartmanni* may have karyosomes which are not central and peripheral chromatin which is unevenly distributed; conversely, *E. coli* trophozoites may have evenly distributed peripheral chromatin or central karyosomes. Thus, no single characteristic is pathognomonic of the nuclei of any of the *Entamoeba* species. The cytoplasm of *E. histolytica* generally has few phagocytized inclusions and is delicately stained, as is that of *E. hartmanni*; however, degenerating organisms may have vacuolated cytoplasm. The cytoplasm of *E. coli* trophozoites typically contains numerous ingested bacteria and yeasts and may be quite vacuolated. The cytoplasm of *E. coli* also tends to stain more intensely than that of *E. histolytica*.

Cysts of *E. histolytica* and *E. hartmanni* are similar in appearance (Fig 59.2, 59.4). Cysts may contain glycogen, which stains reddish-brown in fresh iodine wet mounts. In preparations made from preserved material, the glycogen is removed and only the vacuoles are left. Cysts may contain chromatoid bodies of various sizes and shapes (they generally have rounded ends). Mature cysts contain four nuclei, each of which is approximately one-sixth the diameter of the cyst (10). Immature cysts containing one to three nuclei may also be found. *E. coli* cysts (Fig 59.2, 59.4) may also contain glycogen vacuoles, particularly when immature, and may have chromatoid bodies, but these typically are fibers or have angular or splintered ends. Mature *E. coli* cysts contain eight nuclei, but careful focusing up and down may be required to see them all. Hypernucleate forms containing 16 or even 32 nuclei are occasionally seen. Quadrinucleate *E. coli* cysts are uncommon, and the size of the nuclei in quadrinucleate cysts is generally one-fourth rather than one-sixth the diameter of the cyst (10). The distribution of chromatin on the nuclear membrane and the location of the karyosome are less reliable characteristics for identifying cysts than for identifying trophozoites. Cysts of the *Entamoeba* species are generally round, although there may be some irregularity and indentation, particularly in fixed specimens, possibly as a result of shrinkage.

In saline wet mounts, cysts appear as refractile structures and chromatoid bodies may be evident. Nuclei of unfixed *E. histolytica* cysts are not visible, whereas those of unfixed *E. coli* may be. In formalin-fixed specimens, nuclei of both may be visible. In iodine-stained wet mounts, nuclei are visible, chromatoid bodies do not stain, glycogen stains red-brown (unless glycogen has been washed out by prolonged fixation), and cysts are less refractile.

Identifying non-*Entamoeba* species may also be difficult. The trophozoites of the three species (*D. fragilis, E. nana, I. bütschlii*) overlap in size, and the nuclei share the characteristic of not having peripheral chromatin. The karyosomes of *D. fragilis* nuclei consist of four to eight granules (Fig 59.2, 59.3, 59.4), which may be seen in particularly well-stained organisms; however, in some organisms, the granules may appear to be one large karyosome. If the organism is binucleate, as 80% of *D. fragilis* trophozoites are, identification may still be possible; however, if it is uninucleate, differentiation from other amebae may not be possible unless multiple organisms are examined. The nucleus of *E. nana* typically has a large rounded central karyosome without peripheral chromatin on the nuclear membrane (Fig 59.2, 59.3, 59.4), but there are also *E. nana* nuclei which have triangular-shaped karyosomes, band-shaped karyosomes, and split karyosomes (Fig 59.3) with portions on the nuclear membrane on opposite sides of the nucleus. The presence of such nuclei should make one suspect *E. nana*. *I. bütschlii* also has a large karyosome with no chromatin on the nuclear membrane. In some instances, the nuclei of *I. bütschlii* and *E. nana* cannot be differentiated. However, *I. bütschlii* nuclei typically contain achromatic granules which appear in a group as a crescent on one side of the karyosome or as a circle surrounding the karyosome such that the karyolymph space is hazy (Fig 59.2, 59.3, 59.4). Unfortunately, these may not be demonstrable in many organisms and may make differentiation from *E. nana* difficult. The cytoplasms of the trophozoites of the three species also differ. *I. bütschlii* is a particularly voracious scavenger, with the cytoplasm generally being filled with numerous ingested bacteria, yeasts, and vacuoles. The cytoplasm of *E. nana* often has a similar appearance, although the amount of phagocytized material may be slightly less. The cytoplasm of *D. fragilis* may stain less intensely than that of the other two species, but it also sometimes contains ingested bacteria.

   D. fragilis does not have a cyst stage. Differentiation of the cysts of *I. bütschlii* and *E. nana* (Fig 59.2, 59.4) is usually not difficult. The nucleus of an *I. bütschlii* cyst often has an eccentric karyosome with a crescent of achromatic granules adjacent to it, although variable forms may also be seen (some of which have central karyosomes and some of which do not contain demonstrable achromatic granules). The cyst of *E. nana* when mature contains four nuclei which are smaller than the single nucleus of the *I. bütschlii* cyst. The karyosomes of *I. bütschlii* cysts do not stain with iodine, and those of the *E. nana* cysts stain dark brown with iodine. *I. bütschlii* cysts typically contain a large glycogen vacuole which stains with iodine. Glycogen is washed out in material which has been stored for an extended period or in that stained with permanent stains. It should be emphasized that glycogen vacuoles are also common in cysts of the *Entamoeba* species, and there may be large amounts of glycogen in young *E. nana* cysts; thus, the presence of glycogen alone is not enough to identify *I. bütschlii*. *I. bütschlii* cysts may vary greatly in shape, with elongated or kidney bean-shaped cysts sometimes found. *E. nana* cysts may contain some chromatoid fibrils but generally do not contain the prominent chromatoid bodies associated with the *Entamoeba* species.

Diagnosis of Amebiasis

   Amebiasis in the intestinal tract is usually diagnosed by demonstrating the organisms in fecal specimens or sigmoid aspirates but can be suspected by demonstrating an elevated serologic titer to *E. histolytica*. Hepatic abscess can be strongly suspected if an elevated titer is demonstrated. In addition, if the abscess is aspirated, it may be possible to demonstrate organisms either in the aspirated material or in sections from the margin of the abscess. The material most likely to contain demonstrable amebae is the last material aspirated from the abscess (usually bloody). Cultures of abscess material may be made but require inoculation with *Clostridium perfringens* or another appropriate bacterium to allow growth of *E. histolytica* (22).

   Although new tests are continually being introduced and evaluated, the

indirect hemagglutination test (IHA) introduced in 1961 (17) is the most frequently used procedure for serodiagnosing amebiasis. Details of the procedure
are described by Kagan and Norman (16). The IHA is a highly sensitive and
specific procedure involving a sonic lysate of axenically grown amebae. Several reports (13, 21, 23) have shown that IHA is positive for more than 96% of
patients with amebic liver abscess and for more than 85% of those with acute
amebic dysentery. Specificity was verified by a reactivity rate of less than 6% in
nonamebic diseases and healthy individuals. Antibody can persist for more
than 2 years in some patients (14). Negative amebic serologic results rule out
an amebic liver abscess as the cause of a patient's problem. It has been suggested that serologic tests for amebae be performed for all patients suspected
to have ulcerative colitis to rule out amebiasis before beginning therapy (18).
The Center for Disease Control considers an IHA titer of 1:128 to be clinically
significant (Table 57.2). Because the test is simple, and the reagents are commercially available, serodiagnosis by IHA at the local level is possible.

An alternative procedure which can be performed in the small laboratory
is counterelectrophoresis (CEP). Available from at least two manufacturers,
CEP is a sensitive, simple, and rapid test. Although not quantitative, CEP results correlate well with those of IHA for clinically apparent cases (19). Some
sera produce more than one reactivity band, the significance of which is not
yet known.

An ELISA method which detects *E. histolytica* antigens in fecal specimens
has recently been described (25) and is commercially available (Immunozyme,
Millipore Corp., Bedford, Mass.). It appears promising, with good sensitivity
and specificity.

Atrial Ameba

The atrial ameba, *Entamoeba gingivalis*, occurs only as a trophozoite and
closely resembles *E. histolytica*. The fact that such an organism does exist
should be remembered when attempting to diagnose pulmonary amebiasis
with expectorated sputum specimens, because the two organisms might be
confused. *E. gingivalis* typically contains numerous cytoplasmic inclusions including bacteria, erythrocytes, and leukocytes.

Flagellates

Giardia lamblia

Intestinal flagellates belong to the class Mastigophora. The intestinal
pathogen, *Giardia lamblia*, is recognized more and more often as a source of
disease in the United States and elsewhere in the world (30). It is the most
common pathogen found in fecal specimens in the United States, being present in 3.5% of all specimens submitted to state public health laboratories (7).

Giardiasis is an intestinal parasitic infection of the duodenum and jejunum which causes alternating diarrhea and constipation accompanied by ab-

dominal discomfort. The abdominal discomfort is likely to be described as being above rather than below the umbilicus as is commonly seen with colonic disease. *G. lamblia* has caused several large outbreaks in the United States including those in Rome, New York (26), and Aspen, Colorado (24), and is a continuing problem as a cause of sporadic diarrhea in this country. It has also caused outbreaks in various foreign countries and has particularly been a problem among travelers to Moscow and Leningrad, Russia. It has caused outbreaks in nursery schools (4). Campers in the western United States often acquire giardiasis from contaminated water in lakes and streams. It appears that there may be reservoirs for *G. lamblia* in various animal species (3).

Large outbreaks of giardiasis have generally been traced to water supplies. *G. lamblia* cysts are apparently not killed by the level of chlorine present in many municipal water supplies, and unless filtering systems are adequate to remove organisms, major outbreaks can occur (15).

The trophozoites of this species inhabit the duodenum and jejunum, where they cause inflammation of the mucosa with a malabsorption-type syndrome. The symptoms may vary somewhat from day to day, but giardiasis should be suspected in anyone who has had diarrhea for 10 days or longer.

Diagnosing giardiasis depends on demonstrating the parasites in fecal specimens or in small intestinal contents (28). Studies have shown that the number of organisms present in feces may vary significantly from day to day (11), and it is suggested that obtaining a specimen every second or third day for a total of three specimens might be advisable to assure diagnosis. Occasionally, diagnosis may still not be established, and duodenal aspiration may be required to demonstrate the presence of *G. lamblia*.

Recently, a report by Visvesvara and Healy (29) has indicated the possible usefulness of the IIF test in the serodiagnosis of giardiasis. Using axenically cultured organisms as antigen, the test was positive in 67 percent of proven cases. No cross-reactions were identified in this original article. Still preliminary in nature, the test is being offered on an experimental basis at the CDC.

Morphologic characteristics of intestinal flagellates are illustrated in Figures 59.5 and 59.6 and described in Tables 59.3 and 59.4. Morphologically, *G. lamblia* organisms have a distinctive appearnce. The trophozoite is shaped like half a pear, with a sucking disk occupying the anterior half of the flattened surface. The organism has two nuclei which have large karyosomes, usually central, and no peripheral chromatin. There are typically four pairs of flagella. The two axonemes extend through the organism in the long axis, and there is a median body in the center of the organism. In saline mounts of fresh material, the *Giardia* trophozoites have a movement generally described as a "falling leaf in a stream," which differs markedly from the ameboid movement of *E. histolytica*. Cysts of *G. lamblia* are oval and have two to four nuclei, the quadrinculeate form being mature. Fibrils (axonemes and median body) are visible in wet mounts. Portions of the cytoplasm may have pulled away from the cyst wall. In fecal specimens, there may be some cysts which show degenerative changes, and diagnosis should not be based on cysts which do not contain demonstrable nuclei and fibrils. Finding such organisms should suggest that a careful search be made for typical cysts of *G. lamblia*.

Figure 2
PROTOZOA FOUND IN STOOL SPECIMENS OF MAN

	FLAGELLATES			CILIATE	COCCIDIA
	Trichomonas hominis	*Chilomastix mesnili*	*Giardia lamblia*	*Balantidium coli*	*Isospora* spp.
Trophozoite					immature oöcyst / mature oöcyst
Cyst	No cyst				single sporocyst / double sporocysts

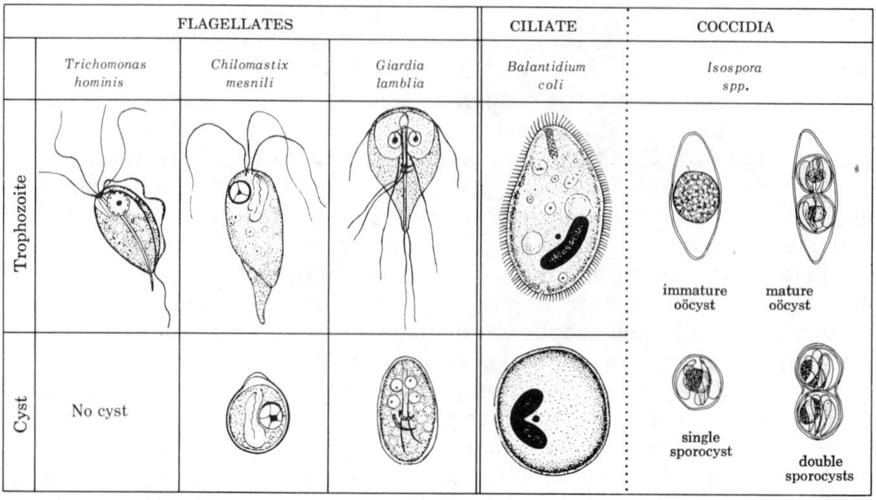

Figure 59.5—Flagellates, ciliate, and coccidia found in stool specimens of man. Adapted with permission from Brooke MM and Melvin DM: Morphology of Diagnostic Stages of Intestinal Parasites of Man, U.S. Department of Health, Education, and Welfare Publ. No. (HSM) 72-8116.

Chilomastix mesnili

This flagellate is non-pathogenic and may be found in stool specimens (Fig 59.5, 59.6; Tables 59.3, 59.4). In saline mounts of fresh material, it exhibits stiff and wobbling movement. It has three anterior flagella, and there is a flagellum in the cytostome. The nucleus usually has a large, granular karyosome, and there may be chromatin on the nuclear membrane which is usually arranged in a "lop-sided" manner (or with a concentration of chromatin along one side). The karyosome may be central. The cytostome—which extends one-third to one-half the length of the body—is present adjacent to the nucleus and can be a helpful diagnostic characteristic. Careful focusing may aid in demonstrating the cytostome. A spiral groove extends the length of the body and is usually visible only as an irregularity of the outline of the organism. The organisms are elongated and have a tapered posterior end and the nucleus located near the anterior end. In stained smears, these organisms may be confused with trophozoites of various species of amebae, but *Chilomastix* should be suspected if nuclei are always present at one end of the organism and the opposite end tapers. Flagella are not generally visible in fresh or stained materials. The type of motion in wet mounts allows these organisms to be differentiated from the amebae and other intestinal flagellates. Cysts of *C. mesnili* are elongated and lemon-shaped, with a nipple-like hyaline structure at one end. The nucleus is generally at the side and resembles the nucleus of the tropho-

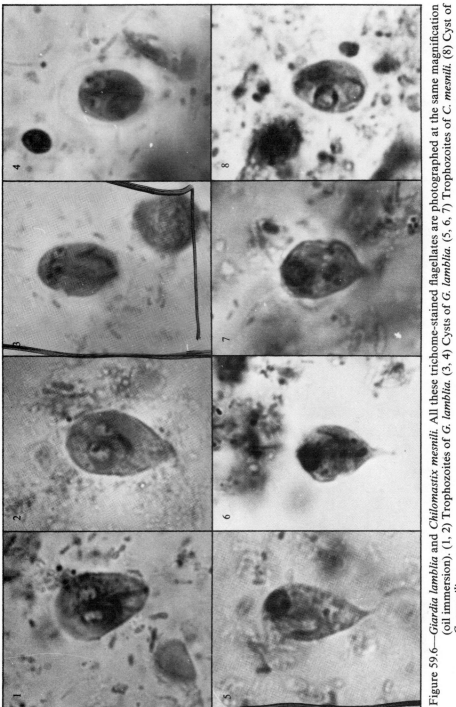

Figure 59.6—*Giardia lamblia* and *Chilomastix mesnili.* All these trichome-stained flagellates are photographed at the same magnification (oil immersion). (1, 2) Trophozoites of *G. lamblia.* (3, 4) Cysts of *G. lamblia.* (5, 6, 7) Trophozoites of *C. mesnili.* (8) Cyst of *C. mesnili.*

TABLE 59.3—MORPHOLOGY OF TROPHOZOITES OF INTESTINAL FLAGELLATES

Species	Size (Length)	Shape	Motility	Number of Nuclei	Number of Flagella*	Other Features
Trichomonas hominis	8-20 μm. Usual range, 11-12 μm.	Pear-shaped.	Rapid, jerking	1 Not visible in unstained mounts.	3-5 anterior. 1 posterior.	Undulating membrane extending length of body.
Chilomastix mesnili	6-24 μm. Usual range, 10-15 μm.	Pear-shaped.	Stiff, rotary.	1 Not visible in unstained mounts.	3 anterior. 1 in cytostome.	Prominent cytostome extending 1/3–1/2 length of body. Spiral groove across ventral surface.
Giardia lamblia	10-20 μm. Usual range, 12-15 μm.	Pear-shaped.	"Falling leaf."	2 Not visible in unstained mounts.	4 lateral. 2 ventral. 2 caudal.	Sucking disk occupying 1/2–3/4 of ventral surface.
Enteromonas hominis	4-10 μm. Usual range, 8-9 μm.	Oval.	Jerking	1 Not visible in unstained mounts.	3 anterior. 1 posterior.	One side of body flattened. Posterior flagellum extending free, posteriorly or laterally.
Retortamonas intestinalis	4-9 μm. Usual range, 6-7 μm.	Pear-shaped, or oval.	Jerking	1 Not visible in unstained mounts.	1 anterior. 1 posterior.	Prominent cytostome extending approximately 1/2 length of body.

* Not a practical feature for identification of species in routine fecal examinations.

Adapted with permission from Brooke MM and Melvin, DM: Morphology of Diagnostic Stages of Intestinal Parasites of Man, U.S. Department of Health, Education, and Welfare Publ. No. (HSM) 72-8116.

TABLE 59.4— MORPHOLOGY OF CYSTS OF INTESTINAL FLAGELLATES

SPECIES	SIZE	SHAPE	NUMBER OF NUCLEI	OTHER FEATURES
Trichomonas hominis	No cyst.			
Chilomastix mesnili	6-10 μm. Usual range, 8-9 μm.	Lemon-shaped, with anterior hyaline knob or "nipple."	1 Not visible in unstained preparations.	Cytostome with supporting fibrils. Usually visible in stained preparation.
Giardia lamblia	8-19 μm. Usual range, 11-12 μm.	Oval or ellipsoidal.	Usually 4. Not distinct in unstained preparations. Usually located at one end. Immature cysts may have two or three nuclei.	Fibrils or flagella longitudinally in cyst. Occasionally may be slightly visible in unstained cysts. Deep-staining fibers or fibrils may be seen lying laterally or obliquely across fibrils in lower part of cyst. Cytoplasm often retracts from a portion of cell wall.
Enteromonas hominis	4-10 μm. Usual range, 6-8 μm.	Elongated or oval.	1-4, usually 2 lying at opposite ends of cyst. Not visible in unstained mounts.	Resembles *E. nana* cyst. Fibrils or flagella are usually not seen.
Retortamonas intestinalis	4-9 μm. Usual range, 4-7 μm.	Pear-shaped or slightly lemon-shaped.	1 Not visible in unstained mounts.	Resembles *Chilomastix* cyst. Shadow outline of cytostome with supporting fibrils extends above nucleus.

Adapted with permission from Brooke MM and Melvin, DM: Morphology of Diagnostic Stages of Intestinal Parasites of Man U.S. Department Health, Education, and Welfare Publ. No. (HSM) 72-8116.

zoite. The primitive cytostome and cytostomal fibrils are evident in wet mounts or in permanently stained smears. The configuration of the cytostomal fibrils has been likened to that of a safety pin.

Trichomonas hominis

This flagellate is a commensal which can inhabit the intestinal tract of man (Fig 59.5, Table 59.3). It does not form cysts and is fairly small. In saline wet mounts, it has quick, jerky motions, and when trapped in fecal material an undulating membrane and flagella may be visible. The undulating membrane arises at the anterior end and runs along the entire length of the organism, ending in a free posterior flagellum. Extending through the center of the organism are an axostyle and a curved rod (the costa), which marks the attachment of the undulating membrane to the organism. *T. hominis* trophozoites generally do not stain well in permanently stained preparations and may be difficult to differentiate from amebae. Organisms are usually delicately stained, and the nucleus varies in appearance—sometimes appearing to have peripheral chromatin. The presence of multiple organisms with nuclei toward one end, the presence of the axostyle, and the lack of a prominent cytostome may lead one to suspect this organism. The undulating membrane is generally not evident in stained preparations or is seen as a wavy line extending down the body.

Two very small, infrequently seen flagellates (*Enteromonas hominis* and *Retortomonas intestinalis*) are not a major problem; their characteristics are shown in Tables 59.3 and 59.4.

Trichomonas vaginalis

This flagellate is a common cause of vaginitis and is similar to *T. hominis*. It may also occasionally cause prostatitis in males, although males are more often asymptomatic carriers who may spread the infection. *T. vaginalis* is larger (30 μm) than *T. hominis*, and the undulating membrane extends only half the length of the body. Because they have different habitats, it is generally not necessary to differentiate *T. hominis* from *T. vaginalis*.

Diagnosis is usually based on detecting organisms with the typical jerky movement in wet mounts of vaginal materials, urine, or urethral material. Culture methods have been developed which are somewhat more sensitive than direct wet mounts and may prove helpful (22).

Ciliate

The only ciliate which parasitizes man is *Balantidium coli*. This organism (Fig 59.5 and Table 59.5) is quite large and is covered with cilia which are slightly longer near the cytostome. Both cysts and trophozoites occur, each of which contains a large macronucleus and a smaller micronucleus. Trophozoites have prominent contractile vacuoles. Infected people have often been associated with swine, a reservoir host of this infection. The disease is similar to amebiasis of the colon, and there may be invasive disease with ulcerations

TABLE 59.5—MORPHOLOGY OF INTESTINAL CILIATE AND COCCIDIA

SPECIES	SIZE (LENGTH)	SHAPE	MOTILITY	NUMBER OF NUCLEI	OTHER FEATURES
Balantidium coli					
Trophozoite	50-70 µm or more. Usual range, 40-50 µm.	Ovoid with tapering anterior end.	Rotary, boring.	1 large, kidney-shaped macronucleus. 1 small, subspherical micronucleus immediately adjacent to macronucleus. Macronucleus occasionally visible in unstained preparation as hyaline mass.	Body surface covered by spiral, longitudinal rows of cilia. Contractile vacuoles are present.
Cyst	45-65 µm. Usual range, 50-55 µm.	Spherical or oval	—	1 large macronucleus visible in unstained preparations as hyaline mass.	Macronucleus and contractile vacuole are visible in young cysts. In older cysts, internal structure appears granular.
Isospora belli *Sarcocystis* sp.	Oocyst: 25-30 µm. Usual range, 28-30 µm.	Ellipsoidal.	Nonmotile.		Mature oocyst contains 2 sporocysts with 4 sporozoites each.
	Sporocyst:	Round or oval.			*I. belli:* Usual diagnostic stage is immature oocyst with single granular mass (zygote) within. *Sarcocystis* sp. Usual diagnostic stage is mature sporocyst.

Adapted with permission from Brooke MM and Melvin DM: Morphology of Diagnostic Stages of Intestinal Parasites of Man, U.S. Department of Health, Education, and Welfare Publ. No. (HSM) 72-8116.

of the colon. Metastatic disease does not occur in other organs. In immature cysts, the cilia may still be evident. It is important to differentiate *B. coli* from some of the free-living protozoa which might be found in pond water, etc., with which they might be confused.

Intestinal Sporozoa

There are two human intestinal sporozoan infections which in many ways are similar to the feline stage of toxoplasmosis (12). They are isosporiasis and sarcocystis. Both organisms parasitize the mucosal cells of the small intestinal tract.

Isosporiasis (5) is caused by the coccidian *Isospora belli,* and the disease is acquired by fecal-oral contamination. Infection in the intestinal mucosa is both asexual, with schizogony, and sexual, with formation of oocysts. In freshly passed feces, there are immature oocysts which contain zygotes. Each zygote then divides to form two sporoblasts; each of these sporoblasts develops a cyst wall and becomes a sporocyst in which there are four curved, sausage-shaped sporozoites. Diagnosis is established by demonstrating the oocysts (Fig 59.5, Table 59.5) by direct examination, by concentration procedures, or occasionally, in peroral small intestinal biopsies. Infection can cause a malabsorption syndrome and is generally self-limited. Cysts of *Isospora* may morphologically resemble hookworm eggs but are much smaller. They can be differentiated by measuring with an ocular micrometer.

Various *Sarcocystis* species which infect the muscle of domestic animals may infect humans who eat undercooked infected meat. Humans develop the sexual stage in the epithelium of the intestinal tract. In sarcocystosis, the form found in fresh feces is mature sporocysts (either singly or in pairs) rather than the immature oocysts that are typically associated with *I. belli* infections. Infections caused by *Sarcocystis* species were formerly called *Isopora hominis* infections.

Nonparasitic Objects

Numerous objects found in feces may be confused with parasites, and many are described in Table 59.6. *Blastocystis hominis,* "the parasitologist's yeast," is a harmless commensal organism of uncertain taxonomy which may be confused with cysts of various amebae (particularly *E. nana*) because of its size and shape. These organisms vary greatly in size and have granules which vary in size and number and which may be misinterpreted as cyst nuclei. *B. hominis* organisms are lysed by water so that concentration procedures (on fresh specimens) which involve water will destroy these organisms. Various blood and tissue cells are also likely to be confused with amebae but generally do not have the detailed structure of amebae and have nuclei which are relatively larger than those of the amebae. Several pseudoepidemics of amebiasis have resulted because of laboratories which misidentified white blood cells as amebae. Yeasts are frequently present in the stool but are not generally difficult to identify.

TABLE 59.6—NONPARASITIC OBJECTS

ARTIFACT	RESEMBLANCE	SALINE MOUNT	DIFFERENTIAL CHARACTERISTICS OF ARTIFACT IN PERMANENT STAIN	
			CYTOPLASM	NUCLEUS
Polymorphonuclear leukocytes (Seen in dysentery and other inflammatory bowel diseases.)	E. histolytica cyst	Usually not a problem Granules in cytoplasm. Cell border irregular.	Less dense, often frothy. Border less clearly demarcated than that of ameba.	More coarse. Large, relative to size of organism. Irregular shape and size. Chromatin unevenly distributed. Chromatin strands may link nuclei.
Macrophages (Seen in dysentery and other inflammatory bowel diseases. May be present in purged specimens.)	Amebic trophozoite, especially E histolytica	Nuclei larger and of irregular shape, with irregular chromatin distribution. Cytoplasm granular, may contain ingested debris. Cell border irregular and indistinct. Movement irregular and pseudopodia indistinct.	Coarse. may contain inclusions.	Large and often irregular in shape. Chromatin irregularly distributed. Many granules. Nucleus may be disintegrated.
Squamous epithelial cells (from anal mucosa)	Amebic trophozoite	Nucleus refractile and large. Cytoplasm smooth. Cell border distinct.	Stains evenly, no inclusions.	Large and single. Large chromatin mass may resemble karyosome.
Columnar epithelial cells (from intestinal mucosa)	Amebic trophozoite	Nucleus refractile and large. Cytoplasm smooth. Cell border distinct.	Variable appearance, may be vacuolated.	Large with heavy chromatin on nuclear membrane. Often large central chromatin mass resembling karyosome.

Table 59.6—(Continued)

Blastocystis hominis (Yeastlike organism that frequency grows in feces. Ruptures in water.)	Protozoan cyst	Spherical to oval. 6-15 μm in length. Central clear area. Peripheral refractile granules (3-7) may resemble nuclei.	Central mass may stain light or dark. Prominent wall.	Peripheral granules may resemble nuclei. Granules vary in size and appearance. True nuclear structure not present.
Yeasts (Normal constituent of feces)	Protozoan cyst	Oval. Thick wall. No internal structure. Budding forms may be seen.	Oval. Little internal structure. Refractile cell wall. Budding forms may be seen.	Not confused with amebic nucleus.
Starch granules	Protozoan cyst	Rounded or angular. Very refractile. No internal structure. Stain pink to purple in iodine mounts.	Not a problem in permanently stained slides.	

Note: Other artifacts, such as contaminating plant cells and pollen grains, are occasionally seen. These should not be difficult to differentiate.
Adapted from Smith JW, McQuay RM, Ash LR, Melvin DM, Orihel TC, and Thompson JH. 1976. Diagnostic parasitology—Intestinal Protozoa. American Society of Clinical Pathologists, Chicago.

References

1. ADAMS EB and MACLEOD IN: Invasive amebiasis. I. Amebic dysentery and its complications. Medicine 56:315–323, 1977
2. ADAMS EB and MACLEOD IN: Invasive amebiasis. II. Amebic liver abscess and its complications. Medicine 56:325–334, 1977
3. BARBOUR AG, NICHOLS CR, and FUKUSHIMA T: An outbreak of giardiasis in a group of campers. Am J Trop Med Hyg 25:384–389, 1976
4. BLACK RE, DYKES AC, SINCLAIR S, and WELLS JG: Giardiasis in day-care centers: Evidence of person-to-person transmission. Pediatrics 60:486–491, 1977
5. BRANDBORG LL, GOLDBERG SB, and BREIDENBACH WC: Human coccidiosis—A possible cause of malabsorption. N Engl J Med 283:1306–1313, 1970
6. BURROWS RB and SWERDLOW MA: *Enterobius vermicularis* as a probable vector of *Dientamoeba fragilis*. Am J Trop Med Hyg 5:258, 1956
7. CENTER FOR DISEASE CONTROL: Intestinal Parasite Surveillance Annual Summary 1976. Atlanta, Ga, 1977
8. CENTER FOR DISEASE CONTROL: Intestinal Parasite Surveillance Annual Summary 1978. Atlanta, Ga, 1979
9. CENTER FOR DISEASE CONTROL. LABORATORY TRAINING & CONSULTATION BRANCH: Amebiasis: Laboratory Diagnosis—A Self-Instructional Lesson, Parts I, II, and III. U.S. Dept. of Health, Education, and Welfare, Washington, DC, PHS Publ. No. 77-8327, 1976
10. COPELAND BE and KIMBER J: Nuclear size in diagnosis of *Entamoeba histolytica* on stained smears. Am J Clin Pathol 50:664–668, 1968
11. DANCIGER M and LOPEZ M: Numbers of *Giardia* in the feces of infected children. Am J Trop Med Hyg 24:237–242, 1975
12. FRENKEL JK: Advances in the biology of sporozoa. Z Parasitenkd 45:125–162, 1974
13. HEALY GR: The use and limitations to the indirect hemagglutination test in the diagnosis of intestinal amebiasis. Health Lab Sci 5:174–179, 1968
14. HEALY GR, VISVESVARA GS, and KAGAN IG: Observations on the persistence of antibodies to *E. histolytica*. Arch Invest Med 5:495–500, 1974
15. JACOBOWSKI W and HOFF JC (eds.): Proceedings National Symposium on Waterborne Transmission of Giardiasis. U. S. Environmental Protection Agency (EPA-600/9-79-001). National Technical Information Service, Springfield, Va, 1979, 306 pp
16. KAGAN IG and NORMAN L: Serodiagnosis of parasitic diseases. *In* Manual of Clinical Immunology. Rose NR and Friedman HF (eds.). American Society Microbiology, Washington, DC, 1976, pp. 382–409
17. KESSEL JF, LEWIS WP, PASQUEL CH, and TURNER JA: Indirect hemagglutination and complement fixation tests in amebiasis. Am J Trop Med Hyg 14:540–550, 1965
18. KROGSTAD DJ, SPENCER HC, and HEALY GR: Current concepts in parasitology—Amebiasis. N Engl J Med 298:262–265, 1978
19. KRUPP IM: Comparison of counter-immunoelectrophoresis with other serologic tests in the diagnosis of amebiasis. Am J Trop Med Hyg 23:27–30, 1974
20. MAHMOUD AAF and WARREN KS: Algorithms in the diagnosis and management of exotic diseases. XVII. Amebiasis. J Infect Dis 134:639–643, 1976
21. MEEROVITCH E and ALI KAHN Z: Preliminary report on the serological response of amebiasis patients from an endemic area in N.W. Saskatchewan. Can J Public Health 58:270–274, 1967
22. MELVIN DM and BROOKE MM: Laboratory Procedures for the Diagnosis of Intestinal Parasites. Bureau of Laboratories, Laboratory Training & Consultation Div., U.S. Dept. of Health, Education, & Welfare, Public Health Service, Atlanta, Ga, 1974
23. MILGRAM EA, HEALY GR, and KAGAN IG: Studies on the use of the indirect hemagglutination test in the diagnosis of amebiasis. Gastroenterology 50:645–649, 1966
24. MOORE GT, CROSS WM, MCGUIRE D, MOLLOHAN CS, GLEASON NN, HEALY GR, and NEWTON LH: Epidemic giardiasis at a ski resort. N Engl J Med 281:402–407, 1969
25. ROOT DM, COLE FX, and WILLIAMSON JA: The development and standardization of an ELISA method for the detection of *Entamoeba histolytica* antigens in fecal samples. Arch Invest Med 9:203–210, 1978

26. SHAW PK, BRODSKY RE, LYMAN DO, WOOD B, HIBLER CP, HEALY GR, MACLEOD KIE, STAHL W, and SCHULTZ MG: A communitywide outbreak of giardiasis with evidence of transmission by a municipal water supply. Ann Intern Med 87:426–432, 1977
27. SMITH JW: Identification of fecal parasites in the special parasitology survey of the College of American Pathologists. Am J Clin Pathol 72:371–373, 1979
28. SMITH JW and WOLFE MS: Giardiasis. Annu Rev Med 31:373–383, 1980
29. VISVESVARA GS and HEALY GR: The possible use of an indirect immunofluorescence test using axenically grown *Giardia lamblia* antigens in diagnosis of giardiasis. *In* Proceedings National Symposium on Waterborne Transmission of Giardiasis. Jacobowski W and Hoff JC (eds.). National Technical Information Service (EPA-600/9-79-001), Springfield, Va, 1979, pp 53–63
30. WOLFE MS: Current concepts in parasitology. Giardiasis. N Engl J Med 298:319–321, 1978
31. YANG J and SCHOLTEN TH: *Dientamoeba fragilis:* A review with notes on its epidemiology, pathogenicity, mode of transmission, and diagnosis. Am J Trop Med Hyg 26:16–22, 1977

CHAPTER 60

INTESTINAL HELMINTHS

James W. Smith, Marilyn S. Bartlett, and Kenneth W. Walls

Introduction

There are three major groups of helminths which infect the intestinal tract of man. They are nematodes (or roundworms), trematodes (or flukes), and cestodes (or tapeworms). The trematode, *Paragonimus,* which infects the lung, and schistosomes, which live in the blood vessels, are also discussed in this chapter because the eggs are often found in feces. Nematode infections are still a significant problem in the United States (1, 4, 25) (Table 57.1), although the incidence and severity of infections have decreased as a result of improved sanitation. Trematode infections usually are acquired outside the United States, although there are endemic foci of schistosomiasis in Puerto Rico. Cestode infections continue to be a problem, and the incidence of *Taenia* infections may have risen during the past 50 years (4). The life cycles vary, ranging from simple ones in which eggs are infective when passed or shortly thereafter, to complex life cycles in which one or sometimes two or more intermediate hosts are required. Many parasitic infections are acquired by ingesting embryonated eggs or infective larvae from appropriate intermediate hosts. Other infections are acquired when larvae penetrate the skin. Some parasites remain localized in the gastrointestinal tract, whereas others migrate through various tissues of the body before finally lodging in the final sites of infection. Most of these helminths are exclusively human parasites, although some may have animal reservoirs.

Signs and symptoms of helminth infections vary and may be caused by adults, larvae, or eggs. Parasitic infections should be included in the differential diagnosis of patients with elevated eosinophil counts. Eosinophilia is particularly common when parasites are in tissue, and at this time diagnostic stages are often not present in feces. Knowledge of geographic distributions, epidemiology, and life cycles is important for ascertaining what infections a patient might develop, who might acquire the infection from an infected patient, and what measures might be effective in controlling the parasite.

Diagnosis is usually based on demonstrating a stage of the parasite in fecal specimens, although demonstrating parasites in tissue or detecting serologic response to the parasites may be effective in some instances. Adult worms, or portions of adult worms, may be passed in fecal specimens and can be identified by careful examination and comparison to characteristics described and illustrated in atlases and standard textbooks on parasitology. It is also important to differentiate human parasites from free-living helminths, insect larvae, and fragments of tissue and foreign debris.

The principal means of diagnosing intestinal helminth infection is identifying eggs. Identification should be approached systematically using the following characteristics. Size of eggs is particularly important (Fig 60.1 and 60.2). The eggs of different parasites vary in size, and careful measurement of eggs with a calibrated ocular micrometer allows differentiation of those which are similar in overall configuration but different in size. The shape of the egg is important, as are the thickness and structure of the shell. The presence of specialized structures such as hooks, spines, opercula, and shoulders on the shell may be an aid in identification. A mammillated albuminoid outer covering is present on *Ascaris lumbricoides* eggs, and polar plugs are present in the eggs of *Trichuris trichiura* and some related organisms. The contents of the eggs should be examined to determine the level of development. Some eggs contain undeveloped ova when passed, whereas others are dividing, and still others are embryonated and contain larvae. If these features are considered and if the examiner is familiar with the appearance of fecal background material, there should be no difficulty in identifying eggs in fecal specimens.

Nematodes

Nematodes are the most common helminths which parasitize the intestinal tract of man, and infections are usually diagnosed by finding eggs or larvae in feces.

Enterobius vermicularis

This parasite causes enterobiasis (oxyuriasis, pinworm infection), which is the most common helminth infection in the United States and affects people of all social strata, particularly children. The infection rate is not known, though there are estimates that 30% of all children and 16% of all adults are infected, with rates exceeding 50% in some institutions (25). The adult pinworms live in the caecum and adjacent areas. The female measures 13 mm long, has a sharply pointed posterior end, and has cephalic alae. The gravid female migrates to the anus, usually when the patient is sleeping, and deposits eggs in the perianal folds or ruptures, releasing numerous embryonated eggs. The eggs are infective when passed or shortly thereafter, and infection is acquired by ingesting them. Eggs are distributed in clothing, bed linen, etc., and other persons may become infected by accidentally ingesting infective eggs from these objects. Symptoms ascribed to pinworm infections include pruritus ani and irritability, but in most cases, no symptoms are evident. Occasionally, *Enterobius* is found in ectopic sites such as the vagina or peritoneal cavity and may even lead to the formation of granulomas (5, 20).

Infection is diagnosed by demonstrating the typical eggs by the cellophane-tape or Vaseline-swab techniques. Because the eggs are deposited outside the anus, fecal specimens are generally not satisfactory for diagnosis (it is estimated that only 5%-10% of cases will be diagnosed on fecal examination).

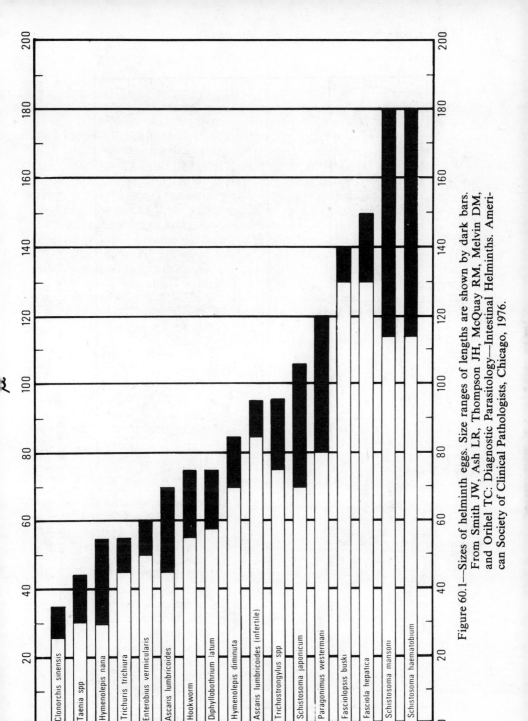

Figure 60.1—Sizes of helminth eggs. Size ranges of lengths are shown by dark bars. From Smith JW, Ash LR, Thompson JH, McQuay RM, Melvin DM, and Oribel TC: Diagnostic Parasitology—Intestinal Helminths. American Society of Clinical Pathologists, Chicago, 1976.

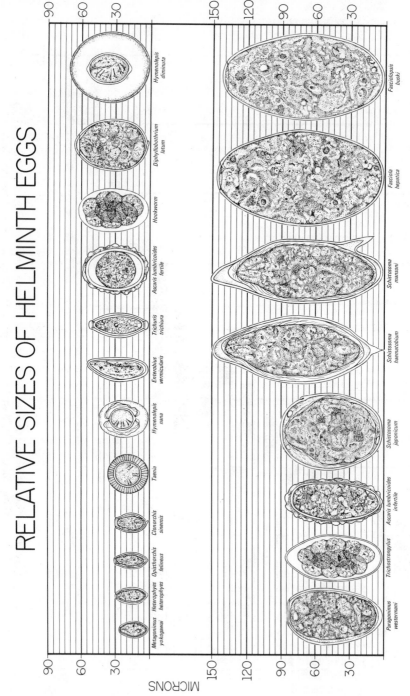

Figure 60.2—Relative sizes of helminth eggs. From parasitology training materials, Parasitology Training Branch, Center for Disease Control, with permission.

The frequency of positive cellophane-tape examinations is an index of the severity of infection (18). If examinations are done daily for 6 days, persons with the lightest infections will be positive on only 1 or 2 days, whereas those with severe infections will be positive every day. Approximately 90% of infections will be detected if three specimens are examined.

The egg of *E. vermicularis* (Fig 60.2, 60.3) is elongated, measures 50–60 μm long and 20–30 μm wide, and has a moderately thick shell. The shell is flattened on one side and contains a folded larva. Sometimes gravid female worms may be found in the perianal area or in feces; they are identified on the basis of their gross morphology and on the morphology of the eggs contained in the uteri. They measure up to 13 mm long and have a thin, sharply pointed tail.

Trichuris trichiura

This parasite causes trichiuriasis (whipworm infection), which is a common helminth infection, worldwide in distribution, and especially prevalent in tropical and subtropical areas. The adult worm measures up to 50 mm long, and has a long slender anterior portion and a shorter thick posterior portion thus leading to the common name "whipworm." The adults infect the colon, with their anterior portions entwined in the intestinal mucosa where they apparently remain attached for their entire lifetime (4–5 years). Most infections are asymptomatic, but heavy infections (150 or more worm pairs) may be accompanied by diarrhea and very heavy infections by dysentery (10). The unembryonated eggs are passed in the stools and require a maturation period of several weeks (3 weeks under optimal conditions) before infective larvae develop. Infection is acquired by ingesting the embryonated eggs which hatch in the intestine where the larvae mature to adults and complete the cycle.

Diagnosis is established by finding the typical elongated, undeveloped eggs (Fig 60.2, 60.3), measuring 52–57 by 22–23 μm, with distinctive refractile polar plugs. The shell is moderately thick. A simple method of estimating worm burden is to prepare a standard smear (equivalent to 2 mg of stool). Infections are designated as light when there are fewer than 5 eggs per coverslip and heavy when there are more than 25 eggs. Atypical eggs may be found in specimens from patients receiving anthelmintic therapy.

Ascaris lumbricoides

This parasite is the largest nematode which parasitizes the intestinal tract of humans and causes ascariasis (roundworm infection), which is found worldwide. The female measures up to 35 cm long by 6 mm in diameter; the male is slightly smaller. The posterior end of the male has a copulatory organ and tends to be curled. The adults live in the upper small intestine and are not attached to the mucosa. The female lays approximately 200,000 eggs per day. The eggs are undeveloped when passed but develop and contain infective larvae after 2–4 weeks when deposited in a satisfactory environment. When infective eggs are ingested, the larvae are released in the small intestine, penetrate the intestinal mucosa, and enter the blood stream, which carries them to

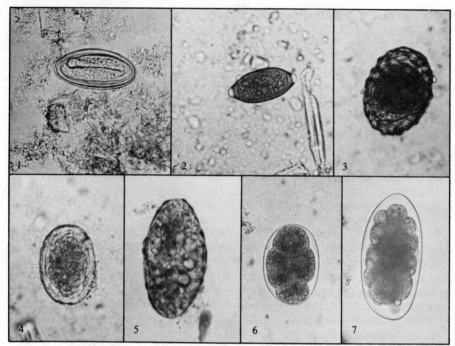

Figure 60.3—Nematode eggs. These eggs in wet mount were photographed at the same
magnification. (1) *Enterobius vermicularis*. (2) *Trichuris trichiura*. (3) *Ascaris lumbricoides*, fertile. (4) *A. lumbricoides*, fertile, decorticate. (5) *A. lumbricoides*, unfertilized. (6) Hookworm. (7) *Trichostrongylus* sp.

the lungs. They undergo some maturation in the lungs, and migrate upward in
the respiratory tree, are swallowed, and finally reach the small intestine where
they grow to maturity. Time from ingestion of the embryonated egg to presence of an egg-laying adult is approximately 2 months. The migration phase
may cause a Löeffler syndrome (peripheral eosinophilia and diffuse pulmonary infiltrates) or peripheral eosinophilia alone.

Adult worms can cause various symptoms (16, 26). They are not attached
to mucosa and can migrate up and down the intestine. Migration is often stimulated by fever or drug therapy—especially anesthetics. With severe infections, worms in the intestine may cause various symptoms including intestinal
obstruction. Worms may migrate into the bile duct and cause obstruction or
cholangitis or may migrate into the lumen of the appendix and cause appendicitis. Adult worms occasionally migrate into the stomach and may be vomited
out or they may be passed in feces.

Diagnosis is established by identifying the adult worm, or more commonly by finding eggs in stool specimens. One adult female can produce
enough eggs to provide approximately five eggs per coverslip containing 2 mg
of feces. Infections with more than 100 eggs per coverslip are considered
heavy. Any number of *Ascaris* worms can cause serious disease because of
their propensity to migrate.

Fertile *Ascaris* eggs are round to slightly oval and have an irregular albuminoid mammillated covering which is stained yellow-brown by bile. They measure 45–70 by 35–50 µm and have a very thick shell. The undivided ovum is rounded, and there is usually a clear area between the ovum and the shell at each end of the egg (Fig 60.2, 60.3). Occasionally, eggs lose the mammillated covering (decorticated) (Fig 60.3), and in such instances, the thick shell is quite prominent. Decorticated eggs must be differentiated from the thin-shelled eggs of hookworm—especially in older fecal specimens in which *Ascaris* eggs may be segmented. Infertile eggs may also be found; they are generally larger and more elongated than fertile eggs (Fig 60.3), measuring up to 94 µm long by 44 µm wide. The external mammillated layer is more irregular and the egg contains irregular globules of yolk material which fill the egg so that there are no clear areas at the ends. *Ascaris* eggs can survive in 5% Formalin for extended periods and may become embryonated.

In general, serologic tests for ascariasis in humans are unimportant except in the differential diagnosis of *A. lumbricoides* larval migration from *Toxocara* spp. larval migration (visceral larva migrans, VLM). Although a combination of indirect hemagglutination (IHA) and bentonite flocculation (BFT) tests have been the procedures of choice, the recent introduction of a highly sensitive enzyme linked immunosorbent assay (ELISA) procedure (6, 9) with an *Ascaris* egg antigen has contributed significantly to the improvement of serologic tests for ascariasis and VLM. This development is discussed more thoroughly under visceral larval migrans. An ELISA titer of 1:32 is considered significant (Table 57.2).

Hookworms

Hookworm infections are caused by two species, *Ancylostoma duodenale* (the so-called Old World hookworm), and *Necator americanus* (the so-called New World hookworm). Infections are most prevalent in tropical and subtropical areas, but they also occur in temperate areas. This parasite infects the small intestine, where the adults attach to the intestinal mucosa and cause blood loss estimated at 0.15–0.25 ml of blood per day per adult *A. duodenale* and 0.03 ml per day per adult *N. americanus*. The female worm measures up to 12 mm long; the male is slightly shorter. The male has a fan-shaped copulatory bursa at the posterior end. The female lays eggs which are passed in the feces. Under appropriate conditions, the eggs embryonate and produce rhabditiform larvae which hatch and develop to the filariform infective stage in about 7 days. If filariform larvae contact the skin of an appropriate host, as when someone steps on feces with bare feet, the larvae penetrate the skin, gain access to the host's circulation, travel to the lungs, and penetrate into the alveoli. They then migrate through the tracheo-broncheal tree to the epiglottis, are swallowed, and finally reach the small intestine. During the initial invasion and migration stage, there may be marked inflammation around the area of larval penetration (a condition known as ground itch), particularly in sensitized individuals. Larvae migrating through the lungs, if particularly numerous, may cause Loeffler syndrome. Gastrointestinal symptoms are usually minimal, although severe infections may be accompanied by diarrhea, abdominal pain, and nausea. The major manifestation of infection is iron deficiency anemia casued by blood loss. An estimate of the number of worms present may give some indication as to whether anemia is caused by hookworms and whether the infection needs to be treated (11).

The diagnosis is established by finding the oval eggs (Fig 60.2, 60.3, 60.5), which measure 58–76 by 38–40 μm and have a thin shell. The egg is usually in the four- to eight-cell segmented stage when passed but may vary from unsegmented in diarrheic specimens to embryonated in specimens from severely constipated patients. In direct exams of 2 mg of feces, more than 25 eggs per coverslip indicate heavy infection. Unfixed older specimens may contain embryonated eggs and larvae. In such instances, the larvae must be differentiated from those of *Strongyloides stercoralis*. Hookworm rhabditiform larvae (Fig 60.4) have a long buccal cavity and an inconspicuous genital primordium. Hookworm filariform larvae (Fig 60.4) have an esophagus (approximately one-fourth the length of the larva) and a pointed tail. In addition, the larvae must be differentiated from those of free-living nematodes, and the eggs must be differentiated from those of *Trichostrongylus* spp. (Fig 60.3, 60.5) and *Meloidogyne (Heterodera)* spp. (Fig 60.5). The latter are parasitic nematodes of plants whose eggs are ingested when eating incompletely washed root vegetables such as carrots.

The eggs of various hookworm species cannot be differentiated, and species identification must be based on the examination of adult worms. Adults are occasionally found in feces and can be identified on the basis of mouth parts and on the configuration of the copulatory bursa of male worms.

Trichostrongylus

These parasites are small nematodes of various species which parasitize the small intestine of humans and various animals. Infections are particularly common in the Far East, India, and Russia, but there have been sporadic cases in Latin America and the United States (13). Females lay eggs which are passed in the segmented stage in stools, become embryonated, and then hatch. The infective larvae crawl on vegetation and infect a new host when ingested with contaminated food or water. Adults develop in the intestine without migrating through the lung. The disease is usually asymptomatic, although unusually heavy infections may produce abdominal pain and diarrhea.

The diagnosis is established by finding the typical eggs (Fig 60.2, 60.3, 60.5) which measure 79–98 μm by 40–50 μm and have somewhat pointed ends. Eggs of the different species cannot be differentiated. Their larger size and tapered ends help to differentiate them from hookworm eggs.

Strongyloides stercoralis

This parasite is a small nematode which lives buried in the mucosa of the upper small intestine. Infection is most common in warm climates but also occurs in temperate areas. The parasitic female is only 2 mm long and reproduces parthenogenetically (there is no parasitic male). The embryonated eggs are laid in the mucosa and hatch just before or as they reach the lumen. The

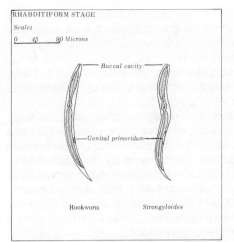 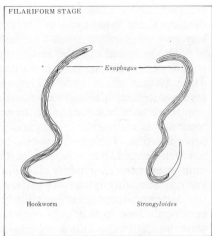

Figure 60.4—Nematode larvae. Comparison of rhabditiform and filariform larvae of hookworm and *Strongyloides stercoralis*. Adapted with permission from Brooke MM and Melvin DM: Morphology of Diagnostic Stages of Intestinal Parasites of Man. U.S. Department of Health, Education, and Welfare Publication No. (HSM) 72-8116, 1969.

rhabditiform larvae find their way to the intestinal lumen and are passed in the feces. The larvae mature to infective filariform larvae in a short time, and upon contact with the skin of a susceptible host penetrate and migrate through the circulatory system to the lungs and on to the small intestine. This process is

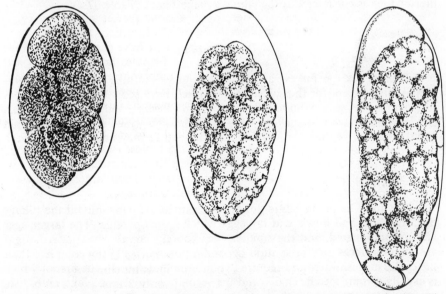

Figure 60.5—Comparison of eggs of hookworm (left), *Trichostrongylus* species (center), and *Meloidogyne (Heterodera)* species (right).

similar to the migration of hookworm. Under certain conditions, larvae may develop a free-living cycle in the soil with male and female adults, eggs, and larvae.

The infection may be accompanied by skin lesions at the site of penetration or Loeffler syndrome while the parasites migrate through the lungs. The intestinal phase is usually asymptomatic or mild; however, patients with severe infections may have diarrhea.

Rhabditiform larvae sometimes develop into the infective filariform stage while still in the intestinal tract and then can penetrate the mucosa and cause a superinfection. The exact conditions which predispose to superinfection are not well-defined, but it is seen particularly among severely malnourished or immunosuppressed patients (17). Patients with superinfections may have larvae migrating through a wide variety of tissues, and the infection may be fatal.

Diagnosis is generally established by detecting larvae in feces (eggs are very rarely seen in feces). *Strongyloides* rhabditiform larvae (Fig 60.4) have a short buccal cavity and a prominent genital primordium. *Strongyloides* filariform larvae have a notched tail and an esophagus approximately one-half the length of the body. Occasionally, larvae may not be found even with repeated fecal examination. In such instances organisms can be demonstrated in duodenal aspirates or with the Baermann concentration technique (14). Superinfection should be suspected when filariform larvae are present in freshly passed specimens (7).

Strongyloidiasis is sometimes difficult to differentiate from ascariasis; serologic tests can sometimes be useful. The IHA uses an extract of adult worms. Cross-reactions with ascariasis occur in about 15% of sera tested, but the homologous titer is usually considerably higher than the heterologous. A titer of 1:64 is considered to be clinically significant (Table 57.2).

Trematodes

Trematodes, or flukes, are flattened dorso-ventrally and all are hermaphroditic except for the schistosomes which have separate sexes. The mature worms vary greatly in length from 1 mm (*Metagonimus*) to 70 mm (*Fasciolopsis*) and have two suckers—one oral, through which the digestive tract opens, and one ventral, for attachment. The cuticle may be smooth or rough depending on the species.

Hermaphroditic Flukes

The adult hermaphroditic flukes which infect humans inhabit the biliary tree, intestine, and lungs, and lay eggs which have opercula. The larger eggs are unembryonated, and the smaller eggs contain larvae when passed. Eggs are found in feces and/or sputum depending on species. They complete their life cycles in freshwater and require two intermediate hosts—the first of which is usually certain specific snails, and the second of which is a plant, crab, fish, ant, etc. Feces must reach the water to allow the larval stages to enter the appropriate first intermediate host. Dietary custom must allow the second intermediate host to be ingested in order for the life cycle to be completed.

Most trematode infections occur in tropical and subtropical areas of the world with specific trematodes being present in specific areas. Dams and irrigation systems are particularly important in the epidemiology of the diseases. Diagnosis is usually established by demonstrating eggs in fecal specimens by direct mount or Formalin-ether concentration. Zinc sulfate methods are unsatisfactory unless the specimens are first fixed in Formalin to prevent the opercula from popping.

Although serologic tests for most hermaphroditic trematodes are being evaluated—particularly *Fasciola, Clonorchis,* and *Paragonimus*—none are used routinely. In the United States, the prevalence, even among travelers, does not justify providing diagnostic procedures for these infections even in large centers, although such new "universal" tests as ELISA may make the tests practical.

Fasciolopsis buski

This large intestinal fluke measures up to 70 mm long by 20 mm wide and 3 mm thick. This worm attaches to the mucosa of the upper small intestine. Eggs mature in freshwater and release larvae, which invade the tissues of a particular species of snail. In the snail, large numbers of larval forms are produced, which leave the snail, and encyst on water plants. When these water plants are ingested by appropriate hosts, the parasites excyst and grow to adulthood in the small intestine. The infections are usually asymptomatic but there may be diarrhea, epigastric pain, and eosinophilia. Diagnosis is established by finding the large operculate eggs (Fig 60.2, 60.6), which measure 130–140 by 80–85 μm in feces. The eggs are unembryonated and are filled by the large ovum. The eggs cannot be reliably differentiated from those of *Fasciola hepatica*.

Heterophyes species and Metagonimus species

These parasites are minute worms (1–3 mm long) of numerous species which can infect the intestine of humans. The first intermediate hosts are various molluskan species, and the second intermediate hosts are freshwater fish. Infection is acquired from ingesting uncooked fish and is generally asymptomatic, but occasional patients may have symptoms similar to those associated with *Fasciolopsis* infection. The diagnosis is established by finding the embryonated operculate eggs in feces. These small eggs (Fig 60.2), which measure less than 30 by 17 μm, may be difficult or impossible to differentiate from those of *Clonorchis* and *Opisthorchis* species, although the former generally do not have an abopercular knob or hook and are wider at the opercular end.

Fasciola hepatica and Fasciola gigantica

These parasites may infect the biliary tract of various domestic and wild animals such as cattle, sheep, and goats, and may occasionally parasitize man. *Fasciola hepatica* is distributed worldwide, whereas *Fasciola gigantica* is restricted to Africa and the Orient. Both parasites live in the biliary tree, and the eggs are passed in feces. Life cycles are similar to that of *Fasciolopsis,* and the second intermediate host is an aquatic plant such as water cress. Ingested infective larvae are released from their cysts to penetrate through the intestinal wall and reach the liver, where they bore through the capsule into the liver parenchyma and finally reach the bile ducts. There they mature and live. The young larvae produce little or no symptomatology, but there may be eosinophilia during migration. The adult worms may cause fibrosis of the bile ducts with hyperplasia of the epithelium and may contribute to stone formation and development of cirrhosis. Diagnosis is established by finding the operculate eggs (Fig 60.2, 60.5) measuring 130–150 μm by 60–90 μm in the stool. Eggs cannot be reliably distinguished from those of *Fasciolopsis*. Occasionally, eggs may be present after infected liver of other hosts is ingested. If such a situation is suspected, the patient should not eat liver for 3 to 5 days, after which additional stools can be examined. If eggs are still found, the person is actually infected.

Clonorchis sinensis and Opisthorchis

These species are closely related. It has been proposed that *Clonorchis sinensis* should be in the genus *Opisthorchis*. *C. sinensis* is sometimes known as the Chinese liver fluke. These parasites inhabit the biliary tree of man and those of such animals as cats and dogs. *Clonorchis* is found in the Orient, whereas *Opisthorchis* is usually found in Central and Eastern Europe but has been found sporadically in the Orient. The adult parasites measure as long as 25 mm. The life cycle is similar to that of other trematodes, with freshwater fish being the second intermediate host. Infection is acquired by eating uncooked fish. The infective larvae migrate through the ampulla of Vater into the bile ducts of the liver where they mature and live. Infection is generally asymptomatic although heavy infections are sometimes accompanied by various gastrointestinal disturbances (19). Infection is diagnosed by demonstrating the embryonated eggs (23–35 μm by 12–20 μm) (Fig 60.2, 60.6) in stools. Eggs of these two genera cannot be reliably differentiated, and it is acceptable to report a generic identification of *Clonorchis/Opisthorchis* species. The eggs of *Clonorchis/Opisthorchis* often have a hook on the abopercular end and are narrower at the end with the flattened operculum than are the eggs of *Heterophyes/Metagonimus* species.

Paragonimus species

Several species may parasitize the lungs of humans and other carnivores. *Paragonimus westermani* is the most common and is found in Asia. Occasionally, human infections with *Paragonimus* have been reported from Africa and South and Central America. Some have been caused by species other than *P. westermani*. The adult parasites measure up to 12 mm long by 6 mm wide and live in the lungs, where they are encapsulated by the host's fibrous reaction. Capsules usually communicate with the bronchi, and eggs are passed into the respiratory tree, where they may be expectorated in sputum or swallowed and passed in the stools. The life cycle is similar to that of other trematodes, with infection following ingestion of encysted larvae in muscles of the second intermediate hosts—i.e., crayfish or crabs. Larvae migrate through the intestinal wall, across the peritoneal cavity, and bore through the diaphragm to reach the lungs. Symptoms may accompany migration. The presence of adult worms in the lungs leads to the production of large amounts of mucus and to episodes of hemoptysis. Parasites occasionally do not reach the lungs and have been found

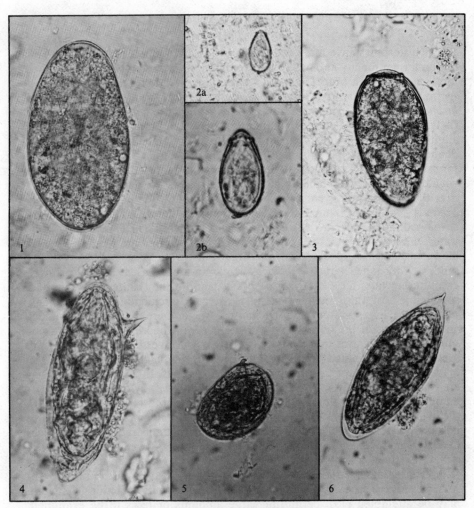

Figure 60.6—Trematode eggs. Except for 2b, these eggs in wet mount were photographed at the same magnification. (1) *Fasciola hepatica* or *Fasciolopsis buski*. (2a, 2b) *Chlonorchis sinensis*; 2b is an oil immersion photomicrograph to show the structure of this small egg. (3) *Paragonimus westermanni*. (4) *Schistosomal mansoni*. (5) *S. japonicum*. (6) *S. haematobium*.

in various ectopic locations. Diagnosis is established by finding the operculate unembryonated eggs (Fig 60.2, 60.6), which measure 80–120 by 48–60 µm and have a moderately thick shell. The operculum is fattened and is usually set off from the rest of the shell by prominent shoulders. The abopercular end may be thickened but does not have a knob. Measuring eggs with a properly calibrated ocular micrometer aids in distinguishing them from the eggs of *Diphyllobothrium latum* and *Fasciola* or *Fasciolopsis*.

Schistosomes

Schistosomes have male and female worms and inhabit the blood vessels of humans and many animals. They are the most important trematodes which infect man in terms of incidence and severity of infection. The species that infect man are *Schistosoma mansoni, Schistosoma japonicum,* and *Schistosoma haematobium.* The incidence of infection is rising in many areas of the world (24), although control efforts in mainland China seem to be successful (3). The adult parasites are slender—females measure up to 26 mm long and 0.5 mm in diameter. Males are slightly shorter and have a folding of the body which forms a gynecophoral canal in which the female resides. Adults live in small venules and elicit little inflammatory reaction. Eggs are deposited in venules near the mucosa and eventually find their way into the lumen of the viscus. There is significant inflammatory reaction around the eggs. The eggs are fully developed when they are passed in feces or urine. When exposed to freshwater, the larvae escape from the eggs and find appropriate freshwater snail intermediate hosts. In the snail, the organisms proliferate, and many thousands of fork-tailed larvae known as cercariae are released. These cercariae swim in the water for a short period of time, and if they contact the skin of a susceptible host, they actively penetrate, enter the circulation, establish themselves in the liver, and develop. During this stage, there may be enlargement and tenderness of the liver which may be accompanied by urticaria and eosinophilia. The worms then migrate to the system of vessels to which they are specialized, reach sexual maturity, and begin laying eggs. The disease in humans is caused by inflammatory reaction to the eggs. In addition, some eggs are carried to the liver by the portal vein or to the lungs by the systemic circulation and cause granulomatous inflammation and fibrosis in these organs. In the liver, they can cause fibrosis and the eventual development of cirrhosis and portal hypertension. Diagnosis is established by demonstrating eggs in feces *(S. mansoni, S. japonicum)* or urine *(S. haematobium).* The eggs can be demonstrated in direct mounts or with Formalin-ether or acid-ether concentrations (15). Zinc sulfate flotation is not satisfactory for the heavy schistosome eggs. In some instances, especially patients with light or chronic infections, hatching may be attempted (15), permitting large amounts of feces to be examined. Feces are mixed with distilled water in a flask (usually a side-arm flask) which is painted or covered to keep out light. The eggs hatch, and the swimming larvae (micracidia) seek light in the neck or the side arm. They can be detected with a hand lens, removed with a capillary pipette, and examined microscopically. Because larvae of the species are indistinguishable, species differentiation cannot be accomplished with this technique. Eggs can sometimes be demonstrated in crush preparations or sections of material from biopsies of rectal or bladder tissue. Movement of larvae in unfixed eggs shows that they are alive and that the infection is active.

Schistosoma mansoni

Infection with this parasite occurs in tropical Africa, the Nile valley, Brazil, Venezuela, West Indies, and Puerto Rico. In the United States, the infection is generally seen in Puerto Ricans who have moved to the United States. *S. mansoni* adults live in the mesenteric veins of the large intestine, and in the early stages infection can cause abdominal pain and diarrhea with blood and mucus in the stools. These symptoms usually subside, and the chronic phase begins. There may be fistulas in the perianal area, and hepatic cirrhosis may develop.

Diagnosis is usually made on the basis of identifying the large eggs (116–180 μm by 45–58 μm), which are oval and have a large distinctive lateral spine protruding from the side near one end (Fig 60.2, 60.6). If the spine is not readily evident, the egg can be rotated by tapping the coverslip.

Schistosoma japonicum

This parasite is found primarily in China, Korea, and the Philippines, and causes a disease similar to that associated with *S. mansoni* but is generally more severe because more eggs are laid per worm. The eggs readily reach the liver, and liver problems are common in people infected with this parasite. The eggs (Fig 60.2, 60.6) are slightly oval, measuring 70–105 by 50–65 μm, and characteristically have a short rudimentary lateral spine which may be difficult to demonstrate even with tapping of the coverslip.

Schistosoma haematobium

This parasite is found primarily in Africa, particularly along the Nile River delta, although there are foci in the Middle East and Madagascar. Parasites migrate from the liver through the hemorrhoidal veins to the venous plexes of the urinary bladder, prostate, uterus, and vagina, and the initial symptom is often hematuria, most commonly at the end of micturition. The host's reaction to eggs in the bladder wall causes fibrosis and hyperplasia of the epithelium. Association between *S. haematobium* infections and squamous cell carcinoma of the urinary bladder has been noted but is not conclusively proven. Diagnosis is usually established by finding eggs in urinary sediment. The eggs (Fig 60.2, 60.6) measure 112–180 μm by 40–70 μm and have a prominent terminal spine. Mid-day urine specimens are usually best.

Cercarial Dermatitis

Swimmer's itch, also known as schistosomal cercarial dermatitis, is a skin infection caused by the cercariae of non-human schistosomes such as those which infect birds. The disease occurs after a person's skin is exposed to fresh or salt water containing cercariae. In hosts other than the natural ones, the cercariae are unable to penetrate to the circulatory system and may cause erythema and urticaria and sometimes papules in the skin. Some degree of prior sensitization is required. Reaction is most intense 2 or 3 days after the initial contact and subsides spontaneously. It has been described in many parts of the world including the United States, and diagnosis is established on clinical grounds.

Serology

Even though the immunology of schistosomiasis has been extensively studied, the available serologic tests are inadequate. A number of tests have been suggested. Buck and Anderson (2) evaluated the complement fixation (CF) and cholesterol-lecithin tests and found each lacking. Tanaka et al. (21) reported that CF is highly sensitive and specific for detecting *S. japonicum* infections. Fiorillo et al. (8) reported that indirect hemagglutination (IHA) is sensitive in acute infections. Wilson et al. (27) demonstrated that indirect immunofluorescence (IIF) test with cryostat sections of adult worms was highly sensitive and specific. Earlier tests showed marked cross-reactions with sera from patients with trichina infections, but the IIF test reacted less frequently, and visual evaluation of the distribution of fluorescence frequently allowed the false-positives to be detected.

In general, residents of endemic areas who have clinical problems caused by schistosomiases will have a constant low antibody level and acute infections often cannot be differentiated from chronic infections. Lunde (12) has reported the use of ELISA with adult and cercarial antigens to differentiate early from late schistosomiasis. Maddison (personal communication) has failed to confirm this result with sera from patients with chronic infections in Egypt. Until ELISA can be further evaluated and clearly demonstrated as effective, IIF remains the test of choice because of its specificity and sensitivity. However, due to the lack of correlation with type of clinical disease (27), titers are of no value, and results should be reported simply as "positive" or "negative" (Table 57.2). Serology is most useful for ruling out schistosomiasis as a diagnosis.

Cestodes

Cestodes (23) are flattened parasites with an anterior portion known as the scolex (which has structures for attachment to the intestinal mucosa) and a body or strobila composed of a chain of segments. The individual segments, proglottids, develop from the neck; each proglottid has both male and female organs. The point at which the male and female sex organs meet is known as the genital pore. The proglottids develop from immature to mature egg-producing proglottids, with those farthest from the scolex being most fully developed. With some species, eggs are laid from the individual proglottids, but with most the eggs are stored in the uterus. Such proglottids filled with eggs are known as gravid proglottids. Adult and larval stages of cestodes contain basophilic laminated bodies known as calcareous corpuscles which aid in recognizing tissue as cestode tissue. Eggs or gravid proglottids are passed in feces. Eggs of most species contain larvae, though some species are undeveloped. An intermediate host(s) is (are) required for the asexual larval stages to develop. The infective stage develops in the tissues of the intermediate host, and the life cycle is completed when the infective larva is ingested.

Humans sometimes serve as intermediate hosts for cestode larval stages which cause such diseases as hydatid disease, cysticercosis, coenurosis, and sparganosis. (These infections are discussed in Chapter 58.)

Taenia spp.

Two *Taenia* species cause human infections. Man is the sole definitive host for *Taenia saginata,* the beef tapeworm, and *Taenia solium,* the pork tapeworm. *Taenia solium* is most common in Eastern Europe, Latin America, China, Pakistan, and India; most cases in the United States are imported. *Taenia saginata* is more widely distributed and prevalent in the Middle East, Africa, Europe, and Latin America, but is occasionally seen in the United States. The frequency with which *Taenia* infections were found with stool examinations in 1976 was approximately twice that in previous surveys in 1931-35 and 1963-67, but the reason for this increase (4) is not known.

Both *Taenia* species live in the small intestine and produce worms with a strobila up to 7 meters long. The eggs are stored in the uterus and reach the outside when gravid proglottids drop from the strobila and either rupture in the intestine freeing the eggs or pass intact in the stools. In the latter instance, the proglottids may move in the fashion of an inchworm and may sometimes be present in specimens submitted to the laboratory. The appropriate intermediate hosts (cattle for *T. saginata* and pigs for *T. solium)* swallow the eggs, and larval cysts (cysticerci) develop in the tissues. Infection is acquired by ingesting cysticerci in poorly cooked meat. Usually there is only one adult worm in each infection.

Symptoms in humans are minimal, and the disease is usually discovered by observing proglottids in the fecal specimens. Humans may be an intermediate host for *T. solium* and develop a disease known as cysticercosis; they cannot be an intermediate host of *T. saginata.*

Diagnosis is based on finding eggs or proglottids. Eggs can be detected in stools with direct wet mount examination or concentration techniques, or found in perianal folds using the cellophane-tape technique. The eggs (Fig 60.2, 60.7) are spherical (31–43 μm in diameter), have a thick radially striated shell, and contain a six-hooked embryo. Eggs of the two species cannot be differentiated. Passed proglottids can be cleared overnight in cooled glycerol to allow the uterine branches to be counted and a specific identification to be made. Alternatively, proglottids can be cleared in carbol-xylol (1:3), or the uterus can be injected with India ink through the genital pore. The gravid proglottids of *T. saginata* have 15–20 lateral branches, and those of *T. solium* have 7–13 (Fig 60.8). The worm will not be passed intact with some treatments but will with others. Species can also be differentiated by the morphology of the scolex. The scolex of each species has four suckers. That of *T. solium* has a rostellum with two rows of hooks, whereas that of *T. saginata* has no restellum and no hooks (Fig 60.9).

Hymenolepsis nana

This dwarf tapeworm of humans causes the most prevalent tapeworm infection in the United States (4). The adult has a delicate strobila which measures up to 40 mm long, and the scolex has a prominent rostellum with hooks.

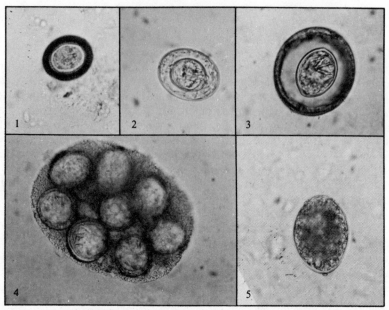

Figure 60.7—Cestode eggs. These eggs in wet mounts were photographed at the same magnification. (1) *Taenia* sp. (2) *Hymenolepis nana*. (3) *H. diminuta*. (4) *Dipylidum caninum* egg packet (5) *Diphyllobothrium latum*.

Humans are usually infected by ingesting freshly passed eggs. The larvae are released from the eggs, penetrate the mucosal villi, and develop into infective larvae. The larvae then emerge into the lumen and develop into adults in direct proportion to the number of eggs ingested. The tissue larval stage, which only lasts for a few days, is apparently sufficient to confer strong immunity to the host. *H. nana* is a common parasite of the house mouse, and its eggs may develop into infective larvae in various intermediate arthropod hosts. When

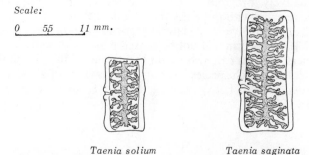

Figure 60.8—Proglottids of *Taenia* and *T. saginata*. Adapted with permission from Brooke MM and Melvin DM: Morphology of Diagnostic Stages of Intestinal Parasites of Man, U.S. Department of Health, Education, and Welfare Publication No. (HSM) 72-8116, 1969.

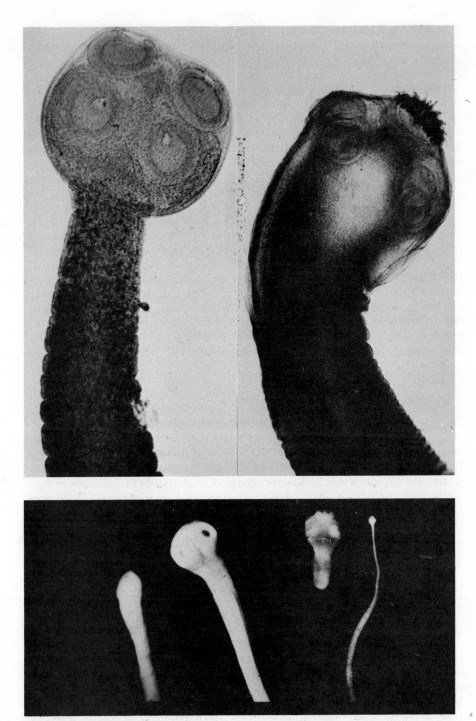

Figure 60.9—Cestode scolices: 1 and 2 are photomicrographs of carmine-stained scolices of *Taenia saginata* (1) and *Taenia solium* (2). 3 is a photomacrograph
of scolices of (L to R) *D. latum, T. saginata, T. solium,* and *H. nana.*

infection develops by accidentally ingesting an infected arthropod, immunity is not developed to the tissue phase, and eggs from adult worms may hatch in the small intestine of the same host to produce a hyperinfection. This is felt to be the pathogenesis in the occasional individuals in whom large numbers of worms are found. Patients with large numbers of worms may have gastrointestinal symptoms. Diagnosis is established by finding the oval colorless eggs (Fig 60.2, 60.7), which measure 30–55 μm in the greatest dimension. These eggs typically have prominent polar thickenings from which four to eight long, thin filaments project. The size and the presence of polar filaments are particularly helpful in differentiating *H. nana* from *H. diminuta*.

Hymenolepsis diminuta

This parasite usually infects rats, mice, and other rodents, but sporadic human infections may occur. The embryonated eggs are ingested by fleas or other arthropods, and infective larvae develop in their tissues. Humans are infected by accidentally ingesting infected arthropods. Adult tapeworms measure up to 60 cm long, and the scolex has no hooks. Infected humans are usually asymptomatic. Eggs are released when the gravid proglottids detach from the body of the adult worm and disintegrate in the intestine. Diagnosis is based on finding the oval or round eggs (Fig 60.2, 60.7), which measure 60–82 by 72–86 μm. These eggs have an inner membrane with two rudimentary polar thickenings but do not have polar filaments. They contain a six-hooked embryo.

Dipylidium caninum

This is primarily a parasite of dogs and is distributed worldwide. The life cycle involves a flea intermediate host which ingests the egg and in which the infective larva develops. The definitive host is infected by ingesting an infected flea. The larva attaches itself to the small intestinal mucosa and matures to the adult parasite which measures approximately 70 cm long. Proglottids are barrel shaped and have a genital pore and sex organs on each side. The gravid proglottid contains numerous small capsules or packets, each containing 8–20 eggs. Humans are usually accidental hosts and remain asymptomatic. Diagnosis is based on finding gravid proglottids or packets of embryonated eggs (Fig 60.7) in the feces. The spherical eggs measure 20–40 μm in diameter.

Diphyllobothrium latum

The broad fish tapeworm is widely distributed in temperate climates including the lakes of the northern United States and Canada, northern and central Russia and Europe, Manchuria, and Japan. Occasionally, infections have been reported in other areas. The parasite attaches to the small intestine and can grow to be as long as 10 meters. The scolex is elongated and has two long lateral grooves called bothria which are for attachment. The proglottids have active oviposition, and the eggs are passed unembryonated. The eggs must reach freshwater in which to embryonate and release swimming larvae. The first intermediate host is a small aquatic arthropod, and the second intermediate host is a small fish which ingests the arthropod. The third intermediate host is a larger fish which ingests the smaller fish (22). In the muscles of the larger fish, a larva known as a sparganum or plerocercoid develops to the infective stage. The life cycle is completed when a larva is ingested in raw or inadequately cooked fish by any of the definitive hosts. Human infections are usually caused by *Diphyllobothrium latum,* but other species of *Diphyllobothrium* occasionally infect humans. (Species cannot be differentiated on the basis of egg morphology.) Infected humans are usually asymptomatic, with the passage of a portion of the strobila usually causing a patient to seek medical attention. Occasionally, patients develop Vitamin B_{12} deficiency because the parasite selectively competes for it.

Diagnosis is based on finding the characteristic eggs (Fig 60.2, 60.7), which measure 58-76 μm long by 40-51 μm wide. The eggs are operculate and unembryonated, in contrast to those of other cestodes infecting man. They may have a small nipple-like protrusion (abopercular knob) on the posterior pole. There are no shoulders adjacent to the operculum.

References

1. BLUMENTHAL DS: Intestinal nematodes in the United States. N Engl J Med 297:1437-1439, 1977
2. BUCK AA and ANDERSON RI: Validation of the complement fixation and slide flocculation tests for schistosomiasis. Geographic variations of test capacities. Am J Epidemiol 96:205-214, 1972
3. BUEDING E (chairman): Report of the American schistosomiasis delgation to the Peoples Republic of China. Am J Trop Med Hyg 26:427-457, 1977
4. CENTER FOR DISEASE CONTROL: Intestinal Parasite Surveillance Annual Summary 1976. Atlanta, Ga, 1977
5. CHANDRASOMA PT and MENDIS KN: *Enterobius vermicularis* in ectopic sites. Am J Trop Med Hyg 26:644-649, 1977
6. CYPESS RH, KAROL MH, ZIDIAN JL, GLICKMAN LT, and GITLIN D: Larva specific antibodies in patients with visceral larva migrans. J Infect Dis 135:633-640, 1977
7. EVELAND LK, KENNEY M, and VALENTIN Y: Laboratory diagnosis of autoinfection in strongyloidiasis. Am J Clin Pathol 63:421-425, 1975
8. FIORILLO AM, COSTA JC, and PASSOS J: Identification of hemagglutinating antibodies in chronic schistosomiasis. Rev Inst Med Trop (Sao Paulo) 15:371-376, 1973
9. GLICKMAN LT, SCHANTZ PM, DEMBROSKE R, and CYPESS RH: Evaluation of serodiagnostic tests for visceral larva migrans. Am J Trop Med Hyg 27:492-498, 1978
10. JUNG RC and BEAVER PC: Clinical observations on *Trichocephalus trichirus* (Whipworm) infestation in children. Pediatrics 8:548-557, 1951
11. LAYRISSI M and ROCHE M: The relationship between anemia and hookworm infection. Results of surveys of rural Venezuelan population. Am J Hyg 79:279-301, 1964
12. LUNDE MN, OTTESEN EA, and CHEEVER AW: Serological differences between acute and chronic schistosomiasis mansoni detected by enzyme-linked immunosorbent assay (ELISA). Am J Trop Med Hyg 28:87-91, 1979
13. MARKELL EK: Pseudohookworm infection—Trichostrongyliasis. N Engl J Med 278:831-832, 1968
14. MARKELL EK and VOGE M: Medical Parsitology, 4th Edition. W.B. Saunders Co, Philadelphia, 1976
15. MELVIN DM and BROOKE MM: Laboratory Procedures For the Diagnosis of Intestinal Parasites. Laboratory Training & Consultation Div., Bureau of Laboratories, Center for Disease Control, U.S. Dept. of Health, Education & Welfare, Public Health Service, Atlanta, Ga, 1974

16. PIGGOTT J, HANSBARGER EA, and NEAFIE RC: Human ascariasis. Am J Clin Pathol 53:223–234, 1970
17. PURTILO DT, MEYERS WM, and CONNOR DH: Fatal strongyloidiasis in immunosuppressed patients. Am J Med 56:488–493, 1974
18. SADUN EH and MELVIN DM: The probability of detecting infections with *Enterobius vermicularis* by successive examination. J Pediatr 48:438–441, 1956
19. STRAUSS WG: Clinical manifestations of clonorchiasis. A controlled study of 105 cases. Am J Trop Med Hyg 11:625–630, 1962
20. SYMMERS WSTC: Pathology of oxyuriasis. Arch Pathol 50:475–516, 1950
21. TANAKA H, DENNIS DT, KEAN BH, MATSUDA H, and SASA M: Evaluation of a modified complement fixation test for schistosomiasis. J Exp Med 42:537–542, 1972
22. VIK R: The genus *Diphyllobothrium.* An example of systematics and experimental biology. Exp Parsitol 15:361–380, 1964
23. WARDLE RA and MCLEOD JA: The Zoology of Tapeworms. Univ of Minnesota Press, Minneapolis, 1952
24. WARREN KS: Regulation of the prevalence and intensity of schistosomiasis in man. Immunology or ecology. J Infect Dis 127:595–609, 1973
25. WARREN KS: Helminthic disease endemic in the United States. Am J Trop Med Hyg 23:723–730, 1974
26. WARREN KS and MAHMOUD AAF: Algorithms in the diagnosis and management of exotic diseases. XXII Ascariasis and toxocariasis. J Infect Dis 135:868–872, 1977
27. WILSON M, SULZER AJ, and WALLS KW: Modified antigens in the indirect immunofluorescence test for schistosomiasis. Am J Trop Med Hyg 23:1072–1076, 1974

CHAPTER 61

ARTHROPOD ECTOPARASITES

Harry D. Pratt and James W. Smith

Introduction

Arthropods affect human health in many ways. Some are involved in the mechanical transmission of pathogens. Others play important roles in the biological transmission, development, and survival of viruses, bacteria, protozoa, and metazoa that cause human disease. Arthropods also injure humans directly by envenomization, vesication, blood sucking, irritation and invasion of the tissues, and stimulation of allergic responses.

Mosquitoes, certain flies, fleas, bed bugs, spiders, ticks, and mites bite with their mouthparts. Bees, wasps, and scorpions sting with an appartus at the posterior end. For most people, such bites or stings cause only temporary local swellings and itching which are usually treated with calamine or other soothing lotions, although some become secondarily infected from scratching. A few persons become sensitized to protein from the insect saliva or sting (9). If they are bitten at a later date, when the body has had time to develop antibodies to these foreign proteins, these people develop larger, more severe welts around each bite. A person repeatedly infested with scabies mites may develop a generalized rash and intense itching over much of the body and not simply in the area of the scabies mite lesions. The most severe reactions affect a few persons who are sensitized by the stings of bees, wasps, or hornets. If these people are stung again, they may have a severe reaction to this same foreign protein and may die from anaphylactic shock, respiratory edema, vascular occlusion, or damage to the nervous system. Such deaths usually occur rapidly, often within an hour after the sting (9).

Arthropods are very widespread in the environment, and excrement and fragments of arthropods are present in soil and dust. Persons may become hypersensitive to these arthropod materials and develop allergic manifestations such as asthma and hay fever.

It is beyond the scope of this chapter to deal with all of the arthropods of medical importance or the therapy and control of arthropod infestations. The most common ectoparasites submitted to laboratories for identification in the United States are discussed, and pictorial keys are presented which show the principles of identification. More detailed information on arthropods of medical importance and their identification, treatment, and control is available in various references (5, 8, 10, 11, 12, 21).

Phylum Arthropoda

Class Insecta

Order Hemiptera, Family Cimicidae (bed bugs)
    The bed bug *(Cimex lectularius)*
Order Anoplura, Family Pediculidae (human lice)
    The head louse *(Pediculus capitis)*
    The body louse *(Pediculus humanus)*
    The crab louse *(Pthirus pubis)*
Order Siphonaptera, Family Pulicidae (fleas)
    The Oriental rat flea *(Xenopsylla cheopis)*
    The cat flea *(Ctenocephalides felis)*
    The dog flea *(Ctenocephalides canis)*
Order Diptera (flies)
    Fly maggots—many species of the families Calliphoridae,
    Gasterophilidae, Hypodermatidae, Muscidae, Piophilidae,
    Sarcophagidae, Stratiomyiidae, and Syrphidae.

Class Arachnida

Order Acarina, Family Ixodidae (hard ticks)
    The American dog tick *(Dermacentor variabilis)*
    The Rocky Mountain wood tick *(Dermacentor andersoni)*
    The lone star tick *(Amblyomma americanum)*
    The brown dog tick *(Rhipicephalus sanguineus)*
Order Acarina, Family Argasidae (soft ticks)
    Relapsing fever ticks *(Ornithodoros* spp.)
Order Acarina, Family Sarcoptidae (Scabies mites)
    Scabies mite *(Sarcoptes scabiei)*
Order Acarina, Family Demodecidae (Follicle mites)
    Follicle mite *(Demodex folliculorum)*
Order Acarina, Family Trombiculidae (Chiggers)
    Chigger (larva of a Trombiculid mite)

These arthropods can be identified by using the characters in the pictorial key (Fig 61.1) or specialized literature (5, 8, 13, 21).

Specimens of ectoparasites should be preserved and shipped for identification in 70% ethyl alcohol, rather than formalin, which is irritating to the eyes of the identifier. Fly larvae may have to be washed in water to remove debris, particularly those collected from fecal samples or wounds. After they are washed in clean water, fly larvae should be killed in hot (not boiling) water, about 80 C for a few mintues, so that they do not become black when placed in 70% alcohol.

Most ectoparasites can be identified with a dissecting microscope with magnifications of 25 to 75 power. Some fleas, fly larvae, and mites may have to be treated overnight with cold 10% potassium or sodium hydroxide to remove the internal flesh and permit better visibility of key characters. Such specimens can then be washed in water, dehydrated in 70% ethyl alcohol, cellosolve, and clove oil, and mounted in Canada balsam as permanent slides.

PICTORIAL KEY TO GROUPS OF HUMAN ECTOPARASITES

Chester J. Stojanovich and Harold George Scott

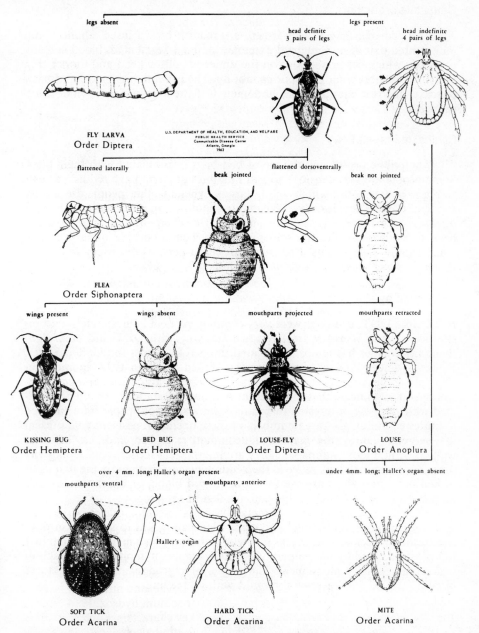

Figure 61.1—Pictorial key to groups of human ectoparasites. From reference 5 by permission.

Bed Bug

Causative organism

The bed bug *(Cimex lectularius)* is a reddish-brown insect about 5 mm long, with a pair of 4-segmented antennae, and a 3-segmented, blood-sucking proboscis which lies in a groove on the underside of the head and thorax (Fig 61.1). It has short wing pads but cannot fly. The pronotum is broad and has a concave anterior margin. The abdomen is flattened and somewhat heart-shaped.

Clinical manifestations

The public health importance of bed bugs is associated with their bites. Some people are very sensitive to bed bug bites and will have reddish wheals as big as a half dollar which itch intensely, whereas other people are hardly aware of them. Theoretically, the bed bug should be an ideal vector of human diseases since it feeds repeatedly on man. However, these insects have not been incriminted in the transmission of any communicable disease despite many careful experiments. Bed bugs can cause nervous disorders and sleeplessness among sensitive children and adults (10, 12, 21).

Epidemiology

Before DDT, bed bugs were very common pests in homes, hotels, and institutions. Since World War II residual spraying with DDT and other synthetic insecticides has almost eradicated the bed bug from the United States. However, since DDT was banned in the United States in 1972, sporadic reports of bed bugs have been more numerous. Health authorities and pest control operators indicate that these recent bed bug infestations are often associated with shipping of infested furniture or movement of people from infested to unifested buildings. Large numbers of these nocturnal pests may be present in a bedroom. During the day, they hide in mattresses, bedsteads, cracks in the wall, or behind loose wallpaper. They are intermittent feeders on sleeping victims and, when surfeited, retire to their hiding places. Frequently the first signs of bed bug infestations are the tiny spots of red blood, or the flattened dead insects which were killed as the victim rolled in his sleep.

Bed bugs develop by gradual metamorphosis with three stages in their life cycle: egg, nymph, and adult. The eggs, which are glued to surfaces in daytime resting places such as cracks in a wall or buttons on a mattress, hatch in 1 to 7 weeks depending on temperature. There are five nymphal stages, each of which must follow a blood meal. The adults, which can live as long as 9 to 18 months, can survive for several months without feeding.

Human Lice

Three types of sucking lice in the order Anoplura are specific parasites of man. They are usually, but not always, confined to a certain part of the body.

They are named according to the region of the body that they infest and/or for their general appearance: head louse, body louse, and pubic or crab louse. In other parts of the world, particularly before synthetic insecticides such as DDT were used, the body louse was involved in outbreaks of epidemic or louse-born typhus, trench fever, and louse-borne relapsing fever. Fortunately these diseases do not occur in the United States today. However, increasing numbers of louse infestations have been reported in the United States in recent years, particularly of head lice in school children (3, 4, 8, 10–12, 15, 18–20).

Causative Organisms (See Figure 61.2)

For many years it has generally been accepted that the head and body lice are subspecies of *Pediculus humanus*. The head louse was called *Pediculus humanus capitis* and the body louse, *Pediculus humanus humanus*. However, Busvine (3) studied a number of cases of double infestations of head and body lice on the same individuals and found no evidence of intermediates although it is known that mating between these two lice can produce intermediates. He, therefore, concluded that, since the two populations remain separated in spite of their proximity to each other, these lice are distinct species. The head louse should be called *Pediculus capitis* and the body louse, *Pediculus humanus*.

The head louse *(Pediculus capitis)* is 1 to 2 mm long, with the 3 pairs of legs of approximately equal size and an elongate abdomen with slightly darkened margins but without lateral hairy tufts. The adults and immatures called nymphs are found on the head and neck, particularly behind the ears and on the back of the neck. The eggs, called "nits," are glued to the hairs (Fig 61.3).

The body louse *(Pediculus humanus)* is usually 2 to 4 mm long, with the three pairs of legs of approximately equal size and an elongate abdomen with pale margins and no lateral hairy tufts. The adults and immatures are found on the hairy parts of the body below the neck and frequently rest on clothing when they are not feeding. Typically the eggs are laid on clothing, particularly along the seams.

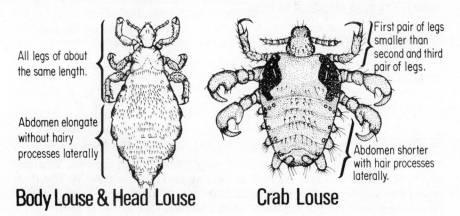

All legs of about the same length.

Abdomen elongate without hairy processes laterally

First pair of legs smaller than second and third pair of legs.

Abdomen shorter with hair processes laterally.

Body Louse & Head Louse   Crab Louse

Figure 61.2—Lice commonly found on man. From reference 5 by permission.

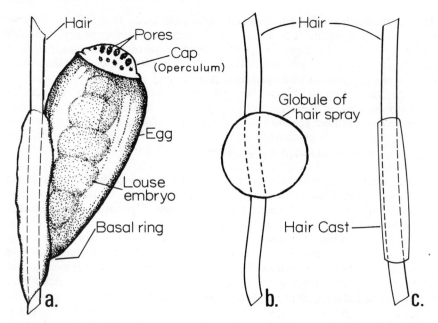

Figure 61.3—Egg of head louse, hair spray globule, and hair cast. From Pratt HD and
Littig KS: Lice of Public Health Importance, Center for Disease Control,
Atlanta, Ga, 1973.

The pubic or crab louse *(Pthirus pubis)* is 0.8 to 1.2 mm long, with the
first pair of legs much smaller and more slender than the second and third
pairs of legs and a short, crab-like abdomen with lateral hairy tufts. The adults
and immatures are typically found on the pubic (hence the species name
"pubic louse") and anal areas of the body or on other parts of the body with
widely spaced hairs (e.g., chest, armpits, moustache, beard, eyebrows, or eye-
lashes). The eggs are glued to hairs.

Clinical Manifestations

Infestations of human lice are called pediculosis from the generic name of
the head and body lice, *Pediculus.* Frequently such infestations lead to scratching, secondary infections, and scarred, hardened, or pigmented skin—the classic signs of pediculosis.

Epidemiology

Pediculosis usually occurs among people who live in crowded locations
and have limited facilities for regular bathing and laundering (18). The three
types of human lice grow by a process known as gradual metamorphosis, with
three stages in their life histories: eggs, nymphs, and adults (Fig 61.4). The
eggs, frequently called "nits," are attached to hairs (head and crab lice) or

clothing (body lice). The immature nymphs suck blood and molt three times before becoming adults. The adults may live for a month or more. They can live 24 to 48 hr away from their human host. Eggs of the body lice laid on clothing can survive for a longer time. However, infested clothing not worn for a month would probably be free of both living lice and viable eggs (4). Lice are transmitted from an infested person to an uninfested by direct contact and indirectly by infested materials such as clothing or bedding. Head lice (which are the major problem species in the United States) can be acquired from infested garments such as coats, caps, and scarves, from such items piled together (particularly in school cloak rooms), from infested combs and brushes, from lying on infested carpets or beds, or from having the head come in contact with upholstered furniture that has been used by an infested person. Hairs with nits attached may be blown considerable distances and serve as a means of transmission. Usually one person will have only 10 to 20 head lice, but infestations with hundreds or thousands of body lice have been reported (4, 12, 15, 17). The distribution of head lice is influenced by such factors as age, sex, crowding at home, family size, method of closeting clothes, socioeconomic status, and race. In the United States, recent studies (19, 20) suggest that blacks are less frequently infested than whites. Crab lice are usually spread by sexual contact. Rarely, they may be picked up from toilet seats.

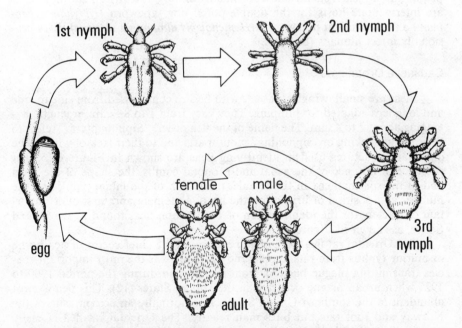

Figure 61.4—Life cycle of the head louse. From Pratt HD and Littig KS: Lice of Public Health Importance, Center for Disease Control, Atlanta, Ga, 1973.

Diagnosis

Head louse infestations are diagnosed by directly inspecting the head and neck, particularly behind the ears and the back of the neck, for crawling forms and nits. Body crab louse infestations are diagnosed by examining for lice and their eggs those hairy parts of the body below the neck, particularly the chest, armpits, and pubic and anal areas. Body lice and their eggs are often found on clothing, especially the seams of collars, waists, and armpits. Care should be taken to differentiate between an active infestation—live adults or nymphs— and an inactive infestation—the presence of empty egg cases. Pseudo-epidemics, particularly of head lice in school children, have been reported (16) in which globules of hair spray or hair casts have been misidentified as nits (Fig 61.3). It is best to remove the hairs and examine them under a microscope to confirm the presence of eggs glued to hairs. Live eggs contain an embryo and have a cap with pores; empty eggs usually do not have the cap.

Fleas

Fleas are among the most common ectoparasites which affect humans in the United States. Fleas cause irritation, loss of blood, and extreme discomfort. Public health workers are concerned with fleas as vectors of bubonic plague and flea-borne or murine typhus from rats to man and as vectors of sylvatic plague among wild rodents and occasionally among humans. In addition, fleas are intermediate hosts for the double-pored dog tapeworm *(Dipylidium caninum)* and two rodent tapeworms *(Hymenolepis diminuta* and *nana)* that occasionally infect humans (8, 10, 12).

Causative Organisms

Fleas are small, wingless insects with bodies compressed from side to side and long legs adapted for jumping. They vary from 1 to 8.5 mm in length, averaging about 2 to 4 mm. The name of the flea order, "Siphonaptera," refers to their blood-sucking or "siphoning" mouthparts and to their lack of wings. The important structures used in identifying fleas are shown in Figure 61.5. The presence or absence of the genal and pronotal combs, the shape of the head and of the spermatheca in the female, the length of the labial palpi, and the number and position of bristles on the head, abdomen, and tarsi offer important characters for the identification of 10 common fleas found in the United States, as shown in Figure 61.6.

The Oriental rat flea *(Xenopsylla cheopis)* is the chief vector of flea-borne or murine typhus from rats to man and probably was the most important species transmitting plague bacteria from rats to man during the period 1900 to 1925 when urban plague occurred in the United States (12). This flea is most abundant in the southern United States. It is normally an ectoparasite of the Norway and roof rats but bites man readily. The Oriental rat flea is easily identified by the characters shown in the pictorial key (Fig 61.6). It has no genal or pronotal combs, the front margin of the head is rounded and the thorax is of normal length, the mesopleuron is divided by a vertical thickening, the ocular bristle is inserted in front of the eye, and the female has a large, dark, C-shaped spermatheca.

The cat flea *(Ctenocephalides felis)* and the dog flea *(Ctenocephalides canis)* both have a genal comb and a pronotal comb, each with about seven or eight pointed black teeth on each side of the body. As shown in the pictorial key (Fig 61.6), the head of the cat flea is about twice as long as high and the first two spines of the genal comb are about the same length, whereas the head of the dog flea is less than twice as long as high and the first spine of the genal comb is definitely shorter than the second. It is usually not necessary to distinguish between these two closely related species because they have similar habits. Both species attack cats, dogs, rats, and man. In many parts of the United States, the cat flea is more abundant than the dog flea.

A number of other species of fleas do attack man, particularly the human flea *(Pulex irritans)* in the San Francisco Bay area and the sticktight flea *(Echidonophaga gallinacea)* in the southern United States. Other species of fleas not included on the pictorial key can be identified with specialized literature (5, 10, 21).

Clinical Manifestations

Flea bites are almost unbearable for some persons; others are relatively undisturbed by them. People who are bitten by fleas have reactions ranging from small red spots (where the mouthparts of the flea have penetrated the

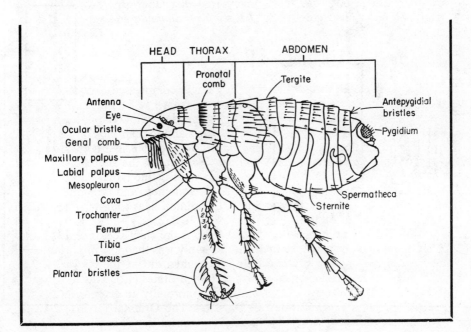

Figure 61.5—Flea. From reference 5 by permission.

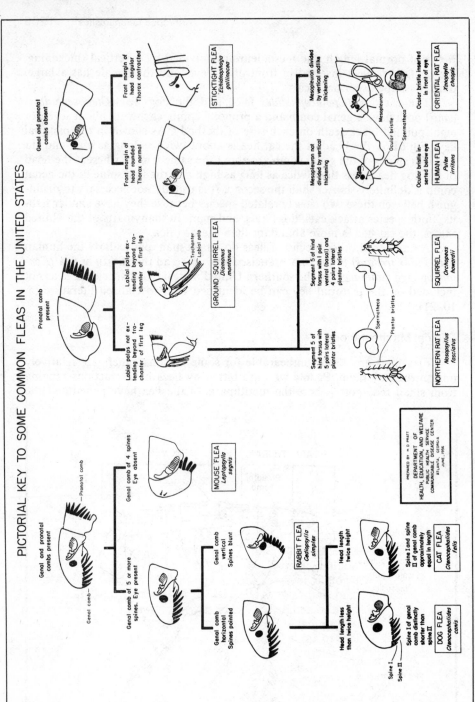

Figure 61-6.—Pictorial key to some common fleas in the United States. From reference 5 by permission.

skin), surrounded by a slight swelling and reddish discoloration, to a very severe generalized rash. The development of sensitivity to flea bites requires an initial sensitization by the insect. Thus, a latent period occurs between the time of the first exposure and the time when subsequent flea bites elicit skin reactions.

Epidemiology

Fleas are bloodsucking insects seldom found far from their host animals—often cats, dogs, or rats. Fleas develop by a process known as complete metamorphosis through four life stages: eggs, larva, pupa, and adult. The adult fleas suck blood from warm-blooded animals and usually mate on the host. The eggs of many fleas are not sticky or attached to the host, so they drop onto the ground, carpet, or bedding material of the host. This explains the large number of fleas in dog or cat boxes, in kennels, or in carpets on which a pet sleeps. Depending on the flea species, temperature, and moisture, the eggs hatch in a few days or weeks, and the larvae develop—sometimes as rapidly as in 2 weeks—and molt to become pupae. Then, the adults emerge from the pupal cocoons, ready for a blood meal. Many human infestations occur in homes with heavy infestations of cat or dog fleas. As long as the cat or dog is present, the newly emerged adult fleas simply hop onto and feed on these pets, and complaints of people being bitten by fleas are infrequent. However, if people leave their homes and take their pets with them, or board their cats and dogs for 2 to 4 weeks or longer, numerous fleas may mature in the vacant houses or apartments. Such fleas have had no opportunity for a blood meal. When people enter such a dwelling, they may be attacked by hundreds of hungry fleas and suffer excruciating pain.

Fly Maggots

Causative Organisms

Flies belong to the insect order Diptera, or two-winged insects. Flies develop by complete metamorphosis and have four stages in their life cycle: egg, larva, pupa, and adult. Fly larvae are frequently called maggots. A brief discussion of fly maggots is included in this manual because some species are found in wounds and sinuses or in the umbilical area of newborn babies, and because fly larvae are sometimes found in stool and urine samples submitted to laboratories for examination. More thorough discussions of fly larvae and keys and illustrations to aid in identification are included in James (13) and in a number of general references (5, 10, 21).

A typical muscoid fly larva is legless and somewhat cone-shaped, with a narrow anterior end bearing the mouthparts and anterior spiracles and a broader posterior end with two prominent posterior spiracles. The structures of the mouthparts and the anterior and posterior spiracles are characters used in identification. Most muscoid fly larvae are rather similar and are classified using characters shown in Figure 61.7. Two types easily recognized with the

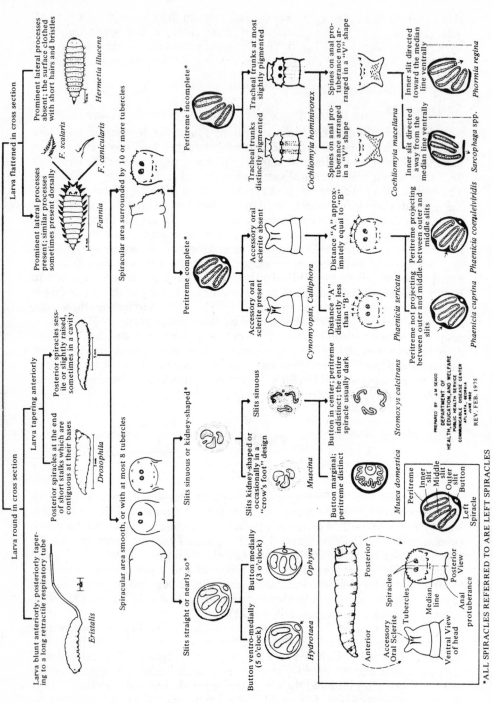

PICTORIAL KEY TO MATURE LARVAE OF SOME COMMON FLIES

*ALL SPIRACLES REFERRED TO ARE LEFT SPIRACLES

naked eye are the lesser house fly and latrine fly (*Fannia* spp.), which have prominent lateral processes, and the rat-tailed maggot (*Eristalis tenax*), which has a long, telescopic, respiratory tube.

Clinical Manifestations and Epidemiology

Infestation with fly maggots causes a condition known as "myiasis," in which the fly larvae feed on living, necrotic, or dead tissues of humans or on the food in the human alimentary canal. Depending on the location of the fly larvae, a number of terms have been used to describe the various types of myiasis as gastrointestinal or enteric (digestive tract); dermal, subdermal, or cutaneous (skin); auricular (ear); ocular (eye); nasopharyngeal (nose); and urinary or urogenital (urogenital tract) (13).

Enteric myiasis

Maggots in the digestive tract may cause queasiness, nausea, pain in the abdomen, diarrhea, dysentery (with actual discharge of blood resulting from injury to the intestinal mucosa), and nervousness. Fifty species of fly larvae have been reported, either positively or questionably, from cases of "enteric myiasis" among humans (10). The flies involved are usually species which lay their eggs or larvae on cold meats, fish, cheese, ripe fruit, and other foods. Most of the eggs and larvae are undoubtedly destroyed by normal digestive juices in the human alimentary tract. However, there apparently is documentation of living larvae which were expelled either in the stool or vomit, or both. Some of these cases involved children who drank "dirty water" from a ditch containing rat-tailed maggots (*Eristalis tenax*) and children and adults who ate meat or fish containing larvae of the flesh flies (*Sarcophaga* spp.) or ripe fruits with soldier fly larvae (*Hermetia illucens*).

Laboratory workers should be very careful in reporting enteric myiasis. Stool samples can easily be contaminated in the laboratory, particularly by species of flesh flies (*Sarcophaga* spp.) which are strongly attracted by the smell of feces. These insects lay larvae rather than eggs, and the first two larval instars are often completed in a day, so that it is possible to find third instar larvae in stool samples only a day old. Female *Sarcophaga* have been observed laying larvae on a cardboard carton containing a fresh stool sample on a laboratory bench one day, and third instar larvae were found in the material when it was examined the following day. In such cases of questionable "enteric myiasis," a second stool sample should be passed in a fly-free room and the material examined at once.

Dermal and subdermal myiasis

The infestation of cuts and open sores by living calliphorid and sarcophagid larvae that feed on bleeding, festered, or malodorous tissues has been known for many years—most often in wounded persons on battlefields. Civilian cases following snagging on barbed wire, gun-shot wounds, and open sores on the scalp and other parts of the body have been reported (10, 13). Many of these cases should be considered as facultative myiasis—caused by species of green-bottle flies (*Phaenicia*), black blowflies (*Phormia regina*), or flesh flies

(*Sarcophaga*) that are attracted by the smell of blood or diseased tissues and that normally lay their eggs or larvae on dead animals. Sometimes such infestations are benign or even beneficial in "cleaning up" suppurating wounds. Several infestations by larvae of the green-bottle fly (*Phaenicia sericata*) have been reported in the umbilical region of newborn babies, the flies having been attracted by the smell of blood of the tied-off cord.

Other more serious cases of dermal myiasis in humans are caused by larvae of the primary screw-worm (*Cochliomyia hominivorax*) or *Wohlfahrtia magnifica*, whose larvae are normally obligatory parasites of mammals. Their larvae can cause very painful, serious wounds in living tissues—particularly in the eye, nose, mouth, and vaginal regions (10, 13).

Ticks

Ticks are bloodsucking arachnids that are ectoparasites of many vertebrates including humans. Ticks have a four-stage life cycle: egg, 6-legged larva, 8-legged sexually immature nymph, and 8-legged sexually mature adult. Usually a blood meal is necessary for the larva to molt to become a nymph, and another blood meal for the nymph to molt to become an adult. Hard ticks have only one nymphal stage, whereas soft ticks may have four or five.

There are two families of ticks (Fig 61.8)—hard ticks in the family Ixodidae and soft ticks in the family Argasidae. Hard ticks have a hard dorsal plate or scutum and the mouth parts are located at the anterior end, clearly visible from above. Soft ticks have a leathery body but no hard plate on the dorsal part of the body, and the mouthparts are located ventrally and are not visible from above. Both hard and soft ticks can bite man and can cause painful, itching lesions.

Causative Organisms

The three most important species of hard ticks in the United States are the American dog tick (*Dermacentor variabilis*), the Rocky Mountain wood tick (*Dermacentor andersoni*), and the lone star tick (*Amblyomma americanum*). Ticks in the genera *Dermacentor* and *Amblyomma* are often called "ornate" ticks because they have whitish markings on the scutum easily seen with the naked eye, a hand lens, or a stereoscopic microscope. The ticks in the other genera of North American ticks do not have these whitish markings and are called "inornate" ticks.

The American dog tick (*Dermacentor variabilis*) is found in most of the eastern United States and in limited area on the Pacific Coast, in northern Idaho, and in eastern Washington. Small males of these brownish ticks may be only 3 mm long, whereas engorged females may grow from 5 mm to 13 mm or more long. As shown in the pictorial key (Fig 61.8), the mouthparts (palpi and hypostome) are about as long as the basis capituli, and the sides of the basis capituli are parallel. The scutum has diffuse whitish markings that may be faint or well-defined. The fine punctuation, called "goblets," on the spiracular plates on the underside of the abdomen, behind and lateral to the fourth pair

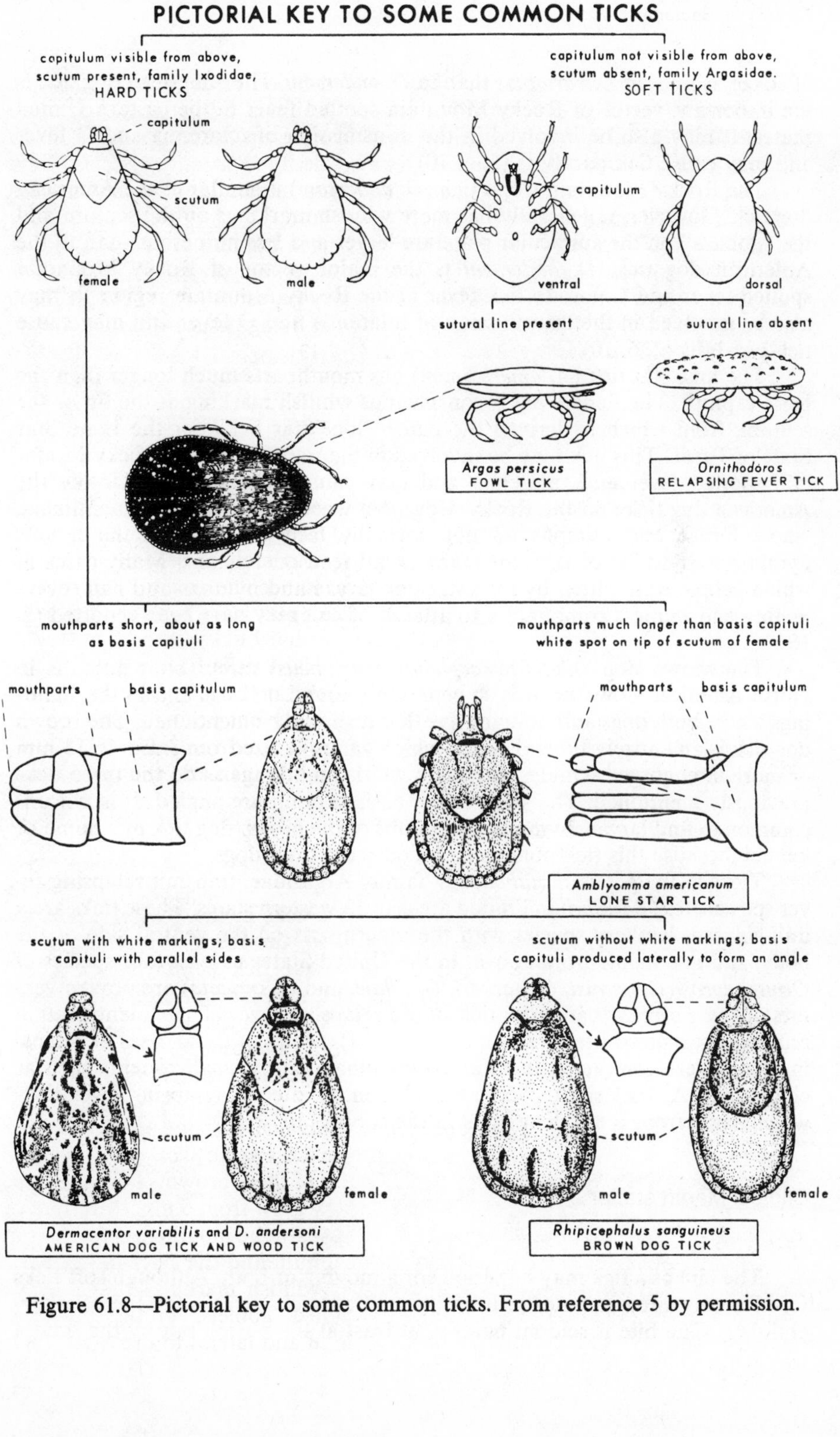

PICTORIAL KEY TO SOME COMMON TICKS

copitulum visible from above, scutum present, family Ixodidae, HARD TICKS

capitulum not visible from above, scutum absent, family Argasidae. SOFT TICKS

capitulum

scutum

female

male

capitulum

ventral

dorsal

sutural line present

sutural line absent

Argas persicus FOWL TICK

Ornithodoros RELAPSING FEVER TICK

mouthparts short, about as long as basis capituli

mouthparts much longer than basis capituli white spot on tip of scutum of female

mouthparts   basis capitulum

mouthparts   basis capitulum

Amblyomma americanum LONE STAR TICK

scutum with white markings; basis capituli with parallel sides

scutum without white markings; basis capituli produced laterally to form an angle

scutum

male

female

scutum

male

female

Dermacentor variabilis and *D. andersoni* AMERICAN DOG TICK AND WOOD TICK

Rhipicephalus sanguineus BROWN DOG TICK

Figure 61.8—Pictorial key to some common ticks. From reference 5 by permission.

of coxae, is finer in *D. variabilis* than in *D. andersoni*. The American dog tick is the important vector of Rocky Mountain spotted fever in the eastern United States. It may also be involved in the transmission of tularemia and Q fever and may cause tick paralysis (2, 6, 10).

The Rocky Mountain wood tick (*D. andersoni*) is similar to the American dog tick. However, it generally has more whitish markings on the scutum and the "goblets" on the spiracular plate are larger and less numerous than in the American dog tick. *D. andersoni* is the major vector of Rocky Mountain spotted fever and Colorado tick fever in the Rocky Mountain region. It may also be involved in the transmission of tularemia and Q fever and may cause tick paralysis (2, 6, 10).

The lone star tick (*A. americanum*) has mouthparts much longer than the basis capituli. The female has a conspicuous whitish marking at the tip of the scutum, from which is derived the name "lone star tick" for the Lone Star State of Texas. This tick may be involved in the transmission of Rocky Mountain spotted fever and tularemia and may cause tick paralysis. Unlike the American dog tick and the Rocky Mountain wood tick previously mentioned, whose larvae and nymphs do not normally feed on humans, the larvae, nymphs, and adults of the lone star tick all feed on humans. Many cases in which people were bitten by lone star tick larvae and nymphs and had severe itching and redness comparable to attacks of chiggers have been reported (2, 10).

The brown dog tick (*Rhipicephalus sanguineus*) rarely bites humans in North America. However, it is so commonly found on dogs and in the buildings where both dogs and humans live that it should be mentioned. The brown dog tick is an entirely brownish tick which varies in size from 3 mm to 13 mm or more in engorged females. It has no whitish markings as do the three ticks previously mentioned. The sides of the basis capituli are angled. It is not uncommon to find larvae, nymphs, and adults of the brown dog tick in a home or kennel, because this tick obtains its blood meal from dogs.

Ticks in the genus *Ornithodoros*, family Argasidae, transmit relapsing fever spirochetes (*Borrelia*) in limited areas in 13 western states. These ticks are a dull-colored, leathery species with the mouthparts on the ventral side of the body, and not visible from above. In the United States at least four species of *Ornithodoros* (*O. hermsi, O. parkeri, O. talaje*, and *O. turicata*) are proven vectors of the *Borrelia* that cause tick-borne relapsing fever. Their identification requires specialized literature (5, 7, 10, 12, 21). Many of these cases of relapsing fever were contracted in rural cabins inhabited by small rodents such as chipmunks. As they slept, people were bitten by infected relapsing fever ticks which came from the rodent nests in the cabins (10, 22).

Clinical Manifestations

Tick bites

The bite of a tick may be serious or annoying or both. Although soft ticks feed for only a few minutes or hours, some hard ticks remain fastened for several days. The bite is seldom painful, at least at the outset, but by the time a person notices it, the tick may have done considerable damage. Tick bites often heal slowly and itch intensely—leading to scratching, redness, and sometimes secondary infections. Some patients have allergic manifestations with blister formation at the site of the bite.

Tick paralysis

In some cases, if a tick remains fastened and engorged for several days, patients develop a peculiar flaccid paralysis beginning at the extremities and gradually spreading to other parts of the body. If the tick is not removed, the muscles of respiration are affected, and the patient may die of respiratory insufficiency. If the tick is found and removed, the patient usually recovers spontaneously within a few hours—suggesting that the paralysis is caused by a toxic substance in the tick's saliva (8, 10, 12).

Epidemiology

People usually encounter ticks in grassy or brushy areas where ticks find their normal hosts among small mammals, such as field mice, dogs (*D. variabilis*), large mammals (*D. andersoni*), or deer (*A. americanum*). The rising incidence of Rocky Mountain spotted fever in the eastern United States may be associated with the fact that more people live in suburbs with brushy areas infested with ticks or may indicate that more dogs in homes are infected with ticks (2). Most of the cases of relapsing fever in the West are associated with people sleeping in rustic cabins infested with small rodents and soft ticks (*Ornithodoros*) (22).

Control

If a tick becomes attached, the simplest method of removing it is slowly and steadily pulling with forceps so as not to break off the mouthparts and leave them in the wound. Sometimes touching the tick with the lighted end of a ciagarette, a drop of chloroform, ether, benzene, or vaseline will cause it to release its hold. An antiseptic should be applied to the tick wound. If the hands have touched the tick during removal, they should be washed thoroughly with soap and water, because tick secretions may be infective. Tick control in the home usually requires treating both the animal and the building with various insecticides.

Mites

Scabies

The scabies, mange, or itch mite (*Sarcoptes scabiei*) causes an infectious skin disease called scabies, mange, or "the itch." Diagnosis is confirmed by locating a mite in the epidermis in papules or vesicles or in a tiny burrow containing the female and her eggs. Mellanby (14) recommended cutting a tiny bit of skin from a papule with a safety razor blade or removing the mite from the burrow with a teasing needle and confirming the diagnosis with a compound microscope having a magnification of at least 50 diameters. The mites are oval,

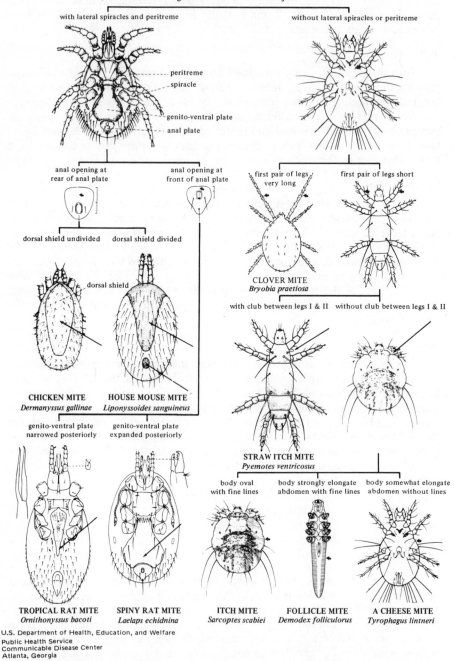

MITES: PICTORIAL KEY TO SOME COMMON SPECIES OF PUBLIC HEALTH IMPORTANCE
Harold George Scott and Chester J. Stojanovich

with lateral spiracles and peritreme

without lateral spiracles or peritreme

peritreme
spiracle
genito-ventral plate
anal plate

anal opening at rear of anal plate

anal opening at front of anal plate

first pair of legs very long

first pair of legs short

dorsal shield undivided

dorsal shield divided

CLOVER MITE
Bryobia praetiosa

with club between legs I & II   without club between legs I & II

dorsal shield

CHICKEN MITE
Dermanyssus gallinae

HOUSE MOUSE MITE
Liponyssoides sanguineus

STRAW ITCH MITE
Pyemotes ventricosus

genito-ventral plate narrowed posteriorly

genito-ventral plate expanded posteriorly

body oval with fine lines

body strongly elongate abdomen with fine lines

body somewhat elongate abdomen without lines

TROPICAL RAT MITE
Ornithonyssus bacoti

SPINY RAT MITE
Laelaps echidnina

ITCH MITE
Sarcoptes scabiei

FOLLICLE MITE
Demodex folliculorum

A CHEESE MITE
Tyrophagus lintneri

U.S. Department of Health, Education, and Welfare
Public Health Service
Communicable Disease Center
Atlanta, Georgia

Figure 61.9—Pictorial key to some common species of mites of public health importance. From reference 5 by permission.

saclike, and less than 1 mm long. Females average 400 μm $\times$ 300 μm, and males 250 μm $\times$ 150 μm. The mouthparts at the anterior end contain chelicerae and paired palps. The body surface is finely wrinkled, and has a number of rather conspicuous blunt spines and many backward-projecting triangular scales on the dorsal surface. The legs are short and stocky, and the two anterior pairs are widely separated from the two posterior pairs. The anus is located at the posterior end (Fig 61.9).

Clinical manifestations

Scabies mites are found in papules around the finger webs, anterior surfaces of the wrists and elbows, anterior axillary folds, belt line, thighs, and external genitalia in men, and nipples, abdomen, and low portion of the buttocks in women. Itching is intense, especially at night, but complications are rare except as lesions become secondarily infected by scratching. The mites are often present on a person for several days to weeks before itching begins (14, 15). Mellanby (14) has shown that the "scabies rash" has a characteristic distribution particularly in the armpits, waist, buttocks, inner thigh, and ankle areas that does not correspond with the location of the mites, primarily in the webbing of the fingers and the folds of the wrists. Moreover, Mellanby believes that a true sensitization occurs with scabies. If the first infestation with scabies mites is eradicated with treatment, the rash will appear with reinfestation, sometimes within a matter of hours and even with the skin penetration of only a single mite.

Epidemiology

Since 60 percent of the mites have been reported in lesions on the hands or wrists (14), touching or shaking the hands of infested people appears to be one of the primary methods of transmitting scabies mites. Female mites are transferred from one person to another by simple contact and less commonly from undergarments or soiled bedclothes freshly contaminated by infested persons. Scabies is often considered to be a "family disease"—with mites transferred from husband to wife or from one child to another, particularly if more than one child sleeps in the same bed. The disease is frequently acquired through sexual contact, particularly by military personnel and other groups of people. Scabies epidemics occur particularly during time of war, poverty, or social upheaval when facilities for bathing and laundering are limited. The disease occurs among certain groups who bathe or launder their clothing infrequently, but scabies is uncommon among persons who bathe daily and regularly launder clothing and bedding. If one member of a family or group of persons has scabies, it is advisable to treat all close contacts (14, 15).

Demodex folliculorum

Demodex folliculorum is an elongated mite with stubby legs (Fig 61.9) which infests hair follicles or sebaceous glands (particularly of the face); it is widespread and probably infects over half of middle-aged adults. The infestation is usually asymptomatic but may be associated with blackheads. The mites are often an incidental finding in histologic sections of facial skin.

Trombiculid mites (chiggers)

Trombiculid mites infest grasses and bushes, and their six-legged larvae, i.e., chiggers (red bugs, harvest mites), may attack humans. The larvae attach to the skin, usually in areas where clothing is tight, such as the part of the ankle at the top of the socks or skin touched by belts and elastic bands. Sensitive individuals react to the secretions of the larvae with swollen itching areas at the sites of attachment which persist for days. Excoriations may become secondarily infected.

References

1. BENENSON AA: Control of Communicable Diseases in Man, 12th Edition. American Public Health Association, Washington, DC, 413 pp, 1975
2. BURGDORFER W: Ecology of tick vectors of American spotted fever. Bull WHO 40:375-381, 1969
3. BUSVINE JR: Evidence from double infestations for the specific status of human head lice and body lice (Anoplura). Systematic Entomology 3:1-8, 1978
4. BUXTON PA: The Louse, 2nd Edition. Williams and Wilkin Co, Baltimore, 164 pp, 1946
5. CENTER FOR DISEASE CONTROL: Pictorial Keys: Arthropods, Reptiles, Birds and Mammals of Public Health Importance. USDHEW, CDC, Atlanta, Ga, 192 pp, 1967
6. COOLEY RA: The Genera Dermacentor and Otocentor (Ixodidae) in the United States, with Studies in Variation. Natl Inst Health Bull No. 171, 89 pp, 1938
7. COOLEY RA and KOHLS GM: The Argasidae of North America, Central America, and Cuba. Am Midland Naturalist Mon No. 1, 152 pp, 1944
8. FAUST EC, RUSSELL PF, and JUNG RC: Craig and Faust's Clinical Parasitology, 8th Edition Lea and Febiger, Philadelphia, 890 pp, 1970
9. FRAZIER CA: Insect Allergy. Allergic and Toxic Reactions to Insects and Other Arthropods. W. H. Green Co., St. Louis, Mo, 493 pp, 1969
10. HARWOOD RF and JAMES MT: Entomology in Human and Animal Health, 7th Edition. MacMillan Co, New York, 548 pp, 1979
11. HORSFALL WR: Medical Entomology: Arthropods and Human Disease. Ronald Press Co., New York, 467 pp, 1962
12. HUNTER GW III, SCHWARTZWELDER JC, and CLYDE DF: Tropical Medicine, 5th Edition W. B. Saunders, Philadelphia, 900 pp. 1976
13. JAMES MT: The Flies that Cause Myiasis in Man. USDA Misc. Publ. 631, 175 pp, 1948
14. MELLANBY K: Scabies. E.W. Classey Ltd., Hampton, Middlesex, England, 81 pp, 1972
15. ORKIN M, MAILBACH HL, PARISH LC, and SCHWARTZMAN RM: Scabies and Pediculosis. J.B. Lippincott Co, Philadelphia, 224 pp, 1977
16. OSGOOD SB, JELLISON WL, and KOHLS GM: An episode of pseudopediculosis. J Parasitol 47:985-986, 1961
17. PAN-AMERICAN HEALTH ORGANIZATION: Proceedings of the International Symposium on the Control of Lice and Louse-Borne Diseases. Sci. Publ. No. 263. Pan-American Health Organization, Washington, DC, 311 pp, 1973
18. SHOLDT LL, HOLLOWAY ML, and FRONK WD: The Epidemiology of Human Pediculosis in Ethiopia. Special Publication. Navy Disease Vector Ecology and Control Center, Naval Air Station, Jacksonville, Fla, 150 pp, 1979
19. SLONKA GF and McKINLEY TW: Controlling Head Lice. USDHEW, PHS, CDC, Atlanta, Ga, 16 pp, 1975
20. SLONKA GF, McKINLEY TW, McCROAN JE, SINCLAIR SP, SCHULTZ MG, HICKS F, and HILL N: Epidemiology of an outbreak of head lice in Georgia. Am J Trop Med Hyg 25:739-743, 1976
21. SMITH FGV (ed.): Insects and Other Arthropods of Medical Importance. British Museum (Natural History), London, 561 pp, 1973
22. THOMPSON RS, BURGDORFER W, RUSSELL R, and FRANCIS BJ: Outbreak of tick-borne relapsing fever in Spokane County, Washington. J Am Med Assoc 210:1045-1050

INDEX

A

Absidia, identifying characteristics, 980
Acanthamoebae, infections caused by, 1139, 1140
Accidents in the laboratory, 52-53
Accreditation of Hospitals, Joint Commission on, 42
Acetate utilization test, 792
N-Acetyl-L-cysteine-sodium hydroxide procedure, 680-681
reagent, 804
Achromobacter
differentiation from other genera, 566
infections caused by, 568, 572
Acidaminococcus, classification, 173, 205
Acid-fast stain for *Nocardia,* 848
Acinetobacter
antimicrobial susceptibility, 576
differentiation from other genera, 566, 573
infections caused by, 568
Acremonium
characteristics, 1035-1037
cutaneous infections caused by, 920
Actinobacillus, 413-417
antimicrobial susceptibility, 416
biochemical reactions, 415
characteristics, 413
clinical manifestations, 413
diagnostic procedures, 414-416
epidemiology, 413-414
evaluation of laboratory findings, 417
specimen collection and processing, 414
Actinomadura madura, classification and characteristics, 1033, 1034
Actinomadura pelletieri, characteristics, 1033, 1034
Actinomyces cultures, special seals for, 802
Actinomyces israelii
frequency of isolation, 176
habitats in endogenous infections, 173
Actinomyces species
appearance, 144, 145, 151, 152, 153, 154
classification and characteristics, 143-144, 149, 150, 173

differentiation of, 206
frequency of isolation, 176
Actinomycetes, differentiation from fungi, 858
Actinomycosis, 143-158
antimicrobic susceptibility, 156
causative organisms, 143-144
clinical manifestations, 144-145
diagnostic procedures, 147-156
epidemiology, 146
public health significance, 146-147
specimens for diagnosis, 147
Aeromonas hydrophila, differentiation from *Chromobacterium,* 399
Agar dilution test, 755-757
Agar disk diffusion test, 749-755
Agglutination tests, principles of, 82-84
AIM-4 system for identifying *Enterobacteriaceae,* 355
Alcaligenes
antimicrobial susceptibility, 576
differentiation from other genera, 565, 566, 573
infections caused by, 568
Alkaline peptone water, formula and preparation, 813
Allescheria boydii, 983
$ALLO_3$, proposed classification, 444
$ALLO_4$, proposed classification, 444
Alternaria
cutaneous infections caused by, 920
diagnostic characteristics, 1016, 1023
Amebae
diagnosis of amebiasis, 1161-1162
incidence in clinical specimens, 1096
infections caused by, 1139-1140, 1153-1154
morphology, 1154-1161
nonfecal specimens for diagnosis, 1111
serologic tests for, 1098
American Association for Laboratory Animal Science, 112
American Industrial Hygiene Association, 43
D-Aminolevulinic acid reagent, 804
Amphotericin B

M

N

O

U

V

W

X

Y

Z